FOUNDATIONS IN
Neonatal and
Pediatric
Respiratory Care

Teresa A. Volsko, MBA, MHHS, RRT, CMT-E, FAARC
Director, Respiratory Care
Transport, and the Communication Center
Akron Children's Hospital

Sherry L. Barnhart, RRT, RRT-NPS, AE-C, FAARC
Respiratory Care Discharge Planner
Arkansas Children's Hospital

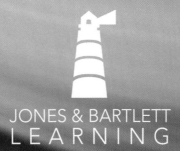

JONES & BARTLETT
LEARNING

World Headquarters
Jones & Bartlett Learning
5 Wall Street
Burlington, MA 01803
978-443-5000
info@jblearning.com
www.jblearning.com

Jones & Bartlett Learning books and products are available through most bookstores and online booksellers. To contact Jones & Bartlett Learning directly, call 800-832-0034, fax 978-443-8000, or visit our website, www.jblearning.com.

Substantial discounts on bulk quantities of Jones & Bartlett Learning publications are available to corporations, professional associations, and other qualified organizations. For details and specific discount information, contact the special sales department at Jones & Bartlett Learning via the above contact information or send an email to specialsales@jblearning.com.

7827-9

Production Credits

VP, Product Management: David D. Cella
Director of Product Management: Cathy L. Esperti
Product Manager: Sean Fabery
Product Specialist: Rachael Souza
Director of Production: Jenny L. Corriveau
Project Specialist: Brooke Haley
Marketing Manager: Michael Sullivan
VP, Manufacturing and Inventory Control: Therese Connell
Composition: S4Carlisle Publishing Services

Cover Design: Scott Moden
Text Design: Scott Moden
Director of Rights & Media: Joanna Gallant
Rights & Media Specialist: Robert Boder
Media Development Editor: Troy Liston
Cover Image (Title Page, Part Opener, Chapter Opener): © Andriy Rabchun/Shutterstock.
Printing and Binding: LSC Communications
Cover Printing: LSC Communications

Library of Congress Cataloging-in-Publication Data
Names: Volsko, Teresa A., author. | Barnhart, Sherry L., author.
Title: Foundations in neonatal and pediatric respiratory care / Teresa A. Volsko, Sherry L. Barnhart.
Description: First edition. | Burlington, Massachusetts : Jones & Bartlett Learning, [2019] | Includes bibliographical references and index.
Identifiers: LCCN 2018016842 | ISBN 9781449652708 (pbk.)
Subjects: | MESH: Respiratory Tract Diseases--therapy | Respiratory Therapy | Infant, Newborn | Child
Classification: LCC RJ312 | NLM WS 280 | DDC 618.92/2--dc23
LC record available at https://lccn.loc.gov/2018016842

6048

Printed in the United States of America
23 22 21 20 19   10 9 8 7 6 5 4 3 2 1

I dedicate this book to the respiratory care students whose quest for knowledge inspired me to find new and innovative ways to maximize their educational experience and to the credentialed practitioners who share a passion for caring for infants, children, and their families. I also dedicate this book to my family, whose understanding, love, and support allowed me to pursue and fulfill my dreams! ∾

Teresa A. Volsko

This book is dedicated to the children and their families who have taught me about courage and hope and unconditional love; to Dr. Robert H. Warren, whose wisdom and friendship gave me the confidence to pursue teaching and writing; and to Caleb and Gabriel, who will forever be the greatest blessings in my life. ∾

Sherry L. Barnhart

Brief Contents

Contents

Foreword

"If you would achieve extraordinary results, you must live an uncommon life."

~ **R. L. Chatburn**

The textbook you are now holding is extraordinary for several reasons. It is a first edition, meaning that it represents a monumental amount of skill and effort to birth. Revising a book that has seen multiple editions is hard enough, but creating a first edition is a difficult task and a huge responsibility because it must present new information in creative ways to advance the common knowledge of the intended audience. Most textbooks are written by educators, but the editors of this book are much more than that. Just as academic hospitals frequently express their mission statements in terms of serving the tripartite goals of clinical care, education, and research, these editors have served as leaders in all three areas.

Teresa Volsko has had extensive experience as a neonatal and pediatric respiratory therapist, pediatric disease manager, director of a 4-year respiratory care program at a state university, and technical director of both respiratory care and research departments in a major children's hospital. She is also a fellow of the American Association for Respiratory Care. Beyond that, she is one of the most prolific researchers in the field of respiratory care, with over three dozen publications in peer-reviewed medical journals. In addition to this book, Terry is coeditor of a popular respiratory care equipment book, along with multiple chapters in many other academic textbooks.

Sherry Barnhart has extensive clinical experience as a neonatal and pediatric respiratory therapist, home care therapist, supervisor, instructor, education coordinator, asthma educator, and discharge planner. She has served on committees of the American Association for Respiratory care for over 30 years. Her writing experience includes being the editor of a previous book on perinatal and pediatric respiratory care as well as chapters in subsequent editions of that book and other textbooks concerning pediatric respiratory care. Sherry's research experience includes being study coordinator at the Arkansas Allergy & Asthma Clinic. Sherry has earned multiple professional awards and is a fellow of the American Association for Respiratory Care.

These editors have participated in the evolution of the field from the early days, when neonatal/pediatric mechanical ventilation was in its infancy, and long before surfactant, ECMO, high-flow oxygen, care paths, and countless other technologic developments. They both continue to teach at the university level and to hospital staff. To say that they have lived uncommon professional lives would be an understatement.

The planning of the book was also extraordinary. Using their extensive network of colleagues, these editors elicited feedback from educators on opportunities to improve the teaching resources that they currently use for their neonatal and pediatric classes. They used that feedback to map out the book's content (taking advantage of the gaps the educators identified in current resources) as well as the layout of the book (the chapters progress in a logical manner that mirror the way the course is taught). As a result, there are many innovations and unique illustrations that demonstrate how to properly provide care and to use equipment in this specialty area.

Another important feature of this book is that all the contributors are clinicians who are actively practicing in this specialty area. Many of them are national experts. They not only provide the most relevant evidence-based material from the literature but also provide content that has relevant practical application to current practice. This can be seen by the extensive use of figures and illustrations that display graphics (monitoring screen shots and ventilator graphic screenshots), photos of equipment use and setup, and photos of procedures. Patient education materials are provided in the chapters as well.

This book is intended for any clinician involved in neonatal or pediatric health care, as students or as practitioners. This includes respiratory therapists, nurses, physician assistants, nurse practitioners, and physicians. In addition, this book also serves as an exceptional reference for credentialed practitioners who are interested in taking the Neonatal Pediatric Special credentialing exam of the NBRC. Many chapters address the key components of neonatal and pediatric care, including all the elements of the content outline for the exam.

"The wise work without attachment, for the welfare of the society."

~ Bhagavad Gita

Robert L. Chatburn, MHHS, RRT-NPS, FAARC
Professor of Medicine
Lerner College of Medicine of Case Western
    Reserve University
Clinical Research Manager, Respiratory Institute
Director of Medical Simulation Fellowship,
    Education Institute
Cleveland Clinic
Cleveland, Ohio
April 2018

Preface

Children are precious and represent our hopes and dreams for tomorrow. Neonatal and pediatric care have evolved significantly throughout the years. Advances in respiratory care have made a significant impact on the health and well-being of infants, children, and their families. Technologic advances resulted in improved survival for children of all ages. The care a child and family require to support the best outcomes is more than a passion for this specialized area of respiratory care. In this inaugural edition, the authors recognize the importance of sharing the essential elements of care that are unique to children as they grow and develop and provide the clinician with the knowledge needed to effectively communicate recommendations for therapeutic intervention or changes to the plan of care. The authors embraced this work as an opportunity to build a learning community that supports a culture of interdisciplinary professionalism.

The approach or layout of each chapter is standardized, much like the format for scientific papers published in medical journals. Each chapter provides the reader with a the thorough review of the literature on the subject. The chapters addressing specialized equipment provide practical relevance of the equipment, including technologic specifications, indications for use, processes required for application to the patient, limitations, and troubleshooting techniques. These chapters guide the reader through the theoretical constructs to better enable the healthcare professional to distinguish between equipment malfunction and patient intolerance. Understanding this important difference is an essential critical thinking component and helps the clinician to clearly articulate recommendations for the respiratory plan of care with the interdisciplinary team.

Similarly, chapters dedicated to congenital or acquired illnesses are standardized as well. These chapters provide theoretical constructs in addition to summarizing best practices for medical management, and they provide the essential tenants of family-centered care. The outlines for these chapters include etiology, pathophysiology, diagnosis, clinical presentation, medical management, potential complications, and outcomes. Cumulatively, these sections provide the reader with the necessary information to clearly articulate the need to initiate therapy or modify the plan of care.

Section-by-Section Overview

The sections of this text are written progressively, commencing with the basic tenants essential to the care of children of all ages; continuing as a child grows and develops to prenatal, antenatal, neonatal, and pediatric care; and culminating in the specialized care required for diagnosing and managing pediatric disorders.

The text is written in a clear and concise manner. Illustrations, tables, and figures are provided to enhance the learning experience. The supplemental web-based materials provide relevant, evidence-based materials to enhance the reader's current practice.

Caring for Infants, Children, and their Families: Chapters 1 & 2

These chapters address the important elements germane to the care of children of all ages. It begins with a chapter addressing the developmental milestones and the changing needs children and their families have during each period of growth from infancy through adulthood. This section also includes a chapter on family-centered care. This expanded view of how to work with children and families includes information on how to deliver comprehensive care that incorporates the values and attitudes of the child, family, and healthcare team to address the special needs of the infant, child, and family.

Perinatal and Neonatal Care: Chapters 3–11

These chapters begin with an in-depth narrative of the natural history of pulmonary and cardiac development, adaptive developmental characteristics of maternal–fetal circulation, and transitional pulmonary and circulatory events that occur after a child is born. Key factors integral to assessing maternal needs to either provide the best outcomes or prepare for specialized care of the pre- or full-term infant after birth are detailed. The components of a general physical and cardiopulmonary assessment, as well as a laboratory and radiologic testing, are reviewed. Tables complement the text and provide the learner with age-specific normal values for vital signs, blood gases, and analytes. Color illustrations provide the learner with visual examples of common abnormal findings. Acquired and congenital disorders are reviewed, and best practices for managing the cardiopulmonary needs with respect to the specific disorder(s) are shared. This section also addresses the fundamentals of neonatal and infant resuscitation, which includes airway management, vascular access, medication administration, and maintaining adequate circulation as well as techniques used for stabilization in the postresuscitative phase.

Pediatric Care: Chapters 12–18

These five chapters provide a comprehensive review of the history, physical, and diagnostic assessment and care of the pediatric patient. This section begins with the indications for and techniques used to obtain an accurate history, including history of present illness, past medical and surgical history, and family history.

A detailed description of the initial physical examination and assessment of changes in patient status are also provided. The components of a general physical and cardiopulmonary assessment are reviewed, as are laboratory and radiologic testing. Recommendations and procedures required to resuscitate and stabilize the pediatric patient are presented, including cardiopulmonary resuscitation, airway management, and pharmacologic support.

This section details the etiology, diagnosis, and treatment of common acute and chronic pediatric respiratory disorders. A practical approach to evaluating clinical, laboratory, and radiologic imaging information used in the diagnosis and medical management of acute and chronic disorders of the cardiorespiratory system is provided. Acute and neurodegenerative disorders that affect the cardiorespiratory function are also discussed. The learner will gain an appreciation of how respiratory function is compromised and the therapeutic options available to stabilize and improve respiratory function.

Diagnosis, Monitoring, and Management: Chapters 19–32

These chapters focus on the specialized invasive and noninvasive equipment used to assess and monitor cardiopulmonary function and to treat cardiorespiratory disorders in infants and children. The learner will be presented with the theory and operational characteristics for diagnostic, monitoring, and therapeutic equipment commonly used for patients of all ages in a context that addresses the unique use and considerations specific to infants and children.

The chapters within this section will also familiarize the learner with the indications, proper use, and limitations of equipment used for elective and emergent care. Included are the systems and devices used to deliver oxygen, medicated aerosol, specialty gas, and airway clearance therapy as well as the devices used to secure and maintain a patent airway and to provide ventilatory support to infants and children. Evidence-based protocols for the initiation and management of specialty gas mixtures, ECMO, pharmacologic intervention, and mechanical ventilation include algorithms for care to facilitate critical thinking skills and application of best practices.

Transitional Care of Infants, Children, and Their Families: Chapters 33–35

The final chapters in this text address the needs of children and their families as they continue along the continuum of care from acute to subacute and extended care in the home or a long-term care facility. This section provides a comprehensive approach to the critical elements necessary for the safe transition from the acute care or hospital environment. The learner will be presented with the components essential to discharge planning, patient/family education, equipment selection and maintenance, home requirements, and outpatient care. The role of the respiratory therapist in supporting the family and facilitating the transition from acute to home or long-term care is discussed.

This section also addresses the sensitive issues patients and families face when making end-of-life decisions. Information distinguishing palliative care from hospice offers the learner information to assist with providing medical, emotional, and spiritual support to the family, patient, and medical care team.

What's Unique

- This text follows the NBRC matrix and can be used to prepare for the specialty credential examination.
- Case studies conclude every chapter, allowing readers to apply what they have learned.
- Each chapter provides the reader with a thorough review of the literature on the subject.
- Discussion of equipment within the chapters includes the indication and limitations of use, patient application, recommendations for troubleshooting, and technologic specifications.
- Chapters dedicated to neonatal and pediatric respiratory disorders provide not only the best practices for diagnosis and medical management but also discussion of forward-thinking research needs in this patient population.
- Information related to family-centered care is provided that will help the reader develop the necessary skills to work with neonatal and pediatric patients and their families and to better understand the unique needs and stresses that infants, children, and families experience during hospitalizations and when living with a serious illness.

How to Use This Book

Chapter Features

Each chapter of the book begins with a list of **Chapter Objectives** in the NBRC testing format to help you focus on the most important concepts in that chapter.

Each chapter contains **Tables** that highlight important information, such as **Table 18-10**, Behaviors and Responses Evaluated through the Glasgow Coma Scale.

This text is **highly illustrated** with diagrams and photos demonstrating a variety of concepts, including **Figure 19-10** which shows two methods of mixing a capillary blood sample.

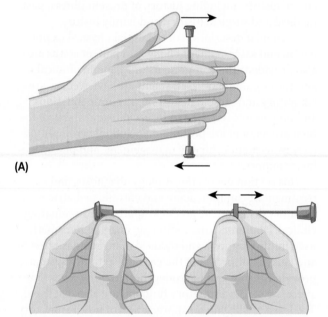

(A)

(B)

FIGURE 19-10 Mixing a capillary sample by (**A**) gently rolling the sample between the fingers and the palm or (**B**) inserting a metal filing, or flea, and using a magnet to move the filing within the blood sample.

Box features such as **Box 6-1** Calculation of Adequate Mean Blood Pressure Using Gestational Age, provide the reader with examples, equations, and numbered lists to clarify various techniques.

TABLE 18-10
Behaviors and Responses Evaluated through the Glasgow Coma Scale[76,80]

Behavior	Response	Score
Eye opening	Spontaneous	4
	Verbal command	3
	Open to pain	2
	Not opening	1
Verbal	Oriented	5
	Consolable but confused	4
	Inconsistent, inconsolable	3
	Inconsolable, agitated	2
	No response	1
Motor	Obeys commands	6
	Localizes pain	5
	Withdraws from pain	4
	Flexes from pain	3
	Extends from pain	2
	No motor response	1

Note: A score is assigned to each of the behaviors depending on the child's response.

Data from Kaplan JL, Porter RS. *Merck Manual of Diagnosis and Therapy.* 19th ed. Whitehouse Station, NJ: Merck Sharp & Dohme; 2011; and Hess D, MacIntyre N, Galvin W, Mishoe S. *Respiratory Care Principles and Practice.* 3rd ed. Burlington, MA: Jones & Bartlett Learning; 2016.

> **BOX 6-1 Calculation of Adequate Mean Blood Pressure Using Gestational Age**
>
> Gestational age in weeks + 5 = adequate mean blood pressure
>
> Example of adequate MBP for a 26 weeks' gestation neonate:
>
> $$26 + 5 = 31 \, mm \, Hg$$

Each chapter concludes with either a **Case Study** or **Critical Thinking** questions to help the reader review and put into practice what they have learned.

Case Study

A male premature infant was born by caesarean section at 27 weeks' gestation with a birth weight of 1100 grams. His Apgar scores were 1 at 1 minute and 6 at 5 minutes. After transfer to the NICU on CPAP 6 cm H_2O and an FiO_2 of 0.40, the patient's respiratory status deteriorated. He was intubated and received mechanical ventilatory respiratory support for 5 weeks for RDS. His first opthalmic examination revealed bilateral changes consistant with Grade 2 ROP. CryoROP criteria, treatment was performed at a corrected gestational age.

The infant responded well to the treatment, and both eyes showed rapid regression of the abnormal vessels.

1. **What are the main risks factors of developing ROP?**
2. **What classification system is used to describe the extent of ROP?**
3. **How many zones are used to define the area of retina covered by physiologic retinal vascularization?**

CRITICAL THINKING QUESTIONS

1. Explain what pulmonary surfactant is and why it is important to the developing fetal lung.
2. Describe the role hormones and growth factors play in fetal lung development.

Instructor and Student Resources

Qualified Instructors will receive a full suite of instructor resources, including the following:

For the Instructor
- A comprehensive chapter-by-chapter PowerPoint deck
- A test bank containing more than 1000 questions on a chapter-by-chapter basis as well as a midterm and a final

For the Students
- A full suite of flash cards to be used as a study tool
- A comprehensive practice exam of 140 new items that follow the detailed content outline for the NBRC Neonatal and Pediatric Specialty Examination
- Case studies are available online as writeable PDFs

About the Authors

Teresa A. Volsko, MBA, MHHS, RRT, CMTE, FAARC, is a fellow of the American Association for Respiratory Care and serves as adjunct faculty for Rush University in Chicago and Northeast Ohio Medical University in Ohio. Currently Terry is the director of Respiratory Care, Transport, and the Communication Center and interim director of the Rebecca D. Considine Research Institute for Akron Children's Hospital. She is the author of over 100 abstract and manuscript publications in peer-reviewed medical journals as well as several book chapters. Terry has served the profession in many capacities and is currently a member of the board of trustees for the American Respiratory Care Foundation, on the board of directors for Lambda Beta, editorial board member of the journal *Respiratory Care,* and on the American Association for Respiratory Care's Evidence-Based Clinical Guidelines Committee.

Born and raised in the Youngstown, Ohio, area, she received her associate degree in respiratory therapy technology, bachelor of science and master of health and human services, and master of business administration from Youngstown State University. Terry's passion for the respiratory care profession and her dedication to mentoring respiratory care students and credentialed professionals spans more than three decades.

Sherry L. Barnhart, RRT, RRT-NPS, AE-C, FAARC, is a fellow of the American Association for Respiratory Care and is currently the Respiratory Care Discharge Planner for Arkansas Children's Hospital. Sherry has previously edited two textbooks and a clinical handbook on perinatal and pediatric respiratory care. She has also authored multiple textbook chapters that are specific to the care of infants and children. Sherry is active in the respiratory care profession, where she has served in numerous leadership roles, including president of the Lambda Beta Society. During her nearly 40 years of experience in the field of neonatal and pediatric respiratory care, Sherry has maintained an unyielding commitment to provide the highest level of care to this patient population, serving as both an educator to respiratory therapy students and clinicians and as an advocate for obtaining advanced specialty credentials in this unique area of respiratory care practice.

Contributing Authors

Linda Allen-Napoli, MBA, RRT-NPS, RPFT
Director, Respiratory Care
The Children's Hospital of Philadelphia
Philadelphia, Pennsylvania

Joyce Baker, MBA, RRT, RRT-NPS, AE-C
Respiratory Therapist V, Asthma Liaison, Pulmonary
    Rehabilitation Therapist
Children's Hospital Colorado
Aurora, Colorado

Pamela Jo Baker, MSN, MBA, RN, PCNS-BC
Chief Nursing Information Officer
Akron Children's Hospital
Akron, Ohio

Melissa Baldwin, BSN, RN, RRT, RRT-NPS
Neonatal Intensive Care
Arkansas Children's Hospital
Little Rock, Arkansas

Ariel Berlinski, MD, FAAP
Professor of Pediatrics
UAMS College of Medicine
Medical Director, Respiratory Care Services
Arkansas Children's Hospital
Director, Pediatric Aerosol Research Laboratory
Arkansas Children's Research Institute
Little Rock, Arkansas

Peter Betit, MBA, RRT, RRT-NPS, FAARC
Director, Respiratory Care & ECMO Program
Boston Children's Hospital
Boston, Massachusetts

Michael T. Bigham, MD, FAAP, FCCM
Medical Director, Transport Services and Chief
    Quality Officer
Akron Children's Hospital
Akron, Ohio

Wendy G. Burgener, MSNc, APRN, CPNP, AC/PC
Pulmonary Pediatric Nurse Practitioner
University of Arkansas for Medical Sciences
Arkansas Children's Hospital
Little Rock, Arkansas

Lisa L. Bylander, BS, RRT, RRT-NPS, AE-C
Patient Care Coordinator, Respiratory Care Services
Arkansas Children's Hospital
Little Rock, Arkansas

April B. Carpenter, MSNc, APRN, CPNP-PC
Pulmonary Pediatric Nurse Practitioner/Coordinator
APRN Council Chair
University of Arkansas for Medical Sciences
Arkansas Children's Hospital
Little Rock, Arkansas

Gulnur Com, MD
Associate Professor of Clinical Pediatrics
University of Florida
Pediatric Pulmonology and Sleep Medicine
Sacred Heart Medical Group
Pensacola, Florida

Robin Connolly, BS, RRT
Respiratory Care Department
Boston Children's Hospital
Boston, Massachusetts

Eve deMontmollin, RN, CPN, CHPPN
Palliative Care Specialty Nurse
Arkansas Children's Hospital
Little Rock, Arkansas

Amanda Dexter, MS, RRT, RCP, CHSE
Clinical Assistant Professor
Global Medical Brigades Faculty Advisor
University of North Carolina at Charlotte
Charlotte, North Carolina

Kimberly L. DiMaria, MSN, CPNP-AC, CCRN
Pediatric Critical Care Nurse Practitioner
Children's Hospital Colorado
Aurora, Colorado

Mohamad El-Khatib, PhD, FAARC
Professor, Department of Anesthesiology
Director, Respiratory Therapy
American University of Beirut
New York, New York

Lee Evey, MHA, RRT, RRT-NPS
Director of Respiratory Care
Director of ECLS
Texas Children's Hospital
Houston, Texas

Katherine L. Fedor, MBA, RRT, RRT-NPS, CPFT
Manager, Pediatric Respiratory Care
Children's Hospital, Cleveland Clinic
Cleveland, Ohio

Kellianne Fleming, MS, RRT, RRT-NPS
Manager, Neonatal Pediatric Section
Rush University Medical Center
Chicago, Illinois

Noel Hairston, MBA/HCF, CRA
Administrative Director of Medical Imaging
Akron Children's Hospital
Akron, Ohio

Emma E. Holland, MSN, APRN, PNP-PC
Pediatric Nursing Faculty
University of Phoenix School of Nursing
Honolulu, Hawaii

M. Barbara Howard, BS, RPFT, AE-C
Clinical Laboratory Scientist
Pulmonary/Exercise Diagnostic Laboratories
Oishei Children's Outpatient Center
Buffalo, New York

James W. Hynson
Respiratory Therapist
Arkansas Children's Hospital
Little Rock, Arkansas

Lisa Johnson, BAS, RRT, AE-C
Pediatric Asthma Program
Vidant Medical Center
Greenville, North Carolina

Farrah D. Jones, BS, RRT, CPFT
Clinical Research Associate
Arkansas Children's Hospital Research Institute
Little Rock, Arkansas

Thomas G. Keens, MD
Professor of Pediatrics, Physiology, and Biophysics
Keck School of Medicine of the University of
    Southern California
Division of Pediatric Pulmonology and Sleep Medicine
Children's Hospital Los Angeles
Los Angeles, California

Pamela K. Leisenring, BS, RRT, RPFT
Supervisor, Pulmonary Laboratory
Arkansas Children's Hospital
Little Rock, Arkansas

Janna Matson, Pharm.D
Pharmacy Manager
Publix Pharmacy
Jacksonville, Florida

Dana Nelson, MSN, RN, CNS
Administrative Director, Maternal Fetal Medicine
Akron Children's Hospital
Akron, Ohio

Tim Op't Holt, EdD, RRT, AE-C, FAARC
Department Chair and Professor
Cardiorespiratory Care
University of South Alabama
Mobile, Alabama

Kendra Paxton, MSN, RN, CMTE
Flight Nurse
MetroHealth Medical Center
Cleveland, Ohio

Iris A. Perez, MD
Associate Professor of Clinical Pediatrics
Keck School of Medicine of USC
Attending, Division of Pediatric Pulmonology and
    Sleep Medicine
Children's Hospital Los Angeles
Los Angeles, California

Michelle Melin Peterson, BA, CCLS
Certified Child Life Specialist, Perianesthesia
Akron Children's Hospital
Akron, Ohio

John Priest, BSRT, RRT, RRT-NPS
ECMO Specialist
Boston Children's Hospital
Boston, Massachusetts

Charlotte V. Reikofski, MSPH, MPA, RRT
Manager
Pediatric Respiratory Therapy
Medical University of South Carolina
Charleston, South Carolina

Kimberly D. Robbins, BS, RRT, RRT-NPS, RPFT
Respiratory Therapist – Pulmonary Lab/Outpatient
Arkansas Children's Hospital
Little Rock, Arkansas

Amanda L. Roby, MHHS, RRT, RPGST, RST
Assistant Professor, Health Professions
Youngstown State University
Youngstown, Ohio

Laura Ryan, MD
Assistant Professor of Anesthesiology
Baylor College of Medicine
Staff Anesthesiologist
Texas Children's Hospital
Houston, Texas

Jamie L. Sahli, BS, RRT, AE-C
Program Director of Respiratory Therapy
Pickens Technical College
Aurora, Colorado

Scott Schachinger, MD
Neonatologist
Division of Neonatology
Akron Children's Hospital
Akron, Ohio

Steven Sittig, RRT, RRT-NPS, CNPT, FAARC
Flight Respiratory Therapist
Stanford Medical Center
Sioux Falls, South Dakota

Andrew South, MD
Neonatologist
Division of Neonatology
Akron Children's Hospital
Akron, Ohio

Stephen Stayer, MD
Professor of Anesthesiology and Pediatrics
Baylor College of Medicine
Associate Chief, Pediatric Anesthesiology
Texas Children's Hospital
Houston, Texas

Jana L. Teagle, BS, CTRS, CCLS, CBIS
Therapeutic Recreation, Child Life, & Brain Injury Specialist
Nemours/A. I. duPont Hospital for Children
Wilmington, Delaware

Kelly G. Thompson-Davis, BS, RRT, RRT-NPS, RN
Cardiovascular Intensive Care
Baptist Health Medical Center
Little Rock, Arkansas

Lisa Tyler, MS, RRT, RRT-NPS, CPFT, ACCS, AE-C
Manager, Respiratory Care Services
The Children's Hospital of Philadelphia
Philadelphia, Pennsylvania

Katherine R. Ward, PA-C
Pediatric Intensive Care Unit
Senior Instructor of Pediatrics
University of Colorado School of Medicine
Aurora, Colorado

Robert H. Warren, MD
Adjunct Clinical Professor
Department of Pediatrics
Pulmonary Medicine Section
University of Arkansas for Medical Sciences
Little Rock, Arkansas

Craig Wheeler, MS, RRT, RRT-NPS
Respiratory Care Supervisor
Boston Children's Hospital
Boston, Massachusetts

David M. Wheeler, MEd, RRT, RRT-NPS
Facilitator of Professional Development
Pediatric Respiratory Therapy
Medical University of South Carolina
Charleston, South Carolina

L. Denise Willis, MS, RRT, RRT-NPS
Research Respiratory Therapist
Arkansas Children's Hospital
Little Rock, Arkansas

Reviewers

Tanya J. Bird, MS, RRT
Director of Clinical Education
Polk State College
Winter Haven, Florida

Mary Beth Bodin, MSN, DNPc, NNP-BC
Faculty NNP Program
University of Alabama School of Nursing
University of Alabama at Birmingham
Birmingham, Alabama

Randy De Kler, MS, RRT
Program Director, Respiratory Care
Miami Dade College
Miami, Florida

Marie A. Fenske, EdD, RRT
Director of Clinical Education/Faculty
GateWay Community College
Phoenix, Arizona

Robert Harwood, MSA, RRT, RRT-NPS
Clinical Assistant Professor
Georgia State University
Atlanta, Georgia

Robert L. Joyner Jr., PhD, RRT, FAARC
Associate Professor and Chair of Health Sciences
Director, Respiratory Therapy Program
Salisbury University
Salisbury, Maryland

Heather Neal-Rice, MEd, RRT, RRT-NPS
Assistant Professor
University of Arkansas for Medical Sciences
Little Rock, Arkansas

Sara Parker, BHS, RRT, RRT-NPS
Clinical Instructor
University of Missouri
Columbia, Missouri

Shawna Strickland, PhD, RRT, RRT-NPS, RRT-ACCS,
  AE-C, FAARC
Associate Executive Director-Member Services
American Association for Respiratory Care
Irving, Texas

1

Growth and Development

Pamela Jo Baker
Michelle Melin Peterson

© Anna Rubak/ShutterStock, Inc.

OUTLINE

OBJECTIVES

1. Explain the benefits of a supportive family structure.
2. List the key concepts of family-centered care.
3. Discuss the developmental milestones that are key at each level of development.
4. Describe the uses for developmental milestones.
5. List the factors that have a profound effect on growth and physical development.
6. Discuss the impact hospitalization has on a child's growth and developmental milestones.
7. Describe interventions that can support a child's and family's psychosocial and emotional needs.

KEY TERMS

bonding
cyberbullying
deformational
   plagiocephaly
developmental milestones

family-centered care
growth charts
guided imagery
parallel play

Introduction

Infants and children experience rapid growth and development until adulthood. Their bodies and minds grow, adapt, and change to meet their ongoing and complex physical and mental needs in preparation for the demands of adult life. This constant change includes the growth of their body in all dimensions, along with the development of cognitive skills in their physical, mental, and emotional domains.

A supportive family structure will encourage the child to attain optimum growth and development through the nurturing of the child in a safe and stable environment. Family involvement and interest in supporting the growth and development of all aspects of life is essential to reach maximum potential as an adult. This support starts with the **bonding** between infant and parent at birth, where the relationship begins to develop, through interactions all through childhood (**Figure 1-1**). These interactions include looking, touching, talking, signing, playing, and taking an active interest in development, with continued progression throughout the child's life.

In 1959, Carl Rogers presented his ideas on client-centered therapy in psychiatric care. He contended that family life and society had implications on therapeutic relations through the mutual influence of the treatment process, family dynamics, and the individual's function and participation in social life.[1] Throughout the 1960s, Rogers's developed these ideas through work with pediatric institutions and parent advocacy efforts to highlight the importance and empowerment of the family in children's well-being. These concepts were developed further with the addition of the Bronfenbrenner model of developmental ecology, which consists of four systems, each operating at different levels but in the same space and time, from the most specific, or micro, level, through the meso, exo, and macro levels.[2] This model lent weight to the idea that the individual is not alone in their development but is influenced by their immediate family, extended family, and larger societal environment systems. The idea that a child's support from and interaction with those various levels influence the child's development and responses to stimuli is a tenet of the family-centered care model. Using the concepts of family-centered care when interacting with children and their family members helps develop a collaborative relationship with the family. The main concepts of family-centered care include the following: (1) recognition of the family as central to and providing the primary source of strength and support in the child's life, (2) acknowledging parents or adult caregivers as bringing expertise about the child, and (3) the concept that families are unique and diverse in their makeup.[1] Any assessment of the child's growth and development throughout their life span is dependent on their familial relationships.

Periods of Growth and Development

Infants and children experience rapid growth and development of their bodies and minds from infancy through adulthood. These changes include the growth of their body in all dimensions, along with the development of cognitive skills in their physical, mental, and emotional domains. The milestones associated with this growth can be measured physically and through the mastery of behaviors and skills.

Infants: Developmental Milestones

Developmental milestones are behaviors and tasks that most children can do by a certain age. Like growth, developmental milestones are built upon the experience and mastery of the behaviors before them. As the child ages, these developmental milestones can be used to gauge the progress of a particular child against the achievements of the average child. Just as a change or delay in growth can signal a health problem, changes in or failure to meet developmental milestones also signals a problem. Depending on the milestone, the problem can signal a problem in musculoskeletal or neurobiologic structure.

Physical Growth

The growth of an infant's body throughout childhood and into adulthood follows a well-documented pattern. There are tools for tracking this growth through sequential height, weight, head circumference, and/or basic metabolic index measurements over time. **Growth charts** are a series of percentile curves in which the selected body measurements of a particular child are plotted against the known percentile of other children. Typically, growth charts are specific to both the age and the sex of the child. Some growth charts are adjusted to compensate for premature birth, which allows for more accurate longitudinal comparisons as the child progresses through infancy into the toddler years. Using

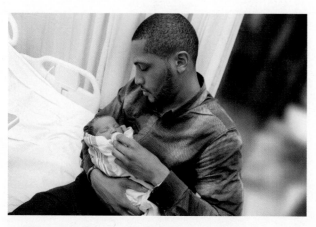

FIGURE 1-1 An illustration of bonding.
© USGirl/iStock/Getty Images Plus.

a sex-specific growth chart to plot the child's growth by age over time can determine the child's pattern of growth; compare their growth to other children of the same sex and age; and help to identify any unexpected lags or changes in their growth pattern, which could signal health issues for the child. The Centers for Disease Control and Prevention (CDC) recommends that the

World Health Organization's (WHO) growth standards be used to monitor the growth for infants and children ages 0 to 2 years, as shown in **Figure 1-2**, and that the CDC growth charts are used for children age 2 years and older in the United States.[3]

The growth and development of infants starts before birth, during the gestation period. The health

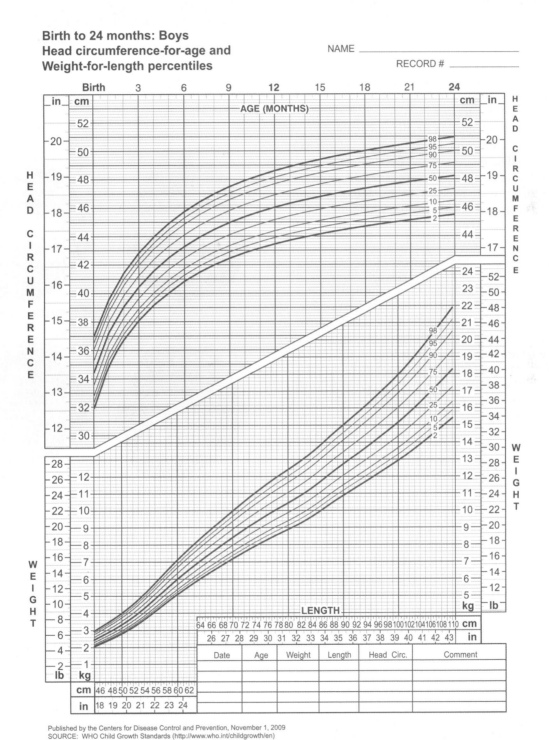

Birth to 24 months: Boys
Head circumference-for-age and
Weight-for-length percentiles

Published by the Centers for Disease Control and Prevention, November 1, 2009
SOURCE: WHO Child Growth Standards (http://www.who.int/childgrowth/en)

FIGURE 1-2 An example of a WHO and CDC growth chart.
Reproduced from the Centers for Disease Control and Prevention.

and genetic makeup of the mother and father, the length of gestation, and the environmental factors related to the pregnancy all influence the status of the infant at birth. Babies born prematurely can experience significant delays in growth and development as their bodies strive to overcome the physical stressors of early birth.

Infants, categorized as children from birth to age 1 year, grow rapidly this first year of life when following normal patterns of growth and development. Through age 6 months, infants will gain 150 to 210 grams (5–7 ounces) per week in weight and 2.54 cm (1 inch) in length per month to double their weight from birth. Growth slows slightly over the next 6 months to 90 to 150 grams (3–5 ounces) per week and half an inch per month. By 12 months of age, an infant has tripled in weight and doubled in length from birth.[4] The infant's nutritional status has a profound effect on growth and development. It is essential for infants to receive proper nutrition to support their growth needs. Sucking, swallowing, and breathing coordination are necessary functions that enable the infant to consume the adequate amount of calories to support growth and development.

In the first few months of life, an infant's activity is limited to sleeping and eating. Typically, an infant eats every 3 to 4 hours. Breast milk from the mother or another human milk donor provides the best source of nutrition, but if breast milk is not available, fortified formulas are an acceptable substitute. An infant who is unable to manipulate their tongue and lips to achieve a seal around the nipple and suck and swallow in coordination with breathing will experience growth and health problems. Growth will slow and the infant may exhibit symptoms of respiratory compromise related to aspiration. Infants with chronic cough or gagging, especially during feedings, need to be assessed for problems with muscle coordination and responses during feeds.

Because an infant spends much of their time sleeping, it is important to educate parents and caregivers on safe sleep practices. During sleep times, infants should be alone in bed, clothed in a safe sleep sack, and positioned supine, or on their back. The bed should be free from any other items (i.e., pillows or toys; see **Figure 1-3**). A single blanket may be used to cover the infant. Safe sleep guidelines were established by the American Academy of Pediatrics to prevent sudden infant death syndrome (SIDS), which usually occurs in previously healthy infants between ages 2 and 4 months.[5] While the "Back to Sleep" guidelines helped to reduce the incidence of SIDS, they have increased the incidence of related physical deformities. Many infants developed **deformational plagiocephaly**, or a physical condition whereby the soft bones of the head become flat on the back of the head as a result of frequently laying supine

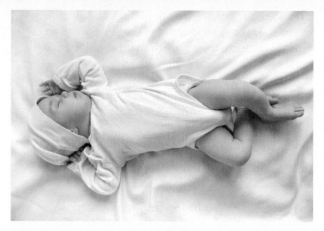

FIGURE 1-3 An example of a baby in a safe sleep position.
© DVAO/Shutterstock.

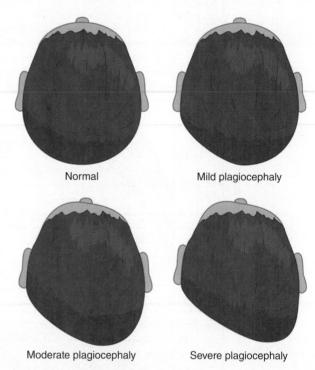

Normal   Mild plagiocephaly

Moderate plagiocephaly   Severe plagiocephaly

FIGURE 1-4 Different degrees or severity of deformational plagiocephaly.

for prolonged periods of time (**Figure 1-4**). In order to encourage the formation of correct skull shape as the infant ages, frequent position changes of the head and body are encouraged. An example is the use of tummy time, which is time when the infant, awake and supervised, is positioned prone (stomach down) on a firm surface and allowed to move independently to develop neck and chest muscles to lift their head and relieve pressure on the back of their skull. Infants can lift their heads with good control by age 3 months (**Figure 1-5**). Helmet therapy is often used to correct the malformation and guide the shape of the cranium as the child grows and develops (**Figure 1-6**).

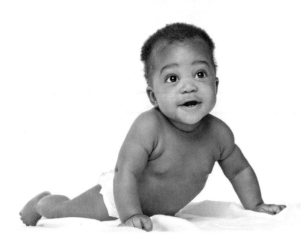

FIGURE 1-5 A child positioned prone, for tummy time.
© Flashon Studio/Shutterstock.

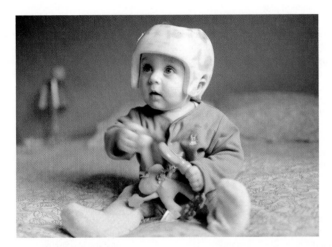

FIGURE 1-6 Helmet therapy may be used to help reshape the skull when a child has a more severe form of deformational plagiocephaly.
© area73/iStock/Getty Images Plus.

Cognitive, Sensory, and Language Growth

At age 6 months, teeth begin to erupt in the mouth, usually preceded by drooling and gumming behavior from age 4 months. Six months of age is considered the earliest time to introduce more solid foods by spoon to an infant. Language development parallels this development of oral skills, with cooing at age 2 months, babbling at age 6 months, and sound repetition at 9 months, such as ma-ma and da-da. By 1 year of age, infants can consistently use two to three words and begin to use gestures with these words, such as waving, shaking head no, and pointing at objects wanted. Infants recognize and understand words well before they have the ability to speak those words.

Motor Growth

An infant's gross motor functions, developing throughout the first year of life, are categorized in 3-month increments. As the muscles develop and strengthen, head control occurs at 3 months of age, sitting independently at 6 months of age, crawling at 9 months of age, and walking by 12 months of age. These skills progress, one after another, and build on the infant's growth in strength and coordination skills as each milestone is reached. The timing of skills to age is a generalization, as some infants achieve some skills sooner or later than average, but the sequence of skills stays the same (see **Table 1-1**).[4]

Social Growth

Social interactions in infancy progress from fixed eye movement and responsive smile to the ability to visually recognize and respond to caregivers by spontaneously smiling. As an infant's growth advances, the infant is awake and alert for longer periods of time. During this

TABLE 1-1
Growth and Developmental Milestones for Infants (Birth to 1 Year of Age)

Age	Physical	Gross Motor	Fine Motor	Sensory	Cognition
1 month	Weekly weight gain averages 150–210 g to double of birth weight by 6 months Monthly length gain of 2.5 cm Monthly head circumference increases by 1.5 cm	Assumes flexed position with pelvis high but knees not under abdomen when prone; turns head from side to side when prone	Strong grasp with hands predominately closed	Able to fixate on moving object in range of 45° when held at a distance of 20–25 cm; quiets when hears a voice	Cries to express displeasure and makes comfort sounds during feeding; watches parent's face intently when talking to infant
2 months	Posterior fontanel closes	Assumes less-flexed position when prone; lifts head up 45° when prone			Crying becomes differentiated; vocalizes to familiar voice; has social smile in response to stimuli

(Continues)

TABLE 1-1

Growth and Developmental Milestones for Infants (Birth to 1 Year of Age) (*Continued*)

Age	Physical	Gross Motor	Fine Motor	Sensory	Cognition
3 months	Primitive reflexes fading		Holds rattle but does not reach for it; holds hands open	Follows objects to periphery (180°); locates sound by turning head side to side and looking in same direction	Squeals to show pleasure and makes sounds to talk when spoken to; less crying during wakeful periods with interest in surroundings
4 months		Has almost no head lag when pulled to a sitting position and balances head when sitting; rolls from back to side	Reaches for objects but overshoots, grasps objects with both hands, plays with hands and pulls clothes over face in play		Laughs aloud and shows excitement with whole body
5 months	Start of tooth eruptions	Turns from abdomen to back	Grasps objects voluntarily, takes objects to mouth directly, plays with toes	Visually pursues dropped objects	
6 months	Has two lower central incisors	Rolls from back to abdomen, may chew and bite as teeth erupt	Holds bottle, secures dropped objects, will drop one item to take another	Adjusts posture to see object	Begins to imitate sounds; babbles one-syllable utterances like ma, da, or di; begins to fear strangers, holds arms up to be picked up
7 months	Upper central incisors erupt Weekly weight gain averages 90–150 g to triple birth weight by 12 months Monthly height gain of 1.25 cm to increase height by 50% from birth length	Sits, leaning forward on both hands	Transfers objects from one to other hand	Can fixate on small objects; responds to name	Produces vowel sounds and chained syllables like mama, dada; has increasing fear of strangers and fretfulness when parent out of sight
8 months		Sits steadily unsupported	Reaches for toys out of reach and begins using pincer grasp		Responds to the word no
9 months	Upper lateral incisors erupt	Pulls self to stand and stands holding on to furniture; creeps on hands and knees	Uses thumb and index finger in pincer grasp	Localizes sound by turning head diagonally and directly toward sound	
10 months		While standing, lifts foot to take step; sits by falling down	Crude release of objects begins		Says dada and mama with meaning; develops object permanence

Age	Physical	Gross Motor	Fine Motor	Sensory	Cognition
11 months	Lower lateral incisors erupt	Cruises or walks holding on to furniture or with both hands held	Drops objects deliberately to be picked up; has neat pincer grasp		Plays games up-down, so big, peek a boo; shakes head for no; may develop habit of security blanket or favorite toy
12 months		Walks with one hand held; attempts to stand alone momentarily	Attempts to build two-block stack but fails; can turn pages in book but many at a time	Discriminates simple geometric shapes, can follow rapidly moving objects	Says 3–5 words besides mama/dada; comprehends meaning of several words; searches for objects even if not hidden but only in last place seen

Data from *Wong's Nursing Care of Infants and Children*, Hockenberry and Wilson, 2015 (pp. 430–433).

period, infants become increasingly able to console and comfort themselves, and they begin exploring their environment and surroundings through their five senses: by reaching for objects; placing objects in their mouth; attending through sound; responding to simple games, such as peek-a-boo; and imitating facial expressions. Temperament, or behavioral tendencies, begins to present at this young age. Language is developing as a means of communication and expression. Older infants learn that specific actions lead to specific responses and can repeat actions. Play consists of exploring self and becoming aware of their environment. Socially, caregivers are the providers of all the child's needs and a firm attachment bond should be established. During this attachment phase, children develop trust. Once trust has been established, children typically begin to experience separation/stranger anxiety around 7 months of age.

Toddlers: Developmental Milestones

Toddlers, ages 12 months to 36 months, are keen explorers of their world as their bodies continue to grow fast but not as rapidly as their infant phase (**Figure 1-7**). As toddlers grow and develop, they master independent movement and thinking.

Physical Growth

A toddler's growth rate is 1.8 to 2.7 kg (4–6 pounds) per year and height growth slows to 7.5 cm (3 inches) per year.[6] Growth in height is more from leg than trunk growth, which occurs in spurts over months; therefore, when plotted on a growth chart, a step-like pattern of growth can be seen.

During the toddler years, their major gross motor development is independent walking and refinement

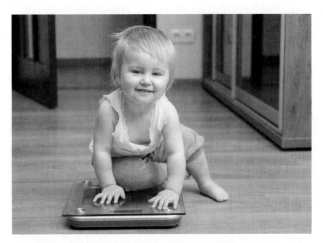

FIGURE 1-7 Toddlers explore their environment.
© Tatyana Vyc/Shutterstock.

of this behavior. By age 1 year, toddlers can walk independently, and at 18 months are attempting to run but fall frequently. By 2 years of age, toddlers are walking well and mastering going up and down stairs one at a time, kicking a ball, and running with fewer falls.[7] By 2.5 years, toddlers can stand on one foot for a few seconds and take a few steps on tiptoe. By age 3 years, these skills are well developed and smoothly completed.[7]

Cognitive, Sensory, and Language Growth

Toddlers are very curious and learn many things from their environment via sight and touch. Vigilant supervision of the toddler's activity is very important for the child's safety. Drowning is the leading cause of injury and death for toddlers, so activities around water,

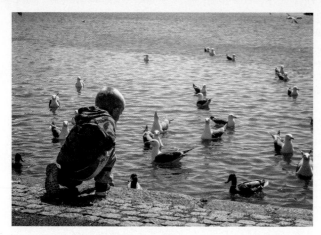

FIGURE 1-8 A child's natural curiosity poses a risk for drowning, especially near pools, ponds, and lakes.
© Edgar9/Shutterstock

including bathtubs, pools, ponds, lakes, whirlpools, or the ocean, must be supervised at all times (**Figure 1-8**). Swimming and water safety lessons should be started as early as possible. Another frequent developmental risk is choking. Toddlers should sit when eating and be instructed to chew food thoroughly to prevent choking. Toys and small items, including pencils, crayons, or lollipops, should not be allowed in mouths while walking or playing.

Motor Growth

Fine motor skills are also developing and refining throughout the toddler years. Toddlers develop these skills through play and practice, such as throwing overhand and retrieving objects when playing catch with others, making intentional circles and straight lines when drawing, and use of utensils while eating. At this age, toddlers can also build towers with four or more blocks and will knock it over and retrieve the objects over and over as they practice these skills. **Table 1-2** provides a summary of the developmental milestones that toddlers experience.

Social Growth

Toddlers move from dependence to independence as they master their newly acquired motor, language, and intellectual skills. Children learn their body parts at this age as well as begin to exhibit control over their body functions. Autonomous behavior is being exhibited as they curiously explore their environment with these skills while still trusting the relationship and bond that has been established with their caregiver(s). Developmentally, older toddlers become egocentric—their world is about them. During which time, they enter into a "me," "I can do it myself" phase. Toddlers can also be possessive. Children in this age group move from watching children play to **parallel play**, which

is playing alongside other children but not engaging. They also begin pretend play at this age. Older toddlers may start to exhibit fearful behaviors in response to stressors.

Preschoolers: Developmental Milestones

The preschool years span from 3 through 5 years of age. A significant period of growth and development occurs during this period as children prepare for a more independent life, which is usually signaled by attending school. During this period, children are mastering their fine and gross motor skills, including control of their bodily systems. A preschooler's cognitive skills include the development of increased attention span and memory. They work more cooperatively and play with others, instead of in parallel. They also are more tolerant of separation from their parents and are able to interact with strangers without much anxiety.

Physical Growth

Physical growth is very similar to toddlers in that the growth rate is approximately 2 to 3 kilograms (4.4–6.6 pounds) per year. Height growth is slower and occurs in spurts.[6] Growth in the long bones of the legs occurs more than in the trunk (**Figure 1-9**).

Cognitive, Sensory, and Language Growth

Preschoolers become more interested in learning about adults and children outside of the family, including gender roles and norms. As they explore their environment more widely, their risk for injuries related to accidental trauma increases; accidents remain their leading causes of injury or death. To prevent injury, it is important to teach preschoolers about traffic safety and to reinforce the use of traffic safety when they play. It is equally important to teach children how to properly use safety gear, such as helmets, car seats, and seat belts; adherence to the use of safety gear requires vigilance by parents, caregivers, and adults

Cognitive development continues with more complex language skills and understanding. Parents and adults interacting with preschoolers should expose them to complete sentences and a wider range of vocabulary words in conversation and reading materials. A preschooler's vocabulary expands from about 300 words at age 2 years to more than 2100 words by the end of age 5 years.[6] Preschoolers, especially 4-year-olds, are very inquisitive; they ask many questions about their observations to increase their understanding. Preschoolers need clear and consistent instructions, in step-by-step explanations that include the expected behaviors for each step. If behavior varies from what is expected, the preschooler should receive feedback on the expected behavior, including an explanation on how to successfully achieve that behavior.[7]

TABLE 1-2
Growth and Developmental Milestones for Toddlers (2–3 Years of Age)

Age	Physical	Gross Motor	Fine Motor	Sensory	Cognition
2 years	Average weight gain 1.8–2.7 kg/year	Runs well; wide stance	Builds tower of 6–7 blocks; aligns 2–4 blocks into train	Able to differentiate geometric shapes and colors	Increasing independence from parents
	Average height gain 10–12.5 cm/year	Kicks ball forward without falling	Turns pages of book one at a time	Finds things even when hidden under two or three covers	Shows defiant behavior (doing what they have been told not to)
	Adult height is approximately twice height at 2 years	Goes up and down stairs alone, one step at a time	Turns doorknob; unscrews lids	Completes sentences and rhymes in familiar books	Dresses self in simple clothes
		Picks up object without falling	Might use one hand more than the other	Plays simple make-believe games	Has 300-word vocabulary and talks in 2- to 3-word phrases
				Follows two-step instructions, such as "Pick up your shoes and put them in the closet."	Uses verbal self-reference (mine, me, I)
					Developing awareness that others have different feelings and desires
3 years	Average height gain 7.3 cm/year	Climbs well	Copies a circle with a pencil or crayon	Shows concern for a crying friend	Copies adults and friends
	Average weight gain 2.5 cm	Runs easily	Can work toys with buttons, levers, and moving parts	Shows affection without prompting	Separates easily from parents
		Pedals a tricycle (three-wheel bike)	Does puzzles with three or four pieces	Shows a wide range of emotions	Understands the idea of mine and his or hers
		Walks up and down stairs, one foot on each step	Builds tower of 9–10 blocks; uses blocks to build bridge	May get upset with major changes in routine	Understands words like in, on, and under
			Feeds self independently	Knows own and others' gender	Follows instructions with two or three steps
					Play is parallel
					Learning simple games but follows own rules

Data from *Wong's Nursing Care of Infants and Children*, Hockenberry and Wilson, 2015 (pp. 499 and 529) (Wilson D., 2015) and (Centers for Disease Control and Prevention, 2016).

The development of children's understanding of others and their own mind has been studied under the concepts developed through Wimmer and Perner's "theory of mind" work.[8] This field of socio-cognitive science dates back to the late 1970s and seeks to explain and predict the development of children's understanding of the mind and how it relates to human actions and interactions. At approximately 4 years of

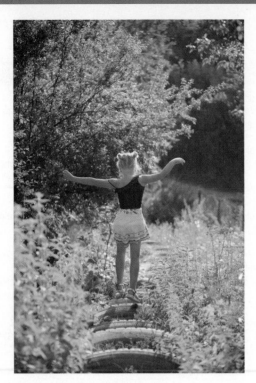

FIGURE 1-9 Preschoolers experience growth in the long bones of the legs during their growth spurts.
© Natalia Kirsanova/Shutterstock.

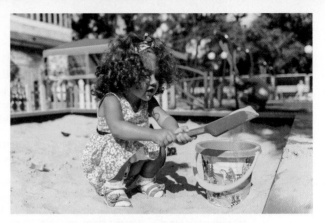

FIGURE 1-10 A preschooler at play.
© Helen Sushitskaya/Shutterstock.

age, children begin to understand that there may be alternative representations of the same object: the literal representation and the figurative representation. This development is the beginning of understanding metaphors and other idioms of speech used to communicate with others.[9] To facilitate and enhance meaningful communication, it is important to recognize where the child is on this continuum of understanding. This development of cognition is similar to the intuitive thought phase from age 4 to 7 years, described in Piaget's cognitive theory. Piaget's cognitive theory explains the development of social awareness and others' points of view from the preconceptional phase (2–4 years of age), which has more egocentric thinking and a self-centered point of view.[10]

Motor Growth

Playing is an important activity and essential to the development of a preschooler's gross motor function. Eye–hand coordination improves during this phase, as the child learns to catch and throw a ball, hop, skip, and jump (**Figure 1-10**). During this phase of growth and development, the child begins to alternate steps while climbing and walking down stairs. **Table 1-3** outlines the normal developmental milestones preschoolers reach.

Social Growth

Preschool-age children experience mastery of their environment and, at this stage, are preoccupied with how they can control it. They begin to show the ability

to separate from caregivers for short periods of time. Self-control behaviors are developed at this stage as well. Preschoolers also begin to develop empathy. Preschoolers may become more fearful and view illness as punishment. Play moves from associative to play that is cooperative as they begin to interact with other children, learning about taking turns and sharing and becoming aware of others' emotions. Preschoolers engage in symbolic play, turning an object into something new or different,[11] as well as increased imaginative play.

School-Age Children: Developmental Milestones

Middle childhood brings many changes in a child's life. By this time, children can dress themselves, catch a ball more easily using only their hands, and tie their shoes. Having independence from family becomes more important to the child during this stage of growth and development. Attending school allows the child to have regular contact with a larger world. Friendships become more and more important. Physical, social, and mental skills develop quickly during this time, making this stage a critical period for a child's development. School-age children develop confidence in all areas of life, including through friends, schoolwork, and sports.

Physical Growth

As the preadolescence period begins, growth rates for girls and boys begin to differ. Girls grow more rapidly and develop their secondary sexual characteristics from 9 to 13 years of age, while boys lag about 2 years behind girls' development.[12] For girls, the most notable characteristics are the onset of public hair and breast development. A recent study addressed the effect that age and ethnicity have on the sexual maturation of children in the United States. The median age for onset of pubic hair among girls varies by ethnicity, with appearance at approximately 9.4 years

TABLE 1-3
Growth and Developmental Milestones for Preschoolers (Age 4–5 Years)

Age	Physical	Gross Motor	Fine Motor	Socialization	Cognition
4 years old	Growth is slower and regular	Skips and hops on one foot	Able to cut out pictures following outline	Would rather play with other children	Starts to understand time
	Height increases 6.5–9 cm annually	Catches ball reliably	Can lace shoes but may not be able to tie bow	Is more creative in make believe; tries role-playing	Remembers parts of a story
	Weight gain is 2–3 kg annually	Throws ball overhand	Can copy more complex shapes, like diamonds	Tells stories to others, sometimes dramatically	Understands the idea of same and different
		Walks down stairs using alternating steps	Draws a person with two to four body parts	Knows simple songs	Names some colors and some numbers
			Starts to copy some capital letters	Tends to be selfish and impatient	Judges others by one dimension (e.g., height, weight, or order)
					Able to run simple errands outside the home
					Very aware of rules but does not always understand what is right or wrong
5 years old	Eruption of permanent dentation may begin	Can do a somersault	Uses fork and spoon, sometimes table knife	Less rebellious, more trustworthy and responsible	Counts 10 or more things
	Handedness is established, with about 90% of children being right handed	Can use the toilet on own	Can draw a person with at least six body parts	Eager to do things correctly and follow the rules	Knows about things used every day, like money and food
		Swings and climbs	Can print some letters or numbers		Speaks very clearly
		Jumps rope	Copies a triangle and other geometric shapes		Tells a simple story using full sentences
		Walks backward			Uses future tense in sentences

Data from *Wong's Nursing Care of Infants and Children*, Hockenberry and Wilson, 2015 (pp. 529–530) (Wilson D., 2015) and Centers for Disease Control and Prevention Important Milestones (Centers for Disease Control and Prevention, 2016).

for non-Hispanic blacks, 10.6 years for non-Hispanic whites, and 10.4 years for Mexican Americans. The median age for the onset of female breast development was found to be approximately 9.5 years for non-Hispanic blacks, 9.8 years for Mexican Americans, and 10.4 years for non-Hispanic whites.[13] Similarly, ethnicity affected the median age for secondary sexual characteristics in males. The median age for the onset of pubic hair development for boys was

approximately 11.2 years for non-Hispanic blacks, 12.0 years for non-Hispanic whites, and 12.3 years for Mexican Americans.

During this period, there is growing awareness of changes in body shape for both sexes as puberty approaches. Body image and eating problems will typically surface during this developmental phase. Body image stress can also occur as children observe their growth pattern differing from others, particularly if the school-age child perceives their growth as earlier than their peers, later than their peers, or occurring at a different rate. It is important to reassure children and to explain that physical changes follow a pattern and occur at a pace that are unique to them.

Cognitive, Sensory, and Language Growth

School-age children are beginning to find their place in the world. They play on teams and work together much more than younger children; they want to be liked and accepted by friends; and they communicate their experiences, thoughts, and feelings much more articulately to others, especially their peers. Although they are very active and engage with others in play, they also investigate their own interests, including starting collections or participating in activities related to a particular topic. Children of this age enjoy joining clubs and being a member of a cohesive group, but a consequence of this engagement with their peers is that children who have physical and/or socioeconomic differences from their peers may experience social pressure to conform to the preferences, activities, and behaviors of the rest of the group. Children experiencing social pressures develop coping behaviors to mask their differences. For example, children with diabetes may find that their diet restrictions, blood testing, and insulin injections make them feel different from their peers, so they start eating like their peers or skipping glucose testing or insulin injections when around others. If a child has a scar, chronic disease, or developmental challenge, for example, there is potential for the child to be a victim of bullying, where they are subjected to repetitive emotional, verbal, or physical abuse by others who want to establish power in their group.[14]

Motor Growth

Independence and increased physical confidence facilitate an exploration of the physical environment and physical development. Typically, there is less adult supervision and an increased propensity for adventure and risk-taking during this developmental phase. Therefore, middle childhood can lead to more adventure injuries. These injuries are typically sports- and/or activity-related and include injuries associated with the use of bikes, scooters, skateboards, skates, and sleds.[15] Boys are more injury prone at this age than girls, which is directly related to the frequency with which risk-taking behavior occurs.[15] Safety guidelines for this age are important for children to follow to decrease the risk to injury. **Table 1-4** provides a summary of growth and developmental milestones common to school-age children.

Social Growth

School-age children move to an industrious phase, wanting to be successful in typical activities, such as

school, as more processes in their growth and development take shape. The development of concrete thought process and the ability to begin to reason mean that school-age children may exhibit misconceptions and fears. Children in this age group are able to separate from parents for longer periods of time; be cooperative; be attentive; and more fully understand directions, relationships, and morals.[11] In this age group, children have a sense of self and are relating to and engaging with peers, who are becoming increasingly important. School-age children will begin to develop same-sex friendships. They learn to collaborate and compete.

Adolescents: Developmental Milestones

As children grow toward their teen years, this next phase of their development completes the transition to adulthood. Adolescence, from approximately 13 to 18 years, is a time filled with biologic maturation and the physical and cognitive changes needed for an independent adult life.

Physical Growth

Puberty is a collective term for this period of physical maturation. It is a sequence of changes started and controlled by hormonal influences. There is no one trigger to the start of puberty. The hypothalamus-pituitary-gonadal system, which developed in the fetal stage of life, matures and releases increasing levels of gonadotropin-releasing hormone, which influences the timing and rate of onset of puberty; these hormonal changes are affected by environment and the body's overall health, physical fitness, and nutritional level.[16]

Female response to this change in hormones includes the development and release of eggs from the ovaries, known as menstruation (the beginning of which is called menarche), in a cyclic pattern approximately every 28 days. The buildup of estrogen in high enough concentrations during puberty causes the growth and development of the vagina, uterus, fallopian tubes, and breasts as well as the development of pubic and axillary hair. Male development is attributed to increased testosterone secretion. Testosterone and other androgens cause growth and development of the male reproductive system, penis, scrotum, prostate, and seminal vesicles of the testicles to produce and deliver sperm. These hormones also influence muscle mass growth, general body and facial hair growth, and the deepening of the voice.[17]

Cognitive, Social, and Emotional Growth

Adolescents also experience emotional growth. During this phase, their sexual identity is established and this manifests in interactions with others. Homosexual, bisexual, or transgender orientation is also known to the person, and their interactions with others will be framed around the positive or negative acceptance they perceive from family and friends.

TABLE 1-4
Growth and Developmental Milestones for School-Age Children (6–12 Years)

Age	Physical	Gross Motor	Fine Motor	Socialization	Cognition
6–7 years	Loses first tooth; jaw begins to expand to accommodate permanent teeth	Able to bathe and achieve bedtime routines without supervision	Likes to draw, paint, cut, fold, and print	Starts to form stronger, more complex friendships and peer relationships; becomes more emotionally important to have friends, especially of the same sex	Understands the concept of numbers
	Increased dexterity		Able to use knife at table	Experiences more peer pressure	Begins to understand time measurements and uses watches and clocks
	Vision reaches maturity				Can be boastful and cheat to win
					Has difficulty acknowledging their misdeeds
8–9 years	Continues to gain height 5 cm per year	Dresses self completely	Reads more, enjoys comics	Is more critical of self	Interested in boy–girl relationships
	Moves constantly with smooth control	Makes use of common tools and is able to be responsible for household chores	Knows dates and calendar progression	Fears failing, especially in school	Explores home and community alone and with friends
			Understands concepts of whole and parts and fractions	Able to run errands	Plays mostly with the same sex but occasionally with the opposite sex
				Able to make choices in purchases	
				Takes music and sport lessons	
10–12 years	Becomes more aware of body as puberty approaches	Washes and dries hair	Writes brief stories	Respects parents	Is more diplomatic in interactions with others
	Male growth slows, weight gain continues	Able to complete all grooming needs but may need to be reminded to do so	Uses telephone for contact with friends and family	Very invested in friends and talks about them constantly	May have a best friend
	Remainder of permanent teeth erupt, except for wisdom teeth			Family connections are important	

Data from *Wong's Nursing Care of Infants and Children*, Hockenberry and Wilson, 2015 (pp. 584–585) (Rodgers, 2015) and Centers for Disease Control and Prevention Important Milestones (Centers for Disease Control and Prevention, 2016).

Romantic relationships start to develop from age 14 years.[16] However, girls and boys experience sexual arousal differently. Boys begin masturbating between 12 and 15 years of age and, in general, practice regularly.[16] As such, boys are more familiar, during adolescence, with their path to pleasure and orgasm prior to intimacy with a partner, while girls are less likely to engage in masturbation and generally experience their first arousal with an intimate partner. Girls' attitudes toward sex, their sexual experience, and the likelihood of adolescent pregnancy are impacted by the focus of their sexual health education. If the education focused on the context of relationships, adolescent girls tend to be more knowledgeable about sex, have less sexual experience, and experience fewer adolescent pregnancies than education that focused on the body.[16]

According to the 2011 Youth Risk Behavior Survey, 47% of adolescents in high school report engaging in sexual intercourse.[18] The 2006–2010 National Survey of Family Growth reports only 78% of adolescent females and 85% of adolescent males 15 to 19 years of age used a contraceptive method for first sexual intercourse.[19] Most pregnancies (88%) among adolescents (15–17 years of age) in the United States are unintended. The birth rate to 15- to 19-year-old females was 39.1 per 1000 female subjects in 2011; however, birth rate statistics underestimate actual adolescent pregnancy rates because they do not include pregnancies that end either through abortion or other fetal loss.

This last phase of childhood adds more freedom of choice in activities and lifestyle as the teen navigates to adult life. This is a time of experimentation and risk taking. Family influences continue to be of importance in the lives of adolescents, even as they turn their attention to friends and partners. Children raised in single-parent families, typically headed by females, experience more behavioral problems and poorer academic achievement, engage in earlier sexual activity, demonstrate poorer psychological well-being, and experience greater life adversity as compared to the children of two-parent families.[20] Friend and family relationships also impact substance use and abuse. The protective effects of family and school connections decrease the risk of substance abuse, in the forms of tobacco use, alcohol binge drinking, and use of cannabis.[21] Peers remain the strongest social factor influencing alcohol, tobacco, and illicit drug use, particularly when the teen's best friend uses these substances.[21]

Risk taking during this period, as with the former years, can result in injuries. Injuries from high-risk behaviors can mask self-harm tendencies. Repeated presentations to emergency rooms for injury may signify an underlying mental health problem that is not being addressed or acknowledged by the teen.[22] Patterns of self-harm may or may not signal suicidal intent. These patterns may also be a means of coping with strong feelings or emotional distress. Self-harm is generally

TABLE 1-5

Common Causes of Intentional and Unintentional Death among Teens

Cause	% of Deaths
Accidents	48
Homicide	13
Suicide	11
Cancer	6
Heart disease	3

differentiated from suicide attempts by the intent of the action: Self-harm is the result of an act of self-injury or self-poisoning that was not intended to result in death.[23] Behavioral health interventions are necessary when self-harm is suspected to prevent escalation of these behaviors to more serious health events or death.

Adolescents are most prone to injury or death related to preventable activities. The leading causes of death in adolescence are unintentional injuries from accidents[24] (see **Table 1-5**). Motor vehicle accidents accounted for almost three-quarters (73%) of all deaths from unintentional injury.[24] A significant contributor to morbidity and mortality in teens is substance use, especially alcohol use. Fatal accidents occur at greater frequency while driving under the influence. Substance use is also a main contributor to accidental poisonings and drownings. Adolescents, who have multiple risk behaviors, have a significant increase in the likelihood of death because of a greater and more frequent exposure to dangerous situations.[25]

Adolescents today have been born into a world with widespread use of technology. These digital natives take technological changes and advances in stride and use these tools easily in their daily lives. They use social media to develop ties outside their family, and sometimes their community, for a more worldly view. Technology and digital media outlets help adolescents form a personal cultural identity, which may differ from their family of origin because their use of technology enables them to reach a more global network of people with viewpoints that may differ from what they are regularly exposed to.[26] Developing their own cultural identity can strain familial patterns, especially with regard to behavior expectations.

The use of technology can also expose the adolescent to other dangers, such as cyberbullying. This behavior is similar to bullying previously discussed with school-age development. **Cyberbullying** is covert psychological bullying conveyed through electronic means and can result in physical and psychological harm with emotional distress, symptoms of depression, and adverse coping mechanisms, such as withdrawal and substance abuse.[27] Other symptoms of bullying include stomachaches, headaches, nausea, insomnia, and anxiety. Open and frank discussions with the adolescent about their interactions with others, in person and electronically, can help to determine if bullying, whether virtual or physical, is occurring. It is important to consider that adolescents may be reluctant to confess to cyberbullying because of the fear that limitations may be placed on their access to electronic media and interactions with others.

Adolescents are discerning "who" they are and are learning how to achieve and communicate their self-identity. Abstract reasoning leads them to more complex, competitive activities, both intellectually and socially. Adolescents also have an increased need for privacy. Achieving independence is the aim in the adolescent years. Peer groups and socialization are paramount and keeping connected is vital. **Table 1-6** provides an overview of the growth and development milestones that adolescents experience.

TABLE 1-6
Growth and Development Milestones for Adolescents (13–18 Years)

Age	Physical	Sexuality	Identity	Sensory	Cognition
12–14 years	Growth accelerates	Starts to explore intimate self with evaluation of development	Tries out different roles as they explore their potential	Increased moodiness	Shows more interest in and influence by peer group
	Secondary sexual characteristics appear	Starts to date, usually in groups	Focus is on themselves; going back and forth between high expectations and lack of confidence	Feels a lot of sadness or depression	Expresses less affection toward parents; sometimes might seem rude or short-tempered
			Concerned about body image, looks, and clothes	Spends time daydreaming	Feels stress from more challenging schoolwork
			Decline in self-esteem		Could develop eating problems
15–17 years	Stature reaches 95% of adult height	Identifies sexual orientation, at least internally, but may not be ready to share with others if outside the perceived norm	Self-centered	Tendency to withdraw when upset	Abstract thinking developing
	Slowing growth in girls	Deep capacity for caring and sharing	Rich fantasy life	Emotional responses fluctuate over time	Concern with philosophic, political, and societal problems
	Secondary sexual characteristics well advanced	Developing more intimate relationships		Sensitive to feeling inadequate and finds it hard to ask for assistance	
18 years and older	Physically mature with growth almost complete	Forms stable relationships and attachments	Body image mostly established	Emotions are more constant	Has established abstract thought
	Comfortable in physical growth and body	May publicly identify as homosexual or bisexual	Mature sexual identity	Able to better regulate external expressions of emotion	Able to view problems systematically
			Increase in self-esteem		Can develop and execute long-term plans

Data from *Wong's Nursing Care of Infants and Children*, Hockenberry and Wilson, 2015 (p. 652) (Ethington, 2015) and Centers for Disease Control and Prevention Important Milestones (Centers for Disease Control and Prevention, 2016).

Hospitalization and the Effect Hospitalizations Have on Growth and Developmental Needs

Infants and children are hospitalized for a variety of reasons. Many are hospitalized shortly after birth and require repeated hospitalizations for conditions or defects present at birth, which are attributed to a complex mix of genetic, environmental, and maternal factors. Acute and chronic illnesses, as well as accidental and nonaccidental injuries, commonly require hospitalization. Suspicious injuries, failure to grow or weight loss, and changes in development should be investigated for the cause, including review of the family support structure for the infant.

Hospitalization, although at times a necessary component of medical care, is a very unfamiliar setting for a child. It is essential for the healthcare staff to provide a supportive environment in which the child's fears are addressed, comfort is provided, and the child is supported in a way that fosters continued growth and development. This is especially important to children with chronic illnesses, such as congenital heart defects, cystic fibrosis, and cancer, where repeated extended hospitalizations may be required throughout their childhood.

Effects of Hospitalization on Growth and Developmental Milestones

Healthy children typically develop on a continuum. Children grow and learn very quickly through these early years, and each milestone a child achieves is typically a building block for all future milestones.

Some healthcare encounters, such as frequent outpatient visits, surgeries, and repeated and/or extended hospitalizations, pose special challenges to a child's typical growth and emotional well-being. Children may experience lapses or regression in physical, emotional, intellectual, or social development. Pain can also influence or impede development. Emma Plank, a pioneer in child life development, recognized the negative impact extended hospitalizations had on children, especially when no parent was present or there was a need for isolation precautions for infection control.[27] Limited emotional support and decreased opportunities for socialization impeded the child's normal growth and development experiences.[27] As a result, programs were established to help children cope and develop more holistically in hospital settings. These programs were specifically designed to address a child's emotional, social, and cognitive needs, with the intent of overcoming the developmental setbacks hospitalization can cause.

TABLE 1-7

Age-Specific Hospitalization Issues and Concerns Based on Erickson's Psychosocial Stages of Development

Age	Psychosocial Concerns in Healthcare Settings
Birth to 1 year	Separation from caregivers; unfamiliar environment, routine, and people; lack of stimulation
1–3 years	Reduced independence; lack of opportunities for self-control; separation anxiety
4–5 years	Limitations on sense of control and independence; magical thinking and egocentric thought resulting in misunderstanding; fear
6–12 years	Separation from normal activities associated with home, school, and peers; concrete literal thought resulting in misconceptions; fear of body mutilation, loss of body function; reduced self-esteem
13–17 years	Limitations related to privacy, peer relationships, independent activity, and decision making; concerns with perception of others, body image

Data from (Rollins, 2005) pp. 22–23; (Thompson, 2009) p. 30.

Children between 9 months and 4 years of age are most vulnerable to the negative effects and stressors of hospitalization.[28] Early hospitalization can affect a child's long-term development and adjustment. Additionally, repeated hospitalizations early in life have been linked to emotional disturbances that may manifest in a child's later years.[29]

Providing support to the family as a unit is equally important. Children will respond to their caregiver's cues. An anxious parent can project anxiety to their child, causing their child to respond to care in an anxious manner. Psychosocial interventions, such as emotional support, preparing the child and family for healthcare procedures, involving the parent as a support to the child during care or procedures, and promoting play facilitate positive coping skills, adaptation to healthcare encounters, and healthy growth and development.[29] **Table 1-7** outlines the fears and concerns children face during hospitalization.

Supporting the Child's and Family's Needs through Family-Centered Care

The first psychosocial intervention and/or provision of emotional support cannot be provided until a trusting, confident relationship between the child and healthcare provider exists. It is important to note that professional boundaries must be established and maintained. Establishing open and clear communication is critical in promoting collaboration with family members. Healthcare providers should use developmentally appropriate language with children. Addressing needs and treating the child and family as a cohesive unit, or providing **family-centered care**, promotes adherence to the plan of care and provides a structure to support continued growth and development. Key concepts of family-centered care include clear and open lines of communication, which keep the child and family informed and actively engaged in the plan of care; involving the child and family in healthcare decisions, which allow care to be tailored to meet the child's and family's priorities, preferences, and values; and having patient needs anticipated and addressed. The aforementioned principles of family-centered care lead to better health outcomes, ensure quality, and promote safety.[28]Additional benefits of family-centered care include the following:

- Greater responsiveness to patient- and family-identified needs and priorities
- Creation of a more supportive workplace environment
- Creation of more effective learning environments for professionals-in-training
- Wiser use of scarce resources, with a reduction in healthcare costs
- A cadre of families able to advocate for quality in health care and the resources to support quality care
- Enhanced competitiveness for the hospital in the marketplace

Overall, family-centered care initiatives will lead to improved medical and developmental outcomes.

The literature reports that children who are prepared for medical procedures experience significantly lower levels of fear and anxiety and have better long-term adjustment to medical challenges.[29,30] "The goal of psychological preparation is to increase children and family members' sense of predictability and control over potentially overwhelming life experiences, allowing them to proceed in these situations with a resulting sense of mastery and with the lowest possible level of distress."[28] Preparation can take place before, during, or after an event and will help the child to better anticipate what they will see, hear, feel, and smell. Allowing children ample opportunities to manipulate, be desensitized to, or "practice" with equipment used for their care enables the child to cope better. Children will benefit from "rehearsing" with equipment on favorite play items. Modeling, via watching instructional videos,

or engaging with others in the activity are useful tools for many age groups. Preparing parents will also have an overall positive effect on the child's coping. Preparation can also consist of promoting the use of coping strategies, such as teaching children to identify coping skills or offering a choice of specific coping strategies, allowing the child to choose what may work. Examples of offerings can include counting; singing ABCs or a favorite song; deep breathing; or the use of **guided imagery** techniques, such as imagining yourself in a peaceful, pleasant place.[28]

Children need numerous opportunities to help maintain and promote their typical growth and development. Children should have strange environments normalized. This normalization comes through knowledge of child development, the skills and training to enter into a supportive relationship with families, and the ability to collaborate with members of the interdisciplinary healthcare team. Age-appropriate toys and books should be available to patients, along with adaptations, such as Braille, large print, or photo or audio books, which accommodate sight and hearing limitations due to illness or injury. The benefits of play in healthcare settings are numerous. Play can help reduce stress, promote expression of feelings, and provide mastery of and effective coping with strenuous events.[31,32] Play and socialization opportunities should be promoted and incorporated into the child's hospital routine. Children will also benefit from opportunities for expressing feelings. Doll play, manipulation toys, "loose parts," medical play, painting, drawing, and journaling may all help children express themselves in the healthcare setting and allow them to assimilate information they have experienced.[31]

Healthcare professionals can also learn from children. Learn the language the individual child uses to communicate needs, how they identify body parts, and how they innately cope. Children's cues are very important, and treatments should capitalize on the child's strengths. Engaging the child by determining what works for them and offering realistic choices will help elicit the child's participation and provide for more effective compliance.

The use of developmentally engaged strategies establishes trust, increases compliance with the plan of care, and facilitates mastery of skills, which in turn positively impact the child's hospital experience. Parental presence and engagement in the child's care buffers the effects of separation and other stressors that can be a concern across the developmental continuum. **Table 1-8** lists a few age-appropriate therapeutic care strategies that can enhance the quality of clinical interventions with patients as well as patient/family satisfaction.

TABLE 1-8
Examples of General Strengths Used to Provide Developmentally Appropriate Therapeutic Care

Developmental Stage	Therapeutic Intervention
Neonate	Cluster care, or provide interventions and hands-on care around the same timeframe, as much as possible Minimize stimulation and avoid quick movements Use a soothing tone
Infants/toddlers	Use simple language Get on the child's level Even though children may not fully understand, use a calm, friendly, confident voice When appropriate, model equipment or process first on parent or self Have play medical kits available for children to see equipment that is primary colored and appears nonthreatening Use comfort positioning to provide supportive, therapeutic care, which can lead to a child coping best with their experience; when a child lies on their back, vulnerability can increase and they may not cooperate as well Partake in the routine the healthcare environment has established
Preschoolers	Use minimal, nonthreatening language Offer a preschooler realistic choices and allow them to participate in their care Provide directions and suggestions in positive manner. Say, "You need to stay very still" as opposed to "Don't move" Reinforce that treatments are not punishment Challenge the preschooler by saying colors, counting, or reciting the alphabet, capitalizing on their strengths and knowledge Allow expression of feelings through play and verbalization; correct misconceptions Allow for manipulation of equipment and use concrete terms, being realistic and truthful
School age	Support concrete thinking/learning, moving toward logical thinking Give specific information, such as the sequence for procedures, and encourage participation Promote medical play and socialization activities to help identify misconceptions Teach coping strategies Offer age-appropriate activities that encourage mastery
Adolescents	Provide an opportunity for involvement in their care and decisions related to their experience and health promotion Communicate honestly, with thorough explanations Promote/allow for independence Help identify and promote coping techniques Respect and maintain privacy Encourage peer interactions

Data from (Rollins, 2005) pp. 56–57; (Thompson, 2009) pp. 189–192; (TenHuisen, 2004); (Victoria State Government, Maternity and Newborn Clinical Network, Department of Health and Human Services, 2017).

Case Study

Alex is a 9-month-old Caucasian baby, born to a gravida 1, para 1 single mother. He was delivered at term (40 weeks' gestation) by normal vaginal delivery. Birth weight was 3.5 kg; at 6 months, his weight was 8 kg, both of which are at the 50th percentile. His medical history was nonsignificant and immunizations are up to date. At 9 months of age, he was evaluated by his primary care physician with a 2-day history of diarrhea and reduced feeding. Upon assessment the following data are available:

Temperature: 37°C
Weight: 7.4 kg (5th percentile)
Normal skin turgor
Heart rate: 110 beats per minute

Respiratory rate: 32 breaths per minute
Blood pressure: 72/37 mm Hg

The mother reports that she feeds him 8 ounces of whole milk approximately five times per day. She has not started him on solid food.

Upon examination, the infant did not engage. He did not smile or laugh, despite efforts to elicit a response, and was nonverbal.

1. **Based on the data presented, which of the following is the most likely diagnosis for Alex?**
   a. Cognitively delay
   b. Failure to thrive
   c. Deformational plagiocephaly
   d. Lactose intolerance

References

1. Bamm EL, Rosenbalm P. Family-centered theory: origins, development, barriers, and supports to implementation in rehabilitation medicine. *Arch Phys Med Rehabil*. 2008;89(8):1618–1624.

2. Christensen J. A critical reflection of Bronfenbrenner's Development Ecology Model. *Problems of Education in the 21st Century*. 2016;69:22–28.

3. Centers for Disease Control and Prevention. (2010, September 9). Growth charts. https://www.cdc.gov/growthcharts/index.htm. Updated September 9, 2010. Accessed May 4, 2017.

4. Wilson D. Health promotion of the infant and family. In: Hockenberry MA, Wilson D, eds. *Wong's Nursing Care of Infants and Children*. St. Louis, MO: Elsevier Mosby; 2015:413–451.

5. American Academy of Pediatrics, Task Force in Sudden Infant Death Syndrome. SIDS and other sleep-related infant deaths: expansion of recommendations for a safe infant sleeping environment. *Pediatrics*. 2011;128(5):e1341–e1346.

6. Wilson D. Health promotion of the toddler and family. In: Hockenberry MA, ed. *Wong's Nursing Care of Infants and Children*. St. Louis, MO: Elsevier Mosby; 2015:488–568.

7. Centers for Disease Control and Prevention. Important milestones: your child by three years. https://www.cdc.gov/ncbddd/actearly/milestones/milestones-3yr.html. Updated August 18, 2016. Accessed May 30, 2017.

8. Pavarini GS. Parental practices and theory of mind development. *J Child Fam Study*. 2013;22:844–853.

9. Caillies S, Le Sourn-Bissaoui S. Children's understanding of idioms and theory of mind development. *Dev Sci*. 2008;11(5):703–711.

10. Monroe, R. Health promotion of the preschooler and family. In: Hockenberry MA, ed. *Wong's Nursing Care of Infants and Children*. St. Louis, MO: Elsevier Mosby; 2015:523–568.

11. Fussell JA. Cognitive development. In: Voigt RG, Macias MM, Myers SM, eds. *Developmental and Behavioral Pediatrics*. Washington, DC: American Acedemy of Pediatrics; 2011:171–200.

12. McCarthy K. Health problems of early childhood. In: Hockenberry MA, Wilson D, eds. *Wong's Nursing Care of Infants and Children*. St. Louis, MO: Elsevier Mosby; 2015:543–650.

13. Sun SS, Schubert CM, Chumlea WC, et al. National estimates of the timing of sexual maturation and racial differences among US children. *Pediatrics*. 2002;110(5):911–919.

14. Rodgers C. Health promotion of the school age child and family. In: Hockenberry MA, ed. *Wong's Nursing Care of Infants and Children*. St. Louis, MO: Elsevier Mosby; 2015:569–650.

15. Schwebel DC, Brezausek CM. Child development and pediatric sport and recreational injuries by age. *J Athl Train*. 2014;49(6):780–785.

16. Scott SM, Walsh AM. Adolescent sexual development: an overview of recent research. *Can J Commun Ment Health*. 2014;35(1):21–29.

17. Ethington MG. Health promotion of the adolescent and family. In: Hockenberry MA, ed. *Wong's Nursing Care of Infants and Children*. St. Louis, MO: Elsevier Mosby; 2015:651–760.

18. Klein JD, American Academy of Pediatrics Committee on Adolescence. Adolescent pregnancy: current trends and issues. *Pediatrics*. 2005;116(1):281–286.

19. Sundaram A, Vaughan B, Kost K, et al. Contraceptive failure in the United States: estimates from the 2006–2010 National Survey of Family Growth. *Perspect Sex Reprod Health*. 2017;49(1):7–16.

20. East L, Jackson D, O'Brien L. Father absence and adolescent development: a review of the literature. *J Child Health Care*. 2006;10(4):283–295.

21. Patton GC, McMorris BJ, Toumbourou JW, Hemphill SA, Donath S, Catalano RF. Puberty and the onset of substance use and abuse. *Pediatrics*. 2004;114(3):e300–e306.

22. Arkins BT. Assessing the reasons for deliberate self harm in young people. *Ment Heath Pract*. 2013;16(7):28–32.

23. Griesbach D. Links between self-harm and attempted suicide in young people. *Mental Health Today*. 2008;23–25.

24. Miniño A. *Mortality among teenagers aged 12–19 years: United States, 1999–2006. NCHS data brief*. https://www.cdc.gov/nchs/data/databriefs/db37.pdf. Accessed May 16, 2017.

25. Feigelman W, Gorman BS. Prospective predictors of premature death: evidence from the National Longitudinal Study of Adolescent Health. *J Psychoactive Drugs*. 2010;42(3):353–361.

26. Shifflet-Chila ED, Harold R, Fitton VA, Ahmedani BK. Adolescent and family development: Autonomy and identity in the digital age. *Children and Youth Services Review*. 2016;10(70):364–368.

27. Carter JM, Wilson FL. Cyberbullying: a 21st century health care phenomenon. *Pediatr Nurs*. 2015;41(3):115–125.

28. Thompson RH. *The Handbook of Child Life: A Guide for Pediatric Psychosocial Care*. Springfield, IL: Charles C. Thomas; 2009.

29. Rollins JH, Bolig R, Mahan CC. *Meeting Children's Psychosocial Needs Across the Health-Care Continuum*. Austin, TX: Pro-ED; 2005.

30. American Academy of Pediatrics Committee on Hospital Care. Child life services. *Pediatrics*. 2000;106(5):1156–1159.

31. Nilsson E, Svensson G, Frisman GH. Picture book support for preparing children ahead of and during day surgery. *Nurs Child Young People*. 2016;28(8):30–35.

32. Gaynard L, Wolfer J, Goldberger J, Thompson R, Redburn L, Laidley L. *Psychosocial Care of Children in Hospitals: A Clinical Practice Manual*. Rockville, MD: Child Life Council; 1998.

2

Family-Centered Care

Jana L. Teagle

OUTLINE

OBJECTIVES

1. Identify the principles of family-centered care.
2. Recognize the needs of hospitalized children in all five developmental levels.
3. List the components of family-centered care that parents need during their child's hospitalization.
4. Discuss the needs of siblings when a brother or sister is hospitalized.
5. Describe the role of the child life specialist in helping a child and family cope with hospitalization.

KEY TERMS

animal-assisted therapy
child life specialists
family-centered care
family-centered rounds

hospitalized children
siblings
transition to adulthood

Introduction

The needs of hospitalized children and their families are great. Each family is unique, consisting of a variety of people: parents, siblings, step-parents, grandparents, partners, aunts, uncles, cousins, and sometimes those who are not related but live close by or with the family. The issues that a family faces during a hospitalization are as diverse as the family themselves. These issues are likely to occur when a child is hospitalized for an extended period, resulting in the need for support and stress management.[1]

Oftentimes, families do not live near the hospital. Getting to and from the hospital, all while juggling work, school responsibilities, and caring for other children and pets, is challenging. Parents may be away from work for a significant period of time during the hospitalization, which can make paying bills and maintaining a home difficult. For siblings, having parents divided between the hospital and home or needing to stay with friends or relatives can be frightening and a deviation from their normal routine. It is important during hospitalization to give families the psychosocial support they need through the help of social workers, pastoral care personnel, child life specialists, psychologists, therapists, nurses, and physicians. Amenities at the hospital, such as showers, places to sleep and do laundry, and accessibility to meals and other resources, are of great assistance to families during this stressful time. Giving families options and control in an environment where they feel they have very little is an essential aspect of assisting families of hospitalized children.

Family-Centered Care

The concept of **family-centered care** is based on the assumption that the family is the constant in a child's life. A child's illness can affect the entire family, and so family-centered care is a respectful partnership between a child's family, specifically the parents or primary caregivers, and the clinical practitioners and professionals caring for that child.[2] According to the National Center for Family and Professional Partnerships, the foundation for this care begins with the family and medical team partnering to provide care that is in the best interests of the child and the family. As children age, they, too, assume a role in this partnership. With trust acknowledged as being fundamental, it is vital that each individual involved in the child's care have respect for the skills and expertise of others—not only those of the medical team but also the family as well. Through open and objective communication, with a willingness to negotiate if needed, decisions concerning the child's care are made together.[3] **Table 2-1** lists essential components of family-centered care.[4]

Every child is a component of a much larger system: The child is part of the family, and the family is part of the larger community. Children and families

TABLE 2-1
Components of Family-Centered Care

Family is recognized as the constant in a child's life.
The strengths of the family and child are unique.
The child participates in care and decision making.
Cultural diversity and family traditions are respected and honored.
Information about a child's care is shared with the family.
Families are referred to community-based services.
Family-to-family support networks are encouraged.
Youth are supported as they **transition to adulthood**.
Family and professionals work together to determine a plan of care.
Programs and policies to support the family are implemented.
Successes are celebrated.

are members of churches, schools, and extracurricular activity networks. With a variety of family and community structures come many unique values and beliefs as well as a mix of understandings and misconceptions about diagnoses and hospitalizations. Sometimes, family members all agree with the medical plan, but other families may have very diverse beliefs, making it difficult for them, and sometimes their child, to make the best decisions regarding medical care. Misconceptions that family members may have can be addressed and clarified in a face-to-face meeting between the family and medical staff.

Communication and coordination are key elements to building successful working relationships with patients and families during their hospitalization.[3] Having family present to discuss the child's medical needs and recommendations of the healthcare team helps facilitate better communication among the family, patient, and medical staff. Verbal and nonverbal communication is critical when families are in stressful environments, such as a hospital or clinic. Healthcare professionals must approach children and their families with respect and an attitude that demonstrates value for feelings, opinions, and individuality.[3]

Trust is a fundamental element of family-centered care. Building rapport and trust is vital for families to feel comfortable with the individuals caring for their child. For some families, this occurs quickly, while other families require more time.

As a result of research surrounding attachment theory, which suggests that children who are separated from their primary caregiver are very likely to experience emotional problems, there has been a change in the attitudes and practices regarding parents staying with their child while in the hospital.[4] Now parents are encouraged and even expected to remain with their child, with many patient rooms at children's hospitals designed to include an area for parents.[4] In addition to staying at the bedside with their child, families are encouraged to be active participants in their child's care, either independently or with the assistance of a nurse or other medical professional. If they feel comfortable doing so, parents are often asked to remain close to their child during a procedure to help the child in coping with the procedure.

Bedside rounding is a prime example of family-centered care. Instead of the child's medical team meeting privately in a conference room to discuss the differential diagnoses, treatment goals, and current plan of care, teams often meet in the child's room where they speak with the family and/or child, incorporating their opinions, questions, suggestions, and beliefs into the plan. Including family in clinical rounds improves communication and shares decision making. It also provides learning opportunities for residents and students.[5] Some hospitals use a system where cards that hang outside a child's room are flipped to denote if parents do or do not want to participate in bedside rounding. This decision can be changed daily based upon the families' needs and desires for that day. Depending on their age, older children may be more involved in their care when medical rounds are held at the bedside. Even though a child's age mandates that parents be the ultimate decision makers, children have the opportunity to ask questions and to share their thoughts about the care they receive. Oftentimes, parents are provided with a notebook to write down questions or concerns to discuss with the medical team during **family-centered rounds**. This also serves as a way for parents to write answers to questions and to share this information later with family members who are not present at the time of rounds. With emerging technology, family members may be able to participate in rounds via speakerphone or video chat.

There are many principles and applications within family-centered care. Not only is family-centered care important to children and their families, but it can be beneficial to hospitals by improving family and staff satisfaction.[1] One study noted that participating in family-centered rounds was associated with increased physician comfort in family participation, a perception of positive impact on staff involvement, and improved patient outcomes.[6]

Needs of the Hospitalized Infant, Child, and Adolescent

A child's reaction to hospitalization or prolonged illness is determined largely by the developmental age of the child, prior hospitalization experiences, the ability to cope with stress, and the degree of security they feel through family support. Sudden illnesses or unexpected hospitalizations are very stressful to children; this stress can affect how they recover from an illness and, in some cases, may prolong the illness and hospital stay.

Infants

From birth to 1 year, infants are constantly growing and changing. Their senses continue to develop. While exploring their environment, they learn through sound, sight, and touch. Infants are securing attachment and are learning to trust that their caregivers will meet their needs. When hospitalized, an infant's normal routine is disrupted, leading to fussiness and difficulty with sleeping and eating. Due to family constraints or procedures during their hospitalization, there may be separation between the infant and their familiar caregivers. This can affect the trusting relationship that has been developing since birth. In situations where the family is unable to be present all the time, having continuity of care among nurses and therapists can aid in the infant developing trusting relationships with medical caregivers. Although it may be difficult to do, attempting to maintain a schedule similar to one the infant uses at home can be beneficial in maintaining sleep, wake, and feeding cycles. Families are encouraged to bring developmentally appropriate play materials from home, which assists in maintaining a stimulating environment and encourages normal growth and development. Comfort items and developmentally appropriate toys for infants include mirrors, black-and-white pictures, rattles, teethers, mobiles, bouncy seats, swings, and swaddlers. As with a child of any age, families are encouraged to participate in the infant's care and to remain in the room. For mothers who are breastfeeding, this may include breastfeeding accommodations and support from a lactation consultant as well as meals to ensure the proper nutrition needed to breastfeed. Additionally, first-time parents of infants can often benefit from education on calming and soothing techniques, feeding and positioning, and safe sleep practices.

Toddlers

Toddlers are children between 1 and 3 years of age. They are busy and constantly learning from the world around them. Toddlers are gaining independence and "believe the world is focused primarily on them."[7] Their motor and verbal skills are increasing rapidly, but their understanding is still quite limited, causing them to become easily frustrated. This frustration is seen in temper tantrums, varying forms of aggression, and even regression in skills that they have recently mastered, such as potty-training. Toddlers have a difficult time distinguishing reality from fantasy, which may contribute to their misunderstanding of medical-related explanations.[8] Many times, especially in an unfamiliar environment like a hospital, toddlers become fearful and develop stranger anxiety when their family is not present.[7] Because the receptive language of a toddler is not as developed as their expressive language, they may better understand medical procedures when a simple explanation is offered in language they are familiar with. Allowing caregivers to stay close; keeping routines as normal as possible; and setting and maintaining rules, limitations, and expectations during hospitalization are important for normalization. Offering choices when applicable and encouraging as much independence as possible will also assist in toddlers' adjustment and ability to cope with a hospitalization. Providing a safe place for play, such as a hospital playroom, allows for continued growth and development in physical and social skills. If toddlers are unable to leave their room due to isolation or medical complexities, it is important to provide developmentally appropriate activities for bedside play.

Preschoolers

Children who are 3 to 6 years of age are considered preschoolers. They have a developing imagination and enjoy participating in make-believe play. Their world is egocentric and filled with "magical thoughts," often feeling like they are the cause of all earthly events.[8] They tend to act older than they are, mimicking caregivers and friends near their age. Like toddlers, hospitalized preschoolers can demonstrate signs of aggression and regression in certain behaviors. Because they fear being away from their family, they may be clingy during their hospital stay. Providing them with opportunities for choices and independence, when appropriate, and keeping a routine are important. If preschoolers are having a difficult time complying with treatments or taking medications, a simple sticker chart with small prizes can assist with encouraging and rewarding them during this difficult period. Encouraging questions and offering simple yet honest answers will assist in alleviating misconceptions and increase the preschooler's understanding about what is happening to them in the hospital. Because it may be difficult for them to verbalize their feelings, allowing preschoolers opportunities for play within the hospital will assist in normalizing the environment and providing them with a means of self-expression. Other means of expression may be through art, music, dramatic play, and medical play. The use of puppets or dolls is effective in explaining medical procedures or devices to preschoolers.

School-Age Children

School-age children are described as children who are ages 6 to 13 years. During this developmental period, they are gaining more and more independence, going to school independently, and often participating in extracurricular activities with peers. Because of this, school-age children often cope well if their family cannot always be at the hospital. They are eager to please but can be self-conscious. Their problem-solving skills are increasing as well. They are able to understand a sequence of events, often leading to their understanding of death and its finality in regard to a pet, friend, or family member. Like children in other stages of development, school-age children benefit from opportunities to play and explore their environment during

a hospitalization. They need a sense of control in the hospital, so when choices are available, it is important to give them options. School-age children have fears of failure, family problems, death, and rejection.[6] They often worry about fitting in with their peers, so a playroom where they can socialize with others who may be going through similar circumstances can be beneficial to them. Asking school-age children for their questions and clarifying any misconceptions they may have assists them in coping with a hospitalization and illness. Because of their imaginative thinking, using puppets or dolls for education concerning a procedure or medical equipment is appropriate for this age.

Adolescents

Adolescence is the period from 13 through 18 years of age, after which age a person is considered an adult. Adolescents think abstractly and work to establish personal identity.[7] They are quite independent and seek separation from family, relying more heavily on their peer groups for support, and so increased dependence on family and separation from peers can be frustrating for hospitalized adolescents. An adolescent's privacy is highly important to them and respecting their privacy in the hospital is vital to their ability to cope. Because they think abstractly, they are more aware of stressors and strains that their illness or hospitalization may place on their families. They often fear that the illness or hospitalization may be affecting their identity and who they are currently. Allowing adolescents the opportunity to ask questions as well as to provide input concerning their treatment plans can assist in maintaining their independence and having a developmentally appropriate level of control in their care. To promote normalization within the hospital environment, visits from friends are encouraged, as are activities with peers. Many hospitals have a teen room or lounge where adolescents can meet, with age-specific activities, such as a karaoke machine, video games, a pool table, and more advanced arts and crafts. Technology and social media allow adolescents to maintain communication with their peers while in the hospital, especially in the event they cannot leave their room. Depending on the diagnosis, there are face-to-face as well as online support groups that help adolescents understand that they are not alone when dealing with their medical complexities.

Needs of the Family

The stress, uncertainty, and fear of the unknown that a family experiences when a child is hospitalized can cause the hospitalization itself to become a traumatic event. Parents may neglect their own health in order to care for their child. Recognizing the needs and concerns of the entire family is important in preventing deterioration and ensuring that they are supported.

Information and Accommodations

Providing families with information about their child's care in terms that they can understand is key to making them feel comfortable and involved in the hospitalization. Many have inadequate knowledge about their child's condition and need details about the diagnosis, plan of care, prognosis, and discharge goals. It is crucial that families are told where they can stay during the hospitalization. In cases where rooms are not private, parents should be directed to sleep rooms or waiting areas where they can stay in the event that the medical staff needs them. Families need information on how to gain access to meals, showers, laundry facilities, and play opportunities for their child and siblings. It is common for social workers to assist families in obtaining community resources, should they need assistance from outside the hospital for their child or themselves. These resources include local pharmacies, restaurants, transportation options, home nursing agencies, and funding sources for home modifications or medical supplies.

Reassurance and Support

Family members often need psychosocial support and assurance that they can continue to care for their child. Often the greatest stressors for a family when their child is hospitalized are not the child's illness or the hospitalization itself but sibling care, job responsibilities, financial strains, and other commitments. Being a good listener for a family is critical, as is guiding them to the member of the multidisciplinary team who can provide them with the resources they need. The family can be referred to community counseling for the ongoing support needed to deal with the stress, anxiety, and guilt that often accompanies having a child with a chronic illness or unexpected injury.

Consistency

Consistency is especially important for families of **hospitalized children**, but it is often difficult because of physician schedules, emergencies, diagnostic testing, and therapies. Many hospitals have one primary physician who follows the child, with other healthcare professionals, based upon diagnosis or service, who also care for the child. Although maintaining the same physicians throughout the hospitalization may be difficult, many hospitals have primary nurses assigned to patients for continuity of care. These nurses become familiar with the family and are better able to get to know the patient and family and can communicate with the team and the family equally, acting as a liaison to assist in the family being comfortable with the care their child is receiving.

Communication

Communicating with families about their child's care in terms that they can understand is crucial in making families feel comfortable and involved during the hospitalization. Parents appreciate honesty when discussing their child's medical condition and needs. Additionally, they need the opportunity to ask questions in a safe forum. If parents are unable to be present with their child, keeping them up-to-date by phone with any changes in their child's medical status and the expected plan of care is important in maintaining family involvement.

Needs of Siblings

Having a sibling who is sick or injured can be a very confusing and upsetting time for children. They may be forced to identify and deal with a wide range of feelings and concerns in the absence of their parents, who are either physically or emotionally unavailable.[3] When a child is hospitalized and parents spend the majority of their time at the hospital, **siblings** are often left in the care of relatives and friends. Although these may be familiar people, it still results in a disruption in the siblings' daily routines. Remaining in the family home keeps the environment familiar, and maintaining school, extracurricular activities, and meal and bedtime routines as much as possible aids in the siblings' ability to cope with the illness and hospitalization. In considering these things, it is important to keep in mind that changes in sleeping patterns, eating habits, school performance, emotions, typical developmental skills (regression), and behavior can all be signs that a sibling is not coping well with the changes in their family and/or living structure. Factors influencing a sibling's response to hospitalization include the sibling's age and developmental level, the nature of the threat, the relationship between the sibling and the ill child, the nature of the changes, and the family's socioeconomic status.[3]

Assistance from a child life specialist, who is trained in developmental theory and with assisting children with coping with hospitalization, can be vital in making a sibling's hospital experience a positive one. If a child life specialist is not available, taking the time to talk with a sibling and explaining the situation and medical equipment in the patient's room, in simple terms, can help alleviate misconceptions and promote a better understanding. Allowing the sibling an opportunity to ask questions and express their feelings is also important. If possible, give the child a means to be involved in their ill sibling's care and hospital experience. This could be helping with a small task, such as getting juice from the refrigerator, making a card to be hung in the hospital room, or bringing a favorite toy or stuffed animal from home. This allows siblings to feel involved in the hospital experience and prevents them from feeling so disconnected from their family.

Role of the Child Life Specialist

Most children's hospitals have **child life specialists** in both inpatient and outpatient areas. These specialists are a vital component in how children and their families cope with hospitalization and how they will perceive future hospital experiences. Child life specialists have many roles, including helping children adjust to procedures, diagnoses, and devices. With their strong background in child development and family systems, they promote effective coping through play, education, preparation, and self-expression activities.[9] They also provide psychosocial support to children and their families.

Providing children and their siblings with opportunities for a variety of types of play is not only normalizing an unfamiliar place but also a means through which children learn and explore their environment. Many child life programs have play spaces throughout the hospital where children are offered a safe place to participate in developmentally appropriate activities with other children going through similar situations. There are unit-based playrooms that provide a quick and safe escape from the hospital room while still being closely monitored by nursing staff. These play areas can be available 24 hours a day, which is beneficial to a child who has difficulty sleeping or finally feels well enough to play in the middle of the night. Other hospitals have large community play spaces where special events are held, such as holiday parties, visits from celebrities, and activities with volunteer groups. These play areas may have sections specific to a developmental level, such as an infant-toddler area with play mats and riding toys. Arts and crafts, video games, pool tables, air hockey tables, board and card games, books, cooking, and musical instruments are some of the activities that may be offered in hospital play spaces. Many of these modalities allow for the child's self-expression in interpreting and experiencing what is occurring during their hospitalization. Some hospitals are fortunate enough to also have a space that is only for adolescents. This allows for socialization with peers and more mature conversations and activities that may be difficult for a child life specialist to facilitate in the presence of younger children.

Through education, child life specialists help children and families cope with hospitalization. Whether preparing the child for a blood draw, accompanying them to interventional radiology for placement of a peripherally inserted central catheter (PICC), or explaining a new diagnosis, child life specialists educate patients and siblings in a way that they can understand based on their developmental level. Dolls, puppets, books, and drawings are used to assist in a child's understanding of their medical condition or the procedure that they will be undergoing. Examples are found in **Figure 2-1** and **Figure 2-2**. Child life specialists provide pre-admission tours and education to children who are scheduled for an upcoming procedure or surgery, allowing the child time to ask questions and to become familiar with the environment. They also provide distractions during painful or anxiety-provoking procedures to help the child find an alternative focus. Relaxation techniques, including deep breathing and guided imagery, are used

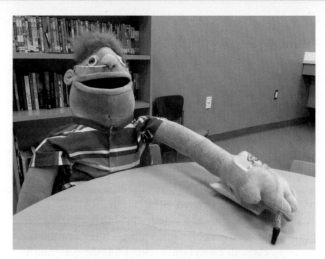

FIGURE 2-1 A puppet is used to explain how an IV will be placed.

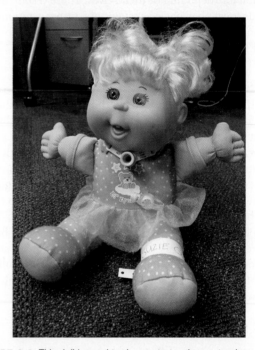

FIGURE 2-2 This doll is used to demonstrate where a tracheostomy tube is placed.

to help a child go through a painful time, such as following surgery.

Child life specialists also support children and their families at the end of life. They often assist with pain management and relaxation techniques, as discussed earlier, and help the child understand changes that are occurring. They assist terminally ill children in having difficult conversations with parents, siblings, or friends, in which they discuss the child's wishes, dreams, and hopes. They provide memory-making activities, such as a family tree with thumbprints, handprints, or footprints, or hand molds. **Figure 2-3** and **Figure 2-4** provide examples of these activities. By participating in these legacy-building activities, the family is given a meaningful opportunity to make memories and have

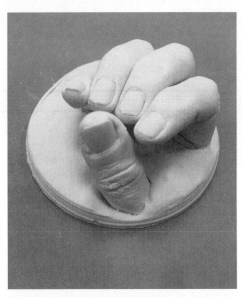

FIGURE 2-3 Hand molds are made to provide a tangible memory for parents and family.

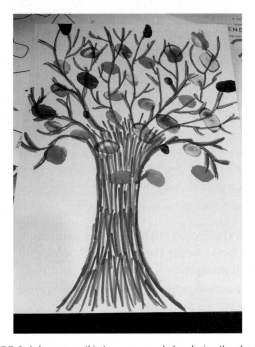

FIGURE 2-4 Leaves on this tree were made by placing thumbprints from family members.

open dialogue about their child. These activities may be done while the child is still alive or after the child has already died, depending on family preference. Child life specialists often collaborate with the palliative care team to provide support to the child and their siblings in the home or in support groups.

Advocating for children and their needs is another role of the child life specialist. This includes speaking and working with the medical team to meet a child's needs—for example, organizing a team of medical professionals to allow a patient who is ventilator-dependent to safely leave their room and participate in normalization activities with peers. Child life specialists also assist with school and community reintegration, in which they work with school personnel or community partners to articulate the physical, social, and emotional needs of the child to allow for a smooth transition from the hospital.

Animal-Assisted Therapy

Animals have been found to calm children and make them feel less frightened. For many children, their pets are a big part of their life at home that they miss when they are in the hospital. Many hospitals have pet therapy programs in which animals visit patients, with certain restrictions based on isolation status and diagnosis. The animals and their handlers are trained and must pass a certification test that assures, as best as possible, that the animal and handler are safe to be in a medical setting. Most pet therapy programs involve dogs, but other animals, including cats, ponies, and rabbits, can be included. **Animal-assisted therapy** can be a one-on-one intervention as well as a group session, depending on the needs of the child and their family.

There are numerous physical, social, and emotional benefits to having animal-assisted therapy in a children's hospital. One study reported that pediatric patients experienced decreased blood pressure and perception of pain following surgery when they spent time with dogs.[10] Animals can be used in conjunction with physical and occupational therapy to assist patients with their gross and fine motor skills. For a child who has been difficult to engage in therapy, adding a dog to the therapy often makes a difference in the child's participation. Children and families who miss seeing their pets may have a more positive affect and mood when an animal is present, as evidenced by smiling and an increase in interaction and conversation. Petting a dog and engaging in conversation with the dog's handler can raise a child's comfort level or serve as a positive distraction during stressful times. During or following animal-assisted therapy, children often discuss their pets at home, which can be an aid in building rapport with staff. Animals can also be used as part of play with children, giving them control in the hospital environment to "play doctor" with the animal, as seen in **Figure 2-5**.

Conclusion

Family-centered care should be in the forefront of pediatric health care. The child's healthcare team is not only made up of medical professionals but also includes the child and their family. Hospitalizations can be extremely stressful times for the child and family. Various professionals within the hospital provide accommodations and psychosocial support to families during their child's stay. Meeting these needs assists in the families' ability to cope and process information during the hospital stay.

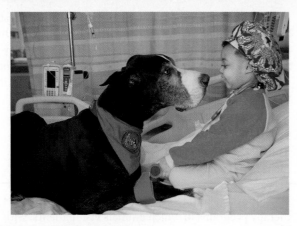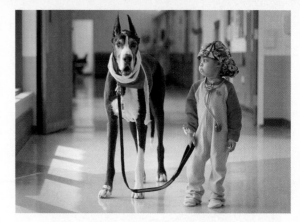

FIGURE 2-5 Animal-assisted therapy.

Case Study

Melissa is a 4-year-old child who sustained a traumatic brain injury (TBI) when her father's car was rear-ended by a semi-truck. She was airlifted to the nearest children's hospital, which was nearly 100 miles from her home. The first 3 weeks of her hospital stay were spent in the pediatric intensive care unit (PICU). While there she became ventilator dependent and a tracheostomy was placed. She also required placement of a gastrostomy tube to assist with nutrition. Melissa eventually transferred to the inpatient rehabilitation unit where she spent several months working to improve daily function. While her parents remained at the hospital to focus on her care and recovery, Melissa's 5-year-old sister and 8-year-old brother were at home under the care of their grandparents. The child life specialist met with the siblings to assist in answering their questions about their sister's condition and the medical equipment. Following the meeting, both siblings wished to visit their sister. The siblings also chose to create posters and to decorate pillowcases with markers and paint for Melissa to use in her room and to remind her of them. Melissa missed her dog at home, so it was arranged for pet therapy to visit her room.

Prior to discharge home, plans were made for Melissa's tracheostomy tube to be removed. She and her family had many questions about the process of decannulation. The siblings were afraid that she would be unable to breathe without the tube. A therapy doll was used to help familiarize them with removing the tube. They were able to take turns pulling the tube out of the doll's neck. Melissa's parents were able to be with her when the tube was removed and assist with distractions and coping during the procedure. Melissa was eventually able to transfer to the hospital's outpatient rehabilitation program. There she participated in a 5-days per week program for 6 months following discharge from the hospital.

1. **What challenges might Melissa's parents have faced during their daughter's extended hospitalization?**
2. **What activities helped Melissa's siblings feel more connected to her?**
3. **What benefits did the animal-assisted therapy provide Melissa?**

References

1. National Center for Family/Professional Partnerships. Family Voices, Inc. http://www.fv-ncfpp.org/quality-health-care1/family-centered-care. Published 2015. Accessed June 13, 2015.
2. American Academy of Pediatrics, Committee on Hospital Care and Institute for Patient- and Family-Centered Care. Patient- and family-centered care and the pediatrician's role. *Pediatrics.* 2012;129:394–404. doi:10.1542/peds.2011-3084.
3. Rollins JH, Bolig R, Mahan CC. *Meeting Children's Psychosocial Needs Across the Health-Care Continuum.* Austin, TX: Pro-Ed; 2005.
4. Kuo DZ, Houtrow AJ, Arango P, et al. Family-centered care: current applications and future directions in pediatric health care. *Matern Child Health J.* 2012;16:297–305.
5. Muething SE, Kotagal UR, Schoettker PJ, et al. Family-centered bedside rounds: a new approach to patient care and teaching. *Pediatrics.* 2007;119:829–832.
6. Children's Hospital of Philadelphia's Child Life Education & Creative Arts Therapy Department. Brothers and sisters, tools to help children when a sibling is sick. Children's Hospital of Philadelphia. http://issuu.com/choppublications/docs/chop=brothers-and-sisters. Published 2012. Accessed October 9, 2015.
7. Berk LE. *Child Development.* 6th ed. Boston, MA: Allyn and Bacon; 2003.
8. Thompson RH, Stanford G. *Child Life in Hospitals: Theory & Practice.* Springfield, IL: Charles C. Thomas; 1981.
9. Child Life Council. Child Life Council website. www.childlife.org. Published 1998. Accessed October 22, 2015.
10. Calcaterra V, Veggiotti P, Palestrini C, et al. Post-operative benefits of animal-assisted therapy in pediatric surgery: a randomised study. *PLoS One.* 2015;10(6):e0125813.

3

Development of the Fetal Lung

Sherry L. Barnhart
James W. Hynson

OUTLINE

OBJECTIVES

1. Describe the respiratory system's development from the endodermal and mesodermal components.
2. Identify the stages of lung development and the major events of each stage.
3. Explain the effect that pulmonary surfactant has on alveolar surface tension.
4. List the major components of pulmonary surfactant.
5. Discuss the factors that influence physiologic maturation of the fetal lung.
6. Differentiate among pulmonary agenesis, pulmonary aplasia, and pulmonary hypoplasia.
7. List the pathophysiologic causes of secondary pulmonary hypoplasia.

KEY TERMS

acinus
amniotic fluid
dipalmitoylphosphatidylcholine (DPPC)
gestational age
laryngotracheal groove
lecithin-to-sphingomyelin (L:S) ratio
lung bud

oligohydramnios
phospholipids
polyhydramnios
pulmonary agenesis
pulmonary aplasia
pulmonary hypoplasia
pulmonary surfactant
surface tension
surfactant protein

Introduction

The primary function of the lungs is to exchange oxygen and carbon dioxide between the alveoli and the blood. However, during intrauterine growth, the fetal lungs do not participate in gas exchange; instead, the mother's placenta provides oxygen and removes carbon dioxide for the fetus. At birth, the lungs must undergo a rapid transition and become the gas exchange organ for the body, making lung maturation essential for an infant's survival and adaptation to extrauterine life. Congenital malformation with inadequate lung development is a major cause of neonatal death and disease. The most common cause, however, is premature birth in which the lung has simply not had sufficient time to grow. Understanding fetal lung development is an essential component in both preventing and treating damage to the lungs.

In discussions of heart and lung development, the term **gestational age** is used to describe the growth and age of a fetus. The American Academy of Pediatrics defines gestational age as the time period between the first day of the mother's last menstrual period and the day of delivery. It is conventionally expressed as completed weeks; for example, a 25-week, 5-day fetus has a gestational age of 25 weeks—the age should not be rounded to 26 weeks. A pregnancy is considered to be full term at 40 weeks of gestation. Postnatal age is the amount of time that has elapsed since birth. Days, weeks, months, and years are used to describe postnatal age.[1]

Stages of Lung Development

The cells of an embryo separate into three layers, which are referred to as germ layers: the ectoderm (outer layer), mesoderm (middle layer), and endoderm (inner layer). Each layer gives rise to specific body tissues; it is from the endoderm that the fetal lungs eventually develop. As illustrated in **Figure 3-1**, lung development proceeds in an organized manner and is typically divided into five distinct stages:

- Embryonic
- Pseudoglandular
- Canalicular
- Saccular
- Alveolar

The first four stages occur prenatally, while the alveolar stage continues after birth. Each stage gradually transitions to the next, with some overlap between stages, and disruption in any stage can profoundly affect lung development and result in a number of pulmonary defects.

Embryonic Stage (3–7 Weeks' Gestation)

During the embryonic stage, which lasts from about 3 to 7 weeks' gestation, the fetal lungs begin in the foregut endoderm as a **laryngotracheal groove**. The groove separates from the primitive esophagus and a pouch, or **lung bud**, appears. Over the next few weeks, the bud divides into two bronchial buds and a primitive trachea is formed. Development of the buds corresponds to the right and left mainstem bronchi and the mature lung lobes; the bud on the right develops into three lobar buds and the one on the left develops into two lobar buds. As the buds elongate, they continue to grow and divide, and by the end of the 6th week of gestation, all segmental bronchopulmonary branches are formed. This patterning process by which the lung bud develops into the bronchopulmonary tree is called branching morphogenesis.

The mesenchyme also develops during the embryonic stage. Originating from the mesoderm, the mesenchyme surrounds the airway branches. It is composed of tissue that will eventually form blood and lymph vessels as well as the cartilage and smooth muscle of the airways. Respiratory epithelial cells that form the

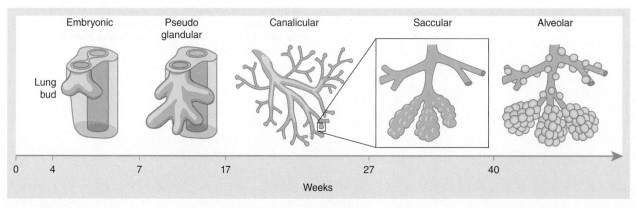

FIGURE 3-1 Stages of fetal lung development.

primitive airways evolve from the endoderm and grow into the surrounding mesenchyme. Central bronchial arteries develop during this stage, and the diaphragm is completely developed by the 7th week of gestation.[2]

Pseudoglandular Stage (7–17 Weeks' Gestation)

The pseudoglandular stage lasts from 7 to 17 weeks' gestation. This stage is marked by formation of the conducting airways with the repeated lateral and terminal branching of airways into the mesenchyme. Although the airways continue to grow in length and diameter, new branches are not formed after this stage. By the end of this stage, the tracheobronchial tree is formed with up to 27 generations of branches, with the final level at the terminal bronchioles.

The airways are thick, hollow tubules and the lungs appear to be glandular, hence the term pseudoglandular. Initially the airways are narrow and thickly lined with pseudostratified columnal epithelium that contains glycogen. As branching progresses, airway diameter increases and the epithelium thins into a tall columnar epithelium. Cilia begin to form on the epithelium of the trachea and mainstem bronchi by 10 weeks' gestation and on the peripheral airway epithelium by 13 weeks' gestation. Mucus-producing glands appear, and goblet cells, which also secrete mucus, develop in the bronchial epithelium by the 14th week. Cartilage, smooth muscle, and connective tissue also develop in the trachea and the airway walls during this stage.[3,4]

It is during the pseudoglandular stage that new bronchial arteries develop as the central bronchial arteries disappear. A network of pulmonary arteries and veins develops in parallel with the conducting airways. As the airways develop, the pulmonary vasculature becomes progressively longer and continues to surround and follow alongside the branching airways. Lymphatic vessels appear in the lung by 10 weeks' gestation.[5]

Canalicular Stage (17–26 Weeks' Gestation)

When the canalicular stage begins at the 17th week of gestation, all nonrespiratory portions of the tracheobronchial tree are present and the airway branching pattern has been completed. As this stage progresses, each terminal bronchiole further differentiates to form a primitive pulmonary **acinus**. This primitive acinus consists only of the bronchioles, ducts, and sac; it does not contain the alveoli that are found in the acinus of the mature lung. The lung periphery epithelium becomes thinner, and the rich capillary network begins to multiply in the interstitial space. This leads to the formation of a functional air–blood barrier that, although inefficient, is thin enough to sustain gas exchange in extremely premature neonates. Evolution of the acinus and the capillaries surrounding it is a critical step in providing a healthy gas-exchange surface for the lungs.[6]

During this state, the airways have developed smooth muscle and now have epithelial cells that produce fetal lung liquid.

By 20 to 22 weeks' gestation, type II and then type I pneumocytes are differentiated and readily identified. The type II pneumocytes synthesize surfactant and store it in unique organelles called lamellar bodies, which are later secreted into the alveolar space. It is during the canalicular stage that lamellar bodies are recognizable in type II pneumocytes. The number and size of lamellar bodies increase as the lungs develop. The canalicular stage continues through 26 weeks' gestation, and it is during the latter part of this stage that the lungs are transformed into a gas-exchanging organ and the fetus becomes viable.[7]

Saccular Stage (27–36 Weeks' Gestation)

The saccular stage, also referred to as the terminal sac stage, begins at the 27th week of gestation and continues until just before term, at 36 weeks' gestation. Previously, it was considered to be the final phase in lung development. This stage begins with the respiratory bronchioles evolving into alveolar ducts and the appearance of terminal alveolar sacs, referred to as saccules. Small crests form on the edges of the saccules; the crests, along with a capillary network, are eventually pulled into the saccules, resulting in a double capillary network that forms the primary septa between the saccules. The saccules continue to branch and grow in number, forming whole clusters of saccules off of the alveolar ducts. As the saccules subdivide into smaller units, primitive alveoli are produced, with the first alveoli appearing by around 32 weeks' gestation.[8]

Type I and type II pneumocytes continue to differentiate during this stage. Type I pneumocytes flatten and become more abundant, causing the epithelium to become thinner. The interstitial tissue between the saccules becomes thinner as well, and the capillaries are brought closer to the type I cells. This results in a reduced distance between the alveolar space and the intravascular space, which enhances the potential for gas exchange and in turn improves the chances for fetal survival. As the type II pneumocytes continue to increase in number and size, there is an increase in lamellar bodies, leading to more abundant storage of surfactant. All generations of conducting airways and respiratory branches are in place by the end of this stage.[7]

Alveolar Stage (36 Weeks' Gestation through Postterm)

Alveoli form in the alveolar stage when secondary septa subdivide the terminal saccules and the double capillary lining of the saccules fuses into a single layer of capillaries. This process, known as alveolarization, leads to greater surface area of the lungs available for gas exchange.

The alveolar stage begins around 36 weeks' gestation and continues postnatally for several years. The most rapid growth occurs in the first 6 months of life; alveoli continue to increase in number until about 8 years of age, with the greatest increase in number occurring in the first 2 years. The diameter of the alveoli also continues to increase until growth of the chest wall is complete. Although estimates vary, the term neonate has 50 to 150 million fully developed alveoli, compared to approximately 400 million alveoli in the lungs of an adult.[9–11]

Development of Surfactant

Surfactant is a complex mixture of lipids and proteins that is secreted into the alveolar space. It functions to lower surface tension at the air-liquid interface in the lung and in turn to stabilize the alveoli. Defective pulmonary surfactant metabolism results in respiratory distress and may lead to severe lung disease in neonates and older infants.

Function

At the end of expiration, when lung volumes are low, **surface tension** of the water layer within the alveoli causes the lungs to have a tendency to collapse. A very thin film of surfactant lines the alveolar surface of the lungs and reduces surface tension, which prevents the alveoli from completely collapsing and allows them to easily expand during inspiration. Without surfactant, alveolar surface tension increases and the alveoli have a tendency to collapse, the residual volume of gas is not maintained, and the alveoli lose their stability and become stiff. As lung compliance decreases, the neonate struggles with each breath to inflate the diffusely atelectatic lung. Lung immaturity and the resultant surfactant deficiency are the primary causes of respiratory distress syndrome in the premature neonate. **Table 3-1** lists the roles of **pulmonary surfactant**.

Production

Surfactant production is carried out in the type II pneumocytes and stored in the lamellar bodies. Lamellar bodies are released into the alveolar space by a process known as exocytosis, where they then appear to be

transformed into a lattice-like structure called tubular myelin. Surfactant is retained by the tubular myelin until forming a monomolecular layer over the alveolar epithelium. The tubular myelin aids in distributing the surfactant along the alveolar surface. Active surfactant secretion is detected by 30 weeks' gestation and can be stimulated by a number of mechanisms, including beta-agonists, adenosine triphosphate, and lung distention.[12] Surfactant has a finite life span and must be removed from the alveolar space. The rate of secretion must be balanced by the rate of removal. Rather than being lost to the airways, the majority of surfactant is recycled: About 85% of the surfactant is taken up by the type II pneumocytes, where it is repackaged in lamellar bodies and eventually secreted back into the alveolar space. The remaining 10% appears to be taken up by alveolar macrophages and less than 5% is cleared through the airways.[13]

Composition

As illustrated in **Figure 3-2**, **phospholipids** are the dominant component of lung surfactants, comprising nearly 80% of the surfactant complex. The remaining 20% is almost evenly split between neutral lipids, mostly cholesterol, and **surfactant proteins**.

Dipalmitoylphosphatidylcholine (DPPC) is the most abundant phospholipid in surfactant. DPPC is often referred to as lecithin and may be used as a marker for fetal lung maturity when compared to the amount of sphingomyelin in amniotic fluid. This evaluation is known as the **lecithin-to-sphingomyelin (L:S) ratio**. Phosphatidylglycerol is the second most abundant phospholipid in surfactant, followed by much smaller amounts of phosphatidylethanolamine, phosphatidylinositol, phosphatidylserine, and sphingomyelin.[14,15]

TABLE 3-1
Function of Pulmonary Surfactant

Lines the alveolar surface
Reduces alveolar surface tension
Prevents alveolar collapse
Facilitates lung expansion
Improves lung compliance
Maintains alveolar inflation at lower pressures

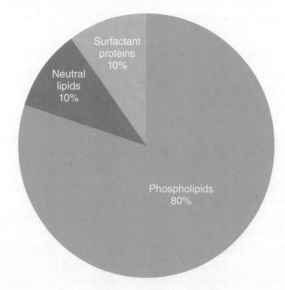

FIGURE 3-2 Composition of surfactant.

Surfactant proteins directly affect the properties of the lipids in surfactant. Four surfactant proteins have been identified:

- Surfactant protein A (SP-A)
- Surfactant protein B (SP-B)
- Surfactant protein C (SP-C)
- Surfactant protein D (SP-D)

SP-A is the most prominent, comprising nearly 50% of surfactant proteins,[16] while SP-D is the largest of the surfactant proteins. Both of these proteins are important in defense against infection and inflammation in the alveoli.[17] They promote bacterial and viral clearance, block inflammatory mediator production, and possess antimicrobial properties. Unlike SP-D, SP-A helps regulate the synthesis, secretion, and recycling of phospholipids and is essential for the production of tubular myelin.[18]

Both SP-B and SP-C are small proteins with similar surface properties that help spread surfactant lipids across the surface of lung tissue. SP-C is the smallest surfactant protein but one of the more abundant.[16] Mutations in genes of the surfactant proteins, often referred to as surfactant protein deficiency, can result in abnormal composition and decreased function of surfactant. This raises the surface tension in the lung. Infants who have mutations in SP-B present with severe respiratory failure that is refractory to conventional therapy, including surfactant replacement.[19] Mutations in SP-C are associated with chronic interstitial lung disease.

Factors That Influence Fetal Lung Development

Fetal lung development consists of both lung growth and lung maturation. Table 3-2 lists the hormones and growth factors that stimulate lung maturity. For lung development to proceed normally, the fetus must have adequate breathing movements and an appropriate amount of fetal lung fluid in the airways. Pulmonary hypoplasia can occur if fetal breathing movement is impaired or fluid production is decreased.

Hormones and Growth Factors

Hormones, especially glucocorticoids, accelerate lung maturity. This understanding has led to the widespread administration of corticosteroids, primarily betamethasone and dexamethasone, to mothers during premature labor. The result is a reduction in complications of prematurity, including respiratory distress syndrome and intraventricular hemorrhage.[20] Table 3-3 lists how growth factors are involved in fetal lung development, although the role that growth factors play in the development of congenital abnormalities or in postnatal conditions is not well understood.[21]

TABLE 3-2
Hormones and Growth Factors That Stimulate Lung Maturity

Glucocorticoids (cortisol)
Thyroid hormones
Estradiol
Vascular epithelial growth factor
Fibroblast growth factor
Prolactin
Thyrotropin-releasing hormone
Catecholamines
Epidermal growth factor

TABLE 3-3
Role of Growth Factors in Fetal Lung Development

Promote lung bud development
Specify patterns of airway branching
Determine airway size
Regulate septation of the terminal saccules to form alveoli

Fetal Breathing Movements

During intrauterine growth, normal distention of the lungs depends upon adequate physical space in the fetal thorax. It also depends upon **amniotic fluid** being brought into the lungs by fetal breathing movements. Fetal breathing movements are detected as early as 10 weeks' gestation, and they include movement of the diaphragm and chest wall, with diaphragmatic movement being much more pronounced. During the early stages of development, fetal breathing movements occur intermittently and are rapid and irregular.[22] As the fetus grows, movements become more organized and increase in strength and frequency. By 30 to 40 weeks' gestation, they are occurring 40% of the time.[23] Diaphragm movement and chest wall excursion may provide a stretching stimulus to the lungs that promotes alveolar development. The movements are also important in building strength and maintaining adequate lung volume in preparation for the first breath.[24]

Fetal Lung Fluid

During intrauterine life, the fetal lungs are filled with fluid. At one time it was believed that this liquid was a result of the fetus inhaling amniotic fluid, but in the 1940s, scientists unexpectedly found that this was not the case and that the liquid is actually produced by the lungs. The fluid is secreted by the pulmonary epithelium at a rate of 4 to 5 mL/kg/hour. For an average neonate, this is approximately 250 to 300 mL of fluid production per day, which compares roughly to the functional residual capacity (FRC). Some of the lung fluid produced moves from the trachea into the pharynx, where about half of it is swallowed and half of it enters the amniotic sac to mix with amniotic fluid. Because pressure in the fetal trachea is normally higher than pressure in the amniotic fluid, most of the fluid remains in the lungs. The presence of fluid in the fetal lung maintains lung expansion and directly affects growth, including the size and shape of the developing airways.[25]

As the fetus grows, fetal breathing movements increase and lung fluid moves into the amniotic sac. It is this mixture with amniotic fluid that allows lung maturity to be predicted by measuring the phospholipid component of surfactant in amniotic fluid. The production of fetal lung fluid slows with gestational age. During active labor and with breathing following delivery, fluid is cleared from the lungs into the interstitial spaces surrounding the alveoli, where it is absorbed into the pulmonary circulation or lymphatic system. Absorption is escalated by the secretion of fetal epinephrine.[26] For the successful transition to extrauterine life, it is critical that fluid be removed from the alveoli, thereby decreasing pulmonary resistance and allowing air to flow into the lungs.

Inadequate Fetal Lung Development

Inadequate development of the fetal lung can range from agenesis to aplasia to hypoplasia. **Table 3-4** defines these abnormalities in lung development. Of these, pulmonary hypoplasia is the most common.[27]

TABLE 3-4
Underdevelopment of the Fetal Lung

Disorder	Definition/Characteristics
Pulmonary agenesis	• Complete absence of the lung tissue, pulmonary vessels, and bronchus • Caused by primitive lung bud's failure to develop • Usually unilateral; right side has poorest prognosis • Bilateral is incompatible with life
Pulmonary aplasia	• Consists of carina and mainstem bronchial stump that ends in a blind pouch • Absence of lung tissue and pulmonary vessels • Usually unilateral • Bilateral is incompatible with life
Pulmonary hypoplasia	• Decreased number of airways, cells, and alveoli • Results in decreased size and weight of lungs • Primary hypoplasia has no obvious cause; is rarest form • Secondary hypoplasia is caused by fetal or maternal condition that limits fetal lung growth; is most common form

Pulmonary Hypoplasia

The hypoplastic lung presents with the following:

- Reduced weight
- Fewer airway generations
- Fewer and smaller alveoli
- Decreased pulmonary vasculature
- Reduced surface area for gas exchange

Although most often presenting as unilateral, hypoplasia may affect both lungs. Hypoplasia is of major concern because without adequate tissue and blood flow for gas exchange, the result is often severe respiratory distress and even neonatal death.[28] Although clinical symptoms may be similar, **pulmonary hypoplasia** is not equivocal to the immature lungs of the premature neonate. As listed in **Table 3-5**, most cases of pulmonary hypoplasia are due to an underlying abnormality.

Pulmonary Agenesis and Pulmonary Aplasia

Abnormal fetal lung development can result in other conditions that occur less often than pulmonary hypoplasia. **Pulmonary agenesis** is a condition in which the lung and all bronchus and pulmonary vessels are completely absent. When the agenesis is unilateral, the trachea essentially acts as a bronchus. **Pulmonary aplasia** is the rare condition in which there is a rudimentary blind-ended main bronchus and complete absence of a lung. When occurring bilateral, both pulmonary agenesis and pulmonary aplasia are incompatible with life.

Lung Compression

Any disorder that causes inadequate intrathoracic space or restricts growth of the chest can result in compression of the lungs in spite of the presence of fetal breathing movements. Congenital diaphragmatic hernia (CDH)

TABLE 3-5
Causes of Secondary Pulmonary Hypoplasia

Lung Compression
Congenital diaphragmatic hernia
Thoracic tumors
Pleural effusion
Osteogenesis imperfecta
Thoracic dystrophy
Dwarfism
Abnormal Fetal Breathing Movements
Spinal muscular atrophy
Congenital myotonic dystrophy
Phrenic nerve agenesis
Inadequate Amniotic Fluid
Oligohydramnios
Renal agenesis
Urinary tract obstruction
Polycystic kidney disease

is the most common condition associated with restricted growth due to lung compression.[29] In CDH, an abnormal opening or hernia in the diaphragm occurs early in fetal lung development. The hernia allows abdominal contents to move into the chest and compress the developing lung.

Absent or Abnormal Fetal Breathing Movements

Absent or decreased fetal breathing movements prevent adequate lung distention and stretch, which are critical for normal lung growth. Movements may be impaired by lesions of the central nervous system, spinal cord, and brain as well as some neuromuscular diseases.

Inadequate Amniotic Fluid

By the 4th week of gestation, the fetus is completely surrounded by a watery fluid, usually clear or light yellow in color, known as the amniotic fluid. The amniotic fluid is essential to the fetus and performs the following functions:

- Provides space for growth and development
- Acts as a cushion that absorbs blows
- Serves as a fluid source
- Provides a barrier against infection
- Maintains a steady temperature around the fetus

After about 11 weeks' gestation, the fetal kidneys produce the majority of the amniotic fluid. The amount of fluid continues to increase with gestational age until around 36 weeks' gestation. **Polyhydramnios**, an abnormally high level of fluid, occurs in approximately 1% of all pregnancies and is associated with preterm labor and delivery and several fetal anomalies.

A decreased amount of amniotic fluid is known as **oligohydramnios**. It occurs in approximately 4% of pregnancies and is detected most often during the last trimester, although it can occur at any time during the pregnancy. The decreased fluid volume may cause the amniotic pressure to fall and result in excess lung fluid being expelled through the larynx. This in turn reduces fluid pressure and fetal lung volume, which are critical to normal lung development. The degree of pulmonary hypoplasia is dependent upon the onset, severity, and duration of oligohydramnios. Prolonged premature rupture of the membranes surrounding the fetus causes early leaking of amniotic fluid and is a common cause of oligohydramnios.[30] Fetal renal problems also contribute to oligohydramnios. Urinary tract malformation and conditions that prevent urine formation or urine entry into the amniotic sac are commonly associated with pulmonary hypoplasia.[31] There is also a higher risk of oligohydramnios in pregnancies that extend 2 or more weeks past the due date. The loss of amniotic fluid during this time is believed to be due to placental insufficiency.[32]

CRITICAL THINKING QUESTIONS

1. Explain what pulmonary surfactant is and why it is important to the developing fetal lung.

2. Describe the role hormones and growth factors play in fetal lung development.

References

1. American Academy of Pediatrics, Committee on Fetus and Newborn. Age terminology during the perinatal period. *Pediatrics*. 2004;114:1362–1364.

2. Joshi S, Kotecha S. Lung growth and development. *Early Hum Dev*. 2007;83:278–794.

3. Jeffery P. The development of large and small airways. *Am J Respir Cell Mol Biol*. 1998;157:S174–S180.

4. Burri PH. Fetal and postnatal development of the lung. *Ann Rev Physiol*. 1984;46:617–628.

5. Hall SM, Hislop AA, Pierce C, Haworth SG. Prenatal origins of human intrapulmonary arteries: formation and smooth muscle maturation. *Am J Resp Cell Mol Biol*. 2000;23:194–203.

6. Hislop A., Reid L. Development of the acinus in the human lung. *Thorax*. 1974;29:90–94.

7. DiFior JW, Wilson JM. Lung development. *Semin Pediatr Surg*. 1994;3:221–232.

8. Cardoso WV, Lu J. Regulation of early lung morphogenesis: questions, facts and controversies. *Development*. 2006;133:1611–1624.

9. Langston C, Kida K, Reed M, Thurlbeck WM. Human lung growth in late gestation and in the neonate. *Am Rev Respir Dis*. 1984;129:607–613.

10. Burri PH. Fetal and postnatal development of the lung. *Annu Rev Physiol*. 1984;46:617–628.

11. Hislop A, Wigglesworth JS, Desai R. Alveolar development in the human fetus and infant. *Early Hum Dev*. 1986;13:1–11.

12. Zuo YY, Veldhuizen RA, Neumann AW, et al. Current perspectives in pulmonary surfactant – inhibition, enhancement and evaluation. *Biochem Biophys Acta*. 2008;1778:1947–1977.

13. Wright JR, Clements JA. Metabolism and turnover of lung surfactant. *Am Rev Respir Dis*. 1986;135:426–444.

14. Hallman M, Kulovich M, Kirkpatrick E, Sugarman RG, Gluck L. Phosphatidylinositol and phosphatidylglycerol in amniotic fluid: indices of lung maturity. *Am J Obstet Gynecol*. 1976;125:613–617.

15. Grenache DG, Gronowski AM. Fetal lung maturity. *Clin Biochem*. 2006;39:1–10.

16. Weaver TE. Pulmonary surfactant-associated proteins. *Gen Pharmacol*. 1988;19:361–368.

17. Haczku A. Protective role of the lung collectins surfactant protein A and surfactant protein D in airway inflammation. *J Allergy Clin Immunol*. 2008;122:861–879.

18. Wright JR. Host defense functions of pulmonary surfactant. *Biol Neonate*. 2004;85:326–332.

19. Hawgood S. Surfactant protein B: structure and function. *Biol Neonate*. 2004;85:285–289.

20. Bizzaro MJ, Gross I. Effects of hormones on fetal lung development. *Obstet Gynecol Clin North Am*. 2004;31:949–961.

21. Kumar VH, Lakshminrusimha S, El Abiad MT, et al. Growth factors in lung development. *Adv Clin Chem*. 2005;40:261–316.

22. Wigglesworth JS, Desai R. Is fetal respiratory function a major determinant of perinatal survival? *Lancet*. 1982;319:264–267.

23. Patrick J, Campbell K., Carmichael L, et al. Patterns of human fetal breathing during the last 10 weeks of pregnancy. *Obstet Gynecol*. 1980;56:24–30.

24. Davis GM, Bureau MA. Pulmonary and chest wall mechanics in the control of respiration in the newborn. *Clin Perinatol*. 1987;14:551–579.

25.   Hooper SB, Harding R. Fetal lung liquid: a major determinant of the growth and functional development of the fetal lung. *Clin Exp Pharmacol Physiol.* 1995;22:235–241.

26.   Inselman LS, Mellins RB. Growth and development of the lung. *J Pediatr.* 1981;98:1–15.

27.   Porter HJ. Pulmonary hypoplasia. *Arch Dis Child Fetal Neonatal Ed.* 1999;81:81–83.

28.   Kotecha S. Lung growth: implications for the newborn infant. *Arch Dis Child Fetal Neonatal Ed.* 2000;82:69–71.

29.   Laudy JA, Wladimiroff JW. The fetal lung 2: pulmonary hypoplasia. *Ultrasound Obstet Gynecol.* 2000;16:482–494.

30.   Hislop A, Reig L. Persistent hypoplasia of the lung after repair of congenital diaphragmatic hernia. *Thorax.* 1976;31:450–455.

31.   Perlman M, Williams J, Hirsch M. Neonatal pulmonary hypoplasia after prolonged leakage of amniotic fluid. *Arch Dis Child.* 1976;51:349–353.

32.   Wallenburg HC, Wladimiroff JW. The amniotic fluid. II. Polydydramnios and oligohydramnios. *J Perinat Med.* 1977;5:233–243.

4

Fetal Gas Exchange and Circulation

David M. Wheeler

Charlotte V. Reikofski

OUTLINE

OBJECTIVES

1. List the three germ layers that develop the different body systems in utero.
2. Describe the stages of cardiac development.
3. Explain the role of the placenta.
4. Describe the fetal blood flow.
5. List the factors that influence the transition from fetal blood flow to that which occurs with extrauterine life.
6. Describe how fetal shunts change when the transition from fetal to extrauterine life occurs.

KEY TERMS

blastocyte
ductus arteriosus
ductus venosus
ectoderm
embryoblast
endoderm
foramen ovale
looping
mesoderm

morula
placenta
placental circulation
septum primum
trophoblast
umbilical artery
umbilical vein
vitelline circulation
zygote

Introduction

This chapter will discuss the common course of circulatory development. This includes the natural history of cardiac development, adaptive developmental characteristics of maternal–fetal circulation, and transitional circulatory events that occur after the child is born.

Embryonic Development

Shortly after conception, the fertilized ovum undergoes rapid cellular proliferation. By the 3rd week of life, three germ layers—the endoderm, ectoderm, and mesoderm—are formed. These germ layers become different body systems as the embryo grows and develops. During fetal development, the heart is the first organ to form; by the 3rd week of life, formation of the heart and the circulatory system begins. It is important to note that the heart and circulatory system may not develop normally. Knowledge of the stages of embryonic heart and major vessel development will provide an understanding of the congenital cardiac defects that can occur. The heart is developed and fully functional by the 8th gestational week.

Early Development

The **zygote**, the single-celled earliest stage of human development, is formed within 12 to 24 hours of fertilization and contains all the genetic material needed to form a human embryo.[1] The zygote undergoes cellular division and forms daughter cells, or blastomeres. By day 3 to 4, between 12 and 32 blastomeres have formed and compacted into a solid ball of cells called a **morula**.[1,2] Fluid enters the intercellular spaces of the morula, and by day 6 the intercellular fluid-filled spaces fuse and create a large fluid cavity, or **blastocyte**.[1,3]

The blastocyte continues to grow and the cells separate into two distinct layers. The outermost layer is known as the **trophoblast,** or trophoectoderm, which contains approximately 80 cells and forms the chorionic sac and fetal components of the placenta.[1,2] The inner layer, known as the inner cell mass, or **embryoblast,** is a compact mass containing approximately 46 cells that forms the embryonic tissues.[1,2] By day 6, the trophoblast superficially implants onto the epithelial wall of the uterus.[1–3]

At the time of implantation, the uterine wall is highly vascularized and edematous, and it secretes both mucus and glycogen to supply the blastocyst with nutrients from the uterine tissues.[1,2] Uteroplacental circulation establishes as the trophoblast fully invades the uterine lining. Specifically, branches of the uterine arteries, called spiral arteries, invade the uterine lining, and the trophoblast cells puncture these arteries and create a conduit between the growing trophoblast and maternal circulation.[5] The blastocyst now receives nutrients directly from maternal blood, which is the initiation of primitive circulation.

After yolk sac development, approximately 3 weeks after fertilization, the blastocyst's inner cell mass divides into a trilayer disk. The central portion, or embryonic disk, forms three layers: the ectoderm, endoderm, and mesoderm.[1,4] The **ectoderm** forms the nervous system, skin or epidermis, glandular tissue, and many of the sensory organs. The **endoderm** produces the cecum, intestine, stomach, thymus, liver, pancreas, thyroid, prostate, and lungs.[1] The **mesoderm** is the last germ layer to form; it contributes to the blood; endothelium; heart; kidneys; reproductive organs; bones; skeletal tissues; and smooth and connective tissue, such as tendons, ligaments, dermis, and cartilage.[1,2]

Between day 18 and 19, blood islands form on either side of the head region of the trilayer disk, which become primitive blood tubes or endocardial tubes (**Figure 4-1**). This stage is the beginning of the embryo's vascular development. A complete timeline of the significant milestones of fetal heart development is found in **Table 4-1**. The trilayer, disc-like embryo undergoes a process of folding, and the heart tubes fold into what will eventually become the thoracic cavity. During this process, the head and lateral regions of the trifold disk fold inward, pushing the heart-forming region into a frontal position. This allows the heart tubes to fuse into a single-chamber heart called the primitive heart tube. By the 21st day, the primitive heart is bilaterally symmetrical and centrally positioned

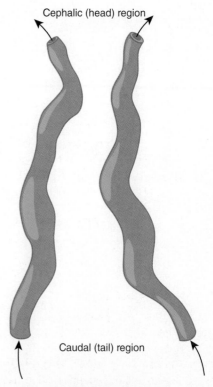

Cephalic (head) region

Caudal (tail) region

FIGURE 4-1 An illustration of the endocardial tubes. The blood flows through the endocardial tubes from the caudal to the cephalic region.

TABLE 4-1
Stages of Fetal Heart Development

Stage	Gestational Week	Day	Developmental Milestones
Early development		16	Blood islands appear
	3	18	Heart tubes form
		21	Heart tubes fuse
Chamber development			Heart tube fusion complete
		22	Heart beats begin
			Bidirectional blood flow starts
		23	Folding, looping, and ballooning begin
	4	25	Septum primum growth begins and atrial separation commences
			Ventricular separation starts
		28	Endocardial cushions form
			Unidirectional blood flow starts
	5	32	Septum secundum begins
	6	37	Foramen ovale development completes
Maturation		46	Ventricular formation completes
	7	49	Four chamber development completes
			Valve formation matures
	8	52	Complete separation of the aorta and pulmonary artery occurs
		56	Valve formation completes

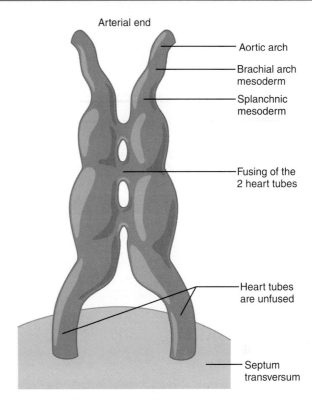

Arterial end

- Aortic arch
- Brachial arch mesoderm
- Splanchnic mesoderm
- Fusing of the 2 heart tubes
- Heart tubes are unfused
- Septum transversum

FIGURE 4-2 An illustration of cellular fusion. The endocardial tubes fuse into one primitive heart tube.

consists of the left **umbilical vein** and **umbilical artery**. The **vitelline circulation**, consisting of the vitelline artery and vein, develops as the precursor to the future liver circulation.[10] The two arms of the caudal end of the primary heart tube link with the developing embryonic, placental, and vitelline circulation.[7] By day 22, peristaltic contractions of the heart tube or cardiac contractions are detectable and bidirectional blood flow begins.[5]

Chamber Development

By the 4th gestational week, the heart undergoes dramatic changes through differential cellular growth in a process called **looping**.[7] The cephalic, aortic root end moves to the right, ventrally, and caudally in respect to the tail end, which moves cranially and dorsally.[7] These movements bring the cephalic and caudal ends of the heart tube together lengthwise while folding the center part of the heart tube into a flattened S-shape (**Figure 4-3**). As the heart tube merges, three recognizable structures form: the bulbus cordis, ventricular bulge, and atrial bulge (**Figure 4-4**). The atrial bulge is inferior to the ventricular bulge at this very early stage of development.[8–9] These structures connect to the sinus venosus, which receives nutrient-rich, oxygenated blood from the placeta.[10] As these structures continue to bend and fold, the truncus arteriosus begins to form (**Figure 4-5**). This structure will eventually connect the heart to the arterial system.[10] Days 23 to 25 are

within the embryo, taking the shape of an elongated X (**Figure 4-2**).[1,6,7]

During this period, the embryonic circulation consists of three veins (the anterior, common, and posterior cardinal veins) and three arteries (the ventral and dorsal aorta and the aortic arch). As the embryo develops, **placental circulation**, or circulation between the mother and fetus, establishes to provide gas exchange necessary to sustain life. Placental circulation

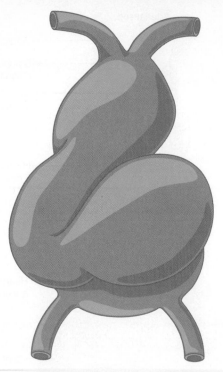

FIGURE 4-3 The process of folding, looping, and ballooning forms the initial structures of the heart. This illustration shows the caudal portion bending dorsally, cranially, and to the left.

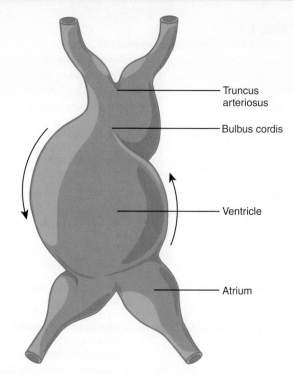

FIGURE 4-5 Chamber formation begins as the cephalic portion bends ventrally, caudally, and to the right, merging the heart tubes and forming the bulbus cordis, ventricular bulge, and atrial bulge.

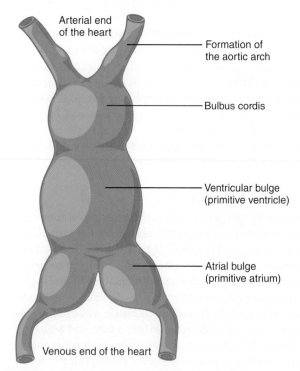

FIGURE 4-4 Development of the primitive heart tube at approximately the 4th gestational week.

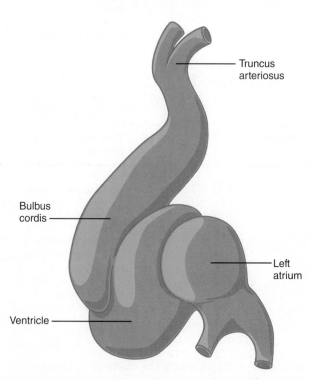

FIGURE 4-6 As the structures continue to bend and fold, the truncus arteriosus develops.

significant because this is when the heart tube begins to fold and loop. A process known as dextral looping occurs between days 23 and 28. During this time, approximately day 28, the heart tube is much larger, and a common atrium, common ventricle, and outflow tract have formed (**Figure 4-6**). Blood flow at this stage of development is unidirectional: It flows into the common atrium, then through a narrow common atrioventricular canal, into a primitive ventricle, and through the outflow tract.[10]

Maturation

As the heart continues to evolve, endocardial cushions encroach upon the common atrioventricular canal, fuse, and ultimately divide the common atrioventricular tract into left and right atrioventricular tracts. The upper common atrium and lower common ventricle are divided by two common atrioventricular canals (**Figure 4-7**). The **septum primum** originates in the roof of the common atria and stretches to connect with the fused endocardial cushion of the atrioventricular canal.[11] As this atrial septum forms, a small opening remains and acts as a conduit between the atria, called the **foramen ovale**. A muscular ventricular septum, the primordial interventricular septum, grows from the floor of the common ventricle upward to divide the ventricles[12] (**Figure 4-8**). Spiral ridges form within the common outflow tract, ultimately creating the aortic root and pulmonary trunk.[12] The mitral and tricuspid valves form from the endocardial cushions in the atrioventricular canals, while pulmonic and aortic valves form from endocardial cushions in the outflow tract (**Figure 4-9**). At the beginning of the 8th gestational week, the formed structure of the heart will persist for the remainder of intrauterine life.[7,12]

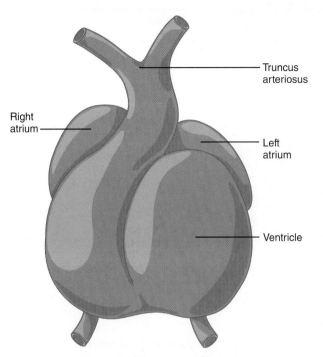

FIGURE 4-7 The partially differentiated heart tube. The upper common atrium and lower common ventricle are divided by two common atrioventricular canals.

Fetal and Transitional Circulation

We now turn our attention to a more thorough examination of maternal–fetal blood flow; the unique shunts that characterize fetal circulation, occurring in utero; and the transitional circulation, occurring after birth when the infant's first breath is drawn.

The Placenta

The natural history of fetal growth and development is contingent upon the functional efficiency, fractal

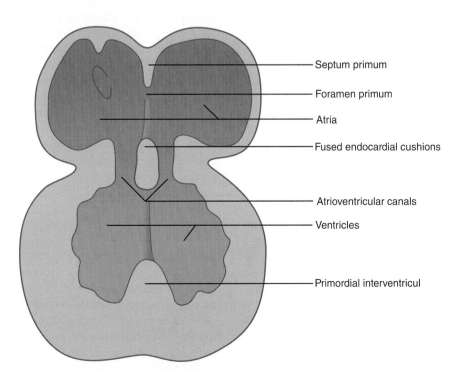

FIGURE 4-8 The development of the heart's four chambers commences with septation. As the septum primum grows, the atria are divided. Growth of the primordial interventricular septum divides the single ventricle.

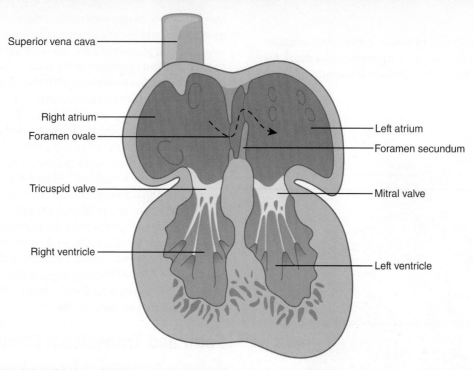

FIGURE 4-9 A frontal view of the heart following growth, which partitions into four chambers. The dotted arrow shows how blood flows from the right to the left atrium through the foramen ovale.

architecture, and adaptability of the **placenta**. The placenta is the hub of maternal–fetal interaction. It provides metabolic, renal, hepatic, immunologic, and gas exchange functions for the fetus in utero.[13] Placental architecture and performance will have immediate and long-term implications for the health both of the developing fetus and of the mother. It has been demonstrated that placental size, shape, and function can affect the overall health of a human throughout their lifespan.[13] In this section, we will focus our attention on the indispensable gas exchange capability of the placenta, fetal circulation, and the transitional events that co-attend the birth of the infant.[13–16]

The human placenta is attached to the maternal uterine wall and communicates with the fetus through the umbilical cord, which is the life-sustaining conduit between mother and developing infant. The umbilical cord derivates from the placental chorionic plate and is the origination point of a network of cotyledon vessels or lobules. The average human placenta weighs 500 grams and is 22 cm in length.[13–16] The placenta is 2 to 2.5 cm thick in the center and thins as it stretches peripherally, and the umbilical cord is 55 to 60 cm in length and contains two umbilical arteries and one umbilical vein (**Figure 4-10**).[13–17]

The human placenta is hemochorial, in that maternal blood interacts with the chorionic membrane of the infant, which, in turn, interacts directly with fetal circulation and blood flow. Therefore, under normal circumstances, there is no mixing of maternal

and fetal blood. Oxygenated blood flows to the fetus through the umbilical vein, while deoxygenated blood travels from the fetus back to the placenta through the umbilical arteries.[13,16,18]

Deoxygenated fetal blood flows to the placenta through the umbilical arteries, which bifurcate to configure the network of chorionic arteries. Chorionic arteries, in turn, branch into cotyledon arteries that further bifurcate and feed the fundamental unit of exchange: the chorionic villi, which eventually branch to form a substantial arterio-venous capillary system. This network of conducting vessels efficiently transports gases and nutrients to the developing fetus (Figure 4-10).[17,19]

Fetal blood shares an intimate proximity to maternal blood. The chorionic villus fetal vascular endothelial cells segregate maternal from fetal blood while transporting molecular gases, nutrients, and immune agents and removing fetal waste.[13,15,17]

Fetal Circulation

Fetal circulation is characterized by a sophisticated architecture. There are three shunts that serve to enhance the efficacy and distribution of blood flow to the developing fetus: the **ductus venosus, ductus arteriosus,** and foramen ovale. Together, these three shunts regulate the flow of fundamental resources (nutrients and molecular gases) for intrauterine life.[20,21]

The ductus venosus is a shunt, connecting the intra-abdominal umbilical vein to the inferior vena

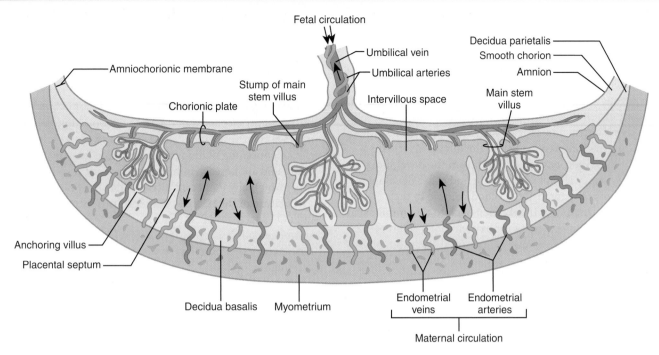

Fetal circulation

Umbilical vein
Umbilical arteries
Decidua parietalis
Smooth chorion
Amnion

Amniochorionic membrane
Stump of main stem villus
Chorionic plate
Intervillous space
Main stem villus

Anchoring villus
Placental septum

Decidua basalis   Myometrium
Endometrial veins   Endometrial arteries

Maternal circulation

FIGURE 4-10 A cross-section of the placenta showing the vascular network.

cava at its inlet to the heart. However, the ductus venosus channels 70% to 80% of umbilical blood through the liver before entering the inferior vena cava. The low degree of shunting through the ductus venosus indicates the higher growth-related urgency for the liver.[22] However, the oxygen extraction of the developing liver is a relatively modest 10% to 15%; the well-oxygenated blood from both the ductus venosus and the liver move to the inferior vena cava and the right atrium **(Figure 4-11)**.[20–23]

From the right atrium, approximately 80% of blood flow is directed through either of two adaptive anatomical shunts: the foramen ovale or the ductus arteriosus. These structures serve to selectively shunt blood from the pulmonary circulation and the developing lung field. It is critical to remember that the growing lung has attenuated gas and metabolic requirements and is quite well served with approximately 20% of fetal blood flow.[20,24]

The foramen ovale is an aperture-like opening of the atrial septum between the right and left atria. This shunt is a low-resistance passage to the left atrium, then to the left ventricle, which pumps blood through ventricular contraction to the aorta. Additionally, the well-oxygenated blood from the ductus venosus has a higher kinetic energy in the inferior vena cava and will maintain the patency of the unidirectional valve in the foramen ovale that selectively opens to the left atrium (Figure 4-11).[17,20,24]

The ductus arteriosus is the third important anatomic shunt; it connects the trunk of the pulmonary artery to the aorta. The blood volume pumped to the

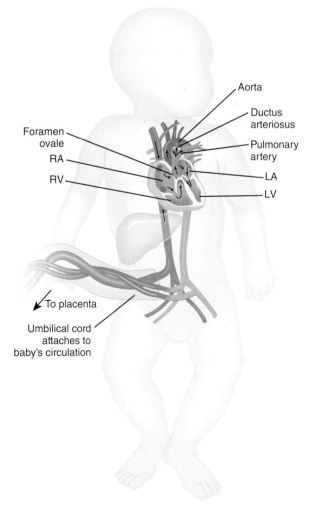

Aorta
Ductus arteriosus
Pulmonary artery
Foramen ovale
RA
RV
LA
LV

To placenta

Umbilical cord attaches to baby's circulation

FIGURE 4-11 Blood flow through the three structural shunts.

pulmonary trunk encounters the highly resistive vessels of the collapsed fetal lungs. The high pulmonary vascular resistance serves a protective function, defending the developing lung from volume overload while selectivity shunting the flow of oxygenated blood through the ductus arteriosus to the caudal aorta. This pattern of flow from the ductus arteriosus selectively favors aortic flow to the brain and upper extremities. Both the foramen ovale and the ductus arteriosus shunt oxygen-enriched blood from the developing pulmonary circuit to the brain and other developing systems. The majority of blood volume to the aorta flows to the lower trunk, then back to the umbilical arteries and the placenta for oxygenation (**Figure 4-12**). At term, or approximately 40 weeks' gestation, blood flow within the placenta and subsequently to the fetus is 500 to 700 mL/min.[17,20,24]

Transitional and Neonatal Circulations

The first breath is said to generate a massive negative inspiratory force that is required for initial lung expansion. This opening of the lung creates an astounding amplification in pulmonary blood flow, which replaces umbilical venous return as the source of preload for the left ventricle, and a dramatic reduction in pulmonary vascular resistance. This is primarily the result of a triad consisting of lung field expansion; increasing PaO_2; and an increase in native pulmonary vasodilators, principally PGI2 and nitric oxide. The pulmonary vasculature of the neonate is very sensitive to changes in PaO_2. Increasing PaO_2 with the first breath may also stimulate endogenous nitric oxide release. The significant swing in pulmonary vascular resistance from very high in utero to relatively low at birth is due to the

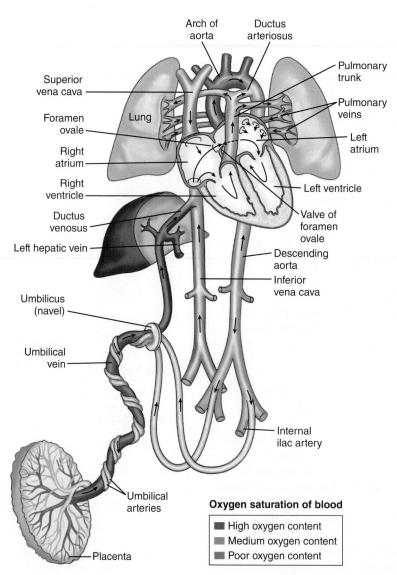

FIGURE 4-12 Fetal circulation.

TABLE 4-2
Comparison of Functional and Anatomical Shunt Closure after Transition to Extrauterine Life

Type of Shunt	Occurrence of Functional Closure	Occurrence of Anatomical Closure
Ductus venosus	Immediately following umbilical cord clamping	Up to 14 days after birth
Foramen ovale	Within 1 minute of the first breaths after birth	May take days to months; 15–20% of adults still have a patent foramen ovale
Ductus arteriosus	10–15 hours	2–3 months

expansion of the lungs, increased oxygenation, and molecularly mediated vasodilation. These changes create a circuit that will reverse pressure/flow relationships and close the adaptive shunts so vital for fetal growth and development.[17,20,24–27]

Fetal shunts will transform functionally with a greater urgency than anatomically (**Table 4-2**). The ductus venosus closes functionally with the clamping of the umbilical cord due to the absence of flow/pressure required to maintain patency. However, anatomic closure may take up to 14 days.[17,20,24,26,27] It is important to note that all transitional timetables are extended in infants born prematurely.

The functional closure of the foramen ovale occurs within minutes following lung expansion due primarily to the dramatic reversal of the fetal atrial pressure gradient. Within minutes after birth, the pressure gradient between the right and left circuit changes, with the left-sided pressure now greater than the right. This is predominantly due to decreasing pulmonary vascular resistance, increasing oxygenation, and increasing systemic vascular resistance. Within this new pressure relationship, right atrial pressure is now significantly lower than left atrial pressure, causing the unidirectional flap that opened into the left atrium in utero to shut, functionally closing the foramen ovale. However, the anatomic closure of the foramen ovale may take longer.[16,21] Approximately 15% to 20% of adults manifest some residual foramen ovale flow.[24–27]

The ductus arteriosus is functionally closed by 10 to 15 hours after birth. In the changing architecture of the newborn cardiopulmonary circuit, flow and pressure gradients change. After birth, pressures on the left side of the heart far exceed those on the right. With the pressure changes in the pulmonary and systemic circulatory circuits, blood flow through the ductus arteriosus decays and this shunt begins to close. Anatomic closure occurs within 2 to 3 months when the structure of the ligamentum arteriosus is completed.[25–27]

CRITICAL THINKING QUESTIONS

1. Why are the cardiopulmonary transitions co-attendant with the first breath important for the respiratory care professional?

2. What is the primary site of gas exchange for the fetus?

References

1. Pansky B. *Review of Medical Embryology*. New York, NY: MacMillan; 1982.
2. Hardy K, Handyside AH, Winston, RML. The human blastocyst: cell number, death, and allocation during late preimplantation development in vitro. *Development*. 1989;107(1):597–604.
3. Hardy K, Hooper MAK, Handyside AH, Rutherford AJ, Winston, RML, Leese HJ. Non-invasive measurement of glucose and pyrivate uptake by individual human oocytes and preimplantaton embryos. *Hum Reprod*. 1989;4(3):188–191.
4. Edwards RG, Purdy JM, Steptoe PC, Walters DE. The growth of human pre-implementation embryos in vitro. *Am J Gynecol*. 1981;14(1):408–416.
5. Dangel J. Changing physiology in the first-to third-trimester fetal circulation. *Cardiol Young*. 2014;24(Suppl 2):13–18.
6. Itskovitz-Eldor J, Schuldiner M, Karsenti D, et al. Differentiation of human embryonic stem cells into embroid bodies comprising the three embryonic germ layers. *Mol Med*. 2000;6(2):88–95.
7. Moorman A, Webb S, Brown N, Lamers W, Anderson R. Development of the heart: (1) formation of the cardiac chambers and arterial trunks. *Heart J*. 2003;89(7):806–814.
8. Makikallio K, Tekay A, Jouppila P. Yolk sac and umbilicoplacental hemodynamics during early human embryonic development. *Ultrasound Obstetr Gynecol*. 1999;14(3):175–179.
9. Risau W. Mechanisms of angiogenesis. *Nature*. 1997;386(6626):671–674.
10. Harrison GL. *The Shaping of Life: The Generation of Biological Pattern*. New York, NY: Cambridge University Press; 2006.
11. Webb S, Kanani M, Anderson RH, et al. Development of the human pulmonary vein and its incorporation in the morphologically left atrium. *Cardiol Young*. 2001;11(6):632–642.
12. Anderson RH, Webb S, Brown BA, Lamers W, Moorman A. Development of the heart: (2) septation of the atriums and ventricles. *Heart*. 2003;89(8):949–958.
13. Kaufmann P, Scheffen I. Placental development. In: Polin RA, Fox WW, Abman SH, eds. *Fetal and Neonatal Physiology*. 2nd ed. Philadelphia, PA: W.B. Saunders; 2004:95–97.
14. Cunningham FG, Gant NF, Leveno KJ. *Williams Obstetrics*. 21st ed. New York, NY: McGraw-Hill; 2001.
15. Faber JJ, Thornburg KL. *Placental Physiology*. New York, NY: Raven Press; 1983.
16. Khong TY. Placental vascular development and neonatal outcome. *Semin Neonatol*. 2004;9(4):255–267.
17. Fox H. *Pathology of the Placenta*. 2nd ed. Philadelphia, PA: W.B. Saunders; 1997.
18. Rosenfeld CR. Regulation of placental circulation. In: Polin RA, Fox WW, Abman SH, eds. *Fetal and Neonatal Physiology*. 2nd ed. Philadelphia, PA: W.B. Saunders; 2004:114–120.
19. Blackburn ST. *Maternal, Fetal and Neonatal Physiology: A Clinical Perspective*. Philadelphia, PA: W.B. Saunders; 2003.
20. Kiserud T, Acharya G. The fetal circulation. *Prenat Diagn*. 2004;24(13):1049–1059.
21. Kiserud T, Rasmussen S, Skulstad S. Blood flow and degree of shunting through the ductus venosus in the human fetus. *Am J Obstet Gynecol*. 2000;183(1 pt 1):147–153.
22. Kiserud T. The ductus venosus. *Semin Perinatol*. 2001;25(1):11–20.

23. Borrell A. The ductus venosus in early pregnancy and congenital anomalies. *Prenat Diagn*. 2004;24(9):688–692.

24. Friedman AH, Fahey JT. The transition from fetal to neonatal circulation: normal responses and implication for infants with heart disease. *Semin Perinatol*. 1992;17(2):106–221.

25. Wilson AD, Rao PS, Aeschlimann S. Normal fetal foramen ovale flap and transatrial Doppler velocity pattern. *J Am Soc Echocardiogr*. 1989;3(6):491–494.

26. Lakshminrushimha S, Steinharn RH. Pulmonary vascular biology during neonatal transition. *Clin Perinatol*. 1999;26(3):601–619.

27. Rudolph AM. Fetal circulation and cardiovascular adjustments after birth. In: Rudolph AM, Rudolph CD, eds. *Rudolph's Pediatrics*. 21st ed. New York, NY: McGraw-Hill; 2003:1749–1753.

5

Maternal and Fetal Assessment

Dana Nelson

Sherry L. Barnhart

OUTLINE

OBJECTIVES

1. Describe the key components of a maternal medical history.
2. Identify maternal medical and social issues that may result in a high-risk pregnancy.
3. Discuss the role of prenatal care in identifying and reducing complications during pregnancy.
4. Differentiate between gravida and parity.
5. List infections that can impact maternal health and perinatal transmission.
6. Explain the risk of developing premature rupture of membranes.
7. Describe placenta previa and placental abruption.
8. Differentiate between preeclampsia and eclampsia.
9. Explain the differences between pregestational and gestational diabetes.
10. List the complications common to infants of a diabetic mother.
11. Define polyhydramnios and oligohydramnios and the disorders associated with each.
12. Identify indications for antepartum fetal monitoring.
13. Describe a nonstress test and a contraction stress test.
14. Explain the uses for ultrasound.
15. Recognize the risk factors for a high-risk pregnancy and delivery.
16. List medications used to stop preterm uterine contractions.
17. Discuss the risks to the fetus when a pregnancy is postterm.

KEY TERMS

advanced maternal age (AMA)
amniocentesis
contraction stress test (CST)
eclampsia
fetal biophysical profile (BPP)
gestational diabetes mellitus (GDM)
gravida
HELLP syndrome
high-risk delivery
high-risk pregnancy
multiple gestation
nonstress test (NST)

nuchal cord
oligohydramnios
parity
placental abruption
placenta previa
polyhydramnios
postterm pregnancy
preeclampsia
prenatal care
premature rupture of membranes (PROM)
preterm labor
tocolytic agents
umbilical cord prolapse (UCP)

Introduction

A pregnancy is considered high-risk when complications develop during the pregnancy, the mother is pregnant with multiples (e.g., twins, triplets), or conditions are present in the mother or fetus that can adversely affect the outcome of the pregnancy. Maternal history, fetal assessment, and intrapartum monitoring provide valuable information that enables the healthcare team to provide timely and appropriate care during the pregnancy and delivery. This chapter will provide a foundation for the clinician to obtain facts, recognize risk factors, and take the appropriate steps in preparing for a **high-risk pregnancy** and delivery.

Identifying the High-Risk Pregnancy

When certain factors are present, a pregnancy is considered at high-risk for the mother or infant having problems during the pregnancy, at birth, or following delivery. High-risk pregnancies should be closely monitored. In some cases, the mother is referred to a facility that specializes in these pregnancies. Predicting and preparing for a **high-risk delivery** can improve perinatal outcome and prevent death.

Maternal Medical History

Obtaining an accurate medical history is essential in identifying a high-risk pregnancy. It should include information about the current and any previous pregnancies, past and present medical history, family surgical histories, medication intake, and prenatal care. Maternal history is usually obtained through a combination of medical record review and an interview with the mother. It is typically followed by a thorough physical assessment.

Health Disorders

A high-risk pregnancy may occur because of a medical condition that exists before the mother becomes pregnant. As listed in **Table 5-1**, there are many

health disorders, both acute and chronic, that affect a pregnancy. A number of chronic conditions, such as asthma, diabetes, hypertension, anemia, and autoimmune disease, are associated with premature birth. Acute disorders, such as shock or trauma, can lead to pregnancy complications. Poor nutrition, low maternal weight, and obesity also contribute to a high-risk pregnancy.[1]

Complications encountered in past pregnancies often become risk factors for future pregnancies. A premature birth in the past puts a mother at higher risk of experiencing preterm labor and delivery again. Likewise, a mother who had a previous pregnancy that resulted in miscarriage or multiple gestations is at higher risk of those occurring again.[2] In most cases, however, a pregnancy will be uncomplicated if the mother's medical problem is well controlled and she receives good prenatal care.

Prenatal Care

Prenatal care is the comprehensive medical care and monitoring that a woman receives during pregnancy. It involves the physical assessment of the mother and fetus, screening and treatment for medical conditions, and emotional support and counseling. The focus of prenatal care is early identification and treatment of potentially serious problems that can harm the mother or fetus. Women who do not receive prenatal care or whose care is delayed until late in the pregnancy have an increased risk of preterm birth, low birthweight, and neonatal death.

Obtaining an accurate pregnancy history and estimate of the infant's due date is critical. Terms used to indicate details of this history include **gravida**, which refers to the number of times the mother has been pregnant, and **parity**, which refers to the number of pregnancies that went beyond 20 weeks' gestation or to viability. The number of fetuses does not affect the parity. A more descriptive history of pregnancy outcomes or parity is provided with the TPAL acronym,

---

TABLE 5-1
Maternal Factors Contributing to a High-Risk Pregnancy

Chronic Conditions	Past Pregnancies	Maternal Age	Infection	Pregnancy Complications
Asthma	Cesarean delivery	Younger than 18 years	Viral infections	Preterm labor
Hypertension	Preterm delivery	Older than 35 years	Bacterial infections	Postterm pregnancy
Anemia	Multiple gestation		Sexually transmitted diseases	Preeclampsia
Autoimmune disease	Stillbirth			Gestational diabetes
Kidney disease	Miscarriage			Cervical insufficiency
Cardiac disease	Placenta previa			Placenta previa
Epilepsy	Placental abruption			Placental abruption
Obesity	Low birthweight			Polyhydramnios
				Intrauterine growth restriction
				Antepartum hemorrhage
				Multiple gestation
				Breech presentation at delivery

where the mother is assigned a four-digit number determined by the following:

- T represents the number of term births regardless of their outcome.
- P represents the number of preterm births occurring before 37 weeks' gestation.
- A represents the number of abortions, both elective and miscarriages.
- L represents the number of living children at the time the history is obtained.

Box 5-1 provides examples of using this terminology.

A mother's prenatal care is somewhat standardized into monthly visits for the first 28 weeks of pregnancy, then moving to every 2 weeks until 36 weeks of pregnancy, and then weekly leading up to the point of delivery. This course of care will vary greatly depending on the needs and risk status of the mother and fetus. Prenatal lab testing for the lower-risk patient generally includes an initial panel of bloodwork with the complete blood count (CBC), blood type and screen, antibodies, viral testing, and testing for chlamydia and gonorrhea. Additional testing and screening for diabetes and hypertension will follow, as they may develop over the months of pregnancy.[1] Education and counseling are also a large part of prenatal care. Table 5-2 lists topics often discussed during visits.

Maternal Age

A mother's age at the time of pregnancy may increase the risk of having unfavorable maternal and fetal outcomes. A maternal age of younger than 19 years and an **advanced maternal age (AMA)**, which is defined as older than 35 years, are associated with greater odds of complications. Both age groups are at higher risk of having preterm labor and delivery, preeclampsia, poor fetal growth, fetal distress, postpartum hemorrhage, and intrauterine fetal demise. There is an increased incidence with young mothers of having intrauterine

TABLE 5-2
Topics of Discussion and Education during Prenatal Care

Fetal growth and development
Nutrition
Weight gain
Exercise
Occupational hazards
Medication use
Prescription
Over-the-counter
Illicit drugs
Depression
Breastfeeding
Sexual relations
Risks of cesarean section delivery

infections that can harm the fetus, while the mother with AMA is at significant risk of placenta previa, placental abruption, and the need for cesarean delivery.[3]

AMA has long been associated with the risk of fetal genetic concerns. Over the past 30 years, the incidence of pregnancy among women with AMA has increased from approximately 5% to 15% of all births.[4] Age is a factor in fertility reduction. Advances in reproductive medicine have improved the ability for women older than age 35 years to achieve pregnancy. One of the most common risks associated with fertility treatment is multifetal pregnancies, which carry a greater risk for maternal morbidity and fetal morbidity and mortality.

Age is noted to have an impact upon preexisting or new medical diagnosis during pregnancy. Both hypertension and diabetes have an increased risk of development as a mother ages. Age also diminishes the body's normal ability to adapt to physiologic change. Cesarean delivery is more common among these mothers, especially if there has been a previous cesarean delivery or if there is multifetal gestation.[4]

Because of the increased risk for preterm births and intrauterine fetal demise, antenatal surveillance is important with young mothers and those with AMA. Although there are increased risks of complications, pregnancy outcome is generally good, especially when prenatal care is optimum.

Infections

Infections are major contributors to both maternal and fetal morbidity and mortality. Transmission can occur transplacentally, intrauterine, or during the postnatal period, causing low birthweight, developmental abnormalities, or congenital disease. While infection can severely impact the mother, the risk of transmission to the fetus is critical. The timing of infection is important in assessing risk, as the danger of some viral infections varies depending on whether they occur early in pregnancy, late in pregnancy, or at the time of delivery.

BOX 5-1 Examples of Classifying a Pregnancy History

- A mother has had 3 previous pregnancies and delivered 2 term children and 1 child at 30 weeks' gestation. She is Gravida 3 with a TPAL of 2-1-0-3.
- A mother is pregnant for the 6th time; she has delivered 3 term children, 2 preterm children, and has had 1 miscarriage. She is Gravida 6 with a TPAL of 3-2-1-5.
- A mother is pregnant for the 2nd time and has had 1 abortion. She is Gravida 2 with a TPAL of 0-0-1-0.

Viral Infections

Hepatitis is a viral infection with the potential for life-long impact on the fetus. Although there are numerous types of hepatitis, hepatitis B (HBV) results in maternal and neonatal consequences, and infection can be severe. Mothers infected with HBV may or may not be symptomatic; their disease may be acute, with no sequelae, or chronic, with liver cirrhosis or liver failure. Transmission occurs through fluid contact at birth. Because an untreated neonate has a 70% to 90% risk of infection, with nearly a 90% risk of developing a chronic HBV infection, prenatal identification of maternal hepatitis B surface antigen is critical.[1]

Human immunodeficiency virus (HIV) type 1 is a viral infection relevant to maternal health and perinatal transmission. It is estimated that of the approximately 50,000 new HIV infections each year, 150 will be in newborns as a result of mother-to-infant transmission.[5] All pregnant women should be screened for HIV early in the pregnancy. Identification of the virus requires treatment, as early treatment lowers viral loads and can impact viral transmission to the fetus. Medication given early to HIV-positive mothers and to the newborn after delivery can reduce transmission.[5] Rapid HIV testing is an option offered to laboring mothers who were not tested during the pregnancy. To reduce transmission risk, infants born to HIV-infected mothers and those whose status is unknown should have a rapid antibody test done as soon as possible after delivery and receive antiretroviral medications within 12 hours.

Bacterial Infections

Group B streptococci (GBS) have long been a noted cause of morbidity and mortality for neonates in the perinatal period. Approximately 25% of pregnant women are colonized with the bacteria and should be treated with antibiotics. Neonatal transmission is possible during labor and delivery and can result in newborn sepsis, pneumonia, or, less commonly, meningitis.[1]

IV antibiotics are administered during labor to mothers with positive cultures, to those who have a history of a previous baby with a GBS infection, to mothers with rupture of membranes greater than 18 hours before delivery, and to mothers who present with fever during labor.[6] Although there is also a late onset GBS infection, there is currently no prevention strategy.

Sexually Transmitted Diseases

Diseases transmitted through sexual contact cause problems during pregnancy and disproportionately affect women throughout their childbearing years. Sexually transmitted diseases (STD) can impair fertility, cause chronic disease, and contribute to neonatal morbidity. Screening and treatment of the mother and sexual partner(s) are important, as most re-infections after treatment are due to an untreated or new sexual partner or poor adherence to the treatment regimen.[7] Moreover, identification of one STD places the mother at risk for multiple diseases and warrants additional screening.

One of the most common viral infections that causes problems during pregnancy is genital herpes, or herpes simplex 2 (HSV-2). When the mother has a primary outbreak of HSV-2 in late pregnancy, the risk for fetal transmission is 30% to 50%. Transmission in the absence of lesions, in mothers with a known history of HSV-2, or in those who are infected in the early months of pregnancy, is less than 1%.[8] Identifying a history of HSV-2 during prenatal care and monitoring for symptoms is important. Suppressive therapy with antivirals is usually recommended at 36 weeks' gestation.[9] Mothers in labor should be examined for the presence of lesions. If no signs exist, then vaginal delivery is appropriate; to reduce transmission risk, a cesarean delivery is recommended if lesions are present.[8]

Human papillomavirus (HPV) is a prevalent viral infection that can be transmitted to the fetus. Infection is usually mild and may be asymptomatic and as such often unrecognized.[10] Pregnancy may exacerbate HPV infections, and although there are medications that can be used, many have fetal teratogenic effects and cannot be safely administered during pregnancy. Exposure to the virus during delivery poses lower risk to the neonate and routine cesarean section is not necessary.

Chlamydial infection from *Chlamydia trachomatis* is one of the most common infections in sexually active women younger than 25 years of age, and annual screening is recommended for this population.[11] It is associated with pelvic inflammatory disease (PID), which can impact fertility, and neonatal transmission at birth. Oral antibiotics are given to treat chlamydial infections during the pregnancy. Some medications, including doxycycline, have teratogenic concerns for the fetus and are not recommended for use, especially in the second and third trimesters.[11] Infection occurs through contact during a vaginal delivery: Close to one-half of the neonates born to women with untreated chlamydial infection will develop the infection. Colonized neonates will develop symptoms at sites that involve the mucous membranes of the eye, oropharynx, urogenital tract, and rectum, resulting most commonly in conjunctivitis 5 to 12 days postdelivery. More severe infection can lead to pneumonia. The current standard of care for neonates is administration of erythromycin ophthalmic ointment immediately after delivery.[11] Antibiotic treatment is required for neonates diagnosed with chlamydial infection.[1]

Gonorrhea, caused by the bacteria *Neisseria gonorrhoeae*, is another common STD in women younger than 25 years. Prevalence is higher in women of African American, American Indian, Hispanic, and Alaska Native ethnicity. It is also more common in women with previous STD infections or multiple partners.[1] Infected mothers are often asymptomatic. Gonorrhea can cause PID, infertility, arthritis, and dermatitis. Screening is done during an initial prenatal visit and antibiotic treatment given if results are positive. Transmission of infection to the neonate occurs during delivery and results in ophthalmia neonatorum with a risk of sight impairment, sepsis, and meningitis. Preventive prophylaxis is routine after delivery and consists of erythromycin ophthalmic ointment applied to each eye immediately after delivery, regardless of whether the delivery was vaginal or cesarean.[12]

Syphilis, caused by *Treponema pallidum*, can be transmitted to the fetus through the placenta and result in congenital syphilis or stillbirth.[13] Pregnant women are screened at the initial prenatal visit and, if syphilis is confirmed, are treated with antibiotics.[1] If the infant tests positive for syphilis or if the mother received late or no treatment, then penicillin is given for 10 days.

Trichomoniasis is caused by infection with the parasite *Trichomonas vaginalis*. It is the most common nonviral STD. Trichomoniasis can lead to infertility and adverse pregnancy outcomes. Racial disparities exist, with African American women demonstrating higher exposures than white, non-Hispanic women.[14] Identification in pregnancy is important to reduce the associated risk of **premature rupture of membranes (PROM)** and subsequent preterm delivery. Trichomoniasis should be suspected with any complaint of vaginal discharge during a pregnancy. Perinatal transmission to the fetus is rare.[14]

Substance Abuse

The dangers of maternal smoking during pregnancy have long been a focus in public health. Maternal smoking is associated with several complications, including IUGR, placental abruption, PROM, placenta previa, ectopic pregnancy, and low birthweight. It is also associated with events beyond the pregnancy and delivery, including sudden infant death syndrome (SIDS), increased risk of infant colic, childhood asthma, and childhood obesity.[15] The home environment, specifically one with secondhand smoke, increases the risk of a low birthweight. Smokeless tobacco use also increases the risk of preterm delivery and low birthweight. It is recommended that all clinicians address the issue of tobacco use at the first prenatal visit. If maternal use is identified, then smoking cessation is addressed at every visit. Smoking cessation before the third trimester can greatly reduce the incidence of low birthweight. While the use of nicotine replacement products is sometimes offered in pregnancy, there are no clear studies to ascertain safety or benefit and close follow-up care is recommended. Family members and support persons should be reminded that smoking in the home and around the pregnant mother will increase her health risks and is

not supportive of her cessation efforts. Unfortunately, 50% to 60% of the mothers who quit smoking during pregnancy return to the habit within a year.[16]

Because caffeine crosses the placental barrier, maternal caffeine intake during pregnancy can be of concern. Fetal impact includes an increased risk of miscarriage, low birthweight, and preterm delivery. Moderate intake, around 200 mg or less daily, does not appear to contribute to pregnancy risk.[17,18]

Alcohol is one of the most studied substances of concern in pregnancy, with research documenting the teratogenic effects on the fetus dating back to 1968.[19] Alcohol passes from the mother through the placenta to the fetus. Drinking alcohol during pregnancy has profound effects on fetal development, with effects on the brain being the most significant. Additionally, it can cause miscarriage, stillbirth, growth restrictions, and multiple other defects.[20] The term Fetal Alcohol Spectrum Disorder (FASD) is used to describe the range of disabilities that a child can face throughout life.[21] An ultrasound may identify some of the physical abnormalities related to this spectrum. Early detection will allow for best intervention. While the effects of prenatal exposure are known, the amount of alcohol ingested to predict the impact on the fetus is not. As there is no established minimum dose for impact, mothers should be told to avoid all alcohol intake for the duration of the pregnancy. **Table 5-3** lists the characteristics and behaviors that may be found in the child with FASD.

Marijuana, also known as cannabis sativa, contains tetrahydrocannabinol (THC), which crosses the placental barrier and appears to also cross into breast milk. Studies have not conclusively shown an increased morbidity or mortality related to marijuana use during pregnancy or clinically significant withdrawal symptoms.[22]

TABLE 5-3
Effects of Prenatal Exposure to Alcohol

Distinctive facial features: smooth ridge between the nose and upper lip, small eyes, thin upper lip
Birth defects with joint, limb, and finger deformities
Growth delays with small head circumference, microcephaly, and short stature
Low bodyweight
Vision or hearing difficulties
Cardiac anomalies
Renal hypoplasia or agenesis
Brain and neurologic disorders
Neural tube defects
Poor coordination and balance
Developmental, speech, and language delays
Learning disabilities
Poor reasoning, judgement, and emotional control
Attention-deficit/hyperactivity disorder
Depression and anxiety
Irritability
Poor memory
Low IQ scores

As there are many unknowns, mothers should be encouraged to discontinue marijuana use, including medical marijuana, while pregnant.[23]

Use of the central nervous system stimulant amphetamine during pregnancy may result in low birthweight. Infants exposed to recent amphetamine use may also be lethargic and difficult to arouse after birth and may feed poorly. Amphetamines may also reduce the mother's breast milk supply.[24,25]

Cocaine is a powerful stimulant and has been associated with numerous risks to the mother and fetus. It is a potent vasoconstrictor that can constrict maternal blood vessels and cause severe impairment of fetal–maternal circulation and fetal death. Hypoxia to the placental bed may result in placental abruption. It also increases the risk of PROM, preterm labor and delivery, uterine rupture, and spontaneous abortion. Maternal health can also be impacted by cocaine use, with an increased risk of heart attack, stroke, seizures, respiratory failure, and changes in taste and smell that cause weight loss and appetite changes.[26] Because cocaine crosses the placenta, it rapidly spreads to the fetal tissues and organs. Toxic effects include hydronephrosis, cleft palate and lip, and gastroschisis. It can also cause significant fetal heart arrhythmias and decreased cardiac output. After delivery, although cocaine withdrawal is not fatal, it can be uncomfortable, with the infant exhibiting agitation.[22]

Opioid use in pregnancy is an area of great concern due to the highly addictive potential and the impact on maternal health and the newborn. Drugs classified as opioids include the prescription medications codeine, Percocet, morphine, and oxycodone; the illicit drug heroin; and treatment maintenance drugs methadone and buprenorphine (Subutex). Prescription use is generally for pain control but can be abused for nonmedical use or used for chronic pain in patients who then become pregnant. Heroin and methadone are the most commonly used opioids among pregnant women. Opioids rapidly transfer to the placenta, within 60 minutes of use. Maternal overdose can cause respiratory failure and death.[26] Maternal opioid withdrawal can impair fetal growth and lead to IUGR.[27] Neonatal abstinence syndrome (NAS) is the neonatal impact of maternal opioid abuse; it is characterized by irritability, high-pitched cry, poor feeding, jittery reflexes, and temperature instability. Seizures can also occur.[26] Care of the neonate with NAS includes a low-stimulation environment and, if needed, oral morphine or methadone.[22]

Complications during Pregnancy

Complications during pregnancy may involve the mother's health, the infant's health, or both. They can stem from preexisting medical conditions or ones that the mother acquires during the pregnancy. Complications can occur at any stage of the pregnancy, including

TABLE 5-4
Complications during Pregnancy
Placental abruption (abruptio placentae)
Placenta previa
Preeclampsia
Eclampsia
Gestational diabetes
Maternal infection
Premature labor
Prolonged rupture of membranes (PROM)
Intrauterine growth restriction (IUGR)
Gestation longer than 42 weeks
Twin to twin transfusion

during labor and delivery. **Table 5-4** lists the more common pregnancy complications.

Placental and Cord Disorders

The placenta and umbilical cord are vital to the healthy development of the fetus. The placenta is a pancake-shaped organ that, during pregnancy, attaches to the wall of the mother's uterus (**Figure 5-1**). Implantation is usually, but not always, on the upper posterior portion of the uterine wall. It is bathed in the mother's blood and uses the umbilical cord to supply the fetus with blood rich in oxygen and nutrients. The umbilical cord also transfers waste products, including carbon dioxide, from the fetus to the mother's blood. Most umbilical cords have one vein and two arteries. The vein brings oxygenated blood from the mother's placenta to the fetus, while the arteries take deoxygenated blood from the fetus back to the placenta, without the two blood supplies mixing. The placenta also secretes hormones, including those that promote and stimulate growth of the uterus and mammary glands.

Placenta Previa

Placenta previa is a condition in which the placenta is implanted abnormally low in the uterus, partially or completely covering the cervix. As the fetus grows, the walls of the uterus become thinner and the placenta stretches, pulling away from the uterine wall. The mother will often have sudden vaginal bleeding, with or without cramping. Complete bed rest is advised to minimize complications.[28] A cesarean section delivery is necessary if the bleeding is excessive or if the cervix is completely covered, as vaginal delivery may further tear the placenta and cause hemorrhaging. However, if the pregnancy progresses and the placenta moves into a position away from the cervix, then the mother can plan for a vaginal delivery.

Mothers at risk of placenta previa are those with AMA; multifetal gestation; and those with a history of cesarean delivery, uterine surgery, multiparity, multifetal gestation, in vitro fertilization, and smoking. Complications of placenta previa are listed in **Table 5-5**.

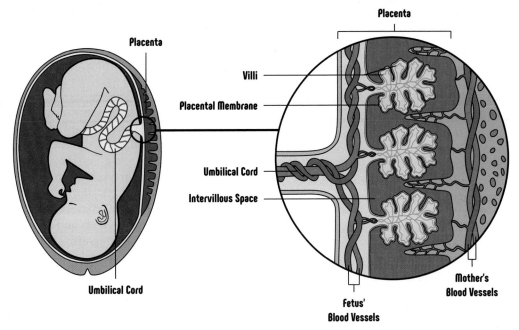

FIGURE 5-1 Fetus and placenta anatomy. Diagram illustrating how the umbilical cord moves blood from the mother's placenta to the fetus.
© udaix/Shutterstock.

TABLE 5-5
Complications of Placenta Previa

Maternal Complications	Fetal Complications
Hemorrhage	Insufficient blood supply to the fetus
Preterm delivery	Intrauterine growth restriction (IUGR)
Shock	Hypoxia
Blood clots	Anemia
Infection	Death
Death	

Placental Abruption

Placental abruption, also known as abruptio placentae, is a condition in which the placenta either partially or completely separates from the uterine wall. Total abruption is a catastrophic event with high morbidity and mortality for the fetus and mother. Because the placental blood supply is the source of oxygen and nutrition for the fetus, any degree of interruption places the fetus at risk of preterm delivery and death. Early recognition of the abruption with appropriate treatment may prevent fetal asphyxia and reduce the risk of fetal and maternal death.

The most common symptoms of abruption are vaginal bleeding with abdominal pain and uterine contractions. As bleeding progresses, or in the case of total abruption, there may be maternal shock, disseminated intravascular coagulation, and signs of fetal distress, including fetal bradycardia. Bleeding may not be a good marker of severity, however, as it is not always present

externally, as is the case with a concealed abruption where blood loss initially occurs behind the placenta.

Treatment of placental abruption depends upon the severity of the abruption and the stability of the mother and fetus. The prognosis is bleak if the abruption occurs before 24 weeks' gestation. If the fetus is between 24 and 34 weeks' gestation, then the mother is given IV corticosteroids to promote fetal lung maturity. Because total placental separation with severe hemorrhage and death can occur suddenly, fetal monitoring is required in all suspected abruptions. Emergent care and resources for blood transfusion must be available for optimal outcomes. In the presence of maternal or fetal decompensation, delivery of the fetus is accomplished by the most expeditious route, usually cesarean section. If the fetus is stillborn, vaginal delivery is an acceptable option.

At risk for abruption are mothers with AMA; previous placental abruption; and a history of PROM, hypertension, including preeclampsia, cesarean delivery, abdominal trauma, cocaine use, and smoking.[29] Complications of placental abruption are listed in **Table 5-6**.

TABLE 5-6
Complications of Placental Abruption

Maternal Complications	Fetal Complications
Hemorrhage	Insufficient blood supply to the fetus
Preterm delivery	
Shock	Hypoxia
Acute renal failure	Death
Death	

Umbilical Cord Abnormalities

Evaluation of the umbilical cord is a routine part of the obstetric ultrasound examination. It usually contains three blood vessels: two smaller arteries and one larger vein. The most common umbilical cord abnormality is a single umbilical artery (SUA), sometimes referred to as a two-vessel cord, in which there is only one artery and one vein. It is associated with organ anomalies, most often in the renal, cardiovascular, gastrointestinal, and central nervous systems, and chromosomal abnormalities, mainly Trisomy 13 and 18. A single umbilical artery may be detected on an ultrasound. When a prenatal diagnosis is made, it should prompt further sonographic evaluation with echocardiography to rule out associated anomalies.[30]

Umbilical cord prolapse (UCP) is an obstetric emergency in which the umbilical cord passes through the cervix in front of or alongside the fetal presenting part. As the infant moves through the birth canal, it places pressure on the cord. Prolonged compression of the cord restricts blood flow and oxygen to the fetus and, if not delivered quickly, can lead to perinatal hypoxic ischemic encephalopathy or death. Doppler studies can detect the position of cord loops. Fetal bradycardia during labor may also indicate that a prolapsed cord is compressed.

A **nuchal cord** is an umbilical cord that becomes coiled around the fetus's body, usually the neck. They are common, occurring in up to 30% of all births. It may be suspected prior to delivery if there are fetal heart decelerations or through color Doppler imaging. A cord that is loose around the neck can be slipped over the infant's head during delivery. If not detected and left untreated, the cord may quickly prolapse, restricting blood flow and oxygen.

Other cord issues include cord braiding in utero, knots in the cord, and umbilical cord cysts. Management is generally increased antepartum surveillance to detect problems early on, with most issues becoming apparent as the pregnancy progresses. A cesarean section may be necessary to reduce fetal morbidity or death.

Hypertensive Disorders

Hypertension is a major cause of morbidity, complicating 5% to 10% of pregnancies.[31] Chronic hypertension is defined as a blood pressure above 140/90 mm Hg, existing prior to pregnancy or manifesting before the 20th week of gestation. Sometimes hypertension is present before the mother becomes pregnant and, when well controlled, the pregnancy is often normal. Women with preexisting hypertension are more likely to develop complications during pregnancy. It is important to identify this condition early in pregnancy and to routinely assess its impact on maternal health.

If left untreated, hypertension can decrease uteroplacental blood flow and progress to IUGR. The use of antihypertensive therapy reduces the maternal risk of stroke and organ damage, but it is essential to avoid medications that can harm fetal development, as some antihypertensive agents impact uterine blood flow by lowering pressures and altering placental perfusion. Treatment must be a balance of maternal care and blood pressure stabilization, use of appropriate medications with impact monitoring, and delivery of the baby when there is an inability to improve maternal or fetal care.

Hypertension that presents in pregnancy without proteinuria is known as gestational hypertension. This condition may either progress to preeclampsia or remain as elevated pressures and disappear after delivery. Elevated blood pressures after the postpartum time frame would define the condition as chronic hypertension.

Preeclampsia

As many as 25% of pregnancies complicated by chronic hypertension develop preeclampsia. Unique to pregnancy, **preeclampsia** is the condition in which the mother develops elevated blood pressures and proteinuria after the 20th week of pregnancy. Blood pressures associated with preeclampsia are generally a systolic pressure >140 mm Hg and diastolic pressure >90 mm Hg. **Table 5-7** lists the risk factors for developing preeclampsia. Maternal symptoms of preeclampsia include severe headache, blurry vision, stomach pain, irritability, malaise, and excessive weight gain or swelling that occurs over a short period of time.[32]

Treatment of preeclampsia focuses on minimizing maternal and fetal morbidity and mortality. The only known cure and reversal of this condition is delivery of the pregnancy, which is not always the optimal fetal solution. If the pregnancy is at or near term, then delivery is the intervention of choice. If severe preeclampsia is present and the pregnancy is remote from delivery, the mother and fetus are monitored closely and considerations for care are based on maternal health risk as well as fetal conditions, such as IUGR <5%, oligohydramnios, and nonreassuring fetal testing. Treatment aimed at maternal symptoms can have consequences for the fetus. For

TABLE 5-7
Maternal Risk Factors for Developing Preeclampsia

Chronic hypertension
Prior pregnancy with preeclampsia
First pregnancy
Young mother
Advanced maternal age (AMA)
Multifetal pregnancy
Diabetes
Obesity
Connective tissue disorder
Chronic renal disease

example, medication that lowers maternal blood pressure may further reduce perfusion and increase vascular resistance, which will negatively impact uterine blood flow and fetal perfusion. At any time up to 34 weeks' gestation, if preeclampsia becomes severe and maternal or fetal conditions deteriorate, delivery is indicated.[33] Close postpartum evaluation of the mother should continue for at least the first 24 to 48 hours after delivery, as seizures commonly occur within that time frame.

Eclampsia and HELLP Syndrome

Preeclampsia can progress to eclampsia. **Eclampsia** is defined as hypertension with the presence of seizures, after other seizure disorders or causative factors have been ruled out. **HELLP syndrome** can be difficult to diagnose as it may present in the absence of preeclampsia. It was named after its clinical characteristics:

H – hemolysis
EL – elevated liver enzymes
LP – low platelets

HELLP presents serious morbidity concerns and is managed similarly to preeclampsia. Maternal mortality rate is as high as 25%, with the most common reasons for death being liver rupture, stroke, and cerebral hemorrhage.[34]

Diabetes during Pregnancy

Diabetes complicating pregnancy presents a special set of risks for maternal and fetal health. The prevalence of diabetes is on the rise, and it is currently estimated that at least 7% of all pregnancies are complicated by diabetes.[35] The classifications of diabetes as published by the American Diabetes Association are found in **Box 5-2**.

Pregestational Diabetes

Pregestational diabetes is defined as type 1 or type 2 diabetes that is present prior to the pregnancy. Mothers with this preexisting condition are at the highest risk for morbidity and, although not usually permanent, they experience some worsening of disease during pregnancy. Because diabetes is a disease of vascular involvement, virtually every system in the body is at risk for complications.

Poorly controlled diabetes during the first trimester of pregnancy increases the risk of congenital anomalies and a spontaneous abortion. Excess glucose from the mother acts as a fetal teratogen in a developing fetus, with damage often occurring during the first 6 weeks of development. Because of this risk, many high-risk pregnancy centers have programs for counseling and management of women with diabetes who are planning a pregnancy. The goal of preconception care is to achieve normoglycemia prior to pregnancy.

Gestational Diabetes

Gestational diabetes mellitus (GDM) is diabetes that first occurs during a pregnancy. It is estimated that approximately 2% to 9% of pregnant women will develop GDM.[36] This form of diabetes relates more strongly to type 2 form, with insulin resistance increasing throughout pregnancy in response to pregnancy hormones. There is also a relationship to genetics, with family members often reporting a type 2 diagnosis.[37] Current practice is to screen all mothers for GDM between 24 and 28 weeks' gestation. The mother who had GDM in a previous pregnancy has a 60% to 70% chance of developing it in future pregnancies.[38] **Table 5-8** lists the risk factors associated with developing gestational diabetes.

BOX 5-2 Classification of Diabetes

Type 1 Diabetes
Due to destruction of insulin-producing β-cells
Accounts for 5–10% of diabetes cases
Requires insulin for survival
Formerly referred to as insulin-dependent diabetes or juvenile-onset diabetes

Type 2 Diabetes
Due to progressive insulin secretory defect
Reduced insulin sensitivity/increased insulin resistance
Accounts for 90–95% of diabetes cases
Late onset
Formerly referred to as non-insulin-dependent diabetes or adult-onset diabetes
Managed through diet and oral hypoglycemics

Gestational Diabetes
Occurs in 2–9% of all pregnancies
Diagnosed in the second or third trimester of pregnancy
Relates more strongly to type 2 diabetes
Usually resolves on its own after pregnancy

Diabetes Due to Other Causes
Genetic defects of β-cells of the pancreas
Monogenic diabetes syndromes
Diseases of the exocrine pancreas (e.g., cystic fibrosis)
Drug- or chemical-induced diabetes
Immune-mediated diabetes

TABLE 5-8
Maternal Risks for Developing Gestational Diabetes

Asian, Hispanic, African American, Native American race
Obesity
Advanced maternal age (AMA)
History of gestational diabetes
Family history of diabetes mellitus
Previous pregnancy with infant weight >9 pounds
Polycystic ovarian disease

TABLE 5-9
Complications Associated with a Diabetic Pregnancy

Maternal Complications	Fetal Complications
Spontaneous abortion	Congenital defects
Preeclampsia	Macrosomia
Preterm labor	Intrauterine growth restriction (IUGR)
Polyhydramnios	
Pyelonephritis	Stillbirth
Infection	Delayed lung maturity
Ketoacidosis	Asphyxia
Cesarean delivery	
Hypoglycemia	

TABLE 5-10
Conditions Associated with Abnormal Amniotic Fluid Volume

Polyhydramnios	Oligohydramnios
Maternal diabetes	Maternal diabetes
Multiple pregnancy	Preeclampsia
Maternal substance abuse	Kidney or urinary tract defects
Fetal anemia	
Congenital infections	Placental abruption
Twin to twin transfusion syndrome	Intrauterine growth restriction (IUGR)
Congenital anomalies	Leaking amniotic sac
Genetic disorders	Rupture of membranes
Preterm labor	Postterm pregnancy
Placental abruption	Miscarriage
Umbilical cord prolapse	
Postpartum hemorrhage	
Miscarriage	

Complications of Diabetes during Pregnancy

The mother with diabetes is at significant risk of certain complications, as listed in **Table 5-9**. Unlike pregestational diabetes, in which there is high risk of IUGR, the mother with gestational diabetes is at risk of delivering an infant with macrosomia, which is defined as fetal weight greater than 4000 grams or the 90th percentile. This may be related to poor maternal glucose control with fetal production of insulin that acts as an in utero growth hormone. There is an increased incidence of cesarean delivery in this population due to fetal size.[39]

Abnormal Amniotic Fluid Volume

The amount of amniotic fluid present is an important factor in monitoring fetal health and development. An ultrasound is used to estimate the fluid volume. High or low fluid levels may indicate certain conditions of concern: **Polyhydramnios** is the condition where too much amniotic fluid is surrounding the fetus, and **oligohydramnios** is defined as a lower than normal amount of amniotic fluid.[40] Because abnormal amniotic fluid levels are sometimes associated with fetal anomalies, a detailed ultrasound to identify structural defects is important in prenatal management. **Table 5-10** lists reasons for abnormal amniotic fluid volume.

Twin to Twin Transfusion Syndrome

Twin pregnancy can be complicated by a syndrome where one twin, the donor, provides a blood supply to the second twin as the recipient. This change in blood volume and nutrients results in the donor twin becoming anemic and growth restricted, while the recipient twin experiences fluid overload and polycythemia. This is known as twin to twin transfusion syndrome (TTTS); it is usually diagnosed when one twin begins to accumulate high amniotic fluid levels, or polyhydramnios, and the other twin falls behind on growth and the amniotic fluid levels become low, or oligohydramnios. The twin with polyhydramnios may develop heart failure and hydrops. The twin with oligohydramnios has a reduced ability to move in utero and is at risk of developing contractures and pulmonary hypoplasia. This prognosis is risky, with outcomes including prematurity, brain damage, and death of one or both twins.[41]

Antenatal Fetal Assessment

The purpose of fetal assessment during the antepartum period is to identify fetuses who are at risk for premature birth, stillbirth, or complications in utero or at delivery. Predicting and preparing for a high-risk delivery can improve perinatal outcomes and prevent neurologic impairment and death. Several devices and techniques are available to assess the fetus. These include ultrasound, electronic fetal monitoring, and amniocentesis. Depending on the clinical situation, more than one modality is often used to assess fetal status. **Table 5-11** lists conditions that indicate a need for fetal assessment.

Ultrasound

First used in the 1950s as an obstetric tool, ultrasound provides real-time imaging and the ability to assess uterine and fetal structure and activity. It is a noninvasive procedure commonly used to evaluate the level of amniotic fluid and to identify placental location, fetal anomalies, and fetal size and position. An ultrasound can assist in intrauterine care and prepare for a complicated delivery. Recent technology includes Doppler flow studies and four-dimensional (4D) imaging, which allow for clear views of fetal structure and function.

TABLE 5-11
Indications for Antenatal Fetal Assessment

Maternal Conditions	Complications of Pregnancy
Hypertension	Preeclampsia
Diabetes	Polyhydramnios
Heart disease	Oligohydramnios
Renal disease	Premature rupture of membranes (PROM)
Systemic lupus erythematosus	Intrauterine growth restriction (IUGR)
	Multiple gestation
	Postterm pregnancy
	Decreased fetal movement
	Previous high-risk pregnancy
	Previous miscarriage

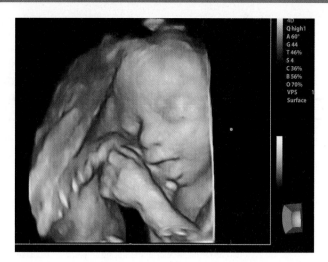

FIGURE 5-2 Four-dimensional (4D) ultrasound.
© whitetherock photo/Shutterstock.

Figure 5-2 illustrates the detailed view of a fetus obtained from 4D ultrasound.

The safety of ultrasound during pregnancy has been studied, with few reported safety concerns for the mother or fetus.[42] More than three generations have been exposed to ultrasound with no known adverse effect; in fact, current technology has reduced the energy exposure to the fetus.

Fetal Heart Rate Monitoring

Monitoring the fetal heart rate (FHR) is another modality used to assess fetal well-being. **Figure 5-3** illustrates how electronic fetal monitoring is used during pregnancy, labor, and delivery to monitor the fetus's heart rate as well as the strength and duration of uterine contractions.

Nonstress Test

The **nonstress test (NST)** is a noninvasive test in which a monitor measures the FHR in response to fetal movement, generally over a 20-minute period, and records a tracing of the FHR and uterine activity. It is performed after 28 weeks' gestation and is based on the premise that a healthy fetus's heart rate will accelerate when the fetus is spontaneously moving.[43] The test is described as "nonstress" because it is done during a period where there are no uterine contractions and the fetus is moving spontaneously. **Table 5-12** explains how results from a NST are interpreted.

Contraction Stress Test

The **contraction stress test (CST)** measures the FHR response to uterine contractions. The purpose of this test is to evaluate the fetus's ability to tolerate changes in blood flow and oxygenation during contractions. The CST is conducted in a manner similar to the NST. A fetal heart rate monitor and a uterine contraction monitor are placed on the mother's abdomen while an IV infusion of oxytocin is used to induce contractions. When the placenta is healthy, there is adequate blood flow and transport of oxygen to the fetal blood, even during a contraction. However, when the placenta

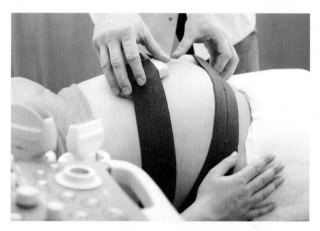

FIGURE 5-3 Fetal heart rate monitoring. Photo of abdominal belts in place. One will monitor the fetal heart rate and the other will monitor uterine contractions.
© Doro Guzenda/Shutterstock.

is compromised, the blood vessels in the placenta are compressed during a contraction and the fetus does not receive adequate blood flow and oxygen. The fetus responds to the hypoxia with a decreased heart rate.

For adequate interpretation, a CST must be conducted for at least 10 minutes and have a minimum of three contractions that last 40 to 60 seconds each.[43] Because of the risks involved in inducing contractions, caution should be used when testing mothers prior to 37 weeks' gestation who are at risk for preterm labor; mothers with placenta previa, placental abruption, incompetent cervix, or premature rupture of membranes; and mothers who have had a previous cesarean delivery. Table 5-12 explains how results from a CST are interpreted.

Fetal Biophysical Profile

The **fetal biophysical profile (BPP)** is a noninvasive test that uses observations obtained during an ultrasound and the results of a NST to evaluate the well-being of a fetus and to determine if a fetus is at risk of fetal death.[44] An ultrasound is observed for 30 minutes and a scoring

TABLE 5-12
Interpretation of Fetal Heart Rate Monitoring

Test	Result	Interpretation	Assumptions
Nonstress test	FHR accelerations two or more times during a 20-minute period	Reactive	Fetus is receiving adequate oxygen and blood flow Normal fetal survival
	Insufficient FHR accelerations after 40 minutes	Nonreactive	Fetus is sleeping Fetus has impaired oxygenation Fetus is acidotic Requires further evaluation
Contraction stress test	Normal baseline FHR with no late FHR decelerations during contractions	Negative	Fetus is receiving adequate oxygen and blood flow Fetus is capable of sustaining heart rate under stressed conditions Normal fetal survival
	Late FHR decelerations during at least 50% of contractions	Positive	Fetus has impaired oxygenation Fetus is unable to sustain normal FHR under stress Adverse fetal outcome Increased risk of fetal death Requires further evaluation
	Abnormal baseline FHR or intermittent late FHR decelerations during less than 50% of contractions	Suspicious	
	Fewer than three contractions during a 10-minute period	Unsatisfactory	

FHR = fetal heart rate

system is used to assess five indicators that a fetus is healthy:

- Fetal tone: Flexion and extension of limbs
- Fetal breathing movements
- Fetal body movements
- Amniotic fluid volume
- Results of the nonstress test

Each parameter is given a score of 2 or 0; a score of 2 is given when a criterion is met, indicating a normal finding, and score of 0 is given when a criterion is not met, indicting an abnormal finding. With five parameters being scored, 10 is the maximum score that can be given: A total score of 8 to 10 is normal, 6 is equivocal, and 4 or less is abnormal. If the ultrasound is performed and all the indicators are normal, then the NST may not be performed. An abnormal score warrants further evaluation and even delivery if the infant is close to term. **Table 5-13** summarizes the BPP scoring system.

Amniocentesis

Amniocentesis is the most common invasive diagnostic test in pregnancy. It is used most often to identify chromosome abnormalities; however, it can also be used to determine lung maturity, analyze amniotic fluid, test for infection, and release amniotic fluid from fetuses with polyhydramnios.

An amniocentesis can be performed between 16 and 18 weeks' gestation. An ultrasound is used to confirm the gestational age of the fetus, the location of the placenta, the position of the fetus, and the location of the optimum amniotic fluid pocket. The mother's abdomen is numbed using a local anesthetic. As illustrated in **Figure 5-4**, a needle is inserted through the abdomen and into the uterus, using the ultrasound to guide it to an amniotic fluid pocket, where fluid is aspirated.[45] Although it is relatively safe, complications may occur, including bleeding, amnionitis, rupture of the amniotic sac, and fetal loss.

High-Risk Labor and Delivery

Most pregnancies progress routinely and labor and delivery occurs without any problems. Regular prenatal care improves the chances of identifying conditions early and referring the mother to a team of specialists who can determine the best treatment strategies and provide advanced care. This team is present during delivery and often consists of a neonatologist, neonatal nurse practitioner, and respiratory therapist. Planning appropriate interventions during labor and delivery can minimize the risk of maternal and fetal complications. However, in spite of early monitoring, serious problems that place both the mother's and infant's health at risk can develop suddenly and unexpectedly.

Preterm Labor and Delivery

Labor is considered to be **preterm labor** when uterine contractions occur between 20 and 37 weeks' gestation and they are of sufficient frequency and intensity to

TABLE 5-13
Biophysical Profile Scoring

Observation	Score of 0 Given	Score of 2 Given
Nonstress test	Nonreactive: 1 or less FHR accelerations within 40 minutes	Reactive: 2 or more FHR accelerations within 20 minutes
Fetal breathing movements	No FBM ≥30 seconds within 30 minutes	1 or more rhythmic FBM of ≥30 seconds within 30 minutes
Fetal body movements	Two or fewer body movements within 30 minutes	Three or more body or limb movements within 30 minutes
Fetal tone	Slow limb extension or absent fetal movement	One or more episodes of limb extension with return to flexion
Amniotic fluid index	No fluid pocket or pocket is 1 cm or less	AFI >5 cm or a pocket of amniotic fluid measuring at least 2 cm

FHR, fetal heart rate; FBM, fetal breathing movements; AFI, amniotic fluid index

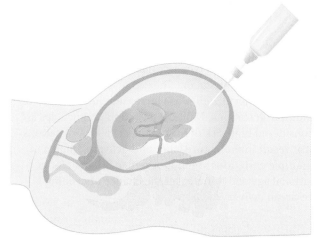

FIGURE 5-4 Amniocentesis. Illustration of an amniocentesis being performed.
© ellepigrafica/Shutterstock.

TABLE 5-14
Risk Factors Related to Preterm Labor and Delivery

History of prior preterm delivery	Cervical insufficiency
Surgery involving uterine entry	Cervical tissue removal
Cervical trauma: Elective abortion, surgery for cervical dysplasia, obstetric trauma	Urinary tract infection
Cervical length ≤25 mm	Smoking
Periodontal disease	Prepregnancy low bodyweight
Illicit drug use	Infections: Bacterial, viral, sexually transmitted
Pregnancy interval less than 18 months	Polyhydramnios
Chorioamnionitis	Placenta previa
Multiple gestations	Fetal anomalies
Placental abruption	Low socioeconomic status
Nonwhite race	

cause effacement and dilation of the cervix. A preterm delivery is defined as one occurring after 20 weeks' gestation but prior to 37 weeks' gestation. Labor and delivery may occur spontaneously or be induced due to maternal or fetal complications. Neonatal morbidity and mortality are the consequences of preterm delivery, with extreme prematurity and very low birthweight accounting for much of the mortality. Survivors of preterm delivery are at an increased risk of chronic lung disease, vision and hearing deficits, intracranial hemorrhage, motor and learning deficits, and cerebral palsy, to name some complications.[46]

Although it is often difficult to predict preterm delivery, a variety of maternal, obstetric, and fetal characteristics are known to increase the risk. The largest predictor of preterm labor and delivery is a history of previously having a preterm birth. The number of prior preterm deliveries and the gestational age of the infant at delivery also impact this risk.[47] A cervical length of 25 mm or shorter, measured with a transvaginal ultrasound as part of the prenatal care, has been demonstrated to be the most sensitive predictor of preterm birth between both high- and low-risk mothers.[48] Risk factors related to preterm labor and delivery are listed in **Table 5-14**.

Preterm Labor Symptoms

Identifying preterm labor is difficult for mothers who are pregnant for the first time, as they have no frame of reference. Some mothers report little to no discomfort with contractions, which may delay seeking help. Symptoms of preterm labor include the following:

- Uterine cramping or contractions
- Increase in vaginal discharge: Watery, bloody, or with mucus

- Increased vaginal pressure sensation
- Low backache

Management of Preterm Labor

Management of preterm labor involves a thorough assessment of medical history, clinical symptoms, and measures to prevent an early delivery.[49] Tocolysis is the treatment in which medication is used to reduce uterine contractions. The primary purpose of tocolytic therapy is to delay delivery for 48 hours and to allow glucocorticoids to improve lung maturity. **Tocolytic agents** are given to mothers in whom the fetus has reached a point of viability, which is usually by 24 weeks' gestation, but by 34 weeks' gestation, the risk of neonatal morbidity and mortality is low and tocolytic therapy is not generally recommended due to risk for maternal complications. Therefore, tocolytic therapy is believed to outweigh the risk of maternal and fetal complications between 24 and 33 weeks' gestation and is recommended as part of the care plan, provided no contraindications exist.

Which agent is given depends upon maternal comorbid conditions and the gestational age of the fetus. The most common agents used are magnesium sulfate, indomethacin, and nifedipine. At one time terbutaline was the agent of choice; however, in 2011, the Food and Drug Administration issued a Black Box Warning after reports of serious adverse effects, including death. Magnesium sulfate reduces smooth muscle contractility and tends to be the primary agent used today. Use is limited to 5 to 7 days, however, as longer use has been associated with hypocalcemia in the fetus, resulting in neonatal skeletal abnormalities, including osteopenia.[50] Indomethacin, a prostaglandin, is recommended for short-term use and not used after 32 weeks' gestation. When used for more than 48 hours, it can decrease renal blood flow in the fetus and cause oligohydramnios. Nifedipine is a calcium channel blocker and may be associated with more successful prolongation of pregnancy and fewer admissions to the neonatal intensive care unit.[49,51]

Tocolytic agents are relatively contraindicated when there is evidence that delaying labor could place the mother or fetus at risk, as may be the case with the following conditions:

- Placental abruption
- Maternal hemorrhage
- Oligohydramnios
- Nonstress test that is nonreactive
- Contraction stress test that is positive
- Repetitive severe FHR decelerations

Antenatal corticosteroids accelerate type 1 and type 2 pneumocyte development, which increases surfactant production, enhancing lung maturation and reducing fetal morbidity and mortality. Administration is an intramuscular injection given to the mother for a fetus that is between 24 and 34 weeks' gestation and at risk of preterm delivery. When betamethasone is used, it is given as two doses of 12 mg, waiting 24 hours between doses. If dexamethasone is the chosen steroid, then four doses of 6 mg are given 12 hours apart.

Progesterone is a hormone produced naturally during pregnancy that reduces contractions of the uterus and plays an important role in maintaining pregnancy. Progesterone supplementation may be given to women at high risk for preterm delivery, as it appears to reduce preterm birth in mothers who have had a previous spontaneous preterm singleton birth and in mothers with a short cervix in the current pregnancy. Supplementation is usually started around 16 to 20 weeks' gestation and continued through the 36th week of gestation. It appears to be safe for the mother and fetus with no major adverse events.[52,53]

The risk of GBS sepsis is elevated with preterm labor, even without premature rupture of membranes. Antibiotics should be given prophylactically and maintained until delivery.

Multiple Gestation

The pregnancy with twins, triplets, or more is referred to as a **multiple gestation**. The use of fertility drugs and in vitro fertilization has increased the incidence of multiple gestations. Multiple gestation pregnancies are considered high risk of having maternal complications that result in premature labor and delivery. Infants of multiple gestations are more likely to be small for gestational age and it increases the chance of needing a cesarean delivery.

Postterm Pregnancy

Normally, a pregnancy lasts 37 to 42 weeks and is referred to as a term pregnancy. When the pregnancy extends past 42 weeks, then it is considered a **postterm pregnancy**. Mothers at risk of a postterm delivery include those with a prior postterm pregnancy; maternal obesity; increasing maternal age; nulliparity, which is the term used to describe a woman who has never delivered a child; and mothers who were themselves born postterm. **Table 5-15** lists the maternal and fetal risks of postterm pregnancies.

TABLE 5-15
Maternal and Fetal Risks of Postterm Pregnancies

Maternal Risks	Fetal Risks
Cesarean delivery	Stillbirth
Dysfunctional labor	Macrosomia
Infection	Shoulder dystocia
Postpartum hemorrhage	Neonatal seizures
	Meconium aspiration syndrome
	Lower Apgar scores
	Oligohydramnios
	Umbilical cord compression
	Fetal heart rate abnormalities
	Fetal acidosis
	Uteroplacental insufficiency
	Encephalopathy

Case Study 1

A 29-year-old G4P2 Hispanic woman, with a history of gestational diabetes mellitus (GDM), presents to her OB/GYN office for a routine prenatal visit at 24 weeks' gestation. Her physical examination is unremarkable, and her fetal well-being is reassuring. Because of her previous history of GDM, she is at high risk of developing GDM during this pregnancy and the doctor recommends a glucose challenge test, which is the most common method of screening for GDM. Test results reveal that her 1-hour glucose loading test (GLT) is 179 mg/dL (normal value <140 mg/dL). Because her GLT value is high, she then undergoes a 3-hour glucose tolerance test (GTT), which is used for a definitive diagnosis of GDM. The patient is positive for GDM when all of her plasma glucose values are elevated. Treatment recommendations include beginning a diabetic diet, participating in moderate exercise sessions three times a week, daily home glucose monitoring, and weekly antepartum visits to monitor glycemic control. The doctor explained to the mother that GDM poses little risk to her at this time; however, it is associated with an increase in infant birth trauma and perinatal morbidity and mortality with the risk to her fetus directly related to its size. The goal of antepartum treatment of GDM is to prevent fetal macrosomia, which is defined as an estimated fetal weight of ≥ 4500 grams, and its resultant complications by maintaining desirable maternal blood glucose levels throughout gestation. It was explained that if diet alone did not maintain blood glucose at desirable levels, then hypoglycemic therapy with insulin injections given several times a day may be required.

1. **Why was this patient considered to be at high risk for GDM and tested at 24 weeks' gestation?**
2. **Who is at greatest risk when the mother has GDM?**
3. **What are two testing methods for GDM?**
4. **What is the primary treatment for GDM?**

Case Study 2

A 35-year-old woman presented to the prenatal clinic after missing her last two menstrual cycles. Her home pregnancy test was positive and an ultrasound confirmed the pregnancy. Gestational age was calculated to be at 10 weeks. An initial assessment of the woman's medical and obstetric history included the following: She smoked tobacco for 15 years and currently smokes one pack per day; she had recently used cocaine but stated it is not frequent; she denied alcohol use. Her obstetric/gynecologic history included an uncomplicated spontaneous vaginal delivery at 35 weeks' gestation 4 years ago and 2 years later a cesarean section at 36 weeks' gestation for nonreassuring fetal heart tones. Her medical history included chronic hypertension and a history of asthma, for which she had never been intubated or hospitalized. Her vital signs were as follows: temperature 36.7°C, respiratory rate of 20 breaths per minute, heart rate of 86 beats per minute, BP 142/79 mm Hg. Lab results: hemoglobin 13.0 g/dL, hematocrit 37%, white blood cell count 8000, blood type A−, Rh antibody screen positive. She was negative for gonorrhea, chlamydia, and HIV.

1. **What puts this patient at high risk for pregnancy complications?**
2. **What fetal complications are associated with this patient's presentation?**
3. **At this time, what recommendations would you give this patient to improve her health?**

References

1. American Academy of Pediatrics, American College of Obstetricians and Gynecologists. *Guidelines for Perinatal Care.* 7th ed. Elk Grove Village, IL: AAP, Washington, DC: ACOG; 2012.
2. American College of Obstetricians and Gynecologists. ACOG Committee Opinion #313, September 2005. The importance of preconception care in the continuum of women's healthcare. *Obstet Gynecol.* 2005;106:665–666.
3. Cavazos-Rehg PA, Krauss MJ, Spitznagel EL, et al. Maternal age and risk of labor and delivery complications. *Matern Child Health J.* 2015;19:1202–1211.
4. Canterino JC. Advanced maternal age and risks for adverse outcomes. *Maternal Fetal Medicine, The Female Patient.* 2012;37:25–32.
5. American College of Obstetricians and Gynecologists. ACOG Committee Opinion #635, June 2015. Prenatal and perinatal human immunodeficiency virus testing: expanded recommendations. *Obstet Gynecol.* 2015;125:1544–1547.
6. Cagno CK, Pettit JM, Weiss BD. Prevention of perinatal group b streptococcal disease: updated CDC guideline. *Am Fam Physician.* 2012;86:59–65.
7. American College of Obstetricians and Gynecologists. ACOG Committee Opinion #632, June 2015. Expedited partner therapy in the management of gonorrhea and chlamydial infection. *Obstet Gynecol.* 2015;125:1526–1528.
8. Centers for Disease Control and Prevention. 2015 Sexually transmitted diseases treatment guidelines. Genital HSV infections. Atlanta, GA: US Department of Health and Human Services, Centers for Disease Control and Prevention; 2015.
9. American College of Obstetricians and Gynecologists. ACOG Practice Bulletin #82, June 2007. Management of herpes in pregnancy. *Obstet Gynecol.* 2007;109:1489–1498.

10. Centers for Disease Control and Prevention. Sexually transmitted diseases treatment guidelines. Human papillomavirus (HPV) infection. Atlanta, GA: US Department of Health and Human Services, Centers for Disease Control and Prevention; 2015.

11. Centers for Disease Control and Prevention. Sexually transmitted diseases treatment guidelines. Chlamydial infections. Atlanta, GA: US Department of Health and Human Services, Centers for Disease Control and Prevention; 2015.

12. Centers for Disease Control and Prevention. Sexually transmitted diseases treatment guidelines. Gonococcal infections. Atlanta, GA: US Department of Health and Human Services, Centers for Disease Control and Prevention; 2015.

13. Centers for Disease Control and Prevention. Sexually transmitted diseases treatment guidelines. Syphilis. Atlanta, GA: US Department of Health and Human Services, Centers for Disease Control and Prevention; 2015.

14. Centers for Disease Control and Prevention. Sexually transmitted diseases treatment guidelines. Trichomoniasis. Atlanta, GA: US Department of Health and Human Services, Centers for Disease Control and Prevention; 2015.

15. Varner MW, Silver RM, Rowland Hogue CJ, et al. Association between stillbirth and illicit drug use and smoking during pregnancy. *Obstet Gynecol*. 2014;123:113–125.

16. American College of Obstetricians and Gynecologists. ACOG Committee Opinion #471, November 2010. Smoking cessation during pregnancy. *Obstet Gynecol*. 2010;116:1241–1244.

17. Maslova E, Bhattacharya S, Lin S, Michels KB. Caffeine consumption during pregnancy and risk of preterm birth: a meta-analysis. *Am J Clin Nutr*. 2010;92:1120–1132.

18. American College of Obstetricians and Gynecologists. ACOG Committee Opinion #462, November 2010. Moderate caffeine consumption during pregnancy. *Obstet Gynecol*. 2010;116:467–468.

19. Lemoine P, Harousseau H, Borteyru JP, Menuet JC. Children of alcoholic parents – observed anomalies; discussion of 127 cases. *Ther Drug Monit*. 2003;25:132–136.

20. Ornoy A, Ergaz Z. Alcohol abuse in pregnant women: effects on the fetus and newborn, mode of action and maternal treatment. *In J Environ Res Public Health*. 2010;7:364–379.

21. Centers for Disease Control and Prevention. Fetal alcohol spectrum disorders: alcohol use in pregnancy. http://www.cdc.gov/ncbddd/fasd/alcohol-use.html. Accessed July 28, 2017.

22. Hudak M, Tan RC. Committee on Drugs; Committee on Fetus and Newborn; American Academy of Pediatrics. Neonatal drug withdrawal. *Pediatrics*. 2012;129:e540–e560.

23. American College of Obstetricians and Gynecologists. ACOG Committee Opinion #637, June 2015. Marijuana use during pregnancy and lactation. *Obstet Gynecol*. 2015;126:234–238.

24. Oei J, Abdel-Latif ME, Clark R, et al. Short-term outcomes of mothers and infants exposed to antenatal amphetamines. *Arch Dis Child Fetal Neonatal Ed*. 2010;95:F36–F41.

25. American College of Obstetricians and Gynecologists. ACOG Committee Opinion #479, March 2011. Amphetamine abuse in women of reproductive age. *Obstet Gynecol*. 2011;117:751–755.

26. Bhuvaneswar CG, Chang G, Epstein LA, Stern TA. Cocaine and opioid use during pregnancy: prevalence and management. *Prim Care Companion J Clin Psychiatry*. 2008;10:59–65.

27. American College of Obstetricians and Gynecologists. ACOG Committee Opinion #524, May 2012. Opioid abuse, dependence, and addiction in pregnancy. *Obstet Gynecol*. 2012;119:1070–1076.

28. Zlatnik MG, Cheng YW, Norton ME, et al. Placenta previa and the risk of preterm delivery. *J Matern Fetal Neonatal Med*. 2007;10:719–723.

29. Oyelese Y, Ananth CV. Placental abruption. *Obstet Gynecol*. 2006;108:1005–1016.

30. Geipel A, Germer U, Welp T, et al. Prenatal diagnosis of single umbilical artery: determination of the absent side, associated anomalies, Doppler findings and perinatal outcome. *Ultrasound Obstet Gynecol*. 2000;15:114–117.

31. American College of Obstetricians and Gynecologists, Task Force on Hypertension in Pregnancy. Hypertension in pregnancy. Report of the American College of Obstetricians and Gynecologists' Task Force on Hypertension in Pregnancy. *Obstet Gynecol*. 2013;122:1122–1131.

32. American College of Obstetricians and Gynecologists. ACOG Committee Opinion #638, September 2015. First trimester risk assessment for early-onset preeclampsia. *Obstet Gynecol*. 2015;126:e25–e27.

33. Sibai BM, Publications Committee, Society for Maternal-Fetal Medicine. Evaluation and management of severe preeclampsia before 34 weeks' gestation. *Am J Obstet Gynecol*. 2011;205:191–198.

34. Barton JR, Sibai BM. Diagnosis and management of hemolysis, elevated liver enzymes, and low platelets syndrome. *Clin Perinatol*. 2004;31:807–833.

35. American Diabetes Association. Diagnosis and classification of diabetes mellitus. *Diabetes Care*. 2014;37:Supplement 1.

36. Crowther CA, Hiller JE, Moss JR, et al. Effect of treatment of gestational diabetes mellitus on pregnancy outcomes. *N Engl J Med*. 2005;352:2477–2486.

37. American Diabetes Association. Gestational diabetes mellitus. *Diabetes Care*. 2004;27 Suppl 1:S88.

38. Philipson EH, Super DM. Gestational diabetes mellitus: does it recur in subsequent pregnancy? *Am J Obstet Gynecol*. 1989;160:1324–1331.

39. Kamana KC, Shakya S, Zhang H. Gestational diabetes mellitus and macrosomia: a literature review. *Ann Nutr Metab*. 2015;66(Suppl 2):14–20.

40. Harman CR. Amniotic fluid abnormalities. *Semin Perinatol*. 2008;32:288–294.

41. Duncombe GJ, Dickinson JE, Evans SF. Perinatal characteristics and outcomes of pregnancies complicated by twin-twin transfusion syndrome. *Obstet Gynecol*. 2003;101:1190–1196.

42. Lyons EA, Dyke C, Cheang M. In utero exposure to diagnostic ultrasound; a six year follow-up. *Radiology*. 1988;166:687–690.

43. Devoe LD. Antenatal fetal assessment: contraction stress test, nonstress test, vibroacoustic stimulation, amniotic fluid volume, biophysical profile, and modified biophysical profile – an overview. *Semin Perinatol*. 2008;32:247–252.

44. American College of Obstetricians and Gynecologists. ACOG Practice Bulletin #145, July 2014. Antepartum fetal surveillance. *Obstet Gynecol*. 2014;124:182–192.

45. American College of Obstetricians and Gynecologists. ACOG Committee Opinion #643, September 2015. Identification and referral of maternal genetic conditions in pregnancy. *Obstet Gynecol*. 2015;126:e49–e51.

46. Werner EF, Han CS, Pettker CM, et al. Universal cervical-length screening to prevent preterm birth: a cost-effectiveness analysis. *Ultrasound Obstet Gynecol*. 2011;38:32–37.

47. American College of Obstetricians and Gynecologists. ACOG Practice Bulletin #130, October 2012. Antepartum fetal surveillance. *Obstet Gynecol*. 2012;120:964–973.

48. Ross MG. Preterm labor. http://emedicine.medscape.com/article/260998. Accessed July 28, 2017.

49. American College of Obstetricians and Gynecologists. ACOG Practice Bulletin #127, October 2012. Management of preterm labor. *Obstet Gynecol*. 2012;119:1308–1317.

50. American College of Obstetricians and Gynecologists. ACOG Committee Opinion #573, September 2013. Magnesium sulfate use in obstetrics. *Obstet Gynecol*. 2013;122:727–728.

51. Flenady V, Wojcieszek AM, Papatsonis DN, et al. Calcium channel blockers for inhibiting preterm labour and birth. *Cochrane Database Syst Rev*. 2014;CD002255.

52. Iams J. Prevention of preterm parturition, clinical practice. *N Eng J Med*. 2014;370:254–261.

53. Iams J. Identification of candidates for progesterone: why, who, how and when? *Obstet Gynecol*. 2014;123:1317–1326.

6

Evaluation of the Neonate

Melissa Baldwin

Kelly G. Thompson-Davis

© Anna Rubak/ShutterStock, Inc.

OUTLINE

OBJECTIVES

1. Describe how gestational age can be determined before and after delivery.
2. Discuss the importance of determining gestational age and how it is determined using the New Ballard Scale.
3. Define periodic breathing in a neonate.
4. Recognize abnormal vital signs in a neonate.
5. Given a neonate's gestational age, calculate an adequate value for mean blood pressure.
6. Define macrocephaly and microcephaly.
7. Describe normal findings when assessing the neonate's chest.
8. List and describe the signs of respiratory distress.
9. Identify the location of retractions in the neonate.
10. Explain the general components of the cardiac examination of a neonate.
11. Understand how the neurologic assessment assists in identifying disorders in the neonate.
12. Identify the laboratory tests recommended for the critically ill neonate.

KEY TERMS

acrocyanosis	nasal flaring
apnea	New Ballard Score
capillary refill time	occipitofrontal
ductus arteriosus	circumference (OFC)
gestational age	pectus carinatum
grasp reflex	pectus excavatum
grunting	periodic breathing
heart murmur	postductal
large for gestational	preductal
age (LGA)	retractions
macrocephaly	rooting reflex
mean blood pressure (MBP)	Silverman Score
microcephaly	small for gestational
Moro reflex	age (SGA)

Introduction

The timely assessment of the neonate can greatly affect neonatal outcomes. Careful assessment of the neonate's gestational age, weight, size, and respiratory function assists the respiratory care practitioner in determining appropriate interventions.

Determining Gestational Age

Assessment of the neonate should begin immediately after delivery, although in most cases it begins prior to birth through ultrasound and fetal heart rate monitoring. Accurately estimating the **gestational age** is important in assessing fetal growth and making decisions regarding obstetric management. The interpretation of antenatal tests, such as the nonstress test and the biophysical profile, often depend upon gestational age. Prenatal assessment of gestational age is most often based upon maternal history and ultrasound measurements. During the first trimester, gestational age is estimated by measuring both the gestational sac and the length between the crown (head) and the rump of the fetus. Measurements made during this time have the least variability and are likely to be the most accurate. Ultrasounds performed later in the pregnancy estimate gestational age through measurements of the circumference of the fetal head and abdomen and the length of the femur, which is the longest fetal bone.[1]

True gestational age, however, is determined at birth. The **New Ballard Score** is a system that determines gestational age of a neonate through the assessment of six physical and six neuromuscular features. The system works on the presumption that fetal skin, subcutaneous tissues, and the neuromuscular system mature at predictable rates, and a numeric score is determined for each of the 12 features. Using a table, as seen in **Figure 6-1**, the cumulative score correlates with a maturity rating, or gestational age.[2] Gestational age can be determined in infants as young as 20 weeks' gestation and should be measured within the first 48 hours of life to ensure accuracy.

Physical Assessment

The initial physical assessment begins in the delivery room immediately following birth while drying, warming, positioning, and suctioning the neonate. Typically, physical assessment follows a head-to-toe sequence, but with neonates the assessment is prioritized to allow for critical information to be obtained first—for example, auscultation of the heart and lungs should be done immediately if a neonate is quiet and not crying following delivery.

Vital Signs

Vital signs are established early in the assessment. **Table 6-1** shows the normal values for vital signs in a neonate.

Respiratory Rate

A normal, term neonate has an average respiratory rate of 40 to 60 breaths per minute. The younger the gestational age, the higher the expected respiratory rate; because the fetal lungs are not fully developed, it is not uncommon for a 25 weeks' gestational age neonate to breathe 70 breaths per minute. All neonates have an irregular breathing pattern; therefore, breathing should be assessed over a 1-minute period to determine the respiratory rate.

An abnormal respiratory rate can indicate various problems. If the neonate is tachypneic with a respiratory rate greater than normal, then hypoxemia, acidosis, anxiety, or pain should be suspected. Bradypnea, a respiratory rate of fewer than 30 breaths per minute, may occur when the neonate has received certain medications, is hypothermic, or is neurologically impaired. Premature neonates usually display a breathing pattern known as **periodic breathing**. This is described as an irregular pattern of intermittent respiratory pauses that last longer than 5 seconds. A neonate who presents with **apnea**, which is the absence of spontaneous breathing lasting longer than 20 seconds, often has cyanosis, hypotonia, pallor, or bradycardia. The neonate who is apneic or who has tachypnea or bradypnea should be supported until the cause can be determined and corrected.

Heart Rate

The normal range of heart rate for a neonate varies from 100 to 160 beats per minute. The neonate's clinical state should be considered when assessing the heart rate. Sleeping neonates generally have a slower heart rate than one who is crying or hungry. The premature neonate (fewer than 35 weeks' gestation) has less variability in heart rate compared to a near-term or term newborn. Heart rate can be assessed at the point of maximal impulse (PMI), located at the fifth intercostal space, midclavicular line. Alternate sites to obtain a pulse are over the brachial or femoral artery and the umbilical stump if the neonate is newly delivered. A neonate's heart rate will normally increase with stimulation. If this does not occur, then electrolyte levels should be assessed. An abnormal heart rate or rhythm suggests cardiorespiratory compromise and warrants further investigation. A persistent tachycardia above 160 beats per minute may indicate hypoxia, hypovolemia, anemia, or sepsis. Persistent bradycardia of fewer than 80 beats per minute occurs most often with complete heart block. Both tachycardia and bradycardia are cause for an electrocardiogram and further diagnostic tests.

Blood Pressure

Normal blood pressures vary based on a neonate's weight and gestational age. Hypertension commonly

Neuromuscular maturity

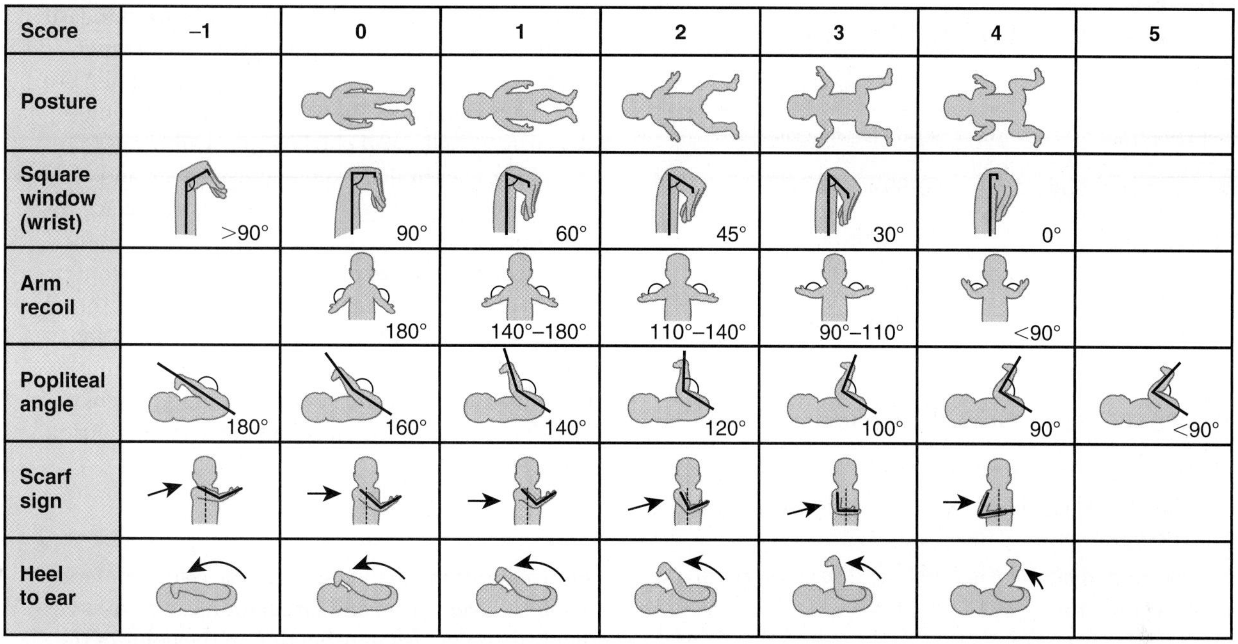

Score	−1	0	1	2	3	4	5
Posture							
Square window (wrist)	>90°	90°	60°	45°	30°	0°	
Arm recoil		180°	140°–180°	110°–140°	90°–110°	<90°	
Popliteal angle	180°	160°	140°	120°	100°	90°	<90°
Scarf sign							
Heel to ear							

Physical maturity

							Maturity rating	
Skin	Sticky, friable, transparent	Gelatinous, red, translucent	Smooth, pink; visible veins	Superficial peeling and/or rash; few veins	Cracking, pale areas; rare veins	Parchment, deep cracking; no vessels	Leathery, cracked wrinkled	
Lanugo	None	Sparse	Abundant	Thinning	Bald areas	Mostly bald	**Score**	**Weeks**
Plantar surface	Heel-toe 40–50 mm: −1 <40 mm: −2	>50 mm, no crease	Faint red marks	Anterior transverse crease only	Creases anterior 2/3	Creases over entire sole	−10	20
							−5	22
							0	24
Breast	Imperceptible	Barely perceptible	Flat areola, no bud	Stippled areola, 1–2 mm bud	Raised areola, 3–4 mm bud	Full areola, 5–10 mm bud	5	26
							10	28
Eye/Ear	Lids fused loosely: −1 tightly: −2	Lids open; pinna flat; stays folded	Slightly curved pinna; soft; slow recoil	Well curved pinna; soft but ready recoil	Formed and firm, instant recoil	Thick cartilage, ear soft	15	30
							20	32
							25	34
Genitals (male)	Scrotum flat, smooth	Scrotum empty, faint rugae	Testes in upper canal rare rugae	Testes descending, few rugae	Testes down, good rugae	Testes pendulous, deep rugae	30	36
							35	38
							40	40
Genitals (female)	Clitoris prominent, labia flat	Clitoris prominent, small labia minora	Clitoris prominent, enlarging minora	Majora and minora equally prominent	Majora large, minora small	Majora cover clitoris and minora	45	42
							50	44

FIGURE 6-1 New Ballard Score to determine gestational age.

Reproduced from Ballard JL, Khoury JC, Wedig K, et al. New Ballard Score, expanded to include extremely premature infants. *J Pediatrics.* 1991;119:417–422.

occurs in neonates with renal problems and those with a history of an indwelling umbilical artery catheter. It is also associated with cardiac and pulmonary disorders, including patent ductus arteriosus, coarctation of the aorta, and bronchopulmonary dysplasia.[3] An adequate **mean blood pressure (MBP)** value can be calculated if the neonate's gestational age is known. This calculation is explained in **Box 6-1.**

TABLE 6-1
Normal Ranges for Vital Signs of the Neonate

Heart rate	100–160 beats/min
Respiratory rate	30–60 breaths/min
Blood pressure – diastolic	60–90 mm Hg
Blood pressure – systolic	30–60 mm Hg
Temperature	36.5–37.5°C

BOX 6-1 Calculation of Adequate Mean Blood Pressure Using Gestational Age

Gestational age in weeks + 5 = adequate mean blood pressure

Example of adequate MBP for a 26 weeks' gestation neonate:

$$26 + 5 = 31 \text{ mm Hg}$$

Size and Weight

Most examinations begin with an evaluation of neonatal size, including measurements of weight, length, and head circumference. These measurements, along with the gestational age, are plotted on a growth chart that will indicate a percentile. An example of this chart is shown in **Figure 6-2**. This percentile compares the measurements with neonates of the same gestational age.[4] For example, a growth chart indicating that a neonate is in the 25th percentile for gestational age means that the neonate is larger than 25 neonates and smaller than 75 neonates, if compared with 100 neonates of the same gestational age. Lower percentages indicate a smaller neonate, while larger percentages indicate a larger neonate. From these percentiles a neonate is then classified as small, average, or large for gestational age. Neonates who are **small for gestational age (SGA)** have birth weights that are below the 10th percentile. This can be the result of growth restriction during the pregnancy, often caused by congenital infections, placental insufficiency, and congenital disorders. Neonates who are above the 90th percentile for birth weight are considered **large for gestational age (LGA)**. This is most often due to maternal diabetes.

Measurement of head circumference, also known as **occipitofrontal circumference (OFC)**, is critical in the evaluation of the neonate. Proper measurement is illustrated in **Figure 6-3**. **Macrocephaly** is defined as a head circumference that is greater than two standard deviations above the mean for a given age, gender, and gestation. It is often a feature of congenital syndromes as well as increased intracranial pressure, enlarged bones in the skull, and brain tumors. **Microcephaly** is a head circumference that is two or more standard deviations below the mean for a given age, gender, and gestation, most often the result of the brain failing to grow at a normal rate. Prenatal infections, including the Zika virus, rubella, and chicken pox, can result in microcephaly. Cerebral anoxia, maternal drug and alcohol abuse, and exposure to toxic chemicals also place the fetal brain at risk.

The weight and size of a neonate are important indicators of health. Neonates who are SGA and those who are LGA are both at greater risk of presenting with or developing problems. Most neonatal intensive care units use the metric system to monitor weight. **Box 6-2** contains information on converting metric measurements.

Skin

Abnormalities in a neonate's skin are often immediately obvious. Oxygenation and circulation can be assessed quickly through visual inspection of the color of the neonate's skin and oral mucous membranes.

Pallor in a neonate with respiratory distress is often an indication of hypoxia, reduced peripheral perfusion due to shock or congenital heart disease, or acute blood loss, such as occurs with fetal–maternal hemorrhage in placental abruption. In neonates without respiratory distress, pallor often indicates anemia.

As illustrated in **Figure 6-4**, **acrocyanosis** is cyanosis of the hands, feet, and around the mouth. It is a sign of peripheral vasoconstriction and is common in most neonates at birth; as oxygenation and circulation improve, usually within 72 hours of delivery, acrocyanosis will disappear and the skin quickly begins to turn pink. If the neonate is not oxygenating well, the skin will have a pale pallor and the skin and mucous membranes will remain cyanotic or turn a dark color of blue-gray. This indicates central cyanosis due to hypoxemia, which is often the result of congenital heart defects with right-to-left shunting, persistent pulmonary hypertension, or lung disorders, including respiratory distress syndrome. Cyanosis may also be a result of blood lost during labor. A significant amount of blood loss may be the result of external hemorrhage from a placental abruption or ruptured umbilical cord. Bruising from birth trauma may also present as bluish discoloration of the skin, so the infant's mucous membranes should be assessed to determine if it is true cyanosis.

Stimulation at birth will cause a neonate to cry and gasp. As the transition from fetal to neonatal life occurs postdelivery, the oxygen saturation will begin to rise and the skin color will improve. In the normal neonate, the oxygen saturation should steadily rise toward 90% in the first 5 minutes of life; it usually reaches 95% within 10 to 15 minutes, although in some healthy neonates it may

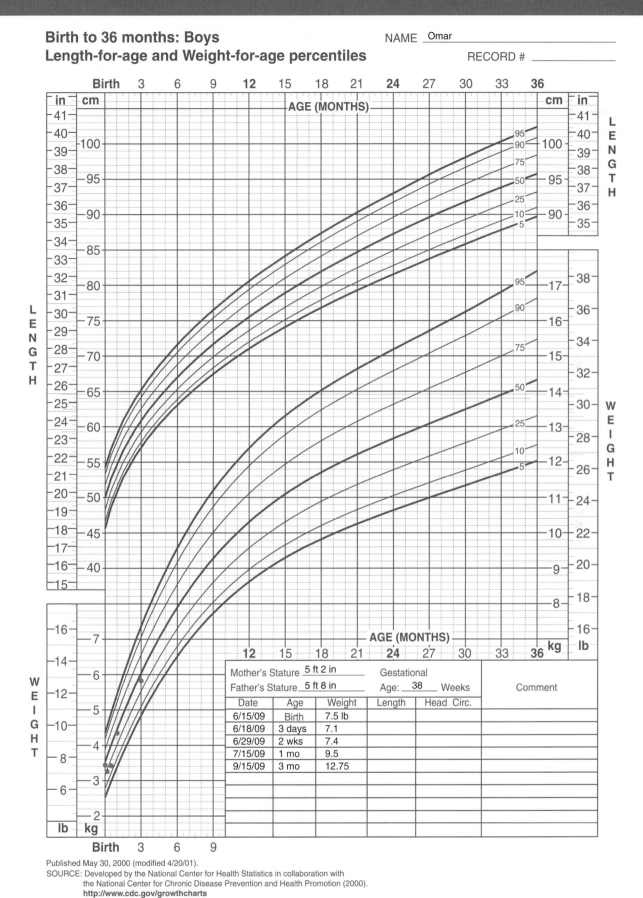

Birth to 36 months: Boys
Length-for-age and Weight-for-age percentiles

NAME Omar

RECORD # _____

Mother's Stature	5 ft 2 in		Gestational		
Father's Stature	5 ft 8 in		Age: 38 Weeks		Comment
Date	Age	Weight	Length	Head Circ.	
6/15/09	Birth	7.5 lb			
6/18/09	3 days	7.1			
6/29/09	2 wks	7.4			
7/15/09	1 mo	9.5			
9/15/09	3 mo	12.75			

Published May 30, 2000 (modified 4/20/01).
SOURCE: Developed by the National Center for Health Statistics in collaboration with
the National Center for Chronic Disease Prevention and Health Promotion (2000).
http://www.cdc.gov/growthcharts

FIGURE 6-2 Growth chart to plot length and weight. By plotting the weight, the infant was in the 10th percentile at birth. By 3 months of age, he has moved to between the 25th and 50th percentile for weight. There are no measurements for length plotted.

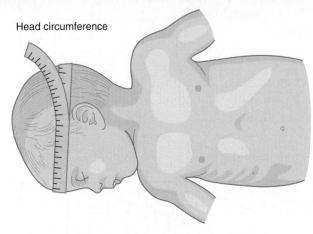

Head circumference

FIGURE 6-3 Measurement of head circumference in a neonate.

BOX 6-2 Converting Measurements

1 kilogram = 2.2 pounds

1 kilogram = 1000 grams

1 pound = 453.5 grams

1 pound = 16 ounces

1 ounce = 28.35 grams

1 inch = 2.54 cm

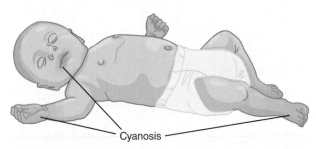

Cyanosis

FIGURE 6-4 Acrocyanosis. Notice the bluish discoloration/cyanosis of the neonate's hands and feet and around the mouth.

take up to 60 minutes.[5] If the neonate does not appear to be "pinking up," vigorous stimulation should be applied. If cyanosis continues, then underlying congenital abnormalities should be suspected and a pulse oximeter used to evaluate the oxygenation status.

It is normal for jaundice to occur during the 2nd or 3rd day following delivery and then disappear within a week. However, jaundice within the first 24 hours of birth is considered abnormal and further evaluation is indicated. Yellowish-green staining of the skin or fingernails indicates that the neonate was exposed to meconium-stained amniotic fluid while in utero.

Abdomen

Careful examination of the neonate's abdomen can detect anomalies, birth injuries, and disorders that often result in respiratory compromise. The neonate with a sunken or hollowed appearance of the abdominal cavity is described as having a scaphoid abdomen. This is highly suggestive of congenital diaphragmatic hernia (CDH), a defect in which the diaphragm allows the abdominal contents to enter the chest cavity. CDH compromises early lung development, leading to pulmonary hypoplasia and persistent pulmonary hypertension. A distended abdomen suggests an obstruction, often due to meconium ileus.

Abdominal wall defects are usually diagnosed prenatally. Gastroschisis is a defect in which the large and small intestines protrude or bulge out of the abdominal wall, usually to the right of the umbilical cord. The intestines are fully exposed with no membrane covering them and may have tissue damage due to having direct contact with the amniotic fluid. It typically affects preterm neonates, those who are SGA, and neonates of mothers who are younger than 30 years of age and have had few pregnancies. An omphalocele occurs when there is an opening where the umbilical cord meets the abdominal wall and the abdominal contents, typically the intestines, liver, and stomach, herniate through the umbilical base. Unlike gastroschisis, the herniated organs are covered by the membrane that covers the umbilical cord. Neonates born with omphaloceles often have congenital heart defects, neural tube defects, or chromosomal anomalies, including Trisomy 13, 18, or 21.

Umbilical cord abnormalities are important to note. A normal umbilical cord has three blood vessels: two umbilical arteries and one umbilical vein, with the vein being the larger of the vessels. When the umbilical cord has only one artery and one vein, it is referred to as a two-vessel cord or a single umbilical artery (SUA). This condition occurs in about 1% of pregnancies and is associated more often with chromosome abnormalities and congenital anomalies, with renal anomalies occurring most often.[6]

Respiratory Assessment

Thoracic assessment of the neonate begins with a general overview of the size and shape of the chest and evaluation of respiratory effort and work of breathing. Findings from this assessment often lead to further evaluation and diagnostic testing.

Examination of the Chest

The neonate's chest is normally symmetric. A small chest is suggestive of pulmonary hypoplasia, while a barrel chest may be present in neonates with air-trapping disorders, such as meconium aspiration syndrome. Rib deformities, absence of chest muscle, and widely spaced nipples are often associated with various syndromes and a genetic consultation is warranted. Common malformations of the sternum include pectus excavatum and pectus carinatum.

Pectus excavatum, sometimes referred to as funnel chest, is the depression of a part or all of the sternum. **Pectus carinatum** is the anterior or outward protrusion of the sternum. These conditions normally have no clinical significance for the neonate but may have implications as the child ages.

Evaluation of Respiratory Distress

Respiratory distress occurs frequently in neonates and can quickly progress to respiratory failure if not promptly recognized and managed. The clinical signs of respiratory distress in the neonate are listed in **Table 6-2**.

Nasal flaring, as illustrated in **Figure 6-5**, is the term used to describe the widening of the nares or nostrils with each breath during inspiration. It is a sign of respiratory distress and is the result of the neonate attempting to move more air through the nares and decrease airway resistance.

Grunting is heard during expiration when the neonate is breathing against a glottis that is partially closed. This increases the functional residual capacity of the lungs, causing an increase in pressure at the end of expiration and helping maintain alveolar patency. It can vary from being mild and only audible with a stethoscope to severe where it is audible with the naked ear. Grunting is commonly associated with respiratory distress syndrome and other disorders where there is alveolar collapse.

Seen during inspiration, **retractions** are the inward movement or sucking in of the skin covering the chest.

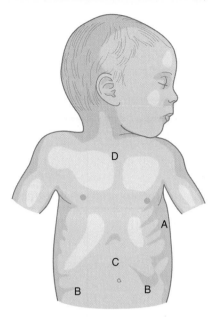

FIGURE 6-6 Location of retractions observed in a neonate: **A.** Intercostal retractions; **B.** Subcostal retractions; **C.** Substernal retractions; and **D.** Suprasternal retractions.

They may be observed in various areas of the chest, as illustrated and described in **Figure 6-6**. They are caused by reduced lung compliance or increased airway resistance. As compliance or resistance worsens in a neonate, retractions become more prominent. Retractions are more easily observed in neonates as compared to older children.

In a normal chest exam, there should be synchronized thoracic and abdominal effort without retractions or grunting. Paradoxical respirations are asynchronous respiratory efforts of the thoracic and abdominal walls. During inspiration, the chest wall will draw in as normal, but the abdominal wall will push out. It is typically referred to as "seesaw" breathing, and it indicates severe respiratory distress. Repositioning the airway may be warranted if the neonate appears to be struggling while breathing. Moving the neonate to a supine position with the head and neck extended can improve respiratory effort.

The **Silverman Score**, shown in **Figure 6-7**, is a tool used to quantify respiratory distress and lung disease.[7] It has five areas to assess and grade or score the neonate. The lowest grade in each area is a 0, indicating minimal, if any, problems, and the highest grade is a 2, in which the neonate is having more difficulty. The grades given are totaled, and the sum determines the degree of respiratory distress: A grade of 0 indicates no respiratory distress, while a grade of 7 or more indicates severe distress.

Auscultation of the Chest

Auscultation of the neonate's chest is an integral part of the physical assessment. Because the chest is small,

TABLE 6-2
Clinical Signs of Respiratory Distress in the Neonate

Nasal flaring
Grunting
Tachypnea
Retractions

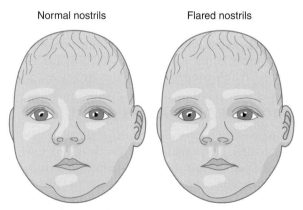

Normal nostrils   Flared nostrils

FIGURE 6-5 Nasal flaring in which the neonate's nostrils widen with each breath in an attempt to move more air into the lungs. This is a clinical sign of respiratory distress.

Silverman score

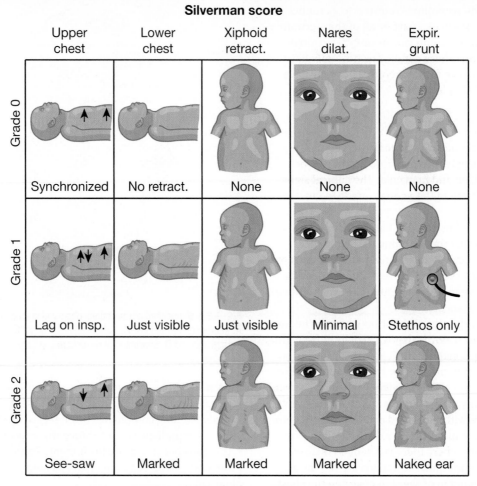

FIGURE 6-7 Silverman scoring system to evaluate the degree of respiratory distress. Following assessment, the grades are totaled with the sum determining the degree of respiratory distress: 0 = no distress, 1 to 3 = mild distress, 4 to 6 = moderate distress, 7 to 10 = severe distress.

Data from Silverman WA, Anderson DH. A controlled clinical trial of effects of water mist on obstructive respiratory signs, death rate and necropsy findings among premature infants. *Pediatrics.* 1956;17:1–6.

sounds can be easily transmitted from one area to another. Breath sounds should be compared between the right and left lungs. Asymmetric or diminished breath sounds are indicative of various disorders, including but not limited to respiratory distress syndrome, pneumothorax, pneumonia, and meconium aspiration syndrome. Rhonchi are coarse breath sounds heard over the large airways and usually indicate that the neonate needs to be suctioned. An airway obstruction resulting from excessive oral secretions during delivery may be present, requiring the use of bulb suction and/or wall suction to remove the fluid and clear the neonate's airway. Large amounts of secretions may have been swallowed, and the need to monitor for further respiratory compromise should be done. Wheezes emit from the smaller airways and are commonly heard during the expiratory phase. Rales or crackles are caused by air moving through fluid in the smaller airways and alveoli are not uncommon shortly after birth. Stridor is a high-pitched inspiratory sound that is audible by stethoscope or ear. It usually indicates an upper airway obstruction.

Chest Radiograph

A chest radiograph may be necessary to assist in the diagnosis of a neonate with respiratory distress. Examination of the lung fields can reveal lung processes, such as parenchymal lung disease or pneumonia, and lung abnormalities, including pulmonary hypoplasia due to congenital diaphragmatic hernia. The size and shape of the heart may also be assessed to rule out or confirm congenital heart disease. Locations of the stomach, liver, and heart are noted to rule out dextrocardia and situs inversus.

Cardiovascular Assessment

A neonate with respiratory distress who rapidly deteriorates often has an underlying cardiac disorder. Assessing cardiovascular function is critical in identifying life-threatening congenital heart defects and providing treatment. Areas of focus include the intensity and timing of upper and lower extremity pulses, capillary refill, preductal and postductal oxygen saturation, and measurement of blood pressure in all four extremities.

Cardiac Murmurs

A **heart murmur** is due to turbulent blood flow in or around the heart. They are a common finding in neonates and usually resolve within the first 48 hours following birth. Murmurs are evaluated for their intensity or loudness, with descriptions that range from barely audible, soft, loud, to loud enough to hear with the stethoscope off of the chest. They are also evaluated for their timing in the cardiac cycle. Systolic murmurs are associated with ventricular ejection, usually benign, and due to the turbulent blood flow that occurs with the closure of fetal shunts at birth. When they are accompanied by normal oxygen saturation and no abnormal clinical findings, no further workup is required. Diastolic murmurs occur during ventricular relaxation and filling and are due to abnormal flow patterns in the heart and vessels. Continuous murmurs occur throughout the cardiac cycle, both during contraction and relaxation of the heart. Both diastolic and continuous murmurs are most often associated with congenital heart defects. There may be multiple murmurs heard when a neonate has a combination of heart defects. Regardless of the type of murmur, further testing is required if the neonate presents with cyanosis, respiratory distress, or signs of cardiovascular compromise. It is important to note that not all neonates with a heart murmur have a congenital heart lesion. Likewise, the absence of a heart murmur does not necessarily rule out congenital heart disease.

Peripheral Pulses

The axillary, radial, brachial, femoral, and posterior tibial pulses are palpated to assess for rate, regularity, and character. Weak or absent pulses are a sign of inadequate perfusion due to the reduced cardiac output that occurs in shock or hypotension. Certain congenital heart defects, such as aortic stenosis and hypoplastic left heart syndrome, also present with weak or absent pulses. Bounding peripheral pulses are often found with a patent **ductus arteriosus** or in right-to-left shunt defects that result in fluid volume overload in the systemic circuit. A pulse that is more prominent in the arm than the leg is associated with coarctation of the aorta.

Capillary Refill Time

Capillary refill time is a widely accepted method to assess cardiac output and peripheral circulation in a neonate. It is checked by pressing on the skin over the chest or an extremity just until the area blanches, then counting the number of seconds it takes until the color returns. Normal capillary refill time in neonates is fewer than 3 seconds. Several conditions can cause a delay in refill time, including hypoxia, sepsis, shock, dehydration, and reduced cardiac output.

Preductal and Postductal Oxygen Saturation

Obtaining preductal and postductal oxygen saturation measurements can provide information about blood shunting and help determine the need for further cardiac evaluation. A pulse oximeter probe placed on the neonate's right hand is measuring oxygen saturation proximal to the aortic opening of the ductus arteriosus. This is considered to be a **preductal** measurement—the blood has left the heart but has not reached the ductus arteriosus in the aorta. Placing a pulse oximeter probe on the neonate's left hand or either foot measures oxygen saturation distal to the aortic opening of the ductus arteriosus—a **postductal** measurement. Simultaneous measurement of preductal and postductal oxygen saturation, as illustrated in **Figure 6-8**, allows detection of ductal shunting, which is present with congenital heart defects. A preductal saturation that is higher than the postductal saturation is indicative of left heart abnormalities that include coarctation of the aorta, aortic stenosis, and interrupted aortic arch. It is also found in the normal heart with persistent pulmonary hypertension. In a neonate with transposition of the great arteries, the postductal saturations are higher than the preductal saturations.

Neurologic Assessment

The neurologic assessment is usually completed alongside the physical assessment. It includes observation of the neonate's alertness, activity, and tone as well as response to stimuli. Alertness depends upon several factors, including gestational age, maternal exposure

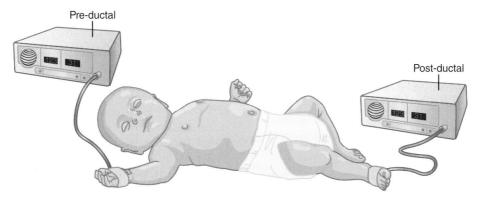

FIGURE 6-8 Placement of pulse oximeter probes for monitoring preductal and postductal oxygen saturation.

to anesthesia or narcotics during labor, prenatal exposure to drugs, placental insufficiency, and infection. Observing how neonates spontaneously open their eyes and move their faces and extremities helps determine their level of alertness. Neonates will respond to bright lights by shutting their eyes tightly, although this is highly dependent upon age. The neonate's response to stimuli should be determined, noting whether the response is appropriate or if the neonate is irritable or lethargic. An irritable neonate is agitated and cries and is unable to be soothed with even minimal stimulation, which is often seen with hypoglycemia or drug withdrawal. A lethargic neonate is unable to remain alert.

Movement of all extremities and symmetry and smoothness of the movement is important to note during assessment. Extremity weakness may indicate a difficult birth or neurologic impairment. Normal-toned neonates can easily be picked up with adult hands placed under the armpits. The arms and legs will flex and the neonate will maintain the flexed position when at rest. Neonates who are hypotonic are more difficult to pick up when adult hands are placed under their armpits because the arms do not stay flexed, causing the neonate to slip through the hands. Hypotonia often indicates hemorrhage, encephalopathy, sepsis, metabolic imbalance, or congenital anomalies.

Reflex presence and strength are important signs of neurologic development and brainstem function. To assess the **Moro reflex**, the neonate is held and the head allowed to drop slightly but suddenly. A normal response is for the neonate to be startled, with the arms extended and abducted outward and the palms open. This is quickly followed by the neonate bringing the arms inward in an embracing posture with the hands clenched into fists and is often associated with a momentary cry. A Moro reflex that is depressed or asymmetric is abnormal and often indicates a brachial plexus injury or fractured clavicle due to birth trauma. The **grasp reflex** is tested by placing a finger in the neonate's open palm. A normal response is for the neonate's hand to close around the finger and the grasp tightened when the finger is moved within the palm. An abnormal grasp reflex may also indicate injury to the brachial plexus. A **rooting reflex** occurs when the cheek is stroked and the neonate turns toward the stroked side and begins making sucking motions. This is a normal reflex that is present until about 4 months of age.

Diagnostic Tests

The public health program in the United States mandates that newborns be screened for congenital disorders. The tests screen for genetic disorders that may not be apparent at birth but if not detected soon can lead to severe illness, chronic disability, or death. These include sickle cell anemia, hemoglobinopathies, phenylketonuria (PKU), galactosemia, and cystic fibrosis. The newborn screen can provide early detection of treatable diseases before symptoms occur, lead to treatment that can prevent serious problems, such as severe developmental delay or death, and detect carriers of certain genetic disorders.[8]

A complete blood count (CBC) is often obtained to evaluate the neonate for anemia, infection, or thrombocytopenia. The CBC may be obtained through a capillary, venous, or arterial sample. The maternal and perinatal history assessment must be included when interpreting the results of a CBC. The red blood cell (RBC) count is a measurement of the number of circulating erythrocytes. Anemia and polycythemia can be identified by evaluating the RBC count. Neonatal anemia can be caused by acute or chronic blood loss, decreased erythrocyte production, increased erythrocyte destruction, or shortened erythrocyte survival. Polycythemia is present when the venous hematocrit is greater than 65%. Symptoms include lethargy, irritability, and hypotonia.[9]

Leukocytes, or white blood cells (WBC), are the neonate's primary defense system against foreign organisms, tissues, and substances. An elevated WBC is known as leukocytosis and may indicate infections or leukemia. A decreased WBC, referred to as leukopenia, may indicate a viral or bacterial infection. It also occurs in neonates born to a mother with pregnancy-induced hypertension (PIH). Neutrophils are the predominant WBC type circulating in the blood. They defend the body by phagocytosis. Neutrophilia, which is an increase in the number of neutrophils in the blood, is the result of inflammation, certain malignancies, or the presence of corticosteroids. Neutropenia, a decrease in the neutrophil count, results from infection, impaired bone marrow production, or abnormal distribution and is indicative of neonatal sepsis. It is also associated with PIH, birth asphyxia, intrauterine growth restriction (IUGR), Rh hemolytic disease, and periventricular hemorrhage.

Thrombocytes, or platelets, are responsible for coagulation, hemostasis, and blood thrombus formation. One of the most common hematologic problems of the neonate is thrombocytopenia, or reduced platelets. It is caused by the decreased production or increased destruction, sequestration, or loss of platelets. **Table 6-3** lists conditions associated with thrombocytopenia in the neonate. Thrombocytosis is rare and may be physiologic or caused by infection, inflammation, iron or vitamin E deficiency, congenital neoplasms, Down syndrome, or congenital adrenal hyperplasia.[9]

In the critically ill neonate, laboratory testing is directed toward a suspected etiology. However, in neonates in which there is no clear etiology, a battery of tests are conducted to assist in determining the diagnosis and treatment. **Table 6-4** lists the tests typically conducted in the laboratory workup of a critically ill neonate.[10] It is important to note that the blood loss that occurs during laboratory testing is the primary cause of anemia during the first weeks immediately after birth, especially in the very low birthweight neonate. Although multiple laboratory tests may be necessary, it is essential to remain aware of the amount of blood being sampled and to avoid excessive blood draws.

TABLE 6-3
Conditions Associated with Thrombocytopenia in the Neonate

Sepsis, bacterial and viral
Disseminating intravascular coagulation (DIC)
Necrotizing enterocolitis
Persistent pulmonary hypertension of the newborn (PPHN)
Erythroblastosis fetalis
Polycythemia
Congenital infections
Congenital anomalies and syndromes
Neonatal alloimmune thrombocytopenia
Maternal immune thrombocytopenic purpura
Preeclampsia

TABLE 6-4
Laboratory Tests for Assessment of the Critically Ill Neonate

Complete blood count (CBC) with differential
Electrolytes
Blood glucose
Ionized calcium
Blood culture
Urine culture
Urinalysis, including organic acids and ketones
Blood urea nitrogen
Creatinine
Arterial blood gas
Magnesium
Phosphorus
Blood ammonia
Lactate
Pyruvate
Cerebrospinal fluid

Case Study 1

A 2000 gram male infant was delivered at 34 weeks' gestational age by cesarean section due to breech presentation, premature labor, and rupture of membranes. On physical examination the infant was non-dysmorphic, appeared vigorous, had spontaneous respirations, and the skin was pink and well perfused. Apgar scores were 7 and 9 at 1 and 5 minutes, respectively. One hour after admission to the neonatal intensive care unit, the infant developed tachypnea and nasal flaring with moderate subcostal and substernal retractions. Bronchial breath sounds that were slightly diminished in intensity were present. Analysis of umbilical arterial blood revealed a pH of 7.37, a PaO_2 of 50 mm Hg, and a $PaCO_2$ of 30 mm Hg. To improve work of breathing, continuous positive airway pressure (CPAP) of + 6 cm H_2O was initiated via nasal prongs. One hour later the infant's vital signs were as follows: temperature 37.6°C under radiant heat, blood pressure 60/42 mm Hg, heart rate 130 beats per minute, oxygen saturation 94% to 96% while breathing 40% oxygen with CPAP, and blood glucose 70 mg/dL. The remainder of the examination was normal for the gestational age.

The infant's respiratory status gradually improved, and over the next 3 days he was weaned from CPAP and transitioned to a nasal cannula and then to room air. Two days later, the infant was discharged home.

1. **What are important components of the initial neonatal assessment?**

2. **What was concerning about this patient's respiratory status, and what should the healthcare team continue to monitor?**

3. **What intervention would you consider if the CPAP + 6 did not improve the infant's work of breathing?**

Case Study 2

A 3070 gram female infant was delivered via cesarean section at 39 weeks' gestational age for failure to progress. Apgar scores were 7 and 8 at 2 and 5 minutes, respectively. The infant was admitted briefly to the neonatal intensive care unit for a sepsis evaluation due to suspected maternal chorioamnionitis where she received antibiotics as treatment. On day 3 of life, the infant developed respiratory distress with marked

(continues)

Case Study 2 (*continued*)

subcostal and intercostal retractions. On physical exam, the infant had cyanotic extremities, decreased breath sounds on the left side of the chest, and a scaphoid abdomen. Vital signs were as follows: respiratory rate of 65 breaths per minute, heart rate of 163 beats per minute, blood pressure of 90/50, and pulse oximetry of 91% on room air. At this time, an arterial blood gas was drawn, with the following results: pH 7.31, $PaCO_2$ 53, PaO_2 37, and base excess + 1. CBC showed the following: white blood cell count 11,000; hematocrit 39.1%; platelets 225K; and a differential of segmented cells, 33 lymphocytes, and 11 monocytes. A chest radiograph was obtained and demonstrated a left-sided congenital diaphragmatic hernia. Oxygen was provided with a nasal cannula, and the infant was transported to the operating room. Upon surgical exploration, a 20-mm by 15-mm defect in the posterolateral diaphragm was discovered. Herniated transverse colon and small bowel were reduced, and the defect was primarily closed. The infant had an uneventful hospital course and, on day 12 of life, she was discharged home.

1. **What was an obvious sign that may have suggested that the infant had an undiagnosed congenital diaphragmatic hernia?**

2. **How was the congenital diaphragmatic hernia definitively diagnosed in this infant?**

3. **What type of respiratory interventions could have been used to stabilize this infant with respiratory distress before a definitive diagnosis was made?**

References

1. Kalish RB, Thaler HT, Chasen ST, et al. First- and second-trimester ultrasound assessment of gestational age. *Am J Obstet Gynecol.* 2004;191:975–978.

2. Ballard JL, Khoury JC, Wedig K, et al. New Ballard Score, expanded to include extremely premature infants. *J Pediatrics.* 1991;119:417–423.

3. Nickavar A, Assadi F. Managing hypertension in the newborn infants. *Int J Prev Med.* 2014;5:S39–S43.

4. Centers for Disease Control and Prevention. Using the WHO growth charts to assess growth in the United States among children ages birth to 2 years. http://www.cdc.gov/growthcharts/clinical_charts.htm. Published April 15, 2015. Accessed January 9, 2018.

5. Toth B, Becker A, Seelbach-Göbel B. Oxygen saturation in healthy newborn infants immediately after birth measured by pulse oximetry. *Arch Gynecol Obstet.* 2002;266:105–107.

6. Murphy-Kaulbeck L, Dodds L, Joseph KS, et al. Single umbilical artery risk factors and pregnancy outcomes. *Obstet Gynecol.* 2010;116:843–850.

7. Silverman WA, Anderson DH. A controlled clinical trial of effects of water mist on obstructive respiratory signs, death rate and necropsy findings among premature infants. *Pediatrics.* 1956;17:1–6.

8. Kaye C. Introduction to the newborn screening fact sheets. *Pediatrics.* 2006;118:1301–1314.

9. Milcric TL. The complete blood count. *Neonatal Netw.* 2009;28:109–115.

10. Kim UO, Brousseau DC, Konduri GG. Evaluation and management of the critically ill neonate in the emergency department. *Clin Ped Emerg Med.* 2008;9:140–148.

7

Neonatal Stabilization and Resuscitation

Steven Sittig
Teresa A. Volsko

OUTLINE

OBJECTIVES

1. List the key elements needed to prepare for a high-risk delivery.
2. Describe the equipment needed to achieve and maintain a patent airway and to support ventilation following delivery.
3. Explain methods of preventing heat loss during stabilization of an infant following birth.
4. Describe how an Apgar score is assigned.
5. Discuss the importance of judicial oxygen use in the delivery room following birth.
6. Explain the role of CPAP during stabilization of a newborn.
7. List the indications for bag-mask ventilation.
8. Explain the method for selecting the appropriate-sized endotracheal tube during resuscitation.
9. Describe the two methods for performing chest compressions.
10. List the routes for emergency medication administration.
11. List the indications for epinephrine and volume expanders.
12. Explain the components of postresuscitative care.
13. List the ethical considerations related to resuscitation of a newborn.

KEY TERMS

acrocyanosis
Apgar score
chest compressions
epinephrine
intraosseous (IO)
sniffing position
STABLE
umbilical venous
    catheter (UVC)
volume expander

Introduction

In 2013, there were approximately 448,265 premature births, accounting for 11.4% of the total births in the United States for that year.[1] According to the American Heart Association, approximately 10% of newborns require some type of intervention at birth to initiate spontaneous respirations, fewer than 1% require extensive resuscitation,[2] and a significant number may require some degree of resuscitation.[3] Three screening questions may be useful in identifying whether a newborn will require delivery room resuscitation:

- Is the newborn term or 40 weeks' gestation?
- Does the newborn have good tone?
- Is the newborn breathing or crying?

If the answer to all three questions is yes, there is generally no need for resuscitation and routine care (the infant is dried, placed skin to skin with the mother, and covered with dry linen to maintain a normal temperature) can be provided in the delivery room. Observation of breathing, activity, and color must be ongoing.

If the answer to any of these assessment questions is no, then the infant should be moved to a radiant warmer to receive initial stabilization and care. In the event resuscitation is required, a well-trained and specially equipped team must be available at all times to attend at-risk deliveries or deliveries where more than routine care is anticipated.

A maternal history may help predict the need for resuscitation in the delivery room. Perinatal asphyxia and extreme prematurity are the two complications of pregnancy that most frequently necessitate complex resuscitation by skilled personnel. However, only 60% of asphyxiated newborns can be predicted antepartum, with the remaining newborns identified at the time of birth. Birthweight is another predictor of the need for resuscitation: Nearly 80% of low-birthweight infants require resuscitation and stabilization at delivery.[4]

Preparing for a High-Risk Delivery

Preparing for a high-risk delivery, or the delivery of an infant who may require more than routine care, provides the direct care team with all of the tools needed to work effectively together. Preparation involves ensuring the following: (1) that a team skilled in neonatal assessment and resuscitation is present to provide care; (2) that equipment essential to assess, intervene, and stabilize the patient is available for use; and (3) that essential equipment is functioning properly.[5]

Environmental Preparation

During the transition from intra- to extrauterine life, the infant will be covered with amniotic fluid, or the fluid that supported the infant in utero. This wet infant, taking their first breaths, does not have the physiologic capabilities to keep warm. Specifically, infants have a limited amount of subcutaneous fat and an increased surface-area-to-weight ratio, which contributes to rapid heat loss. Additionally, infants are not effectively able to shiver. These capabilities are even more limited when the infant is born prematurely. Therefore, it is important to assess and provide care to an infant in an environment that will minimize hypothermia.

A radiant warmer provides a stable surface upon which to evaluate and provide care to the patient in a warm environment. Performance steps related to environmental preparation include preheating the radiant warmer and gathering and laying out towels or blankets to dry the infant. The temperature for a radiant warmer is generally set at 35.6°C and adjusted after the infant is dried and their temperature assessed.

A clock or timer mounted to or near the radiant warmer is helpful for timing assessments and interventions and tracking the length of time resuscitation efforts are employed. A cardiorespiratory monitor and pulse oximeter provide noninvasive assessment of vital signs and oxygenation status.

Equipment and Supplies

Equipment and supplies needed to secure and maintain a patient airway and support ventilation must be readily available and assessed to ensure proper working order. It is much easier to troubleshoot an equipment malfunction before it is needed for use; ensuring the equipment is available and working properly avoids delays in care and the risk of adverse events. Although less frequently used, vascular access supplies and medications to support resuscitation efforts during collapse must also be readily available.

Suction

Suction equipment and supplies are instrumental to clearing the airway. A bulb syringe may be helpful for clearing visible secretions form the nares and oropharynx. A mechanical suction source, secretion collection canister, and suction catheters should also be readily available and tested to ensure proper function. If the suction apparatus has intermittent and continuous modes available for use, select the "continuous" mode. Evaluate the negative pressure of the suction apparatus by occluding the end suction tubing used to attach a suction catheter. While occluded, suction pressure should range between 80 and 100 mm Hg, and pressure should return to 0 when the occluded end of the tubing is released. **Table 7-1** provides a complete list of suction supplies.

Ventilation Equipment

Equipment should be available to assess breathing and to provide assisted ventilation if needed. Devices

TABLE 7-1
Suction Equipment and Supplies

Type of Equipment	Supplies
Bulb syringe	

Mechanical suction	Suction source
	    Electrically powered device
	    Wall suction with regulator
	Supplies
	    Canister and connector tubing
	Suction catheters
	    5 or 6 F, 8 F, 10 F, 12 or 14 F
	Meconium aspirator

may require manual use, or they can be automatically programmed to deliver a set pressure and FiO_2. Flow-inflating, self-inflating, or T-piece resuscitators can be used in the delivery room. It is important to factor in the skill levels of care providers when selecting the type of resuscitator used, as some require more training and finesse for use. Regardless of the type of resuscitator selected, all staff responsible for the care of an infant in the delivery room must have adequate training in the use of the device.

Flow-inflating resuscitators lack a nonrebreathing valve and are capable of providing free-flow oxygen, assisted ventilation, or continuous positive airway pressure (CPAP). Flow-inflating bags require an oxygen source to function, while self-inflating resuscitators, or bag-valve resuscitators, incorporate a nonrebreathing valve between the patient connector and self-inflating compressible unit. Although an oxygen source is not required for this device to function, supplemental oxygen is required during resuscitation. The nonrebreathing valve prevents the delivery of free-flow oxygen or CPAP to an infant. When needed, a different device or oxygen tubing connected to a source gas must be used to provide CPAP or free-flow oxygen, respectively, to the infant.

An oxygen blender should be available to provide variable concentrations of oxygen to the manual resuscitators or to connect to tubing, to provide free-flow oxygen, if needed. A T-piece resuscitator connects to a high-pressure oxygen source and has an adjustable FiO_2. Small-bore tubing and a source must be available to provide free-flow oxygen if a self-inflating resuscitator is used to provide ventilation.

A T-piece resuscitator has an adjustable pressure setting and can provide positive pressure ventilation, CPAP, or free-flow oxygen to the patient. There are two types of T-piece resuscitators to choose from; both the Neo-Tee Infant T-Piece Resuscitator (Mercury Medical, Clearwater, FL) and the Neopuff Infant T-Piece Resuscitator (Fisher & Paykel Healthcare, East Tamaki, New Zealand) connect directly to an oxygen flowmeter.

These devices have an adjustable pressure setting and manometer built in to monitor delivered pressures during manual ventilation or CPAP. Table 7-2 compares the three most common devices used in a delivery room to provide oxygen and ventilatory support.

Resuscitation masks are available in a variety of sizes to accommodate the facial size of a range of infants. One of each size—small, medium, and large—should be available for use. Table 7-3 lists the equipment required to provide oxygen and to assess and support ventilation.

Intubation Equipment

Although equipment used to establish and maintain an airway may not be needed, it is important to anticipate and plan for its use. In addition to a laryngoscope, blades, and an artificial airway or endotracheal tube (ETT), it is important to have supplies to verify tracheal placement and to secure the ETT. Table 7-4 outlines the equipment needed to perform and support postintubation care. The availability of disposable laryngoscope blades and handles may minimize the need to have extra bulbs for the blades or batteries for the handle on hand.

Vascular Access Supplies

It may be necessary to administer medications to an infant in cardiopulmonary collapse. The umbilical vein provides an accessible vessel for cannulation; the equipment necessary to catheterize and secure umbilical vessels is found in Table 7-5.

Resuscitative Drugs

A small number of medications need to be readily available for resuscitation in the delivery room. Table 7-6 lists these medications, along with the rationale for their use and concentrations. The list is limited to medications that increase the rate and force of cardiac contractions, reverse narcotic-induced respiratory failure, and treat hypovolemia.

Transport Equipment

Following delivery room care or resuscitation, infants needing more than routine postnatal care require a vehicle for transport to a special care or neonatal intensive care unit. Either a transport isolette or a radiant warmer with a transport trolley can be used. During equipment preparation, the compressed gas source must be assessed to ensure an adequate gas supply is available for use. The units should also contain a cardiorespiratory monitor and pulse oximeter. The transport device should be connected to an electrical outlet, turned on, and warmed to minimize heat loss and prevent hypothermia during transport to a definitive care unit.

TABLE 7-2
Equipment Used to Achieve and Maintain Ventilatory Support

Feature	Type of Resuscitator		
	Self-Inflating	Flow-Inflating	T-Piece
	Courtesy of SunMed.	Courtesy of SunMed.	Courtesy of Mercury Medical. Courtesy of Fisher & Paykel Healthcare.
Requires a gas source to function	No	Yes	Yes
Delivers exact concentrations of oxygen from the blended gas source	No	Yes	Yes
Monitors delivered pressures with a built-in manometer	Not all brands	Not all brands	Yes
Delivers free-flow oxygen	No	Yes	Yes
Provides reliable control of peak inspiratory pressure (PIP) and positive end-expiratory pressure (PEEP)	No	No	Yes
Provides CPAP	No	Yes	Yes
Requires a proprietary circuit to connect to the mask or endotracheal tube	No	No	Yes
Requires ventilating pressures to be set before use	No	No	Yes

TABLE 7-3
Equipment Required to Provide Oxygen, Assess, and Ventilate an Infant in the Delivery Room

Equipment Type	Rationale for Use
Stethoscope	Auscultate the presence and characteristics of breath sounds
Blender	Provides precise FiO_2 control
Oxygen tubing	For delivery of free-flow oxygen when a self-inflating resuscitator is available for use
Flow-inflating, self-inflating, or T-piece resuscitator Appropriate-size resuscitation bag has a volume of 450–750 mL	Provide ventilatory assistance Flow-inflating and T-piece resuscitators also provide CPAP and free-flow oxygen
Resuscitation mask	Provides a patient interface to facilitate resuscitator use
8 F feeding tube and 20-mL syringe	Allows for decompression of the stomach during ventilatory support with a resuscitator and mask

TABLE 7-4
Equipment and Supplies Needed for Endotracheal Intubation

Equipment	Specifications
Laryngoscope and blades	Number 00 for micro-preterm infants Number 0 blade for preterm infants Number 1 blade for term infants
Endotracheal tubes (mm internal diameter)	2.5 3.0 3.5 4.0
CO_2 detector	Colormetric device Capnography
ETT-securing device	Tape Commercially available ETT-securing device
Laryngeal mask airway	Sizes vary by brand and manufacturer
Ancillary supplies	Scissors Alcohol wipes Extra batteries (for the laryngoscope handle) Extra bulbs if nonfiberoptic blades are used

TABLE 7-5
Umbilical Vessel Catheterization Supply List

Sterile gloves
Scalpel
Scissors
Antiseptic solution to prepare the skin
Umbilical catheters (sized 3.5 and 5.0 F)
Three-way stop cock
Syringes of various sizes (1, 3, 5, 10, 20, and 50 mL)
Needles and IV tubing or a needleless tubing set
Umbilical tape

Neonatal Stabilization

A detailed perinatal history is helpful in determining the need for intervention in the delivery room. Chapter 5 reviews the maternal risk factors that compromise the health of an infant at birth. There may be occasions where there is insufficient time to collect a detailed maternal history, or a detailed history cannot be obtained. Information regarding the approximate gestational age of the infant, length of time membranes were ruptured, administration of antenatal steroids, presence (oligohydramnios, polyhydramnios) and characteristics of the amniotic fluid (foul smelling, meconium stained, etc.), and number of infants to be delivered helps the direct care team anticipate the interventions needed.

The initial steps, outlined next, are listed separately. However, it is important to note that care to the infant should be provided as a continuous, coordinated process.

Preventing Heat Loss and Cold Stress

Providing warmth is the first step in an infant's resuscitation. The infant should be placed on a preheated radiant warmer to help prevent heat loss and to allow the resuscitation team the ability to constantly assess the infant. Preventing heat loss in the newborn is vital because cold stress can increase oxygen consumption and impede effective resuscitation.[6,7] Hypothermia also contributes to perinatal respiratory depression.[8,9] The temperature of newly born, nonasphyxiated infants should be maintained between 36.5°C and 37.5°C after birth during resuscitation or stabilization.[10,11]

Warmed blankets or towels used to dry the infant should be quickly removed, as wet linen contributes to heat loss. Polyethylene bags may be used as an additional measure to reduce the risk of heat loss and mortality

TABLE 7-6
Resuscitative Drugs

Drug Class/Description	Medication	Use	Preparation
Adrenergic agonist	Epinephrine	Increase rate and force of cardiac contractions	Ampules (3 or 5 mL) of a 1:10,000 solution
Isotonic saline solution	Normal saline (0.9% NaCl)	Treat hypovolemia from indirect blood loss Intravenous flush	250 mL
Crystalloid balanced electrolyte solution	Lactated Ringer's	Treat hypovolemia from indirect blood loss Replenish electrolytes	250 mL
Opioid antagonist	Naloxone	To reverse narcotic-induced respiratory depression Used in the postresuscitation phase, if needed	1 mg/mL

in infants weighing less than 1500 grams.[12] Exothermic mattresses or warming mattresses can also be used to reduce the risk of heat loss. However, the literature reports that the use of a warming mattress in conjunction with a polyethylene bag does not improve outcomes; rather, more infants had body temperatures outside the target range of 36.5 and 37.5°C when a warming mattress was used in addition to a polyethylene bag.[13]

Continuous temperature monitoring is important to the ongoing care of the infant. This can be accomplished through serial axillary temperature readings or a skin temperature monitoring system connected to the radiant warmer. Many radiant warmers have systems to automatically control the heat output of the warmer based on the infant's skin temperature.

Securing and Maintaining a Patent Airway

Assessing the respiratory status is an important element of care. Properly positioning the infant on the warming table is a crucial first step. Achieving and securing a patent airway and maintaining adequate ventilation may minimize the need for additional resuscitative efforts.

Positioning to Prevent Airway Obstruction

The infant should be positioned supine with the neck slightly extended, as illustrated in **Figure 7-1**. The **sniffing position**, or positioning the infant supine with the neck slightly extended, aligns the posterior pharynx, larynx, and trachea. This position prevents airway obstruction and facilitates the initiation of assisted ventilation if needed. Neck flexion or hyperextension may partially or fully restrict air from entering the trachea from the upper airway.

Visual inspection of the infant's face and neck will identify craniofacial conditions that may make it challenging to achieve and maintain a patent airway (**Figure 7-2**). Infants with macroglossia or large tongues are prone to airway obstruction, as the tongue may inherently obstruct air from moving into the trachea by virtue of its size. Infants with Pierre Robin syndrome

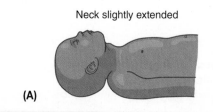

Neck slightly extended

(A)

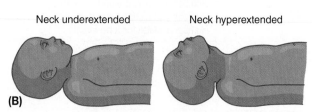

Neck underextended   Neck hyperextended

(B)

FIGURE 7-1 Comparison of head positions in infants. (**A**) Correct or sniffing position. (**B**) Incorrect position showing hyperextension and flexion.

have a short chin and a posteriorly positioned trachea, making it difficult to align the upper airway structures and trachea and minimize airway obstruction. Although airway obstruction may not be a concern with an infant with a cleft palate, it may be more difficult to provide supplemental oxygen or ventilatory support. Ineffective respiratory effort may be a sign of airway obstruction. Caregivers should reposition the infant's head and reassess respiratory effort.

Clearing Airway Secretions

Amniotic fluid, secretions, and, in some instances, meconium must be cleared from the upper airway. A bulb syringe or suction catheter can be used to gently clear the airway and to prevent airway obstruction or aspiration. Secretions in the mouth should be cleared first, followed by suctioning of the nares (**Figure 7-3**). When using a suction catheter, vacuum pressures should not exceed 100 mm Hg.[2] To avoid laryngeal spasms, bradycardia, pharyngeal or laryngeal epithelial injury, or atelectasis, limit the time of each suction pass to

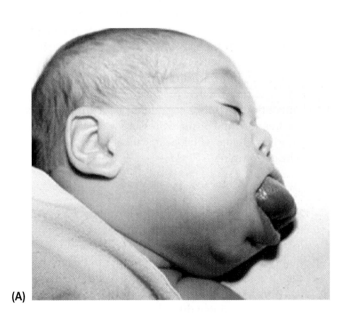

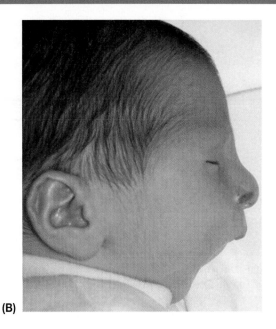

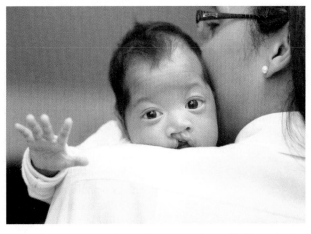

FIGURE 7-2 Conditions that make it challenging to secure and maintain a patent airway. (**A**) Macroglossia. (**B**) Pierre Robin Syndrome. (**C**) Cleft palate.

(**A**) Courtesy of Cleft and Craniofacial Center at Cincinnati Children's Hospital Medical Center; (**B**) Sesenna E, Magri A, Magnani C, Brevi B, and Anghinoni M. Mandibular distraction in neonates: Indications, techniques, results. *Italian Journal of Pediatrics.* 2012;38:7. Courtesy of Dr. E. Sesenna; (**C**) © Peoplelmages/iStock/Getty Images Plus.

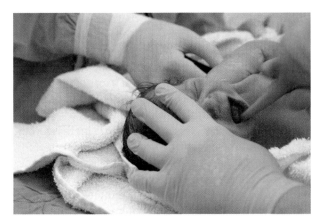

FIGURE 7-3 Suctioning with a bulb syringe gently removes secretions and amniotic fluid from the airway.

© Voorheis/iStock/Getty Images Plus.

3 to 5 seconds. The American Heart Association and the American Academy of Pediatrics made substantial changes to suctioning and airway management guidelines for neonatal resuscitation based on available evidence in the literature. The changes were based on the lack of evidence to support the benefit of some routine suctioning practices in the delivery room. Routine intrapartum suctioning and intubation to suction secretions for nonvigorous infants is no longer recommended.[2]

Should the infant require direct laryngotracheal suctioning, intubate the trachea with an ETT and directly apply suction to the ETT. There are commercially available adaptors that enable the suction source to easily attach to the ETT. **Figure 7-4** illustrates how a meconium aspirator adaptor can be used to connect the tubing from the suction source to the ETT. The meconium

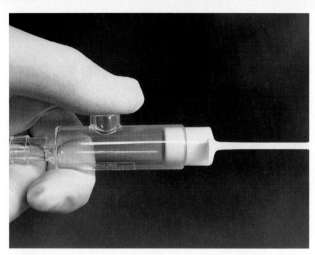

FIGURE 7-4 A meconium aspiratory adaptor can be used to connect the ETT to the suction tubing from the suction source.
Courtesy of Neotech Products.

aspirator adaptor has an opening that, when occluded by the thumb, applies suction pressure to the airway. Vagal stimulation can occur during suctioning, so it is important to closely monitor the infant's heart rate.

Assessing the Neonate

Assessment of an infant during the transition to extra-uterine provides caregivers with the information needed to direct care. Primary evaluation of an infant following delivery consists of appraising respiratory effort, heart rate, and skin color.

Respiratory Effort

Evaluation of the infant's respiratory effort is also an ongoing process. Assess the rate, depth, and ease of respiratory effort. When ineffective respiratory efforts are noted, reposition the infant's head and neck to a sniffing position. Mild stimulation may be needed to increase the rate and depth of respiration by rubbing the infant's back or flicking the bottom of the feet. However, it should not be necessary to continue to stimulate an infant in order to restore a normal respiratory rate. Infants requiring stimulation only to restore a normal or near-normal respiratory rate will respond quickly; therefore, provide stimulation for a maximum of two efforts. Infants with apnea, frequent apneic spells, or gasping respiratory efforts require assisted ventilation to reduce hypoxemia during their transition to extra-uterine life.[2] After birth, infants with ineffective respiratory rate and effort will seldom have a heart rate within the normal range.

Heart Rate

The heart rate can be assessed several ways: (1) lightly grasping the base of the umbilical cord and feeling for a pulse, (2) listening over the heart with a stethoscope for the heartbeat, or (3) palpating the brachial or femoral pulse. An infant should have a heart rate faster than 100 beats per minute.

However, if the heart rate is less than 100 beats per minute, initiate positive pressure ventilation with a T-piece resuscitator or bag and mask.[2] External cardiac compressions and positive pressure ventilation are required for infants with a heart rate of fewer than 60 beats per minute.[2]

Skin Color

During the first few breaths after birth, the infant's circulatory system will transition from fetal circulation. As the lungs begin to provide oxygen to the blood supplied systemically, changes in the color of the newborn infant's skin from a bluish to pinkish color will occur. Assessing an infant's central perfusion can be accomplished by examining the color of the mucous membranes: An uncompromised newborn infant will have pink mucous membranes, while central cyanosis or a bluish color of the face, trunk, and mucous membranes is a sign of tissue hypoxemia.

Often, for the first few minutes of life, **acrocyanosis**, or a bluish color of the hands and feet, is present. Acrocyanosis is usually a normal finding at birth caused by decreased extremity circulation and is not a reliable indicator of low oxygen levels. However, it may indicate other conditions, such as cold stress. Continuous noninvasive monitoring can be helpful; noninvasive temperature monitoring can alert clinicians to cold stress and provides additional data to differentiate a normal from an abnormal finding, such as in the case of acrocyanosis. Pulse oximetry is a reliable method of assessing oxygenation in the delivery room and is an adjunct to the skin assessment for signs of central cyanosis.

Apgar Score

The **Apgar score**, first described in the early 1950s, is the oldest and most commonly used assessment tool for the evaluation of the newborn in the delivery room.[14] This scoring system evaluates the presence and characteristics of five parameters: heart rate, respiratory rate, skin color, reflex irritability, and muscle tone (**Table 7-7**). Total scores range from 0 to 10. The score was designed to provide a systematic way to evaluate newborns and to guide clinical care. Infants with lower scores, such as scores less than 5, require more rigorous clinical intervention. The first score is assigned at 1 minute of age, and the newborn is rescored at 5 minutes of age to evaluate their ability to adapt to extrauterine life. Infants scoring less than 7 at 5 minutes of age are generally reassessed every 5 minutes until a score of 7 or greater is obtained.

Infants who are significantly compromised at birth require prompt intervention. It is important to note that

TABLE 7-7
The Apgar Scoring System

Acronym Letter	Parameter (Description)	Apgar Score		
		0	1	2
A	Skin color (Appearance)	Pale Blue	Body pink, extremities blue	Body and extremities pink
P	Heart rate (Pulse)	None	<100 beats/min	>100 beats/min
G	Reflex irritability in response to stimuli (Grimace)	No response	Grimace	Cry Cough Sneeze
A	Muscle tone (Activity)	Limp	Some flexion	Well flexed
R	Respiratory effort	None	Weak Irregular	Strong cry

Data from Apgar V. A proposal for a new method of evaluation of the newborn infant. *Curr Res Anesth Analg.* 1953;32(4):260–267.

interventions should never be delayed or interrupted to obtain a score. A low Apgar score (0–3) at 5 minutes of age is strongly associated with the risk of infant death.[15] The likelihood of mortality was highest among newborns whose score remained at 0 after 10 minutes of resuscitation efforts.[16]

The use of this tool to predict outcomes for newborn infants may be limited. Depending on the gestational age, premature infants lack the developmental maturity to receive a higher score and will inherently score lower.[17] For example, an infant born at 25 weeks' gestation will not have the lung maturity to support an effective respiratory rate and effort and will also lack irritability reflexes and muscle tone. Modifications of the Apgar score are reported in the literature; these tools assess the newborn's condition independent of gestational age and interventions. The score assigned by modified Apgar scoring tools represents the medical interventions and the neonatal condition.[18] These modified Apgar scores range from 0 to 17 points: A score of 17 describes a newborn with a clinical condition that does not require intervention, and a score of 0 describes an infant failing to respond to aggressive resuscitative interventions.

Neonatal Resuscitation

Delivery room management requires skill and a coordinated interdisciplinary team effort. Routine care encompasses drying the infant, removing wet linens, and providing a warm environment that minimizes cold stress during transition to extrauterine life. Assessing

the newborn is also an important component of routine care. During the initial assessment, assuring the infant is in the sniffing position helps to maintain a patent airway. However, routine care may not be sufficient to stabilize some infants in the delivery room and additional interventions, such as resuscitation, may be needed. When the assessment indicates the need, resuscitation should begin immediately. Resuscitative interventions an infant receives in the delivery room are assessment-based and include oxygen delivery, assisted ventilation, external cardiac compressions, or medications.

Administering Oxygen

For many years, the use of 100% oxygen was recommended in newborn resuscitation to quickly improve oxygen saturation. However, in 2010, the American Academy of Pediatrics and the American Heart Association amended this long-held tenet because of the growing evidence in the literature for the potential for lung injury due to prolonged oxidative stress, which may last up to 12 weeks in a term infant.[19] Administering 100% oxygen to hypoxic newborns immediately after birth delays cardiopulmonary recovery and causes a fourfold increase in the risk of mortality. The literature also reports an increased risk for iatrogenic lung injury due to oxygen toxicity in preterm infants receiving 100% oxygen during delivery room resuscitation.[20,21]

Judicious use of oxygen in the delivery room, guided by monitoring of preductal oxygen saturations, is recommended. The recommendations are based on the normal physiologic changes that occur during the transition from fetal to extrauterine circulation shortly after birth. The American Heart Association and the American Academy of Pediatrics recommend frequent preductal oxygen assessments by pulse oximetry, at 1 minute intervals for the first 5 minutes of life, followed by an assessment at 10 minutes. To obtain a preductal saturation, attach the pulse oximeter probe to the infant's right hand or wrist. The timing of assessments and targeted preductal oxygen saturations are outlined in **Table 7-8**.[2]

Supplemental oxygen delivered by an oxygen blender can be delivered through a face mask and flow-inflating bag, an oxygen mask, or a hand cupped around oxygen tubing. The oxygen source should deliver a flow of at least 5 L/minute, and the delivery device should be held close to the face to maximize the inhaled concentration. If supplemental oxygen is to be provided for a prolonged period, heated and humidified oxygen should be delivered to the newborn. Self-inflating bags should not be used to passively deliver oxygen because flow cannot be delivered until the bladder of the resuscitation bag is squeezed.

The goal of oxygen therapy during resuscitation is to provide sufficient oxygen delivery to the tissues. Clinically, the ideal oxygen concentration for use during resuscitation remains unknown. To prevent harm associated with hyperoxia and/or hypoxia, oxygen delivery

TABLE 7-8
Neonatal Resuscitation Program (NRP) Guidelines for Targeted Preductal Oxygen Saturations Following Delivery

Timing of Assessment (minutes after birth)	SpO$_2$
1	60–65%
2	65–70%
3	70–75%
4	75–80%
5	85–90%
10	90–95%

Data from Wyckoff MH, Aziz K, Escobedo MB, et al. Part 13: Neonatal resuscitation 2015 American Heart Association guidelines update for cardiopulmonary resuscitation and emergency cardiovascular care. *Circulation.* 2015;132(suppl 2):S543–S560.

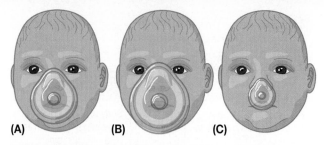

(A)   **(B)**   **(C)**

FIGURE 7-5 (**A**) A properly fitting resuscitation mask will cover the nose and mouth but will not cover the eyes. (**B**) Masks that are too large will cover the eyes. (**C**) Masks that are too small will not adequately cover the nose and mouth.

should be titrated according to the Neonatal Resuscitation Program (NRP) target levels outlined in Table 7-8.

CPAP and Positive Pressure Ventilation

Infants may need respiratory support that extends beyond administration of supplemental oxygen. The type and amount of support depends on the infant's respiratory effort.

CPAP Administration

The lungs of infants born prematurely, fewer than 36 weeks' gestation, are surfactant-deficient and may have difficulty achieving adequate functional residual capacity (FRC) and maintaining acceptable alveolar ventilation. Administration of CPAP, at a minimum of 4 to 5 cm H$_2$O, in the delivery room assists with lung expansion, establishes FRC, and improves oxygenation for infants in mild to moderate respiratory distress who may not be able to generate sufficient negative intrathoracic pressure to achieve or maintain adequate ventilation. CPAP can be applied through the use of a T-piece resuscitator or flow-inflating bag connected to a resuscitation mask. When a flow-inflating resuscitation bag is used to provide CPAP, a manometer should always be used to monitor applied pressures. Oxygen delivery in conjunction with CPAP therapy should follow the aforementioned NRP guidelines.

Bag-Mask Ventilation

Positive pressure ventilation is indicated when the infant is apneic, has ineffective respiratory effort, and/or has a heart rate below 100 beats per minute despite administration of 100% oxygen.[2] Assisted ventilation should be delivered at a rate of ventilation of 40 to 60 breaths per minute. Although positive pressure ventilation can be provided with various interfaces, bag-mask ventilation is the quickest and is an essential skill in resuscitation. Mask selection is very important to ensure a proper fit: The mask should cover the nose and mouth, without covering the eyes. **Figure 7-5** illustrates proper and improper mask fit.

Manual ventilation may be provided by a flow-inflating resuscitation bag, self-inflating resuscitation bag, or T-piece resuscitator. During manual ventilation, care must be taken to avoid delivery of excessive ventilating pressures, which can cause pulmonary injury. NRP guidelines recommended initially delivering positive pressure ventilation at an inspiratory pressure of 20 cm H$_2$O.[2] Providing effective bag-mask ventilation will result in an improvement in heart rate (i.e., increase in heart rate to greater than 100 beats per minute), skin color, and oxygen saturation. Observing chest rise is not a reliable method of determining the adequacy of ventilation because the chest may rise when inadequate or excessive pressures are delivered to the newborn.

If positive pressure ventilation does not result in an increase in heart rate and/or oxygen saturations within 5 to 10 breaths, corrective action must be taken. Assess the fit of the mask on the newborn's face to assure the seal is adequate. Reapply the mask on the infant's face and lift the jaw forward slightly to keep the mouth slightly open and to maintain the head in a sniffing position. Commonly, a leak in the mask seal will occur between the cheek and the bridge of the nose. Take care when reapplying the mask to avoid applying excessive pressure to the newborn's face. The fingers of the clinician ventilating the newborn should rest on the lower jaw; be certain to avoid touching the neck or soft tissue under the chin while holding the mask in place, as pressure to these areas will contribute to upper airway obstruction (**Figure 7-6**). Reattempt ventilation. If the infant's heart rate, oxygen saturation, and color still

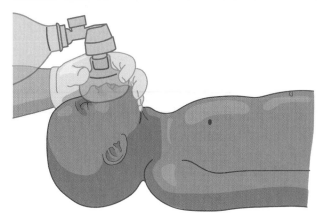

FIGURE 7-6 An illustration of proper hand position during bag-mask ventilation.

TABLE 7-9
Troubleshooting Techniques to Improve Manual Ventilation

Reapply the mask to the infant's face.
Reposition the head to the sniffing position.
Suction the mouth and nose if secretions are present.
Open the newborn's mouth slightly and lift the jaw forward.
Increase pressure gradually every few breaths until the heart rate and oxygen saturations improve.
Consider inserting an airway, such as a laryngeal mask airway or an endotracheal tube.

---

do not improve, increase the amount of positive pressure delivered with each breath. Although a majority of patients will respond to lower ventilating pressures, it is occasionally necessary to ventilate with higher pressures; however, pressures greater than 30 cm H_2O are rarely required. A list of troubleshooting techniques can be found in **Table 7-9**. Ideally, the manual resuscitator should have the ability to deliver postive end-expiratory pressure (PEEP). A flow-inflating resuscitation bag and T-piece resuscitator have the ability to deliver PEEP without an external attachment. An external PEEP value should be used when a self-inflating resuscitation bag is used for manual ventilation.

Ventilation with an Endotracheal Tube or Airway Adjunct

The majority of newborns can be adequately managed with a T-piece resuscitator or bag-mask ventilation. When these methods are not adequate, however, it is time to move to a more secure airway. If the current bedside staff is unfamiliar or does not have experience with intubating infants, continue mask ventilation until more-experienced help arrives. Expertise in neonatal

airway management requires an understanding of early human anatomical development as well as a set of clinical skills to provide safe tracheal intubation, especially in a preterm newborn.

The decision to intubate or to use an alternative airway depends on the condition of the newborn. The proper equipment must always be available and ready for immediate use. Endotracheal intubation or an alternate airway should be considered in the following instances:

- Tracheal suctioning for meconium is required
- Bag-mask ventilation is ineffective or prolonged
- Chest compressions are performed
- Tracheal administration of medications, such as surfactant, is necessary
- Special resuscitation circumstances, such as congenital diaphragmatic hernia or extremely low birthweight

The proper ETT size for newborns can be roughly estimated by dividing the gestational age by 10; for example, a clinician would select a 3.5-mm ID ETT for a newborn at 35 weeks' gestation. Endotracheal intubation is typically completed orally, using a laryngoscope with a straight blade. Chapter 22 outlines the intubation procedure. Confirmation that the ETT is placed correctly is essential. A colorimetric CO_2 detector or capnography can be used to differentiate an esophageal from a tracheal intubation. Observing symmetrical chest wall motion and listening for equal breath sounds, especially in the axillae, and for the absence of breath sounds over the stomach are secondary measures. However, a chest radiograph is currently the only method of verifying the depth of tracheal tube placement.

When a clinician skilled in endotracheal intubation is not readily available and bag-mask ventilation is ineffective, an airway adjunct, such as a laryngeal mask airway, may be inserted to facilitate ventilation.[22,23] Recent international resuscitation guidelines recommend the use of a laryngeal mask airway when bag-mask ventilation is ineffective and endotracheal intubation is unsuccessful or not available in newborns at or older than 34 weeks' gestation. Data are limited for their use in preterm infants delivered at fewer than 34 weeks of gestation or who weigh less than 2000 grams. Use of the laryngeal mask has not been evaluated during chest compressions or for administration of emergency medications.[2]

Provide Chest Compressions

Chest compressions are indicated in newborns with a heart rate of fewer than 60 beats per minute after stimulation and 30 seconds of positive pressure ventilation have been provided. Newborns with a heart rate of fewer than 50 beats per minute are likely hypoxic and acidotic, which can lead to depressed myocardial function and a

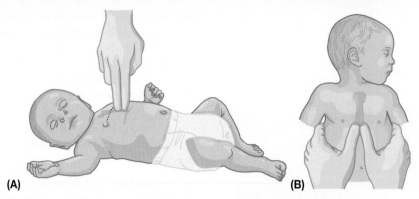

FIGURE 7-7 CPR can be performed using the (**A**) two-finger method or the (**B**) two-thumb technique.

decrease in cardiac output. Effective chest compressions must be coordinated with assisted ventilation.

Two different methods can be used to perform chest compressions in the newborn: the two-thumb technique and the two-fingers method;[2,13] the literature reports that use of the two-thumb technique generates higher blood pressures and coronary perfusion pressure and reduces rescuer fatigue.[24–26] To perform the two-thumb technique, place the thumbs of both hands on the lower third of the infant's sternum, cradle the fingers around the infant's back and chest, and compress the sternum toward the spine with the thumbs. To perform the two-finger method, place the fingertips of the index and middle fingers of one hand on the lower third of the sternum and compress the sternum toward the spine. Most clinicians prefer to use their dominant hand for the compressions, while the other hand is placed under the infant along the thoracic spine to provide a firmer surface to compress against. **Figure 7-7** illustrates the hand position for both techniques. Compress the chest a distance equal to one-third of the anterior-posterior diameter of the chest. Allow the chest to re-expand fully during relaxation, without removing the thumbs or fingers, depending on the technique used, from the chest. External cardiac compressions are performed at a rate of 120 per minute, accompanied by manual ventilation at 30 breaths per minute.[2,27,28] The cadence for newborn compression to ventilation is usually verbalized by the clinician performing the cardiac compressions as "One and Two and Three (compressions) and breath," with manual ventilation performed each time the word "breath" is spoken.

Obtain Vascular Access

During resuscitation, medications may be administered either by endotracheal instillation or intravenously, though intravenous administration remains the most reliable route for medication delivery. For newborns, cannulation of the umbilical vein provides easy direct vascular access. An umbilical stump contains two arteries and one vein; the umbilical vein is the largest of the three vessels and has thinner walls, compared to the umbilical arteries. **Figure 7-8** shows the location of the umbilical vessels. The vein is located at the 11 or 12 o'clock position, compared to the arteries, which lie in close proximity to each other at the 4 and 8 o'clock positions. The umbilical vein remains patent and viable for cannulation until approximately 1 week after birth.

During cannulation of term or near-term infants, the tip of the catheter should lie a short distance from the insertion point, or approximately 1 to 2 cm beyond the point at which good blood return is obtained. Catheter malposition has been associated with morbidity and mortality. Low-lying venous catheters are associated with an increased incidence of intraventricular hemorrhage and death in preterm infants who are less than 29 weeks' gestation.[29] Catheters inserted too high may cause hepatic damage by infusing medications directly into the liver.[30] Following resuscitation, the **umbilical venous catheter (UVC)** may either be removed or secured in place for continued venous access. If secured in place, a chest radiograph should be obtained to confirm placement.

Intraosseous (IO) access also provides an acceptable route for vascular access. Vascular access by this method may be easier and faster during newborn resuscitation if the direct care team lacks experience with umbilical venous placement.[31]

Administer Medications

Neonatal resuscitation drugs should be available in locations where births take place, including labor and

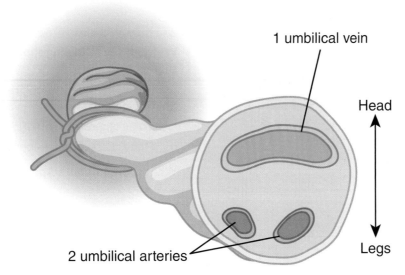

1 umbilical vein

Head

2 umbilical arteries

Legs

FIGURE 7-8 Position of the umbilical vein and arteries.

delivery rooms, operating rooms, and the emergency department (ED). Personnel responsible for the direct care of the newborn must be familiar with medications and their concentrations, dosages, and routes of administration. Resuscitation drugs currently recommended include epinephrine (1:10,000) and isotonic sodium chloride solution (0.9%) as an intravascular volume expansion agent. During cardiopulmonary resuscitation of a newborn, as medications are prepared for administration, positive pressure ventilation and chest compressions should remain uninterrupted.

Epinephrine

Epinephrine remains the primary vasopressor for use in neonatal resuscitation. Epinephrine is recommended for a heart rate of fewer than 60 beats per minute after 30 seconds of adequate positive pressure ventilation with 100% oxygen and chest compressions. Epinephrine increases coronary perfusion pressure primarily through peripheral vasoconstriction, which increases blood flow to the brain and coronary arteries.

Current neonatal resuscitation guidelines recommend prompt IV administration of epinephrine in a dose of 0.01 to 0.03 mg/kg (1:10,000 solution) by umbilical venous catheter or IO.[2] Endotracheal administration results in unpredictable absorption and may require higher doses than those administered by an IV route.[32] High-dose epinephrine poses additional risks to premature and asphyxiated newborn infants and does not result in better long-term survival than conventional doses.[33]

Volume Expanders

Volume expansion (using crystalloids or red blood cells) is recommended when blood loss is suspected. Typically, these infants will have poor perfusion and present as pale, with a weak pulse or low heart rate despite effective resuscitation.[2]

Isotonic saline may also be used as a **volume expander**. Volume expanders are administered at the recommended dose of 10 mL/kg.[2] It may be necessary to administer additional boluses of either crystalloids or red blood cells. During the resuscitation of a premature infant, care should be taken to avoid rapid administration of volume expanders, as rapid infusion of large volumes of fluid have been associated with intraventricular hemorrhage.[2,3]

Postresuscitation Care

Newborns receiving delivery room resuscitation require frequent assessment, cardiopulmonary monitoring, and comprehensive care to support their nutritional, hemodynamic, and ventilatory needs. The mnemonic **STABLE** is used to represent the six parameters essential to newborn assessment in the aftermath of resuscitation. The core assessment parameters include blood **S**ugar monitoring and treatment, **T**emperature stabilization and maintenance, maintaining a patent **A**irway, normalizing **B**lood pressure, obtaining **L**ab work to assess acid–base and electrolyte balance, and providing the family with **E**motional support.[34] The essential elements of assessment and comprehensive care should be provided in preparation for, during transport to, and during admission to a neonatal care unit.

Case Study

A respiratory therapist is called to attend the delivery of a term infant. The mother has had no prenatal care and reports that her "water broke" several days ago.

Immediately following vaginal delivery, the infant was placed on a preheated radiant warmer and dried with warmed towels. The infant was placed in a sniffing position and assessed. The following data are available at 1 minute of age:

- Respiratory rate: 15 breaths per minute, with weak, irregular effort
- Color: Pale, with central cyanosis
- Response to stimuli: Grimace
- Muscle tone: Limp
- Heart rate: 97 beats per minute

1. **Which of the following should the respiratory therapist do first?**
   a. Provide 100% free-flow oxygen
   b. Intubate the trachea
   c. Provide bag-mask ventilation
   d. Initiate chest compressions

2. **What is the 1-minute Apgar score?**
   a. 0
   b. 1
   c. 3
   d. 5

References

1. Centers for Disease Control and Prevention. *National Vital Statistics Reports*. 2015;64(1):1–68. https://www.cdc.gov/nchs/data/nvsr/nvsr64/nvsr64_01.pdf

2. Wyckoff MH, Aziz K, Escobedo MB, et al. Part 13: Neonatal resuscitation: 2015 American Heart Association guidelines update for cardiopulmonary resuscitation and emergency cardiovascular care. *Circulation*. 2015;132:S543–S460.

3. Kattwinkel J, Perlman JM, Aziz K, et al. Part 15: neonatal resuscitation: 2010 American Heart Association guidelines for cardiopulmonary resuscitation and emergency cardiovascular care. *Circulation*. 2010;122(suppl 3):S909–S919.

4. Tudehope D, Papadimos E, Gibbons K. Twelve-year review of neonatal deaths in the delivery room in a perinatal tertiary centre. *J Paediatr Child Health*. 2013;49(1):E40–E45.

5. Clifford M, Hunt RW. Neonatal resuscitation. *Best Pract Res Clin Anaesthesiol*. 2010;24(3):461–474.

6. Gandy GM, Adamson SK Jr, Cunningham N, Silverman WA, James LS. Thermal environment and acid-base homeostasis in human infants during the first few hours of life. *J Clin Invest*. 1964;43:751–758.

7. Dahm LS, James LS. Newborn temperature and calculated heat loss in the delivery room. *Pediatrics*. 1972;49:504–513.

8. Perlman JM. Maternal fever and neonatal depression: preliminary observations. *Clin Pediatr*. 1999;38:287–291.

9. Lieberman E, Lang J, Richardson DK, Frigoletto FD, Heffner LJ, Cohen A. Intrapartum maternal fever and neonatal outcome. *Pediatrics*. 2000;105:8–13.

10. Escobedo M. Moving from experience to evidence: changes in US Neonatal Resuscitation Program based on International Liaison Committee on Resuscitation Review. *J Perinatol*. 2008;28(Suppl 1):S35–S40.

11. American Academy of Pediatrics. Neonatal Resuscitation Program instructor update (Fall/Winter 2015). https://www.aap.org/en-us/Documents/NRP_Instructor_Update_Fall_Winter_2015_final.pdf. Accessed February 17, 2016.

12. Leadford AE, Warren JB, Manasyan A, et al. Plastic bags for prevention of hypothermia in preterm and low birth weight infants. *Pediatrics*. 2013;132(1):e128–e134.

13. McCarthy LK, Molloy EJ, Twomey AR, Murphy JF, O'Donnell CP. A randomized trial of exothermic mattresses for preterm newborns in polyethylene bags. *Pediatrics*. 2013;132(1):e135–e141.

14. Apgar V. A proposal for a new method of evaluation of the newborn infant. *Curr Res Anesth Analg*. 1953;32(4):260–267.

15. Iliodromiti S, Mackay DF, Smith GC, Pell JP, Nelson SM. Apgar score and the risk of cause-specific infant mortality: a population-based cohort study. *Lancet*. 2014;384(9956):1749–1755.

16. Pasupathy D, Wood AM, Pell JP, Fleming M, Smith GC. Rates of and factors associated with delivery-related perinatal death among term infants in Scotland. *JAMA*. 2009;302(6):660–668.

17. Rüdiger M, Küster H, Herting E, et al. Variations of Apgar score of very low birth weight infants in different neonatal intensive care units. *Acta Paediatr*. 2009;98(9):1433–1436.

18. Rüdiger M, Aguar M. Newborn assessment in the delivery room. *Neoreviews*. 2012;13;e336.

19. De Felice C, Bechelli S, Tonni G, Latini G, Hansmann G. Systematic underestimation of oxygen delivery in ventilated preterm infants. *Neonatology*. 2010;98(1):18–22.

20. Vento M, Moro M, Escrig R, et al. Preterm resuscitation with low oxygen causes less oxidative stress, inflammation, and chronic lung disease. *Pediatrics*. 2009;124:439–449.

21. Mendoza-Paredes A, Liu H, Schears G, et al. Resuscitation with 100% vs. 21% oxygen following brief repeated apnea selectively protects vulnerable neonatal brain regions from hypoxic injury. *Resuscitation*. 2008;76(2):261–270.

22. Szyld E, Aguilar A, Musante GA, et al.; Delivery Room Ventilation Devices Trial Group. Comparison of devices for newborn ventilation in the delivery room. *J Pediatr*. 2014;165:234–239.

23. Yang C, Zhu X, Lin W, et al. Randomized, controlled trial comparing laryngeal mask versus endotracheal intubation during neonatal resuscitation—a secondary publication. *BMC Pediatrics*. 2015;16:17.

24. Huynh TK, Hemway RJ, Perlman JM. The two-thumb technique using an elevated surface is preferable for teaching infant cardiopulmonary resuscitation. *J Pediatr*. 2012;161(4):658–661.

25. Christman C, Hemway RJ, Wyckoff MH, Perlman JM. The two-thumb is superior to the two-finger method for administering chest compressions in a manikin model of neonatal resuscitation. *Arch Dis Child Fetal Neonatal Ed*. 2011;96:F99–F101.

26. Whitelaw CC, Slywka B, Goldsmith LJ. Comparison of a two-finger versus two-thumb method for chest compressions by healthcare providers in an infant mechanical model. *Resuscitation*. 2000;43: 213–216.

27. Hemway RJ, Christman C, Perlman J. The 3:1 is superior to a 15:2 ratio in a newborn manikin model in terms of quality of chest compressions and number of ventilations. *Arch Dis Child Fetal Neonatal Ed*. 2013;98:F42–F45.

28. Kattwinkel J, ed. *Textbook of Neonatal Resuscitation*. 5th ed. Dallas, TX: American Heart Association; 2006.

29. Kurtom W, Quast D, Worley L, Oelberg DG. Incorrect umbilical vein catheterization is associated with severe periventricular hemorrhages and mortality in extremely premature newborns. *J Neonatal Perinatal Med*. 2016;9(1):67–72.

30. Grizelj R, Vukovic J, Bojanic K, et al. Severe liver injury while using umbilical venous catheter: case series and literature review. *Am J Perinatol*. 2014;31(11):965–974.

31. Keith K, Abe KK, Blum GT, Yamamoto LG. Intraosseous is faster and easier than umbilical venous catheterization in newborn emergency vascular access models. *Am J Emerg Med*. 2000;18(2): 126–129.

32. Barber CA, Wyckoff MH. Use and efficacy of endotracheal versus intravenous epinephrine during neonatal cardiopulmonary resuscitation in the delivery room. *Pediatrics*. 2006;118(3):1028–1034.

33. Weiner GM, Niermeyer S. Medications in neonatal resuscitation: epinephrine and the search for better alternative strategies. *Clin Perinatol*. 2012;39(4):843–855.

34. O'Neill N, Howlett AA. Evaluation of the impact of the S.T.A.B.L.E. Program on the pretransport care of the neonate. *Neonatal Netw*. 2007;26(3):153–159.

CHAPTER

8

Respiratory Diseases of the Newborn

Linda Allen-Napoli

Lisa Tyler

OUTLINE

OBJECTIVES

1. Discuss the neonatal expiratory diseases and associated respiratory distress.
2. Identify and differentiate causes of neonatal respiratory distress.
3. Discuss clinical symptoms and differential diagnosis for apnea of prematurity, transient tachypnea of the newborn, respiratory distress syndrome, neonatal pneumonia, meconium aspiration syndrome, and persistent pulmonary hypertension of the newborn.
4. Understand management techniques for respiratory diseases of the newborn.
5. Describe outcomes associated with respiratory diseases of the newborn.

KEY TERMS

air leak syndrome
apnea
apnea of prematurity
bronchopulmonary
   dysplasia (BPD)
chronic lung disease
   (CLD)
meconium aspiration
   syndrome (MAS)

neutral thermal
   environment
persistent pulmonary
   hypertension of the
   newborn (PPHN)
respiratory distress
   syndrome (RDS)
transient tachypnea of
   the newborn (TTN)

Introduction

In the immediate newborn period, neonatal respiratory disorders are the most common reason for an infant to be admitted to the intensive care unit. Respiratory distress affects up to 7% of all newborn infants and is more common as the level of prematurity increases. Newborns with respiratory distress must be evaluated promptly, as they can progress to respiratory failure and cardiopulmonary arrest.

There are several different respiratory disorders that can cause respiratory distress, insufficiency, and failure. Outcomes are directly related to the accuracy and timing of the differential diagnosis as well as to the implementation of appropriate management. Neonatal respiratory diseases can affect infant survival or mortality and the occurrence of chronic disorders that may have a significant effect on the developing infant and their family.

Apnea of Prematurity

Apnea of prematurity is a developmental disorder common to infants born before term, or before 40 weeks' gestation, that results from immature respiratory control. Apnea of prematurity is defined as apneic events that last more than 20 seconds or shorter apneic periods associated with oxygen desaturation and/or bradycardia.[1] Approximately 70% of infants born prior to 34 weeks' gestational age will have clinically significant apnea, bradycardia, and oxygen desaturations.[1] The frequency and severity is inversely proportional to gestational age, with almost all infants born at less than 28 weeks' gestation and extremely low birthweight infants (birthweight less than 1000 grams) being affected.[1] Periodic breathing with short breathing pauses of 5 to 10 seconds are normal in preterm infants and some full-term infants.[1] Periodic breathing is different from apnea of prematurity because it is not pathologic, is not associated with significant hypoxia or bradycardia, and will resolve without the need for intervention.[1]

Etiology and Incidence

In utero, fetal breathing is intermittent. In healthy infants, breathing becomes continuous immediately after birth. The regulatory neurologic mechanisms responsible for this transition are not completely understood; however, the immaturity of breathing response associated with apnea of prematurity affects all levels of respiratory control.[2] Most apneic spells in preterm infants are central, with absent inspiratory efforts, or mixed, with upper airway obstruction that precedes or follows a central apnea.[3]

Pathophysiology

The factors that affect central **apnea** in preterm infants are associated with hypercapnia due to a blunted

TABLE 8-1
Factors Associated with Apnea of Prematurity

Factors Associated with Central Apnea	Factors Associated with Mixed Apnea
Hypercapnia	Factors associated with central apnea
Hypoxia	Hypopharyngeal muscle tone
Hyperbilirubinemia	Upper airway reflexes
	Nasal obstruction
	Laryngeal edema

ventilatory response to CO_2; hypoxia due to a biphasic response of hyperventilation followed by hypoventilation; and hyperbilirubinemia, a condition where there is too much bilirubin in the blood, which can cross the blood–brain barrier and cause a further decrease in response to hypercarbia or hypoxia.

The mixed apnea is affected by the factors associated with central apnea as well as those associated with obstructed apnea. Pharyngeal tone is poor in preterm infants and can cause airway collapse, especially during rapid eye movement (REM) sleep. During REM sleep, hypotonia of the chest wall and upper airway muscles, as well as reductions in pharyngeal tone, often occur. Head position also affects an infant's ability to maintain a patent airway, as flexion of the neck makes the airway susceptible to collapse. Upper airway reflexes may also contribute to apnea, but the mechanism is poorly understood. Newborn infants are obligate nose breathers, so they depend on nasal patency for adequate ventilation. Apnea may also be stimulated with nasal swelling or obstruction.[4] **Table 8-1** outlines the factors associated with central and mixed apnea.

Clinical Presentation

Apnea in preterm infants breathing spontaneously without respiratory support will appear within the first 2 to 3 days of life. The apnea will usually be accompanied by bradycardia and hypoxemia.[5] Preterm infants receiving mechanical ventilatory support may have episodic desaturation and bradycardia; however, this may not be considered apnea of prematurity until the neonate is liberated from respiratory support. Independent of the need for mechanical ventilation, the frequency of episodic desaturation usually increases in frequency after the 2nd or 3rd week of life and persists for several weeks. Apnea of prematurity typically resolves before 37 weeks' postmenstrual age in infants born after 28 weeks' gestation. In infants born at or before 28 weeks' postmenstrual age, the apnea will frequently persist until term (40 weeks') postmenstrual age.

Diagnosis

Other causes of apnea need to be excluded before the diagnosis of apnea of prematurity is made as apnea is a common symptom of many other conditions. The following disorders should be considered: respiratory distress syndrome, other pulmonary conditions, hypoglycemia, other metabolic diseases, infections, and central nervous system pathology.

When all other causes are ruled out, then the diagnosis of apnea of prematurity can be made. If infection is suspected, laboratory studies, such as complete blood count, urinalysis, and spinal fluid analysis, are performed. Hypoglycemia and metabolic disorders can be confirmed or eliminated by obtaining glucose and electrolyte levels. Chest radiographs are used to evaluate the presence of underlying pulmonary conditions. There may be additional studies performed to determine if a pathologic condition associated with the upper airway exists.

Management

Cardiorespiratory monitoring should be used for any patient at risk of apnea. Treatment of apnea of prematurity should be instituted if the apneic spells are frequent, prolonged, or associated with bradycardia and frequent desaturations or if they require interventions with bag-mask ventilation and frequent tactile stimulation.[6,7] There are no conclusive studies to indicate how the severity of apnea should be measured; therefore, each clinical center needs to develop a system to measure severity. Factors often used to measure the severity of apnea include the number of events per day and the amount of intervention that is needed to relieve each event. Clinical guidelines or protocols are helpful in defining a system for escalating treatments, if necessary.

There are three major treatment approaches for apnea of prematurity, which are used either alone or in combination: (1) general measures to reduce risk of apnea and hypoxemia, (2) methylxanthine therapy, and (3) nasal continuous positive airway pressure (CPAP). General measures should be applied to any infant born at less than 37 weeks' gestational age. The goal is to decrease factors contributing to the increased risk for apnea and associated hypoxemia. Body temperature fluctuations can also precipitate apnea episodes; as such, preterm infants should be cared for in an environmentally controlled setting by placing the infant in a radiant warmer or incubator.

When a new onset of apnea or increased severity occurs, other diagnoses that are highly associated with apnea, such as neonatal sepsis, should be considered. Infants should be positioned to avoid extreme flexion or extension and to maintain upper airway patency. Nasal patency is maintained through bulb suctioning of the nares as indicated. Pulse oximetry is used to monitor SpO_2 and supplemental oxygen is administered to avoid hypoxemia.

Methylxanthines cause stimulation of the respiratory neural output and are the primary pharmacologic therapy used to treat apnea of prematurity. Theophylline and caffeine have both been studied and effectively used as well. Studies comparing methylxanthines to placebo demonstrated that methylxanthine treatment resulted in fewer apneic episodes.[8] Caffeine, however, has become the preferred drug because it has a longer half-life, wider margin of safety, and lower frequency of adverse effects.[8] Treatment with therapeutic caffeine is usually reserved for those patients who require intervention with bag-mask ventilation or multiple episodes of tactile stimulation. Some newer but limited data suggest that early prophylactic caffeine for very preterm infants may be beneficial.[8] Caffeine is given as a loading dose of 20 mg/kg caffeine citrate, followed in 24 hours by a daily maintenance dose of 5 to 10 mg/kg, administered intravenously or orally. Therapeutic levels of caffeine are measured 5 to 7 days after the drug is started. The acceptable therapeutic range is 5 to 25 mg/L, although continued monitoring of serum caffeine levels is not considered helpful in management.[9] Discontinuation of caffeine is individualized because the data to support a standardized approach are not available. A common plan is to discontinue the caffeine when the infant reaches a postmenstrual age of 32 to 34 weeks if there have been no apneic periods requiring intervention for 5 to 7 days.[9]

Nasal CPAP with pressures of 4 to 6 cmH$_2$O may be initiated if the apnea is significant. The suggested advantage is that the CPAP splints the upper airway open and reduces obstruction.[10] CPAP is typically used in conjunction with methylxanthines. Some centers are using a heated high-flow nasal cannula to provide supplemental oxygen and CPAP. Current studies have shown that CPAP levels are unpredictable with a heated high-flow nasal cannula and further studies are needed to validate its use for CPAP administration. An infant who continues to have apnea may need to progress to noninvasive ventilation (NIV) or intubation and mechanical ventilatory support.[11] Some infants will need to continue to receive methylxanthines after discharge. In these cases, adequate discharge education needs to be provided, to include cardiopulmonary resuscitation and stimulation techniques. The infants will be placed on an impedance monitor at home, which will alarm for apnea and bradycardia events and can store event data to be downloaded and reviewed by the medical team to help decide further treatment needs.

Complications and Outcomes

Infants with obstructive apnea exceeding 20 seconds have an increased incidence of intraventricular hemorrhage, hydrocephalus, prolonged mechanical ventilation, and abnormal neurologic development after their first year of life.[1] Apnea of prematurity resolves in 98% of infants by 40 weeks' postmenstrual age.

Preterm infants are known to have an increased risk of sudden infant death syndrome, but there is no evidence to link this with apnea of prematurity. Caffeine therapy has been shown to decrease the risk of cerebral injury and bronchopulmonary dysplasia and to decrease the length of mechanical ventilation.

Respiratory Distress Syndrome

Respiratory distress syndrome (RDS), formally known as hyaline membrane disease (HMD), remains a significant problem for premature infants born at fewer than 28 weeks' gestation. Although management has evolved over the years, which has improved survival rates for the smallest infants, the potential for comorbidities, such as **bronchopulmonary dysplasia (BPD)** in this patient population, is at risk to increase.[12] The main cause of RDS in premature infants is a surfactant deficiency resulting from pulmonary insufficiency soon after birth. However, not all infants born prematurely develop RDS, suggesting that there may be susceptibility factors. Because multiple factors can contribute to the pathogenesis of RDS specifically in premature infants, the etiology is considered to be multifactorial.[13]

In the United States, RDS has been estimated to occur in 20,000 to 30,000 newborn infants annually, which accounts for approximately 1% of all pregnancies.[14] Approximately 60% to 80% of the neonates born at 26 to 28 weeks' gestation develop respiratory distress syndrome, whereas fewer than 30% of premature neonates born at >32 weeks' gestation develop the condition.[14]

Etiology and Incidence

The incidence and severity of RDS are inversely related to the gestational age of the newborn infant. In one report, the National Institute of Child Health and Human Development Neonatal Research Network showed that the overall incidence rate of RDS was 42% in infants weighing 501 to 1500 grams; within that range, the highest rate, at 71%, was reported in infants weighing 501 to 750 grams, with rates of 54%, 36%, and 22% reported in infants weighing 751 to 1000 grams, 1001 to 1250 grams, and 1251 to 1500 grams, respectively.[15] Antenatal corticosteroid administration to mothers in preterm labor accelerates maturation of the neonate's lung and significantly reduces the incidence of RDS and mortality.[16]

Pulmonary surfactant is a lipoprotein complex substance (90% lipids, 10% proteins) produced by alveolar type II cells. Surfactant is essential to normal pulmonary function. It is responsible for reducing surface tension and pressures of the alveolar air–liquid interface, which in turn prevents pulmonary collapse during exhalation.[17] Preterm newborns are unable to produce surfactant of adequate quality and quantity due to pulmonary immaturity, the primary etiology of RDS. In utero, the fetal lung is filled with fluid. In preparation for birth and transition to air breathing, surfactant is expressed into the lung starting around the 20th week of gestation. Most surfactant is produced after 30 weeks' gestation, with accelerated surfactant production starting around week 36 in the prenatal period.[18]

Pathophysiology

In preterm infants, the immature pulmonary system impairs surfactant, contributing to the development of RDS. Surfactant deficiency causes high surface tension within the lung and decreased compliance. The low lung volumes lead to atelectasis, ventilation-perfusion (V/Q) mismatch, and hypoventilation, which result in hypoxemia and hypercarbia. Surfactant deficiency also causes inflammation and subsequent respiratory epithelial injury, which can lead to pulmonary edema and increased airway resistance.[19] Respiratory and metabolic acidosis occur and cause pulmonary vasoconstriction and impaired endothelial and epithelial integrity. As a result, proteinaceous exudates leak into the alveoli and form hyaline membranes. In the absence of lung protective strategies and oxygen management, progressive atelectasis, barotrauma or volutrauma, and oxygen toxicity damage the endothelial and epithelial cells lining these distal airways and result in exudation of fibrinous matrix. The presence of hypoxia, acidosis, hypothermia, and/or hypotension may further impair surfactant production and/or secretion. Oxygen toxicity, barotrauma, and volutrauma will occur in up to 25% of neonates with RDS, which causes damage to their structurally immature lungs and leads to BPD.[20] Antioxidant deficiency and free-radical injury worsen lung injury and contribute to **chronic lung disease (CLD)** (**Figure 8-1**).

Macroscopic evaluation reveals that the lungs of affected newborns appear airless, requiring an increased critical opening pressure to inflate (**Figure 8-2**). Diffuse atelectasis of distal airspaces, along with distension of distal airways and perilymphatic areas, are observed microscopically. In larger premature infants, the epithelium begins to heal at 36 to 72 hours after birth and endogenous surfactant synthesis begins. The recovery phase is characterized by regeneration of alveolar cells, including type II cells, with a resultant increase in surfactant activity.

Clinical Presentation

RDS typically presents within minutes of birth. Signs frequently include cyanosis, nasal flaring, grunting, retractions, and tachypnea or apnea. In some cases, infants may not appear ill immediately after delivery but will develop respiratory distress within the first few hours of life. If untreated, RDS progressively worsens over the first 48 hours of life, leading to respiratory failure and, in some cases, multiple organ failure. On physical examination, auscultated breath sounds are decreased, and infants appear pale with diminished peripheral pulses. Urine output often is low in the first 24 to 48 hours and peripheral edema is common.

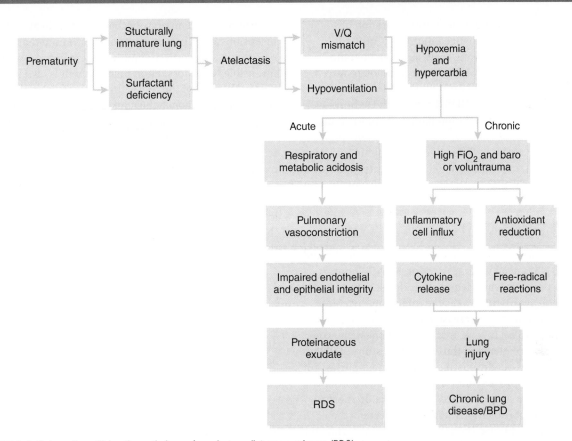

FIGURE 8-1 Schematic outlining the pathology of respiratory distress syndrome (RDS).

Infants may recover completely or develop chronic lung damage, resulting in bronchopulmonary dysplasia (BPD). FIO2 = fraction of inspired oxygen; HMD = hyaline membrane disease; V/Q = ventilation/perfusion.

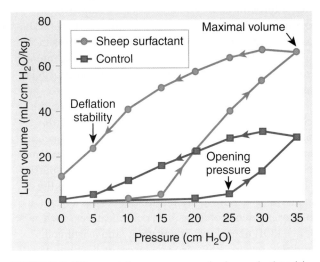

FIGURE 8-2 Difference in lung pressure opening in an animal model. The orange outline pressure volume curve represents sheep lungs with surfactant and the blue outlined pressure volume curve represents surfactant-deficient lungs.

Reproduced from Jobe AH. Lung development and maturation. In: Martin RJ, Fanaroff AA, Walsh MC, eds. *Fanaroff & Martin's Neonatal Medicine—Diseases of the Fetus and Infant.* 9th ed. St. Louis: Elsevier; 2011.

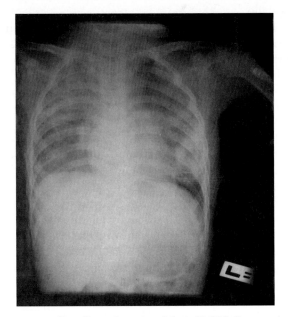

FIGURE 8-3 Chest X-ray of a preterm infant with RDS. Decreased lung volumes and a diffuse reticulogranular "ground-glass" appearance of the lungs with air bronchograms are seen.

© Santibhavank P/Shutterstock.

Diagnosis

The diagnosis of RDS is based on a clinical assessment of progressive respiratory failure immediately or shortly after birth, exhibited by increases in the work of breathing and oxygen requirement. The chest radiographic demonstrates low lung volume and diffuse reticulogranular "ground-glass" appearance with air bronchograms (**Figure 8-3**).[21] This radiographic pattern results from alveolar atelectasis contrasting with aerated airways.

It is important to note that early administration of surfactant therapy has changed the classic "ground-glass appearance of the lungs with air bronchograms" radiologic presentation of RDS from common to rare.[22]

The lecithin-to-sphingomyelin ratio (L:S) test is a standard for confirming RDS. Lecithin and sphingomyelin are phospholipids found in the amniotic fluid; lecithin levels increase as the lung matures and begins to produce surfactant while typically the sphingomyelin remains constant. A L:S ratio of 2.0 or greater indicates that RDS is unlikely because there is a sufficient amount of surfactant.[23]

Management

Prior to the use of exogenous surfactant, uncomplicated or mild RDS typically progressed for 48 to 72 hours. When hypoxemia was adequately addressed, respiratory function began to improve as the infant's endogenous surfactant production increased, with complete resolution of the RDS by 1 week of age. Treatment with exogenous surfactant changed the expected history of RDS. Within minutes of administration, exogenous surfactant dramatically improves pulmonary function, improves work of breathing, and reduces hypoxemia. In most cases, the use of exogenous surfactant shortens the clinical course of RDS. There are two types of surfactant used clinically: natural and synthetic. Although both types effectively treat RDS, research shows that natural surfactant is better at reducing pulmonary air leaks and mortality.[24]

The use of CPAP and/or NIV also improves the clinical course of RDS, even in infants who did not receive surfactant therapy.[25] Early intervention with NIV can reduce the need for mechanical ventilation. The use of NIV with early extubation also reduces the need for re-intubation.

Mechanical ventilatory support is used to recruit and stabilize surfactant-deficient alveoli, either by establishing the appropriate mean airway pressure using high-frequency oscillatory ventilation or optimal recruitment using adequate positive end-expiratory pressure (PEEP) while avoiding overdistention.[26] Permissive hypercapnia (pH <7.22) is an acceptable practice and can lead to a reduction in ventilator days.[26] Supplemental oxygen therapy with hyperoxemia is linked to the development of retinopathy of prematurity (ROP).[27] In very low birthweight babies, SpO_2 should be maintained between 85% and 92% and the partial arterial oxygen pressure (PaO_2) maintained between 50 and 80 mm Hg. Wider fluctuations in SaO_2 should be avoided because they are also associated with increased incidence of ROP.[28]

Supportive care for babies with RDS is essential. Radiant warmers should be used in the delivery room and in the neonatal intensive care unit to maintain the infant on their **neutral thermal environment**, or the environmental temperature that prevents heat and insensible water loss. It is important to note that incubators are superior to radiant warmers in preventing insensible water loss. Fluid management is also important in the care of the premature infant but does not significantly influence the course of RDS.[22] Nutritional support should start at birth in order to reduce weight loss and to minimize long-term postnatal growth restrictions. Low systemic blood flow and treatment for hypotension are important predictors of poor long-term outcomes. In patients with RDS, low systemic blood pressure may be due to hypovolemia, a large left-to-right ductus, or an atrial shunt. Understanding the cause of a low systemic blood pressure can indicate the most appropriate treatment plan. A patent ductus arteriosus (PDA) may cause clinical problems for the very preterm infant with RDS. Although there is limited evidence to support a specific recommendation, when there is poor perfusion due to the existence of a left-to-right shunt and weaning from respiratory support is difficult, prophylactic indomethacin has been shown to be efficacious.[29] **Table 8-2** summarizes current recommendations for the management of infants with RDS.

Complications and Outcomes

There have been significant improvements in the prognosis of RDS. However, acute complications can occur and include pneumothorax, pulmonary interstitial emphysema, intraventricular hemorrhage, necrotizing enterocolitis, PDA, and sepsis. To improve outcomes and minimize the presence or severity of RDS, administration of antenatal steroids to mothers in preterm labor and the use of surfactant replacement, volume-targeted mechanical ventilation, and/or NIV are recommended.

It is also essential to optimize supportive care, including maintenance of normal body temperature, proper fluid management, sufficient nutritional support, appropriate management of the ductus arteriosus, and circulation support to maintain adequate tissue perfusion.[22] Advances in medical care have increased the survival of extremely premature infants. As a result, a higher incidence of long-term complications, such as CLD, ROP, neurologic impairment, and learning disabilities, occurs. RDS also increases the likelihood of developing pulmonary abnormalities, such as asthma, reactive airway disease, and respiratory infection, as the infant matures.[30]

Transient Tachypnea of the Newborn

Transient tachypnea of the newborn (TTN) was first described in 1966 by Avery and colleagues.[31] It has also been known as transient RDS, type II RDS, wet lungs, and retained fetal lung liquid syndrome.

TABLE 8-2
A Summary of the Management of Infants with RDS

Prenatal care	• Babies at risk should be born in centers where appropriate care can be delivered, including mechanical ventilation. • Birth should be delayed to allow for maximum benefit of prenatal corticosteroid therapy.
Delivery room stablization	• Stabilize baby with warmer to prevent heat loss. • Avoid excessive tidal volumes and exposure to 100% oxygen. • For extreme preterm infants, consider intubation for prophylactic surfactant administration if antenatal steroids have not been given; administer CPAP early.
Respiratory support and surfactant	• Surfactant should be given as early as possible in the course of RDS. • Repeat doses of surfactant may be required. • Older babies can often be extubated to NIV following surfactant administration; assessment should be made to determine the course of care. • For preterm infants who require mechanical ventilation, avoid hyperoxia, hypocarbia, and volutrauma. • Caffeine therapy should be used to minimize the need for mechanical ventilation. • Babies should be maintained on NIV instead of mechanical ventilation when possible.
Supportive care	• Antibiotics should be started until sepsis has been ruled out, unless risk of infection is low. • Maintain body temperature in the normal range. • Careful fluid balance is required with early aggressive nutritional support. • Blood pressure should be monitored regularly, aiming to maintain normal tissue perfusion; if necessary, use inotropes. • Consideration should be given to whether pharmacologic closure of the ductus arteriosis is indicated.

Etiology and Incidence

TTN is considered a parenchymal lung disease, caused by pulmonary edema, resulting from a delay in the clearance and reabsorption of fetal lung fluid. The incidence of TNN is 5.7 per 1000 live births in term deliveries of 37 to 42 weeks' gestation.[31] There is a higher incidence of TTN among term infants born by cesarean section without active labor.[31] Macrosomia, maternal diabetes, maternal asthma, and multiple gestations have also shown an increased risk for TTN. It is considered a self-limiting disease because the fetal lung fluid is eventually absorbed and the symptoms disappear.

Pathophysiology

Fetal lung fluid clearance normally begins before term birth and continues during labor and postnatally. In late gestation, the lung epithelium switches from secreting chloride and fluid into the air sacs to reabsorption in response to catecholamine and other hormones. Increased oxygen tension at birth augments the capacity of the epithelium to transport sodium. Fluid is passively reabsorbed after birth due to changes in the oncotic pressures in the alveoli, interstitium, and blood vessels.[32]

A disruption in any of the aforementioned normal mechanisms will delay reabsorption and lead to a failure to remove fluid, which will result in fluid accumulation in the alveolar spaces and interstitium. Lung fluid can pool into perivascular tissues and interlobar fissures until it is eventually cleared by the lymphatic system or absorbed into small blood vessels. The excess lung fluid decreases compliance and increases the work of breathing. Tachypnea develops to compensate for the increased work of breathing that occurs with changes in pulmonary compliance. Fluid accumulation can also result in partial collapse of the bronchioles, air trapping, and ventilation/perfusion mismatch. Clinically, ventilation/perfusion mismatch manifests in hypoxemia and potentially hypercapnia.

Clinical Presentation

The onset of symptoms usually occurs at the time of birth or within 2 hours after delivery. Infants present with tachypnea (respiratory rates of 60–100 breaths per minute) and an increased work of breathing manifested by nasal flaring, mild intercostal and subcostal retractions, and expiratory grunting.[34] Blood gas analysis often reveals hypoxemia and respiratory acidosis.[34] The anterior-posterior diameter of the chest will be increased when air trapping is present. Breath sounds in affected infants are typically clear. Infants with mild to moderate TTN are symptomatic for 12 to 24 hours, but symptoms can last up to 72 hours in severe cases.

Diagnosis

The diagnosis of TTN is made clinically after other common neonatal diseases have been ruled out. Clinical and radiographic presentation for TTN overlaps with other neonatal disorders. However, symptoms associated with TTN generally last for fewer than 72 hours. Additionally, infants with TTN do not frequently require an FiO_2 above 0.60 or mechanical ventilatory support.

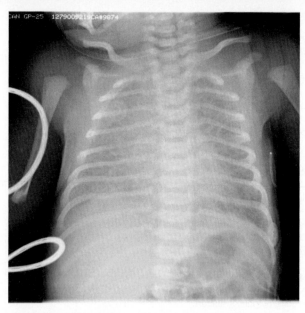

FIGURE 8-4 Chest radiograph showing streaky markings and mild cardiomegaly as seen in TTN.

Case courtesy of Radswiki, Radiopaedia.org, rID: 12032.

Characteristic findings on chest radiograph include increased lung volumes with flattened diaphragms, interstitial edema appearing as fluffy infiltrates, and prominent vascular markings with streaky perihilar markings (**Figure 8-4**).[33] Pleural effusions and mild cardiomegaly can also be present. Radiologic findings are symmetrical and typically resolve in approximately 48 hours.[33]

Management

Because TTN is a benign, self-limiting condition, management is supportive, and treatment is directed at preventing hypoxemia and hypercapnia. In most cases, supplemental oxygen by a nasal cannula at low flows can be used; rarely does an infant with TTN require supplemental oxygen concentrations greater than 0.40. Some patients may require the use of noninvasive nasal CPAP. If the infant is found to require more respiratory support than previously described, TTN is most likely not the diagnosis.

Supportive measures include maintaining a neutral thermal environment. Infants with a high work of breathing should be provided nutritional support through intravenous fluids or orogastric tube feedings. In order to rule out pneumonia, a complete blood count is often performed.

Complications and Outcomes

TTN is self-limiting. Symptoms generally resolve within 24 to 72 hours, and patient outcomes are good. Air trapping may pose the risk of developing air leaks. There is newer evidence to suggest that TTN is associated with wheezing (asthma) later in life.[35]

Neonatal Pneumonia

Neonatal pneumonia is an infection of the lung in a newborn. This inflammatory pulmonary process can originate in the lung or be a focal complication of a systemic inflammatory process. It is estimated that neonatal pneumonia accounts for up to 10% of childhood mortality worldwide, with the highest case mortality rates in developing countries.[36] Early-onset pneumonia is associated with generalized sepsis and first manifests at or within hours of birth. Late-onset pneumonia usually occurs after 7 days of age, most commonly in neonatal ICUs among infants who require prolonged invasive ventilation for unresolved lung issues and is often a result of a hospital-acquired infection, such ventilator-associated pneumonia.[37]

Etiology and Incidence

The incidence of neonatal pneumonia varies according to gestational age, intubation status, race, and socioeconomic status. Other factors influencing incidence include the diagnostic criteria used to detect the pneumonia, the setting in which the infant receives care (i.e., level designation of the neonatal ICU), and the standard of care delivered to the infant. In resource-rich settings, the estimated incidence of pneumonia is <1% among full-term infants and approximately 10% in preterm infants.[38] In resource-limited settings, pneumonia is a major contributor to infant mortality. In 2015, the World Health Organization estimated that pneumonia caused >900,000 deaths worldwide in children younger than 5 years of age, with the majority of deaths occurring in infants younger than 1 year of age.[39] Group B streptococcus (GBS) accounts for most cases of early-onset pneumonia. Conversely, the most common bacteria causing late-onset pneumonia are gram-negative bacilli, such as *Escherichia coli* or *Klebsiella*.[40] Pneumonia from GBS may progress quickly and lead to shock or death; mortality in this patient population is high at 20% to 50%.[41] Congenital pneumonia is a common cause of mortality among extremely low birthweight infants (<1000 grams), with the literature reporting a 30% mortality rate.[36] Pneumonia caused by maternal enteric organisms frequently accompanies chorioamnionitis and/or funisitis and is considered a congenital infection. **Table 8-3** lists the bacterial organisms that are commonly found in early- and late-onset neonatal sepsis and pneumonia.

Pathophysiology

Neonatal pneumonia can be acquired in a variety of ways: intrauterine or congenital (infection transmitted through the placenta or as the infant ascends through the birth canal), intrapartum (aspiration of infected amniotic fluid), or postnatal (environmental, healthcare-acquired infection) routes. The pathologic changes vary with the type of organism. Bacteria most frequently are the causative agent (i.e., GBS, *E. coli*), followed

TABLE 8-3
Bacterial Organisms Responsible for Early- and Late-Onset Neonatal Pneumonia

Early Onset (7 or fewer days)	Late Onset (more than 7 days)
• Group B streptococcus (g+) • *Escherichia coli* (g–) • *Staphylococcus aureus* (g+) • *Listeria monocytogenes* (g+) • *Enterococcus* spp. (g+) • *Ureaplasma urealyticum* (g+)	• *Escherichia coli* (g–) • *Staphylococcus epidermidis* (g+) • *Klebsiella* or *Enterobacter* species (g–) • *Pseudomonas aeruginosa* (g–) • *Chlamydia trachomatis*

g+: Gram positive; g–: Gram negative

by viruses, then fungi (i.e., *Candida, Chlamydia trachomatis*).

Bacterial pneumonia is characterized by pulmonary inflammation, injury of bronchopulmonary tissue, and leakage of proteinaceous exudate into the alveoli, bronchi/bronchioles, and interstitium.[37] Viruses typically cause an interstitial pneumonia, characterized by infiltration of mononuclear cells and lymphocytes. The literature suggests that respiratory insufficiency in neonatal pneumonia is likely due to the inhibition of surface tension–lowering properties of surfactant rather than surfactant deficiency.[37] Extensive inflammation occasionally occurs with hyaline membrane formation, followed by varying degrees of interstitial fibrosis and scarring.[37]

Clinical Presentation

Neonatal pneumonia is commonly classified as either of early or late onset. Early-onset pneumonia occurs within the first 7 days of life while late-onset occurs after the 7th day of life. Clinical signs include respiratory distress beginning at or soon after birth. Tachypnea is present in a majority of the cases (60–89%). Infants may have associated lethargy, apnea, tachycardia, and poor perfusion. Their clinical course may progress to septic shock. Other signs include cough, temperature instability, poor feeding, metabolic acidosis, and abdominal distention.[37] Persistent fever has been reported in neonates with viral pneumonia. Chest radiographic appearance can vary depending on the infectious agent; reticulogranular-nodular infiltrates appearing as streaky or hazy are commonly associated with viral disease while patchy parenchymal infiltrates and consolidations are more common when a bacterial infection is present (**Figure 8-5**). There may also be hyper-aeration in areas of the lung that are free of infiltrates.[37]

Diagnosis

Because signs of pneumonia are nonspecific, the diagnosis can be challenging. Neonates with sudden onset of respiratory distress or other signs of illness should be

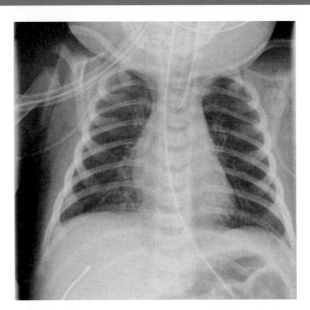

FIGURE 8-5 A chest X-ray of neonatal pneumonia showing consolidation, especially in the right upper lobe.
Case courtesy of Dr. Jeremy Jones, Radiopaedia.org, rID: 23898.

evaluated for pneumonia in addition to a complete sepsis evaluation. The diagnosis of neonatal pneumonia is based on a combination of clinical, radiographic, and microbiologic findings, including chest X-ray, pulse oximetry, blood cultures, gram stain, and culture of tracheal aspirate.

Management

In early-onset pneumonia, broad-spectrum antibiotics are administered intravenously, mirroring the antimicrobial therapy used to treat neonatal sepsis. Vancomycin is frequently the initial treatment of choice for most late-onset healthcare-associated pneumonia. Local patterns of infection and bacterial resistance should always be used to help guide empiric antimicrobial choices. The antimicrobial agent may be changed once the pathogen is identified and sensitivity results are available.

Complications and Outcomes

The prognosis of neonatal pneumonia depends upon the severity of disease, the gestational age of the infant, underlying medical conditions, and the infecting organism. Increased mortality is associated with preterm birth, preexisting CLD, or immune deficiencies. Most term neonates managed in resource-rich settings recover well without long-term consequences.

Meconium Aspiration Syndrome

Meconium is fetal bowel content, which is normally passed by a newborn within 48 hours after birth. This viscous, sticky, odorless, dark-green substance is composed of intestinal secretions, mucosal cells, solid elements of swallowed amniotic fluid, and water. **Meconium aspiration syndrome (MAS)** occurs when the infant passes meconium prior to or during birth.

Etiology and Incidence

Meconium passed prior to birth or during the birth process will cause the amniotic fluid to have a green discoloration. Depending on the amount of meconium passed, the color of amniotic fluid can range from light to dark green and is often referred to as meconium-stained amniotic fluid (MSAF). The presence of MSAF signals a concern at delivery because there is the potential for the infant to aspirate the fluid. Meconium passed prior to birth can be associated with fetal hypoxic distress, precipitated by placental insufficiency, maternal hypertension, preeclampsia, oligohydramnios, and maternal drug abuse. Fetal hypoxic distress not only stimulates the passage of meconium in utero but also stimulates fetal gasping movements, which can result in meconium movement into the lung. In postterm infants, MSAF is considered a physiologic occurrence due to maturation of the gastrointestinal tract.

Fetal gasping movements increase the likelihood that the infant will aspirate MSAF, which can lead to MAS. There are a variety of factors that increase the risk for MAS, including the presence of MSAF, fetal hypoxic distress, gestational age greater than 41 weeks, and African American and Pacific Islander descent.

It is uncommon for meconium to be found in the amniotic fluid prior to 34 weeks' gestation because the gastrointestinal tract does not mature prior to that gestational age. Therefore, MSAF is primarily seen in near-term or term infants, with a marked increase in incidence after 41 weeks' gestation. The reported incidence of MSAF as a percentage of live births and MAS as a percentage of infants with MSAF varies with gestational age. The incidence of MSAF and MAS significantly increases at term (40 weeks' gestation) and postterm (41-42 weeks' gestation).[42]

The timing of the initial insult resulting in MAS is controversial. Some studies have suggested that chronic in utero insult may be responsible for the development of severe MAS, while the infant who suffers an acute insult during the birth process may develop mild to moderate MAS.[43] MAS occurs in an estimated 25,000 to 30,000 cases per year, with 1000 deaths, or an overall mortality of 1.2%, attributed to MAS annually in the United States.[44] Thirty percent of patients with MAS require intubation and ventilation. Risk factors associated with mortality include myocardial dysfunction, lower birthweight, and a higher oxygen requirement.[45]

Pathophysiology

There are three major pathophysiologic effects associated with MAS: acute airway obstruction, surfactant dysfunction, and chemical pneumonitis.

Acute airway obstruction occurs because of the presence of thick meconium in the airways. The viscosity and amount of meconium aspirated have an effect on

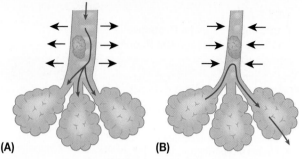

FIGURE 8-6 An illustration of the ball-valve effect. (**A**) During inspiration, because the airways expand, the inspired gas is able to pass through the airway. (**B**) During expiration, the airways return to their resting state; air is unable to pass around the obstruction, causing air trapping and air leaks.

Data from Harris TR, Herrick BR. *Pneumothorax in the Newborn*. Biomedical Communications, Arizona Health Sciences Center: Tucson, AZ, 1978.

whether partial or complete airway obstruction occurs. When a partial obstruction is present, a ball-valve mechanism occurs in the airway. This is due to changes in thoracic pressures with breathing. During inspiration, the airway diameter increases, and airways elongate, which allows inspired gas to flow around the obstruction (**Figure 8-6a**). When expiration occurs, the airway diameter decreases, causing gas to be trapped (**Figure 8-6b**).[46] As the trapped gas increases, **air leak syndrome** with pneumothorax, pneumomediastinum, and/or pneumopericardium can occur. Because meconium aspiration causes regional atelectasis, air leaks can complicate an already existing ventilation/perfusion mismatch. The presence of meconium in the alveoli also decreases the production of and inactivates surfactant, which increases surface tension and decreases lung compliance and inspired tidal volumes.

Meconium is an irritant to the lung tissue and causes chemical pneumonitis. It also increases interleukins and tumor necrosis factors, which induce an inflammatory response. Hypoxia often ensues, which plays a significant role in exacerbating the inflammatory response seen in MAS infants.

Clinical Presentation

The clinical presentation initially occurs in the delivery room. The key is to observe the presence of MSAF with or without meconium staining of the infant upon delivery. The severity of MAS depends on the amount and viscosity of the meconium the infant aspirates. Often there is a history of fetal stress during the pregnancy. When chronic fetal stress occurs, babies may be small for gestational age and present with lower birthweights and lengths. There is early onset of respiratory distress, either depression at birth, which can occur in up to 33% of infants born through MSAF, or within 2 hours of birth. Symptoms of respiratory distress include tachypnea, cyanosis, grunting, accessory muscle use, and nasal flaring. Blood gas analysis can show hypoxemia, and in patients with significant respiratory distress, hypercarbia and acidosis will be present. Blood gas analysis is generally used to manage care rather than to diagnose disease, as the presence of metabolic acidosis will depend upon the severity of hypoxia prior to birth. Rales and rhonchi are the most common adventitious breath sounds heard.

Infants with severe MAS have up to a 57% chance of developing **persistent pulmonary hypertension of the newborn (PPHN)**.[48] When fetal asphyxia is associated with MAS, there can be a failure of transition to extrauterine circulation, which predisposes the infant to PPHN.

Diagnosis

The diagnosis is primarily based on the presence of meconium in the amniotic fluid and an infant with the signs and symptoms of respiratory distress at or shortly after birth. Presence of meconium in the trachea during intubation would further support a diagnosis of MAS. The initial chest X-ray typically shows streaky, linear densities. As the disease progresses, the lungs typically appear hyperinflated with a flattening of the diaphragms. Regional atelectasis can be seen as diffuse patchy infiltrates, alternating with areas of expansion. When the disease is severe, the lungs develop an appearance of homogeneous density (**Figure 8-7**). If pulmonary air leaks exist, pneumothorax, pneumomediastinum, and/or pneumopericardium can be seen.[47] Chest X-ray findings are similar to other neonatal diseases and are used to support the diagnosis and guide disease management. Therefore, the diagnosis of MAS must be differentiated from other causes of neonatal respiratory distress. **Table 8-4** outlines the other diseases that also occur for infants born through MSAF. In order to rule out cardiac disease or pulmonary hypertension, an echocardiograph is often performed.

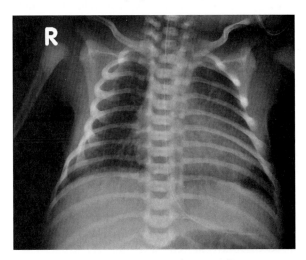

FIGURE 8-7 A chest radiograph showing patchy infiltrates, hyperinflation, and flattened diaphragms representative of MAS.

Case courtesy of Dr. Shailaja Muniraj, Radiopaedia.org, rID: 49835.

TABLE 8-4
Differential Diagnoses for Infants Born with Meconium-Stained Amniotic Fluid

- Transient tachypnea of the newborn
- Delayed transition from fetal circulation
- Sepsis or pneumonia
- Persistent pulmonary hypertension of the newborn

TABLE 8-5
Pathways for Meconium Aspiration Syndrome

Mild MAS	Requires <40% oxygen for <48 hours
Moderate MAS	Requires >40% oxygen for >48 hours without air leak
Severe MAS	Requires assisted ventilation for >48 hours; often associated with persistent pulmonary hypertension of the newborn

Management

The most important aspect of management of MAS is prevention. Since 1990, the rate of MAS has decreased dramatically due to changes in obstetric practice, specifically reduced postterm deliveries, improvements in fetal monitoring, and a quicker response to an abnormal fetal heart rate.[44] The rate of MAS is higher in developing countries, where the availability of prenatal care is less. Historically, all infants born with MSAF were intubated after delivery of the head and suctioned to remove meconium in the airway before delivery of the infant's body continued. However, research demonstrated that this practice did not improve outcomes when compared to oropharyngeal suction with appropriate resuscitation postdelivery.[49]

Management varies based on clinical presentation. MAS can be divided into mild, moderate, and severe pathways (**Table 8-5**).[50] Appropriate postdelivery assessment of the infant should be performed, which directs the course of treatment. The American Academy of Pediatrics Neonatal Resuscitation Steering Committee and the American Heart Association have established guidelines for the postdelivery treatment of the infant with MSAF (**Table 8-6**).[51] Resuscitation should follow the same principles for infants with MSAF as for those with clear fluid.[51] Research does not support the use of intrapartum intubation and suction until clear of meconium, intrapartum nasopharyngeal or nasopharyngeal suction, administration of corticosteroids, or amnioinfusion, which have not been proven to provide benefit or improve outcomes.

The treatment of mild MAS may only involve supplemental oxygen therapy to minimize hypoxemia.

TABLE 8-6
Current Resuscitation Guidelines for Infants with Meconium-Stained Amniotic Fluid at Birth

Presentation/Assessment	Action
Baby is vigorous (defined as normal respiratory effort, normal muscle tone, and heart rate >100 beats/min)	Allow the baby to stay with the mother for normal newborn care. Gently suction the mouth and nose with a bulb syringe.
Baby is not vigorous (defined as depressed respiratory effort and poor muscle tone)	Place the baby on the radiant warmer, clear secretions from the mouth and nose with a bulb syringe.
If after these initial steps baby is still not breathing or the heart rate is <100 beats/min	Administer positive pressure ventilation.

TABLE 8-7
A Review of Supported and Unsupported Therapeutic Interventions for the Treatment of MAS

Supported Interventions	Unsupported Interventions
Surfactant lavage	Intrapartum intubation and suctioning to clear meconium
HFV	Intrapartum oropharyngeal or nasopharyngeal suctioning
Nitric oxide	Corticosteroids
ECMO	Amnioinfusion

The targeted SpO_2 is as high as 99% to help in the prevention of hypoxia and associated airway obstruction and vascular remodeling of the pulmonary bed. If the infant develops respiratory distress and hypoxemia, intubation and mechanical ventilation are required. Every attempt should be made to keep the peak inspiratory pressure low, inspiratory time short, expiratory time long, PEEP moderate, and rates high.[52]

High frequency ventilation (HFV) is often used. The delivery of tidal volumes, which are less than dead space, results in less barotrauma and increased mobilization of secretions. Although there have been no prospective randomized trials comparing conventional ventilation to HFV, the use of lower mean airway pressures and higher rates with HFV would theoretically minimize barotrauma and potentially reduce air leak syndrome.

Because meconium interferes with surfactant by altering and inactivating it, surfactant replacement therapy can be used to replenish inactivated or altered surfactant and can work to help remove meconium. Surfactant replacement therapy reduces the severity of disease and prevents the need for extracorporeal membrane oxygenation (ECMO), but it has not been shown to improve mortality.[53] Studies did not show a significant decrease in mortality, hospital stay, length of ventilation, supplemental oxygen use, or lung injury with the use of surfactant replacement but did show a decrease in the need for ECMO.[50]

As meconium presence induces an inflammatory response in the lung, multiple clinical trials have investigated the potential benefits of administering steroids to these infants. Presently, the evidence is not conclusive and further research needs to be performed.[54]

Severe MAS may lead to PPHN. Administration of inhaled nitric oxide (iNO) to decrease pulmonary hypertension has led to a small decrease in the need for

ECMO in these infants.[55] ECMO is used in patients when all other therapies have failed and has a high survival rate for infants with MAS, at 90%.[52] Table 8-7 summarizes the current treatment for MAS and provides a list of unsupported practices that should not be used to treat this condition.

Complications and Outcomes

MAS has a clinical course dependent on the severity of illness. When MAS is mild, it typically resolves in 2 to 4 days; in more severe cases, the disease course and complications from treatment may last much longer. Older studies have shown a wide range of mortality for MAS, from 5% to 40%, with newer studies reporting rates of <15%.[56] Complications associated with MAS can include air leak associated with volutrauma or the ball-valve effect producing air trapping. The need for mechanical ventilation and ECMO increases the occurrence of CLD, with the degree dependent upon the extent and duration of volutrauma and need for supplemental oxygen. The presence of hypoxia, either prenatally or postnatally, and acidosis increase the risk of neurologic deficits that can last through life. Despite the improvements in avoiding meconium passage prior to birth, those infants presenting with meconium staining have a higher mortality than those without.[57]

Persistent Pulmonary Hypertension of the Newborn

At birth, fetal circulation is required to transition to postnatal circulation. The transition to postnatal circulation depends on the removal of the placenta, the catecholamine surge associated with birth, the initial filling of the lungs with air during the first breath(s), adjustment to a cold extrauterine environment, successful clearance of fetal lung fluid, and the infant's ability to achieve and maintain adequate alveolar ventilation and oxygenation. When conditions interfere with the change to postnatal circulation, the transitional circulation will continue and persistent pulmonary hypertension of the newborn will result.

Etiology and Incidence

PPHN occurs in approximately 2 in 100 live births affecting near-term (greater than 34 weeks' gestational age) to full-term infants.[58] It is rarely seen in preterm infants but has a higher risk in these infants when there is fetal growth restriction and after prolonged rupture of membranes before birth. Epidemiologic studies have demonstrated black and Asian maternal race and male sex are associated with a significantly higher risk for PPHN.[59] Maternal high body mass index or diabetes mellitus; maternal use of aspirin, nonsteroidal anti-inflammatory drugs (NSAIDs), or selective serotonin reuptake inhibitors (SSRIs); and cesarean delivery are also risk factors associated with PPHN.[59]

There are three major abnormalities associated with the pulmonary vasculature that are understood to precipitant the delay in full transition to postnatal circulation: underdevelopment or structural anomalies of the pulmonary vasculature, idiopathic PPHN or PPHN that occurs in the absence of lung disease, and hypoxia associated with parenchymal lung disease.[60,61]

Underdeveloped pulmonary vasculature causes a reduction in the cross-sectional area and will elevate pulmonary vascular resistance (PVR). Underdevelopment is associated with conditions responsible for pulmonary hypoplasia, such as congenital diaphragmatic hernia, congenital pulmonary (cystic adenomatous) malformation, renal agenesis, oligohydramnios, and fetal growth restriction. There is a limitation to development after birth and therefore a limit to the degree of postnatal pulmonary vasodilatation that can occur, resulting in the highest mortality rate for infants with the aforementioned conditions responsible for pulmonary hypoplasia.[62]

Maldevelopment of the pulmonary vasculature occurs in lungs that are structurally normal, having the correct amount of alveolar development and pulmonary vessels. In these patients, there is an abnormal thickening of the muscle layer of the pulmonary arteries (PPHN4), resulting in an increased PVR at birth. There appears to be vasculature remodeling occurring over the first 7 to 14 days of life, which decreases PVR. Vascular mediators, including the cyclic NO/cGMP pathway, are thought to be the cause.[63] Conditions associated with maldevelopment include postterm delivery, meconium staining, and meconium aspiration syndrome. Disorders that produce excessive circulation may also influence vascular maldevelopment. These would include premature closure of the ductus arteriosus, which can be caused by the mother consuming NSAIDs, aspirin (prostaglandin inhibitor), and SSRI antidepressants during the second half of pregnancy. When premature closure of the ductus is the cause of PPHN, it is termed idiopathic PPHN.

Maladaptation of the pulmonary vascular bed occurs in a normally developed vasculature. Perinatal conditions cause active vasoconstriction and compromise the normal fall in PVR that occurs postnatally. The conditions associated with maladaptation include perinatal depression, pulmonary parenchymal diseases, and bacterial infections, especially those caused by GBS.

The most common cause of PPHN is hypoxia associated with parenchymal lung disease, such as RDS and bronchopulmonary dysplasia.

Pathophysiology

In fetal life the placenta performs the functions associated with gas exchange. The lungs are filled with fluid and the fetal PaO_2 is low with a resultant high PVR. In the late gestational period, the fetus will prepare for the birth transition by increasing factors that promote pulmonary vasodilation, including the NO/cGMP pathway and the prostacyclin pathway. At the time of birth, the placenta is clamped, elevating systemic vascular resistance, and the lungs become air filled, the PaO_2 and pH increase, and vasoactive substances are released, resulting in a reduction of PVR. These changes happen rapidly, with 80% of the transition occurring by 24 hours of age and the remainder completing within another 2 weeks. **Figure 8-8** illustrates the circulator transition occurring with the adaptation form uterine to

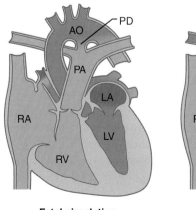
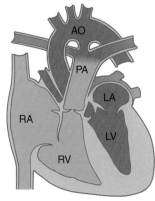
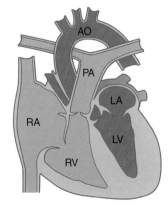

Fetal circulation   **8 Hours old**   **24–72 Hours**

FIGURE 8-8 An illustration of the circulatory changes that occur as an infant transitions from uterine to extrauterine life.

extrauterine life. If the PVR fails to fall, this can result in significant hypoxemia, hypercapnia, acidosis, and PPHN. Right atrial pressure is high, causing the foramen ovale to stay open with right-to-left shunting to the left atria and further decreased pulmonary blood flow. The ductus arteriosus will stay open in response to hypoxia and alterations in normal vasoactive substances, creating an additional right-to-left shunt.

Clinical Presentation

Some infants will have a delay in transition from fetal circulation and will usually only present with mild PPHN, manifested by mild hypoxemia and no respiratory distress. As the transition to extrauterine life continues in this group of infants, their clinical course will improve.

PPHN will usually present within 12 hours of birth and, when severe, will worsen rapidly, with significant hypoxemia and cardiopulmonary instability. PPHN is associated with signs of respiratory distress, tachypnea, cyanosis, grunting, nasal flaring, and retractions. More than half of the infants will be born with low Apgar scores and will need immediate intervention in the delivery room.[63] Typically, cyanosis and hypoxemia respond poorly to normal interventions and require continued escalations in care (labile hypoxemia). The majority of infants will have other respiratory conditions associated with PPHN. **Table 8-8** lists the conditions most frequently associated with PPHN.[63]

Diagnosis

PPHN should be considered when the infant has a history that includes the associated risk factors listed in **Table 8-9**.[62] Risk factors combined with hypoxemia that is unresponsive to oxygen therapy and mechanical

TABLE 8-8
Conditions Commonly Associated with PPHN and Their Relative Frequencies

Condition	Relative Frequency of Occurrence
MAS	41%
Idiopathic with no respiratory condition observed	17%
Pneumonia	14%
Combined or indistinguishable RDS/pneumonia	14%
RDS	13%
Congenital diaphragmatic hernia	10%
Pulmonary hypoplasia	4%

TABLE 8-9
Conditions That Predispose an Infant to PPHN

Prenatal Conditions
Fetal hypoxia
Maternal asthma
Maternal obesity
Maternal diabetes
Poor prenatal care
Cesarean delivery
Maternal use of SSRIs
Maternal use of NSAIDs
Abnormal fetal heart rate
Term or near-term gestation
Maternal tobacco smoke exposure
Maternal use of prostaglandin inhibitors

Antenatal Conditions
Sepsis
Pneumonia
Hypothermia
Polycythemia
Pneumothorax
Hypoglycemia
Birth asphyxia
Myocardial failure
Low Apgar score
Pulmonary hypoplasia
Large for gestational age
Respiratory distress at birth
Meconium aspiration syndrome
Transient tachypnea of the newborn

Reproduced from Barnhart S. Neonatal and pediatric respiratory care. In: Hess D, McIntyre NR, Galvin WF, Mishoe SC, ed. *Respiratory Care Principles and Practice.* 3rd ed. Boston, MA: Jones & Bartlett Learning: 1073-1112.

ventilation should raise the level of suspicion, especially when it is out of proportion to the level of pulmonary disease. Clinically, PPHN is most often recognized in term or near-term neonates, but it can infrequently occur in premature neonates.

The definitive diagnosis of PPHN is made by echocardiography: The echocardiogram will show normal heart structure and eliminate the differential diagnosis of cyanotic congenital heart disease. Doppler studies will show right-to-left shunting through the patent ductus arteriosus and/or foramen ovale.

Although dependent on the cause of PPHN, often the infant will have an initial period where the PaO_2 does reach >100 mm Hg. After birth, or generally within 12 hours, arterial blood gas analysis will show a low PaO_2, frequently even with high FiO_2 administration. Preductal (right radial artery) and postductal (umbilical artery and arteries in lower extremities) blood gas analysis that shows a greater than 10- to 20-mm Hg difference will confirm the presence of a ductal shunt. SpO_2 monitoring comparing the right hand with either foot may also be used, and a difference of 5% to 10% is considered significant and consistent with ductal shunting. Use of the left upper

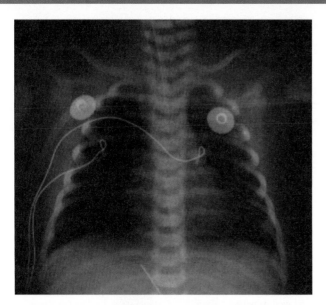

FIGURE 8-9 A chest radiograph of an infant with idiopathic PPHN. Note that the lungs appear black with no vascular markings.

Reproduced with permission from Stevenson D, Cohen RS, and Sunshine MD. *Neonatology: Clinical Practice and Procedures.* New York, NY: McGraw-Hill; 2015. Figure 26-1, p. 363. © McGraw-Hill Education.

extremity must be avoided because it can represent either pre- or postductal values.

Chest X-rays will generally not be helpful in diagnosis of PPHN, as it will be consistent with the underlying condition resulting in PPHN, but are more helpful in the management of the disease process. When the infant has idiopathic PPHN, the X-ray will be radiolucent with a lack of vascular markings (**Figure 8-9**).

Management

The treatment strategy for PPHN is aimed at maintaining adequate systemic blood pressure, decreasing pulmonary vascular resistance, ensuring adequate oxygenation, and minimizing complications caused by high levels of inspired oxygen and ventilator high-pressure settings. General cardiorespiratory management principles include the following: (1) continuous monitoring of oxygenation, blood pressure, and perfusion; (2) maintaining a normal body temperature; (3) correcting metabolic acidosis and electrolyte and glucose abnormalities; (4) nutritional support; (5) clustering care to minimize stimulation and/or handling of the newborn; and (6) minimal use of invasive procedures, such as suctioning.

The oxygenation index (OI) assesses the severity of PPHN and helps to guide the timing of interventions. The OI is calculated by the following formula: $OI = (MAP \times FiO_2 / PaO_2) \times 100$. A high OI will indicate severe hypoxemic respiratory failure. A term or late-term infant with an OI of >25 should be receiving care in a center that has HFV, iNO,[64] and ECMO

available.[62] An OI of >25 has a 50% risk of requiring ECMO and mortality if pulmonary vasodilators are not used.[65] High concentrations of supplemental oxygen delivery should be administered to help relieve hypoxemia and reduce PVR. Preductal SpO_2 should be targeted at >95% and continuous pre- and postductal monitoring of saturations will identify if ductal shunting continues. Mechanical ventilation is initiated in an attempt to resolve hypercarbia and acidosis in order to decrease PVR. $PaCO_2$ is targeted at 35 to 45 mm Hg. The ventilator strategy used will depend on the underlying cause of PPHN and the infant's response to therapy. Idiopathic PPHN will usually not require high mean arterial pressure (MAP) or PEEP levels. In contrast, infants with parenchymal lung disease may require high MAP and PEEP. HFV is often needed to achieve higher MAP while reducing potential lung injury caused by volutrauma. High-frequency oscillatory ventilation also has been shown to improve the treatment outcomes and response to iNO.[66]

iNO is a powerful pulmonary vasodilator with the advantage of having minimal systemic effects that improve oxygenation and reduce the need for ECMO in infants with PPHN.[66] Exogenous nitric oxide regulates vascular tone by relaxing the vascular smooth muscle. iNO is normally started at a concentration of 20 ppm and is lowered as quickly as possible to the lowest concentration that achieves effect. In patients who respond, there is typically a 20% increase in PaO_2 or arterial saturation within 15 to 20 minutes. Higher doses have not been associated with improved effect but have resulted in elevated methemoglobin levels and nitrogen dioxide levels. Measurement of methemoglobin levels is no longer routinely performed as studies have verified safety with the use of <20 ppm. Approximately 30% of infants will not respond to iNO. If lung recruitment and hemodynamic stability are achieved and iNO is still not effective, ECMO should be considered.[67] Rebound pulmonary hypertension has been reported after removal of iNO after prolonged administration but usually reverses after 60 minutes. Studies have shown that weaning iNO gradually will prevent the rebound effect.[67]

Other vasodilatory agents have been studied and used. Sildenafil is a phosphodiesterase inhibitor that has been shown to selectively reduce PVR and has been successful in treating infants with PPHN.[68]

Treatment for any associated disease process should also be provided. Surfactant therapy can be effective in infants with parenchymal lung disease associated with surfactant inactivation or deficiency but is not effective if PPHN is the primary diagnosis. Sedation and analgesia with opioids are often necessary to achieve adequate mechanical ventilation and should be used after appropriate ventilator synchronization has been achieved.

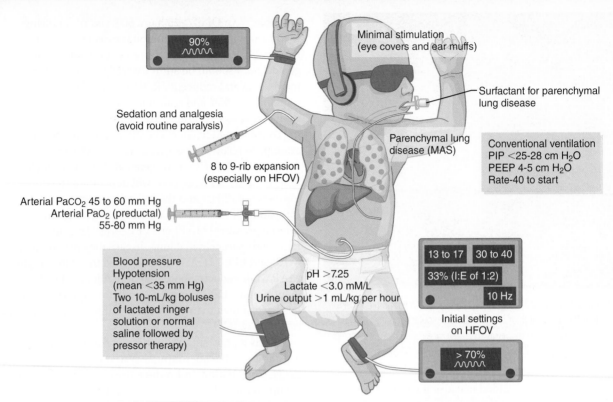

FIGURE 8-10 General principles used for the management for PPHN.

Reproduced with permission from Lakshminrusimha, S, Keszler, M. (2015) Persistent Pulmonary Hypertension of the Newborn. NeoReviews. 2015;16(12). Figure 5. Copyright ©2018 by the AAP.

Neuromuscular blockade is avoided but may be needed when asynchronous breathing and severe hypoxemia persist. Cardiac output is maintained with the use of inotropic agents and with judicious volume replacement.

When mechanical ventilation and iNO are not sufficient to improve oxygenation and ventilation and the OI is >40, ECMO should be considered. ECMO will prevent further induced lung injury, provide oxygenation, relieve acidosis, and allow time for the lung and pulmonary vasculature to heal. **Figure 8-10** highlights the general management principles for PPHN.

Complications and Outcomes

The mortality rate of PPHN has improved with the use of iNO and ECMO. Mortality rates were nearly 40% in the early 20th century, but the use of iNO and ECMO have resulted in survival rates overall of approximately 80%.[63,64] The range of survival varies based on the underlying pathophysiologic cause—diaphragmatic hernia survival is near 50% and MAS is near 90% with the use of ECMO. Neurodevelopmental disabilities have been reported in up to 60% of infants. In a report of 109 school-age survivors of PPHN (77 of whom received iNO and 12 who required ECMO), 24% had chronic respiratory problems, 60% had abnormal chest X-rays, and 6.4% had some degree of hearing loss.[69] Neurodevelopmental outcomes were very encouraging, with no difference seen between these PPHN survivors and the control group in IQ, behavior, or academic achievement.[69]

Case Study 1

A 28-year-old mother gave birth to a 2.8 kg female by cesarean section at 36 weeks' gestation. Apgar scores were 6 at 1 minute and 9 at 5 minutes. The baby developed tachypnea with a respiratory rate of 93 breaths per minute soon after birth and had moderate work of breathing with mild nasal flaring and retractions. The patient was placed on 1 L/min of oxygen by nasal cannula and was transferred to the neonatal intensive care unit. The assessment revealed: heart rate 158 beats per minute; respiratory rate 80 breaths per minute; blood pressure 65/45 mm Hg. The infant was well perfused and breath sounds were clear to auscultation. The remainder of the exam was unremarkable. A chest radiograph was obtained which revealed normal lung expansion, fluid in the horizontal fissures and increased pulmonary vascularity. Differential diagnosis of transient tachypnea of the newborn was made. Over the next 24 hours the infant's respiratory status worsened. Supplemental oxygen by high-flow nasal cannula was initiated at an FiO_2 of 40% to maintain oxygen saturations >92%. By day 3 the patient's status improved, a high-flow nasal cannula therapy was ordered. Within 6 hours the infant did not require any additional oxygen support. Vital signs were as follows: heart rate 145 beats per minute; respiratory rate 50 breaths per minute; blood pressure 60/40 mm Hg; and oxygen saturation >95% on room air. There were no further complications with respiratory function, and the patient was discharge to go home.

1. How can differential diagnosis of transient tachypnea of the newborn be confirmed?

2. How soon does TTN present after birth?

3. What are the typical clinical symptoms that present in the newborn?

4. What are possible predictors of TTN?

Case Study 2

A 30-year-old P1G1 female, whose pregnancy had been uncomplicated, was admitted to the hospital for induction of labor at 41 weeks' gestation. Induction was successful; artificial rupture of the membranes produced thick, meconium-stained amniotic fluid. An amnioinfusion was performed to relieve fetal heart decelerations. However, no change in the frequency of fetal heart rate decelerations was noted and a cesarean section was performed. A 3.6 kg female infant was delivered. The baby was limp at birth and was covered by yellow-green meconium. Little respiratory effort was noted and the infant's respiratory rate was 20 breaths per minute. The heart rate was 90 beats per minute, the baby's color was dusky, and she had poor peripheral perfusion. Positive pressure ventilation was given with 100% oxygen. Apgar scores were 3 at 1 minute and 6 at 5 minutes. The infant was intubated and suctioned for a significant amount of particulate meconium. Heart rate and oxygen saturations improved, and the patient was mechanically ventilated and transferred to the NICU. Chest radiograph revealed the ETT tip was 2 cm from the carina, hyperinflation and perihilar opacities in the lung. The patient continued to receive supportive care with mechanical ventilation and then was weaned to CPAP +6 cm H_2O day 3. She was extubated on day 4 and placed in an incubator with 25% oxygen. Her condition continued to improve with no additional complications, and she was discharged 2 weeks postpartum.

1. What MAS pathway would this patient fall into?

2. What supportive care options are there for patients who are in the severe MAS pathway?

3. What are the risk factors for MAS?

References

1. Eichenwald EC, Committee on Fetus and Newborn, American Academy of Pediatrics. Apnea of prematurity. *Pediatrics*. 2016;137(1): doi:10.1542/peds.2015-3757.

2. Bloch-Salisbury E. Hall MH, Sharma P. Heritability of apnea of prematurity: a retrospective twin study. *Pediatrics*. 2010;126(4): e779-e787.

3. Finer NN, Barrington KJ, Hayes BJ, Hugh A. Mixed, and central apnea in the neonate. Physiologic correlates. *J Pediatrics*. 1992;121(6):943-950.

4. Martin R. Pathogenesis, clinical presentation and diagnosis of apnea of prematurity. Up to Date. 2016. http://www.uptodate .com/contents/pathogenesis-clinical-presentation-and-diagnosis-of -apnea-of-prematurity. Accessed December 17, 2017.

5. DiFiore JM, Arko MK, Miller MJ, et al. Cardiorespiratory events in preterm infants referred for apnea monitoring studies. *Pediatrics.* åå 2001;108(6):1304-1308.

6. Walther-Larsen S, Rasmussen LS. The former preterm infant and risk of post-operative apnoea: recommendations for management. *Acta Anaesthesiol Scand.* 2006;50(7):888-893.

7. Gladstone IM, Katz VL. The morbidity of the 34- to 35-week gestation: should we reexamine the paradigm? *Am J Perinatol.* 2004;21(1):9-13.

8. Henderson-Smart DJ, De Paoli AG. Prophylactic methyl xanthine for prevention of apnea in preterm infants. *Cochrane Database Syst Rev.* 2010;12:CD000432.

9. Mohammed S, Nour I, Shabaan AE, Shouman B, Abdel-Hady H, Nasef N. High versus low-dose caffeine for apnea of prematurity: a randomized controlled trial. *Eur J Pediatr.* 2015;174(7):949-956.

10. Miller MJ, Carlo WA, Martin RJ. Continuous positive airway pressure selectively reduces obstructive apnea in preterm infants. *J Pediatr.* 1985;106(1):91-94.

11. Katz ES, Mitchell RB, Dambrosio CM. Obstructive sleep apnea in infants. *Am J Respir Crit Care Med.* 2012;185(8):805-816.

12. Stoll BJ, Hansen NI, Higgins RD, et al. Very low birth weight preterm infants with early onset neonatal sepsis: the predominance of gram-negative infections continues in the National Institute of Child Health and Human Development Neonatal Research Network, 2002-2003. *Pediatr Infect Dis J.* 2005;24(7):635-639.

13. Clark H, Clark LS. (2005) The genetics of neonatal respiratory disease. *Semin Fetal Neonatal Med.* 2005;10(3):271-282.

14. Carlo WA, Ambalavanan N. Respiratory distress syndrome (Hyaline membrane disease). In: *Nelson Textbook of Pediatrics.* Philadelphia, PA: WB Saunders; 2012: 831-834.

15. Fanaroff AA, Stoll BJ, Wright LL, et al. Trends in neonatal morbidity and mortality for very low birthweight infants. *Am J Obstet Gynecol.* 2007;196(2):147.e1-8.

16. Roberts D, Dalziel S. Antenatal corticosteroids for accelerating fetus lung maturation for women at risk for preterm birth. *Cochrane Database Syst Rev.* 2006;3:CD004454.

17. Isayama T, Chai-Adisaksopha C, McDonald SD. Noninvasive ventilation with vs without early surfactant to prevent chronic lung disease in preterm infants: a systematic review and meta-analysis. *JAMA Pediatr.* 2015;169(8):731-739.

18. Yehya N, Thomas NJ. Disassociating lung mechanics and oxygenation in pediatric acute respiratory distress syndrome. *Crit Care Med.* 2017;45(7):1232-1239.

19. Holme N, Chetculi P. Pathophysiology of RDS in neonates. *Pediatr Child Health.* 2012;22(12):507-512.

20. Ribeiro-Lyra PP, de Albuquerque-Diniz EM. The importance of surfactant on the development of neonatal pulmonary disease. *Clinics (Sao Paulo).* 2007;62(2):181-190.

21. Dewhurst CJ, Harrison RF, Harvey DR, Parkinson CE. Prediction of respiratory-distress syndrome. *Lancet.* 1973;2(7824):332-333.

22. Sweet DG, Carnielli V, Greisen G, et al. European Consensus Guidelines on the management of respiratory distress syndrome. *Neonatology.* 2017;111(2):107-125.

23. McGinnis KY, Brown JA, Morrison JC. Changing patterns of fetal lung maturity testing. *J Perinatol.* 2008;28(1):20-23.

24. Soll RF, Blanco F. Natural surfactant extract versus synthetic surfactant for neonatal respiratory distress syndrome. *Cochrane Database Syst Rev.* 2001;2:CD000144.

25. Morley CJ, Davis PG, Doyle LW, et al. COIN trial investigators: nasal CPAP or intubation at birth for very premature infants. *N Engl J Med.* 2008;358(7):700-708.

26. Ryu J, Haddad G, Carlo WA. Clinical effectiveness and safety permissive hypercapnia. *Clinical Perinatol.* 2012;39(3):603-612.

27. Chen M, Citil A, McCabe F, et al. Infection, oxygen, and immaturity: interacting risk factors of retinopathy of prematurity. *Neonatalogy.* 2011;99(2):125-132.

28. Chow LC, Wright KW, Sola A. Oxygen Administration Study Group: can change in clinical practice decrease the incidence of severe retinopathy of prematurity in very low birth weight infants? *Pediatrics.* 2003;111(2):339-345.

29. Schmidt B, Davis P, Moddemann D, et al. Trial of indomethacin prophylaxis in preterm investigators: long-term effects of indomethacin prophylaxis in extremely low birth weight infants. *N Engl J Med.* 2001;344:1966-1972.

30. Kovisto M, Marttila R, Saarela T. Wheezing, illness and re-hospitalization in the first two years of life after neonatal respiratory distress syndrome. *Pediatrics.* 2005;147(4):486-492.

31. Avery ME, Gatewood OB, Brumley G. Transient tachypnea of the newborn. *Am J Dis Child.* 1966;111(4):380-385.

32. Johnson K, Garcia-Prats J, Kim M. Transient tachypnea of the newborn. *Am J Dis Child.* 2016. https://www.scribd.com/document/336423659/Transient-Tachypnea-of-the-Newborn. Accessed November 14, 2017.

33. Rawlings JS, Wilson JL, García J. Radiological case of the month. Wet lung syndrome (transient tachypnea of the newborn). *Am J Dis Child.* 1985;139(12):1233-1234.

34. Avery ME, Gatewood OB, Brumley G. Transient tachypnea of newborn. Possible delayed resorption of fluid at birth. *Am J Dis Child.* 1966;111(4):380-385.

35. Liem JJ, Hug SL, Ekuma O, Becker AB, Kozyrsky AL. Transient tachypnea of the newborn may be an early clinical manifestation of wheezing symptoms. *J Pediatr.* 2007;151(1):29-33.

36. Duke T. Neonatal pneumonia in developing countries. *Arch Dis Child Fetal Neonatal Ed.* 2005;90(3):F211-F219.

37. Nissen MD. Congenital and neonatal pneumonia. *Pediatr Resp Rev.* 2007;8(3):195-203.

38. Stoll BJ, Hansen NI, Bell EF, et al. Trends in care practices, morbidity mortality of extremely preterm neonates (1993-2012). *JAMA.* 2015;314(10):1039-1051.

39. Sinha A, Yokoe D, Platt R. Epidemiology of neonatal infections: experience during and after hospitalization. *Pediatr Infect Dis J.* 2003;22(3):244-251.

40. World Health Organization (WHO). Pneumonia fact sheet. http://www.who.int/mediacentre/factsheets/fs331/en/. Accessed November 2017.

41. Seale AC, Blencowe H, Bianchi-Jassir F, et al. Stillbirth with group B streptococcus disease worldwide: systematic review and meta-analyses. *Clin Infect Dis.* 2017;65(Suppl 2):S125-S132.

42. Singh BS, Clark RH, Powers RJ, Spitzer AR. Meconium aspiration syndrome remains a significant problem in the NICU: outcomes and treatment patterns in term neonates admitted for intensive care during a ten-year period. *J Perinatol.* 2009;29(7):497-503.

43. Velaphi S, Vidyasagar D. Intrapartum and postdelivery management of infants born to mothers with meconium-stained amniotic fluid: evidence-based recommendations. *Clin Perinatol.* 2006;33(1):29-42.

44. Yoder BA, Kirsch EA, Barth WH, Gordon MC. Changing obstetric practices associated with decreasing incidence of meconium aspiration syndrome. *Obstet Gynecol.* 2002.99(5 Pt 1):731-739.

45. Louis D, Sundaram V, Mukhopadhyay K, Dutta S, Kumar P. Predictors of mortality in neonates with meconium aspiration syndrome. *Indian Pediatr.* 2014;51(8):637-640.

46. Goldsmith JP. Continuous positive airway pressure and conventional mechanical ventilation in the treatment of meconium aspiration syndrome. *J Perinatol.* 2008;28(Suppl 3):S49-S55.

47. Flores MT. Understanding neonatal chest x-rays part II: clinical and radiological manifestations of selected lung disorders. *Neonatal Netw.* 1993;12(8):9-15.

48. Velaphi S, Kwawegen AV. Meconium aspiration syndrome requiring assisted ventilation: perspective in a setting with limited resources. *J Perinatol.* 2008;28(Suppl 3):S35-S42.

49. Halliday HL. Endotracheal intubation at birth for preventing morbidity and mortality in vigorous, meconium-stained infants born to term. *Cochrane Database Syst Rev.* 2001;1:CD00500.

50. Cleary GM, Wiswell TE. Meconium-stained amniotic fluid and the meconium aspiration syndrome: an update. *Pediatr Clin North Am.* 1998;45(3):511-529.

51. Roehr CC, Hansmann G, Hoehn T, Bührer C. The 2010 Guidelines on Neonatal Resuscitation (AHA, ERC, ILCOR): similarities and differences—what progress has been made since 2005? *Klin Padiatr.* 2011;223(5):299-307.

52. Swarnam K, Soraisham AS, Sivanandan S. Advances in the management of meconium aspiration syndrome. *Int J Pediatr.* 2012;2012:359571.

53. El Shahed AI, Dargaville PA, Ohlsson A, Soll R. Surfactant for meconium aspiration syndrome in term and late preterm infants. *Cochrane Database Syst Rev.* 2014;12:CD002054.

54. Mokra D, Mokry J, Tonhajzerova I. Anti-inflammatory treatment of meconium aspiration syndrome: benefits and risks. *Respir Physiol Neurobiol.* 2013;187(1):52-57.

55. Yeh TF. Core concepts: meconium aspiration syndrome: pathogenesis and current management. *NeoReviews.* 2010;11(9):e503-e512.

56. Singh BS, Clark RH, Powers RJ, Spitzer AR. Meconium aspiration syndrome remains a significant problem in the NICU: outcomes and treatment patterns in term neonates admitted for intensive care during a ten-year period. *J Perinatol.* 2009;29(7):497-503.

57. Nair J, Lakshminrusima Update on PPHN: mechanisms and treatment. *Semin Perinatol.* 2014;38(2):78-91.

58. Nakwan N, Pithaklimnuwong S. Acute kidney injury and pneumothorax are risk factors for mortality in persistent pulmonary hypertension of the newborn in Thai neonates. *J Matern Fetal Neonatal Med.* 2016;29(11):1741-1746.

59. Delaney C, Cornfield DN. Risk factors for persistent pulmonary hypertension of the newborn. *Pulm Circ.* 2012;2(1):15-20.

60. Sharma V, Berkelhamer S, Lakshminrushimha S. Persistent pulmonary hypertension of the newborn. *Matern Health Neonatol Perinatol.* 2015;3:1-14

61. Nakwan N, Nakwan N, Wannaro J. Predicting mortality in infants with persistent pulmonary hypertension of the newborn with the Score for Neonatal Acute Physiology-Version II (SNAP-II) in Thai neonates. *J Perinat Med.* 2011;39(3):311-315.

62. Puthiyachirakkal M, Mhanna MJ. Pathophysiology, management, and outcome of persistent pulmonary hypertension of the newborn: a clinical review. *Front Pediatr.* 2013;2:1–23

63. Walsh-Sukys MC, Tyson JE, Wright LL, et al. Persistent pulmonary hypertension of the newborn in the era before nitric oxide: practice variation and outcomes. *Pediatrics.* 2000;105(1 Pt 1):14-20.

64. Committee on Fetus and Newborn: American Academy of Pediatrics. Use of inhaled nitric oxide. *Pediatrics.* 2000;106(2 Pt 1):344-345.

65. Kinsella JP, Truog WE, Walsh WF, et al. Randomized, multicenter trial of inhaled nitric oxide and high-frequency oscillatory ventilation in severe, persistent pulmonary hypertension of the newborn. *J Pediatr.* 1997;131(1 Pt 1):55-62.

66. Christou H, Van Marter LJ, Wessel DL, et al. Inhaled nitric oxide reduces the need for extracorporeal membrane oxygenation in infants with persistent pulmonary hypertension of the newborn. *Crit Care Med.* 2000;28(11):3722-3727.

67. Keller RL, Hamrick SE, Kitterman JA, Fineman JR, Hawgood S. Treatment of rebound and chronic pulmonary hypertension with oral sildenafil in an infant with congenital diaphragmatic hernia. *Pediatr Crit Care Med.* 2004;5(2):184-187.

68. Lakshminrusimha S, Keszler M. Persistent pulmonary hypertension of the newborn. *NeoReviews.* 2015;16(12).

69. Rosenberg AA, Lee NR, Vaver KN, et al. School-age outcomes of newborns treated for persistent pulmonary hypertension. *J Perinatol.* 2010;30(2):127-134.

© Anna Rubak/ShutterStock, Inc.

OUTLINE

OBJECTIVES

1. Describe the abnormalities underlying major congenital malformations of the lungs.
2. Discuss the etiology and pathophysiology of the various congenital disorders in newborns and infants.
3. Recognize and manage choanal atresia or other upper airway disorders.
4. Define the complications and outcomes primarily associated with the development of choanal atresia.
5. Examine the etiology and pathophysiology of a tracheoesophageal fistula.
6. Identify and manage a tracheoesophageal fistula.
7. Explain the complications and outcomes primarily associated with the development of a tracheoesophageal fistula.
8. Review the development, etiology, and pathophysiology of a congenital diaphragmatic hernia.
9. Understand and manage a congenital diaphragmatic hernia.
10. Describe the complications and outcomes primarily associated with the development of a congenital diaphragmatic hernia.
11. Understand the etiology, diagnosis, and management of surfactant protein deficiencies.
12. Explain the complications and outcomes of surfactant protein deficiencies.
13. Distinguish and manage various congenital pulmonary anomalies.

KEY TERMS

anastomosis
atretic plate
bronchogenic cyst
choanal atresia
congential diaphragmatic
    hernia (CDH)
congenital pulmonary
    airway malformation
congenital pulmonary
    anomalies
distraction osteogenesis
esophageal atresia
glossoptosis
macroglossia
mandibular hypoplasia
mitomycin C
oligohydramnios

paradoxical cyanosis
Pierre Robin syndrome
polyhydramnios
pseudomacroglossia
pulmonary agenesis
pulmonary aplasia
pulmonary hypoplasia
pulmonary sequestration
stridor
surfactant
surfactant protein
    deficiencies
tracheoesophageal
    fistula (TEF)
Treacher Collins
    syndrome (TCS)

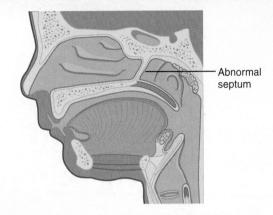

—Abnormal septum

FIGURE 9-1 An illustration of the lack of continuity between the nasal cavity and the pharynx that occurs with choanal atresia.

Introduction

In order to provide effective patient care to neonates, it is fundamental for clinicians to have knowledge of the etiology and pathophysiology of various congenital disorders of the respiratory system. Recognizing, managing, and treating these disorders requires an understanding of how the disorder presents, the predisposed clinical condition, and the treatment options available.

This chapter will focus on the etiologic and pathophysiologic characteristics of the most common congenital disorders of the respiratory system. It will focus on providing information on several complex disorders and engage the reader in management strategies designed to improve clinical outcome.

Choanal Atresia

Choanal atresia, which occurs in approximately 1 in 7000 live births and is more predominant among females, has been recognized for more than 200 years.[1,2] It is a congenital disorder in which there is a narrowing of the back of the nasal cavity (choanae), resulting in a lack of continuity between the nasal cavity and the pharynx (Figure 9-1). Choanal atresia is the most common form of congenital nasal obstruction, and infants often present with difficulty breathing.

Very few risk factors have been identified for this disorder. Two suspected risk factors for the development of choanal atresia are molecular models, including abnormalities in vitamin A metabolism and prenatal drug treatments for hyperthyroidism, and genetic causes.[1] Newborn infants are commonly described as obligate nasal breathers, as they prefer breathing through their noses rather than their mouths. Evidence suggests that there is potential loss of nasal humidification in infants who mouth breathe, which can lead to alterations in lung surfactant and mucociliary clearance as well as decreased lung compliance.[3]

Because mouth breathing is not a normal response in newborn infants, this anatomical closure or obstruction of the nasal cavity could result in immediate respiratory distress or potential death. Choanal atresia may be unilateral or bilateral, meaning it can affect one or both sides of the nasal airway. Because partial or complete obstruction is a potential outcome, close attention must be paid on screening, management, and treatment for all infants at risk.

Etiology

Choanal atresia causes unilateral or bilateral blockage or obstruction of the posterior nasal cavity. This disorder is the leading cause of nasal surgery among infants, although its etiology is largely unknown. Recently, molecular model theories have been developed.

Vitamin A metabolism abnormalities have been associated with choanal atresia. Retinoic acid is metabolized from vitamin A, and maternal deficiency in retinoic acid during the gestational period has been linked to craniofacial malformations in many clinical cases.[2] A simple prenatal treatment plan to restore vitamin A levels was effective in preventing choanal atresia.[2]

Choanal atresia cases have also been identified in thionamide-exposed infants. Thionamides are most often used to treat overactive thyroids. Pregnant women diagnosed with hyperthyroidism and the prenatal use of anti-thyroid medication increase the risk for choanal atresia.[2]

Genetic causes for choanal atresia were first described in 1979. These genetic causes, also known as the CHARGE association (Table 9-1),[2] describe multiple congenital anomalies, including choanal atresia, that affect many areas of the body. Infants with CHARGE syndrome have a cluster or combination of anomalies, including coloboma, heart defects, choanal atresia, retarded growth and development, genital hypoplasia, and ear deafness.[2] Many infants with bilateral choanal atresia have other associated CHARGE congenital

TABLE 9-1
Major and Minor Characteristics Associated with CHARGE Syndrome

Major Factors	Minor Factors
Ocular coloboma	Cardiovascular malformations
Choanal atresia	Genital hypoplasia
Characteristic ear abnormalities	Cleft lip/palate
Cranial nerve abnormalities, including sensorineural hearing loss (SNHL)	Tracheoesophageal fistula
	Hypothalamo-hypophyseal dysfunction
	Distinctive CHARGE facies
	Developmental delay

defects as well, so the CHARGE mnemonic can be used to alert clinicians to look for these other potential abnormalities. Tracheostomy is often used in the course of treatment. Although early tracheotomies in patients with CHARGE syndrome cause nonnegligible morbidity and mortality, this treatment option is often preferred to delay hypoxic events and to lessen developmental disturbances.[4]

Pathophysiology

Choanal atresia is a developmental problem of the neonatal airway. This condition can consist of a bony obstruction, a membranous obstruction, or, as in the majority of cases, a combination of the two. Recent evidence suggests that mixed bony/membranous obstructions occur in 70% of infants diagnosed with choanal atresia while pure bony obstructions occur in 30% of infants.[2] The exact pathophysiologic origin of choanal atresia is unknown, but it is postulated that failure of the oronasal membrane to rupture or the misdirection of mesodermal flow leads to malrotation of nasal pits in the developing fetus.[5] The nasal openings are not formed, which causes lack of communication between the nasopharynx and the remainder of the infant's airway. There are four main anomalies associated with this congenital disorder: (1) narrowing of the nasal cavity, (2) lateral obstruction by the atretic plate, (3) medial obstruction by the vomer (nasal septum), and (4) membranous obstruction.[5]

Diagnosis

Choanal atresia can be diagnosed by a comprehensive examination of the nose. Appropriate delivery room management, including assessment of and support to the infant's airway, breathing, and circulation, must

be provided before diagnostic evaluation for this disorder occurs. During initial airway management, choanal atresia may be suspected when there is an inability to pass a nasogastric tube (NG) or suction catheter through each nare. Additionally, placing a shiny metal object or mirror under the nose to observe fogging is a frequently used tool; lack of nasal fogging suggests a unilateral or bilateral obstruction of flow from the airway through the nasopharynx and/or nares.

The definitive diagnosis is established through more sophisticated tests, including computed tomography (CT) scan or nasal endoscopy.[1] A CT scan of the paranasal sinuses and skull base helps to identify the extent, type, and severity of the disorder as well as the estimated size of the nasopharynx (**Figure 9-2**).[1] A CT scan can also differentiate unilateral nasal obstructions, such as a nasal foreign body, septal deviation, or nasal tumor, and may also be helpful in identifying secondary anomalies. However, awareness of potential imaging pitfalls can help to avoid misdiagnoses or unnecessary surgery. Scanning at an angle that defines the permanence of the choanae with the nasopharynx will help to differentiate choanal atresia from other potential diagnoses.[6] Proper imaging skills, knowledge of the disease process, and awareness of the normal ossification sequence of facial structures can play a pivotal role. Disadvantages to using CT in infants include high potential for radiation exposure and the need for sedation to prevent movement artifacts. Local contrast is useful and helps to augment the thickness of the atretic plate and vomer in addition to defining the condition of the nasal mucosa.[6]

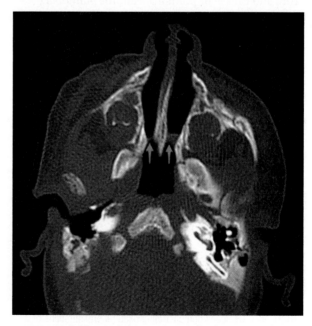

FIGURE 9-2 A CT scan demonstrating a lack of communication of the nasopharynx as indicated by the red arrows.

Case courtesy of Dr. Jeremy Jones, Radiopaedia.org, rID: 12385.

Nasal endoscopy is also described as both a diagnostic and a therapeutic tool for the evaluation and treatment of choanal atresia. Endoscopic imaging provides exceptional visualization of the nasal area. Research has shown that endoscopic examination is able to accurately define nasal malformations, facilitating efficient surgical procedure planning.[7]

Clinical Presentation

Nasal or airway obstruction is not easily diagnosed prenatally. Infants with choanal atresia often present with respiratory distress and **stridor**. Stridor, an abnormal, high-pitched breathing sound caused by a blockage or narrowing in the upper airways, can occur during inspiration, expiration, or both. Upon examination, an infant with this malformation will present with an increase in work of breathing, severe stridor, or cyanosis, which are signs of impending airway obstruction.[8]

The presentation of choanal atresia depends on three factors: whether the obstruction is unilateral, bilateral, or associated with other craniofacial abnormalities (**Figure 9-3**).

Infants with unilateral obstruction often present with symptoms later (between 5–24 months of age) with persistent nasal discharge, nasal obstruction, or occasional ear infections.[1] Occasionally, the diagnosis of unilateral choanal atresia can be acknowledged after unsuccessful septal surgery in adulthood. Chronic upper airway obstruction in infants can also present as obstructive sleep apnea syndrome.[3] In severe cases, nasal obstruction causes hypoxemia and hypercarbia, which can lead to changes in the pulmonary vasculature and cause cor pulmonale and/or pulmonary hypertension.[3]

Bilateral obstruction presenting at birth causes airway compromise. As infants are obligate nasal breathers, more than 50% of those with bilateral obstruction due to choanal atresia will have oxygen desaturation.[1] The occurrence of bilateral nasal obstruction

presents as a neonatal airway emergency, and resuscitation efforts are often needed to stabilize the infant. The clinical presentation of bilateral choanal atresia includes obvious airway obstruction, stridor, and **paradoxical cyanosis** (the relief of airway obstruction when crying occurs).[1] Establishing and protecting an airway is often required prior to definitive management of this disorder.

Craniofacial abnormalities make up a minor, but critical, subgroup of the infants and children with choanal atresia. These complex patients have defective skull bases, abnormal cranial cavities, and thickened choanae tissues.[1] Important discussions surrounding related abnormalities, additional airway obstruction sites, muscle tone, and feeding concerns need to be considered in this subgroup.[1]

Management

A variety of care strategies are available for the management of choanal atresia. A patent nasal cavity is the ultimate outcome measure for surgical management strategies. Although there is substantial literature published on the surgical management of choanal atresia, the intervention or technique used to alleviate the obstruction depends on clinician preference and the thickness of the atretic plate.

There are four "classical" surgical approaches: (1) trans-nasal endoscopy and puncture, (2) trans-palatal resection, (3) trans-septal approach, and (4) sub-labial approach, each with varying degrees of success. More recently, the trans-nasal endoscopic procedure has been reported as the best possible treatment option for choanal atresia.

Trans-nasal puncture is a traditional and safe technique to establish a patent airway. The trans-nasal puncture technique consists of making a perforation in the **atretic plate**,[1] or the anatomical thin tissue plate that separates the nasal cavity from the pharynx. The major disadvantage associated with this approach is the limited field of vision, which often results in inadequate removal of bone/membrane.[7] This treatment technique lost favor due to a high recurrence rate of restenosis,[1] so, when used, it is useful to combine this method with other techniques.

Trans-palatal resection provides excellent exposure of the abnormality, allowing for direct correction of the area with a surgical drill. Unfortunately, increases in operating times, growth disturbance complications, and subsequent orthodontic abnormalities are associated with the use of this technique.[1] As a result, this repair technique is rarely used today.

The trans-septal and sub-labial approaches have been used specifically in patients with craniofacial deformities. These methods allow for the preservation of the nasal septum and maxillary crest, which minimizes the propensity for nasal bone growth disruption.[5]

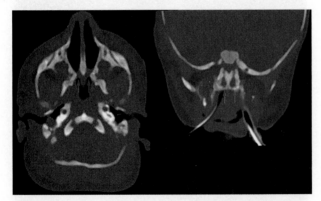

FIGURE 9-3 CT scans demonstrating bilateral presentations of choanal atresia. The arrows point to the bony structures causing the obstruction.

Hellerhoff, used under CC BY-SA 3.0.

Technical advances allow for enhanced visualization, providing more opportunity to use the trans-nasal endoscopic instrument route (**Figure 9-4**). Recently, endoscopic resection has become a popular surgical repair technique. This technique uses an endoscope to visualize and perforate the atretic plate. Once a passage is created, dilators are used to enlarge the area. The advantages to this approach include clear visualization of the nasal field; accurate removal of the atretic plate; the ability to perform the technique in a wide variety of patients, from infants to adults; and a shorter recovery time.[7]

Stenting is often used after performing a surgical procedure to keep the nasal cavity patent. However, it is not clear whether the use of stents following endoscopic surgery prevents stenosis from reoccurring after their removal.[1] In neonates with bilateral choanal atresia, however, stents are essential and recommended in order to maintain a sufficient airway in the early periods following surgery.

Complications and Outcomes

Major complications can occur following surgical repair of choanal atresia and include cerebrospinal fluid leaks, midbrain trauma, and palate perforation.[5] The use of more advanced surgical equipment has reduced the incidence of major complications. Minor complications can often be seen following stent placements.

Postoperative stenosis is the most common complication encountered with surgical repair, occurring in up to 50% of patients. The literature suggests that the presence of gastroesophageal reflux disease (GERD), patient age (<10 days old), and insufficient postoperative revisions are predictive factors for restenosis.[9] **Mitomycin C** is a topical agent aid used intra-operatively

to prevent the formation of scar tissue and restenosis following choanal atresia repair.[5] Mitomycin C is an antibiotic that inhibits cell division, protein synthesis, and fibroblast proliferation, resulting in reduced granulation formation in patients undergoing nasal reconstruction.[5] Although it is recommended as an adjunct therapy for choanal atresia repair, its efficacy outcomes remain controversial.

Postoperative care of these infants should include, as needed, prophylactic oral antibiotics, patient/family education on nasal irrigation for cleansing the nasopharynx, and proper use of home suction devices.[10] Follow-up care consists of nasal breathing assessments and comprehensive examinations of the nose and nasopharynx patency. Surgery is considered successful when bilateral normal nasal breathing is restored and there is no evidence of airway obstruction during feeding or rest.[10] Patient prognosis after nasal reconstruction is excellent.

Mandibular Hypoplasia

Mandibular hypoplasia is a frequently encountered craniofacial disorder in neonates, occurring in approximately 14,000 live births per year.[11] This congenital syndrome, also known as micrognathia, strawberry chin, or hypognathia, is characterized by an undersized facial jaw, specifically a small mandible and receding chin. There are varying degrees of severity, which are shown in **Figure 9-5**. This disorder also involves abnormal or arrested development of the mandible. Infants with markedly hypoplastic mandibles are at high risk for potential abnormalities, including **glossoptosis**, or retraction of the tongue, and upper airway obstruction. Because mandibular hypoplasia not only causes facial disfigurement but also significant functional impairments, care must be used when treating these children.

Etiology

Genetic conditions and environmental factors make the mandible a common location for fetal deformities. In utero, the complex, multistep formation process makes the development of the mandible highly vulnerable to genetic mishaps.[12] Infants born with mandibular hypoplasia were also found to have decreased fetal movement.[12] In addition to jaw abnormalities, the infant's mouth may also be paralyzed.[12]

Pathophysiology

The pathophysiology of mandibular hypoplasia may include such conditions as chromosomal or neuromuscular abnormalities, gene disorders, and other syndromes.[13] The mandibular changes likely follow a hereditary pattern and often occur in conjunction with other congenital diseases.

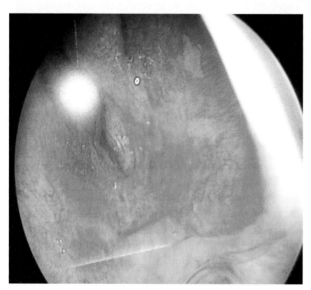

FIGURE 9-4 An endoscopic view of unilateral choanal atresia. The nasal passage in this image is completely obstructed.

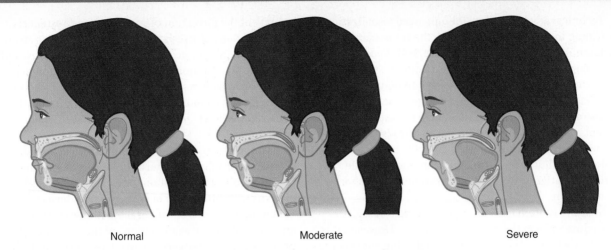

Normal   Moderate   Severe

FIGURE 9-5 An illustration of the varying degrees of severity associated with mandibular hypoplasia.

Diagnosis

Any syndrome associated with abnormal cranio-facial anatomy can lead to airway difficulties and life-threatening problems in infants. Prenatal screening by ultrasound imaging helps identify mandibular hypoplasia and can distinguish it from other malformations, which better prepares clinicians to present the parent(s) with treatment options.[14] With the fetal head in a favorable position, the mandible can be studied by ultrasonography as early as 10 weeks' gestation.[12] Both subjective and objective diagnoses of the fetal mandible can be made. A subjective diagnosis can be conducted by assessing the mandible in relation to the rest of the face via a midsagittal facial profile.[12] Two methods have also been reported to assist in objective diagnosis: the inferior facial angle and the jaw index measure ratios of the facial profile.[12] Both are proven effective in diagnosing mandibular hypoplasia.

Polysomnography (sleep study) is another standard assessment tool used to determine the presence and severity of airway obstruction in children with mandibular hypoplasia. Polysomnography is useful in determining the presence of hypoxemia and CO_2 retention and is often used to compliment clinical and radiologic assessment of children diagnosed with mandibular hypoplasia or similar syndromes.[15]

Important steps to consider when diagnosing mandibular hypoplasia include assessing for the presence of other associated anomalies; determining if there are any abnormal structure arrangements, such as Pierre Robin syndrome; and determining the risk of recurrence.[12]

Clinical Presentation

In addition to the mandibular abnormality, infants and children present with loud snoring, daytime somnolence, oxygen desaturations (<85%), and an elevated apnea/hypopnea index (>5).[15] Clinical morbidities result from the airway obstruction and hypoxemia and often include failure to thrive, developmental delays, GERD, feeding difficulties, CO_2 retention, heart failure, brain damage, and sudden infant death syndrome.[11] There are many other syndromes associated with impaired mandibular development in infants. Mandibular hypoplasia is commonly found in conjunction with such anomalies as Pierre Robin syndrome or Treacher Collins syndrome.

Pierre Robin syndrome is a set of facial abnormalities consisting of mandibular hypoplasia, cleft palate, and glossoptosis (**Figure 9-6**). This triad of deformities may potentially contribute to respiratory distress, airway obstruction, and hypoxia. This condition is now being described as a "sequence" to reflect the developmental succession of these three anomalies. Diagnosis is made through physical examination of signs and symptoms. Possible management or treatment alternatives include glossopexy (tongue-lip adhesion), nasoesophageal intubation, tracheostomy, or use of a modified airway with a Kirschner wire (K-airway).[16] Placing the infant in the prone position with dorsiflexion (upward direction) of the head provides a short-term medical management option.[16]

Treacher Collins syndrome (TCS) is a genetic disorder that affects the ears, eyes, cheekbones, and chin of infants. **Figure 9-7** illustrates the facial abnormalities associated with TCS. This congenital deformity alters the development of facial bones and tissues and is generally associated with a bilateral cleft and craniofacial disease. The primary clinical characteristics of Treacher Collins syndrome include prominent eye dysmorphia, middle and external ear deformity, distinctive midfacial malformations, and maxilla-mandibular abnormalities.[17] In addition to having backward displacement, the

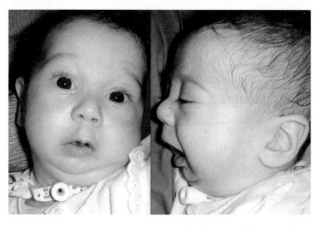

FIGURE 9-6 A frontal and lateral view of an infant with Pierre Robin syndrome.

Sesenna E, Magri A, Magnani C, Brevi B, Anghinoni M. Mandibular distraction in neonates: Indications, techniques, results. *Italian Journal of Pediatrics*. 2012;38. 7. 10.1186/ 1824-7288-38-7. Courtesy of Dr. E. Sesenna.

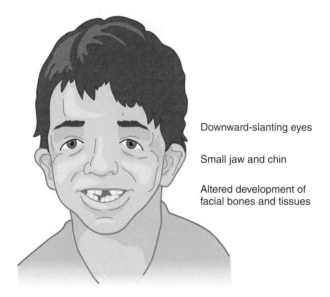

Downward-slanting eyes

Small jaw and chin

Altered development of facial bones and tissues

FIGURE 9-7 An illustration of the facial abnormalities seen with Treacher Collins syndrome.

mandible can be significantly underdeveloped and malformed. CT imaging demonstrates a diminished mandibular size and shape.[17] Treacher Collins syndrome can be also diagnosed using three-dimensional ultrasound imaging. Surgical treatments include palatoplasty to repair the cleft palate, oral surgery, ear reconstruction, and eyelid correction.[17] Midface tissue resuspension may also be considered as the child grows and develops.[17] Bone-assisted hearing aids may be necessary, as auditory loss results in a majority of children with Treacher Collins syndrome.[17]

Management

Diseases associated with anatomical restriction of the upper airway, including mandibular hypoplasia, Pierre Robin syndrome, and Treacher Collins syndrome, can affect upper airway musculature and promote airway obstruction.[3] Management options include stabilizing the airway, waiting for normal growth to resolve, or performing facial advancement surgery.[8]

Ongoing assessment includes evaluation of airway patency, feeding and/or swallowing difficulties, and growth and development milestones. Initially, infants and children require continuous apnea monitoring, oxygen-saturation monitoring, prone positioning, nasopharyngeal tubes, and in some cases continuous positive airway pressure (CPAP).[11,17] Airway suctioning and positioning are part of the infant's and child's routine care. Parenteral nutrition should begin as soon as possible, and parents should be educated on appropriate feeding techniques, patient assessment skills, and strategies to minimize the likelihood for aspiration.[17]

A tracheostomy may be an effective chronic management option for infants with mandibular hypoplasia. Despite its effectiveness, high costs, increased morbidity, speech delays, and psychological problems often accompany tracheostomy tube use. Therefore, it is important for clinicians to investigate alternatives and to provide the parents or caregivers with options.

Surgical procedures, such as lip-tongue adhesion, suture transfixion, various sling procedures, and distraction osteogenesis, are performed to correct the underlying defect.[15] **Distraction osteogenesis** is a fairly common and important treatment option to correct mandibular hypoplasia by making a longer bone out of a very short bone. A distractor is used to pull the two pieces of bone apart slowly and, over time, new bone grows to fill in the gap and allows the tongue to move away from the posterior hypopharynx, relieving upper airway obstruction.[18] **Figure 9-8** shows how the distractor is slowly moved and the angle of the jaw changed as the bone is lengthened. This procedure is intended to improve oral and craniofacial deformity and also helps to maintain a patent airway in patients, especially in those with obstructive sleep apnea syndrome (OSAS).[18] During sleep, patients with mandibular hypoplasia tend to have difficulty maintaining a patent airway, and hypopnea or apnea usually results.[18] The small mandible obstructs the airway by pushing the tongue closer to the pharyngeal wall.[19] A noncontrast CT scan can be done to assess bone stock and facial structure prior to surgery.[11] Correcting the mandible and improving airway patency can help to prevent growth retardation and prolonged need for a tracheostomy tube as well as improve quality of life. Evidence has shown that distraction osteogenesis is the best method for mandibular lengthening.[18] One of the most essential aspects in mandibular reconstruction is preoperative planning. It is important to assess the extent of the mandible defect, determine proper

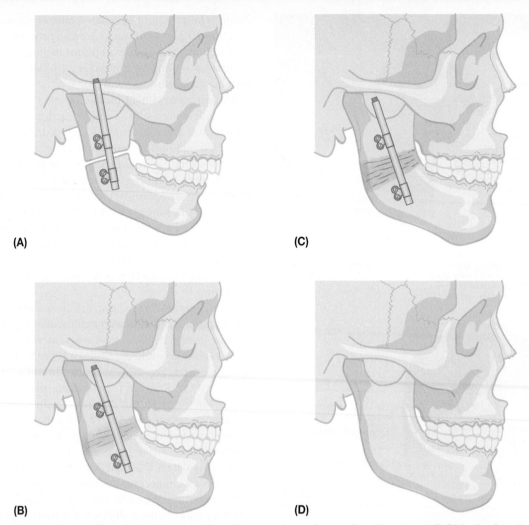

(A)   (C)

(B)   (D)

FIGURE 9-8 (**A**) An illustration of how the distractor is used to pull the two pieces of surgically cut bone apart. (**B–D**) As the distractor is slowly moved, the angle of the jaw changes and the bone is lengthened.

orientation to the site, and perform a skeletal assessment to gain a better understanding of the type of reconstruction that needs to be performed.[20] Distraction osteogenesis has a 92% to 100% success rate in treating mandibular hypoplasia.[11]

Additionally, the presence of OSAS in patients with mandibular hypoplasia may also warrant the potential management with nasal CPAP (nCPAP).[19] The successful use of this noninvasive therapy may avoid the need for more aggressive surgical intervention. Quality of life is much improved for infants and children undergoing surgical reconstructive or mandibular growth treatment.

Complications and Outcomes

Aplasia of the mandibular condyles, a rare orthopedic abnormality that results in the underdevelopment or nondevelopment of various craniofacial structures, is a complication associated with distraction osteogenesis.[17]

In some children, distraction may need to be delayed until later childhood, with a tracheostomy used in the interim to achieve and maintain a patent airway. Additionally, despite surgical efforts to correct facial abnormalities, there is a possibility of relapse. This complication can lead to latent airway obstruction and repeat distraction may be necessary.[17] The presence of secondary airway anomalies, such as tracheomalacia, subglottic stenosis, or tracheal rings, may reduce surgical success; these can be detected by laryngoscopy and/or bronchoscopy.[11] The average complication rate for the treatment of mandibular hypoplasia is 34%, with the majority being minor or moderate incidents.[11] The most common complications include infections, scarring, and dental or nerve injury.[11] Effective interventions and the use of validated evaluation protocols are essential for standardizing care and improving patient outcomes.

Determining the pathology of these complex disease processes is an important step in the plan of care.

Macroglossia

Macroglossia, or an enlarged tongue, can create chewing, speech, and airway management problems (**Figure 9-9**). Macroglossia can be associated with dentomusculoskeletal deformities as well as with other disorders, including Beckwith Wiedemann and Down syndrome.[21] The incidence of macroglossia is unknown. **Pseudomacroglossia** is another condition in which the tongue may be normal in size but is forced to sit in an abnormal position due to anatomical associations.[21] Pseudomacroglossia must be distinguished from true macroglossia because the clinical management strategies vary. However, clinicians need to understand the signs and symptoms associated with both of these congenital disorders in order to improve airway function, facial aesthetics, and the overall health of those affected.

Etiology

There are two etiologic classifications currently used today: true macroglossia and relative macroglossia.[22] True macroglossia may be caused by a wide array of congenital and acquired conditions, including infant muscular hypertrophy (enlargement), glandular hyperplasia, hemangioma (noncancerous skin growths), lymphangioma (lymphatic system lesions), and, most commonly, muscular enlargement.[21] Acquired causes include but are not limited to amyloidosis (amyloid buildup), dental cysts or tumors, and neurologic injury.[21]

Pathophysiology

The pathophysiologic classification of macroglossia is divided into generalized and localized disease groupings.[23] The pathophysiologic classifications are further subdivided into congenital, inflammatory, traumatic, metabolic, and neoplastic categories.[23] This taxonomy is distinguished through physiologic exam and is usually the result of tissue abnormality or from the presence of abnormal development of the oropharynx.[23] Molecular and chromosomal analyses, as well as thyroid function testing, are also used in the pathophysiologic evaluation of macroglossia.[24] Thyroid dysfunction, abnormal genetic testing, and unique familial syndromes have contributed to characteristics seen in infants with macroglossia.[24] Evaluation includes a careful history and thorough physical examination in order to identify potential underlying syndromes.

Diagnosis

Clinical, radiographic, and functional assessments are used in the evaluation and diagnosis of macroglossia. The evaluation should begin with a medical history, including a family history of at least three generations.[22] A complete physical examination of the infant should also be performed and include an evaluation of the site and severity of the oral impendence.[22] In addition to an inspection of the oropharynx, airway fluoroscopy and magnetic resonance imaging (MRI) are both helpful in the diagnosis (**Figure 9-10**).[23] Functional tests to identify variations in speech, chewing, and airway patency should also be performed.[22] Polysomnography should be used to evaluate the degree of the airway obstruction and the urgency for intervention.[23] Laboratory analysis, including thyroid function, metabolic screening, and expanded lab studies, will help to support the diagnosis and are essential in guiding clinical intervention.[22]

Clinical Presentation

There are several clinical and radiographic features that can help clinicians recognize macroglossia. All these features are not always present, and their existence

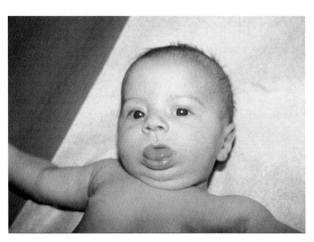

FIGURE 9-9 A child with macroglossia.

Courtesy of Cleft and Craniofacial Center at Cincinnati Children's Hospital Medical Center.

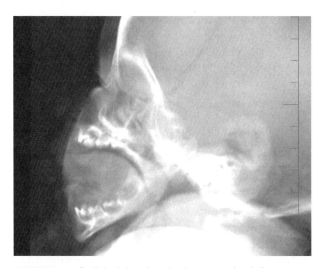

FIGURE 9-10 Radiologic imaging showing macroglossia in a small child.

Courtesy of Dr. Javier Salguero, Radiopaedia.org, rID: 22204.

does not guarantee confirmation of this congenital malformation. Clinical features include a grossly enlarged tongue, open bite, mandibular protrusion, teeth misalignment, speech problems, difficulty eating and chewing, drooling, airway difficulties, and obstructive sleep apnea.[21] Radiographic findings may include the tongue filling the oral cavity, mandibular protrusion, disproportional mandibular growth, and a decreased size of the oropharyngeal airway.[21]

Management

Macroglossia management is intricate. Conservative management measures may be used to reduce inflammation, bleeding, and trauma in patients. These management actions try to correct complications while preserving tongue abilities.[22] The type and size of the malformation will dictate medical or surgical management. Surgical intervention is indicated to alleviate airway obstruction. Various surgical methods can be used to reduce the size of the tongue and include tongue resection surgery (reduction glossectomy), tongue excision, and orthognathic (corrective jaw) surgery.[21] Indications for surgery can include repeated airway or chewing distress, psychological concerns, and impedance of orthodontic appliances.[21] Surgical sequencing through partial resection of the tongue, in combination with orthognathic surgery, has several advantages and is the preferred and most common management option.[21,23] Reducing the size of the tongue while maintaining functional oral abilities is the main goal of this technique.[23] The optimal age for surgical management is between 4 and 7 years; however, high risk associated with some complications may require earlier correction.[22]

Complications and Outcomes

Macroglossia-associated morbidity includes feeding difficulties, respiratory distress, laryngomalacia, tracheomalacia, speech disturbances, and developmental delay.[24] Potential postsurgical complications include excessive bleeding, airway obstruction, loss of taste, motor dysfunction, tongue mobility deficiency, salivary duct injury, and speech and chewing problems.[21] The most common complication associated with reduction glossectomy is incision breakdown:[23] The more muscle removed, the greater the potential for tongue mobility restriction. Postoperative symptoms may be exacerbated before patient improvement occurs. Close patient monitoring is necessary, and possible short-term intubation may be required.[23] Severe surgical complications appear to be very infrequent.[21] Postoperative airway assessment of the patient is important. Substantial improvement in functional (airway, speech, chewing) and aesthetic outcomes can be expected following surgical correction.[21]

Tracheoesophageal Fistula

Tracheoesophageal fistula (TEF) is a congenital miscommunication between the trachea and the esophagus.[25] The prevalence of this congenital deformity is roughly 1 in 3500 live births.[25]

Etiology

The etiology of TEF is largely unknown but is thought to be multifactorial, involving genetic and environmental factors.[25] Environmental risk factors include exposure to certain medications (i.e., anti-thyroids) and infections during pregnancy and maternal diabetes mellitus.[26] Many infants born with TEF are also diagnosed with chromosomal anomalies as well as with abnormalities of the vertebra, gastrointestinal tract, cardiovascular system, renal system, or limbs (known as VACTERL; **Table 9-2**).[25]

Pathophysiology

An unknown in utero malformation best characterizes TEF. During the development of the fetus, the digestive tract separates from the trachea; however, if these structures remain fused, tracheoesophageal irregularities occur. Anatomical classifications are used to describe the presence or absence of **esophageal atresia**, or incomplete communication of the esophagus, and whether an associated fistula is present.[27] **Figure 9-11** provides an illustration of the different types or configurations the defect can take. The most common combination is esophageal atresia with a distal TEF, with the fistula connecting between the lower pouch of the esophagus and the trachea.[25] An isolated esophageal

TABLE 9-2
Anomalies Associated with VACTERL

Potential Problem	Tests Performed
V: Vertebral abnormality (butterfly vertebrae, hemi-vertebrae)	Spinal ultrasound, spinal X-rays
A: Anal anomaly (anal atresia)	Physical examination
C: Cardiac/heart abnormality (ventricular septal defect [VSD], atrial septal defect [ASD], patent ductus arteriosis [PDA])	Cardiac echocardiogram
TE: Tracheoesophageal abnormality	Physical examination
R: Renal/kidney abnormality (solitary kidney, horseshoe kidney)	Renal ultrasound
L: Limb deformity	Physical examination, X-rays

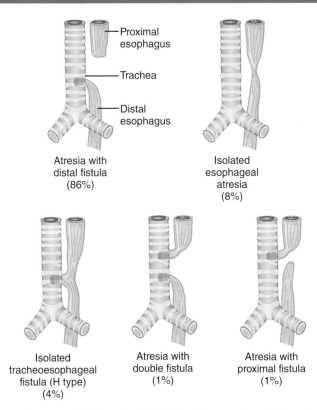

Atresia with
distal fistula
(86%)

Isolated
esophageal
atresia
(8%)

Proximal
esophagus

Trachea

Distal
esophagus

Isolated
tracheoesophageal
fistula (H type)
(4%)

Atresia with
double fistula
(1%)

Atresia with
proximal fistula
(1%)

FIGURE 9-11 An illustration of the different types or forms TEF and esophageal atresia can take and the defect prevalence.

atresia with no TEF may also occur.[27] Esophageal atresia is not present with the H type tracheoesophageal fistula, in which the lateral connection between the tracheal and esophagus gives the appearance of the letter H.[27] Children with an H-type defect are often diagnosed later in infancy; these infants are able to swallow but often choke and cough during the process.[27] Esophageal atresia with proximal and distal TEF is also known as dual TEF because TEF connections are present at the upper and lower pouches of the esophagus and trachea.[27] Esophageal atresia can also occur with an isolated proximal TEF; this involves a TEF connecting the upper pouch of the esophagus and trachea, which allows gastric contents to easily travel directly into the lungs.[27]

Diagnosis

Detection of TEF is complex. The importance of early diagnosis and referral cannot be overstated. Prenatally, **polyhydramnios** of excess amniotic fluid, along with a small or invisible stomach on ultrasound, often suggests the presence of TEF.[25] More recently, ultrasound imaging improvements enhance the provider's ability to detect developmental disorders and congenital malformations, including esophageal atresia and tracheoesophageal fistula, in early pregnancy.[25] Diagnosis

by prenatal ultrasonography is more accurate later in pregnancy when the defective features are better visualized.[28] A new ultrasound technique allows for visualization of the fetal esophagus between the trachea and the aorta, which is helping to improve TEF detection rates.[25]

Postnatally, the presence of oropharyngeal secretions, respiratory difficulties, or the inability to pass a nasogastric tube may raise suspicions for a TEF diagnosis.[25] Chest radiography can also help to confirm a postnatal diagnosis. A lateral chest X-ray and anterior posterior (AP) film also provide valuable insight into the status of the lungs.[29] Radiography often confirms obstruction, the location of the nasogastric tube (either in the blind pouch of the esophagus or in the trachea), and the presence or absence of a gas bubble.[29] Changes to the mediastinal structure as well as the aortic arch position are extremely relevant and help guide physician preference as to the surgical approach. Lastly, echocardiography helps detect or rule out cardiac defects.[29]

Clinical Presentation

TEF is the most common neonatal disorder resulting in respiratory distress, which is caused by flooding of the tracheobronchial tree with aspiration of saliva and/or gastric contents.[29] Shortly after birth, infants present with frothing at the mouth, drooling, choking during attempted feeds, or signs of aspiration pneumonia.[29] Episodes of cyanosis and associated respiratory distress may be severe and progressive. If symptoms are noted, an immediate assessment is required. An isolated TEF or H-type fistula may also present later in life with subtle symptoms, including wheezing and recurrent respiratory infections.[27] Upon physical examination, there is noteworthy abdominal distention caused by excessive air movement.[26] Murmurs or decreased breath sounds may be heard during auscultation of the chest.[26]

Management

The management of esophageal atresia and TEF is challenging. The surgical approach chosen should be individualized to each patient based on the type of defect and the infant's or child's clinical stability. If severe respiratory distress presents, intubation and mechanical ventilation are warranted. Timely surgical intervention is required in order to avoid tracheal aspiration and intestinal overdistention.[27]

The two most common surgical options are immediate transpleural TEF ligation, postponing the esophageal repair until the infant is older, and immediate transpleural TEF ligation in combination with an esophageal **anastomosis**.[28] A surgical anastomosis is a new connection between two body structures. It is vital to ligate the TEF as soon as possible because it poses a great risk for continued pulmonary sequelae if left un-treated.[28] Dramatic improvements in infant respiratory status occur after TEF ligation.[28] More recently, there has been a rise in the number of minimally invasive sur-gical procedures performed in infants with TEF, which often provide better aesthetic results and decreased postoperative complications.[30] Surgical goals are aimed at disconnecting or ligating the communication be-tween the trachea and esophagus and reestablishing esophageal permanence.

Postoperative care should emphasize maintaining good pulmonary hygiene, which includes nasopharyn-geal suctioning, position changes, head elevation, and bronchoscopy if needed.[31]

Complications and Outcomes

Morbidity results from postoperative complications of the airway, additional congenital malformations, and prematurity.[25] Postoperative complications may include anastomotic constriction or leaks, recurrent TEF, GERD, and post-thoracotomy scoliosis or tho-rax asymmetry.[25] Infants with severe GERD may have recurring aspiration pneumonias and need additional medical treatment. Persistent tracheomalacia may also result.[32] Recurrent or undiscovered fistulas are com-monly the source of repeated respiratory compromise.[32] Determinants of overall survival in infants with TEF are birthweight, preoperative ventilator dependence, and associated anomalies.[28] Term and near-term infants and those with fewer associated anomalies have a better chance of survival.[31] A multidisciplinary team approach and parental counseling are ongoing important compo-nents of care.

Congenital Diaphragmatic Hernia

Congenital diaphragmatic hernia (CDH) is a complex congenital disorder with high mortality. Incidence of CDH is roughly 1 in 2500 live births.[33,34] The primary characterization of CDH is a hole in the diaphragm that allows abdominal organs to move into the chest, which hinders lung development (**Figure 9-12**).[34] As a result, CDH infants suffer a combination of various degrees of insufficient lung growth and pulmonary hypertension.[34]

Etiology

During normal gestation, the diaphragm is fully formed by the 12th week. In infants with CDH, a portion of the diaphragm does not form correctly, resulting in a defect that causes the contents of the abdomen to enter the thoracic cavity.[33] Classification of CDH is based upon the anatomical location of the defect: posterolateral, anteriorlateral, or central.[33] Posterolateral defect, also termed a Bochdaleck hernia, makes up 90% of CDH cases, with the remaining 10% comprising anteriolateral defects (Morgagni hernias) and relatively rare forms of total diaphragm absence.[35] The majority of CDH cases occur on the left side, with fewer incidences on the right side or bilaterally.[34,35]

Pathophysiology

CDH has a very complex pathophysiology that remains weakly understood. The literature demonstrates incom-plete growth of the lungs, or **pulmonary hypoplasia**, that occurs prior to diaphragm shortcomings.[33] This demon-strates that lung growth is already affected prior to the development of the diaphragmatic hernia.[36] The dual-hit hypothesis postulates that CDH is the result of devel-opmental compromises. The first hit, or compromise, affects both lungs and occurs before diaphragm develop-ment as a result of genetic and environmental factors.[36] The second hit affects only the ipsilateral lung and oc-curs after development of the defect, causing herniation of organs into the thorax.[36] Retinoid signaling distur-bances, or signaling disturbances in compounds chem-ically related to vitamin A, may play a significant role in the pathophysiology of CDH.[33] Studies have also shown

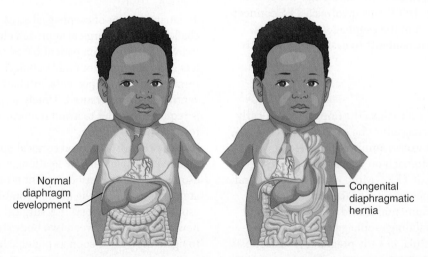

Normal diaphragm development

Congenital diaphragmatic hernia

FIGURE 9-12 An illustration of the lungs and gastrointestinal system in a healthy infant and an infant with congenital diaphragmatic hernia.

an increased risk for CDH in association with various maternal factors, including alcohol use, smoking, low intake of retinol, obesity, and consumption of antimicrobial drugs.[33] Genetics may also play a role, as genetic syndromes, chromosome abnormalities, and congenital anomalies have all been identified in CDH infants.[33]

Diagnosis

Prenatally, CDH is diagnosed by an ultrasound examination. Polyhydramnios is commonly present in pregnancies complicated by CDH.[37] Postnatally, the diagnosis of CDH is confirmed by radiographic imaging. Chest radiography will show abdominal organs in the thorax as well as an abnormal cardiac axis or mediastinal shift away from the defect (**Figure 9-13**).[33,37] Pulmonary hypoplasia can be measured by the severity of fetal breathing movements.[37]

Clinical Presentation

Postnatal clinical symptoms soon after birth also help in the diagnosis and management of CDH. The onset of symptoms may differ depending on the volume of organs in the thorax and the severity of pulmonary hypoplasia present.[29] Undiagnosed patients may present with acute respiratory distress, barrel-shaped chest, concave abdomen, absence of breath sounds, shifted cardiac sounds, and bowel sounds in the chest.[33] Some infants with CDH remain asymptomatic and present later in life with gastrointestinal symptoms.[37] Prenatal diagnosis is advantageous as it can help in better postnatal management of the infant and mother through individualized patient education and planned delivery at a tertiary care facility.[33,37]

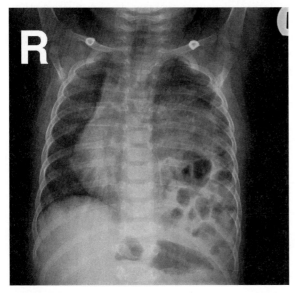

FIGURE 9-13 Chest radiograph of an infant with CDH. There are multiple gas locules within the lower left chest, and the majority of the rest of the left lung has been opacified. The left hemidiaphragm cannot be seen. The mediastinum and the heart are deviated to the contralateral right side.

Courtesy of Dr. Hani Salam, Radiopaedia.org, rID: 9512.

Management

Parental counseling is an essential component in family-centered care. It is important for the parents to understand the severity of the disorder, disease process expectations, and potential outcomes. Prenatal management consists of routine ultrasound surveillance, which can diagnose this disorder and other potential complications.[33]

Postnatal management has evolved to include lung protective strategies during invasive ventilation; permissive hypercapnia; and the use of inhaled nitric oxide (iNO), high frequency ventilation (HFV), or extracorporeal membrane oxygenation (ECMO) to stabilize the infant prior to surgical repair.[33] Delivery room management is aimed at achieving adequate oxygenation and ventilation. A nasogastric tube should be placed to prevent further bowel enlargement.[37] Infants with severe respiratory distress should be immediately intubated and mechanically ventilated. Ventilatory strategies should consist of lung protection principles, maintaining a SpO_2 of at least 85%, allowing for permissive hypercapnia, and stimulating spontaneous breathing.[33] Bag-mask ventilation should be avoided because it can lead to bowel distension and further respiratory distress.[33,37] Arterial blood gas values should be used as ventilatory management determinants.[29]

Once the cardiopulmonary functions are stabilized, usually in the 1st week of extrauterine life, surgical repair can be accomplished. The operating approach consists of either an open or minimally invasive surgical technique.[33] The transabdominal approach is preferred and is the standard technique for repair of the CHD.[38] If the abdominal cavity is inadequate, the transthoracic approach can be used, which typically allows the surgeon adequate exposure to the defect.[38] Generally, the closure method depends on the size and severity of the defect. Smaller diaphragmatic defects are repaired with permanent sutures, whereas larger defects require a patch.[33,37] In recent years, experimental surgical treatment approaches for CDH have been developed and used. Fetal tracheal occlusion therapy is an improved technique of fetal surgery.[33,39] Outcomes vary, with some studies reporting reduced pulmonary hypoplasia while others fail to show improved survival.[33,39] HFV and ECMO can be used as rescue therapies when conventional ventilation fails, with some studies reporting improved survival rates when these therapies are used.[33,37] Recent advancements in neonatal intensive care unit protocols have significantly helped to reduce CDH mortality in hospital centers.[36]

Complications and Outcomes

Despite the continuous improvement in knowledge and management of this disease, CDH still carries a mortality rate of greater than 50%. Pulmonary hyperplasia and persistent pulmonary hypertension of the newborn are chief complications following the repair of CDH.[37] Histologically, there is increased musculature in the pulmonary vasculature.[36] Continued contraction of the vasculature produces chronic constriction of the arterioles, resulting in pulmonary hypertension.[36] Traditional therapies, including pulmonary vasodilators, pharmacologic paralysis, HFV, and ECMO, have all shown potential but have made no noteworthy impact on the pulmonary hypertension issues facing these patients.[37] Presently, iNO therapy, a potent pulmonary vasodilator, is the most common treatment for pulmonary hypertension in CDH infants.[33] However, the benefits of blood pressure enhancement are debatable.

The long-term outcomes and quality of life of infants with CDH varies. Those who survive surgical intervention are at risk for long-term morbidities, including pulmonary diseases, gastrointestinal disorders, growth failure, neurologic impairment, and chest wall deformities.[33] Because morbidity prevalence rates are high, close follow-up and long-term care are required for infants who survive surgical correction of the defect.

Surfactant Protein Deficiencies

Pulmonary **surfactant** is a mixture of lipids and proteins that reduces surface tension at the alveolar interface in the lung. Surfactant is composed of phospholipids and four surfactant proteins: A, B, C, and D.[40] Congenital disorders that disturb normal surfactant transformation cause respiratory insufficiency and failure in infants and children.[41] The disorders are known as **surfactant protein deficiencies** and are caused by mutations in the gene proteins that are critical for the production and function of pulmonary surfactant.[41] Surfactant deficiency is one of the principal causes of respiratory distress in premature infants. Although uncommon, these deficiencies can cause significant morbidity and mortality.

Etiology

This genetic disorder involves the surfactant protein B gene, surfactant protein C gene, and the ABCA3 gene, all of which are critical for surfactant production and proper function of the infant lung.[41,42] As a result of this genetic dysfunction, there is abnormal quantity, composition, and metabolism of surfactant as well as surfactant inactivation, which collectively contribute to respiratory distress and acute lung injury.[42] Clinical studies addressing alterations in surfactant composition report a reduction in overall surfactant proteins, a marked decrease in phosphatidylglycerol levels, as well as significant reduction in the quantities of phosphatidylcholine, both of which are indicators of fetal lung maturity.[43] Animal models suggest that surfactant metabolism may also be affected in acute lung injury as evidenced by poor surface tension properties, increased levels of peptidases, and alterations in surfactant density.[43] Inactivation of pulmonary surfactant is the most common surfactant disorder seen in acute lung injury. Surfactant dysfunction results from the abnormal presence of competitive proteins displacing surfactant, which impairs its ability to reduce surface tension and adversely affects gas exchange.[44] Substances that can cause surfactant inactivation include albumin, hemoglobin, proteases, meconium, and bilirubin.[44] These substances are strong inactivators of surfactant and lead to diminished lung compliance, increase intrapulmonary shunting, and atelectasis.[44]

Pathophysiology

Surfactant protein B deficiency has become increasingly recognized as the most common cause of severe respiratory distress in infants.[45] This deficiency is caused by a genetic disorder, congenital alveolar proteinosis, in which an error occurs during surfactant metabolism that leads to the buildup of surfactant-derived matter in the lung.[46] The incidence of this congenital deficiency is roughly 1 in 100,000 live births.[45] Diagnosis is confirmed through lung biopsy, bronchoalveolar lavage analysis, and DNA testing.[46]

Diagnosis

The lung disorders associated with these gene mutations may have significant overlap in clinical and histologic presentation. Genetic analysis may be helpful in distinguishing these genetic disorders and is a definitive diagnostic tool.[41] High-resolution CT may also be used to aid in the diagnosis. Radiographic characteristics are similar to those found with interstitial lung disease and include the appearance of ground-glass opacities, septal thickening, scarring, and irregular aeration (**Figure 9-14**).[45] Chest radiographs can also aid confirmative diagnosis. Common findings include pulmonary interstitial emphysema and atelectasis (**Figure 9-15**).[43] Histologic findings include interstitial inflammation throughout the lung, pulmonary edema, interstitial pneumonitis, and diffuse alveolar damage.[43,44]

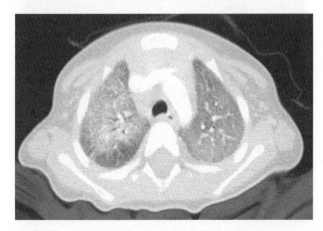

FIGURE 9-14 Surfactant protein C deficiency in an 8-month-old girl presenting with respiratory distress syndrome. CT scan shows extensive ground-glass appearance of the lungs.
Courtesy of Dr. Maurizio Zompatori.

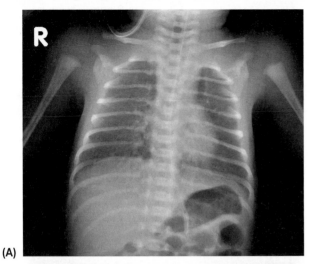

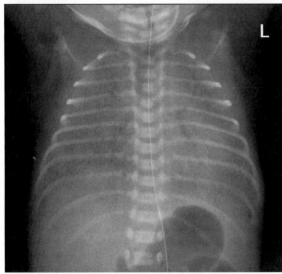

FIGURE 9-15 Chest radiographs of infants with respiratory distress secondary to surfactant deficiency. (**A**) Changes consistent with mild respiratory distress syndrome. Diffuse ground-glass opacities can be seen. The pulmonary vasculature appears normal and the borders of the heart and diaphragm can be seen. (**B**) A chest radiograph showing changes consistent with severe surfactant deficiency. There is a diffuse ground-glass opacification of the lungs. The heart borders and diaphragm are silhouetted.

(**A**) Courtesy of Dr. Shailaja Muniraj, Radiopaedia.org, rID: 50267.; (**B**) Courtesy of Dr. Jeremy Jones, Radiopaedia.org, rID: 56411.

Clinical Presentation

Affected infants experience respiratory insufficiency and respiratory distress shortly after birth, which often advances to respiratory failure.[43] Infants typically present with an increased work of breathing, decreased aeration is noted on auscultation of the lungs, cyanosis, and poor peripheral perfusion.[47]

Management

Infants presenting with respiratory distress require intubation and mechanical ventilatory support. Ventilatory strategies include the use of high levels of positive end-expiratory pressure, higher respiratory rates, and low tidal volumes. HFV has also been successful in

supporting infants until pulmonary transplantation can occur.[45]

Lung transplantation offers the most viable option for infants born with this congenital anomaly. Outcomes following lung transplantation in surfactant-deficient patients are similar to those in infants requiring lung transplant for other indications.[45] Severe bronchomalacia, rejection, and pulmonary venous obstruction are posttransplant complications, which may result in infant death.[45]

Exogenous surfactant has a recognized role in the management of infants with respiratory distress syndrome (RDS) and in neonates diagnosed with surfactant inactivation.[48] Many large clinical trials have demonstrated that the use of exogenous surfactant is effective in the prevention and treatment of RDS due to surfactant inactivation.[49] FDA-approved surfactants currently available for use in the United States include surfaxin, beractant, poractant alpha, and calfactant.[50] Surfactants can be administered by direct instillation, or lavage, and aerosolization.[49] Surfactant directly instilled into the lungs should be administered slowly. The infant should be monitored during surfactant replacement therapy and observed for adverse effects, such as transient hypoxia, bradycardia, reflux, and mucus plugging.[49] Clinical trials have shown that preventive surfactant treatment has reduced the incidence of RDS and well as neonatal mortality.[51] Early rescue surfactant therapy reduces the need for mechanical ventilation and reduces morbidity, such as the incidence of bronchopulmonary dysplasia (BPD) and pneumothoraces.[52] Until recently, infant RDS due to surfactant inactivation was managed with a combination of surfactant therapy and mechanical ventilation. Noninvasive ventilation (NIV), such as nCPAP, has more recently been recognized as an alternative to surfactant instillation after birth. Research comparing conventional methods to noninvasive methods showed decreased risk of BPD and mortality with the use of early nCPAP in infants.[53]

Complications and Outcomes

Surfactant has revolutionized the management process of respiratory diseases that affect the neonatal lung. Surfactant deficiency diseases, as well as RDS, are now uncommon causes of death in infants as a result of advances in medical management and surgical (lung transplantation) techniques. Prognosis has improved in recent years with the increased early use of surfactant therapy, use of lung protective strategies, and developments in lung transplant surgery techniques.[49] Surfactant replacement therapy offers promise to infants with disorders contributing to surfactant inactivation (i.e., premature birth, meconium aspiration).

Congenital Pulmonary Anomalies

Congenital pulmonary anomalies affect the structural development of the lung in utero. They represent a collection of uncommon lung deformities that affect the airway, parenchyma, and vasculature of infants.[54] The lung abnormalities discussed in this section represent ~15% of all congenital anomalies.[54] Most of these lung malformations are discovered during prenatal ultrasounds. Sometimes these congenital abnormalities cause no abnormal clinical symptoms and only require monitoring at predetermined or regular intervals. However, in most cases, pulmonary complications result, requiring intervention at birth or later in life.

Pulmonary Hypoplasia

Pulmonary hypoplasia, or incomplete development of the lung tissue, is a common lung abnormality occurring secondary to a number of other disorders.[55] This disorder is characterized by underdeveloped bronchioles and reduced amounts of lung tissue. It can present unilaterally or bilaterally and results in a decrease in lung cells, airways, or alveoli, impairing gas exchange.[55] A deficiency in thoracic space, breathing movement, or amniotic fluid volumes can lead to pulmonary hypoplasia.[56] Intrathoracic causes can include lung lesions, congenital diaphragmatic hernia, or decreased arterial perfusion.[56] Extrathoracic causes can include renal dysplasia, ascites, osteogenesis imperfecta, and neuromuscular conditions.[57]

Lung compression in utero inhibits proper development of the conducting airways, terminal airways, or both.[55] This reduces the weight and size of the affected lung, most frequently by nearly half. An inadequate amniotic fluid is another common cause of poor neonatal lung growth. Oligohydramnios, or too little amniotic fluid, is commonly caused by early leaking from premature rupture of the membranes surrounding the fetus.[56,57] Prenatal ultrasonography provides early predictors of pulmonary hypoplasia and is the preferred diagnostic examination.[58] MRI, CT scanning, and radiography show disease progression and are used to assess lung volume and vascular abnormalities.[58] Doppler testing may also be used to measure blood flow velocities, as pulmonary arterial resistance is often elevated in pulmonary hypoplasia.[58]

Respiratory distress, including tachypnea, hypoxia, hypercapnia, and acidosis, is the main clinical presentation of infants with pulmonary hypoplasia. Prenatal interventions can include delaying labor to allow for lung maturation.[57] Following birth, the infant will need respiratory support, which, depending on the extent of the disease, ranges from supplemental oxygen administration to ECMO.[57] Treatment and prognosis of pulmonary hypoplasia in infants will significantly depend on the severity level as well as the presence of underlying anomalies.[56]

Pulmonary Aplasia

Pulmonary aplasia, or absence of lung tissue, is a rare congenital malformation and is usually associated with other congenital abnormalities, mainly cardiovascular.[59] It is characterized by the presence of a bronchus without any lung tissue. It usually occurs unilaterally. However, bilateral pulmonary aplasia can occur, but the infant will not be viable.

Abnormal blood flow due to the absence of the pulmonary artery during gestation causes pulmonary aplasia.[59] Prenatal ultrasound screening will reveal lung cavity abnormalities as well as prominent mediastinal shifts.[60] Postnatal chest radiography can be used to evaluate the lung. Pulmonary aplasia presents radiologically as a hemithorax whiteout, substantial lung volume loss, or contralateral lung hyperinflation.[60] A CT scan can confirm the absence of lung tissue. Pulmonary aplasia clinically presents as neonatal respiratory distress with variable intensity.[60] It can also predispose infants to subsequent pulmonary infections.

Pulmonary Agenesis

Pulmonary agenesis, or complete absence of bronchus, lung tissue, and vasculature, is a very rare congenital anomaly of the lung that is also commonly associated with other congenital malformations of the cardiovascular, skeletal, gastrointestinal, or urinary systems.[61] It is characterized by the total absence of bronchus and lung and has no vascular supply to the affected area. Figure 9-16 illustrates the various ways that this disorder may affect the lung and pulmonary vasculature. Diagnosis can be difficult depending on the side of the absent lung. Chest radiography often reveals hemithorax opaqueness, vertebral anomalies, dextrocardia, crowding of ribs, and a deviated trachea and mediastinum.[61,62] Bronchoscopy can confirm the malformation's severity.[62] Additionally, cardioangiography can be used to determine anomalies of the pulmonary artery and remains the gold standard for diagnosis of pulmonary artery agenesis.[61]

The onset of clinical symptoms is remarkably variable. Upon physical examination, flattening of the chest on the affected side accompanied by impaired airway movement can be observed.[62] Chest asymmetry may become more noticeable later in life. Other signs and symptoms include cyanosis at birth, dyspnea, markedly diminished breath sounds, and recurrent respiratory infections.[62]

Pulmonary agenesis can be managed medically and surgery is rarely required. The side of the agenesis affects prognosis. Pulmonary agenesis has a poorer prognosis when the right lung is absent, typically due to the associated system anomalies.[62]

Bronchogenic Cysts

A bronchogenic cyst is an abnormal growth of lung tissue characterized as a malformation of the bronchial tree. Although rare, it represents the most common cystic lesion in the mediastinum.[63] Lung bud cysts arise from abnormal budding of the tracheobronchial tree during fetal development.[63] Bronchogenic cysts are usually single but may multiply and can be filled with fluid, mucus, or blood products.[63] Cysts can originate either

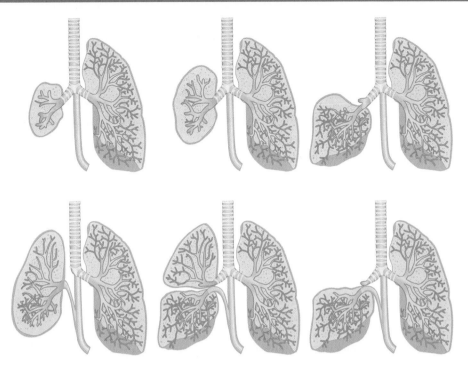

FIGURE 9-16 An illustration of the various ways pulmonary agenesis may present and affect the lung and pulmonary vasculature.

within or outside the thoracic cavity.[63] Intrathoracic cysts can be found in the bronchial wall, the pleura, the mediastinum, or the parenchyma of the lung.[63] They present as masses that may enlarge and cause compression of the infant's lung.[63]

Infants are usually asymptomatic, but diagnosis may be evident radiographically in infants presenting with respiratory distress.[64] An alternative clinical presentation may arise if the cyst enlarges or becomes infected.[63] Diagnostic tools may include a plain radiograph, CT scan, or MRI testing (**Figure 9-17**). Typically the cyst appears as a dense, circular mass with smooth edges. Occasionally, lung compression occurs, which can lead to air trapping or a hyperlucent hemothorax.[64]

Management is somewhat controversial. Some research advocates for surgical excision, and the location of the cyst(s) will determine the extent of resection performed.[65] More recently, percutaneous drainage by imaging guidance is used to treat the cyst(s).[65] Complications can include fistula formation, infection recurrence, or severe pulmonary hemorrhage.

Congenital Pulmonary Airway Malformation

Congenital pulmonary airway malformation, formally known as congenital cystic adenomatoid malformation, is a rare, disorganized overgrowth of fetal lung tissue.[65] The entire lung lobe is replaced by a nonfunctional lung mass, which results from a maturation defect with a proliferation of pulmonary tissues.[65] Pathology progresses with multicystic communications that, unlike bronchogenic cysts, can have a connection to the tracheobronchial tree.[65] In most cases, congenital

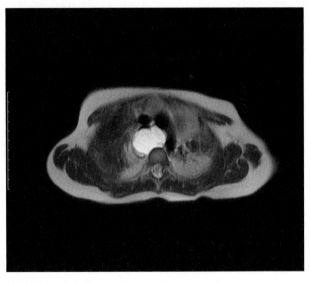

FIGURE 9-17 A CT scan showing a bronchogenic cyst.
Case courtesy of Dr. Mohammad A. ElBeialy, Radiopaedia.org, rID: 28198.

pulmonary airway malformation is usually unilateral and involves a single lobe.

Prenatal ultrasonography may be used to detect the malformation, which appears as an isolated cyst or solid intrathoracic mass.[65] Accumulation of fetal fluid and excessive amniotic fluid volume may also be detected on the prenatal ultrasound.[65] Postnatally, chest radiography and CT scans play significant roles in the diagnosis and presurgical evaluation of the defect by depicting mass location and extent of lesion.[65]

Clinical presentation is similar to that of a bronchogenic cyst. Larger lesions, depending on their extent, may be associated with pulmonary hypoplasia, hypertension, and cardiomyopathy.[65,66] Surgery, usually a lobectomy and occasionally a pneumonectomy, is the treatment option of choice. Unless there are unusual operating complications, postsurgical prognosis is excellent.[66]

Pulmonary Sequestration

Pulmonary sequestration, or accessory lung, is lung tissue that has no connection to the bronchial tree or pulmonary arteries.[67] This disorder is divided into two types: intralobar sequestration and extralobar sequestration.[67] Intralobar sequestration is normal lung tissue without its own visceral pleura neighboring the adjacent normal lung; extralobar sequestration has its own distinct visceral pleura and is completely separated from the adjacent normal lung (**Figure 9-18**).[67] Additionally, with intralobar sequestrations, venous drainage commonly occurs through the pulmonary veins, and with extralobar sequestrations, venous drainage is usually into the systemic (azygos) veins.[67]

The etiology of sequestrations is described as the formation and migration of accessory lung buds prior to the separation of the systemic and pulmonary circulations.[68] Generally, pulmonary sequestrations favorably affect the lower lobe regions. Ultrasound is recommended as the first diagnostic tool to evaluate the pulmonary sequestration. Chest radiography often shows triangular opacities, cystic spaces, and air bronchograms.[68] Doppler ultrasound can be used to define arterial anatomy.[68]

Surgical resection is the traditional treatment method of pulmonary sequestration.[68] Extralobar

sequestrations can be extracted without removing normal lung tissue; however, an intralobar sequestration may require segmental resection or even a lobectomy.[68]

Conclusion

Precise and timely recognition of congenital disorders often makes a profound difference in outcome for infants affected with congenital pulmonary anomalies. These respiratory system deficiencies illustrate the importance of why clinicians must carefully choose appropriate diagnostic modalities and properly assess symptoms in order to effectually and appropriately diagnosis and determine a medical and/or surgical plan of care.

Intralobar sequestration   Extralobar sequestration

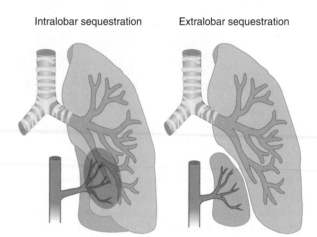

FIGURE 9-18 An illustration of intralobar and extralobar sequestrations.

Case Study 1

A 1000-gram, 28 weeks' gestational age male neonate was born following a premature labor. The infant did not have a respiratory rate of effort at birth despite resuscitation efforts. An orogastric tube was placed to decompress the stomach, the infant was intubated, mechanically ventilated and transferred to the NICU. Upon admission mechanical ventilation was provided. On day 2 of life, the patient was noted to have significant abdominal distension. Chest radiograph revealed a pneumoperitoneum and the orogastric tube was noted to terminate in the proximal stomach. On day 3 of life, significant distention was noted on examination. An abdominal X-ray demonstrated persistent intraperitoneal air. The stomach was distended, and air was seen to be leaking from the stomach with each mechanical breath delivered. A TEF was suspected. Bronchoscopy was then performed which confirmed the diagnosis. A bedside thoracotomy was then performed, with the infant placed in the

left lateral position. The infant was found to have a proximal esophageal atresia through which the initial orogastric tube had perforated and was lying on top of the diaphragm. The TEF was identified and ligated. A primary esophageal anastomosis was performed over a 5 Fr feeding tube. The area between the anastomosis and the tracheal fistula closure was reinforced surgically. The patient received ventilatory assistance and supportive care in the NICU post-operatively. The patient was weaned from mechanical ventilatory support on day 95 of life, and was discharged home on day 110 of life with a weight of 2830 grams. He was doing well and tolerating full feeds through a gastrostomy tube.

1. **Describe a tracheoesophageal fistula.**

2. **What are the two types of surgical options for TEF?**

3. **Explain the clinical manifestations of TEF.**

Case Study 2

A newborn female with a gestational age of 37 weeks and weighing 3.05 kg had a prenatal diagnosis of a left-sided congenital diaphragmatic hernia with bilateral fetal lung hypoplasia. At birth, the baby had a right pneumothorax. The infant was intubated and mechanically ventilated. A nasogastric tube was inserted and a chest tube placed in the right hemithorax. She was transported to the neonatal intensive care unit. Shortly after birth, she had persistent pulmonary hypertension of the newborn (PPHN), for which she needed increasing ventilatory support from the mechanical ventilator. Nitric oxide was administered for treatment of her PPHN. Ultimately she required placement on ECMO cannulation for stabilization while awaiting repair of the CDH. On day 4 of life, the CDH was repaired while still on full ECMO support. During surgery with a subcostal incision, the abdominal viscera, including multiple loops of small bowel, spleen, stomach, and part of the colon, were easily reduced into the peritoneal cavity. In repairing the diaphragmatic hernia, it was determined that the defect was too large to stitch, so a patch was used to close the hole. The baby did well postop and was weaned from ECMO on day 10 of life, 6 days after the CDH repair. She was later extubated on day 17 of life to a nasal cannula at 2 L/min. There were no postextubation complications.

1. **What is CDH?**
2. **What are the postnatal treatments for CDH?**
3. **How is CDH diagnosed?**

References

1. Ramsden JD. Choanal atresia. *Curr Pediatr Rev.* 2011;7(1):9-14.
2. Ramsden JD, Campisi P. Choanal atresia and choanal stenosis. *Otolaryngol Clin N Am.* 2009;42(2):339-352.
3. Blum RH, McGowan FX. Chronic upper airway obstruction and cardiac dysfunction: anatomy, pathophysiology and anesthetic implications. *Paediatr Anaesth.* 2004;14(1):75-83.
4. Naito Y, Higuchi M, Koinuma G, Aramaki M, Takahashi T, Kosaki K. Upper airway obstruction in neonates and infants with CHARGE syndrome. *Am J Med Genet A.* 2007;143A(16):1815-1820.
5. Keller JL, Kacker A. Choanal atresia, CHARGE association, and congenital nasal stenosis. *Otolaryngol Clin North Am.* 2000;33(6):1343-1351.
6. Al-Noury K, Lotfy A. Role of multislice computed tomography and local contrast in the diagnosis and characterization of choanal atresia. *Int J Pediatr.* 2011;2011:280763.
7. Deutsch E, Kaufman M, Eilon A. Transnasal endoscopic management of choanal atresia. *Int J Pediatr Otorhinolaryngol.* 1997;40(1):19-26.
8. Lyons M, Vlastarakos PV, Nikolopoulos TP. Congenital and acquired developmental problems of the upper airway in newborns and infants. *Early Hum Dev.* 2012;88(12):951-955.
9. Kim H, Park JH, Chung H, et al. Clinical features and surgical outcomes of congenital choanal atresia: factors influencing success from 20-year review in an institute. *Am J Otolaryngol.* 2012;33(3):308-312.
10. Ibrahim AA, Magdy EA, Hassab MH. Endoscopic choanoplasty without stenting for congenital choanal atresia repair. *Int J Pediatr Otorhinolaryngol.* 2010;74(2):144-150.
11. Flores RL. Neonatal mandibular distraction osteogenesis. *Semin Plast Surg.* 2014;28(4):199-206.
12. Paladini D. Fetal micrognathia: almost always an omnious finding (editorial). *Ultrasound Obstet Gynecol.* 2010;35(4):377-384.
13. Morokuma S, Anami A, Tsukimori K, Fukushima K, Wake N. Abnormal fetal movements, micrognathia and pulmonary hypoplasia: a case report. Abnormal fetal movements. *BMC Pregnancy Childbirth.* 2010;10:46.
14. Neuschulz J, Wilhelm L, Christ H, Braumann B. Prenatal indices for mandibular retrognathia/micrognathia. *J Orofac Orthop.* 2015;76(1):30-40.
15. Sadakah AA, Elshall MA, Farhat AA. Bilateral intra-oral distraction osteogenesis for the management of severe congenital mandibular hypoplasia in early childhood. *J Craniomaxillofac Surg.* 2009;37(4):216-224.
16. Gershanik JJ, Nervez C. Nasoesophageal intubation in the Pierre Robin syndrome. Success in an infant with mandibular hypoplasia, cleft palate, and glossoptosis. *Clin Pediatr (Phila).* 1976;15(2):173-175.
17. Chang CC, Steinbacher DM. Treacher Collins syndrome. *Semin Plast Surg.* 2012;26(2):83-90.
18. Aoki A, Prahl-Andersen B. Mandibular distraction osteogenesis for treatment of extreme mandibular hypoplasia. *Am J Orthod Dentofacial Orthop.* 2007;132(6):848-855.
19. Miller SDW, Glynn SF, Kiely JL, McNicholas WT. The role of nasal CPAP in obstructive sleep apnoea syndrome due to mandibular hypoplasia. *Respirology.* 2010;15(2):377-379.
20. Chung MT, Levi B, Hyun JS, et al. Pierre Robin sequence and Treacher Collins hypoplastic mandible comparison using three-dimensional morphometric analysis. *J Craniofac Surg.* 2012;23(7):1959-1963.
21. Wolford LM, Cottrell DA. Diagnosis of macroglossia and indications for reduction glossectomy. *Am J Orthod Dentofacial Orthop.* 1996;110(2):170-177.
22. Núñez-Martinez PM, Garcia-Delgado C, Morán-Barroso VF, Jasso-Gutiérrez L. Congenital macroglossia: clinical features and therapeutic strategies in pediatric patients. *Bol Med Hosp Infant Mex.* 2016;73(3):212-216.
23. Shott SR. Surgical management of macroglossia in children. *Arch Otolaryngol Head Neck Surg.* 1996;122(3):326-329.
24. Prada CE, Zarate YA, Hopkin RJ. Genetic causes of macroglossia: diagnostic approach. *Pediatrics.* 2012;129(2):e431-e437.
25. de Jong EM, de Haan MAM, Gischler SJ, et al. Pre- and postnatal diagnosis and outcome of fetuses and neonates with esophageal atresia and tracheoesophageal fistula. *Prenat Diagn.* 2010;30(3):274-279.
26. Scott DA. Esophageal atresia/tracheoesophageal fistula overview. In: Adam MP, Ardinger HH, Pagon RA, et al. *Gene Reviews* (Internet). Seattle, WA: University of Washington, Seattle; 1993-2017.
27. Aschcraft KW, Holder TM. The story of esophageal atresia and tracheoesophgeal fistula. *Surgery.* 1969;65(2):332-340.
28. Zani A, Wolinska J, Gobellis G, Chiu PPL, Pierro A. Outcome of esophageal atresia/tracheoesophageal fistula in extremely low birth weight neonates (<1000 grams). *Pediatr Surg Int.* 2016;32(1):83-88.

29. Kumar A, Bhatnagar V. Respiratory distress in neonates. *Indian J Pediatr.* 2005;72(5):425-428.

30. Rothenberg SS. Thoracoscopic repair of esophageal atresia and tracheoesophageal fistula in neonates, first decade's experience. *Dis Esophagus.* 2013;26(4):359-364.

31. Holder TM, Cloud DT, Lewis JE, Pilling GP. Esophageal atresia and tracheoesophageal fistula. A survey of its members by the surgical section of the American Academy of Pediatrics. *Pediatrics.* 1964; 34(4):542-549.

32. Davies MRQ, Cywes S. The flaccid trachea and tracheoesophageal congenital anomalies. *J Pediatr Surg.* 1978;13(4):363-367.

33. Leeuwen L, Fitzgerald DA. Congenital diaphragmatic hernia. *J Paediatr Child Health.* 2014;50(9):667-673.

34. Greer JJ. Current concepts on the pathogenesis and etiology of congenital diaphragmatic hernia. *Respir Physiol Neurobiol.* 2013;189(2):232-240.

35. McHoney M. Congenital diaphragmatic hernia. *Early Hum Dev.* 2014;90(12):941-946.

36. Keijzer R, Puri P. Congenital diaphragmatic hernia. *Semin Pediatr Surg.* 2010;19(3):180-185.

37. Arora M, Bajpai M, Soni TR, Sai Prasad TR. Congenital diaphragmatic hernia. *Indian J Pediatr.* 2000;67(9):665-670.

38. Sakai H, Tamura M, Hosokawa Y, et al. Effect of surgical repair on respiratory mechanics in congenital diaphragmatic hernia. *J Pediatr.* 1987;111:432-438.

39. Tsao K, Lally KP. Congenital diaphragmatic hernia and eventration. In: Holcomb GW III, Murphy JP, eds. *Pediatric Surgery.* 5th ed. Philadelphia, PA: Saunders; 2010:304-321.

40. Williams GD, Christodoulou J, Stack J, et al. Surfactant protein B deficiency: clinical, histological and molecular evaluation. *J Paediatr Child Health.* 1999;35(2):214-220.

41. Wert SE, Whitsett JA, Nogee LM. Genetic disorders of surfactant dysfunction. *Pediatr Dev Pathol.* 2009;12(4):253-274.

42. Jobe AH, Ikegami M. Surfactant and acute lung injury. *Proc Assoc Am Physicians.* 1998;110(6):489-495.

43. Günther A, Ruppert C, Schmidt R, et al. Surfactant alteration and replacement in acute respiratory distress syndrome. *Respir Res.* 2001;2(6):353-364.

44. Taeusch HW, Keough KMW. Inactivation of pulmonary surfactant and the treatment of acute lung injuries. *Pediatr Pathol Mol Med.* 2001;20(6):519-536.

45. Newman B, Kuhn JP, Kramer SS, Carcillo JA. Congenital surfactant protein B deficiency—emphasis on imaging. *Pediatr Radiol.* 2001;31(5):327-331.

46. Stuhrmann M, Bohnhorst B, Peters U, Bohle RM, Poets CF, Schmidtke J. Prenatal diagnosis of congenital alveolar proteinosis (surfactant protein B deficiency). *Prenat Diagn.* 1998;18(9):953-955.

47. Doan ML, Guillerman RP, Dishop MK, et al. Clinical, radiological and pathological features of ABCA3 mutations in children. *Thorax.* 2008;63(4):366-373.

48. Lacaze-Masmonteil T. Exogenous surfactant therapy: newer developments. *Semin Fetal Neonatal Med.* 2003;8(6):433-440.

49. Bissinger RL, Carlson CA. Surfactant. *Newborn Infant Nurse Rev.* 2006;6(2):87-93.

50. Pfister RH, Soll RF. New synthetic surfactants: the next generation? *Biol Neonate.* 2005;87:338-344.

51. Morley CJ. Systematic review of prophylactic vs rescue surfactant. *Arch Dis Child Fetal Neonatal Ed.* 1997;77(1):F70-F74.

52. Brix N, Sellmer A, Jensen MS, Pedersen LV, Henriksen TB. Predictors for an unsuccessful INtubation-SURfactant-Extubation procedure: a cohort study. *BMC Pediatr.* 2014;14:155.

53. Shim GH. Update of minimally invasive surfactant therapy. *Korean J Pediatr.* 2017;60(9):273-281.

54. Nadeem M, Elnazir B, Greally P. Congenital pulmonary malformation in children. *Scientifica (Cairo).* 2012;2012:209896.

55. Swischuk LE, Richardson CJ, Nichols MM, Ingman MJ. Primary pulmonary hypoplasia in the neonate. *J Pediatr.* 1979;95(4):573-577.

56. de Waal K, Kluckow M. Prolonged rupture of membranes and pulmonary hypoplasia in very preterm infants: pathophysiology and guided treatment. *J Pediatr.* 2015;166(5):1113-1120.

57. Cotton CM. Pulmonary hypoplasia. *Semin Fetal Neonatal Med.* 2017;22(4):250-255.

58. Roberts A. Prenatal diagnosis of pulmonary hypoplasia. *Prenat Diagn.* 2001;21(4):304-307.

59. Ryland D, Reid L. Pulmonary aplasia—a quantitative analysis of the development of the single lung. *Thorax.* 1971;26(5):602-609.

60. Hussain Z, Jan M. Unilateral pulmonary aplasia. *JK-Practitioner.* 2014;19(1-2):46-48.

61. De A. Agenesis of the lung—a rare congenital anomaly of the lung. *Acta Med Iran.* 2013;51(1):66-68.

62. Booth JB, Berry CL. Unilateral pulmonary agenesis. *Arch Dis Child.* 1967;42(224):361-374.

63. Sarper A, Ayten A, Golbasi I, Demircan A, Isin E. Bronchogenic cyst. *Tex Heart Inst J.* 2003;30(2):105-108.

64. Kanemitsu Y, Nakayama H, Asamura H, Kondo H, Tsuchiya R, Naruke T. Clinical features and management of bronchogenic cysts: report of 17 cases. *Surg Today.* 1999;29(11):1201-1205.

65. Bolde S, Pudale S, Pandit G, Ruikar K, Ingle SB. Congenital pulmonary airway malformation: a report of two cases. *World J Clin Cases.* 2015;3(15):470-473.

66. Downward CD, Calkins CM, Williams RF, et al. Treatment of congenital pulmonary airway malformations: a systematic review from the APSA outcomes and evidence based practice committee. *Pediatr Surg Int.* 2017;33(9):939-953.

67. Corbett HJ, Humphrey GME. Pulmonary sequestration. *Paediatr Respir Rev.* 2004;5(1):59-68.

68. John PR, Beasley SW, Mayne V. Pulmonary sequestration and related congenital disorders: a clinico-radiological review of 41 cases. *Pediatr Radiol.* 1989;20(1-2):4-9.

Scott Schachinger

Andrew South

© Anna RubaK/ShutterStock, Inc.

OUTLINE

OBJECTIVES

1. Describe a risk factor primarily associated with the development of retinopathy of prematurity.
2. List the factors contributing to the development of bronchopulmonary dysplasia.
3. Describe the diagnostic criteria for bronchopulmonary dysplasia.
4. Explain the strategy used for management of bronchopulmonary dysplasia.
5. List the mechanisms that contribute to the pathogenesis of pulmonary artery hypertension.
6. Differentiate among pneumothorax, pneumomediastinum, pneumopericardium, and pulmonary interstitial emphysema.
7. Describe the risk factors associated with pulmonary air leaks.
8. Explain the role of chest radiography in the diagnosis of pulmonary air leaks.

KEY TERMS

bronchopulmonary
  dysplasia (BPD)
permissive hypercapnia
pneumomediastinum
pneumopericardium
pneumothorax
pulmonary air leak

pulmonary artery
  hypertension (PAH)
pulmonary interstitial
  emphysema (PIE)
retinopathy of
  prematurity (ROP)
transillumination

Introduction

Medical advances enable us to provide safer and more effective care of our most fragile patients. However, acute complications still occur when caring for infants born prematurely. Complications range from spontaneously life-threatening events, such as pulmonary air leaks and pulmonary artery hypertension, to subacute complications, such as retinopathy of prematurity and chronic lung disease. This chapter will present the complications associated with providing critical care to infants whose cardiorespiratory and nervous systems are still developing after birth.

Retinopathy of Prematurity

Retinopathy of prematurity (ROP), formerly known as retrolental fibroplasia, is an aberrant development of the blood vessels supplying the retina within the eye. The primary risk factor for the development of ROP is prematurity and the subsequent incomplete vascularization of the retina at the time of birth.[1] Additionally, oxygen has been shown to play a critical role in the growth response of the retinal vasculature after birth.[2] Approximately 66% of infants weighing ≤1250 grams at birth develop some degree of ROP, and among infants weighing ≤750 grams, 90% develop disease, with severity inversely proportional to birthweight.[3] Because complete, irreversible loss of vision is a potential outcome of ROP, much attention is focused on screening and treatment, as well as prevention, for all infants at risk.

Etiology

In the 1940s and 1950s, oxygen was routinely used at what would now be considered to be excessive levels to treat apnea of prematurity. Although the use of oxygen therapy contributed to survival, a landmark study published in 1956 provided evidence that excessive oxygen use was responsible for the development of ROP.[4] Subsequent changes in practice, namely decreased use of supplemental oxygen, led to a near complete eradication of ROP. It was not until technologic and medical practice advances allowed for survival of progressively more premature infants that use of oxygen increased, and therefore ROP returned as a significant concern among infants with respiratory disease.[1]

Pathophysiology

Retinal vascular development is incomplete in infants born prematurely. Early in gestation, the developing retina receives oxygen and nutrients through diffusion from the adjacent choroid. However, at the 16th week of gestation, this source becomes insufficient for the increasing demand of the retina and capillaries begin to form at the optic disk, or the most posterior portion of the retina.[5] Over time, capillary growth proceeds anteriorly and symmetrically from the posterior retina. Three-dimensionally, this could be imagined as vascular development initiating at one pole of a globe and advancing on multiple longitudinal lines toward the opposite pole. Retinal vascularization is generally complete by 35 weeks' gestation at the nasal ora serrata and by 44 weeks' gestation at the temporal ora serrata.

For infants born prematurely, retinal vascular development must then proceed in an environment of hyperoxia relative to the in utero environment. Additionally, multiple other potential insults, including sepsis, compromised perfusion, necrotizing enterocolitis, and intraventricular hemorrhage, frequently complicate the postnatal medical course. Any of these medical challenges results in a delay in the normal vascular proliferation. This insult and subsequent delay are identified as the primary stage of ROP development. Beginning at 31 weeks' gestation, the primary stage is followed by abnormal hypergrowth or neovascularization (second stage).[6] This phase of excessive vascular proliferation results in an increase in the number of vessels as well as prohibition of the forward progression of the vessels within the retina. In order for the neovascularization phase to be initiated, adequate levels of vascular endothelial growth factor (VEGF) and insulin-like growth factor-1 (IGF-1) must be present within the avascular retina. VEGF is produced within the avascular retina in response to the hypoxic environment created by an insufficient nutrient supply. Although IGF-1 levels are initially low in preterm infants, with maturation IGF-1 levels increase to reach a critical threshold, after which new vascular development is signaled. Unfortunately, the vascular development can be excessive, with the new vessels growing out of the developing retina and into the vitreous, forming a vascular "ridge" on the surface of the retina, or forming dilated, tortuous vessels. This aberrant blood vessel development is the initial step in the development of ROP. If appropriate treatment is not initiated at this point, retinal detachment and blindness could develop.[6]

The role of oxygen in the development of ROP has been studied in both animal models and humans. In fact, the earliest randomized multicenter trial involving neonates was designed to determine the role of oxygen in the subsequent development of ROP.[7] In the 1950s, when the study was initiated, supplemental oxygen was used to counter the effects of apnea of prematurity. In the study arm, the use of oxygen for apnea of prematurity at ~50% FiO_2 for 28 days was compared with an experimental group in which supplemental oxygen was used only to treat clinical cyanosis. Results of this study showed a dramatic decrease in the presence and severity of ROP in those infants exposed to a restricted oxygen regimen. Subsequent changes in clinical practice led to a near extinction of ROP. However, as changes in technology in the 1970s allowed for survival of smaller and less mature infants, ROP re-emerged and with higher prevalence than had previously been seen. New-found concern for ROP led to focused efforts on determining etiology and risk factors. Important associations between ROP and low birthweight, low gestational age, high severity of illness, and longer duration of oxygen use were uncovered and verified.[7]

Diagnosis

Diagnosis of ROP is made through visualization of the retinal vasculature using indirect ophthalmologic examination. The International Classification of ROP (ICROP) is the accepted classification system used to describe the location, severity, and extent of abnormal blood vessel development.[8]

In order to describe the location or zone of retinal vascular development, the retina can be divided into three zones, which are formed by concentric circles (**Figure 10-1**). Vascular development is first seen in zone 1, which is the most posterior portion of the retina. The center of zone 1 is the optic nerve and has a radius that is twice the distance from the optic nerve to the macula. Zone 2 completely encircles zone 1, extending anteriorly from the border of zone 1. On the nasal side of the orbit, zone 2 extends to the edge of the retina or ora serrata. On the lateral side, zone 2 extends approximately half the distance between the lateral border of zone 1 and the lateral ora serrata. Zone 3 includes the space anterior to zone 2, extending to the ora serrata. During vascularization of the retina, vessels are first seen in zone 1, extending into zone 2, and then zone 3 with further development. Mature vascular development is seen only when vessels extend through zone 3.

The stage of retinopathy is used to describe the severity of abnormal vascular development. **Figure 10-2** shows the appearance of ROP as the retina is visualized by indirect ophthalmologic examination. As ROP advances, severity progresses from stage 1 through stage 5. Stage 1 is the first stage of vascular maldevelopment and is typically described as a line of demarcation separating the normally developing vascular retina from the avascular retina. This line is flat, without three-dimensionally rising from the surface of the retina. Mildly abnormal vessel growth is characteristic of stage 1. With stage 2 ROP, the line of demarcation develops height and width, rising from the surface of the retina. Stage 2 represents moderately abnormal vessel growth. The onset of extraretinal fibrovascular proliferation marks the onset of stage 3 ROP and can be visualized as the extension of abnormal blood vessels and fibrous tissue into the vitreous within the center of the eye. In stage 3, vascular growth is severely abnormal. As the fibrous tissue and vessels grow further from the surface of the retina, physical traction can cause partial detachment of the retina, the hallmark of stage 4. Complete detachment of the retina marks stage 5, with resulting severe visual impairment or blindness.

Clock hours are used to describe both the position of abnormal vessel development within any of the zones and the extent of disease. The extent of disease is typically described as the number of clock hours affected. By ICROP convention, clock hours are used to describe the most severely abnormal portion of the retina. Although not currently used as criteria for treatment, the number of clock hours is essential to understand the extent and progression of disease.

The final component used to describe retinopathy of prematurity is the presence or absence of plus disease. Plus disease is a tortuous and dilated appearance of the

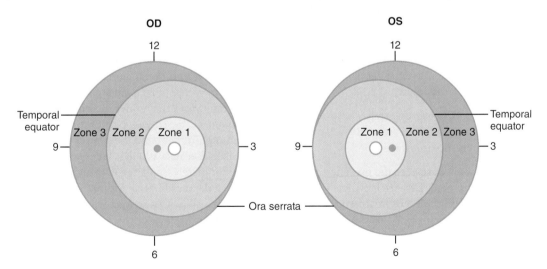

FIGURE 10-1 An illustration of the retina, divided into three concentric circles or zones centered on the optic disc. The zones define the area of retina covered by physiologic retinal vascularization The lower the zone, the more severe the disease.

The three zones seen in this illustration are as follows:
- Zone 1: The posterior pole, consisting of a circle whose radius is twice the distance from the optic disc to the macula.
- Zone 2: A doughnut-shaped area of retina that extends from the edge of zone 1 to a position tangential to the nasal ora serrata and around an area near the temporal anatomic equator.
- Zone 3: The outermost residual crescent of retina anterior to zone 2.

Modified from Kashani AH, Drenser KA, Capone A Jr. Retinopathy of prematurity. In Yanoff M, Duker JS, *Ophthalmology: Expert Consult: Online and Print*. 4th ed. Elsevier Health Sciences; 2013:537, Fig. 6.20-8.

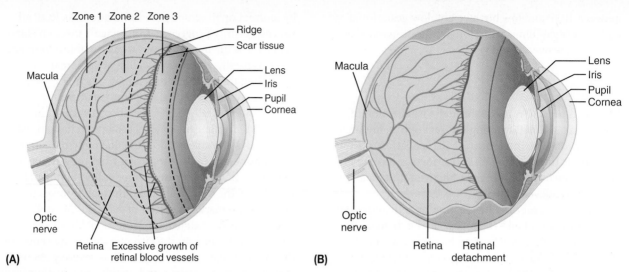

FIGURE 10-2 Stages 3 and 4 of retinopathy of prematurity in preterm infants. The images were obtained with a neonatal retinal imaging system (RetCam, Clarity Medical Systems). (**A**) A thickened ridge with aberrant intravitreal angiogenesis (stage 3); (**B**) Partial retinal detachment (stage 4), which is most evident at the right lower portion of the image where the underlying choroidal vascular detail is out of focus.

Data from The Hospital for Sick Children. (2018). Retinopathy of prematurity (ROP). Retrieved from https://www.aboutkidshealth.ca/Article?contentid=834&language=English.

vessels at the optic disk in zone 1. The presence of plus disease is a mandatory precursor to the development of retinal detachment. Therefore, its identification is critical and demonstrates the need for treatment.

Clinical Presentation

At the time of indirect ophthalmologic examination, infants can be placed in a number of diagnostic categories. Infants described as having immature retinal development have no identified vessel disease. However, because retinal development is incomplete, there is still potential for the identification of abnormality. Continued monitoring of vessel development is essential to ensure appropriate vessel growth.

Type 1 ROP, as described in the CryoROP[3] study, identifies those infants in need of treatment in order to avoid progression of disease to retinal detachment. Criteria for Type 1 ROP are as follows:

1. Zone 1 with plus disease, any stage
2. Zone 1 without plus disease, stage 3
3. Zone 2 with plus disease, stage 2 or 3

"Pre-threshold" disease describes the presence of abnormal vessel development. Disease is typically not severe enough to trigger initiation of treatment; however, infants identified as having pre-threshold disease require frequent monitoring to identify disease progression. Because there are implications to visual development, any retinopathy seen in zone 1 is considered to be pre-threshold, unless qualifications for treatment are met. ROP in zone 2 is also considered pre-threshold when plus disease is identified or when stage 3 is seen.

The timing of the development of ROP is dependent on the gestational age, which provides an estimation of the maturity of the retinal vasculature. Although degree of prematurity at birth is the primary indicator of need

for evaluation, all infants with a birthweight of <1500 grams or a gestational age at birth of less than or equal to 30 weeks are candidates for screening.[9] Additionally, older or larger infants may electively be evaluated if significant risk factors are present, including a need for a high level of respiratory support, or high levels of oxygen, or who have had unstable clinical courses.[9] The timing of the initial ROP evaluation is either at 31 weeks' corrected gestational age, or 4 weeks after birth, with preference given to the later date.[9] The timing of follow-up evaluation is dependent on the findings of the initial exam but typically ranges from 3 weeks to 1 week or less.

Management

The standard of care for ROP is currently in transition. Current traditional management uses diode laser ablation to create burn in all areas of the avascular retina anterior to the border of abnormal vascular development. By destroying part of the retinal tissue, the oxygen requirement and the production of VEGF are decreased. Because VEGF is an essential growth factor to stimulate vascular growth, a decrease in VEGF leads to a decreased drive for further vessel growth, which then allows for more normal subsequent vascular development.[5]

Injection of anti-growth factors directly into the orbit is a treatment option that is rapidly gaining favor. Bevacizumab is a monoclonal antibody that prevents angiogenesis by blocking the effect of VEGF. In a comparison study, bevacizumab showed better outcomes as compared with laser for infants with zone 1 stage 3 ROP with plus disease.[10] There are risks associated with this therapeutic option. Subsequent studies have shown that after anti-VEGF therapy, persistent avascularization of the peripheral retina, recurrent ROP disease, and progression to complete retinal detachment can occur.[11] Additional research is necessary to find options to treat ROP with fewer risks of complications.

Complications and Outcomes

As infants mature, retinal vascular development is assessed. For those who develop ROP, a sequential advancement through the defined stages of ROP is anticipated until progression to the point of needing treatment or spontaneous regression. Infants born at 25 weeks' gestation or fewer have >90% chance of developing ROP. The rate of ROP decreases to approximately 45% for infants born at 30 weeks' gestation.[3] Fortunately, most infants with ROP have mild disease, as fewer than 90% do not progress or require treatment. Progression to advanced disease is best predicted by the presence of abnormalities in zone 1 at the time of initial assessment, presence of plus disease, rapid progression, or extensive (>9 clock hours) stage 3 disease.[3]

Infants with mild ROP (stage 1 or 2, no plus disease) and with spontaneous regression have higher rates of myopia, strabismus, and amblyopia, compared with infants with no history of ROP.[12] Severe myopia and glaucoma are common complications for infants who develop more significant ROP.[13]

Treatment options may affect the complications associated with ROP. Myopia is less frequent after treatment with bevacizumab as compared with laser among those treated for ROP.[14,15] However, there is risk for late occurrence of retinal detachment for those treated with bevacizumab.[11] Progression to retinal detachment is uncommon, less than 2% for both groups combined, after either treatment modality.[15]

Although the exact parameters to be used continue to be a subject of discussion as the risks and balances of competing outcomes are evaluated, it is clear through multiple reports that higher oxygen saturation limits are associated with higher rates of ROP. The SUPPORT Study[16] showed a decrease in ROP from 17.9% to 8.6% for surviving infants <28 weeks' gestation when oxygen saturation targets were decreased from a goal of 91–95% to 85–89%. Unfortunately, the lower targets were also associated with a higher risk for death. The BOOST II Study[17] demonstrated similar risk reduction when lower oxygen saturation levels were targeted. These findings emphasize the importance of avoiding excessively high oxygen saturation targets.

Bronchopulmonary Dysplasia and Chronic Lung Disease

There have been considerable advancements in the field of neonatal-perinatal medicine that have increased the survival of extremely premature infants, yet bronchopulmonary dysplasia continues to be one of the most common complications in these infants.

TABLE 10-1
The Most Common Factors Contributing to the Development of BPD

Prematurity
Ventilator injury
Oxygen toxicity
Fetal and neonatal inflammatory response
Patent ductus arteriosus
Fluid maintenance
Nutrition

Etiology

Bronchopulmonary dysplasia (BPD) is a complication of premature infants originally described over 40 years ago by Northway and colleagues.[18] The initial descriptions and clinical presentation of BPD have evolved, along with improvements in the care of premature infants, resulting in a complex and multifactorial etiology. **Table 10-1** lists the factors contributing to the development of BPD.

Prematurity

Premature birth is the most significant determinant of an infant's risk of developing BPD. The lungs of infants born between 23 and 32 weeks' gestation are in the canalicular and saccular phases of lung development and are surfactant deficient and poorly developed for gas exchange. Birth during this time, along with supportive respiratory therapies, can cause injury and an arrest of normal development.

Ventilator Injury

The use of mechanical ventilation to administer high concentrations of oxygen and peak inspiratory high pressures is one of the most important contributing factors in the development of BPD. Northway and colleagues[18] reported BPD in infants requiring high supplemental oxygen requirements. Increased risk for BPD has been reported in centers with more frequent use of mechanical ventilation.[19] Studies in preterm lambs demonstrate that prolonged mechanical ventilation disrupts lung development and produces pulmonary histopathologic changes that were similar to preterm infants who died with BPD. In a study of human infants who died of BPD, the length of time on mechanical ventilation correlated better with the severity of outcome than did either gestational age at birth or length of time with >60% oxygen.[20,21]

Ventilator-induced lung injury is multifactorial.[22,23] Injury caused by ventilatory support causes damage to the alveolar capillary bed, leading to seepage of fluid, plasma, and blood into airways, alveoli, and the interstitium, inactivating surfactant. Higher ventilator settings are often needed to compensate, leading to an increase in inflammatory mediators and cells in the lung.[22,24]

Barotrauma, volutrauma, and atelectotrauma can occur from mechanical ventilatory support, all of which contribute to lung injury and the subsequent development of BPD. Volutrauma refers to the damage caused by overdistension of the lung by the delivery of high volumes of gas. Barotrauma is caused by the delivery of excessive pressure to the lung. Atelectotrauma refers to the damage caused by continual opening and closing of lung units, or recruitment and de-recruitment of the lung. Animal studies have confirmed that volutrauma is more detrimental to the newborn lung, causing more lung injury compared with barotrauma and atelectotrauma.[24–26] Ventilation with low positive end-expiratory pressure (PEEP) creates atelectotrauma and lung injury in animal models.[27]

Oxygen Toxicity

One of the primary causes of BPD was originally thought to be supplemental oxygen administration. Although it may be a contributing factor, currently it is not identified as a principal inciting factor. Recent investigations identify prenatal factors as a primary cause in the development of BPD before the administration of supplemental oxygen.[28] Not long after Northway et al.[18] first reported their findings of BPD in babies requiring an FiO_2 of 0.80 or greater for as little as 6 days, other investigators noted the development of BPD at lesser amounts of supplemental oxygen administration.[29–31] Recent animal models with chronic oxygen exposure to the developing lung reveal that premature lungs have a reduced capacity to limit oxygen damage, which correlates with increasing immaturity.[32,33]

Studies to determine optimal oxygen saturations have shown that higher saturation targets increased the number of babies requiring oxygen at 36 weeks' gestation[34] and also increased exacerbations of chronic lung disease and the need for oxygen and hospitalization at 3 months of corrected age.[35] These investigations demonstrate a need to carefully expose infants to supplemental oxygen during clinical management.

Fetal and Neonatal Inflammatory Response

An area of recent considerable research is the effect of antenatal and postnatal lung inflammation and the subsequent development of BPD. Just as proinflammatory mediators have been implicated in the onset of preterm labor, they are also considered as a factor associated with fetal onset of lung injury.[36] Infection, which is often undetected in the antenatal period, plays an important role. Forty-five percent of infants delivered after preterm labor have been exposed to low-grade ascending infection.[37] Microorganisms can penetrate intact membranes, leading to asymptomatic bacterial invasion of the amniotic cavity.[38] The fetus can swallow or aspirate the microorganisms, initiating the fetal inflammatory response syndrome.

Numerous investigators have shown direct evidence of an association between the fetal inflammatory response syndrome and the development of BPD.[39–41] Elevated markers of inflammation in amniotic fluid and tracheal aspirates taken soon after birth were associated with a higher incidence of BPD. These mediators induce pulmonary microvascular leakage and cause plasma proteins to flood the airspace, which inactivates surfactant and perpetuates lung inflammation.[42]

Patent Ductus Arteriosus

Patent ductus arteriosus (PDA) occurs in up to 70% of preterm infants before 28 weeks' gestation and is inversely related to gestational age. Left-to-right shunting of blood from the aorta to the pulmonary artery from a persistently patent ductus arteriosus causes an increase in pulmonary blood flow and pulmonary edema. Pulmonary compliance is reduced and airway resistance increases, leading to increased supplemental respiratory needs. PDA has been associated with BPD,[43,44] although a cause-and-effect relationship has not been definitively established. Additionally, there is no evidence that the use of medical treatments for the prevention and treatment of PDA decreases BPD, despite successful closure of the PDA.[45]

Fluid Maintenance

Several studies demonstrate a relationship between excessive fluid and sodium intake as a risk factor for the development of BPD.[46–49] In extremely low birthweight infants, body water content is very high and a large proportion resides in the extracellular fluid compartment. During the 1st week of life, there is a physiologic contraction of the extracellular fluid compartment with negative fluid and sodium balances. Because of this negative fluid balance, newborns have weight loss in the first week of life. The administration of excessive fluid and sodium during this critical period impairs the contraction. Retention of extracellular fluid in addition to the presence of a PDA can lead to worsening lung function and the need for supplemental respiratory support. A meta-analysis showed significant advantages to a restrictive fluid intake strategy for premature infants, with reductions in the risks for PDA and necrotizing enterocolitis; however, there was no significant reduction in the risk for BPD.[50]

Nutrition

Nutrition plays an important role in lung development and maturation. Malnutrition may negatively affect pulmonary function,[51] and it may play a role in the development of BPD. In premature infants, the combination of high caloric needs and low nutritional stores at birth may contribute to the development of BPD. Poor caloric intake during the initial and ongoing respiratory illness may contribute to respiratory muscle fatigue and prolong the duration of mechanical ventilation. In one case-control study, infants who developed BPD had significantly lower mean energy intakes than matched controls.[52] Similar to many other nutritional components, vitamin A stores in premature infants are lower at birth compared to infants born at term.[53,54] The role of vitamin A in the promotion or orderly growth and differentiation of regenerating epithelial tissue makes vitamin A an important nutrient during recovery from lung injury. Vitamin A deficiency causes changes in the lower respiratory tract that are similar to those seen in BPD.[55] Associations have been shown between low levels of vitamin A at birth and 28 days in infants who subsequently developed BPD.[56]

Pathophysiology

The pathology of BPD has changed over time. "Classic" descriptions of BPD encompassed marked cellular necrosis, edema, inflammation, and subsequent fibroproliferation that leads to varying amounts of structural disruption. Maldistribution, obstruction, and air-trapping occur as a result of the widespread fibroproliferative activity, squamous metaplasia of epithelial linings, and accumulation of debris and hypertrophy of smooth muscle in the airways. The final radiographic picture is characterized by atelectasis in close proximity to emphysematous areas (**Figure 10-3**). It is less common to see these severe forms of BPD. Clinical advances, such as prenatal steroids, surfactant therapy, and ventilation strategies, have resulted in a newer, milder form of BPD.[57] This newer form is described as having less inflammation, less structural destruction, minimal

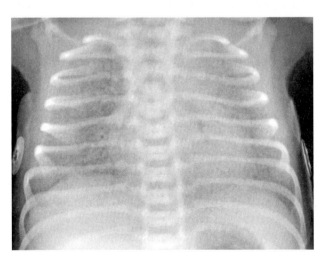

FIGURE 10-3 A chest radiograph showing the classic attributes of BPD. The chest radiograph shows areas of hyperinflation and emphysema with adjacent dense areas of atelectasis.

Published with permission from LearningRadiology.com.

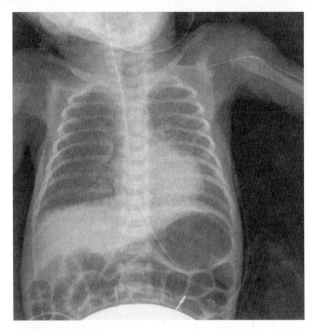

FIGURE 10-4 Chest radiograph of the milder form of BPD, showing diffuse homogenous coarse opacities.

Courtesy of Dr. Benedikt Beilstein, Radiopaedia.org, rID: 52167.

fibrosis, hypoalveolarization, and a radiographic picture of diffuse homogenous coarse opacities (**Figure 10-4**).

Inflammation

Animal models describe the active role that granulocytes play in the pathogenesis of BPD.[57,58] Neutrophils, found in bronchoalveolar lavage fluid of premature infants with respiratory distress syndrome (RDS), peak by the 4th day of life and decline rapidly thereafter in infants who recover uneventfully.[59,60] This fall in neutrophil counts is delayed in infants who later develop BPD.

Proinflammatory mediators are elevated within the first 7 to 10 days after birth in infants who later develop BPD. Elevations in the mediators in umbilical cord blood and tracheal aspirates can be found in premature infants who later develop BPD.[28,41,42,59,61]

Structural Disruption

Granulocyte influx into the lung releases reactive oxygen species and proteases, which can induce cellular injury and cause destruction. The release of protease causes an imbalance between lung protease and anti-protease, shifting the pendulum toward proteolysis. Proteolysis seems to predominate in the lungs of infants who develop BPD. Researchers found high levels of elastase in the lungs of infants who subsequently develop BPD.[59,62] Animal models of BPD also show an increased deposition and abnormal distribution of elastin.[63]

Fibroproliferation

Much of what is known about fibrosis in BPD stems from animal studies, specifically fibrogenic growth factors. In studies conducted with mice, those with an overexpression of fibrogenic growth factors have an arrest of lung development, alveolar enlargement, and fibrosis.[64,65] The literature also reports an increase in smooth muscle actin, a marker for myofibroblasts, in the lung mesenchyme and a rise in collagen I gene expression in the distal airways in mice with BPD.[66] Studies also demonstrate that elevation of fibrogenic growth factors in the lung fluid of premature infants lead to the development of BPD and mice deficient in fibrogenic growth factors are protected from fibrosis.[67-69]

Delayed Development

The arrest of lung development without signs of inflammation or fibrosis is the most prominent finding of the new form of BPD.[70] The first characterizations of the new BPD were based on pathologic findings of infants dying from BPD.[71] The postmortem findings included fewer and larger alveoli, indicating an interference with septation.[72] Septation and alveolarization developmental regulation has been an area to determine the pathology of BPD. There is an imbalance between stimulatory and inhibitory factors, most notably between fibrogenic growth factors and glucocorticoids. At physiologic levels, glucocorticoids encourage the maturation of parenchymal structures and lung functions, such as surfactant production and lung water clearance.[73] In experimental models, a number of factors, such as hyperoxia, hypoxia, mechanical ventilation, and poor nutrition, can decrease lung septation.[74] Despite the beneficial and important maturational effects, animal models have also shown that supraphysiologic doses of glucocorticoids can significantly inhibit alveolarization.[75] These studies demonstrate that alveolarization can be regulated, but more research is needed to understand the signaling pathways involved.

Vascular development is also disrupted in much the same way as septation.[76,77] Lung microvasculature arises *de novo* from the mesenchyme underlying the airways and apposes itself progressively more closely to the epithelium as development progresses. VEGF, which is produced by the epithelium, guides this process.[78] In animal models and humans with BPD, epithelial VEGF expression is reduced.[76,79] Low levels of VEGF in human lung fluid during the first 10 days of life were associated with subsequent development of BPD.[80] Inhibitors of angiogenesis have also shown to impede alveolarization, and it is postulated that angiogenesis is necessary for alveolarization during normal lung development.[81]

Diagnosis

BPD accounts for the vast majority of cases of neonatal chronic lung disease.[82] Over the years, varying definitions of BPD were used in an effort to predict future respiratory illness. BPD was originally diagnosed using a combination of clinical characteristics, radiographic findings, and the prolonged need or use of supplemental oxygen. However, some infants diagnosed with BPD had a full clinical and functional recovery while others developed pulmonary function abnormalities, despite not requiring prolonged supplemental oxygen use.

There is a lack of uniformity in the diagnostic criteria for BPD among clinicians and in the literature. For example, the use of supplemental oxygen as a marker for pulmonary damage and BPD is problematic. The indications for supplemental oxygen vary from center to center because it is difficult to define optimal oxygen levels for these infants. Additionally, supplemental oxygen requirements can be influenced by medications and the need for ventilatory support, which leads to a lack of accurate diagnostic markers for BPD.[83] Making the appropriate diagnosis of BPD helps to identify patients at risk for long-term respiratory problems.

Chest radiographs showing chronic pulmonary involvement plus a clinical course that is compatible with BPD justifies the diagnosis with some degree of consistency. It is important to note that infants with the new form of BPD have a less severe clinical course and that radiographs show diffuse haziness as their hallmark, making it difficult for the diagnosis of BPD.

The National Institutes of Health (NIH) organized a workshop in 2000 to address the inconsistencies in the diagnostic criteria of BPD and to improve the definition of BPD. The workshop's recommendation was to use oxygen for ≥ 28 days and at 36 weeks' postmenstrual age to identify different severities of BPD and also to include oxygen concentration at 36 weeks' postmenstrual age to further define the severity of lung injury. There was also agreement that a minimum of 28 days of supplemental oxygen use was needed to make the diagnosis of BPD.[65] **Table 10-2** outlines these criteria. Other etiologies, such as congenital heart disease, pulmonary lymphangiectasia, chemical pneumonitis from recurrent aspiration, cystic fibrosis, or disorders of surfactant homeostasis, could lead or contribute to lung damage and may be falsely labeled as BPD.

Clinical Presentation

BPD is more commonly seen in extremely low birthweight infants. The majority of infants with RDS experience a mild initial respiratory course because they respond favorably to surfactant administration and are not exposed to aggressive ventilatory support or high concentrations of inspired oxygen. Often a few days of minimal or no requirements for supplemental oxygen or respiratory support follow. Although some infants can be weaned off support, others may require prolonged ventilation due to apnea and poor respiratory effort.

Infants requiring prolonged support due to progressive deterioration in lung function over time are at most risk for the development of BPD. Clinical deterioration

TABLE 10-2
Definition and Diagnostic Criteria for BPD

	<32 Weeks' Gestational Age	>32 Weeks' Gestational Age
Time point of the assessment	36 weeks' postmenstrual age or discharge home, whichever comes first	>28 days' but <56 days' postnatal age or discharge home, whichever comes first
	Treatment with oxygen >21% for at least 28 days plus	
Mild BPD	Breathing room air at 36 weeks' PMA or discharge, whichever comes first	Breathing room air at 56 days' postnatal age or discharge, whichever comes first
Moderate BPD	Need for <30% oxygen at 36 weeks' PMA or discharge, whichever comes first	Need for <30% oxygen at 56 days' postnatal age or discharge, whichever comes first
Severe BPD	Need for >30% oxygen and/or positive pressure (PPV or nCPAP) at 36 weeks' PMA or discharge, whichever comes first	Need for >30% oxygen and/or positive pressure (PPV or nCPAP) at 56 days' postnatal age or discharge, whichever comes first

PMA = postmenstrual age; PPV = positive pressure ventilation; nCPAP = nasal continuous positive airway pressure

Reproduced from Jobe AH, Bancalari E. Bronchopulmonary dysplasia. *American Journal of Respiratory and Critical Care Medicine.* 2001;163(7):1723-1729, Table 1.

can be triggered by systemic or respiratory infections or increased pulmonary blood flow due to a persistently patent ductus arteriosus. Initially, the functional and radiographic lung changes are mild, sometimes showing only diffuse haziness, but in other cases the coarser changes of nonuniform inflation and cystic nature that is observed in the classic form of BPD may develop.

Management

As with all clinical conditions, the "ideal" management strategy for BPD would be to prevent BPD; once established, the treatment for BPD remains mostly supportive. Medical care typically focuses on using respiratory therapies that minimize further lung injury and optimize nutrition and growth, with varying degrees of success. As a result, considerable effort has been devoted to the prevention of the disease. Some therapies may not entirely prevent BPD, but they may lessen the severity of the disease when it does develop. **Table 10-3** lists the strategies used to prevent and/or lessen the severity of BPD.

Prevention of Prematurity

Given the importance of extreme prematurity in the pathogenesis of the new BPD, the obvious and most important preventive measure for BPD is preventing premature births. Maternal injections of 17 alpha hydroxyprogesterone during pregnancy have been shown to reduce the risk of recurrent preterm delivery by about one-third in women with a history of preterm delivery.[84] This prevention strategy is hampered by increasing numbers of multiple pregnancies. Infants in multigestation pregnancies are much more likely to be born earlier and smaller than those born in singleton pregnancies. It is reassuring that the overall preterm

TABLE 10-3
Strategies Used to Prevent and/or Lessen the Severity of BPD

Preventing premature births
Prenatal treatments
Surfactant therapy
Caffeine
Vitamin A administration

Lung-protective strategies
    Oxygen administration guideline use
    Permissive hypercapnia
    Use of noninvasive ventilation

birth rate has slightly declined, although the rate of low birthweight infants is unchanged.[85]

Prenatal Treatments

The prenatal administration of glucocorticoids is the most widely used therapy to accelerate lung maturation in pregnancies at risk for preterm birth. Prenatal glucocorticoids are the standard of care for women at high risk of preterm delivery prior to 34 weeks' gestation. The recommendations come from the 1994 NIH Consensus Conference and were reinforced by a second NIH Consensus Conference in 2000.[86] A recent meta-analysis shows that preterm infants of mothers who received antenatal corticosteroids prior to preterm birth had an overall reduction in RDS.[87] Despite improvements in neonatal morbidity and mortality, antenatal steroids have not been shown to decrease the overall rate of BPD by meta-analysis.[87] Additionally, repeat courses of prenatal glucocorticoids during pregnancy does not appear to further decrease the rate of RDS[88] and may increase the incidence of severe BPD by inhibiting normal lung growth.[89] Nonetheless, based on the latest guidelines, prenatal glucocorticoids should be administered in a single course to any mother at risk of preterm delivery between 24 to 34 weeks' gestation.[86]

Surfactant Therapy

Lack of endogenous surfactant is the primary cause of early respiratory disease in newborn premature infants. Animal studies and early clinical trials with exogenous surfactant for the prevention and treatment of RDS have shown improvements in pulmonary mechanics and protection against ventilator-induced lung damage. Exogenous surfactants have significantly decreased the severity of and mortality from RDS among intubated infants when used very soon after birth.[90] Although prenatal steroids help to accelerate production of surfactant before birth, preterm infants continue to be at risk for RDS.

A reduction in the incidence of BPD was expected after the development of exogenous surfactant. However, recent meta-analyses do not show a reduction in rates of BPD with early surfactant use.[91,92] Two additional strategies were then developed by combining the benefits of early surfactant use and reduced ventilator use. The first method is to administer surfactant during a brief period of intubation without subsequent sustained mechanical ventilation (intubation, delivery of surfactant, immediate extubation). Although some studies with this approach show many benefits, meta-analysis[93] did not demonstrate a decrease in the incidence of BPD at 36 weeks' gestation. The second method was to administer surfactant beyond the first postnatal week to infants in whom a secondary surfactant dysfunction may be present and who are at a high risk for BPD.[94] A randomized controlled trial of this method did show a reduction in mean fraction of inspired oxygen but no difference in the incidence of mortality or BPD between groups.[95]

Caffeine for Apnea of Prematurity

Caffeine is a methylxanthine used to treat apnea of prematurity. A large randomized controlled trial was designed to resolve the long-standing uncertainty about the short- and long-term efficacy and safety of methylxanthine therapy for apnea of prematurity. Initial findings showed a statistically significant reduction in oxygen use at 36 weeks' postmenstrual age (the current consensus definition of BPD) and a reduction in days of positive airway pressure in infants who received early caffeine in the first 10 days of life compared to those who later received caffeine for apnea.[95] The results indicate that caffeine may assist in reducing ventilator-induced lung injury.

Postnatal Anti-Inflammatory Therapies

Systemic corticosteroids affect pulmonary function and lung disease by increasing surfactant synthesis; decreasing recruitment of polymorphonuclear leukocytes to the lung; and reducing the production of prostaglandins, leukotrienes, elastase, and other inflammatory mediators. They also decrease vascular permeability and pulmonary edema formation.[96] Corticosteroids may also regulate lung repair after injury.

Initial studies of premature infants with a high risk for BPD ($\leq$30 weeks' gestation, $\leq$1250 grams, mechanical ventilation at 14 days) showed faster weaning from the ventilator and supplemental oxygen when a 42-day tapering course of dexamethasone was given.[97] There were also significant adverse effects associated with systemic corticosteroid administration, including hypertension, hyperglycemia, gastrointestinal bleeding, hypertrophic cardiomyopathy, and infection.[98] Subsequent studies with corticosteroids for the prevention of BPD continued. Most have demonstrated short-term improvements in pulmonary function. Two meta-analyses, differing on the timing of administration of the corticosteroids, were published to provide information on the effect of treatment with systemic steroids on the incidence of BPD. Early treatment was defined as the initial administration of the corticosteroid course before 8 postnatal days[99] and late treatment was defined as beginning after 7 days' postnatal age.[100]

Benefits of early treatment included lower extubation failure rates and decreased risks of BPD (supplemental oxygen use at 28 days' and 36 weeks' postmenstrual age), death or BPD at 28 days' and 36 weeks' postmenstrual age, patent ductus arteriosus, and ROP, including severe ROP.[99] However, in review of later outcomes, infants were found to have developmental delay, cerebral palsy, and abnormal neurologic examination.[99] Therefore, it was concluded that the benefits of early postnatal corticosteroid treatment ($\leq$7 days) may not outweigh the adverse effects of this treatment.

Infants enrolled in the late treatment trials had fewer extubation failure rates, lower rates of BPD at 28 days' and 36 weeks' postmenstrual age, reduced need for late rescue treatment with dexamethasone, fewer discharges on home oxygen, and a reduction in neonatal mortality at 28 days' postmenstrual age.[100] There was no increase in the risks of blindness, deafness, major neurosensory disability, or cerebral palsy, although there was an increased rate of abnormal neurologic examination.[100] The interpretation of the neurodevelopmental outcomes is difficult. The methodologic quality of the studies determining the long-term outcome is limited in some cases; surviving children were assessed predominantly before school age, which can cause difficulties diagnosing cerebral palsy. No study was sufficiently powered to detect important adverse long-term neurosensory outcomes. The use of late corticosteroids for infants who cannot be weaned from mechanical ventilation after the 1st week of life may be beneficial, but it is important to limit the dose and duration of any course of treatment.[101,102]

Systemic postnatal corticosteroids have significant benefits and risks. Given the adverse long-term neurodevelopmental impairments, it is not recommended to use dexamethasone or hydrocortisone in the 1st week of life. After 7 days of life, dexamethasone was shown to decrease the rate of BPD at 36 weeks' postmenstrual age with less impact on neurodevelopmental outcome. No trials have examined whether the benefits of corticosteroids outweigh the adverse effects for infants at high risk of, or with, severe BPD. Despite the continued risk of long-term neurodevelopmental impairments, there might be some populations of infants in which the benefits outweigh the risks based on the baseline risk of BPD. Infants at high risk of developing BPD treated with corticosteroids were shown to be more likely to survive without neurodevelopmental impairment.[103] This suggests that infants at a certain threshold risk for the development of BPD will have a net benefit (reduction in the risk for BPD without an increase in the risk of cerebral palsy) if corticosteroids are given to prevent BPD.

Inhaled corticosteroids have been evaluated as a prevention strategy for BPD, as there is an association between systemic corticosteroids and serious short- and long-term adverse effects. A meta-analysis examining the effect of early inhaled steroids beginning <2 weeks' postnatal age in ventilator-dependent infants did not find a significant effect on the prevention of BPD or mortality.[104] Evidence does not support the use of inhaled corticosteroids for the prevention or treatment of BPD.

Inhaled Nitric Oxide

Animal studies have shown that inhaled nitric oxide (iNO) decreased early lung inflammation and oxidant stress[105] and improved lung structure in models of BPD.[106] Inhaled nitric oxide may also have anti-inflammatory properties. Based on these observations, numerous studies were done to ascertain the effect of inhaled nitric oxide on the prevention of BPD in premature infants. A meta-analysis evaluated 11 randomized controlled trials of iNO therapy in preterm infants. There was no overall evidence to support a clear role for iNO for the prevention of BPD. However, one of the larger trials, which enrolled intubated infants during the 2nd postnatal week, demonstrated a reduction in BPD but not death. Given these results, it is possible that certain populations of infants with a baseline risk might benefit, but more studies are needed. In 2011, an NIH Consensus on the use of iNO in premature infants concluded that, taken as a whole, the available evidence does not support the use of iNO in the care of premature infants of <34 weeks' gestation who require respiratory support.[107]

Medications

Vitamin A derivatives are critical in the regulation and promotion of growth and differentiation of lung epithelial cells, particularly during repair after lung injury.[108] Preterm infants have low vitamin A levels at birth, and low levels of vitamin A are associated with an increased risk of BPD.[109] Subsequently, vitamin supplementation was established as a strategy to prevent BPD. When extremely low birthweight infants were given vitamin A supplementation, the incidence of BPD was reduced at 36 weeks' postmenstrual age and no risk for neurodevelopmental impairment at 18 to 22 months of age was seen.[110] Therefore, the use of vitamin A supplementation in extremely low birthweight infants may be helpful for the prevention of BPD.

Because pulmonary edema appears to be a significant feature in BPD, diuretics are commonly used to improve lung mechanics, especially in infants on chronic mechanical ventilation or those with established disease. Several small studies in the early 1980s have shown short- and long-term improvements in airway resistance, lung compliance, and oxygenation, and quicker ventilator weaning in infants with BPD, when loop diuretics, such as furosemide, are used.[111,112] Similar to other medications discussed in this chapter, the use of loop diuretics is not without risk. Serious adverse effects are reported in newborn infants due to the excretion of sodium, potassium, and chloride. Hyercalciuria is also prominent with loop diuretics and may lead to nephrocalcinosis and bone demineralization. Despite the widespread use, there are few current studies evaluating the short- and long-term effects in the treatment of infants with BPD. Based on current evidence and the potential complications to loop diuretic use, the routine administration of these agents in infants with (or developing) BPD cannot be recommended.

Diuretic therapy that acts on the distal tubule, such as thiazide-type agents, has also been assessed. Little useful information can be gleaned from the few studies with thiazide diuretics, and their use cannot be recommended based on available evidence.

Bronchodilators have the potential effect of dilating small airways with muscle hypertrophy. However, there are no randomized controlled clinical trials on the use of bronchodilators in the treatment of BPD and little evidence in the literature to support their use in the prevention or treatment of BPD.[113]

Respiratory Support Strategies

There are two important strategies that guide treatment of respiratory conditions in premature infants: provision of appropriate levels of supplemental oxygen to support adequate oxygenation and gentle ventilation with permissive hypercapnia.

The most recent multicenter study identified oxygen saturations (SpO_2) of about 90% to 95% as an optimal target range. This multicenter study, Surfactant, Positive Pressure, and Pulse Oximetry Randomized Trial (SUPPORT), found that lower target ranges of oxygen saturation (85–89%) resulted in an increase in mortality and did not significantly decrease the composite outcome of severe retinopathy.[16] It is challenging to maintain an infant requiring oxygen within a given saturation range because frequent monitoring and manual adjustments in the amount of inspired oxygen may be required to respond to hypoxemic episodes. Close monitoring is essential to avoid increased oxidative stress caused by a hypoxemic event that is followed by hyperoxia.

Permissive hypercapnia (PaCO$_2$ of 45–55 mm Hg, and pH >7.2) is a lung-protective strategy for the management of infants receiving assisted ventilation. Higher levels of PaCO$_2$ are accepted in an effort to avoid the use of high tidal volumes, which contribute to pulmonary overdistention and hypocapnia. Studies implementing this lung injury–minimizing treatment strategy, also referred to as gentle ventilation, demonstrate strong trends for the potential of benefits without increased adverse events.[114,115]

Management of Respiratory Failure

A central tenet in the management of preterm infants with respiratory failure is to support adequate gas exchange with minimum adverse effects on the infant's lungs, hemodynamics, and brain. Long durations of mechanical ventilation are associated with increased likelihood of BPD. Avoidance of mechanical ventilation and successful extubation at the earliest possible time is desirable.

The use of nasal continuous positive airway pressure (nCPAP) has received tremendous recent study as a method to reduce mechanical ventilator exposure. It is less invasive, and cohort comparisons of nCPAP or mechanical ventilation suggested a reduction in the risk of BPD with early nCPAP use compared with intubation and mechanical ventilation. Recent large, multicenter randomized controlled trials evaluated the use of early nCPAP versus intubation and mechanical ventilation and showed that nCPAP reduced the combined outcome of death and BPD by almost 10%.[115–117] Additional important findings with the use of early nCPAP included a trend toward a shorter duration of supplemental oxygen exposure and a significant difference in the duration of mechanical ventilation, supporting the use of nCPAP as an alternative to intubation and invasive ventilatory support.[115–117]

Researchers have sought to avoid the use of invasive ventilation in infants requiring surfactant administration. The INtubation-SURFactant-Extubation (INSURE) approach was developed to administer surfactant to infants with worsening RDS and to reduce invasive ventilatory support by extubating to CPAP or noninvasive positive pressure ventilation (NIPPV). This approach allows infants to benefit from both surfactant and noninvasive respiratory support, such as nCPAP or NIPPV. The available data suggest that minimizing endotracheal ventilation could be achieved by adopting early nCPAP or NIPPV for RDS, and if intubation is required, to use the INSURE approach. This strategy has important short-term advantages in minimizing the use and duration of mechanical ventilation and long term may reduce the rates of BPD.[118]

Complications and Outcomes

The long-term consequences of BPD on the respiratory health of older children and adults are not fully described, as the changes in the care of premature infants has modified the clinical and pathologic characteristics of BPD over the last few decades. BPD improves with age, but lifelong consequences can ensue.

Pulmonary artery hypertension (PAH) is increasingly being recognized as an important complication of BPD because of the association with increased morbidity and mortality.[119] Although PAH is often associated with more severe BPD, not all infants with PAH have severe BPD and not all infants with BPD have PAH. In one series, PAH was diagnosed prior to hospital discharge in 18% of extremely low birthweight infants.[120] Phenotypic variability exists among preterm infants of similar gestational ages, making it difficult to predict which infants are at increased risk of developing PAH. PAH usually resolves when associated with BPD, although mortality rates have been reported to range from 14% to 38% in retrospective studies.[121–123]

Infants with BPD and PAH also have cardiovascular abnormalities, such as pulmonary vein stenosis, atrial septal defects, patent ductus arteriosus, and aorta-pulmonary collateral vessels. Lung structural abnormalities, such as decreased surface area, persistent ventilation-perfusion mismatch, poor gas exchange, and poor airway clearance, are associated with PAH in infants with BPD. PAH can acutely worsen with general anesthesia, positive pressure ventilation, aspiration, gastroesophageal reflux, respiratory infections, and suboptimal nutrition.[121] Mechanisms that contribute to the pathogenesis of PAH include oxygen toxicity, barotrauma, chronic or intermittent alveolar hypoxia along with acidosis, and cardiac dysfunction.

The majority of infants with PAH improve over time with optimizing treatment of BPD and recognizing and preventing factors that exacerbate PAH. This includes avoiding hypoxemic vasoconstriction, improving gas exchange, and optimizing lung growth. Supplemental oxygen administration is the mainstay of treatment, but severe PAH does not respond well to just oxygen therapy and may require inhaled nitric oxide, sildenafil, or bosentan.

Infants and children with a history of BPD are subject to recurrent wheezing episodes that can last from early childhood through adulthood. In the EPICure study of children born before 26 weeks' gestation, 25%

had the diagnosis of asthma at 11 years of age, and 56% had abnormal spirometry.[124] Children with a history of BPD and asthma-like symptoms are more likely to have airway hyperresponsiveness, but only half respond to bronchodilator therapy and inhaled corticosteroids.

Should wheezing worsen with bronchodilator administration, tracheobronchomalacia should be considered and diagnostic measures taken to confirm diagnosis. Infants with BPD can develop tracheobronchomalacia due to prolonged barotrauma, chronic or recurrent infection, chronic aspiration, and endotracheal intubation. This complication of BPD was more common in infants and children with classic BPD who were treated with prolonged periods of high ventilator pressure. Signs of tracheobronchomalacia include "BPD spells" (episodes of abrupt cyanosis with absent airflow) and can be life threatening. Most cases resolve with time and maturity of the tracheal cartilage. Glottic and subglottic damage can occur as a result of chronic endotracheal intubation and is more common in extremely low birthweight infants.

Up to 50% of children with BPD require re-hospitalization during the first two years of life due to respiratory illness.[125,126] Most infections are due to viruses and can interfere with ongoing lung growth and negatively affect lung function in later life.[127] Respiratory syncytial virus (RSV) can cause severe illness in infants and children with BPD, especially those requiring supplemental oxygen, and can be life threatening. RSV infections in the first 2 years of life in children with BPD can contribute to worse lung function at school age compared to those who did not experience an RSV-related hospitalization. Because of the severity of RSV infections, RSV immunoprophylaxis was developed and has been shown to reduce severe RSV infections in infants with BPD.[128] BPD predisposes infants and children to severe lower respiratory tract disease due to *Rhinovirus*, a common infectious virus among the general population that does not typically cause severe disease in healthy individuals.[129] Children who attend day care and have a history of BPD have also been shown to have a two- to threefold increase in emergency department visits, systemic corticosteroid use, antibiotic use, and days with difficulty breathing, presumably due to increased exposure to infectious illnesses.[129]

Supplemental respiratory care of infants with BPD after hospital discharge can range from nasal cannula supplemental oxygen to prolonged mechanical ventilation. Supplemental oxygen should be provided to maintain a target oxygen saturation of >92% in infants who are beyond term with mature retinal development and no pulmonary hypertension.

Infants with severe BPD, with or without obstructive airway disease, require long-term mechanical ventilation for months to years after hospital discharge. Tracheostomy is used to provide these infants with a stable airway for home mechanical ventilation. These infants require high amounts of resources and coordination of care among family members, primary physician, surgeon, pulmonologist, and home care service providers. Additionally, speech, occupational, and physical therapy is needed to ensure that the infant meets developmental milestones.

Children and adults with BPD are seen in many types of clinics throughout the healthcare system. The clinics range from general care offices to multidisciplinary clinics focused on the care of the complications of BPD. Infants discharged from the NICU should be referred to pediatric pulmonologists who are most familiar with the care of these medically fragile patients. Important general measures to reduce the risk for respiratory disease include frequent hand washing and avoidance of exposure to other young children who may have respiratory infections, avoidance of exposure to tobacco smoke, and close adherence to immunization schedules.

Air Leak Syndrome

A **pulmonary air leak** occurs when there is a rupture of the trachea, bronchi, or smaller airways, leading to an escape of air into the surrounding tissue. Air can then be present within the pleural space (**pneumothorax**), mediastinum (**pneumomediastinum**), or pericardium (**pneumopericardium**). When air escapes into the pulmonary interstitium, **pulmonary interstitial emphysema (PIE)** ensues.[130]

Pneumothorax

A pneumothorax develops when air escapes from the airway and enters the space bounded by the parietal pleura of the chest wall and the visceral pleura of the lung.[131]

Pneumomediastinum

The mediastinum includes all space between the bilateral lungs. The mediastinal space includes the heart, esophagus, trachea, and major veins and arteries. A pneumomediastinum occurs when free air traverses from the ruptured alveolus along the pulmonary vasculature to the mediastinum.[132]

Pneumopericardium

Pneumopericardium is the result of air leakage into the pericardial space, which can lead to acute, life-threatening symptoms as air accumulates and comes under tension within the limited pericardial space.[133]

Pulmonary Interstitial Emphysema

An air leak into the pulmonary interstitial space results in pulmonary interstitial emphysema (PIE).[130]

Etiology

Although air leaks can happen spontaneously, they are primarily a complication of mechanical ventilation and

TABLE 10-4
Risk Factors for Air Leaks in the Neonate

Prematurity
Need for delivery room resuscitation
High peak ventilating pressures
Meconium aspiration syndrome
Pulmonary hypoplasia
Surfactant deficiency
Positive pressure ventilation
Long inspiratory time
Pneumonia

the underlying lung pathology that leads to the need for ventilatory assistance. **Table 10-4** outlines the common risk factors associated with air leaks in preterm and term infants.

The primary risk factor for pulmonary air leaks among preterm infants is surfactant deficiency, which results in a poorly compliant lung. Subsequently, high pressure (either from mechanical ventilation or spontaneously produced) is needed to move air into the alveoli. The high pressure predisposes the neonatal airway to injury and subsequent pneumothorax. Infants who receive surfactant treatment for RDS experience rapid improvement in lung compliance upon receiving the treatment. When the same high ventilator pressures needed to ventilate an infant prior to surfactant are used, as pulmonary compliance changes, pneumothorax can occur.[134]

Preterm and term infants can aspirate foreign contents, such as blood, meconium, and amniotic fluid, into the lung, placing them at risk for pneumothorax.[134] Pulmonary hypoplasia associated with congenital diaphragmatic hernia or absence of amniotic fluid is also a predisposing factor. Finally, spontaneous pneumothorax is found in 1% to 2% of healthy term infants and is often asymptomatic. Risk factors are similar to those for pneumothorax, with the addition of direct trauma to the pharynx related to endotracheal intubation.

Pathophysiology

In the neonate, pulmonary air leak occurs when intra-alveolar pressure is high, resulting in alveolar over-distention and rupture of the alveoli. This can happen in the poorly compliant mechanically ventilated lung of a preterm infant or in a term infant who generates significant negative intrathoracic forces to initiate the first breaths immediately after birth. Free air can traverse from the ruptured alveolus along the pulmonary vasculature to the mediastinum and then subsequently to the pleura or pericardium.

There are times when an air leak is severe, such as with a tension pneumothorax. A tension pneumothorax, defined as an increase in intrathoracic pressure on the affected side, can cause the mediastinum to shift away from the affected side, thus displacing heart sounds and cardiac impulse. Additionally, tension pneumothorax can cause an abrupt decrease in cardiac output, which could manifest as a decrease in heart rate and blood pressure.

The primary predisposing factor for PIE is severe lung disease related to RDS. However, PIE can also be seen in the setting of other significant lung disease, such as meconium aspiration syndrome or sepsis. PIE can affect one or both lungs and can affect either the entire lung or a focal respiratory unit. As air accumulates within the interstitial space, lung compliance decreases further, thus further worsening ventilation.

Diagnosis

Transillumination can be performed to assist with the diagnosis of a pneumothorax. **Transillumination** is a noninvasive procedure in which a bright light probe is placed against the infant's chest wall near the axilla. A diffuse bright light illuminating the chest suggests the absence of underlying lung tissue, which is displaced by extrapleural air, suggesting that a pneumothorax is present (**Figure 10-5**). Transillumination is less reliable for large infants due to increased skin thickness or when the air leak is small.

A chest radiograph is most commonly used to determine the presence of pulmonary air leaks. This diagnostic tool allows for differentiation of pneumopericardium, pneumomediastinum, and pneumothorax. A pneumopericardium will classically show visible air crossing the midline on the diaphragmatic border of the heart while a pneumomediastinum appears as lucency on the lateral borders of the heart.

Chest radiographic findings of pneumothorax include hyper-lucency with absence of pulmonary tissue markings (**Figure 10-6**). Small cystic and/or linear lucencies in the affected lung fields are seen if PIE is present (**Figure 10-7**). Typically, an anterior-posterior (A-P)

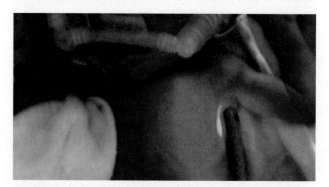

FIGURE 10-5 A small, focused light probe can be used to transilluminate the chest and assess for the presence of a pneumothorax. In this illustration, the chest glows, signifying the presence of free air in the pleural space.

Photo of Astodia courtesy of Futuremed.

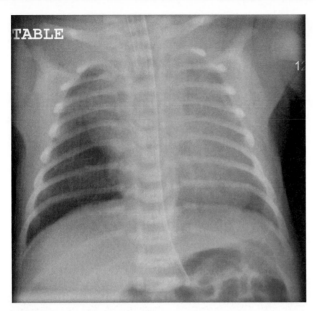

FIGURE 10-6 An A-P chest radiograph showing a pneumothorax.

Case courtesy of Dr. Angela Byrne, Radiopaedia.org, rID: 7589

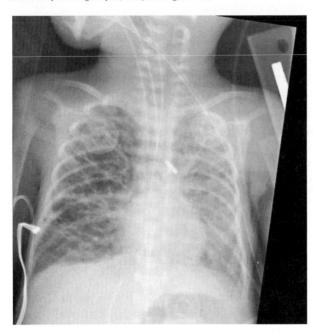

FIGURE 10-7 An A-P chest radiograph showing the cystic lesions characteristic of PIE.

Courtesy of Radswiki, Radiopaedia.org, rID: 11848.

chest radiograph is obtained. However, decubitus or cross-table lateral films can be obtained if the anterior-posterior radiographs do not allow for a definitive diagnosis. Using these diagnostic modalities, free air will be seen in the most superiorly positioned part of the chest.

Clinical Presentation

The size of the air leak often dictates both the clinical presentation and the medical management of the leak. Infants with small air leaks, occupying less than 10% of the affected lung, are typically asymptomatic.

Regardless of gestational age at birth, the primary symptoms of pneumothorax include respiratory distress and cyanosis. Less common symptoms include apnea and bradycardia. On physical exam, decreased breath sounds on the affected side would be expected. If large enough, the pneumothorax could cause an expansion of the affected side, with subsequent increase in the anterior-posterior diameter of the chest. A tension pneumothorax will cause the mediastinum to shift away from the affected side and to displace both heart sounds and the cardiac impulse. A neonate or infant presenting with a tension pneumothorax will have a sudden decrease in cardiac output, which often manifests as bradycardia and hypotension.

Pericardial tamponade occurs secondary to pneumopericardium and typically presents with a decrease in pulses, decrease in blood pressure, and poor peripheral perfusion. On auscultation, heart sounds may sound muffled or distant.

Management

If the infant is asymptomatic, spontaneous resolution of the air leak is anticipated. Typically, management is supportive and includes providing care in a neutral thermal environment, nutritional support, and respiratory care as needed. Small air leaks will often resolve in 24 to 48 hours.

Peak inspiratory and end-expiratory pressures should be decreased to provide tidal volumes within lung-protective strategy ranges when ventilating an infant with a pulmonary air leak. Lowering the set inspiratory time will help reduce mean airway pressure and may aid in patient-ventilator synchrony.

If hemodynamic or respiratory instability is present, action must be taken to remove the extrapleural air. If the infant is symptomatic, needle aspiration, preferably under ultrasound guidance, can be performed to relieve pressure within the pericardium or from the pleural space and allow for return of appropriate cardiac function. Needle aspiration can be effective if the air leak is not ongoing. For continuous air leaks, a chest tube should be placed for continuous removal of accumulated air.

Ventilator management of PIE aligns with lung-protective strategies, decreasing ventilating pressures (peak inspiratory pressure, mean airway pressure) as tolerated. Additionally, high-flow oscillatory ventilation has shown some benefit over conventional ventilation in allowing the injured lung to heal.[135–137]

Complications and Outcomes

Infants with small pulmonary air leaks that resolve spontaneously rarely have an associated morbidity. If untreated, infants with air leaks who are symptomatic may have profound cardiodysfunction, which can cause hypoxia, hypercarbia, and hypotension and lead to cardiopulmonary collapse.

PIE may resolve quickly, within several days of being identified, in some patients. However, in some infants, PIE will persist and contribute to the development of BPD.

Case Study 1

A male premature infant was born by caesarean section at 27 weeks' gestation with a birth weight of 1100 grams. His Apgar scores were 1 at 1 minute and 6 at 5 minutes. After transfer to the NICU on CPAP 6 cm H2O and an FIO2 of 0.40, the patient's respiratory status deteriorated. He was intubated and received mechanical ventilatory respiratory support for 5 weeks for RDS. His first opthalmic examination revealed bilateral changes consistant with Grade 2 ROP. CryoROP criteria, treatment was performed at a corrected gestational age.

The infant responded well to the treatment, and both eyes showed rapid regression of the abnormal vessels.

1. **What are the main risks factors of developing ROP?**

2. **What classification system is used to describe the extent of ROP?**

3. **How many zones are used to define the area of retina covered by physiologic retinal vascularization?**

Case Study 2

A 37-year-old woman with no medical history presented to the hospital at 26 weeks and 3 days of gestation with preterm labor. Her blood pressure was 126/74 mm Hg and her heart rate (HR) was 91 beats per minute. Ultrasound sonography showed the fetus with a breech presentation, a weight of approximately 900 grams, and an HR of 150 beats per minute. The neonate was 830 grams at birth, a female with no abnormalities. The infant was limp with an HR of 80 beats per minute and an SpO_2 of 77% with no breathing effort. The 1-minute Apgar score was 1. Positive pressure ventilation by mask was delivered using a T-piece resuscitator. Peak inspiratory pressure (PIP) was 20 cmH_2O and positive end-expiratory pressure (PEEP) was 4 cmH_2O. SpO_2 continued to fall to 50%, HR was 70 beats per minute, and soft tissue swelling in the right supraclavicular area was observed. The patient was intubated with a 2.5 uncuffed orotracheal tube. However, the neonate's SpO_2 was maintained at 50% even following intubation. On physical examination, worsening of soft tissue swelling in the right neck, axillary, and supraclavicular areas was found

and crepitus was palpable. Abdominal distension and severe cyanosis were observed concurrently. A chest radiograph confirmed the presence of pulmonary air leaks. A needle thoracentesis was performed to treat a right-sided tension pneumothorax. Fifty mL of air was aspirated in the intercostal space of the midclavicular line using a 22-gauge angiocatheter. Following air aspiration, ventilation was achieved for both lungs with the use of the Burnell Jet Ventilator, and the loss of edema in the neck area and reduction of subcutaneous emphysema were observed. The neonate's SpO_2 gradually rose to mid 80s and HR was maintained at 170 beats per minute. The neonate was transferred to the neonatal intensive care unit, where high-frequency jet ventilation was continued.

1. **What are the risk factors for air leaks in the neonate?**

2. **What noninvasive procedure uses a bright light probe placed against the infant's chest wall to diagnose a pneumothorax?**

3. **Name the two techniques for treating air leaks.**

References

1. Fleck BW, McIntosh N. Retinopathy of prematurity: recent developments. *Neoreviews.* 2009;10(1):e20-e29.
2. Penn JS, Henry MM, Tolman BL. Exposure to alternating hypoxia and hyperoxia causes severe proliferative retinopathy in the newborn rat. *Pediatr Res.* 1994;36:724-731.
3. Cryotherapy for Retinopathy of Prematurity Cooperative Group, multicenter trial of cryotherapy for retinopathy of prematurity: three-month outcome. *Arch Ophthalmol.* 1990;108:195-204.
4. Kinsey VE, Jacobus JT, Hemphill FM. Retrolental fibroplasia: cooperative study of retrolental fibroplasia and the use of oxygen. *Arch Ophthalmol.* 1956;56:481-457.
5. Martin RJ, Fanaroff AA, Walsh MC, eds. *Neonatal-Perinatal Medicine, Disease of the Fetus and Infant.* 9th ed. St. Louis, MO: Elsevier Mosby; 2011.
6. Hartnett ME, Penn JS. Mechanisms and management of retinopathy of prematurity. *N Eng J Med.* 2012;367:2515-2526.
7. Phelps DL. Retinopathy of prematurity: history, classification, and pathophysiology. *NeoReviews.* 2001;2(7):e153-e166.
8. International Committee for the Classification of Retinopathy of Prematurity. The International Classification of Retinopathy of Prematurity revisited. *Archs Ophthalmol.* 2005;123:991-999.
9. American Academy of Pediatrics Policy Statement. Screening examination of premature infants for retinopathy of prematurity. *Pediatrics.* 2013;131:189-195.

10. Mintz-Hittner HA, Kennedy KA, Chuang AZ. Efficacy of intravitreal bevacizumab for stage 3+ retinopathy of prematurity. *N Eng J Med.* 2011;364(7):603-615.

11. Hu J, Blair MP, Shapiro MJ, Lichtenstein SJ, Galasso JM, Kapur R. Reactivation of retinopathy of prematurity after bevacizumab injection. *Arch Ophthalmol.* 2012;130(8):1000-1006.

12. Schaffer DB, Quinn GE, Johnson L. Sequelae of arrested mild retinopathy of prematurity. *Arch Ophthalmol.* 1984;102(3):373-376.

13. Quinn GE, Dobson V, Kivlin J, et al. Prevalence of myopia between 3 months and 5 ½ years in preterm infants with and without retinopathy of prematurity. *Ophthalmology.* 1998;105(7):1292-1300.

14. Harder BC, Schlichtenbrede FC, von Baltz S, Jendritza W, Jonas JB. Intravitreal bevacizumab for retinopathy of prematurity: refractive error results. *Am J Ophthalmol.* 2013;155(6):1119-1124.

15. Hwang CK, Hubbard GB, Hutchinson AK, Lambert SR. Outcomes after intravitreal bevacizumab versus laser photocoagulation for retinopathy of prematurity: a 5-year retrospective analysis. *Ophthalmology.* 2015;122(5):1008-1015.

16. SUPPORT Study Group of the Eunice Kennedy Shriver NICHD Neonatal Research Network, Carlo WA, Finer NN, et al. Target ranges of oxygen saturation in extremely preterm infants. *N Eng J Med.* 2010;362(21):1959-1969.

17. The BOOST II United Kingdom, Australia, and New Zealand Collaborative Groups. Oxygen saturation and outcomes in preterm infants. *N Eng J Med.* 2013;368:2094-2104.

18. Northway WH Jr., Rosan RC, Porter DY. Pulmonary disease following respirator therapy of hyaline-membrane disease. Bronchopulmonary dysplasia. *N Eng J Med.* 1967;276(7):357-368.

19. Van Marter LJ, Allred EN, Pagano M, et al. Do clinical markers of barotrauma and oxygen toxicity explain interhospital variation in rates of chronic lung disease? The Neonatology Committee for the Developmental Network. *Pediatrics.* 2000;105(6):1194-1201.

20. Albertine KH, Jones GP, Starcher BC, et al. Chronic lung injury in preterm lambs. Disordered respiratory tract development. *Am J Resp Crit Care Med.* 1999;159(3):945-958.

21. Cherukupalli K, Larson JE, Rotschild A, Thurlbeck WM. Biochemical, clinical, and morphologic studies on lungs of infants with bronchopulmonary dysplasia. *Pediatr Pulmonol.* 1996;22(4):215-229.

22. Dreyfuss D, Saumon G. Ventilator-induced lung injury: lessons from experimental studies. *Am J Resp Crit Care Med.* 1998;157(1):294-323.

23. Attar MA, Donn SM. Mechanisms of ventilator-induced lung injury in premature infants. *Semin Neonatol.* 2002;7(5):353-360.

24. Hernandez LA, Peevy KJ, Moise AA, Parker JC. Chest wall restriction limits high airway pressure-induced lung injury in young rabbits. *J Appl Physiol.* 1989;66(5):2364-2368.

25. Bjorklund LJ, Ingimarsson J, Curstedt T, et al. Manual ventilation with a few large breaths at birth compromises the therapeutic effect of subsequent surfactant replacement in immature lambs. *Pediatr Res.* 1997;42(3):348-355.

26. Wada K, Jobe AH, Ikegami M. Tidal volume effects on surfactant treatment responses with the initiation of ventilation in preterm lambs. *J Appl Physiol.* 1997;83(4):1054-1061.

27. Michna J, Jobe AH, Ikegami M. Positive end-expiratory pressure preserves surfactant function in preterm lambs. *Am J Resp Crit Care Med.* 1999;160(2):634-639.

28. Yoon BH, Romero R, Kim KS, et al. A systemic fetal inflammatory response and the development of bronchopulmonary dysplasia. *Am J Obsetr Gynecol.* 1999;181(4):773-779.

29. Edwards DK, Dyer WM, Northway WH Jr. Twelve years' experience with bronchopulmonary dysplasia. *Pediatrics.* 1977;59(6):839-846.

30. Philip AG. Oxygen plus pressure plus time: the etiology of bronchopulmonary dysplasia. *Pediatrics.* 1975;55(1):44-50.

31. Pusey VA, Macpherson RI, Chernick V. Pulmonary fibroplasia following prolonged artificial ventilation of newborn infants. *Can Med Assoc J.* 1969;100(10):451-457.

32. Varsila E, Pesonen E, Andersson S. Early protein oxidation in the neonatal lung is related to development of chronic lung disease. *Acta paediatrica.* 1995;84(11):1296-1299.

33. Frank L, Sosenko IR. Failure of premature rabbits to increase antioxidant enzymes during hyperoxic exposure: increased susceptibility to pulmonary oxygen toxicity compared with term rabbits. *Pediatr Res.* 1991;29(3):292-296.

34. Network SSGotEKSNNR, Carlo WA, Finer NN, et al. Target ranges of oxygen saturation in extremely preterm infants. *N Eng J Med.* 2010;362(21):1959-1969.

35. Supplemental Therapeutic Oxygen for Prethreshold Retinopathy Of Prematurity (STOP-ROP), a randomized, controlled trial. I: primary outcomes. *Pediatrics.* 2000;105(2):295-310.

36. Yoon BH, Romero R, Yang SH, et al. Interleukin-6 concentrations in umbilical cord plasma are elevated in neonates with white matter lesions associated with periventricular leukomalacia. *Am J Obsetr Gynecol.* 1996;174(5):1433-1440.

37. Romero R, Mazor M, Wu YK, et al. Infection in the pathogenesis of preterm labor. *Semin Perinatol.* 1988;12(4):262-279.

38. Gomez R, Romero R, Ghezzi F, Yoon BH, Mazor M, Berry SM. The fetal inflammatory response syndrome. *Am J Obsetr Gynecol.* 1998;179(1):194-202.

39. Watterberg KL, Demers LM, Scott SM, Murphy S. Chorioamnionitis and early lung inflammation in infants in whom bronchopulmonary dysplasia develops. *Pediatrics.* 1996;97(2):210-215.

40. Hitti J, Tarczy-Hornoch P, Murphy J, Hillier SL, Aura J, Eschenbach DA. Amniotic fluid infection, cytokines, and adverse outcome among infants at 34 weeks' gestation or less. *Obsetr Gynecol.* 2001;98(6):1080-1088.

41. Yoon BH, Romero R, Jun JK, et al. Amniotic fluid cytokines (interleukin-6, tumor necrosis factor-alpha, interleukin-1 beta, and interleukin-8) and the risk for the development of bronchopulmonary dysplasia. *Am J Obsetr Gynecol.* 1997;177(4):825-830.

42. Groneck P, Gotze-Speer B, Oppermann M, Eiffert H, Speer CP. Association of pulmonary inflammation and increased microvascular permeability during the development of bronchopulmonary dysplasia: a sequential analysis of inflammatory mediators in respiratory fluids of high-risk preterm neonates. *Pediatrics.* 1994;93(5):712-718.

43. Rojas MA, Gonzalez A, Bancalari E, Claure N, Poole C, Silva-Neto G. Changing trends in the epidemiology and pathogenesis of neonatal chronic lung disease. *J Pediatr.* 1995;126(4):605-610.

44. Marshall DD, Kotelchuck M, Young TE, Bose CL, Kruyer L, O'Shea TM. Risk factors for chronic lung disease in the surfactant era: a North Carolina population-based study of very low birth weight infants. North Carolina Neonatologists Association. *Pediatrics.* 1999;104(6):1345-1350.

45. Bose CL, Laughon MM. Patent ductus arteriosus: lack of evidence for common treatments. *Arch Disease Child Fetal Neonatal Ed.* 2007;92(6):F498-F502.

46. Hartnoll G, Betremieux P, Modi N. Randomised controlled trial of postnatal sodium supplementation on body composition in 25 to 30 week gestational age infants. *Arch Disease Child Fetal Neonatal Ed.* 2000;82(1):F24-F28.

47. Hartnoll G, Betremieux P, Modi N. Randomised controlled trial of postnatal sodium supplementation on oxygen dependency and body weight in 25-30 week gestational age infants. *Arch Disease Child Fetal Neonatal Ed.* 2000;82(1):F19-F23.

48. Van Marter LJ, Leviton A, Allred EN, Pagano M, Kuban KC. Hydration during the first days of life and the risk of bronchopulmonary dysplasia in low birth weight infants. *J Pediatr.* 1990;116(6):942-949.

49. Costarino AT Jr., Gruskay JA, Corcoran L, Polin RA, Baumgart S. Sodium restriction versus daily maintenance replacement in very low birth weight premature neonates: a randomized, blind therapeutic trial. *J Pediatr.* 1992;120(1):99-106.

50. Bell EF, Acarregui MJ. Restricted versus liberal water intake for preventing morbidity and mortality in preterm infants. *Cochrane Database Syst Rev.* 2014;12:CD000503.

51. Frank L, Sosenko IR. Undernutrition as a major contributing factor in the pathogenesis of bronchopulmonary dysplasia. *Amer Rev Resp Dis.* 1988;138(3):725-729.

52. Wilson DC, McClure G, Halliday HL, Reid MM, Dodge JA. Nutrition and bronchopulmonary dysplasia. *Arch Disease Child.* 1991;66 (1 Spec No):37-38.

53. Shenai JP, Chytil F, Jhaveri A, Stahlman MT. Plasma vitamin A and retinol-binding protein in premature and term neonates. *J Pediatr.* 1981;99(2):302-305.

54. Bauer JM, Verlaan S, Bautmans I, et al. Effects of a vitamin D and leucine-enriched whey protein nutritional supplement on measures of sarcopenia in older adults, the PROVIDE study: a randomized, double-blind, placebo-controlled trial. *J Am Med Dir Assoc.* 2015;16(9):740-747.

55. Shenai JP. Vitamin A supplementation in very low birth weight neonates: rationale and evidence. *Pediatrics.* 1999;104(6):1369-1374.

56. Hustead VA, Gutcher GR, Anderson SA, Zachman RD. Relationship of vitamin A (retinol) status to lung disease in the preterm infant. *J Pediatr.* 1984;105(4):610-615.

57. Carlton DP, Albertine KH, Cho SC, Lont M, Bland RD. Role of neutrophils in lung vascular injury and edema after premature birth in lambs. *J Appl Physiol.* 1997;83(4):1307-1317.

58. D'Angio CT, LoMonaco MB, Chaudhry SA, Paxhia A, Ryan RM. Discordant pulmonary proinflammatory cytokine expression during acute hyperoxia in the newborn rabbit. *Exp Lung Res.* 1999;25(5):443-465.

59. Ogden BE, Murphy SA, Saunders GC, Pathak D, Johnson JD. Neonatal lung neutrophils and elastase/proteinase inhibitor imbalance. *Amer Rev Resp Dis.* 1984;130(5):817-821.

60. D'Angio CT, Basavegowda K, Avissar NE, Finkelstein JN, Sinkin RA. Comparison of tracheal aspirate and bronchoalveolar lavage specimens from premature infants. *Biol Neonate.* 2002;82(3): 145-149.

61. Hitti J, Krohn MA, Patton DL, et al. Amniotic fluid tumor necrosis factor-alpha and the risk of respiratory distress syndrome among preterm infants. *Am J Obsetr Gynecol.* 1997;177(1):50-56.

62. Watterberg KL, Carmichael DF, Gerdes JS, Werner S, Backstrom C, Murphy S. Secretory leukocyte protease inhibitor and lung inflammation in developing bronchopulmonary dysplasia. *J Pediatr.* 1994;125(2):264-269.

63. Pierce RA, Albertine KH, Starcher BC, Bohnsack JF, Carlton DP, Bland RD. Chronic lung injury in preterm lambs: disordered pulmonary elastin deposition. *Am J Physiol.* 1997;272(3 Pt 1):L452-L460.

64. Hardie WD, Bruno MD, Huelsman KM, et al. Postnatal lung function and morphology in transgenic mice expressing transforming growth factor-alpha. *Am J Pathol.* 1997;151(4):1075-1083.

65. Jobe AH, Bancalari E. Bronchopulmonary dysplasia. *Am J Resp Crit Care Med.* 2001;163(7):1723-1729.

66. Zhou L, Dey CR, Wert SE, Whitsett JA. Arrested lung morphogenesis in transgenic mice bearing an SP-C-TGF-beta 1 chimeric gene. *Development Biol.* 1996;175(2):227-238.

67. Lecart C, Cayabyab R, Buckley S, et al. Bioactive transforming growth factor-beta in the lungs of extremely low birthweight neonates predicts the need for home oxygen supplementation. *Biol Neonate.* 2000;77(4):217-223.

68. Kotecha S, Wangoo A, Silverman M, Shaw RJ. Increase in the concentration of transforming growth factor beta-1 in bronchoalveolar lavage fluid before development of chronic lung disease of prematurity. *J Pediatr.* 1996;128(4):464-469.

69. Madtes DK, Elston AL, Hackman RC, Dunn AR, Clark JG. Transforming growth factor-alpha deficiency reduces pulmonary fibrosis in transgenic mice. *Am J Respir Cell Mol Biol.* 1999;20(5):924-934.

70. Jobe AJ. The new BPD: an arrest of lung development. *Pediatr Res.* 1999;46(6):641-643.

71. Husain AN, Siddiqui NH, Stocker JT. Pathology of arrested acinar development in postsurfactant bronchopulmonary dysplasia. *Human Pathol.* 1998;29(7):710-717.

72. Thibeault DW, Mabry SM, Ekekezie II, Truog WE. Lung elastic tissue maturation and perturbations during the evolution of chronic lung disease. *Pediatrics.* 2000;106(6):1452-1459.

73. Ballard PL. Scientific rationale for the use of antenatal glucocorticoids to promote fetal development. *Pediatr Rev.* 2000;1(5):E83-E90.

74. Massaro GD, Massaro D. Formation of pulmonary alveoli and gas-exchange surface area: quantitation and regulation. *Ann Rev Physiol.* 1996;58:73-92.

75. Massaro GD, Massaro D. Retinoic acid treatment partially rescues failed septation in rats and in mice. *Am J Physiol Lung Cell Mol Physiol.* 2000;278(5):L955-L960.

76. Bhatt AJ, Pryhuber GS, Huyck H, Watkins RH, Metlay LA, Maniscalco WM. Disrupted pulmonary vasculature and decreased vascular endothelial growth factor, Flt-1, and TIE-2 in human infants dying with bronchopulmonary dysplasia. *Am J Resp Crit Care Med.* 2001;164(10 Pt 1):1971-1980.

77. Coalson JJ. Experimental models of bronchopulmonary dysplasia. *Biol Neonate.* 1997;71(Suppl 1):35-38.

78. D'Angio CT, Maniscalco WM. The role of vascular growth factors in hyperoxia-induced injury to the developing lung. *Front Biosci.* 2002;7:d1609-d1623.

79. Maniscalco WM, Watkins RH, Pryhuber GS, Bhatt A, Shea C, Huyck H. Angiogenic factors and alveolar vasculature: development and alterations by injury in very premature baboons. *Am J Physiol Lung Cell Mol Physiol.* 2002;282(4):L811-L823.

80. Lassus P, Turanlahti M, Heikkila P, et al. Pulmonary vascular endothelial growth factor and Flt-1 in fetuses, in acute and chronic lung disease, and in persistent pulmonary hypertension of the newborn. *Am J Resp Crit Care Med.* 2001;164(10 Pt 1):1981-1987.

81. Jakkula M, Le Cras TD, Gebb S, et al. Inhibition of angiogenesis decreases alveolarization in the developing rat lung. *Am J Physiol Lung Cell Mol Physiol.* 2000;279(3):L600-L607.

82. Allen J, Zwerdling R, Ehrenkranz R, et al. Statement on the care of the child with chronic lung disease of infancy and childhood. *Am J Resp Crit Care Med.* 2003;168(3):356-396.

83. Bancalari E, Claure N. Definitions and diagnostic criteria for bronchopulmonary dysplasia. *Semin Perinatol.* 2006;30(4):164-170.

84. Meis PJ, Klebanoff M, Thom E, et al. Prevention of recurrent preterm delivery by 17 alpha-hydroxyprogesterone caproate. *N Eng J Med.* 2003;348(24):2379-2385.

85. Osterman MJ, Kochanek KD, MacDorman MF, Strobino DM, Guyer B. Annual summary of vital statistics: 2012-2013. *Pediatrics.* 2015;135(6):1115-1125.

86. Antenatal corticosteroids revisited: repeat courses. *NIH Consens Statement.* 2000;17(2):1-18.

87. Roberts D, Dalziel S. Antenatal corticosteroids for accelerating fetal lung maturation for women at risk of preterm birth. *Cochrane Database Syst Rev.* 2006;3:CD004454.

88. Banks BA, Cnaan A, Morgan MA, et al. Multiple courses of antenatal corticosteroids and outcome of premature neonates. North American Thyrotropin-Releasing Hormone Study Group. *Am J Obsetr Gynecol.* 1999;181(3):709-717.

89. Bolt RJ, van Weissenbruch MM, Lafeber HN, Delemarre-van de Waal HA. Glucocorticoids and lung development in the fetus and preterm infant. *Pediatr Pulmonol.* 2001;32(1):76-91.

90. Soll RF, Morley CJ. Prophylactic versus selective use of surfactant for preventing morbidity and mortality in preterm infants. *Cochrane Database Syst Rev.* 2000;2:CD000510.

91. Soll RF. Prophylactic synthetic surfactant for preventing morbidity and mortality in preterm infants. *Cochrane Database Syst Rev.* 2000;2:CD001079.

92. Soll RF. Prophylactic natural surfactant extract for preventing morbidity and mortality in preterm infants. *Cochrane Database Syst Rev.* 2000;2:CD000511.

93. Stevens TP, Harrington EW, Blennow M, Soll RF. Early surfactant administration with brief ventilation vs. selective surfactant and continued mechanical ventilation for preterm infants with or at risk for respiratory distress syndrome. *Cochrane Database Syst Rev.* 2007;4:CD003063.

94. Merrill JD, Ballard RA, Cnaan A, et al. Dysfunction of pulmonary surfactant in chronically ventilated premature infants. *Pediatr Res.* 2004;56(6):918-926.

95. Laughon M, Bose C, Moya F, et al. A pilot randomized, controlled trial of later treatment with a peptide-containing, synthetic surfactant

for the prevention of bronchopulmonary dysplasia. *Pediatrics.* 2009;123(1):89-96.

96. Schmidt B. Methylxanthine therapy for apnea of prematurity: evaluation of treatment benefits and risks at age 5 years in the international Caffeine for Apnea of Prematurity (CAP) trial. *Biol Neonate.* 2005;88(3):208-213.

97. Bancalari E. Corticosteroids and neonatal chronic lung disease. *Eur J Pediatr.* 1998;157(Suppl 1):S31-S37.

98. Cummings JJ, D'Eugenio DB, Gross SJ. A controlled trial of dexamethasone in preterm infants at high risk for bronchopulmonary dysplasia. *N Eng J Med.* 1989;320(23):1505-1510.

99. Committee on F, Newborn. Postnatal corticosteroids to treat or prevent chronic lung disease in preterm infants. *Pediatrics.* 2002;109(2):330-338.

100. Doyle LW, Ehrenkranz RA, Halliday HL. Early (<8 days) postnatal corticosteroids for preventing chronic lung disease in preterm infants. *Cochrane Database Syst Rev.* 2014;5:CD001146.

101. Doyle LW, Ehrenkranz RA, Halliday HL. Late (>7 days) postnatal corticosteroids for chronic lung disease in preterm infants. *Cochrane Database Syst Rev.* 2014;5:CD001145.

102. Doyle LW, Davis PG, Morley CJ, McPhee A, Carlin JB, DART Study Investigators. Outcome at 2 years of age of infants from the DART study: a multicenter, international, randomized, controlled trial of low-dose dexamethasone. *Pediatrics.* 2007;119(4):716-721.

103. Doyle LW, Davis PG, Morley CJ, McPhee A, Carlin JB, DART Study Investigators. Low-dose dexamethasone facilitates extubation among chronically ventilator-dependent infants: a multicenter, international, randomized, controlled trial. *Pediatrics.* 2006;117(1):75-83.

104. Doyle LW, Halliday HL, Ehrenkranz RA, Davis PG, Sinclair JC. An update on the impact of postnatal systemic corticosteroids on mortality and cerebral palsy in preterm infants: effect modification by risk of bronchopulmonary dysplasia. *J Pediatr.* 2014;165(6):1258-1260.

105. Shah VS, Ohlsson A, Halliday HL, Dunn M. Early administration of inhaled corticosteroids for preventing chronic lung disease in ventilated very low birth weight preterm neonates. *Cochrane Database Syst Rev.* 2012;5:CD001969.

106. Kinsella JP, Ivy DD, Abman SH. Inhaled nitric oxide improves gas exchange and lowers pulmonary vascular resistance in severe experimental hyaline membrane disease. *Pediatr Res.* 1994;36(3):402-408.

107. McCurnin DC, Pierce RA, Chang LY, et al. Inhaled NO improves early pulmonary function and modifies lung growth and elastin deposition in a baboon model of neonatal chronic lung disease. *Am J Physiol Lung Cell Mol Physiol.* 2005;288(3):L450-L459.

108. Cole FS, Alleyne C, Barks JD, et al. NIH Consensus Development Conference statement: inhaled nitric-oxide therapy for premature infants. *Pediatrics.* 2011;127(2):363-369.

109. Veness-Meehan KA. Effects of retinol deficiency and hyperoxia on collagen gene expression in rat lung. *Exp Lung Res.* 1997;23(6):569-581.

110. Kennedy KA. Epidemiology of acute and chronic lung injury. *Semin Perinatol.* 1993;17(4):247-252.

111. Darlow BA, Graham PJ. Vitamin A supplementation to prevent mortality and short- and long-term morbidity in very low birth-weight infants. *Cochrane Database Syst Rev.* 2011;10:CD000501.

112. McCann EM, Lewis K, Deming DD, Donovan MJ, Brady JP. Controlled trial of furosemide therapy in infants with chronic lung disease. *J Pediatr.* 1985;106(6):957-962.

113. Kao LC, Warburton D, Sargent CW, Platzker AC, Keens TG. Furosemide acutely decreases airways resistance in chronic bronchopulmonary dysplasia. *J Pediatr.* 1983;103(4):624-629.

114. Ng G, da Silva O, Ohlsson A. Bronchodilators for the prevention and treatment of chronic lung disease in preterm infants. *Cochrane Database Syst Rev.* 2012;6:CD003214.

115. Hagen EW, Sadek-Badawi M, Carlton DP, Palta M. Permissive hypercapnia and risk for brain injury and developmental impairment. *Pediatrics.* 2008;122(3):e583-e589.

116. Thome UH, Carroll W, Wu TJ, et al. Outcome of extremely preterm infants randomized at birth to different PaCO2 targets during the first seven days of life. *Biol Neonate.* 2006;90(4):218-225.

117. Morley CJ, Davis PG, Doyle LW, et al. Nasal CPAP or intubation at birth for very preterm infants. *N Eng J Med.* 2008;358(7):700-708.

118. Dunn MS, Kaempf J, de Klerk A, et al. Randomized trial comparing 3 approaches to the initial respiratory management of preterm neonates. *Pediatrics.* 2011;128(5):e1069-e1076.

119. Sandri F, Plavka R, Ancora G, et al. Prophylactic or early selective surfactant combined with nCPAP in very preterm infants. *Pediatrics.* 2010;125(6):e1402-e1409.

120. Meneses J, Bhandari V, Alves JG. Nasal intermittent positive-pressure ventilation vs nasal continuous positive airway pressure for preterm infants with respiratory distress syndrome: a systematic review and meta-analysis. *Arch Pediatr Adolesc Med.* 2012;166(4):372-376.

121. Collaco JM, Romer LH, Stuart BD, et al. Frontiers in pulmonary hypertension in infants and children with bronchopulmonary dysplasia. *Pediatr Pulmonol.* 2012;47(11):1042-1053.

122. Bhat R, Salas AA, Foster C, Carlo WA, Ambalavanan N. Prospective analysis of pulmonary hypertension in extremely low birth weight infants. *Pediatrics.* 2012;129(3):e682-e689.

123. An HS, Bae EJ, Kim GB, et al. Pulmonary hypertension in preterm infants with bronchopulmonary dysplasia. *Korean Circ J.* 2010;40(3):131-136.

124. Khemani E, McElhinney DB, Rhein L, et al. Pulmonary artery hypertension in formerly premature infants with bronchopulmonary dysplasia: clinical features and outcomes in the surfactant era. *Pediatrics.* 2007;120(6):1260-1269.

125. Kim DH, Kim HS, Choi CW, Kim EK, Kim BI, Choi JH. Risk factors for pulmonary artery hypertension in preterm infants with moderate or severe bronchopulmonary dysplasia. *Neonatology.* 2012;101(1):40-46.

126. Fawke J, Lum S, Kirkby J, et al. Lung function and respiratory symptoms at 11 years in children born extremely preterm: the EPICure study. *Am J Resp Crit Care Med.* 2010;182(2):237-245.

127. Doyle LW, Ford G, Davis N. Health and hospitalistions after discharge in extremely low birth weight infants. *Semin Perinatol.* 2003; 8(2):137-145.

128. Bhandari A, Panitch HB. Pulmonary outcomes in bronchopulmonary dysplasia. *Semin Perinatol.* 2006;30(4):219-226.

129. Greenough A, Alexander J, Boit P, et al. School age outcome of hospitalisation with respiratory syncytial virus infection of prematurely born infants. *Thorax.* 2009;64(6):490-495.

130. Andabaka T, Nickerson JW, Rojas-Reyes MX, Rueda JD, Bacic Vrca V, Barsic B. Monoclonal antibody for reducing the risk of respiratory syncytial virus infection in children. *Cochrane Database Syst Rev.* 2013;4:CD006602.

131. Chidekel AS, Rosen CL, Bazzy AR. Rhinovirus infection associated with serious lower respiratory illness in patients with bronchopulmonary dysplasia. *Pediatr Infect Dis J.* 1997;16(1):43-47.

132. Greenough A, Bhojnagarwala B. Causes and management of pulmonary air leaks. *Paediatr Child Health.* 2012;22(12):523-527.

133. Jones RM, Rutter N, Cooper AC, Pullan CR. Pneumothorax in the neonatal period. *Anaesthesia.* 1983;38(10):948-952.

134. Cagle KJ. Pneumomediastinum in the neonate. *Neonatal Netw.* 2014;33(5):275-282.

135. Suresh P, Tagare A, Kadam S, Vaidya U, Pandit A. Spontaneous pneumopericardium in a healthy full-term neonate. *Indian J Pediatr.* 2011;78(11):1410-1411.

136. Ramesh Bhat Y, Ramdas V. Predisposing factors, incidence and mortality of pneumothorax in neonates. *Minerva Pediatr.* 2013;65(4): 383-388.

137. Squires KA, De Paoli AG, Williams C, Dargaville PA. High-frequency oscillatory ventilation with low oscillatory frequency in pulmonary interstitial emphysema. *Neonatology.* 2013;104(4):243-249.

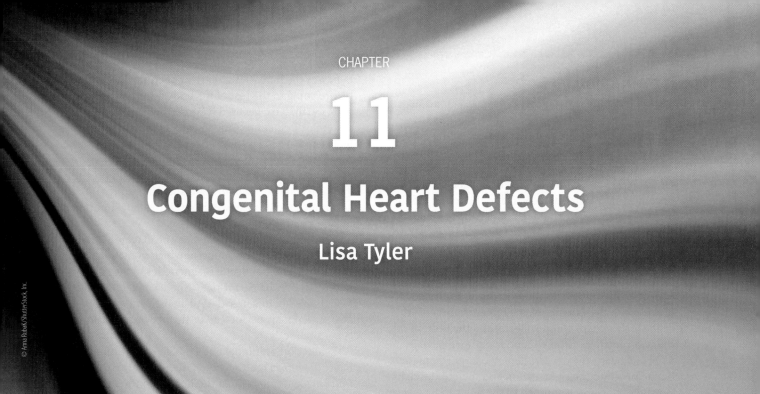

11

Congenital Heart Defects

Lisa Tyler

OUTLINE

OBJECTIVES

1. Provide a general overview of normal cardiac function in children.
2. Discuss acyanotic heart disease versus cyanotic heart disease.
3. Identify and describe acyanotic heart defects with left-to-right shunts.
4. Identify and describe acyanotic heart defects with left ventricular outflow tract obstruction.
5. Identify and describe cyanotic heart defects with decreased pulmonary blood flow.
6. Identify and describe cyanotic heart defects with increased pulmonary blood flow.
7. Identify and describe a single ventricle lesion.
8. Discuss diagnostic intervention and cardiovascular management and outcomes-based data for each defect.
9. Discuss the use of prostaglandins and other specialty gases in this patient population.

KEY TERMS

afterload
aortic stenosis
atrial septal defect (ASD)
atrioventricular canal
    (AVC) defect
cardiomegaly
coarctation of the aorta
cyanotic
Ebstein's anomaly
failure to thrive
foramen ovale
hypoplastic left heart
    syndrome (HLHS)
inhaled carbon dioxide
left ventricular outflow
    tract obstruction
ligation

nitric oxide (NO)
patent ductus
    arteriosus (PDA)
prostaglandin
pulmonary atresia
pulmonary stenosis (PS)
total anomalous pulmonary
    venous return (TAPVR)
transposition of the
    great arteries (TGA)
tricuspid atresia
truncus arteriosus
valvuloplasty
valvulotomy
ventricular septal
    defect (VSD)

Introduction

Congenital cardiac defects are structural abnormalities of the heart, heart valves, or heart vessels that occur during fetal development. They are one of the most common birth defects, accounting for approximately 40,000 births per year, or about 8 in every 1000 births.[1] Of these, 25% are considered a critical defect.[1] Causes of congenital cardiac defects include genetics, medications, drug use, or viral infections during the first trimester of pregnancy.[2] The defects can be minor or severe, may or may not cause symptoms, and may or may not require treatment.

The normal heart has two sides, right and left, separated by an inner wall called a septum. Each side is divided into two chambers; the upper chambers are called atria (where blood collects) and the bottom are the two ventricles (where blood is pumped out). In a normal heart, the oxygen-depleted blood from the body flows into the right atrium and then to the right ventricle, where it is pumped to the lungs to be oxygenated. Oxygen-enriched blood flows into the left atrium, and then to the left ventricle, where it is pumped out to the body through the ascending and descending aorta. There are four valves that control blood flow through the heart (Table 11-1). These valves are like doors that open to allow blood to flow through and then shut to keep blood from flowing backward.

Classification of Congenital Heart Disease: Acyanotic versus Cyanotic Heart Disease

Congenital cardiac defects can be broken down into two general classifications: acyanotic and cyanotic. **Cyanotic** cardiac defects get their name from the bluish appearance of the skin associated with people who have those defects. This occurs because blood either completely bypasses the lungs—therefore not getting oxygenated—before going to the rest of the body or oxygenated blood mixes with deoxygenated blood and goes out into the systemic circulation. Patients with cyanotic cardiac defects will have lower-than-normal oxygen saturations.[3] Acyanotic cardiac disease does not result in lower oxygen saturations but could result in high blood pressure and heart failure.[4] Left-to-right shunting is present in acyanotic cardiac disease while right-to-left shunting is present in cyanotic cardiac disease.[3,4]

Congenital cardiac defects may be detected during routine fetal ultrasounds, at which point a fetal echocardiogram or a fetal magnetic resonance imaging (MRI) may be performed.[5] Some congenital heart defects are not diagnosed until a postnatal pulse oximeter screening is performed or the newborn becomes symptomatic.[6]

Evaluation of infants and children with congenital heart defects is multifaceted. The respiratory therapist must evaluate more than the heart and the lungs to gain an understanding of the hemodynamic stability of the patient (**Figure 11-1**). Mechanical ventilation is the mainstay of therapy for children with cardiac defects. Depending on the type and severity of the defect, mechanical ventilation may be initiated prior to and/or after surgical intervention. The rationale for and use of basic mechanical ventilation principles used for complex care of the cardiac patient include the following points:[7]

- Positive pressure ventilation reduces left ventricular **afterload**, which is beneficial in the presence of poor ventricular function or aortic valve insufficiency. It can also be employed to reduce oxygen consumption.
- A drastic reduction in systemic venous return can occur when positive pressure ventilation is initiated. This can result in cardiac arrest. Preemptive fluid boluses may help avoid this situation.
- Anticholinergics, such as atropine, can be used prior to attempting tracheal intubation to reduce vagal responses in newborns/infants.
- Positive pressure ventilation is effective in the treatment of postoperative atelectasis and diaphragm paralysis and may also be necessary in the presence of vocal cord dysfunction.
- In children with pulmonary hypertension as a result of heart failure, it is important to avoid hypoxia, hypercapnia, acidosis, and atelectasis, all of which can cause vasoconstriction and pulmonary hypertensive crisis.
- Mechanical ventilation can be used in the postoperative period to help optimize oxygen delivery, maintain end organ function, and promote healing.

TABLE 11-1
Location of the Heart Valves

Valve	Anatomical Location
Tricuspid valve	Right side of the heart between the right atrium and the right ventricle
Pulmonary valve	Right side of the heart between the right ventricle and the pulmonary artery
Mitral valve	Left side of the heart between the left atrium and the left ventricle
Aortic valve	Left side of the heart between the left ventricle and the aorta

Cardiovascular status	Respiratory status	Temperature	Fluid status
• Heart rate and rhythm • Heart sounds and peripheral pulses • Blood pressure • Cardiac output • Lab test: glucose, metabolic panel, BUN, creatinine, ALP, ALT, AST, and bilirubin	• Breath sounds • Pulmonary hygiene • Suctioning • Chest radiographs • Chest tubes	• Hypothermia • Hyperthermia	• Intake • Output

FIGURE 11-1 An overview of the physiologic parameters to assess and monitor during the care of patients with congenital cardiac defects.

Along with applying basic ventilation principles, there are also fundamental concepts in the postoperative management of pediatric patients, including maintaining cardiovascular and respiratory status, maintaining normothermia, and strict monitoring of fluid intake and output.[7]

Acyanotic Heart Defects with Left-to-Right Shunts

Acyanotic cardiac disease describes the congenital cardiac anomalies that do not result in lower oxygen saturations. Oxygen saturations are within the normal range because oxygenated blood from the left side of the heart is shunted to the right side.[3] Children with acyanotic heart defects may present with abnormal vital signs, such as an elevated blood pressure, and/or signs of heart failure.[4] Acyanotic heart defects described in this chapter include patent ductus arteriosus, atrial septal defect, ventricular septal defect, and atrioventricular canal defect.

Patent Ductus Arteriosus

The ductus arteriosus is a channel that connects the aortic arch to the pulmonary arteries and is a normal and essential fetal structure. Closure typically occurs within the first few hours to first few days of life. A **patent ductus arteriosus (PDA)** results when the fetal ductus fails to close after birth (**Figure 11-2**).[8]

Etiology and Incidence

During fetal circulation, the ductus arteriosus is open, allowing blood to bypass the lungs and go to the lower portion of the body, exit through the umbilical artery, and return to the placenta for oxygen, while the **foramen ovale** (a small hole located in the septum between the two upper chambers of the heart) allows

Patent Ductus Arteriosus (PDA)

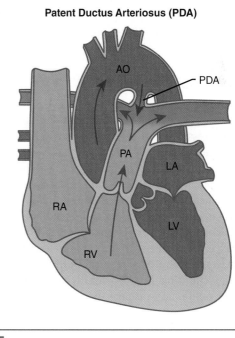

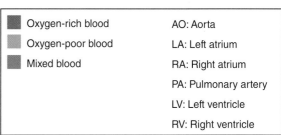

■ Oxygen-rich blood	AO: Aorta
■ Oxygen-poor blood	LA: Left atrium
■ Mixed blood	RA: Right atrium
	PA: Pulmonary artery
	LV: Left ventricle
	RV: Right ventricle

FIGURE 11-2 Schematic of the flow of blood occurring postnatally with a PDA.

Data from The Children's Hospital of Philadelphia.

oxygenated blood to go from the left atrium to the left ventricle to the aorta to supply blood to the brain.[9] Once the baby is born and begins to breathe on their own using the lungs, the partial pressure of oxygen in the arterial blood is increased and there is a decrease in pulmonary vascular resistance. This process causes the ductus arteriosus and foramen ovale to close.[9] When the ductus does not close within 72 hours after birth, it is called a PDA.[10]

PDA is one of the most common congenital heart defects. The reported incidence of PDA in term neonates is only 1 in 2000 births, accounting for 5% to 10% of all congenital heart disease.[8] There is far greater incidence of PDA in preterm neonates; published reports range from 20% to 60% depending on population and diagnostic criteria.[11]

Pathophysiology

A left-to-right shunt occurs through the PDA, resulting in increased pulmonary blood flow. The amount of blood flow and the degree of symptoms are determined by the difference in systemic and pulmonary vascular resistance as well as by the circumference and length of the PDA.

Clinical Presentation

An infant may be asymptomatic if the PDA is small. Symptoms of a persistent PDA include bounding pulses, wide pulse pressure, cardiac hypertrophy, and unexplained metabolic acidosis.[12] A larger PDA will present with signs of heart failure, including poor eating, poor weight gain, tachypnea, tachycardia, and diaphoresis.[12] Aside from heart failure, severely symptomatic PDA may result in pulmonary edema and/or pulmonary hemorrhage requiring ventilator support to provide adequate oxygenation and to deliver increased levels of positive end-expiratory pressure (PEEP) to reduce left-to-right shunting. Infants with PDA are at risk for developing pulmonary vascular disease.

Diagnosis

A patent ductus arteriosus can be diagnosed by physical exam, including auscultation for a heart murmur, along with chest radiograph, which shows **cardiomegaly** and increased vascular markings. A definitive diagnosis is typically made by echocardiography.

Management

There are two main treatment options for PDA: pharmacologic and surgical. Nonsteroidal anti-inflammatory agents (NSAIDs) may be used to treat a PDA because they inhibit **prostaglandin** production within the body.[10] For mechanically ventilated patients, permissive hypercapnia can also be employed to reduce pulmonary blood flow and to improve systemic perfusion. Additionally, PDAs can be closed during a cardiac catheterization with the use of a coil, a specially designed device that expands to the point where it blocks all blood flow. Surgical intervention may also be required. During

surgical closure, there is the placement of sutures or clips to close off the patent channel. Currently, surgical closure, or PDA **ligation**, may be safely and effectively performed within the neonatal intensive care unit. During the surgical procedure, infants are supported through invasive mechanical ventilation. Infants who did not require ventilatory support prior to surgical PDA ligation are typically quickly weaned and extubated postoperatively.

Complications and Outcomes

Potential complications of a persistently patent ductus arteriosus after birth include heart failure, renal dysfunction, necrotizing enterocolitis, intraventricular hemorrhage, and altered postnatal nutrition and growth. A PDA is also a risk factor for the development of chronic lung disease. The clinical implications vary depending on the anatomy of the ductus arteriosus and the underlying cardiovascular status of the patient.[8] Complications of PDA can be prevented or improved by appropriate diagnosis and management.

Atrial Septal Defect

An **atrial septal defect (ASD)** is a hole in the wall (septum) between the upper chambers of the heart, the atria (**Figure 11-3**). At birth, a small ASD may not cause any symptoms, but a larger ASD could lead to heart failure.

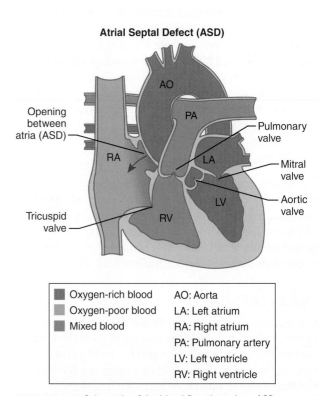

Atrial Septal Defect (ASD)

Opening between atria (ASD)
AO
PA
Pulmonary valve
RA
LA
Mitral valve
Aortic valve
Tricuspid valve
RV
LV

Oxygen-rich blood
Oxygen-poor blood
Mixed blood

AO: Aorta
LA: Left atrium
RA: Right atrium
PA: Pulmonary artery
LV: Left ventricle
RV: Right ventricle

FIGURE 11-3 Schematic of the blood flow through an ASD.
Data from The Children's Hospital of Philadelphia.

TABLE 11-2
The Four Types of ASDs and the Anatomical Location of the Defect or Hole in the Septum

Type	Location of the Defect
Secundum ASD	Middle of the atrial septum
Primum ASD	Lower part of the atrial septum
Sinus venosus	Upper portion of the atrial septum
Coronary sinus	Part of the septum between the coronary sinus and the left atrium is missing

There are four types of ASDs, with the secundum ASD being the most commonly seen type (**Table 11-2**).

Etiology and Incidence

During fetal growth, the atrial septum is formed during the 4th to 6th weeks of gestation. The foramen ovale exists to allow blood to bypass the lungs. After birth, the increase in left atrial pressure should close the foramen ovale; failure of the septum to fuse completely results in an ASD.

Atrial septal defects occur in approximately 13% of all children born with congenital heart disorders, with a prevalence of about 2 per 1000 births.[2] Females have atrial septal defects twice as often as males.

Pathophysiology

In patients with an isolated ASD, blood flow through the defect is dependent on the pulmonary and systemic vascular resistance. Primarily, there is a higher pressure in the left atrium (5–8 mm Hg) than the right atrium (3–5 mm Hg), which causes a left-to-right shunt. When a left-to-right shunt occurs, there is an increase in pulmonary blood flow, as blood is shunted from the left to the right side of the heart, causing volume overload in the right side of the heart (Figure 11-3).

Clinical Presentation

Most ASDs are small and do not cause symptoms during infancy and early childhood. Infants with a large ASD may present with shortness of breath; fatigue; swelling in their hands, feet, or stomach; tiring during feeding; frequent respiratory infections; arrhythmias; and stroke.[13]

Diagnosis

The most common method of detecting an ASD is by auscultation of a murmur. Diagnostic testing can also be used. Confirmation of an ASD can be made by echocardiography. Other tests include MRI and computerized tomography scan (CT scan). Chest radiography is typically unremarkable. However, should congestive heart failure (CHF) develop as a result of the ASD, enlarged pulmonary vascular markings and cardiomegaly may be present.

Management

A small percentage of infants and children with CHF are treated with digoxin and diuretics. Surgical repair includes using sutures or a pericardial patch to close the ASD. This can also be done during cardiac catheterization using a special catheter.

Complications and Outcomes

An unrepaired ASD can lead to right-sided heart failure, atrial arrhythmias, and potentially stroke. Although beta blockers and anticoagulants may be used to treat ASDs, larger ASDs could lead to pulmonary hypertension.[13] The prognosis for children who have ASDs is excellent. Advances in treatment allow most children who have these heart defects to live normal, active, and productive lives with no decrease in lifespan.

Ventricular Septal Defect

A **ventricular septal defect (VSD)** is a hole in the septum between the lower chambers of the heart, the ventricles. The defect may be a single hole, a series of small holes, or an absent septum.

Etiology and Incidence

During the 4th to 6th weeks of gestation, the ventricular septum is formed from muscular and membranous tissues that fuse the endocardial cushion. Insufficient development of these tissues during fetal growth can result in a VSD.

A VSD is the most common form of congenital heart disease in childhood, occurring in 50% of all children with congenital heart disease and in 20% as an isolated defect.[14] Therefore, VSD closure is one of the most commonly performed congenital heart surgeries.

Pathophysiology

Higher pressures in the left ventricle usually cause the blood to move from left to right across the shunt; oxygenated blood goes toward the lungs, causing volume overload in the right side of the heart and increased pressure in the lungs (**Figure 11-4**). Depending on the size and location of the defect, patients with a VSD are at risk for CHF and pulmonary hypertension.

Diagnosis

A murmur is commonly auscultated in patients with a VSD. An echocardiogram is most often used to

Ventricular Septal Defect (VSD)

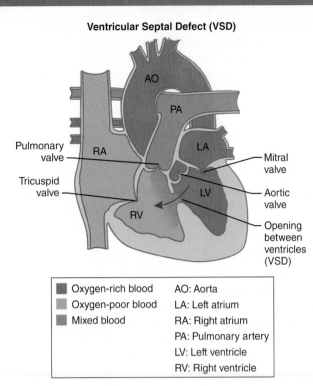

■ Oxygen-rich blood	AO: Aorta
■ Oxygen-poor blood	LA: Left atrium
■ Mixed blood	RA: Right atrium
	PA: Pulmonary artery
	LV: Left ventricle
	RV: Right ventricle

FIGURE 11-4 Schematic of the blood flow through a VSD.

Data from The Children's Hospital of Philadelphia.

diagnose a VSD. As with an ASD, a chest radiograph is unremarkable if the VSD is small, but a large VSD will present radiologically with an enlarged cardiac silhouette and increased pulmonary vascular markings, signifying CHF. Cardiac catheterization may also be used to detect the defect. Pulse oximetry reveals lower oxygen saturations, especially when pulmonary hypertension is present.

Clinical Presentation

Infants with VSDs will typically present with **failure to thrive**, or poor feeding and weight gain. Other symptoms include tachypnea, shortness of breath, and fatigue. Complications caused by VSDs include pulmonary hypertension, heart valve problems, and arrhythmias.

Management

Medications that may be used in the treatment of VSDs include digoxin to increase contractility of the heart muscle, diuretics to decrease volume load on the heart, and beta blockers. Small VSDs may be left unrepaired if the patient is asymptomatic. However, even small VSDs, if left unrepaired, could eventually lead to a leaky aortic valve. Typically, VSDs can be surgically repaired using a patch closure, or they can be closed with mesh during a cardiac catheterization.

Pulmonary artery bands are often used in critically ill infants with multiple VSDs. As a temporary measure, the bands narrow the diameter of the pulmonary artery and reduce pulmonary artery blood flow. Banding is performed by tightly wrapping a strip of Teflon or Dacron around the pulmonary artery to increase the resistance in the pulmonary artery and to reduce the amount of blood that flows through the defect, or reduce the amount of left-to-right shunting. Banding is often performed in children who are very small or hemodynamically unstable. This procedure allows the child time to grow and develop or stabilize, after which time a more comprehensive repair can be performed. When the defect is surgically closed, with sutures, the pulmonary bands are removed.

Complications and Outcomes

Complications may include endocarditis, aortic regurgitation, subaortic stenosis, right ventricular obstruction, heart block, and arrhythmias. Even after surgical closure, a residual VSD may remain.

Small ventricular septal defects that do not close rarely cause long-term difficulties. However, depending on the location of the hole, lifelong follow up may be required. Patients with large VSDs who are diagnosed and managed appropriately can have normal lifespans without restrictions.

Atrioventricular Canal Defect

An **atrioventricular canal defect (AVC)** is a large hole in the middle of the heart involving both atria and both ventricles. This defect allows oxygenated and deoxygenated blood to mix. AVC includes an ASD, VSD, and abnormal mitral and tricuspid valves. This defect is common in infants with Trisomy 21.[15] Classifications of AVCs include a complete AVC (CAVC), partial AVC (PAVC), transitional AVC, and unbalanced AVC. The features of a CAVC include an ASD, nonrestrictive VSD, and a common AV valve with a significant amount of left-to-right shunting. A partial AVC is less severe, with the hole existing only between the atria, requiring a repair of the ASD and mitral valve. A transitional AVC involves an ASD, restrictive VSD, and common AV valve. The right side of the heart and the left side of the heart are not equally involved with an unbalanced AV canal.

Etiology and Incidence

In utero, at 4 to 6 weeks' gestation, the superior and inferior endocardial cushions of the common AV canal fuse and contribute to the formation of the AV valves (mitral and tricuspid) and the AV septum. Failure of the cushions to fuse results in the various AV septal and valvular defects.[16] Atrioventricular canal defects account for about 4% to 5% of all congenital heart defects and occur in about 2 of every 10,000 live births. It occurs equally in boys and girls.[1]

Pathophysiology

Shunting occurs at the atrial and ventricular levels in a left-to-right direction. The right atrium also receives blood from the left ventricle due to a faulty mitral valve and ASD. Blood can also enter the right atrium via the defective tricuspid valve (**Figure 11-5**). The marked increase in volume and load to the right side of the heart and increased blood flow to the lungs create a significant risk for the development of pulmonary hypertension.

Clinical Presentation

Infants with AVC present with dyspnea, poor appetite, poor weight gain, cyanosis, and a heart murmur. They may also present with signs of heart failure, including diaphoresis, fatigue, edema, and wheezing.[16]

Diagnosis

The defect can be seen and characterized, and diagnosis is made with echocardiography and/or cardiac catheterization. An electrocardiogram (ECG) is often used to aid in the diagnosis.

Management

Medical treatment aims to improve the signs and symptoms of CHF. Pharmacologic therapy is based on digitalis, diuretics, and vasodilators.[17] AVC requires surgery within the first 3 to 6 months of life to close the hole(s) between the chambers using patches and to reconstruct or replace the heart valves.

Complications and Outcomes

Following AVC repair, increased pulmonary artery pressure can occur due to pulmonary hypertension. This may be treated using mild hyperventilation and pulmonary vasodilators, including inhaled **nitric oxide (NO)**. Patients with AVC require lifelong follow up with a cardiologist to monitor for problems, such as arrhythmias and leaky valves.

Mechanical Ventilation in Patients with Septal Defects (ASD, VSD, AVC)

Positive pressure ventilation can be used to augment the hemodynamic status of patients with left-to-right shunting as seen in ASD, VSD, and AVC. In these patients, the goal is to avoid increased pulmonary blood flow by avoiding overventilation, respiratory alkalosis, and high FiO_2. Clinicians must monitor the patient carefully when titrating PEEP. PEEP can also increase pulmonary vascular resistance (PVR) and limit pulmonary blood flow.

Acyanotic Heart Defects with Left Ventricular Outflow Tract Obstruction

Left ventricular outflow tract obstruction results from a series of stenotic areas between the left ventricular outflow tract and the descending aortic arch. This can lead to left ventricular hypertrophy and left ventricular failure from increased afterload.

Coarctation of the Aorta

Coarctation of the aorta is a narrowing of the aorta, ranging in severity from mild to severe (**Figure 11-6**). This narrowing or aortic constriction causes increased work of the heart to pump blood to the lower portion of the body. Risk factors for coarctation of the aorta include a bicuspid aortic valve, PDA, aortic valve stenosis, and mitral valve stenosis.

Etiology and Incidence

As the fetus is growing, between the 5th and 8th weeks of gestation, development of the aortic arch occurs. Failure of the aortic arch to develop properly causes a

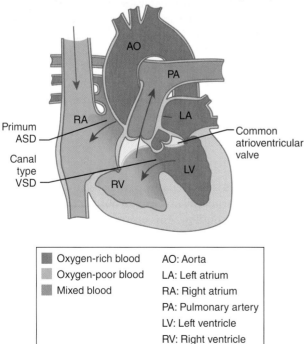

Complete Common Atrioventricular Canal (CAVC)

■ Oxygen-rich blood	AO: Aorta
■ Oxygen-poor blood	LA: Left atrium
■ Mixed blood	RA: Right atrium
	PA: Pulmonary artery
	LV: Left ventricle
	RV: Right ventricle

FIGURE 11-5 Schematic of blood flow through a complete AVC defect.

Data from The Children's Hospital of Philadelphia.

Coarctation of the Aorta

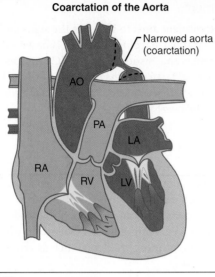

FIGURE 11-6 Schematic of the narrowing that occurs with coarctation of the aorta.

Data from The Children's Hospital of Philadelphia.

restricted opening or lumen in the aorta. Most often this occurs close to where the ductus arteriosus connects the main pulmonary artery to the aorta.

Coarctation of the aorta is a relatively common defect accounting for about 4% to 6% of all congenital heart defects and about 4 per 10,000 live births.[6] This defect occurs more commonly in males than females.

Pathophysiology

Coarctation of the aorta is characterized by an increase in pressure proximal to the narrowing and a decrease in pressure distal to it. The aortic narrowing causes resistance to blood flow through the aorta. As a result, pressures in the left ventricle increase and the proximal aorta dilates, both of which contribute to the development of left ventricular hypertrophy.

Clinical Presentation

Patients with coarctation have higher blood pressures in the upper extremities than in the lower extremities. They also present with weak pedal pulses, a murmur, and an enlarged heart on chest X-ray. If the narrowing is severe enough, the patient will present appearing pale and diaphoretic, with work of breathing and irritability. If the narrowing is not severe, the patient may have shortness of breath along with high blood pressure and colder feet than hands.[18]

Newborns may remain asymptomatic, especially if a PDA is present or if the coarctation is not severe.

Diagnosis

Observation of differential systolic blood pressures between the upper and lower extremities is a distinct feature; blood pressures will be higher when obtained from the upper extremities. As with other cardiac defects, diagnosis of coarctation of the aorta is confirmed with an echocardiogram and/or cardiac catheterization. An ECG is useful in identifying any cardiac arrhythmias that may accompany the defect.

Cardiac catheterization is usually performed in conjunction with a therapeutic intervention, such as balloon dilation. Balloon dilation is a procedure that expands the narrowing so that a stent can be placed. The stent is placed in the narrowed portion of the aorta to keep it open.

Management

There are a few surgical options to treat coarctation of the aorta. Surgery can be performed to remove the narrowed section of the aorta and to perform an end-to-end anastomosis to connect the portion of the aorta prior to the narrowing with the unaffected section after the narrowing. A patch, or aortoplasty, can be performed using part of the left subclavian or synthetic material. Finally, a graft can be used to bypass the coarctation.

Complications and Outcomes

Patients who have had a repair for coarctation of the aorta require long-term monitoring of blood pressure and cardiac function. In most cases, surgical or medical re-intervention is necessary.

Complications may include re-coarctation, stroke, aortic rupture, and cerebral aneurysm. The overall population shows better outcomes in those who reach adolescence, with very good long-term survival to age 60 years.[19]

Aortic Stenosis

Aortic stenosis is a narrowing of the aortic valve. It is a defect that primarily involves an obstruction to the left ventricular outflow. This occurs because the aortic valve, positioned between the left ventricle and the aorta, does not properly open and close, causing blood to leak (**Figure 11-7**). During ventricular contraction, this valve opens and allows blood to flow from the heart to the body. When a poorly working valve traps the blood flowing out from the heart, obstruction of blood flow to the upper and lower body occurs. This obstruction also causes pressure to build inside the left ventricle, causing damage to the left ventricle and ventricular hypertrophy. Congenital aortic stenosis is typically seen

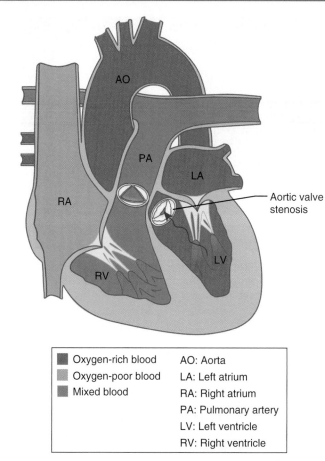

Aortic valve stenosis

Oxygen-rich blood
Oxygen-poor blood
Mixed blood

AO: Aorta
LA: Left atrium
RA: Right atrium
PA: Pulmonary artery
LV: Left ventricle
RV: Right ventricle

FIGURE 11-7 Schematic of the valve narrowing and backflow of blood into the left ventricle that occurs with aortic stenosis.
Data from The Children's Hospital of Philadelphia.

in infants born with a bicuspid aortic valve instead of a tricuspid aortic valve.

Etiology and Incidence

The aortic valve is formed during the 6th to 9th weeks of gestation, when the pulmonary artery and the aorta are formed from the division of the truncus arteriosus.[20] Failure of the cusp to separate causes a valvular aortic stenosis; this is the most common form of the defect, and most often the valve is bicuspid.

Aortic stenosis accounts for approximately 5% to 10% of the total number of congenital heart defects.[1] It occurs more frequently in males than females.[1]

Pathophysiology

Patients with aortic stenosis have increased left ventricular pressures, attributed to the resistance present from the obstructed valve. Eventually, left ventricular hypertension can occur and compromise systemic cardiac output. Increased left ventricular pressures are also associated with left ventricular hypertrophy, aortic insufficiency, and heart failure.

Clinical Presentation

Patients with aortic stenosis may present with chest pain, shortness of breath, fatigue, palpitations, and a murmur. A systolic ejection murmur may be heard best at the second intercostal segment. The child with a severe defect may present in heart failure having poor pulses, hypotension, and tachycardia.

Diagnosis

Differential diagnosis is made by echocardiography or by a transesophageal echocardiogram, which provides more detail and better identifies the presence of left ventricular hypertrophy. MRI may be used to measure the size of the aorta. Patients may undergo cardiac catheterization to identify the degree of severity of the stenosis. Pathology may be seen on chest radiography, which reveals pulmonary congestion from the backflow of blood. The chest X-ray may also show a larger-than-normal left ventricle when ventricular hypertrophy is present.

Management

Symptomatic newborns are started on a prostaglandin E1 infusion to open the ductus arteriosus. Congestive heart failure is treated with digoxin and diuretic therapy until surgery to correct the defect is performed.

Surgical interventions include an aortic valvulotomy or prosthetic valve replacement. Additionally, the balloon angioplasty can be used to dilate the narrow valve. Mechanical valves require anticoagulation to prevent clot formation, while tissue valves may narrow and need to be replaced over time. Aortic stenosis carries a poor prognosis if not treated because it will ultimately lead to heart failure.

Complications and Outcomes

Postoperative complications include persistent stenosis, restenosis of the aortic lumen, and insufficiency of the aortic valve. Long-term complications include the need for aortic valve replacement in adulthood.

Tetralogy of Fallot

Tetralogy of Fallot (TOF) is a heart defect that features four problems (**Figure 11-8**): (1) a hole between the lower chambers of the heart, (2) an obstruction from the heart to the lungs, (3) the aorta (blood vessel) lies over the hole in the lower chambers, and (4) the muscle surrounding the lower right chamber becomes overly thickened.

Etiology and Incidence

TOF is one of the most common forms of cyanotic congenital heart disease, occurring in 4 of every 10,000 live births and constituting 7% to 10% of all congenital

Tetralogy of Fallot (TOF) Interior View

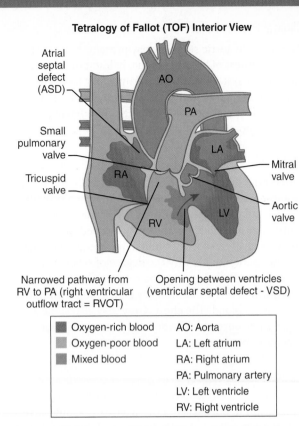

FIGURE 11-8 Schematic of the defects associated with Tetralogy of Fallot.

Data from The Children's Hospital of Philadelphia.

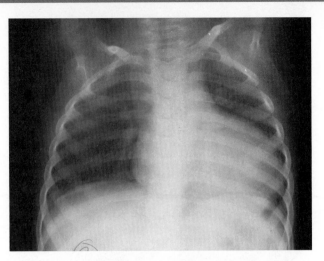

FIGURE 11-9 Chest radiograph of a boot-shaped heart, a finding common with Tetrology of Fallot. The heart with this cardiac malformation takes the shape of a "boot."

Published with permission from LearningRadiology.com.

heart defects.[1] TOF occurs equally in males and females. Approximately 15% of all TOF patients have an associated syndrome, such as Trisomy 21 (Down syndrome) or DiGeorge syndrome (a genetic disorder caused by a defect in chromosome 22 that results in the poor development of several body systems).[21]

Pathophysiology

The degree of cyanosis is directly proportional to the degree of right ventricular outflow tract obstruction (subpulmonary stenosis). If right ventricular outflow tract obstruction is mild, meaning the pressures in the left and right ventricles are equal, blood flow will be determined by the path of least resistance. In this case, blood will shunt from the left ventricle to the right ventricle into the pulmonary bed and the patient will be acyanotic.

If a severe obstruction is present, the resistance to blood flow into the pulmonary bed will increase and cause blood to move from the right ventricle into the left ventricle, then out to the body through the aorta. This right-to-left shunt results in a large amount of deoxygenated blood entering the systemic system. Arterial oxygen desaturation leading to severe hypoxemia and cyanosis will be present. As long as the ductus arteriosus remains open, pulmonary blood flow will be adequate.

Clinical Presentation

The initial presentation of the patient with TOF depends on the degree of right ventricular outflow tract (RVOT) obstruction. Most often, cyanosis is mild at birth and gradually worsens with age as hypertrophy of the right ventricular infundibulum progressively obstructs the RVOT. In some cases, profound cyanosis is significant soon after birth. Hypercyanotic spells, or TET spells, are acute episodes of arterial oxygen desaturation secondary to intermittent worsening of the RVOT obstruction.[22] Infants may become extremely irritable and cyanotic and lose consciousness. Cyanosis is refractory due to the fixed nature of the obstruction to pulmonary blood flow.

Diagnosis

Diagnostic procedures include echocardiogram and cardiac catheterization to identify the defects. ECG is helpful is determining the presence of cardiac arrhythmias, and pulse oximetry is used to assess the degree of hypoxemia and to guide oxygen management. Pathology can also be seen on chest radiography, which reveals a boot-shaped heart (**Figure 11-9**).

Management

Diagnosis of TOF in the neonate before closure of the ductus arteriosus presents the challenging clinical necessity of predicting the degree of pulmonary blood flow once the ductus has undergone spontaneous closure. Neonates with critically restricted antegrade flow and duct-dependent circulation must be started on prostaglandin E1 infusion and considered for a Blalock Taussig (BT) shunt or total repair. A BT shunt is a palliative surgical procedure performed to increase the pulmonary blood flow in patients with whom total repair of the defect cannot be accomplished. In neonatal patients, percutaneous stenting of the PDA is an alternative to surgical palliation, but its use in cases of aortic arch abnormality presents a major technical challenge.

Definitive surgical correction includes closure of the palliative BT shunt if present, opening the RVOT obstruction by resecting the infundibular tissue, and closure of the VSD.[20]

Complications and Outcomes

Potential complications include thrombosis of the BT shunt, which causes heart failure. Other potential complications include dysrhythmias, heart block, and myocardial ischemia.

Some long-term problems can include worsening obstruction due to pulmonic valve dysfunction. Children with repaired TOF also have a higher risk of heart rhythm disturbances. Sometimes these may cause dizziness or fainting. Morality rate is between 5% and 10% within the first 2 years after definitive repair. Generally, the long-term outlook is good, but some children may need medication, heart catheterization, or additional surgery.

Pulmonary Stenosis

Pulmonary stenosis (PS) is a condition characterized by obstruction to blood flow from the right ventricle into the pulmonary artery; stenosis at one or more locations from the right ventricular outflow tract causes the obstruction (**Figure 11-10**). Narrowing of the pulmonary valve is most often present at birth. The stenosis may be subvalvular (before the valve), supravalvular (after the valve), valvular, or in the pulmonary artery. The defect may occur alone or in combination with other heart defects that are present at birth. The stenosis can be mild or severe.

Etiology and Incidence

The pulmonic valve develops between the 6th and 9th weeks of gestation, which is also at the same time the pulmonary artery and aorta develop from the truncus arteriosus. Pulmonary stenosis occurs when the three tubercles in the pulmonary arterial lumen form abnormally, the result of which is a dysfunctional valve. Pulmonary stenosis may be a variant of Noonan syndrome, a genetic condition that affects many areas of the body and is characterized by mildly unusual facial features, short stature, heart defects, bleeding problems, and skeletal malformations.[23] Pulmonary stenosis may also be a variant of William-Beuren syndrome, a rare multisystem genetic disorder characterized by a distinctive "elfin" facial appearance, a low nasal bridge,

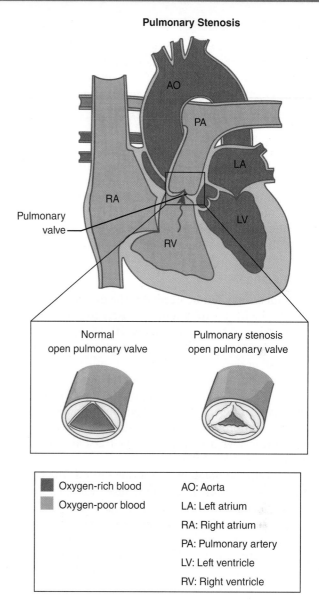

Pulmonary Stenosis

FIGURE 11-10 Schematic of the location and defect associated with pulmonary stenosis.
Data from The Children's Hospital of Philadelphia.

unusually cheerful demeanor, and profound visuospatial impairment.[24]

Pulmonary stenosis accounts for approximately 10% of the total number of congenital heart defects. It is slightly more common in males than females.[25]

Pathophysiology

Severe pulmonary stenosis contributes to increased right ventricular pressure as a result of the increased resistance to blood flow that the valvular stenosis and RVOT obstruction cause. The foramen ovale is patent and a right-to-left shunt occurs. The right ventricle enlarges as its muscular wall hypertrophies in response to the increased afterload, contributing to right-sided heart failure.

Clinical Presentation

Mild or moderate PS may be identified during the routine newborn physical examination. Screening with pulse oximetry may identify infants with severe cases of PS; this method detects oxygen desaturation before it is clinically evident and presents as cyanosis.

Diagnosis

Diagnosis of isolated PS includes other cardiac conditions that present as an incidental finding of a cardiac murmur in asymptomatic children. Although the "click" after a normal heart sound as heard during the cardiac examination is suggestive, echocardiography conclusively distinguishes these conditions from PS.

Management

Treatment may not be needed if the disorder is mild. Children with PS are followed closely to track the progression of function with growth of the valve. For moderate to severe pulmonary stenosis, in the neonatal period a prostaglandin E1 infusion will be started to maintain patency of the ductus arteriosus. Percutaneous balloon pulmonary dilation (**valvuloplasty**) can be performed during cardiac catheterization. Successful valvuloplasty produces a tear in the valve, which widens the track and reduces resistance to blood flow.

A surgical **valvulotomy** is another option. The pulmonary artery is opened and the fused valve leaflets are surgically slit. These slits are large enough to relieve the stenosis yet small enough to prevent regurgitation. If the valve is extremely deformed, part or the entire valve may be removed. If the ventricle is extremely small and the pulmonary flood flow remains compromised, a BT shunt may be created at the time of the valvulotomy.

Complications and Outcomes

Various degrees of pulmonary valve insufficiency and regurgitation may be seen. Long-term outcomes for patients who received a valvulotomy are very good, with survival rates at 93%.[26] Patients with significant right ventricular hypertension and hypertrophy may develop some degree of right ventricular failure postoperatively and/or require re-operation for pulmonary insufficiency.[26]

Pulmonary Atresia

The pulmonary valve is an opening on the right side of the heart that helps prevent blood from leaking back into the heart between beats. In pulmonary atresia, the pulmonary valve does not form correctly: It is sealed and cannot open (**Figure 11-11**).

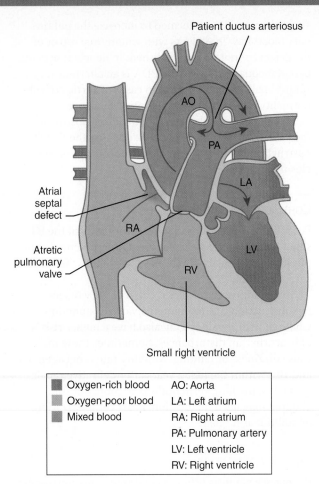

FIGURE 11-11 Schematic of the location and defect associated with pulmonary atresia.
Data from The Children's Hospital of Philadelphia.

Etiology and Incidence

Pulmonary atresia is failure of the pulmonary valve to develop between the 6th and 9th weeks of gestation and results in a valve that is small and lacks an opening. It is a rare congenital heart defect that accounts for only 1% to 3% of the total number of defects and presents in 4 to 8 per 100,000 live births.[20] There is no difference in gender-based incidence.

Pathophysiology

Because there is no opening, blood cannot flow from the right ventricle into the pulmonary artery and on to the lungs. The right ventricle acts as a blind pouch that may stay small and not develop well. The tricuspid valve is often poorly developed as well. Blood can exit through tricuspid regurgitation back into the right atrium. The foramen ovale is typically patent and allows blood to exit the right atrium; as such, deoxygenated blood mixes with the oxygen-rich blood in the left atrium, and the left ventricle pumps this mixture of blood into the aorta and out to the body. The only source of blood flow to the lungs is through the PDA.

Clinical Presentation

Pulmonary atresia symptoms include a blue or purple tint to lips, skin, and nails (cyanosis); shortness of breath; difficulty feeding; and a heart murmur.

Diagnosis

Diagnosis of pulmonary atresia may require some or all of the following: echocardiogram, ECG, chest radiograph, and cardiac catheterization. Pulse oximetry is useful in quantifying the degree of oxygen desaturation.

Management

Initial stabilization includes maintaining a PDA with prostaglandin E1 infusion. The condition is usually treated with cardiac catheterization or surgical intervention. If the right ventricle and right and left pulmonary arteries are of adequate size, correction can be performed by inserting a transanular patch or conduit between the right ventricle and pulmonary artery. If the right ventricle is hypoplastic or underdeveloped and/or the pulmonary arteries are too small for corrective repair, a valvulotomy is performed to provide a connection between the right ventricle and pulmonary artery.

Complications and Outcomes

Possible complications of pulmonary atresia with ventricular septal defect include CHF, infective endocarditis, growth retardation and delayed puberty, arrhythmias, and sudden death. Outcomes and risk factors for the need for additional interventions in these patients are poorly defined.

Tricuspid Atresia

Tricuspid atresia occurs when the tricuspid valve fails to develop. Without a tricuspid valve, there is a complete right-to-left shunt at the atrial level and there is no communication between the right atrium and the right ventricle.

Etiology and Incidence

The tricuspid valve is formed at approximately the 5th week of gestation as a result of the blending of the endocardial cushion tissue and a portion of the ventricular septum and ventricular muscle. A disruption in this process can result in the absence of a communication between the right atrium and ventricle.

Tricuspid atresia occurs in approximately 1% to 3% of children with congenital heart defects, in 2 of every 10,000 live births, and occurs equally in boys and girls.[20]

Pathophysiology

Tricuspid atresia is commonly associated with pulmonary stenosis and transposition of the great vessels. It causes a complete mixing of oxygenated pulmonary venous blood and deoxygenated systemic venous blood in the left side of the heart, which is then ejected by the left ventricle and results in systemic desaturation and variable pulmonary obstruction (**Figure 11-12**). There is increased workload on the heart due to the volume overload.

Clinical Presentation

Symptoms include hypoxemia and tachycardia. Cyanosis is often present in infants and neonates. Digital clubbing is common in older children. Blood flow through the heart will essentially be the same. Systemic venous return in infants allows flow across the atrial septum from the right to the left atrium through a patent foramen ovale (PFO) or an ASD. This shunt must exist because there is no other exit for blood to flow from the right atrium.

Diagnosis

Differential diagnostic considerations depend on the type of presentation. Moderate-to-severe cyanosis may present with decreased pulmonary flow noted on a

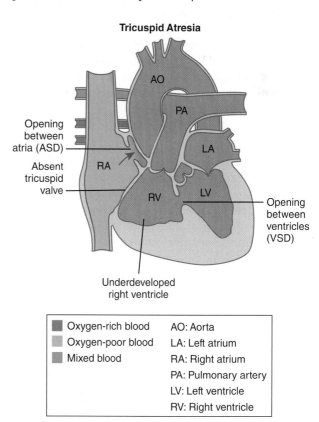

FIGURE 11-12 Schematic of the location and defect associated with tricuspid atresia.

Data from The Children's Hospital of Philadelphia.

chest radiograph. However, a less-severe presentation may also occur with mild cyanosis and increased pulmonary vascular marking on a chest radiograph with or without congestive heart failure. An echocardiogram confirms the presence of tricuspid atresia.

Management

Newborns who are symptomatic require intravenous prostaglandin E1 to maintain ductal patency; additionally, the patient is treated for control of hypoxemia and CHF. Surgical management includes corrective surgery using a modified Fontan procedure. If there is too much blood flowing to the lungs, a pulmonary arterial band may be placed to limit the blood flow.

Complications and Outcomes

Mortality varies and complications include arrhythmias, pleural effusions, and ventricular dysfunction. Later in life, complications include the risk of clot formation that could result in pulmonary embolism or stroke, arrhythmias, lymphatic system complications related to Fontan physiology, lower oxygen saturations, and exercise intolerance.

Ebstein's Anomaly

Ebstein's anomaly is a rare congenital defect in which the tricuspid valve does not properly close (**Figure 11-13**). As a result, blood flow does not move in the right direction, causing the heart to work less efficiently. Blood leaks back from the lower to upper chambers on the right side of the heart. This syndrome also is commonly seen with an ASD.

Etiology and Incidence

The cause of Ebstein's anomaly is still generally unknown. It occurs when the tricuspid valve develops lower than normal on the right ventricle and is characterized by adherence of the septal and posterior leaflets to the underlying myocardium due to the failure of the splitting of the tissue by detachment of the inner layer during embryologic development.[27]

Ebstein's anomaly occurs in approximately 1 per 200,000 live births and accounts for less than 1% of all cases of congenital heart disease.[28]

Pathophysiology

Ebstein's anomaly is a malformation of the right ventricle and the tricuspid valve characterized by the following: (1) adherence of the septal and posterior leaflets to the main myocardium; (2) downward dislocation of the functional valve; (3) dilation of the atrialized portion of the right ventricle, with various degrees of hypertrophy and thinning of the wall; (4) separation, fenestrations, and tethering of the anterior leaflet; and (5) dilation of the right atrioventricular junction.[29]

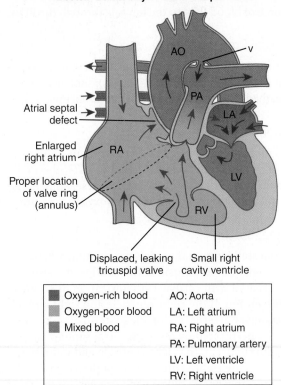

Ebstein's Anomaly of the Tricuspid Valve

Atrial septal defect

Enlarged right atrium

Proper location of valve ring (annulus)

Displaced, leaking tricuspid valve   Small right cavity ventricle

AO
V
PA
LA
RA
LV
RV

Oxygen-rich blood	AO: Aorta
Oxygen-poor blood	LA: Left atrium
Mixed blood	RA: Right atrium
	PA: Pulmonary artery
	LV: Left ventricle
	RV: Right ventricle

FIGURE 11-13 Schematic of the location and defect associated with Ebstein's anomaly of the tricuspid valve.
Data from The Children's Hospital of Philadelphia.

The function of the valve varies widely. The abnormal leaflets result in tricuspid insufficiency or regurgitation, which leads to ineffective blood flow through the right side of the heart. Additionally, during the contractive phase of the atrium, the atrialized portion of the right ventricle balloons out and acts as a passive reservoir, decreasing the volume of ejected blood. There is dilation to the right atrium; this increases the size of the interatrial communication.[29] Right atrial pressure is elevated and the right-to-left shunting of blood occurs through the foramen ovale or an ASD.

Clinical Presentation

Neonates with Ebstein's anomaly may present with cyanosis and CHF caused by regurgitation of the faulty tricuspid valve. Infants may be remarkably fussy or have other symptoms that cannot easily be connected with the rapid heart rhythm. Infants may not feed or grow normally. Symptomatic children may have gradual right-sided heart failure. Children older than 10 years frequently present with arrhythmias, such as supraventricular tachycardia (SVT), and also may have shortness of breath along with fatigue on exertion. An episode of SVT may cause palpitations that can be associated with fainting, dizziness, lightheadedness, or chest discomfort. The symptoms may respond to medications, such as diuretics. In some instances, surgery may be recommended.

Diagnosis

Diagnosis of Ebstein's anomaly is made with echocardiography. An ECG will be useful in detecting the cardiac rhythm disturbances. Chest radiography shows a globe-shaped heart with a narrow waist (**Figure 11-14**).[30] Cardiac catheterization typically is not necessary for diagnosis but may be done for preoperative assessment of the coronary arteries.

Management

Ebstein's anomaly can be mild in many children and surgery is not required. In cases where an abnormal heart rhythm, such as SVT, is present, electrophysiologic evaluation and radiofrequency ablation may be performed. Sometimes the tricuspid valve leaks severely enough to result in heart failure, and surgery may be required.

Several different operations have been used in patients with Ebstein's anomaly. The most common involves a repair of the tricuspid valve.[30] The valve cannot be made normal, but surgery often significantly reduces the amount of leaking. If there is an ASD, it is usually closed at the same time. In some cases, the tricuspid valve cannot be effectively repaired, so it is replaced with an artificial valve. Recurrent SVT may be prevented with medication.

Complications and Outcomes

Complications that may result from Ebstein's anomaly include heart failure, arrhythmias, low oxygen levels, limited physical activity, and, less commonly, sudden cardiac arrest or stroke.

Symptomatic neonates with Ebstein's anomaly have a poor prognosis. Evident cardiac widening, cyanosis, and severe tricuspid regurgitation all predict neonatal death without surgery. Tricuspid valve repair in children demonstrates low early mortality.

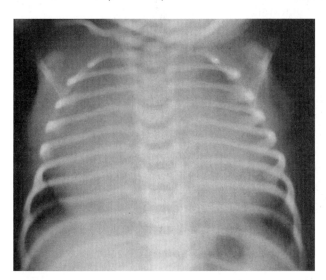

FIGURE 11-14 Preoperative X-ray showing a globe-shaped, wall-to-wall heart that is often present in infants with symptomatic Ebstein's anomaly.

Published with permission from LearningRadiology.com.

Cyanotic Heart Defects with Increased Pulmonary Blood Flow

Cyanotic cardiac defects cause a reduction in blood oxygen saturations, either by causing blood through the heart to completely bypass the lungs before flowing out to the rest of the body or by causing blood oxygenated by the lungs to mix with deoxygenated blood before entering into the systemic circulation.[3] Children with cyanotic heart disease typically have a bluish appearance of the skin.

Transposition of the Great Arteries or Vessels

In **transposition of the great arteries (TGA)**, the pulmonary artery and the aorta are misplaced, or transposed, across the ventricular septum (**Figure 11-15**). Specifically, the pulmonary artery leaves the left ventricle and the aorta rises from the right ventricle, so there is no communication between the systemic and pulmonic circulation. About 50% of infants with a TGA have a coexisting cardiac lesion, most commonly a VSD is present, followed by VSD with PS.

Etiology

Between the 3rd and 4th weeks of gestation, the truncus arteriosus is divided into the PA and the aorta. This results from spiral growth of the truncoconal ridges.

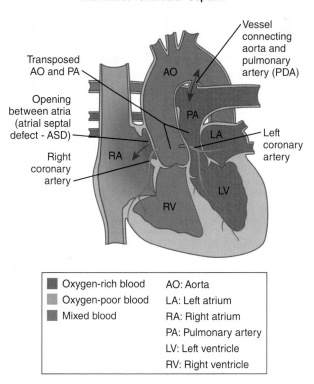

Transposition of the Great Arteries (TGA) with Intact Ventricular Septum

■ Oxygen-rich blood	AO: Aorta
■ Oxygen-poor blood	LA: Left atrium
■ Mixed blood	RA: Right atrium
	PA: Pulmonary artery
	LV: Left ventricle
	RV: Right ventricle

FIGURE 11-15 Schematic of the location and defect associated with transposition of the great vessels.

Data from The Children's Hospital of Philadelphia.

Failure of the truncoconal ridges to rotate completely results in the displacement of the aorta and the pulmonary artery on the ventricles.[20]

Incidence of TGA accounts for approximately 5% to 7% of the total number of congenital heart defects occurring in children. It is more common in males than females.

Pathophysiology

TGA results in two separate circulatory patterns: The right side of the heart manages systemic circulation and the left manages pulmonic circulation. To sustain life, the infant must have an associated defect, such as a patent foramen ovale, ASD, VSD, or PDA, to permit oxygenated blood into the systemic circulation (Figure 11-15). This does cause an increase in cardiac workload.

Clinical Presentation

Manifestations vary depending on the associated defects. If there is no associated defect, there will be severe respiratory depression and cyanosis at birth. Severity is dependent on the amount of intercirculatory mixing through the ASD. The presence of a VSD can result in decreased cyanosis because of improved mixing. Infants have high respiratory rates, greater than 60 breaths per minute. Cyanosis is unaffected by the use of supplemental oxygen, feeding, or crying. There can also be symptoms of heart failure with associated defects, but the cyanosis will be less pronounced.

Diagnosis

Diagnosis of TGA is made with echocardiography, while ECG is useful in displaying any rhythm disturbances. Chest radiography may be normal for the first few days of life. Cardiac catheterization is not required for diagnosis but is often used to assess the coronary arteries.

Management

In the newborn period, management aims to correct metabolic acidosis and to increase arterial oxygenation. A prostaglandin E1 infusion is used to maintain the patency of the ductus arteriosus to achieve adequate arterial oxygenation, or a balloon atrial septostomy is performed during cardiac catheterization to increase mixing and to maintain cardiac output over time.

Two major types of surgery can correct the transposition. The Mustard and Senning repairs are two similar operations for TGA. The Mustard procedure creates a two-way tunnel (a baffle) between the atria.[31] This redirects the oxygen-rich blood to the right ventricle and aorta and the oxygen-poor blood to the left ventricle and pulmonary artery. In a Senning procedure, the surgeon uses the patient's own tissue to create the baffle;

in the Mustard procedure, synthetic material is used. Both procedures are called atrial switch procedures because there is a baffle through the heart's top part, or atria, that allows the blood to reach the ventricles. The procedure is done in the first week of life.

Complications and Outcomes

Many TGA patients have inborn problems with the heart's electrical system. The scarring from previous surgery can also cause electrical problems and sinus node disease (the absence of sinus rhythm with presence of atrial or junctional escape rhythm).[31] This sinus syndrome can cause bradycardia. Pacemakers are used in up to 25% of patients requiring Mustard/Senning procedures by adulthood. Other TGA patients have tachycardia; sometimes they require an ablation to correct fast-beating arrhythmias. Newborns may have lung damage from lack of oxygen to tissues. Complications later in life may include narrowing of the coronary arteries, arrhythmias, heart muscle weakness or stiffness leading to heart failure, and leaky heart valves. TGA has a 90% mortality rate in the 1st year of life if left untreated.

Total Anomalous Pulmonary Venous Return

Total anomalous pulmonary venous return (TAPVR) is a congenital heart defect in the veins leading from the lungs to the heart. More specifically, TAPVR is defined by the failure of the pulmonary veins to return to the left atrium; they either enter the right atrium or another site in the systemic venous system. This causes oxygenated blood to flow into the right atrium instead of the left for systemic circulation and oxygenation. There are four main types of TAPVR: cardiac, supracardiac, infradiaphragmatic, and mixed (**Table 11-3**). **Figure 11-16** shows the defects associated with a supracardiac type of TAPVR.

TABLE 11-3
The Four Main Types of Total Anomalous Pulmonary Venous Return

Type	Description
Cardiac	The pulmonary veins either drain directly into the right atrium or they drain into the coronary sinus
Supracardiac	The pulmonary veins drain into the right atrium through the superior vena cava
Infradiaphragmatic	The pulmonary veins drain into the right atrium through the inferior vena cava and hepatic veins
Mixed	The pulmonary veins split and drain into multiple different areas

Total Anomalous Pulmonary Venous Return (TAPVR) Supracardiac Type

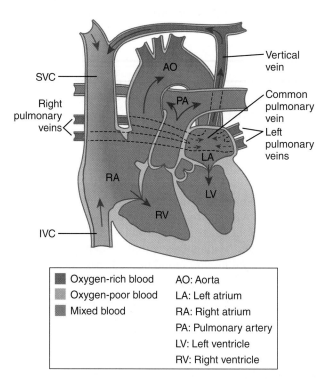

FIGURE 11-16 Schematic of the location and defect associated with the supracardiac type of TAPVR.

Data from The Children's Hospital of Philadelphia.

Etiology and Incidence

During the formation of the lungs in utero, portions of the splanchnic plexus begin to separate into the primitive pulmonary vascular bed. At the same time, the beginning of the left atrium forms and grows to join the pulmonary portion of the splanchnic plexus. Once the connection is made, the primitive pulmonary venous system separates. This then becomes the two right and two left pulmonary veins, each entering the left atrium through a separate opening.[32] TAPVR is the failure of the left atrium to link to the pulmonary venous system.

TAPVR accounts for approximately 1% of the total number of congenital heart defects, or about 0.6 to 1.2 per 10,000 live births.[1]

Clinical Presentation

Infants with TAPVR may present with cyanosis, heart murmur, poor feeding, fatigue, tachypnea, tachycardia, and increased work of breathing. Symptoms may develop soon after birth, or they may be delayed. This partly depends on whether the lung veins are blocked as they drain toward the right atrium. Severe obstruction of the pulmonary veins tends to make infants breathe harder and to look bluer due to lower oxygen levels than infants with little obstruction.

Pathophysiology

There are two pathophysiologic states in TAPVR: obstructed and nonobstructed. In obstructed TAPVR, pulmonary blood flow is reduced due to compression by surrounding structures; this causes cyanosis from the low arterial oxygen saturation. Decreased blood flow and elevated pulmonary venous pressure can result in progressive alveolar edema. In some cases, right heart failure occurs when pulmonary artery pressure is significantly elevated or exceeds system pressure.[33]

In nonobstructed TAPVR, because there is no compression, the entire pulmonary venous blood flow is returned to systemic venous circulation where there is mixing in the right ventricle. Each chamber of the heart contains the same mix of oxygen concentration in the blood.[33] There is typically a left-to-right shunt due to the low resistance of the lungs. The large volume of blood from the heart can lead to overcirculation. The right-to-left shunting across the PFO and ASD is critical for life.

Diagnosis

Diagnostic procedures include ECG, echocardiogram, cardiac catheterization, and MRI. Pulse oximetry is used to noninvasively quantify the degree of hypoxemia. Chest radiography reveals a larger right side of the heart and, depending on the severity, pulmonary edema.

Management

Infants with TAPVR require surgery early in life to remove the connections that should not be present and then to connect the pulmonary veins to the left atrium. If there is a lack of communication, no PFO or ASD, for mixing of blood flow to allow oxygenated blood to get out to the body, a balloon atrial septostomy may be performed in the catheterization lab until surgical repair can be performed. At the time of surgery, any ASD, VSD, PDA, or PFO that exist are closed. Patients who have had a TAPVR repair will require follow-up to monitor for narrowing of the pulmonary veins where the re-connections were established. If this occurs, the patient will likely experience shortness of breath and wheezing and will require placement of a stent or surgical enlargement of the narrowed area.

Complications and Outcomes

When surgical repair is done in early infancy, the long-term survival to adolescence is about 85%.[34] Follow-up is needed to make certain that any remaining problems, such as an obstruction in the pulmonary veins, irregularities in heart rhythm, or sinus node dysfunction, are treated.[34] Some children may need medication, heart catheterization, or additional surgery.

Truncus Arteriosus

A **truncus arteriosus** is the development of a large single vessel that leaves the heart, giving rise to the coronary,

Truncus Arteriosus

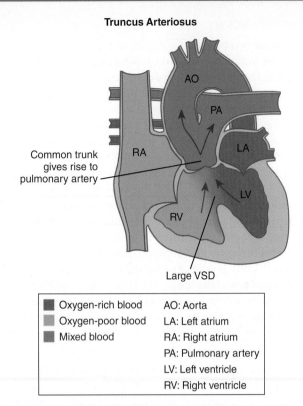

FIGURE 11-17 Schematic of the location and defect associated with truncus arteriosus.

Data from The Children's Hospital of Philadelphia.

systemic, and pulmonary arteries and containing only one valve. With only one artery, there is no specific path to the lungs for oxygen before returning to the heart to deliver oxygen to the body. The truncus arteriosus overlies a VSD; VSD is always seen in conjunction with this defect (**Figure 11-17**).

Etiology and Incidence

Truncus arteriosis is a result of a failure of the primitive arterial trunk to divide into a distinct aorta and pulmonary artery by the end of the 5th week of gestation. This is a rare congenital heart defect, accounting for 1% to 4% of the total number of congenital heart defects and about 6 to 10 per 100,000 live births.[1]

Pathophysiology

Blood ejected from the ventricles enters a common artery and flows either into the lungs or the aortic arch. Pressure in both ventricles is high, and blood flow to the lungs is similar to the systemic cardiac output. Over a couple of weeks, the pulmonary vascular resistance drops, a left-to-right shunt increases, and heart failure occurs.

Clinical Presentation

Infants with truncus arteriosis present with varying levels of cyanosis in the first few days of life. Over the next several days to weeks, symptoms of pulmonary congestion and heart failure develop. Infants demonstrate poor feeding and lethargy, respiratory distress, tachycardia, and hepatomegaly.

Diagnosis

Diagnosis of truncus arteriosis is by echocardiography. An ECG is helpful in demonstrating cardiac rate and rhythm disturbances. Cardiac catheterization is not typically used for diagnosis but rather for therapeutic interventions.

Management

Most neonates and infants need treatment for CHF; this is done with digoxin and diuretic agents. Prostaglandin E1 infusions are usually administered because of the differential diagnosis with duct-dependent systemic or pulmonary blood flow. Positive pressure ventilation and inotropic support are necessary. Surgical repair is necessary within the first few months. A patch is used to close the ventricular defect; the pulmonary arteries are then disconnected from the single great vessel (the truncus) and a tube (a conduit or tunnel) is placed from the right ventricle to the pulmonary arteries. This procedure is sometimes called a Rastelli repair.

Complications and Outcomes

Re-interventions of truncus arteriosis are common; they include replacement of the right ventricle–pulmonary artery conduit (as the patient grows in size, they outgrow the fixed connection). Additionally, truncal valve repair replacements are necessary due to worsening regurgitation.

In patients who had a primary repair, the overall mortality rate was only 11%.[35] Long-term survival following a primary repair is excellent, at 83% to 90%. Uncorrected truncus arteriosis has a poor outcome, with only a 15% survival rate at 1 year.

Single Ventricle Lesions

A single ventricle defect is a congenital heart disorder that affects the heart's ventricles or lower chambers. The chambers can be missing, under developed, or have missing or incomplete development of the ventricular septum. Single ventricle defects have profound affects on oxygenation, pulmonary and systemic circulation.

Hypoplastic Left Heart Syndrome

Hypoplastic left heart syndrome (HLHS) is a complex congenital heart disease in which the left side of the heart does not develop correctly in utero. This leaves the heart without the ability to effectively pump blood to the rest of the infant's body (**Figure 11-18**).

Hypoplastic Left Heart Syndrome (HLHS)

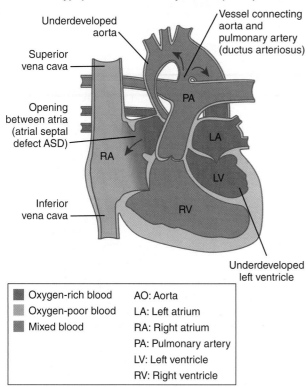

FIGURE 11-18 Schematic of left hypoplastic heart syndrome and associated cardiac defects.

Data from The Children's Hospital of Philadelphia.

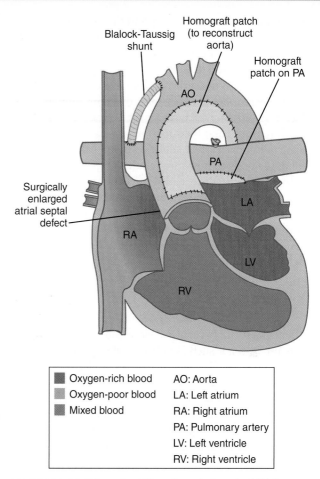

FIGURE 11-19 Schematic of Stage 1 surgical repair of HLHS: Norwood procedure with Sano modification.

Data from The Children's Hospital of Philadelphia.

Etiology and Incidence

The underlying causal mechanism of HLHS is unknown. It is proposed that the embryonic cause of HLHS is a limitation in the left ventricular outflow tract.

HLHS accounts for 2% to 3% of all congenital heart disease, with a prevalence rate of 2 to 3 cases per 10,000 live births in the United States.[36] HLHS is the most common form of functional single ventricle heart disease. A male predominance is observed in most patient populations.[37]

Clinical Presentation

Infants born with HLHS may appear normal at birth but will become seriously ill as the ductus arteriosus begins to close. This will cause cyanosis, tachypnea, tachycardia, feeding intolerance, cold hands and feet due to poor circulation, and lethargy. An infant who goes home undiagnosed with HLHS may present in shock. HLHS is fatal without intervention. Newborns with HLHS require prostaglandin E1 infusions to keep the ductus arteriosis open, allowing oxygenated blood to circulate to the body. These infants will also require a three-surgery palliation.

Diagnosis

HLHS is diagnosed using echocardiography, which is sufficient in most cases to make a diagnosis.

Management

Prior to surgery, it is imperative to keep a fine balance between pulmonary and systemic blood flow. If the newborn has high oxygen saturations and high PaO_2 values, their systemic blood pressure may be negatively impacted. If this is an issue, it may be necessary to intubate the newborn to control ventilation and to allow for mild hypercapnia to limit pulmonary blood flow. If intubation and mechanical ventilation alone do not produce the desired results, adding **inhaled carbon dioxide** (CO_2) to the ventilator circuit can potentially augment this process. Data suggest that the benefits of inhaled CO_2 are mediated through resulting respiratory acidosis. Pulmonary vasoconstriction should result in an improvement in systemic perfusion, an increase in diastolic blood pressure, and a decrease in systemic oxygen saturation.[38]

The first surgery, performed within the first few days of life, is referred to as Stage 1 (**Figure 11-19**). During Stage 1, the small aorta is reconstructed and a BT shunt is placed between the aorta and the right ventricle, allowing the right ventricle to pump blood to both the lungs and the body. Alternatives to the typical Stage 1 are the Sano procedure, in which a conduit is placed between the pulmonary artery and the right ventricle, or a hybrid procedure, which involves stenting the ductus arteriosis and placing a pulmonary artery band to restrict some blood flow to the lungs.

The second in the series of palliative procedures is the bidirectional Glenn or the hemi-Fontan (**Figure 11-20**), in which the shunt from the first surgery is removed and the superior vena cava is connected to the pulmonary artery, allowing blood from the upper half of the body to flow through the lungs.

The final procedure, called the Fontan, connects the inferior vena cava is to the pulmonary artery (**Figure 11-21**). After completion of the Fontan procedure, all blood flows passively through the lungs and then is pumped out to the body by the single right ventricle. If for some reason a three-stage palliation cannot be performed, the infant will require a heart transplant.

Complications and Outcomes

Patients with HLHS require lifelong follow up to monitor for complications, such as fatigue, arrhythmias, stroke, and pulmonary embolism. Fontan patients are also at risk for such conditions as protein-losing enteropathy, which is excessive intestinal protein loss, and plastic bronchitis, which is a lymphatic flow disorder within the lungs. In plastic bronchitis, lymph builds up in the lungs, creating a thick cast that results in respiratory distress.

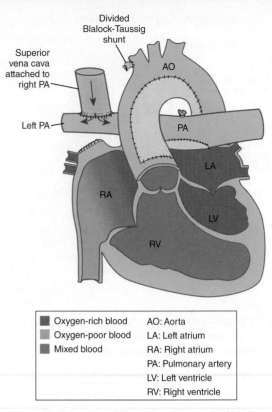

■ Oxygen-rich blood	AO: Aorta
■ Oxygen-poor blood	LA: Left atrium
■ Mixed blood	RA: Right atrium
	PA: Pulmonary artery
	LV: Left ventricle
	RV: Right ventricle

FIGURE 11-20 Schematic of Stage 2 surgical repair of HLHS: bidirectional Glenn.

Data from The Children's Hospital of Philadelphia.

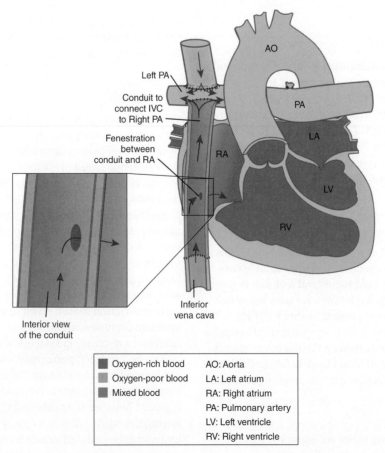

■ Oxygen-rich blood	AO: Aorta
■ Oxygen-poor blood	LA: Left atrium
■ Mixed blood	RA: Right atrium
	PA: Pulmonary artery
	LV: Left ventricle
	RV: Right ventricle

FIGURE 11-21 Schematic of Stage 3 surgical repair HLHS: Fontan.

Data from The Children's Hospital of Philadelphia.

Advancements in both medical and surgical interventions have led to a decrease in the mortality rate of HLHS, from an almost always fatal disease to estimates of 3- to 5-year survival rates of 70% for infants who undergo Stage 1 repair.[39] For children who survive to the age of 12 months, long-term survival is approximately 90%.[40]

Mechanical Ventilation of the Single-Ventricle Patient

In single-ventricle patients, early extubation greatly improves cardiac output. The reason for this is that pulmonary blood flow determines the majority of the cardiac output, and spontaneous ventilation enhances pulmonary blood flow while positive pressure ventilation can significantly decrease pulmonary blood flow. For single-ventricle patients requiring mechanical ventilation, the goal is to avoid high PaO_2 and respiratory alkalosis that lowers PVR. A PaO_2 of 50 to 60 mm Hg is acceptable for this patient population. A mild respiratory acidosis will augment systemic perfusion and help to avoid issues like cerebral ischemia and necrotizing enterocolitis that result from poor systemic perfusion. Negative pressure ventilation via cuirass can be employed in single-ventricle children requiring ventilatory assistance because, like spontaneously breathing, negative pressure ventilation increases pulmonary blood flow. However, negative pressure ventilation via cuirass can be challenging in the face of midsternal incisions and chest tubes.

Conclusion

Congenital heart defects are problems with the heart structure (walls, valves, vessels) that are present at birth. There are many types of cardiac defects; some are isolated and straightforward, and others are incredibly complex and occur in combination with other defects (**Table 11-4**). Medical advances have improved over the past few decades and so has the diagnosis and medical treatment of these patients. As a result, most children with complex disease can survive to adulthood and have active lives as long as they continue the monitor heart condition and needs.

TABLE 11-4
Summary of Cardiac Defects and Corrective Repair Procedures

Defect	Corrective Repair
Patent ductus arteriosus	Coil, clips, or sutures
Atrial septal defect	Patch
Ventricular defect	Patch repair
Complete atrioventricular canal defect	Patch closure and reconstruction or replacement of valves
Coarctation of the aorta	Removal of stenotic area, patch aortaplasty, or graft
Aortic stenosis	Aortic valvulotomy, valve replacement, or balloon angioplasty
Tetralogy of Fallot*	The ductus arteriosus is ligated if patent, patch closure of VSD, RVOT reconstruction, removal of pulmonary infundiblar muscle, pulmonary valvulotmy is performed. Occasionally, the PFO is left open as a "pop-off."
Pulmonary stenosis	Balloon and surgical valvuloplasty
Pulmonary atresia*	Transannular patch or conduit is inserted between the right ventricle and the pulmonary artery. The ASD is closed.
Triscupid atresia*	Modified Blalock-Taussig shunt: This joins the subclavian artery to the right pulmonary artery (systemic to pulmonary shunt).
	Glenn shunt: This joins the superior vena cava to the right pulmonary artery.
	Fontan: This joins the inferior vena cava to the pulmonary artery via a homograft conduit.
Epstein's anomaly*	Repair or replace tricuspid valve if indicated. Patch closure of ASD if one is present.
Total anomalous pulmonary venous return	Anastomosis of the common pulmonary veins to the left atrium, elimination of the anomalous pulmonary venous connection, and closure of any interatrial communication. If a PDA is present, it is ligated.

(continues)

TABLE 11-4
Summary of Cardiac Defects and Corrective Repair Procedures (*Continued*)

Defect	Corrective Repair
Transposition of the great arteries	Arterial switch operation or atrial switch
Truncus arteriosus	Rastelli procedure
Hypoplastic left heart syndrome*	Norwood w/Sano, bidirectional Glenn, Fontan

*Palliative options

Case Study 1

A 4-day-old infant presents to the emergency department. Parents state that the infant has been breathing fast, sweating, and feeding poorly since discharge from the hospital following a normal vaginal delivery.

Upon assessment, vital signs are obtained with the following results:

- Temperature (axillary): 36.7°C
- Heart rate: 160 beats per minute with a murmur
- Respiratory rate: 70 breaths per minute
- SpO$_2$: 95% on room air.
- Breath sounds: Clear to auscultation
- Chest radiograph, which shows cardiomegaly and increased vascular markings

1. **In order to assess this patient, what should the respiratory therapist do first?**
   a. Recommend obtaining electrolytes
   b. Perform a physical assessment
   c. Recommend obtaining a complete blood count
   d. Recommend an ECG

2. **Based on the examination findings, which two steps should the respiratory therapist recommend?**
   i. Echocardiogram
   ii. Blood pressure measurements in all four extremities
   iii. Pre- and postductal oxygen saturation
   iv. Palpating upper and lower extremity pulses
   a. i and iii
   b. ii and iv
   c. i and ii
   d. iii and iv

3. **The diagnosis of patent ductus arteriosus is made by echocardiogram. Which of the following are the treatment options?**
   a. Pericardial patch
   b. Surgical ligation
   c. Administration of beta blockers
   d. Inhalation of nitric oxide

Case Study 2

A 10-day-old infant presents to the emergency department. Parents state that the infant has been very pale, irritable, poorly feeding, tachypneic for the last week, and lethargic for the last 24 hours.

Upon assessment, vital signs are obtained with the following results:

- Temperature (axillary): 36.7°C
- Heart rate: 160 beats per minute
- Respiratory rate: 65 breaths per minute
- Blood pressure: 110/65 mm Hg
- SpO$_2$: 95% on room air
- Breath sounds: Clear to auscultation

Physical examination findings include strong pulses and hypertension in the upper extremities, diminished pedal pulses, and a blood pressure gradient, with low or unreadable blood pressures in the lower extremities. A systolic murmur is present at the upper left

Case Study 2 (*continued*)

sternal border. An apical systolic ejection "click" is present. The physician orders an ECG.

The results of the diagnostic tests are as follows:

- Chest X-ray shows a normal or enlarged heart.
- ECG shows right ventricular hypertrophy.
- ECHO shows a narrowing in the aorta.

A diagnosis of severe coarctation is made, and the infant is admitted to the intensive care unit.

1. In order to assess this patient, what should the clinician obtain?
   a. Electrolytes
   b. Physical assessment
   c. Complete blood count
   d. MRI of the chest

2. Based on the examination findings, what next steps should the clinician consider?

	Blood pressure measurements in all four extremities	Palpating upper and lower extremity pulses	Preductal and postductal oxygen saturation	Auscultating heart sounds
A	Yes	Yes	Yes	No
B	No	Yes	Yes	Yes
C	Yes	No	Yes	Yes
D	Yes	Yes	No	Yes

3. What interventions and/or additional testing should the clinician now consider?
   i. Cardiac catheterization
   ii. Echocardiogram
   iii. Doppler study of the legs
   iv. Chest radiograph

   a. i and iv
   b. ii and iii
   c. i and ii
   d. iii and iv

4. Upon admission to the cardiac intensive care unit, what is the first medical intervention that should be performed?
   a. Initiation of inhaled nitric oxide
   b. Administration of a fluid bolus
   c. Infusion of prostaglandin E
   d. Intubation and mechanical ventilation

5. Corrective actions for coarctation of the aorta include surgery to remove the narrowed area, balloon dilation during cardiac catheterization, and which of the following?
   i. A patch aortoplasty
   ii. Ligation of the ductus arteriosus
   iii. Graft to bypass the coarctation
   iv. Performing a Fontan procedure

   a. i and ii
   b. ii and iv
   c. i and iii
   d. iii and iv

References

1. Reller MSC. Prevalence of congenital heart defects in metropolitan Atlanta, 1998-2005. *J Pediatr.* 2008;153(6):807-813.
2. van der Linde KEH. Birth prevalence of congenital heart disease worldwide: a systematic review and meta analysis. *J Am Coll Cardiol.* 2011;58(21):2241-2247.
3. Waldman JD, Wernly JA. Cyanotic congenital heart disease with decreased pulmonary blood flow in children. *Pediatr Clin North Am.* 1999;46(2):385-404.
4. Teitel D. Recognition of undiagnosed neonatal heart disease. *Clin Perinatol.* 2016;43(1):81-98.
5. Corcoran S, Briggs K, O'Connor H, et al. Prenatal detection of major congenital heart disease—optimising resources to improve outcomes. *Eur J Obstet Gynecol Reprod Biol.* 2016;203:260-263.
6. Hoffman JK, Kaplan S. The incidence of congenital heart disease. *J Am Coll Cardiol.* 2002;39(12):1890-1900.
7. Rimensberger PC, Heulitt MJ, Meliones J, Pons M, Bronicki RA. Mechanical ventilation in the pediatric cardiac intensive care unit: the essentials. *World J Pediatr Congenit Heart Surg.* 2011;2(4):609-619.
8. Schneider DM, Moore JW. Patent ductus arteriosus. *Circulation.* 2006;114(17):1873-1883.
9. Friedman AH, Fahey JT. The transition from fetal to neonatal circulation: normal responses and implication for infants with heart disease. *Semin Perinatol.* 1992;17(2):106-221.
10. Clyman RI. Ibuprofen and patent ductus arteriosus. *N Engl J Med.* 2000;343(10):728-730.
11. El Hajjar M, Vaksmann G, Rakza T, Kongolo G, Storme L. Severity of ductal shunt: a comparison of different markers. *Arch Dis Child.* 2005;90(5):F419-F422.

12. Suzumura H, Nitta A, Tanaka G, Arisaka O. Diastolic flow velocity of the left pulmonary artery of patent ductus arteriosus in preterm infants. *Pediatr Int.* 2001;43(2):146-151.

13. Andrews RT, Tulloh R, Magee A, Anderson D. Atrial defect and failure to thrive in infancy: hidden pulmonary vascular disease. *Pediatr Cardiol.* 2002;23(5):528-530.

14. Minette MS. Ventricular septal defects. *Circulation.* 2006;114(20): 2190-2197.

15. Korenberg JB, Bradley C, Disteche CM. Down syndrome: molecular mapping of the congenital heart disease and duodenal stenosis. *Am J Human Genet.* 1992;50(2):294-302.

16. Wenink AZ, Zevallos JC. Developmental aspects of atrioventriuclar septal defects. *Int J Cardiol.* 1988;18(1):65-78.

17. Calabro RL, Limongelli G. Complete atrioventricular canal. *Orphanet J Rare Dis.* 2006;1:8.doi:10.1186/1750-1172-1-8.

18. Nance JW, Ringel RE, Fishman EK. Coarctation of the aorta in adolescents and adults: a review of clinical features and CT imaging. *J Cardiovasc Comput Tomogr.* 2016;10(1):1-12.

19. Choudhary PC, Canniffe C, Jackson DJ, Tanous D, Walsh K, Celermajer DS. Late outcomes in adults with coarctation of the aorta. *Heart.* 2015;101(15):1190-1195.

20. Curley M., Moloney-Harmon PA. *Critical Care Nursing of Infants and Children.* Philadelphia, PA: W.B. Saunders; 2001.

21. Di Felice VZ, Zummo G. Tetrology of Fallot as a model to study cardiac progenitor cell migration and differentiation during heart development. *Trends Cardiovasc Med.* 2009;19(4):130-135.

22. Kothari S. Mechanism of cyanotic spells in tetrology of Fallot—the missing link? *Int J Cardiol.* 1992;37(1):1-5.

23. Pierpont MB, Basson CT, Benson DW Jr, et al. Genetic basis for congenital heart defects: current knowledge: a scientific statement from the American Heart Association Congenital Cardiac Defects Committee, Council on Cardiovascular Disease in the Young: endorsed by the American Academy of Pediatrics. *Circulation.* 2007;115(23):3015-3038.

24. Pober BR. Williams–Beuren Syndrome. *N Engl J Med.* 2010;362(3):239-252.

25. Armstrong EB, Bischoff J. Heart valve development: endothelial cell signaling and differentiation. *Circ Res.* 2004;95(5):459-470.

26. Roos-Hesselink JW, Meijboom FJ, Spitaels SE, et al. Long-term outcomes after surgery for pulmonary stenosis. *Eur Heart J.* 2006;27(4):482-488.

27. Barbara DW, Edwards WD. Surgical pathology of 104 tricuspid valves (2000-2005) with classic right-sided Ebstein's malformation. *Cardiovasc Pathol.* 2008;17(3):166-171.

28. Perloff, J. *The Clinical Recognition of Congenital Heart Disease.* 5th ed. Philadelphia, PA: WB Saunders; 2003.

29. Attenhofer Jost CH, Connolly HM, Dearani JA, Edwards WD, Danielson GK. Ebsteins anomaly. *Circulation.* 2007;115(2): 277-285.

30. Cherry C, Debord S, Moustapha-Nadler N. Ebstein's anomaly: a complex congenital heart defect. *AJON.* 2009;89(6):1098-1114.

31. Kammeraad JA, van Deurzen CH, Sreeram N, et al. Predictors of sudden cardiac death after Mustard or Senning repair for the transposition of the great arteries. *J Am Coll Cardiol.* 2004;44(5): 1095-1102.

32. Keane JF. *Total Anamalous Pulmonary Venous Return.* Philadelphia, PA: Sauders Elsevier; 2006.

33. Geva T. Anomalies of the pulmonary veins. In: Allen HS, ed. *Moss and Adams Heart Disease in Infants, Children, and Adolescents.* Phildelphia, PA: Lippincott Williams and Wilkins; 2008:761.

34. Tanel RE, Kirshbom PM, Paridon SM, et al. Long-term noninvasive arrhythmia assessment after total anomalous pulmonary venous connection repair. *Am Heart J.* 2007;153(2):267-274.

35. Russell HP, Pasquali SK, Jacobs JP, et al. Outcomes of repair of common arterial trunk with truncal valve surgery: a review of the Society of Thoracic Surgeons congenital heart surgery database. *Ann Thorac Surg.* 2012;93(1):164-169.

36. Gordon BR, Rodriguez S, Lee M, Chang RK. Decreasing number of deaths of infants with hypoplastic left heart syndrome. *J Pediatr.* 2008;153(3):354-358.

37. Karamlou TD, Diggs BS, Ungerleider RM, Welke KF. Evolution of treatment options and outcomes for hypoplastic left heart syndrome over an 18 year period. *J Thorac Cariovasc Surg.* 2010; 139(1):119-126.

38. Jobes DN, Nicolson SC, Steven JM, Miller M, Jacobs ML, Norwood WI Jr. Carbon dioxide prevents pulmonary overcirculation in hypoplastic left heart syndrome. *Ann Thorac Surg.* 1992;54(1): 150-151.

39. Ballweg JD, Dominguez TE, Ravishankar C, et al. A contemporary comparison of the effect of shunt type in hypoplastic left heart syndrome on the hemodynamics and outcome at Fontan completion. *J Thorac Cardiovasc Surg.* 2010;140(3):537-544.

40. Siffel C, Riehle-Colarusso T, Oster ME, Correa A. Survival of children with hypoplastic left heart syndrome. *Pediatrics.* 2015;136(4): e864-e870.

12

Evaluation of the Child

April B. Carpenter
Wendy G. Burgener
Emma E. Holland

OUTLINE

OBJECTIVES

1. Identify key anatomic and physiologic characteristics of children and their role in the development of respiratory distress.
2. Develop basic techniques used for auscultation of the child.
3. Characterize various pediatric airway sounds and recognize their potential causes.
4. Recognize the early and late symptoms of respiratory distress in a child.
5. Use information obtained through the history and physical examination to develop a differential diagnosis and plan of care for a child.

KEY TERMS

chief complaint (CC)
digital clubbing
head bobbing
history of present
  illness (HPI)
kyphoscoliosis
kyphosis
nasal flaring

pectus carinatum
pectus excavatum
Pediatric Assessment
  Triangle (PAT)
retractions
review of systems
scoliosis

Introduction

Respiratory problems are a leading cause of illness and hospitalization among infants and children, accounting for 60% of primary care provider office visits and costing an estimated $129 billion annually.[1,2] Respiratory disorders in infants and children have a wide range of symptoms and severity, ranging from nasal congestion and drainage to complete respiratory failure. Additionally, the anatomy and physiology of infants and children can predispose them to quickly progress to significant respiratory distress when acutely ill.

A complete and accurate medical history and physical examination are invaluable in the evaluation and formation of a diagnosis and treatment plan for the patient. This chapter discusses the examination and respiratory assessment of the child.

Initial Assessment

Respiratory distress must be quickly identified and aggressively treated. Because infants and children have small airways, decreased respiratory reserves and increased metabolic demands, they can quickly decompensate and progress to respiratory failure.

The **Pediatric Assessment Triangle (PAT)**, in **Figure 12-1**, is a rapid, strategic primary assessment of a child's severity of illness.[3] The PAT uses a visual and auditory assessment of the child, including evaluation of the child's appearance, work of breathing, and circulation. It should be completed within the first 30 seconds of evaluating the child. Use of the PAT allows the clinician to quickly form an accurate initial impression of the child as "sick" or "not sick" and, therefore, to prioritize as appropriate.[4]

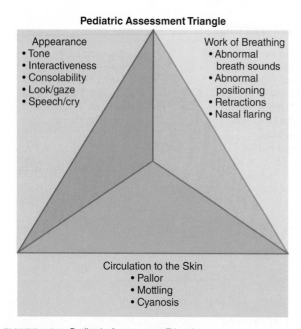

Pediatric Assessment Triangle

Appearance
• Tone
• Interactiveness
• Consolability
• Look/gaze
• Speech/cry

Work of Breathing
• Abnormal breath sounds
• Abnormal positioning
• Retractions
• Nasal flaring

Circulation to the Skin
• Pallor
• Mottling
• Cyanosis

FIGURE 12-1 Pediatric Assessment Triangle.

Used with permission of the American Academy of Pediatrics, Pediatric Education for Prehospital Professionals, © American Academy of Pediatrics, 2000.

History

Once the child has been identified as nonemergent, the clinician can begin to obtain a thorough history. Taking a history is an essential component of assessing a child—some argue it is the most important part of the assessment. A thorough history allows the clinician to gather essential health information, begin development of a relationship between the child and family and medical team, and provide education to the child and family.[5] In the pediatric population, most of the time the history will be obtained from the child's parent, although useful information can be obtained from the young child.

History-Taking Techniques

Obtaining a thorough history begins with setting the interview environment. Ideally, the history should be obtained in an environment that is private, quiet, and free from distractions. The interview environment must ensure that the child's and family's confidentiality are maintained.

Good communication skills are an essential component in obtaining a comprehensive medical history.[6] The clinician should be attuned to both verbal and nonverbal cues. Open-ended questions will generally elicit more information than close-ended questions and will allow the child or parent the opportunity to tell their story in their own words. It is also important to allow them adequate time to express themselves. Pauses in the conversation can sometimes be difficult for the clinician and may feel uncomfortable but are necessary and helpful to ensure that no one feels rushed. Additional communication techniques include clarification, reflection, and summarizing. Clarification, or stating, "I hear you say that . . .," ensures that the clinician understands what the child is saying. Reflecting is paraphrasing and restating what the child or parent has said; it shows them that you are trying to understand what they have said. Summarizing the history allows for an opportunity to ensure accuracy and to develop a shared understanding of the subject matter.

Medical History

The history begins with a discussion of the child's current illness, including the **chief complaint (CC)** and the **history of present illness (HPI)**. The CC is the health problem or concern, described in the child's or parent's own words, which caused the individual to seek medical attention. The HPI is a thorough description of relevant symptoms listed in chronological order and including any previous treatment.

After the HPI, the clinician will elicit the medical history, including general health, accidents/injuries, prior hospitalizations with dates and diagnosis, immunizations, and screening tests. For infants and young children, prenatal and birth history are important to include.

Information to obtain concerning current medications includes the name, dose, route of administration, frequency, duration, reason for taking, and compliance with taking the medication. The patient's allergies must be solicited. If there has been a reaction, it is important to determine what medications and substances caused the reaction and what the specific reaction involved (i.e., rash, hives, edema, difficulty breathing, mental status changes). A history of coughing should be established as well.

The **review of systems** is a list of questions, arranged by organ system, that provides a systematic overview of the child's health. **Box 12-1** lists the areas reviewed.

BOX 12-1 Review of Systems

- General: Weight gain or loss, fatigue, weakness, fever or chills
- Skin: Changes in skin, hair, or nails; itching; rashes; sores; bumps; bruises
- Head: Trauma, headache location, frequency of pain, nausea, vomiting, visual changes
- Eyes: Changes in vision, glasses, contact lenses, blurred vision, tearing, itchiness
- Ears: Infections/treatment, pressure equalization tubes, discharge, vertigo, changes in hearing, hearing screen results
- Nose/Sinuses: Rhinorrhea, congestion, sneezing, itching, allergies, epistaxis
- Mouth/Throat/Neck: Hoarseness, sore throat, *Streptococcus* infections ("strep throat"), dental health, neck swelling
- Cardiac: Murmurs, congenital heart disease, hypertension, palpitations, dyspnea on exertion, edema
- Respiratory: Wheezing, asthma, pneumonia, bronchitis, tuberculosis, cough, sputum production, hemoptysis, shortness of breath
- Gastrointestinal: Appetite, nausea, vomiting, diarrhea, constipation, dysphagia, frequency/change in bowel movements, bleeding, abdominal pain
- Urinary: Frequency (number of wet diapers per day), urgency, hesitancy, polyuria, dysuria, hematuria, nocturia, incontinence, infection, bladder, kidney stones

---

Family and Social History

The family and social history should include information relevant to the health and resources of family members. Family history includes the ages, general health, and cause of death for first-degree relatives, including parents and siblings. The clinician should specifically ask about diabetes, heart disease, stroke, cancer, hypertension, bleeding disorders, asthma, arthritis, tuberculosis, epilepsy, congenital anomalies, chromosomal problems, and mental illness. If any of these are present, age of onset should be included. The social history includes current or highest attained level of education, daycare attendance, living accommodations, persons/pets in the home, and exposure to secondhand tobacco smoke. It is also necessary to ask about the availability of food, electricity, and running water.

Sensitive questions should be asked at the end of the history, taking time to allow for rapport to be established. Older children and teens should be asked about their use of tobacco, alcohol, and illicit drugs, including the type, amount, frequency, duration, any reactions, and previous treatment attempts. Sexual history and risk-taking behaviors should also be assessed.

Physical Assessment

The anatomy of the infant and child contributes significantly to their vulnerability to airway compromise and development of respiratory distress. Infants and toddlers have larger heads with relatively small mouths and large tongues. They also have a floppy epiglottis and narrow airways. Infants are obligatory nose breathers for the first several months of life, and when their nares are obstructed they do not have the reflex to open and breath through their mouths. Newborns have a highly compliant chest wall, making the chest wall suck in paradoxically when the abdomen expands. The ribs in infants and young children are more horizontally oriented, which lessens the intercostal muscles' ability to lift the rib cage, especially when lying flat on the back. The intercostal muscles do not reach full development until school age. Although these are normal characteristics of the child, they can greatly impact the symptoms that appear when the child develops respiratory distress.

Using a systematic approach to physical assessment will ensure a thorough review of all pertinent systems. One approach is to assess the child from head to toe. This begins with a general assessment of hygiene, mental status, and how the child interacts with the environment and caregivers.

Head and Neck

Visual inspection of the head and neck begins with assessing the shape of the head for symmetry. The nares should be patent with moist mucous membranes; if drainage is present, the color and consistency should be noted. **Nasal flaring** is the outward movement or widening of nostrils with inspiratory effort. **Head bobbing** occurs when the sternocleidomastoid muscles, which are also used to stabilize the head, are being used to assist with respiration. Both head bobbing and nasal flaring are signs of increased respiratory effort and accessory muscle use. Facial anomalies can be representative of a specific disease or condition—for example, allergic facies is often seen in the child with asthma.

Drooling or the inability to swallow secretions or liquids can indicate swallowing disorders. It can also be indicative of an impairment or obstruction of the upper airway, either by the presence of a foreign body or swelling within the airway. If a child appears to be in respiratory distress and is drooling, a peritonsillar abscess or epiglottitis could be present. Both can present in this manner and are considered a medical emergency requiring immediate intervention by a specialist.[7] In the normal exam, the lips and mouth are moist. Tooth eruption pattern, cavities, and dentition should be noted, as they are good indicators of overall care and hygiene. The oropharynx should be clear and pink, and the color and consistency of any drainage should be noted.

The trachea should be palpated to determine mobility and position. Deviation of the trachea can indicate a tension pneumothorax or thoracic mass, in which case the trachea will be deviated in the direction opposite the affected lung. Lymph nodes in the neck should be palpated. Crepitations in the neck area may suggest an air leak.

Chest

Inspection of the chest begins with noting the shape and size of the chest wall. A barrel chest indicates air trapping and can be associated with advanced or severe cases of asthma, cystic fibrosis, bronchiectasis, and bronchopulmonary dysplasia. Chest malformations should be noted. The most common is **pectus excavatum**, often referred to as funnel chest: The chest has a sunken appearance and remains sunken even during inhalation. **Pectus carinatum**, also known as pigeon chest, is a condition in which the sternum and rib cartilage protrude from the chest. The vertebrae should be examined for vertebral deformities, most notably **kyphosis**, **scoliosis**, and **kyphoscoliosis**. When these are severe, the rib cage is deformed as well, resulting in restrictive lung disease. The chest should also be inspected both anteriorly and posteriorly for symmetry and expansion. Asymmetrical chest expansion is abnormal and can be due to unilateral lung or pleural disease.

Visual inspection includes evaluation of the respiratory rate and pattern. Although the respiratory rate is an important indicator of pulmonary function, it varies widely based on the child's age and activity level. It is higher in infants, but by adolescence it is the same as an adult. Crying, fever, and increased metabolic rate can raise a child's respiratory rate. Normal values are listed in **Table 12-1**. A child who presents with a sustained respiratory rate over 60 breaths per minute is at risk of tiring, resulting in respiratory failure. A low respiratory rate is also concerning, as it may indicate that the respiratory muscles are becoming fatigued and that, without appropriate intervention, respiratory failure is imminent. Apnea, a pause in breathing lasting more than 20 seconds, requires further investigation. It can be caused by respiratory fatigue, upper airway obstructions, head trauma, narcotic or sedating medications, and infections.

The rate, depth, rhythm, and character of breaths determine the pattern of breathing, which can give important clues to specific etiologies. Note the respiratory rate and movement of the diaphragm and chest wall with quiet breathing and with stronger respiratory effort. Certain illnesses or injuries can cause changes in the breathing pattern. **Table 12-2** describes abnormal breathing patterns that may occur in children.

Assessing the work of breathing includes looking for abdominal or accessory muscle use and the presence of retractions. Use of accessory muscles is an important measure of respiratory distress in children—in general, the greater the degree of accessory muscle use, the greater the degree of distress. **Retractions** are a "sucking in" of the skin in areas overlying the lungs. Retractions should be qualified as mild, moderate, or severe and should be further identified by their location, as described in **Table 12-3**. Severe retractions occurring in multiple locations indicates significant respiratory distress. **Table 12-4** lists findings that indicate both early and late signs of respiratory distress.

TABLE 12-1
Average Respiratory Rates and Heart Rates in Children

Age	<1 year	1–2 years	3–5 years	5–12 years	>12 years
Respiratory rate	30–60	25–40	22–34	18–30	12–16
Heart rate	110–160	100–150	90–140	80–120	60–100

Data from Pediatric Advanced Life Support Manual, American Heart Association. 2015.

TABLE 12-2
Abnormal Breathing Patterns

Pattern	Definition	Causes in Children
Abdominal/paradoxical breathing	An inward motion of the abdomen as the chest wall moves inward during inhalation; asynchrony between the rib cage and abdomen, creating a seesaw-type motion	• Poor muscle tone • Respiratory muscle fatigue • Chest trauma • Multiple rib fractures
Agonal respirations	A pattern of irregular, shallow, and very slow gasping inspirations followed by irregular pauses of apnea	• Cerebral ischemia • Severe hypoxia/anoxia • Cardiac arrest
Apneustic respirations	A prolonged inspiratory phase followed by a prolonged expiratory phase or apnea	• Hypoxic-ischemic injury • Brainstem lesion
Ataxic respirations	Completely irregular breathing frequency and tidal volume with irregular pauses and increasing episodes of apnea	• Head trauma • Stroke • Cerebral palsy • Brain tumor
Biot's breathing	Erratic respiratory pattern with clusters of rapid, tidal volume breaths followed by periods of apnea	• Head trauma • Brainstem lesion • Cervical spine injury
Cheyne-Stokes respirations	Shallow-deep-shallow breathing pattern in which tidal volume begins shallow and progressively increases and then becomes shallow again, followed by apnea, then the cycle starts over	• Stroke • Traumatic brain injury • Brain tumor • Carbon monoxide poisoning • Toxic metabolic encephalopathy
Kussmaul's respirations	Hyperventilation characterized by a consistently labored and increased rate and depth of breathing over a prolonged period	• Severe metabolic acidosis, most often diabetic ketoacidosis

TABLE 12-3
Retractions in the Pediatric Patient

Retraction	Location
Supraclavicular	Directly above the clavicles
Suprasternal	Middle of the neck, just above the sternum
Substernal	Below the end of the sternum
Intercostal	Between the ribs
Subcostal	Below the rib cage

TABLE 12-4
Signs of Respiratory Distress

Early Signs
Tachypnea
Nasal flaring
Head bobbing
Tracheal tug
Grunting on exhalation
Retractions
Prolonged expiratory phase
Stridor
Wheezing
Diminished air entry

Late Signs
Cyanosis
Bradycardia
Inaudible air entry
Apnea/irregular respirations
Changes in level of consciousness

Upon auscultation of the chest, breath sounds should be clear and heard bilaterally with equal intensity. Breath sounds and noisy breathing can be difficult to interpret in the very young child (**Table 12-5**). Sounds vary from fine, high-pitched to low and coarse, depending on the site and nature of the abnormality. A child's chest wall is very thin, making it easy for breath sounds to be transmitted over all lung fields, which is why it can be difficult to determine exactly where in the chest lung sounds are originating. **Box 12-2** describes the procedure used to effectively auscultate breath sounds in a child.

Extremities

Inspection of the child's skin and extremities can add valuable information to the respiratory assessment. The skin should be assessed for birthmarks, rashes, and petechiae. If scars are present, the source should be

TABLE 12-5
Breath Sounds in the Pediatric Patient

Sound	Definition	Common Causes in Children
Wheeze	Continuous musical sounds that typically occur during a prolonged expiratory phase but can occur during inspiration; caused by the air passing rapidly through narrowed airways	• Bronchiolitis • Asthma • Pneumonia • Gastroesophageal reflux • Cystic fibrosis • Foreign body aspiration • Bronchomalacia
Stridor	High-pitched musical sound heard during inspiration or expiration; caused by airway obstruction or narrowing below the level of the larynx	• Laryngotracheobronchitis • Epiglottitis • Laryngomalacia • Tracheitis • Vocal cord paralysis • Subglottic stenosis • Lesions of the larynx • Vascular ring • Foreign body aspiration
Stertor	Low-pitched, wet rattling sound similar to snoring heard during inspiration and while sleeping; caused by airway obstruction or narrowing above the level of the larynx	• Upper airway obstruction • Adenoid hypertrophy • Tonsillar hypertrophy
Crackles	Discontinuous, nonmusical popping sounds heard during inspiration or expiration; caused by air moving through airways narrowed by fluid or mucus	• Pneumonia • Cystic fibrosis • Pulmonary edema • Bronchiolitis • Bronchiectasis • Bronchitis

BOX 12-2 Auscultation of the Pediatric Patient

1. Clear the nasal passages, if needed, to prevent nasal sounds from distorting breath sounds.

2. Perform auscultation on a bare chest, not over clothing.

3. Hold the diaphragm of the pediatric stethoscope against the child's chest.

4. Listen to breath sounds, moving the stethoscope from side to side of the chest, comparing each area. Each lobe of both lungs should be auscultated, listening separately to inspiration and expiration.

5. Listen to breath sounds for at least one full inspiration and expiration in all areas of the chest. You may need to listen longer to differentiate what you are hearing.

determined, as patterns of scars may be suggestive of abuse. Skin color should be noted, as cyanosis, mottling, and pallor are all cause for concern. Examination of the nail beds is necessary to determine the presence of peripheral cyanosis and to assess capillary refill. The fingers and toes are examined for edema and digital clubbing.

The presence of **digital clubbing** strongly suggests a chronic respiratory condition, most likely cystic fibrosis or bronchiectasis. It is also present in children who have certain congenital cardiac defects in which there has been long-term hypoxia.[8] Further evaluation is warranted if clubbing is present.

Summary

The respiratory assessment of a child is different from that of an adult. A thorough, systematic approach to assessment of a child's respiratory status can yield valuable information needed to accurately diagnose and provide effective care. Recognizing respiratory distress while it is in the early stages can help to prevent respiratory failure or cardiac collapse from occurring. When assessing a child's respiratory status, it is important to establish a baseline to compare progress or deterioration against. In order to recognize what is abnormal, it is necessary to be aware of what is normal, keeping in mind that children who have a history of preterm birth or those who have chronic disorders often have a baseline that is not at the normal level.

Case Study 1

A 2-year-old boy presents to the emergency department with a 3-day history of cold symptoms and a CC of waking in the night with trouble breathing. Upon arrival the paramedics report a respiratory rate of 48 breaths per minute, a heart rate of 160 beats per minute, a blood pressure of 60/40 mm Hg, and an oxygen saturation of 90%. A simple oxygen mask with 6 L/min flow is in place. Evaluation of the child begins using the Pediatric Assessment Triangle. The child is awake, alert, and pink in color but is easily agitated. Assessment of work of breathing reveals moderate to severe suprasternal, substernal, and intercostal retractions, high-pitched stridor when upset, and nasal flaring. Additional assessment determines that the child's trachea is midline and chest expansion is symmetrical. Based on the assessment category, treatment should be quickly initiated, including increasing the level of supplemental oxygen to maintain an oxygen saturation >92%, corticosteroids to reduce inflammation, and nebulized racemic epinephrine to treat upper airway obstruction or narrowing.

1. **What is the purpose of the PAT and how quickly should it be performed?**
2. **Which of the vital signs are outside normal limits for this child's age?**
3. **What components of the respiratory examination are suggestive of obstruction or narrowing of the upper airway?**

Case Study 2

A 35-day-old female presents to the emergency department with a 1-day history of slow breathing and decreased feeding. She was well the previous day, breastfeeding 5 to 6 times per day and has had 6 to 8 wet diapers daily. She has been constipated since birth, passing 1 stool every 4 days, and, at the time of presentation, she had not had a bowel movement in 6 days. She was a term infant born via spontaneous vaginal delivery with Apgar scores of 7 at 1 minute and 9 at 5 minutes. The infant is afebrile, with a heart rate of 154 beats per minute, respiratory rate of 20 breaths per minute, blood pressure of 70/50 mm Hg in the right upper extremity, and oxygen saturation of 89% on room air. Her length, weight, and head circumference are in the 60th percentile. Femoral pulses are palpable with capillary refill of 2 seconds. Respiratory examination reveals grunting on exhalation and slow, shallow, and irregular breathing, without wheezing or retractions. Her pupils are small but reactive. The remainder of the physical examination, including cardiac assessment, is normal.

1. **What components of the examination are considered normal for this infant?**
2. **What components of the evaluation indicate respiratory distress?**
3. **What immediate interventions does this infant need?**

References

1. Centers for Disease Control and Prevention. (2014, April 29). Annual number and percent distribution of ambulatory care visits by setting type according to diagnosis group: United States 2009-2010. http://www.cdc.gov/nchs/fastats/physician-visits.htm. Updated April 29, 2014. Accessed February 23, 2018.

2. National Heart, Lung, and Blood Institute. Statistics. 2012. http://www.nhlbi.nih.gov/about/documents/factbook/2012/chapter4. Accessed February 9, 2018.

3. Booth JS, Shirk A, Windle ML. (2014, February 6). Pediatric resuscitation technique. http://emedicine.medscape.com/article/1948389-technique#c2. Updated February 6, 2014. Accessed February 23, 2018.

4. Horeczko T, Eneiquez B, McGrath NE, et al. The pediatric assessment triangle: accuracy of its application by nurses in the triage of children. *J Emerg Nurs*. 2013;39:182-189.

5. Cohen-Cole SA. *The Medical Interview: The Tree-Function Approach*. St. Louis, MO: Mosby Year Book; 1991.

6. Lazare A, Putnam SM, Lipkin M Jr. Three functions of the medical interview. In: Lipkin M Jr, Putnam SM, Lazare A, et al., eds. *The Medical Interview: Clinical Care, Education, and Research*. New York, NY: Springer-Verlag; 1995:6.

7. Savoy NB. Differentiating stridor in children at triage: it's not always croup. *J Emerg Nurs*. 2005;31:503-505.

8. Myers KA, Farquhar DR. The rational clinical examination. Does this patient have clubbing? *JAMA*. 2001;286:341-347.

13

Resuscitation and Stabilization of the Child

Steven Sittig

Teresa A. Volsko

OUTLINE

OBJECTIVES

1. Discuss the components of an initial assessment of the pediatric patient.
2. Define the Pediatric Assessment Triangle.
3. List the symptoms of respiratory distress.
4. Explain the methods to assess neurologic status.
5. Describe vascular access techniques.
6. Describe airway management techniques.
7. List and describe the treatment options for common cardiac arrhythmias.
8. List the essential elements of postresuscitation care.

KEY TERMS

alert verbal painful unresponsiveness (AVPU) algorithm
Broselow tape
capillary refill
central venous line (CVL)
Glasgow Coma Scale (GCS)
grunting

intraosseous (IO) needle
Pediatric Assessment Triangle (PAT)
peripheral IV
primary assessment
pulse pressure
stridor

Introduction

There is an adage that children are like little adults. The truth, however, is quite the contrary. The pediatric population is widely varied in physical size, stages of development and vital signs, and care. A pediatric patient may range from a small infant to a mature teenager. To administer emergency medical treatment based on a "small adult" could lead to ineffective resuscitation and the potential for harm. In 1983, the American Heart Association (AHA) convened a national conference on pediatric resuscitation to develop Cardiopulmonary Resuscitation (CPR) and Emergency Cardiac Care Guidelines for pediatric and neonatal patients. It was in 1988 that the AHA, along with the American Academy of Pediatrics, introduced several pediatric emergency care courses: pediatric basic life support, pediatric advanced life support (PALS), and neonatal resuscitation program (NRP).

Pediatric resuscitation guidelines are intended to address the unique needs of newborn, infants, and children; however, most recommendations are based on expert consensus, studies of pediatric animal models, or extrapolation from adult or neonatal data, as in the case of hypothermia. Prior to the development of the aforementioned courses, pediatric resuscitation was based on modified adult algorithms.[1] The modified adult algorithms did not serve the pediatric population well because the underlying cause of cardiopulmonary arrest is very different in infants and children as compared to adults. The most common cause of cardiopulmonary arrest in adults is underlying coronary artery disease, which often develops into sudden ventricular fibrillation cardiac arrest. This is why early defibrillation in adult cardiac arrest leads to improved survival. The primary cause of pediatric cardiorespiratory arrest, however, is significant hypoxia or circulatory shock as a result of respiratory failure.[2] Early recognition and treatment of respiratory failure, hypoxia, or prolonged shock can help avoid the need for pediatric resuscitation.

Assessment of the Pediatric Patient

In the initial assessment of the pediatric patient, clinicians likely will make quick determinations as to the severity of illness based on direct observation. The plan of care depends on the age of the child and the results of the clinician's assessment of the nature and severity of illness. The initial assessment of the respiratory system should include rate and depth of respirations, presence and severity of retractions, evaluation of inspiratory and expiratory effort, cough characteristics, and alertness.

Pediatric Assessment Triangle

A simple tool called the **Pediatric Assessment Triangle (PAT)** helps to rapidly assess a critically ill child

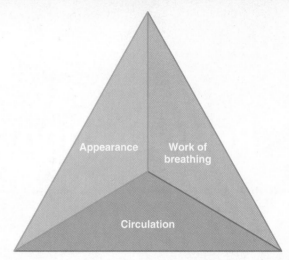

FIGURE 13-1 The PAT, an evaluation of three physiologic points to obtain a baseline assessment of the child, determine the severity of illness, and guide and monitor therapeutic interventions and patient response to therapy.

Used with permission of the American Academy of Pediatrics, Pediatric Education for Prehospital Professionals, © American Academy of Pediatrics, 2000.

(Figure 13-1). Considered an integral part of the general assessment of a sick child, this tool is incorporated into several pediatric emergency courses, including PALS, Pediatric Education for Prehospital Professionals, and Emergency Nursing Pediatric Course. The triangle is designed to be a quick and simple approach to evaluating a child based on visual and auditory clues.[3]

Use of the PAT provides a quick evaluation of the patient and is especially helpful when medical resources are limited. The PAT assists an experienced clinician in visually obtaining data to assess disease severity. It also guides the initial treatment, such as fluid administration and oxygen therapy. A portion of the patient assessment can be performed without such equipment as a stethoscope, pulse oximeter, or blood pressure or cardiac monitor. Rapid assessment, followed by early intervention with appropriate treatment, can avoid respiratory or cardiac arrest in the pediatric patient. The tool uses the acronym ABC to guide the assessment.

Assessing Appearance

The A of the assessment triangle evaluates the child's appearance. As noted in **Table 13-1**, a pediatric patient's appearance is helpful in quickly identifying if the child is very sick. Assessing a child's appearance will provide an indication of the adequacy of ventilation, perfusion to the brain, oxygenation, and central nervous system (CNS) function. For example, a toddler who lies quietly during routine care is an example of an abnormal activity assessment and is at risk for respiratory compromise. Assessment is likely the most sensitive parameter in determining the need for treatment and how the patient responds to initiated therapy.

TABLE 13-1
Signs and Symptoms Associated with Respiratory Compromise

Color	Cyanosis
	Pale
	Ashen/gray
Level of consciousness	Unresponsive to voice
	Diminished responsiveness to pain
	Unable to recognize parents
Activity	Limited extremity movement
	Listlessness
	Limp
Circulation	Capillary refill >2 seconds
	Extremities cool to touch
	Diminished peripheral pulses

TABLE 13-2
Normal Age-Based Values for Respiratory Rate

Description	Age	Breaths per Minute
Infant	Birth to 1 year	30–60
Toddler	1–2 years	25–40
Preschooler	3–5 years	22–34
School-age	6–12 years	18–30
Adolescent	12–18 years	12–16

Assessing Respirations and Characteristics of Breathing

The B of the assessment triangle evaluates the child's respirations and breathing characteristics. Evaluation of work of breathing encompasses the determination of airway patency as well as the child's oxygenation and ventilation status. An evaluation of mental status can provide valuable information about the child's ability to protect and maintain a patent airway. Children who are listless and/or do not respond in an age-appropriate manner when examined are at risk for airway and ventilatory compromise.

The chest wall of infants and small children is very compliant. Increases in airway resistance, and thus increased work of breathing, often manifest as the presence of suprasternal, intercostal, or even substernal retractions. In younger pediatric patients, nasal flaring may be noted as the child attempts to inspire maximal air with each breath; this may be a subtle sign but is indicative of a child in distress. The rate and depth of respirations are also important to note. Normal values for respiratory rate vary with age and are listed in **Table 13-2**.

The sounds an infant or child produces as they breathe can provide the clinician with valuable information. Just as adults perform pursed-lip breathing to open narrowed airways and/or increase functional residual capacity by creating positive end-expiratory pressure, infants often make a **grunting** noise. Grunting describes the sound an infant makes when expiring against a partially closed glottis. Grunting is not a normal finding;

rather, it is a compensatory mechanism to maximize gas exchange and is a hallmark sign of respiratory distress.

Stridor is the sound an infant or child produces on inspiration and is indicative of upper airway edema and/or obstruction. Stridor may be present following extubation or associated with an infectious process or aspiration of a foreign body. Wheezing may be audible as well; this may be present on inspiration or expiration and is typically due to bronchospasm, secretions, or inflammation of the lower airways. Auscultation of breath sounds follows visual assessment of the patient's breathing. The lateral neck and lungs are assessed for the presence and symmetry of air entry as well as occurrence of adventitious breath sounds.

Assessing Circulation

The C of the assessment triangle represents circulation. Rapid assessment of the systemic perfusion is an essential part of pediatric resuscitation. It is accomplished by evaluating mental status, capillary refill, pulses, and blood pressure. The presence and character or volume of peripheral pulses provides an indication of systemic vascular resistance and the degree of shunting that is necessary to maintain blood pressure and end-organ perfusion.[4]

Capillary refill is a valuable initial physiologic parameter. The finger should be lifted slightly above the level of the heart to assure assessment of arteriolar capillary refill and not venous stasis. Light pressure is applied to blanch the fingernail bed. The pressure is released, and the amount of time until color returns is measured. Capillary refill is normal if color returns in less than 2 seconds. Volume depletion or hypotension can cause a delay in capillary refill of more than 3 seconds.[4]

Unfortunately, CPR is often performed poorly in both in-hospital and out-of-hospital settings. More than one-quarter of children requiring resuscitation during hospitalization survive following a cardiac arrest, and 5% to 10% survive following cardiopulmonary arrest and resuscitation out of the hospital setting.[1] This exemplifies the importance of performing high-quality CPR and the link between effective resuscitative efforts and positive patient outcomes. It is reasonable to assume that outcomes can be improved by a greater emphasis on providing prompt, high-quality CPR.[5] Respiratory failure and shock are the most common causes of pediatric cardiopulmonary arrest. Early recognition of these conditions and prompt intervention are key to preventing cardiopulmonary arrest in infants and children. Cardiac arrest in adults is most likely due to underlying cardiac dysrhythmias, the most common of which is ventricular fibrillation, but ventricular fibrillation was found to be present in only 8% of children 1 to 12 years of age and in about one-third of pediatric patients between the ages of 13 and 18 years.[5] Due to the low incidence of shockable dysrhythmias, early, effective CPR is more effective than interrupting CPR for rhythm analysis with a defibrillator in infants and small children.[5]

Primary Assessment

Primary assessment is a systematic approach to determine what life-threatening conditions may exist. The assessment is based on the mnemonic ABCDE, which is as follows:

> A: Airway
> B: Breathing
> C: Circulation
> D: Disability
> E: Exposure

Airway

The tried-and-true assessment airway patency is to "look, listen, and feel" for effective ventilation. This refers to looking at the child's chest for visible movement, as rise and fall of the chest indicates respiratory effort; listening for airflow; and feeling air movement around the child's nose and mouth to evaluate for the presence of air movement. Chest rise and fall without evidence of airflow indicates airway obstruction. Abnormal sounds, such as wheezing, stridor, and snoring, provide the clinician with important information about the condition of the upper and conducting airways. Impaired respiratory effort and ineffective ventilation can result in hypoxemia and hypercapnia. If uncorrected, respiratory acidosis ensues; this can impair cardiac function and lead to cardiac arrest.

Breathing

Assessment of the breathing pattern focuses on how effective the patient is ventilating and oxygenating. Inspect the face, neck, and chest for signs of impaired respiratory mechanics, including nasal flaring, chest wall retractions, or asynchronous breathing. Asynchronous breathing, or seesaw respirations, occurs when the chest and abdomen do not rise and fall together during inspiration and expiration. Instead, the chest rises and the abdomen falls during inspiration while the chest falls and the abdomen rises during expiration, giving a seesaw-like appearance during breathing. This is a hallmark sign of respiratory distress in infants and small children.

One should also note if the respiratory rate is within normal limits for the child's age. Bradypnea is an ominous late sign in the pathway to respiratory arrest. Use of pulse oximetry can determine if hypoxemia is present. Low oxygen saturation, less than 94%, can be corrected with supplemental oxygen. However, it is important for the clinician to collectively evaluate the infant's or child's respiratory status. An infant or child presenting with paradoxical or seesaw breathing and profound tachypnea may require ventilatory support.

Circulation

Assessment of circulation is based on an evaluation of pulse strength, capillary refill, heart rate, skin color, and perfusion. Current AHA recommendations emphasize early initiation of CPR to minimize the time without cardiac flow and to reduce the risk for impaired neurologic function or death.

Pulses in healthy infants and children should be readily palpable under normal ambient temperature conditions at several locations, as shown in **Table 13-3**. Pulses may be more difficult to palpate in obese children or when ambient temperature is low.

Table 13-4 lists normal ranges for heart rate, which are very much age dependent. Typically, the heart rate for a child who is sleeping is approximately 10% lower than the child's awake rate. Heart rates may be higher than normal in response to a variety of conditions, from fairly benign to very serious. Children present with tachycardia in response to pain, anxiety, fever, hypoxemia, hypercapnia, hypovolemia, shock, or an underlying cardiac condition. Very rapid heart rates are typically suggestive of an underlying cardiac condition, and they impair diastolic filling of the atria and ventricles, contribute to low stroke volume, and increase myocardial oxygen demand. Myocardial perfusion is reduced with profound tachycardia because of the combination of increased oxygen demand to the myocardium and reduced left ventricular filling pressures from a shortened diastole.

Pulse pressure is the difference between the systolic and diastolic blood pressures. A narrow pulse pressure occurs when cardiac output is low and there is an increase in systemic vascular resistance.

Disability

A patient's appearance is a sensitive determinant in assessing their need for intervention. The **Glasgow Coma Scale (GCS)** is the most frequently used tool to

TABLE 13-3
Locations of Common Pulses That Can Be Palpated in Healthy Infants and Children

Pulse	Description of the Location	Illustration of the Location
Carotid	On either side of the front of the neck, just below the angle of the jaw	
Brachial	Along the front side of the elbow, in the crease or the antecubital fossa	
Radial	Along the inside surface of the wrist, just below the thumb	
Femoral	In the groin area, below the inguinal ligament and about midway between symphysis pubis and anterior superior iliac spine	 Femoral artery Femoral vein Inguinal ligament

(continued)

TABLE 13-3
Locations of Common Pulses That Can Be Palpated in Healthy Infants and Children (*Continued*)

Pulse	Description of the Location	Illustration of the Location
Posterior tibial	Along the medial portion of the ankle, midway between the posterior border of the medial malleolus and the Achilles tendon	
Dorsalis pedis	Instep of the foot	

TABLE 13-4
Normal Age-Based Values for Heart Rate

Description	Age	Beats per Minute
Infant	Birth to 1 year	110–160
Toddler	1–2 years	100–150
Preschooler	3–5 years	90–140
School-age	6–12 years	80–120
Adolescent	12–18 years	60–100

assess the neurologic status of the pediatric patient. The scale assesses three behaviors: eye opening, verbal response, and motor response.[6] An individual with normal neurologic status can have a maximum score of 15.[7] Modifications to this scale allow it to be applicable to infants, as noted in **Table 13-5**.[8] Scores of less than 8 are associated with the potential for airway compromise and suggest the need for intubation.[9]

The **alert verbal painful unresponsiveness (AVPU) algorithm** is a simpler method of assessing level of consciousness during a neurologic assessment (**Figure 13-2**). This tool was introduced to facilitate rapid neurologic assessment of trauma patients and is based on the level of responsiveness to various types of stimuli.[10] The AVPU is comparable to GCS in assessing level of consciousness and/or deterioration in the mental status of infants and children.[11]

Exposure

Exposure is the final element in a primary assessment series. It serves as a reminder that it is important to remove clothing to conduct a thorough physical exam. Care must be taken to keep the infant or child warm and avoid causing hypothermia, as hypothermia may alter such physical findings as capillary refill and palpating pulses. It is important to be mindful of modesty when removing clothing from adolescent patients.

Pediatric Shock

Cardiac arrest in children is most likely due to prolonged hypoxia and/or hypercarbia from respiratory failure or shock. The PAT is a helpful tool in planning interventions for a critically ill child, and respiratory failure must be quickly addressed and treated to prevent circulatory collapse. Pediatric shock is considered when there is inadequate blood flow and delivery of oxygen to meet tissues' metabolic demands. Shock may present as compensated or uncompensated. In either presentation, no one sign or symptom will confirm the

TABLE 13-5
Glasgow Coma Scale

Behavior	Response	Score	Infant Response Modifications
Eye opening	Spontaneously	4	Spontaneously
	To speech	3	To speech (shouting)
	To pain	2	To pain
	No response	1	No response
Verbal response	Oriented to person, place, and time	5	Babbles, coos appropriately
	Confused	4	Irritable cry
	Inappropriate words	3	Cries in response to pain
	Incomprehensible sounds	2	Moans in response to pain
	No response	1	No response
Motor response	Obeys commands	6	Purposeful movements
	Moves to localized pain	5	Withdraws to touch
	Flexion withdrawal from pain	4	Flexion withdrawal from pain
	Abnormal flexion (decorticate)	3	Abnormal flexion (decorticate)
	Abnormal extension (decerbrate)	2	Abnormal extension (decerbrate)
	No response	1	No response
Interpretation		Total Score	
Best response		15	
Decreased/impaired level of consciousness		<8	
Unresponsive		3	

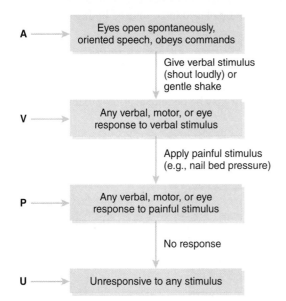

FIGURE 13-2 The alert verbal painful unresponsiveness algorithm.

Reprinted from Kelly CA, Upex A, Bateman N, Comparison of Consciousness Level Assessment in the Poisoned Patient Using the Alert/Verbal/Painful/Unresponsive Scale and the Glasgow Coma Scale. *Annuals of Emergency Medicine.* 2004; 44(2);108-113, with permission from Elsevier.

diagnosis. Infants and children will attempt to maintain blood pressure by increasing heart rate, contractility, and vascular tone. An infant or child presenting in compensated shock will have tachycardia, cool extremities, prolonged capillary refill, weak peripheral pulses compared to central pulses, and normal blood pressure. As the shock state progresses, compensatory mechanisms begin to fail and manifest as signs of inadequate end-organ perfusion. This will result in deterioration of mental status, reduction in urine output, hypotension, apnea, and a metabolic acidotic state. Establishing and maintaining a secure airway, obtaining vascular access, and providing ventilatory and cardiovascular support are essential to reducing morbidity and mortality associated with shock.

Vascular Access

Vascular access should be established as soon as possible for infants and children with suspected respiratory failure and/or shock. However, when a pediatric patient presents with respiratory or cardiopulmonary arrest, vascular access should be obtained after the airway is secured and adequate breathing, gas exchange, and circulation are established. The indication for and duration of vascular access should be carefully considered before placement is attempted to help minimize the number of attempts and the trauma the child and family may experience.

Peripheral Vein Access

In most situations, the insertion of a **peripheral IV** line (peripheral intravenous line) occurs quickly, easily, and with minimal complications. There are limitations to the use of peripheral IVs: Small-bore catheters can be easily occluded; there is the potential for infiltration of IV fluids and/or medications, which may cause local tissue damage;[12] and certain medications, especially antibiotics, are irritating to small veins.

Peripheral IVs are typically placed in the dorsal veins of the hands for toddlers and older children and the dorsal veins of the foot for infants. Peripheral IV insertion in the dorsal veins of the foot should be avoided in toddlers and older children because catheter insertion is more painful and can become easily dislodged. Superficial scalp veins (frontal, superficial temporal, posterior auricular, and occipital veins) are also convenient access

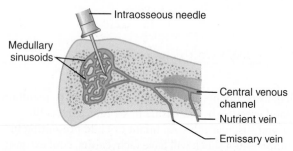

FIGURE 13-3 An illustration of the IO needle entering the bone marrow.

points for infants. However, prior to insertion, it is necessary to shave surrounding hair. It is also important to avoid inadvertent cannulation of the temporal artery or one of its branches when scalp veins are used.

Intraosseous Access

Although acceptable, attempting peripheral IV access may be difficult when end-organ perfusion is inadequate. In this situation, placement of an **intraosseous (IO) needle** can effectively and safely establish a route for fluid resuscitation and/or medication administration. IO access is the recommended vascular access technique to initiate treatment for decompensated shock or during cardiopulmonary arrest.[13]

IO access is accomplished by placing the needle into the noncollapsible network of veins in the medullary sinuses within the bone marrow, as shown in **Figure 13-3**. This venous network drains directly into the central venous circulation and allows for rapid infusion and almost immediate absorption of a variety of drugs. Because the bore of the IO needle is large, crystalloid solutions and medications used for cardiopulmonary resuscitation may be administered.[14] The large-bore needle also enables blood products to be given without lysing red blood cells.[14]

Figure 13-4 shows the three most frequently used sites for IO insertion: the distal femur and the proximal and distal tibia. The proximal tibia is the primary choice for IO insertion in infants and small children while the distal femur and tibia are more commonly accessed in older children and adolescents.[15] Other insertion sites used in older children include the sternum and distal radius. It is important to assess the access site, as an IO should not be placed in an injured limb.

Central Venous Line Placement

A **central venous line (CVL)** is not recommended as a form of initial vascular access in an emergency. Although it may be beneficial after initial resuscitation,

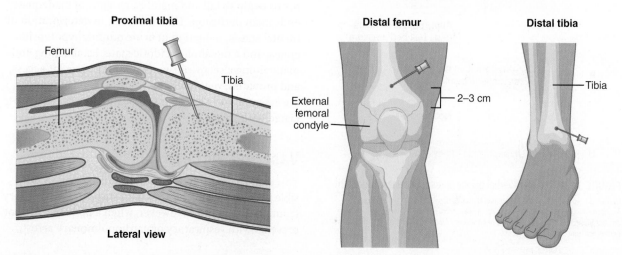

FIGURE 13-4 An illustration of the three most frequently used sites for IO insertion.

the placement of a CVL is time consuming and could significantly delay management of life-threatening conditions. A CVL is preferred in children who require long-term IV access but in whom peripheral access could not be obtained. It may be inserted into the femoral, subclavian, or internal jugular vein; placement of a CVL in the subclavian vein affords the patient the greatest mobility while the internal jugular vein can be cannulated by a cut-down procedure or percutaneous access and is amenable to ultrasound-guided placement.

During cardiopulmonary resuscitation, there may be occasions where no form of vascular access can be obtained in a timely manner. Some resuscitation medications may be administered by endotracheal instillation. The mnemonic LEAN can be used to remember the four medications that can be delivered by endotracheal instillation: lidocaine, epinephrine, atropine, and naloxone. This is not a preferred route of administration, however, because absorption varies widely.

Airway Management

Securing and maintaining a patient airway is a key component in the care of critically ill children. Airway management and effective ventilatory support may prevent circulatory collapse.

Bag-Mask Ventilation

Bag-mask ventilation is an effective, safe method for providing assisted ventilation during respiratory arrest. The literature reports that bag-mask ventilation is an alternative to endotracheal tube ventilation for short periods during prehospital resuscitation in infants and children.[16]

Effective bag-mask ventilation begins with selecting the correct-size mask. The mask should cover the mouth and nose without extending over the chin or putting pressure on the eyes, as illustrated in **Figure 13-5**.

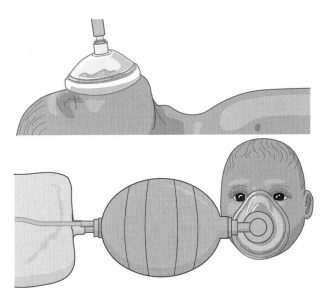

FIGURE 13-5 Illustration of correct placement of the mask during bag-mask ventilation.

A rolled towel under the shoulders of children younger than 2 years and a towel under the head of children aged 2 to 5 years helps to keep the airway open and provides an optimal position for intubation. The chest will rise during manual ventilation when the airway is patent and a mask-to-face seal is obtained. Ventilating with excessive pressure increases the risk of gastric insufflation, which can lead to emesis and aspiration. Ventilating with excessive volume and/or pressure contributes to lung injury.

Intubation

In the prehospital setting, emergent intubation may be required when transport to a tertiary care center is lengthy or the infant/child is at risk for airway obstruction from airway edema (i.e., burns to the face and neck) or airway trauma. Infants and children with impending respiratory failure, decompensated shock, CNS depression, rapid deterioration of the level of consciousness, severe neuromuscular weakness, or lack of airway protection require intubation and assisted ventilation.

Prior to intubation, it is important to assemble the airway equipment needed and to ensure that the equipment is working properly. **Table 13-6** lists the necessary equipment. Before attempting intubation, suction the mouth and hypopharynx to clear secretions that may obscure the view of the vocal cords and reduce the likelihood for aspiration. Hypnotics and sedatives are helpful and may be necessary when a child in need of intubation is awake and alert. Paralytics may also be administered; however, this medication should never be given without the use of a sedative or hypnotic. **Table 13-7** provides a list of medications commonly administered prior to intubation.

Assessing ETT Placement by Carbon Dioxide Monitoring

Capnography confirms tracheal intubation rapidly and reliably. The capnograph provides a numeric value for end-tidal carbon dioxide (CO_2) as well as a waveform, which is of diagnostic value. Colorimetric devices may also be used to confirm tracheal placement. These devices display a color change, typically from purple to yellow, when CO_2 is detected. However, there are conditions that can lead to false positive or false negative readings. Bag-mask ventilation often causes some CO_2 to enter the stomach. Care should be taken when interpreting a slight color change following intubation, which may occur with esophageal intubation. After a few manual ventilations, this color change will quickly disappear, suggesting esophageal intubation. If a capnograph is used to confirm tracheal tube placement and the esophagus is intubated, the device will display a low numeric value of CO_2, which will precipitously drop to near zero with subsequent manual ventilations. False negatives may also occur during cardiac arrest, where

TABLE 13-6
SOAPPIM Mnemonic for Equipment Required for Endotracheal Intubation

S	Suction	1. Assemble suction canister. 2. Set suction pressure to setting appropriate for age. 3. Test suction to verify proper working order. 4. Have tonsil tip and open suction catheters available and ready for use.
O	Oxygen source	1. Verify that there is a flow of gas from the oxygen source to the resuscitation device.
A	Airway(s)	1. ETT sized appropriately for age/size ([Internal diameter for children >2 years of age = Age in years + 4/16]). 2. ETT 0.5 mm smaller than age-appropriate size 3. Laryngoscopy equipment: laryngoscope blade(s) and handle and videolaryngoscope
P	Pharmacy	1. Pharmacologic agents used for rapid sequence intubation
P	Personnel	1. Staff skilled in intubation
I	Intravenous access	1. Peripheral, IO, or central access
M	Noninvasive monitors	1. Cardiorespiratory monitor 2. Noninvasive blood pressure monitoring device 3. Pulse oximeter 4. Colormetric CO_2 detector or capnograph

ETT = endotracheal tube

TABLE 13-7
Medications Commonly Administered Prior to Intubating an Alert and/or Awake Child

Classification	Medication	Dose	Onset (seconds)	Duration (minutes)	Advantages	Disadvantages
Sedatives and hypnotics	Ketamine	1–2 mg/kg/dose IV	45–60	10–20	Sympathomimetic actions Useful with intubation associated with acute severe asthma exacerbation and/or shock	May increase secretions
	Etomidate	0.2–0.4 mg/kg/dose IV	5–15	5–15	May maintain central perfusion pressure May decrease intracranial pressure Useful for patients with isolated head injury	May cause adrenal insufficiency Should not be used in patients with septic shock
	Propofol	1.5–3 mg/kg/dose IV	15–45	5–10	Quick onset Short duration	Decreases blood pressure Decreases central perfusion pressure
	Midazolam	0.3 mg/kg/dose IV	60–180	Dose dependent	Reliable	Contraindicated for shock and overdose associated with barbiturates, alcohol, narcotics, or other CNS depressants
Paralytics	Succinylcholine	1–2 mg/kg IV	30–60	3–5	Rapid onset Short duration of action	Contraindicated in patients with motor neuron disease, burns, or crush injuries
	Rocuronium	0.6–1.2 mg/kg IV	60–90	25–35	Rapid onset	Longer duration of action

there is no pulmonary blood flow and no CO_2 delivered to the alveoli.

Additionally, capnography can be used to determine the effectiveness of CPR. A higher CO_2 value indicates adequate pulmonary blood flow and therefore better cardiac output.[17]

Assessing ETT Placement by Auscultation

Other markers of tracheal intubation, although less reliable than CO_2 detection, include bilateral auscultation of breath sounds, auscultation over the abdomen, "fog" or condensation in the ETT during expiration, symmetric chest rise, and the absence of gastric insufflation. During auscultation, it is best to listen for breath sounds in the axilla and apices to determine if there is endobronchial intubation. Because breath sounds in children are transmitted, auscultating over the anterior chest is a less reliable method of assessing for equal aeration. Likewise, air entry into the stomach, especially in small children, can often be heard over the anterior chest and can fool the examiner. The gold standard for determining optimal positioning of the ETT is plain chest radiography, which should be obtained as soon as possible after tracheal intubation and stabilization of the infant or child.

Circulation

External cardiac compressions provide circulatory support in infants and children with cardiopulmonary collapse. Prior to beginning chest compressions, clinicians should assess the child for the presence of a pulse, which should not exceed 10 seconds. Begin chest compressions when no pulse can be palpated. High-quality chest compressions generate blood flow to vital organs and increase the likelihood of the return of spontaneous circulation. Gently placing the child on a firm, flat surface will help chest compression quality.

The AHA provides guidelines for the depth and rate of external cardiac compressions. The chest is compressed at a rate of at least 100 compressions per minute with sufficient force to depress at least one-third of the anterior-posterior diameter of the chest, or approximately 1½ inches (4 cm) for infants and 2 inches (5 cm) in children. During administration of compressions, it is important to allow complete chest recoil after each compression to allow the heart to refill with blood. It is also important to minimize interruptions of chest compressions. As illustrated in **Figure 13-6**, the heel of one hand can be used to compress the chest of small children while two fingers can be used to compress the chest of an infant.

To prevent deterioration in the quality of CPR, rescuers should switch every 2 minutes, even if the rescuer denies fatigue, as fatigue can lead to decreased rate and depth of compressions and chest wall recoil.[18] In order to maintain adequate cardiac output, when this switch occurs, compressions should resume in fewer than 5 seconds. When a cardiorespiratory monitor is available to analyze the patient's rhythm and a "shockable" rhythm determined, all care providers must stop care and stand clear of the patient as the defibrillation is delivered. Chest compressions should be reinitiated immediately following the shock and should be continued for 2 minutes before another pulse check and rhythm analysis.

Medication Administration

Knowledge of appropriate emergency medications prior to or during resuscitation is paramount. Dosage is based on the child's weight in kilograms. There are situations when obtaining an accurate weight may be difficult, and even experienced personnel may not be able to estimate it accurately.[19] A **Broselow tape** is a commercially available, color-coded, length-based tape that can be used to guide the proper dosage of emergency medications in the pediatric patient.[20] **Figure 13-7** illustrates the use of a Broselow tape.

In contrast to adults, who suffer cardiac arrest from underlying cardiac disease, pediatric patients' hearts

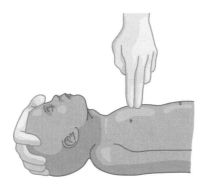
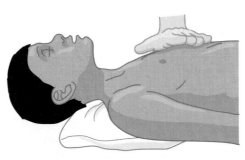

Infant   Child

FIGURE 13-6 Illustration of the hand position used to perform external cardiac compressions on an infant and child.

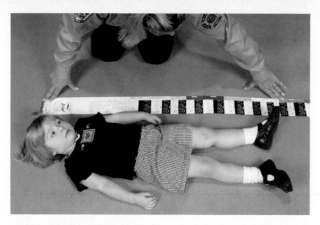

FIGURE 13-7 An illustration of the use of a Broselow tape to estimate height-based weight.

© Jones & Bartlett Learning. Courtesy of MIEMSS.

are for the most part physiologically normal unless a congenital cardiac defect exists. Pediatric heart rhythms can be classified into three easy-to-recognize categories: too fast, too slow, or absent. Many of the medications administered during resuscitation are rhythm dependent. It is also important to assess if the rhythm is stable or unstable. Cardiac output is dependent on heart rate and stroke volume. Cardiac arrhythmias typically affect either heart rate or stroke volume and include bradycardia, pulseless electromechanical activity, supraventricular tachycardia, pulseless ventricular tachycardia, and ventricular fibrillation. **Table 13-8** outlines the medication used to treat common arrhythmias. The AHA and AAP provide guidelines for pediatric resuscitation. Algorithms for the response to respiratory failure, shock, and arrhythmias are outlined in the PALS course.

TABLE 13-8
Common Arrhythmias and Medications Used in Their Treatment

Arrhythmia	Description	Common Causes	Effect of Cardiac Output	Effect on Stoke Volume	Medications Used for Unstable Arrhythmia	Defibrillation/ Synchronized Cardioversion Indicated
Bradycardia	Slower than normal heart rate for age	Vagal stimulation Hypoxia Hypercarbia	Decreases	No effect	Epinephrine Atropine	No
Pulseless electromechanical activity	An electrical signal is present on electrocardiogram, but there is no mechanical contraction of the heart in response to the electrical signal	Hypovolemia Hypoxia Hydrogen ion (acidosis) Hypo/hyperkalemia Hypoglycemia Hypothermia Toxins Tamponade Trauma Thrombosis Tension pneumothorax	Decreases	Decreases	Volume expanders Vasopressors Atropine (if bradycardia is displayed on the monitor)	No
Pulseless ventricular fibrillation	Uncoordinated contraction of the cardiac muscle of the ventricles in the heart, in which the ventricles quiver rather than contract	Degeneration of other malignant arrhythmias, such as ventricular tachycardia	Decreases	Decreases	Epinephrine Amiodarone (with repeated defibrillations) Lidocaine Magnesium	Yes: Defibrillation at 2 J/kg for the first shock, followed by 4 J/kg for subsequent shocks if defibrillation is not achieved with the first dose
Supraventricular tachycardia (SVT)	Fast heart rate involving the heart's upper and lower chambers	Reentrant electric pathway in the heart in which accessory pathway–mediated tachycardia involves two distinct pathways between the atria and ventricles, which create an electrical reentry circuit proceeding down the AV node and then up an accessory pathway outside the AV node	Decreases with unstable	Decreases with unstable	Valsalva maneuvers, such as ice to the face or breath holding and bearing down for stable SVT Adenosine should be administered before subsequent synchronized cardioversions	Yes: Synchronized cardioversion with starting dose of 0.5 J/kg

AV = atrioventricular

Postresuscitation Care

Stabilization is one of the most basic principles of postresuscitation care. The primary goals are to preserve neurologic function and to minimize or prevent end-organ damage. Reassessment and maintenance of cardiorespiratory needs is essential. Diagnostic testing will be dependent upon the condition that precipitated the cardiopulmonary collapse. Chest radiography is useful in confirming the position of the ETT, lines, and drains. Laboratory assessments of acid–base and electrolyte status are used to guide medical and ventilator management. Cardiovascular support includes securing more permanent IV access, especially if IO access was used to obtain blood for laboratory analysis and to administer medications during the resuscitation. Evaluation for fluid resuscitation, vasopressors, and/or inotropes is essential.

The direct care team should provide support to the patient's family during the resuscitation and throughout the postresuscitative care. Family presence during cardiopulmonary resuscitation and postresuscitation care is an important component of family-centered care. The literature reports that family presence during resuscitation and invasive procedures increases parental satisfaction with the care provided to their child and improves their coping mechanisms.[21]

Case Study

You are working in the emergency department when a 12-year-old boy presents with chest pain and shortness of breath. History includes 4 days of cold and cough symptoms. He has missed a week of school and states that he has no energy despite being inactive; the patient is an athlete, so he is generally very active. He has been well except for a viral infection during the winter and has no previous history of asthma or other health issues. His mother is very concerned about his breathing and pain. PAT assessment is completed with abnormal findings for appearance, breathing, and circulation. Vital signs are taken: heart rate is 135 beats per minute, respiratory rate is 45 breaths per minute, blood pressure is 90/65 mm Hg, temperature is 38.0°C, oxygen saturation is 89% on room air. Patient appearance is thin and pleasant in nature; he can speak in complete sentences without difficulty. He has tachypnea with mild retractions. He is slightly pale in color with dusky nail beds, capillary refill >2 seconds.

Initial assessment:

- A: Patent
- B: Intermittently shallow and rapid respiratory rate
- C: Pale; pulse rapid, thready, and weak
- D: Awake/alert, GCS 15
- E: No signs of injury

1. **What is your general impression of this patient?**

2. **What are your initial management priorities and important next actions?**

Oxygen by nonrebreathing mask at 12 L/minute was initiated. A cardiac monitor and an IV were placed, and blood was drawn for laboratory analysis. A chest radiograph revealed cardiomegaly and prominent vasculature. Laboratory studies were nonspecific. The echocardiogram revealed poor cardiac contractility. It is thought that he may have an acquired cardiac problem due to secondary myocarditis from his winter illness.

3. **What is your impression of this patient now?**

Two weeks later he recovered and was sent home. He will need to be monitored in the future to assess cardiac function.

References

1. Sahu S, Kishore K, Lata I. Better outcome after pediatric resuscitation is still a dilemma. *J Emerg Trauma Shock*. 2010;3(3):243-250.
2. Bagnall RD, Weintraub RG, Ingles J, et al. A prospective study of sudden cardiac death among children and young adults. *N Engl J Med*. 2016;374(25):2441-2452.
3. Ludwig S, Lavelle JM. Resuscitation-pediatric basic and advanced life support. In: Fleisher GR, Ludwig S, Henretig FM, eds. *Textbook of Pediatric Emergency Medicine*. 5th ed. Philadelphia, PA: Lippincott Williams & Wilkins; 2006:3.
4. Carcillo JA. Capillary refill time is a very useful clinical sign in early recognition and treatment of very sick children. *Pediatr Crit Care Med*. 2012;13(2):210-212.
5. Rodríguez-Nunez A, López-Herce J, García C, et al. Effective and long-term outcome of cardiopulmonary resuscitation in paediatric intensive care unit in Spain. *Resuscitation*. 2006;71(3):301-309.
6. Teasdale G, Jennet B. Assessment of coma and impaired consciousness. *Lancet*. 1974;ii:81-84.
7. Teasdale G, Allen D, Brennan P, McElhinney E, Mackinnon L. The Glasgow Coma Scale: an update after 40 years. *Nurs Times*. 2014;110:12-16.
8. Durham SR, Clancy RR, Leuthardt E, et al. CHOP Infant Coma Scale ("Infant Face Scale"): a novel coma scale for children less than two years of age. *J Neurotrauma*. 2000;17(9):729-737.
9. Moulton C, Pennycook AG. Relation between Glasgow Coma Score and cough reflex. *Lancet*. 1994;343(8908):1261-1262.

10. Kelly CA, Upex A, Bateman N. Comparison of consciousness level assessment in the poisoned patient using the alert/verbal/painful/unresponsive scale and the Glasgow Coma Scale. *Ann Emerg Med.* 2004;44(2):108-113.

11. Raman S, Sreenivas V, Puliyel JM, Kumar N. Comparison of alert verbal painful unresponsiveness scale and the Glasgow Coma Score. *Indian Pediatr.* 2011;48(4):331-332.

12. Stovroff M, Teague WG. Intravenous access in infants and children. *Pediatr Clin North Am.* 1998;45(6):1373-1393.

13. Smith R, Davis N, Bouamra O, Lecky F. The utilization of intraosseous infusion in the resuscitation of paediatric major trauma patients. *Injury.* 2005;36(9):1034-1038.

14. de Caen AR, Reis A, Bhutta A. Vascular access and drug therapy in pediatric resuscitation. *Pediatr Clin North Am.* 2008;55(4):909-927.

15. Horton MA, Beamer C. Powered intraosseous insertion provides safe and effective vascular access for pediatric emergency patients. *Pediatr Emerg Care.* 2008;24(6):347-350.

16. Ehrlich PF, Seidman PS, Atallah O, Haque A, Helmkamp J. Endotracheal intubations in rural pediatric trauma patients. *J Pediatr Surg.* 2004;39(9):1376-1380.

17. Hartmann SM, Farris RW, Di Gennaro JL, Roberts JS. Systematic review and meta-analysis of end-tidal carbon dioxide values associated with return of spontaneous circulation during cardiopulmonary resuscitation. *J Intensive Care Med.* 2015;30:426-435.

18. Sugerman NT, Edelson DP, Leary M, et al. Rescuer fatigue during actual in-hospital cardiopulmonary resuscitation with audio-visual feedback: a prospective multicenter study. *Resuscitation.* 2009;80(9):981-984.

19. Lubitz DS, Seidel JS, Chameides L, et al. A rapid method for estimating weight and resuscitation drug dosages from length in the pediatric age group. *Ann Emerg Med.* 1988;17:576-581.

20. Lowe CG, Campwala RT, Ziv N, Wang VJ. The Broselow and Handtevy resuscitation tapes: a comparison of the performance of pediatric weight prediction. *Prehosp Disaster Med.* 2016;31(4):364-375.

21. McAlvin SS, Carew-Lyons A. Family presence during resuscitation and invasive procedures in pediatric critical care: a systematic review. *Am J Crit Care.* 2014;23(6):477-484.

14

Acute Respiratory Disorders

Mohamad El-Khatib

© Anna Rubak/ShutterStock, Inc.

OUTLINE

OBJECTIVES

1. Explain how bronchiolitis, respiratory syncytial virus (RSV), and influenza can be transmitted or spread.
2. Describe the pathophysiology of bronchiolitis.
3. List the therapies used in the prevention and treatment of bronchiolitis.
4. Describe the mainstay treatment for RSV.
5. List the pathogens that typically cause laryngotracheobronchitis.
6. Explain the differences in the radiologic findings for larygotracheobronchitis and epiglottitis.
7. Discuss the treatment options for larygotracheobronchitis and epiglottitis.
8. List the factors that increase a child's risk for pulmonary air leak syndromes.
9. List the procedures used to identify a pulmonary air leak.
10. Discuss the options for treating pulmonary air leaks.
11. Differentiate between transudate and exudate.
12. Explain the options for treating a pleural effusion.
13. Explain the methods used to diagnose chylothorax.
14. Discuss the testing used to diagnose a hemothorax.
15. List the options for treating a hemothorax.

KEY TERMS

avian influenza
bronchiolitis
chylothorax
epiglottitis
exudate
hemothorax
influenza
laryngotracheobronchitis (LTB)
paradoxical respirations

pleural effusion
pleurodesis
pulmonary air leak syndromes
respiratory syncytial virus (RSV)
swine flu (H1N1)
thoracentesis
transillumination
transudate

Introduction

Viral and bacterial infections are common in children and cause disorders that affect the airways and lung parenchyma. These conditions may cause mild symptoms in some children and can be treated effectively on an outpatient basis or at home. For others, especially children with preexisting conditions, symptoms are more severe. In this subset of patients, hospitalization and treatment in a pediatric ICU is essential to patient outcomes.

This chapter will review the etiology of disorders commonly seen in young children and the therapeutic modalities used to treat these disorders in the acute and ambulatory care settings.

Bronchiolitis

Bronchiolitis is an acute inflammatory disease of the lower respiratory tract, resulting in obstruction of the small airways, or bronchioles.[1] It is a common seasonal viral infection, with incidence peaking in the winter, that causes wheezing and congestion in infants up to 2 years of age.[2]

Bronchiolitis presents with symptoms similar to a common cold; however, as the disease progresses, coughing, wheezing, and dyspnea often occur. Only a small percentage of children with bronchiolitis will require hospitalization, and of those a few will require treatment in the intensive care unit. A majority of children with bronchiolitis will respond well to supportive care and remain at home.

Etiology

The majority of cases with bronchiolitis result from a viral pathogen, such as respiratory syncytial virus (RSV; most common), influenza and parainfluenza viruses, human metapneumovirus, or adenovirus (**Table 14-1**).[2,3] A majority, approximately 90%, of children are infected with RSV in the first 2 years of life,[4] 40% of which will experience lower respiratory tract infection during the initial infection.[5]

Bronchiolitis is highly contagious, easily spreading from person to person through direct contact with nasal secretions, airborne droplets, and fomites. A combination of two or more infectious organisms can result in severe bronchiolitis; combined RSV and human metapneumovirus infections are strongly associated with severe bronchiolitis, with a 10-fold increase in pediatric intensive care unit admission.[6,7]

Pathophysiology

Infection is spread by direct contact with respiratory secretions. Once acquired, the virus spreads from the upper respiratory tract to the medium and small bronchi and bronchioles. Within 24 hours of acquiring the infection, necrosis of the respiratory epithelium, one of the earliest lesions in bronchiolitis, occurs and triggers an inflammatory response.[8] Infants are quickly affected because of their small airways, high closing volumes, and insufficient collateral ventilation. Bronchial obstruction and airflow restriction develop as a result of increased mucus secretion, edema, and **exudate** (**Figure 14-1**). The obstruction is most pronounced on expiration and can lead to alveolar air trapping and development of intrinsic positive end-expiratory pressure. Complete obstruction can lead to absorption atelectasis and increased ventilation/perfusion mismatch. Bronchoconstriction has not been reported in patients with bronchiolitis.

Complex immunologic mechanisms play a role in the pathogenesis of bronchiolitis. Allergic reactions mediated by immunoglobulin E may account for some clinically significant bronchiolitis.[9,10] Cytokines and chemokines, released by infected respiratory epithelial cells, amplify the immune response by increasing cellular recruitment into infected airways.[11,12]

TABLE 14-1
Prevalence of Pathogens Most Commonly Associated with Bronchiolitis

Etiology	Prevalence
Respiratory syncytial virus (RSV)	20–40% of all cases 70–75% of all hospitalized children younger than 2 years
Influenza virus	10–20% of all cases
Parainfluenza virus	10–30% of all cases
Human metapneumovirus	10–20% of all cases
Adenovirus	5–10% of all cases
Mycoplasma pneumoniae	5–15% among older children and adults

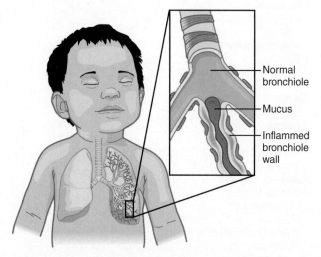

FIGURE 14-1 Increased mucus secretion, edema, and exudate obstruct the lower airways and restrict airflow.

Diagnosis

The diagnosis is based on adequate and thorough history, physical examination, consideration of the patient's age, season in which the viral infection occurs, and the patient's clinical presentation. Common clinical manifestations include tachypnea, tachycardia, fever, diffuse fine expiratory wheezing on chest auscultation, and possibly hypoxia.[13]

Laboratory tests and radiologic studies are of limited value for routine diagnostic use, but further diagnostic tests might be necessary to confirm (or exclude) in patients at high risk for severe disease, including infants younger than 12 weeks of age, those with a history of prematurity, infants with underlying cardiopulmonary disease, or the immunocompromised (Table 14-2).[14] Laboratory tests may also be of value to guide care for patients with more severe forms of bronchiolitis or those who develop complications. Chest radiographs reveal the presence of hyperinflation, peribronchiolar thickening, and, in some, patchy atelectatic areas (Figure 14-2).

Assessment scores may be helpful in quantifying the severity of the disease and in monitoring a patient's response to therapy and progress during hospital care. The severity of bronchiolitis is best determined by assessing the presence and degree of hypoxia. Although there are many different scores that can be used, assessing the infant's respiratory rate is a very useful parameter and can be used to assess the degree of hypoxia. Tachypnea, or a respiratory rate greater than 50 breaths per minute, correlates best with the degree of hypoxia.

Clinical Presentation

Clinical manifestations of bronchiolitis are initially subtle. Infants may become increasingly fussy with lack of appetite. A low-grade fever (<38.6°C) may also be present. Infants younger than 1 month may present with hypothermia. If the viral infection progresses from the upper to the lower respiratory tract, the patient will develop cough, dyspnea, wheezing, and feeding difficulties. Infants and young children with severe cases of bronchiolitis present with obvious respiratory distress characterized by tachypnea, nasal flaring, chest wall retractions, marked wheezing and irritability, and possibly cyanosis.[15] During breathing, thoracoabdominal asynchrony or **paradoxical respirations** can be noted (Figure 14-3). Paradoxical breathing correlates with the degree of airway obstruction, which can be seen radiographically by the presence of hyperinflation or air trapping in the majority of patients.

Patients with bronchiolitis may also have episodes of apnea. In a systematic review, Ralston et al. found that the overall incidence of apnea ranged from 1.2% to 23.8% in infants hospitalized with RSV bronchiolitis.[16] Common nonrespiratory manifestations of bronchiolitis include otitis media, myocarditis, and supraventricular and ventricular dysrhythmias.[17,18]

Complications of bronchiolitis vary and may be associated with the disease or caused by therapy. In most cases, the disease is mild and self-limited, with no serious complications. However, in infants who are younger than 12 weeks of age, are immunosuppressed, or have preexisting heart or lung disease, bronchiolitis can result in serious complications (Table 14-3).[19,20]

TABLE 14-2
Laboratory Tests Indicated for Children at High Risk for Severe Bronciolitis or Complications

- Viral antigen testing of nasopharyngeal secretions for the presence of RSV
- C-reactive protein level
- Blood cultures
- Complete blood count
- Arterial blood gas analysis
- Urine analysis and culture

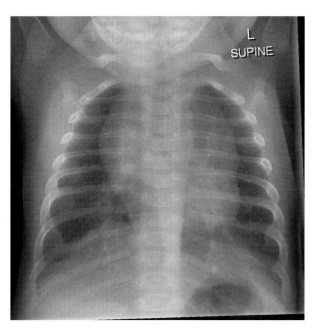

FIGURE 14-2 AP and lateral chest radiographs demonstrating peribronchiolar thickening and some patchy atelectatic areas.
Courtesy of Dr Jeremy Jones, Radiopaedia.org, rID: 35357.

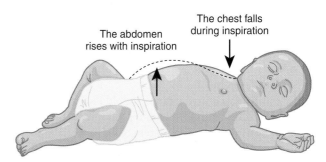

FIGURE 14-3 An illustration of paradoxical or seesaw breathing. Asynchronous movement of the chest and abdomen are noted with this breathing pattern.

TABLE 14-3
Complications of Bronchiolitis

- Acute respiratory distress syndrome
- Bronchiolitis obliterans
- Chronic lung disease
- Apnea
- Myocarditis
- Congestive heart failure
- Arrhythmias

As they age, patients who suffered from bronchiolitis have an increased likelihood of developing asthma.[21] Additionally, as many as 1% of previously healthy children and 3% of developmentally impaired children with bronchiolitis experience some neurologic complications, such as seizures, encephalopathy with hypotonia, irritability, and abnormal tone.[22]

Treatment

Due to the lack of evidence-based support for the treatment of bronchiolitis, treatment strategies vary widely, particularly during the initial management in the emergency department. A survey of the American Academy of Pediatrics (AAP) Emergency Section found that 96% recommended bronchodilators and 8% recommended steroids.[23] Hospital admission is mainly based on the degree of hypoxia: Twice as many pediatric emergency physicians would admit a child with an oxygen saturation of 92% on pulse oximetry than would admit a child with a saturation of 94%.[23]

Due to differences and variations among practices, the AAP published the following recommendations in 2014:[24]

- Bronchodilators, such as albuterol or salmuterol, and epinephrine should not be routinely administered to infants with the diagnosis of bronchiolitis.
- Nebulized hypertonic saline may be administered to hospitalized patients but should not routinely be used as treatment in the emergency department.
- Corticosteroid medications should not be used routinely in the management of bronchiolitis.
- Ribavirin should not be used routinely in children with bronchiolitis.
- Antibacterial medications should be used only in children with bronchiolitis who have specific indications of the coexistence of a bacterial infection. When present, bacterial infection should be treated in the same manner as in the absence of bronchiolitis.

- Clinicians should assess hydration and ability to take fluids orally.
- Supplemental oxygen is indicated if oxyhemoglobin saturation (SpO_2) falls persistently below 90% in previously healthy infants. If the SpO_2 does persistently fall below 90%, adequate supplemental oxygen should be used to maintain SpO_2 at or above 90%. Oxygen may be discontinued if SpO_2 is at or above 90% and if the infant is feeding well and has minimal respiratory distress.
- As the child's clinical course improves, continuous measurement of SpO_2 is not routinely needed.
- Infants with a known history of hemodynamically significant heart or lung disease and premature infants require close monitoring as the oxygen is being weaned.
- Clinicians may administer palivizumab prophylaxis to selected infants and children with chronic lung diseases, a history of prematurity (fewer than 35 weeks' gestation), or congenital heart disease.
- When given, prophylaxis with palivizumab should be given in five monthly doses, usually beginning in November or December, at a dose of 15 mg/kg per dose administered intramuscularly.
- Hand decontamination is the most important step in preventing nosocomial spread of RSV. Hands should be decontaminated before and after direct contact with patients, after contact with inanimate objects in the direct vicinity of the patient, and after removing gloves
- Alcohol-based rubs are preferred for hand decontamination. An alternative is hand washing with antimicrobial soap.
- Clinicians should educate personnel and family members on hand sanitation.
- Infants should not be exposed to passive smoking, and parents should be educated on the hazards associated with exposure to secondhand smoke.
- Breastfeeding is recommended to decrease a child's risk of having lower respiratory tract disease.

After introduction of the AAP guidelines in 2006, the use of bronchodilators to treat pediatric bronchiolitis was reduced from 70% in 2007 to 58% in 2010 by a network of hospitals in 14 U.S. states.[25] Also, significant percentage decreases were seen in admissions (29%), length of stay (17%), nasopharyngeal washings for RSV antigen (52%), chest radiography (20%), all respiratory therapies (30%), beta-agonist administrations (51%), cost of all services (37%), and cost of respiratory therapy services (77%).[26] These changes continued in the 3-year and 4-year follow-up investigations[27] and are aligned with the most recent recommendations published in 2014.[24]

Viral Infections

Viral infections can be caused by different kinds of viruses that can be found in various places in the body, such as the airways, lungs, and gastrointestinal system. Although viral infections can be bothersome, they usually are not serious; however, infants and children with preexisting pulmonary or cardiac conditions may require close observation and admission to a healthcare facility. RSV and the influenza virus are the most common types of viral infections in infants and children.[28]

Respiratory Syncytial Virus (RSV)

Respiratory syncytial virus (RSV) is the leading cause of lower respiratory tract infections in young children in the United States and worldwide and is the most common cause of bronchiolitis and pneumonia in children younger than 1 year of age. In the United States, 4 to 5 million children younger than 5 years acquire an RSV infection yearly; on average, RSV infections lead to more than 125,000 hospitalizations and more than 2 million outpatient visits among children younger than 5 years old.[29] RSV infections occur primarily during the fall, winter, and spring seasons.

Etiology

A child is commonly exposed to the virus by an older sibling or another child who is demonstrating cold-like symptoms. Common modes of transmission are cough and direct physical contact from infected individuals. A number of factors, such as childcare attendance, older siblings in school, crowding and lower socioeconomic status, exposure to environmental pollutants, and minimal breastfeeding, have been associated with an increased risk of acquiring RSV.[30]

Some children are more susceptible to a more severe form of this viral infection and require hospitalization for more comprehensive care. Factors that have been correlated with a more severe form of RSV include prematurity (<35 weeks' gestation), age younger than 3 months at the time of infection, preexisting chronic lung disease, congenital heart disease, congenital immunodeficiency, respiratory rate greater than 60 breaths per minute on room air, oxygen saturation less than 95% on room air, atelectasis or pneumonitis on chest radiography, and family history of asthma.[30]

Pathophysiology

RSV infection is limited to the respiratory tract. Inoculation of the virus occurs in respiratory epithelial cells of the upper respiratory tract, then moves down the respiratory tract by cell-to-cell transfer along intracytoplasmic bridges (syncytia), causing bronchiolitis and later atelectasis and pneumonia.[31]

The illness may begin with upper respiratory symptoms and progress rapidly over 1 to 2 days to the development of diffuse small airway disease. RSV infection causes peribronchiolar mononuclear infiltration and necrosis of the epithelium of the small airways, which leads to edema of the small airways and increased mucus production. The combination of sloughing necrotic tissues, airway edema, and mucus accumulation decreases the airway lumen and causes a partial or complete obstruction of the airway. Partial airway obstruction contributes to air-trapping and alveolar hyperinflation while complete airway obstruction leads to alveolar collapse and pneumonia.

In very young infants, apnea may be present;[32] in infants younger than 6 weeks, a relatively nonspecific sepsis-like clinical presentation has been described.[33]

Reinfection with RSV can occur at any age, but it is more likely to be limited to the upper respiratory tract when it recurs later in life. Upper respiratory tract infection due to RSV is usually more severe than the common cold.

Diagnosis

Patients with RSV infections who are comfortable while breathing room air, are well hydrated, and are feeding well generally might not require any laboratory tests. However, nonspecific laboratory tests, such as a complete blood count, serum electrolytes, urinalysis, and arterial blood gas analysis, might be warranted when the infant or child is at risk for a more severe form of the disease.

Specific diagnostic tests for confirming RSV infection include sputum culture, antigen testing, polymerase chain reaction (PCR) assay, and molecular probing. These tests are usually indicated for therapeutic decision making, isolation of patients, and educating parents and healthcare staff.[34]

Chest radiography is frequently obtained in children with a severe RSV infection. However, the findings are neither specific to RSV infection nor predictive of the course or outcome.

Clinical Presentation

Children with an RSV infection initially present with cold-like symptoms,[35] such as cough, nasal congestion, sneezing, and a low-grade fever. As the infection affects the lower respiratory tract, airway obstruction occurs, causing respiratory distress characterized by tachypnea, chest wall retractions, and wheezing. In severe cases, cyanosis might be present. In very young infants infected with RSV, a sepsis-like presentation or apneic episode might occur.

As many as 40% of children with an RSV infection have an associated otitis media, which may be viral, bacterial, or both.[36] Signs of dehydration secondary to loss of appetite and difficulty in feeding might also be present.[37]

The role of RSV in causing subsequent reactive airway disease remains controversial. Infants hospitalized for RSV and lower respiratory tract infections or bronchiolitis are at higher risk for subsequent wheezing and abnormal pulmonary function tests.[38] This increased risk may persist for more than 10 years after the infection.

Treatment

The mainstay of therapy for RSV infection is supportive care. There is a general lack of evidence-based practices for treatment of RSV infections, although the following pharmacologic therapies have been used for RSV infection:[39]

- Bronchodilators in patients with RSV-related lower respiratory tract infection
- Alpha agonists (nebulized epineprine) in acute RSV bronchiolitis episodes
- Ribavirin (Virazole), a broad-spectrum antiviral agent in vitro, is primarily reserved for patients with significant risk factors and severe acute RSV disease (e.g., transplant recipients). The recommended dose is 6 g of ribavirin in 300 mL of distilled water via a small-particle aerosol generator over 12 to 20 hours per day for 3 to 7 days, depending on clinical response.

Palivizumab has been used in passive immunization to protect against RSV infection in children at high risk for severe RSV disease. According to AAP guidelines for RSV prophylaxis,[39] palivizumab prophylaxis for RSV should be limited to infants born before 29 weeks' gestation and to infants with chronic illness, such as congenital heart disease (cyanotic or acayanotic) or chronic lung disease. Other recommendations include the following:

- Give infants who qualify for prophylaxis in the first year of life no more than five monthly doses of palivizumab (15 mg/kg per dose) during the RSV season.
- In the second year of life, palivizumab prophylaxis is recommended only for children who needed supplemental oxygen for 28 days or more after birth and who continue to need medical intervention (supplemental oxygen, chronic corticosteroid, or diuretic therapy).
- Clinicians may consider prophylaxis for children younger than 24 months if they will be profoundly immunocompromised during the RSV season.

Other treatment modalities can also include oxygen therapy to treat hypoxemia, decrease the work of breathing, and decrease myocardial work and bronchial hygiene to enhance the mobilization of bronchial secretions.

Influenza

Influenza is an extremely contagious respiratory illness caused by influenza A or B viruses.[40] Commonly known as "flu," it spreads through the upper and/or lower respiratory tract and appears most frequently in winter and early spring.

Etiology

Influenza results from infection by any of three basic types of influenza viruses: A, B, or C.[41] Influenza A is more common and generally more pathogenic, causing the most serious disease. Wild aquatic birds are the primary reservoir for the influenza A viruses, although it is also found in many different animals, including pigs and horses. Scientists hypothesize that almost all mammalian influenza A viruses are derived from the avian reservoir. Influenza B affects people only, is usually associated with the mild form of the disease, and is more common in the pediatric population. Influenza C is not as commonly seen, but epidemics of influenza C have been reported, especially in young children.[42]

Influenza A causes larger seasonal outbreaks and more serious respiratory symptoms while types B and C usually cause milder respiratory symptoms. Influenza viruses are constantly changing, with new strains of influenza appearing every few years. **Avian influenza** (H5N1 influenza virus) is transmitted to humans primarily through direct contact with diseased or deceased birds infected with the virus. Contact with excrement from infected birds or contaminated surfaces or water are also considered mechanisms of infection. **Swine flu (H1N1)** was first recognized in humans in 2009 and resulted in increased H1N1-related illnesses in much of the world. Currently, H1N1 is still circulating as a seasonal flu virus, with protection included in the 2015–2016 flu vaccine.

Influenza viruses are spread by contact or by air. They enter the body when someone touches their nose, eyes, or mouth with contaminated hands or inhales contaminated droplets. The spread of influenza viruses can occur up to 7 days after the symptoms start, and young children can still spread the influenza virus even into the second week of illness.

There are several factors that contribute to the winter seasonality of influenza infection. More time is spent indoors during the winter months, leading to a higher probability of having closer contact with others, which makes it easier for the virus to spread. Also, the lower air humidity in the winter allows the virus to survive longer in the air and on surfaces, increasing the chances of contact.

Pathophysiology

Influenza viruses are encapsulated, negative-sense, single-stranded RNA viruses. The A, B, and C types of influenza viruses are distinguished based on the core nucleoproteins. The RNA core consists of 8 gene segments surrounded by a coat of 10 (influenza A) or 11 (influenza B) proteins.[43] Hemagglutinin (H) and neuraminidase (N) are the most significant surface proteins. The various combinations of H and N yield 144 potential subtypes of influenza. Subtyping of influenza A occurs through identification of both H and N proteins; for example, influenza A subtype H1N1 expresses hemagglutinin 1 and neuraminidase 1. Because the viral RNA polymerase lacks error-checking mechanisms, the year-to-year antigenic drift is sufficient to ensure that there is a significant susceptible host population each year.[43]

In addition to humans, influenza also infects several animal species. More than 100 types of influenza A infect most species of birds, pigs, horses, dogs, and seals. Influenza B has also been reported in seals, and influenza C has been reported in pigs. New strains of influenza may spread from animal species to humans, or an existing human strain may pick up new genes from a strain that usually infects birds or pigs.

Influenza A is a genetically labile virus, with mutation rates as high as 300 times that of other microbes.[44] Its major functional and antigenic proteins change by either antigenic drift, which gives the virus the ability to evade annually acquired immunity in humans, or antigenic shift, which permits the reassortment of two strains of viruses. Although less frequent than antigenic drift, antigenic shift can result in a virulent strain of influenza that possesses the triad of infectivity, lethality, and transmissibility in a much greater population of susceptible individuals in whom more severe disease is possible, thus causing a pandemic.

Influenza viruses spread from human to human by aerosols created when an infected individual coughs or sneezes. Infection occurs after an immunologically susceptible person directly inhales the aerosol or touches the deposited aerosols on surfaces, which then allows for a point of entry via the eyes, nose, or mouth. Once the virus is within host cells, cellular dysfunction and degeneration occur and release inflammatory mediators. The incubation period of influenza ranges from 1 to 4 days. Transmission of influenza from poultry or pigs to humans appears to occur predominantly as a result of direct contact with infected animals or through exposure to water and surfaces contaminated by animal droppings.[44]

Viral shedding, the expulsion and release of virus progeny following successful reproduction during a host-cell infection, occurs at the onset of symptoms or just before the onset of illness (0–24 hours). Viral shedding generally continues for 7 to 10 days, but young children may shed influenza viruses for a longer duration, placing others at risk for contracting infection. In highly immunocompromised persons, shedding may persist for weeks to months.[45,46]

Diagnosis

In most cases, influenza A or B infection is diagnosed based on symptoms, which include headache, fever, chills, muscle aches, weakness and fatigue, nasal congestion, sore throat, and cough. However, depending only on the clinical symptoms to diagnose influenza infections may not be very reliable. Other viruses associated with upper respiratory tract infection, such as adenoviruses, enteroviruses, and paramyxoviruses, have a similar clinical presentation. Testing for influenza infection is optimally performed within 48 hours of the onset of symptoms, when a greater amount of the virus is present to be detected. Testing is recommended in particular for people who are hospitalized, have weakened immune systems, or are otherwise at an increased risk of serious complications.[47]

A number of tests are available to detect influenza viruses and include the rapid influenza diagnostic test, viral cultures, and real-time RT-PCR molecular tests. The rapid influenza diagnostic test (RIDT) is one of the most common methods used to diagnose influenza infection, based on detecting the virus in nasal secretions.[48] It may be completed in the doctor's office in less than 15 minutes or be sent to a laboratory, with the results available the same day. This test is best used within the first 48 hours of the onset of symptoms and will generally detect 40% to 70% of influenza cases. None of the available tests can differentiate among the strains of influenza, such H1N1. The main disadvantage of RIDTs is the high rate of false-negative results; RIDTs can also occasionally be positive even when the virus is not present. Viral cultures are considered the gold standard for diagnosing influenza and can be used as confirmation of a RIDT.[49] They can identify both the presence of the virus and the strains of virus present. However, it can take 3 to 10 days to obtain the results.

Real-time RT-PCR and other molecular tests are the most sensitive tests, which detect viral genetic material in respiratory samples, such as a nasal or throat swab.[50] These tests can distinguish between A and B viruses as well as among different strains of influenza A virus.

Clinical Presentation

The classical signs and symptoms of influenza infection come on abruptly and include high-grade fever, headache, maliase, fatigue, body aches, cough, sore throat, runny or stuffy nose, and diarrhea and vomiting, the last of which are more common in infants and children.[51] Most of these symptoms are similar to cold symptoms; the major difference is that symptoms of influenza infection are felt sooner than cold symptoms and with much greater intensity (**Table 14-4**). Even without treatment, most influenza infections will go away within 1 to 2 weeks, although fatigue and a cough may last longer. However, serious secondary complications may develop just as influenza symptoms resolve.

TABLE 14-4
Comparison between Cold and Influenza Symptoms

Symptom	Presentation in a Cold	Presentation in Influenza
Fever	Rare	High (37.7–38.8°C), lasting 3–4 days
Headache	Rare	Prominent
General aches	Slight	Frequent, often severe
Pain	Mild	Usually
Fatigue	Very mild	Prolonged, can last up to 2–3 weeks
Extreme exhaustion	Never	Early and prominent
Stuffy, runny nose	Common	Sometimes
Sore throat	Common	Sometimes
Sneezing	Usually	Sometimes
Cough	Mild to moderate	Common and can become severe

Anyone may be susceptible to complications from influenza, but young children (6 months to 4 years of age), the elderly (older than 65 years of age), pregnant women, nursing home residents, the immunocompromised (HIV/AIDS), or those with preexisting heart and lung disease are at increased risk. Complications, such as viral or bacterial pneumonia, sepsis, pericarditis, myocarditis, and encephalitis, can be very serious and may require immediate medical treatment. Influenza infection can also worsen long-term conditions, such as congestive heart failure or diabetes.

Treatment

Prevention is the most effective strategy. The Advisory Committee on Immunization Practices (ACIP) of the Centers for Disease Control and Prevention (CDC) recommends routine annual influenza vaccination for all persons aged 6 months or older, preferably before the onset of influenza activity in the community.[51] For pregnant women, the CDC recommends that the influenza vaccine be administered during all trimesters of the pregnancy, which is shown to decrease the risk of illness in the mother as well as the risk of influenza and influenza hospitalization in their infants during the first 6 months of life.[52]

Each year in the United States, a vaccine containing antigens from the strains most likely to cause infection during the winter flu season is produced. Trivalent vaccines include two strains of influenza A and one strain of influenza B while the quadrivalent flu vaccines have an additional B virus strain.[53] Both injectable and nasal spray vaccines are available; FluMist, the nasal spray vaccine, is usually indicated for healthy individuals who are 2 to 49 years old and not pregnant.[54] The vaccination becomes effective 10 to 14 days after administration and usually has 50% to 60% efficacy against influenza A viruses and 60% to 70% efficacy against influenza B viruses.[54] No avian influenza vaccine is currently available to the public; however, the U.S. Department of Health and Human Services has purchased a recently developed avian flu adjuvanted vaccine for addition to the Strategic National Stockpile of drugs and medical supplies and, if warranted, subsequent distribution by public health officials.

Whenever there is a surge in severe influenza illness, it is imperative to implement and organize some proven effective guidelines and measures through surveillance and diagnostic services, information sharing and dissemination, community support, hospital and physician capacity, and the supply and delivery of vaccines and drugs.[55]

The ACIP also published recommendations on the use of antiviral agents for prevention and treatment of influenza.[56] When indicated, antiviral agents significantly reduce the severity and duration of illness as well as the secondary complications of influenza infection.[56] However, potential adverse effects (headache, nausea, vomiting, bronchospasm) and higher costs are associated with these antiviral agents. In the United States, five prescription antiviral drugs are approved for chemoprophylaxis and treatment of influenza (Table 14-5). To be effective, oseltamivir, zanamivir, peramivir, amantadine, and rimatadine must be administered within 48 hours of symptom onset. Cases of suspected severe influenza infection should be treated early and aggressively, even before diagnostic tests can be confirmed. The literature reports that in critically ill patients with H5N1 infection, the initiation of oseltamivir therapy up to 6 to 8 days from onset of symptoms may reduce mortality.[57]

TABLE 14-5
Common Prescription Antiviral Drugs Approved for Chemoprophylaxis and Treatment of Influenza

Drug	Description
Oseltamivir	Activity against influenza A and B, including H1N1 Resistance emerged during the 2008–2009 season
Zanamivir	Activity against influenza A and B, including H1N1
Peramivir	Approved by the U.S. Food and Drug Administration in December 2014 Activity against influenza A and B, including H1N1
Amantadine	Activity against influenza A only Resistance emerged to influenza A (H3N2) virus strains
Rimantadine	Activity against influenza A only Resistance emerged to influenza A (H3N2) virus strains

Patients diagnosed with influenza should be educated about potential complications and encouraged to return for evaluation if concerned. This is especially true of patients with underlying chronic disease or those who are immunocompromised. Laninamivir octanoate, an investigational antiviral agent for influenza infection, has been approved in Japan but is not yet available in the United States.[58]

The CDC has made the following recommendations regarding the use of antiviral drugs in influenza:[56]

- Antiviral treatment is recommended as soon as possible for patients with confirmed or suspected influenza who have severe, complicated, or progressive illness or who require hospitalization.
- Antiviral treatment is recommended as soon as possible for outpatients with confirmed or suspected influenza who are at higher risk for influenza complications based on their age or underlying medical conditions. Clinical judgment should be an important component of outpatient treatment decisions.
- Currently recommended antiviral medications include oseltamivir and zanamivir.
- Oseltamivir may be used for treatment or chemoprophylaxis of influenza among infants younger than 1 year of age, when indicated.
- Antiviral treatment also may be considered on the basis of clinical judgment for any outpatient with confirmed or suspected influenza who does not have known risk factors for severe illness if treatment can be initiated within 48 hours of illness onset.
- Because antiviral resistance patterns can change over time, clinicians should monitor local antiviral resistance surveillance data.

Public health measures, such as enhanced surveillance with daily temperature taking and prompt home isolation whenever indicated, have been reported to be effective in limiting influenza transmission in closed environments.[58] Patients most often require hospitalization when influenza exacerbates underlying chronic diseases, particularly in vulnerable patients. Most patients with influenza recover in 3 days; however, malaise may persist for weeks.

Prehospital care for patients with influenza infection is predominantly supportive. Respiratory symptoms, including hypoxia, are managed with supplemental oxygen. More serious manifestations of respiratory distress/failure will require intubation and mechanical ventilation. Hemodynamic stability should be maintained with intravenous administration of crystalloids. Strict attention should be given to the appropriate use of personal protective equipment.

Laryngotracheobronchitis

Laryngotracheobronchitis (LTB) affects the lower laryngeal (L) area, trachea (T), and occasionally the bronchi

(B). It is used as a synonym for classic subglottic croup (**Figure 14-4**). LTB is a common pediatric viral respiratory tract illness and is the most common etiology for hoarseness, cough, and onset of acute stridor in febrile children. It is an inflammatory process that causes edema and swelling of the mucous membranes.[59,60]

Because the subglottic area is the narrowest region of the larynx in infants and children, a slight degree of edema can cause a significant reduction in the cross-sectional area. Morbidity occurs secondary to narrowing of the larynx and trachea below the level of the glottis (subglottic region), causing the characteristic audible inspiratory stridor. **Figure 14-5** shows the steeple sign, a classic radiologic sign associated with LTB.

Etiology

Viral infections are the most common causes of LTB, which is most typically seen in children between 3 months and 3 years of age. The parainfluenza viruses 1, 2, and 3 are the most frequently identified etiologic agents, found in nearly 80% of cases, with type 1 being the most prevalent.[61] Influenza A and B viruses, RSV, rhinovirus, and adenoviruses may also cause LTB in children. These viruses are spread through either direct inhalation from a cough and/or sneeze or by

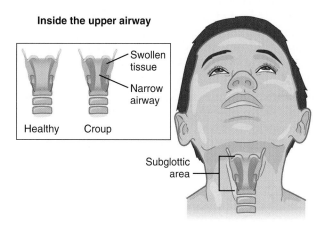

Inside the upper airway

Swollen tissue

Narrow airway

Healthy   Croup

Subglottic area

FIGURE 14-4 An illustration of the pathology occurring with LTB. The subglottic of a child with LTB is significantly narrowed compared to that of an unaffected child.

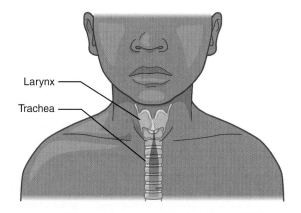

Larynx

Trachea

FIGURE 14-5 The steeple sign, a radiologic indicator of LTB.

contamination of hands from contact with fomites and subsequent touching of the mucosa of the eyes, nose, and/or mouth. *Mycoplasma pneumoniae*, a bacterial pathogen, has also been identified in a few cases of LTB.[62] LTB occurs most often during the late fall and winter seasons.

Pathophysiology

Viral upper respiratory tract infection causes nasopharyngeal inflammation that spreads to the larynx and trachea and occasionally to the mainstem bronchi. The subglottic inflammatory process produces edema, reduces the cross-sectional area of the airway, and compromises the airway at its narrowest portion. Airway resistance markedly increases and leads to excessive work of breathing. Airway inflammation and edema impair vocal cord movement, leading to the characteristic cough.[63] It is thought that some children who experience recurrent bouts of spasmodic croup have a primarily allergic rather than infective etiology.[64]

Diagnosis

The diagnosis of LTB is usually made clinically, based on the classical signs and symptoms (barking cough and stridor), especially during a typical community epidemic of one of the causative viruses. A seal-like barking-type cough and stridor are most commonly associated with LTB. An anterioposterior and lateral radiographic view of the neck might be needed to confirm the diagnosis of LTB and to rule out epiglottitis. The classic steeple sign will be seen in the case of LTB (Figure 14-5). No laboratory tests are necessary to make a diagnosis, although testing for the causative virus might be indicated when the results will influence decisions regarding treatment and contact precautions.

Clinical Presentation

Initially, infants and children with LTB present with nonspecific respiratory and cold-like symptoms. Sore throat, cough, and low-grade fever often precede LTB-specific symptoms by 1 to 3 days. The signs and symptoms of LTB include hoarseness, a seal-like barking cough, and inspiratory stridor. Varying degrees of respiratory distress may also be present. Most children have very mild cases and merely present with a croupy cough and a hoarse cry. Upper airway stridor might only be evident upon activity or agitation except in severe cases, where audible stridor along with some degree of respiratory distress is evident at rest.[65] Signs of severe LTB include tachypnea; tachycardia; visible suprasternal, intercostal, and subcostal retractions with poor air entry; hypoxemia; and hypercapnia. Sudden respiratory arrest may occur during an episode of severe coughing. LTB symptoms are usually worse at night.

Spasmodic croup (recurrent croup) typically presents at night with the sudden onset of "croupy" cough and stridor. Spasmodic croup is mostly allergic in nature but has been reported in children with gastroesophageal reflux.[66] Children will recover fully from recurrent croup within 3 to 6 hours.

Croup severity assessment scores have been developed for use during research and clinical practices. The Westley score evaluates the severity of LTB by assessing five factors: inspiratory stridor, retractions, air entry, cyanosis, and level of consciousness.[67] Each of the factors is assessed and given a score of 0 if the assessment finding is normal to a score of 2, 3, or 5. Any score higher than 0 indicates an abnormal finding (**Figure 14-6**). Another clinically useful LTB severity scoring system is the Alberta Clinical Practice Guideline Working Group.[68]

Complications in LTB are rare, and the vast majority of children recover without consequences or sequelae.

Westly Croup Scoring System						
	Score Associated with the Assessment of the Finding					
Finding	0	1	2	3	4	5
Stridor	None	Audible with a stethescope (at rest)	Audible without a stethescope (at rest)			
Retractions	None	Mild	Moderate	Severe		
Air Entry	Normal	Decreased	Severely decreased			
Cyanosis	None	With agitation	At rest			
Level of Consciousness	Normal					Altered

FIGURE 14-6 An example of a croup severity assessment score. The Westley score evaluates the severity of LTB by assessing inspiratory stridor, retractions, air entry, cyanosis, and the infant's level of consciousness.

Data from Westley CR, Cotton EK, Brooks JG. Nebulized racemic epinephrine by IPPB for the treatment of croup. *Am J Dis Child.* 1978;132:484-487.

The need for endotracheal intubation and mechanical ventilation remain the most severe complication, occurring in about 3% to 6% of patients.[69] Patients intubated secondary to LTB should be extubated as soon as the airway inflammation has decreased and when pulmonary secretions are minimal to prevent possible risks and complications related to endotracheal intubation and invasive mechanical ventilation. Death occurs in approximately 0.5% of intubated patients with LTB.

Treatment

Many patients with viral LTB will need only supportive care. Keeping the patient calm and nonagitated to prevent increased respiratory efforts is paramount. Medications for soothing the swollen airways are helpful. Symptoms typically resolve within 3 to 7 days but can last as long as 2 weeks.

Urgent care of LTB depends on the degree of respiratory distress. In mild LTB, a child may require nothing more than parental reassurance, education regarding the course of the disease, and supportive homecare guidelines.[69] However, in severe LTB, a thorough clinical evaluation should be performed to ensure airway patency and effective oxygenation and ventilation.[69] Agitation and crying of the patient with LTB should be avoided as these might lead to respiratory distress. It is important to closely monitor vital signs, such as heart rate, blood pressure, and temperature. Assessment of respiratory parameters, including respiratory rate, respiratory mechanics, work of breathing, and pulse oximetry, is also imperative in patients with LTB. Patients with evidence of severe respiratory distress may initially require high concentrations of oxygen and ventilatory support. Children requiring tracheal intubation and invasive mechanical ventilation should be intubated with an endotracheal tube that is 0.5 to 1 mm smaller than predicted for the patient's age.

Pharmacologic treatment with corticosteroids and nebulized racemic epinephrine is the cornerstone in the treatment of mild, moderate, and severe LTB.[70] However, the use of corticosteroids should be carefully evaluated in children with diabetes, who are immunocompromised, and who have been recently exposed to or diagnosed with varicella or tuberculosis due to the potential risk of exacerbating the systemic disease process.[69] A single dose of dexamethasone (0.3–0.6 mg/kg) is usually sufficient for reducing the overall severity of LTB, particularly if administered within the first 4 to 24 hours after the onset of illness.[71]

Nebulized racemic epinephrine is also used to alleviate upper airway edema. This aerosolized alpha adrenergic bronchodilator is typically reserved for moderate to severe LTB patients with signs of respiratory distress in the hospital setting. Nebulized racemic epinephrine works by fluid resorption from the interstitium to decrease laryngeal mucosal edema and by bronchial smooth muscle relaxation and bronchodilation.

Evidence of therapeutic benefit is usually apparent within 30 minutes, with an effect that can last for 90 to 120 minutes. Antibiotics are not required unless there is evidence of a secondary bacterial infection or in patients who appear toxic and do not adequately respond to corticosteroid administration and nebulized racemic epinephrine.

Intravenous fluid hydration may be required to stabilize the fluid volume in patients with LTB who fail to maintain adequate oral intake and have increased insensible fluid loss.

Cool mist administration was once the mainstay of treatment for patient with LTB, but randomized studies of children with moderate to severe croup reported no difference in outcome between those who received cool mist therapy and those who did not.[72] Several clinical trials have shown that heliox (a helium and oxygen mixture) delivered by a nonbreathing mask was equally effective to racemic epinephrine in patients with moderate to severe LTB.[73,74]

Epiglottitis

Epiglottitis is a serious airway emergency and can be life threatening. It results from a bacterial infection that causes acute inflammation of the supraglottic region of the oropharynx and is seen in children between 2 and 5 years of age.

Etiology

In children, *Haemophilus influenzae* type B is the most common organism that causes acute epiglottitis (>80%). Other causative agents include group A *Streptococcus pneumoniae* and *H. parainfluenzae*. Less common infectious etiologies include *Staphylococcus aureus*, *Escherichia coli*, *Klebsiella pneumoniae*, and herpes simplex virus. *Candida* and *Aspergillus* may be the cause of epiglottitis in immunocompromised patients. Epiglottitis results from bacteremia and/or direct invasion of the pathogenic organism.[68,75] It is transmitted by aerosol droplets.

Noninfectious causes of epiglottitis are not uncommon but include thermal injuries and throat burns affecting the epiglottis of bottle-fed infants, caustic insults with ingestion of dishwasher soaps, and foreign body ingestion. Also, epiglottitis may occur as a reaction to head and neck chemotherapy.[76, 77]

Pathophysiology

Swelling of the supraglottic structures, including the epiglottis, vallecula, arytenoids, and aryepiglottic folds, occurs. The increased edema in the supraglottic region reduces the caliber of the upper airway and causes turbulent flow during inspiration.[78] As the epiglottis swells, the lateral borders curl and the tip of the epiglottis protrudes posteriorly and inferiorly. The dysmorphic shape of the epiglottis in the narrowed superglottic area acts as a ball-valve mechanism that may produce partial to complete airway obstruction. Airway resistance and work of breathing are significantly increased. The inflamed and enlarged epiglottis may partially cover the esophageal opening and lead to dysphagia. Severe airway obstruction may cause cardiopulmonary arrest.

Diagnosis

Epiglottitis should be suspected when the child presents with signs of bacterial septicemia and an acute onset of upper airway obstruction. Children often present with signs of airway obstruction and increased work of breathing, including tachypnea, tachycardia, stridor, intercostal and suprasternal retractions, and cyanosis.[79] Additional clinical features include tripod positioning, anxiety, drooling, dysphagia, and respiratory distress.

Chest radiographs may be used to make a diagnosis of epiglottitis. Findings on a lateral neck radiograph include the classic thumb sign of an enlarged epiglottis, loss of the vallecular air space, thickened aryepiglottic folds, a distended hypopharynx, and straightening of the cervical spine (**Figure 14-7**).

However, radiography is not as sensitive and specific as direct laryngoscopy or flexible fiberoptic bronchoscopy in diagnosing epiglottitis, which is confirmed when an erythematous and edematous epiglottis is seen (**Figure 14-8**). However, direct visualization or a

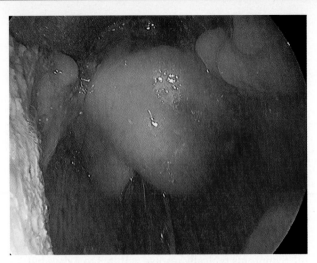

FIGURE 14-8 A view of the epiglottis by flexible fiberoptic bronchoscopy. The epiglottis is erythematous and edematous, suggesting epiglottitis.

Reproduced from Abdallah C. Acute epiglottitis: Trends, diagnosis and management. *Saudi Journal of Anaesthesia.* 2012;6(3):279-281. Reproduced with permission from Wolters Kluwer Medknow Publications.

bronchoscopic view of the epiglottis should be done in the setting where the airway can be secured immediately if necessary.

To determine the pathogenic organism causing the infection, cultures from the blood and/or the surface of the epiglottis may be obtained. However, if such culturing is necessary, it should be performed only after the airway is secured to avoid additional irritation and edema, which can further compromise the airway and cause significant danger to the patient.[80]

Clinical Presentation

The initial clinical presentation of epiglottitis is usually mild but may progress rapidly over 2 to 4 hours. Mostly all children, 95%, will complain of a sore throat. Within a few hours, a high-grade fever will be noted, and the child will have difficulty swallowing and clearing secretions. The child is usually pale and either lethargic or irritated. The supraglottic area becomes swollen, and breathing becomes noisy as swelling occurs in this area. The tongue will thrust forward during inspiration, and the difficulty swallowing will cause the child to drool. The voice and cry are usually muffled. The child will appear air hungry and assume an upright tripod sitting position for leverage to maximize accessory muscle use during inspiration.[81] Cough is not common in epiglottitis. As the condition progresses, suprasternal retractions, tachycardia, tachypnea, and nasal flaring may be present, and the patient will appear toxic. Cyanosis might not appear until complete airway obstruction is impending.

Complete airway obstruction and cardiopulmonary arrest are the most significant complications of epiglottitis.[81] Other complications of epiglottitis include meningitis, epiglottic abscess, cervical adenitis, vocal granuloma, cartilaginous metaplasia of the epiglottis, pneumonia, pulmonary edema, empyema, cellulitis, and septic shock.[81]

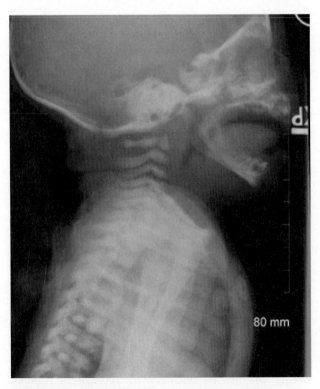

FIGURE 14-7 Radiologic findings from a lateral neck X-ray consistent with epiglottitis include the thumb sign, an indication that the epiglottis is enlarged.

Reproduced from Noble, J et al. Aphonia and epiglottitis in neonate with concomitant MRSA skin infection. *Respirol Case Rep.* 2014;2(3),116–119. Licensed under CC BY 3.0, https://creativecommons.org/licenses/by/3.0/.

Treatment

Children with epiglottitis should be kept as calm as possible; any unnecessary tests, therapies, and causes for the child's agitation should be avoided. Examination of the child's mouth and upper airway should not be started until all personnel are present with the proper equipment to perform tracheal intubation or emergency cricothyroidectomy if needed. Temperature should be measured with a tympanic rather than an oral thermometer. Because hypoxemia is associated with epiglottitis, supplemental oxygen may be required. Ideally, the parents can be involved and may need to hold the oxygen delivery device or oxygen tubing near the child's face if proper placement of the device causes agitation.[82]

During assessment of the child's airway by direct laryngoscopy or bronchoscopy, the most skilled pediatrician, anesthesiologist, or ears, nose, and throat specialist should be present. If needed, an endotracheal tube one size smaller than normal is typically placed nasally. If intubation cannot be done, a tracheostomy must be performed. Percutaneous transtracheal jet ventilation may also be considered to ventilate the patient temporarily if the airway cannot be secured with an endotracheal or tracheostomy tube. Subsequently, these children need mechanical ventilation and appropriate monitoring, preferably in the pediatric intensive care unit. Pharmacologic treatment with sedatives and antibiotics should be started,[82] with antibiotic treatment adjusted based on the results of cultures.

Children with epiglottitis usually require intubation for 24 to 48 hours until no evidence of supraglottic swelling is observed. This is usually assessed with repetitive direct laryngoscopy. An assessment for the presence of air leaks is vital before the decision for extubation is made.

Pulmonary Air Leaks

Pulmonary air leak syndromes are common complications of positive pressure applied during mechanical ventilation, especially with high alveolar pressures and/or volumes. However, a pulmonary air leak may also occur spontaneously.[83] Pulmonary air leaks occur more frequently in the newborn period than at any other time of life. The most common risk factors of pulmonary air leaks include lung immaturity, respiratory distress syndrome, aspiration syndromes, and congenital diaphragmatic hernia.[84] Pulmonary air leaks occur when air escapes from the lung into extra-alveolar spaces where it is not normally present. The resulting disorders depend upon the location of the air. The most common conditions are pneumothorax and pneumomediastinum.

Etiology

Pulmonary air leaks frequently occur in children who receive invasive mechanical ventilatory support. The propensity for air leaks to occur is increased in children with a pulmonary pattern of atelectatic alveoli adjacent to normal alveoli, where high peak alveolar pressures and/or tidal volume are required to maintain acid–base balance. Pneumothorax and pneumomediastinum have also been associated with high positive end-expiratory pressure (PEEP), prolonged inspiratory time, and inverse ratio ventilation. Although prolonged inspiratory time and inverse ratio ventilation are used to improve oxygenation by increasing mean airway pressure (MAP), significant intrinsic PEEP or auto-PEEP results. Spontaneous pneumothorax may also occur in full-term infants as a result of the very high negative intrathoracic pressure created with the first breaths the infant takes after delivery.

Pathophysiology

Almost all pulmonary air leak syndromes follow a common pathophysiologic pathway. When high transpulmonary pressures or tidal volumes are applied to an infant's lungs, the distal airways and alveoli become overdistended or stretched and ruptured. Air from the ruptured alveoli will leak into the interstitium. Air continues to spread peripherally by dissecting along the peribronchial and perivascular spaces toward the visceral pleura and pulmonary hila, causing a pneumothorax with rupture of the visceral pleura.[84] In some cases, air continues to accumulate, moves medially, and dissects out from the hila, causing a pneumomediastinum (**Figure 14-9**).[84,85]

The effect of pneumothorax depends on its size and on the resulting air pressure in the pleural space. Pneumothorax causes compression of the great veins and increases pulmonary vascular resistance. As a result, venous return and cardiac output decrease.

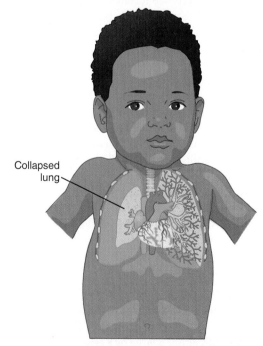

Collapsed lung

FIGURE 14-9 An illustration of a pneumothorax, the presence of air in the space between the parietal and visceral pleurae.

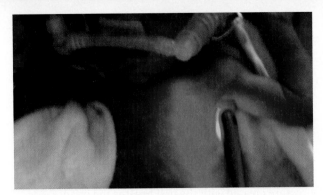

FIGURE 14-10 Use of translumination to detect a pneumothorax in an infant. An area of increased lucency, or spreading of the light source, will occur when air is in the pleural space.

Photo of Astodia courtesy of Futuremed.

A pneumothorax also causes losses in lung volumes and capacities that result in significant shunting and hypoxemia. A large pneumothorax is a life-threatening condition that necessitates immediate intervention and evacuation of the extraneous air.[86,87]

A pneumomediastinum may cause significant shunting and hypoxemia as air collecting above the diaphragm compresses the alveoli and restricts/prevents adequate inflation of the lung.[85,88]

Diagnosis

Pneumothorax should be suspected in any newborn with the sudden onset of respiratory distress. **Transillumination**, a procedure in which a high-intensity light is placed against the chest wall, can be used to identify the free air. Typically, this is done in a darkened room. As the light is placed against the chest wall, an area of increased lucency, or spreading of the light source, will occur when air is in the pleural space (**Figure 14-10**). Transillumination is a valuable tool for rapid and bedside detection and evaluation for the presence of a pneumothorax. However, a definitive diagnosis requires radiologic evidence of air leak; a dense dark area with absent lung markings that separates the lung from the chest wall is usually indicative of a pneumothorax. The affected side may appear hyperlucent because air accumulates anteriorly when the infant lies in the supine position (**Figure 14-11**). A large pneumothorax is associated with tracheal deviation to the opposite side of the pneumothorax; however, this X-ray finding would not be present when bilateral pneumothoraces are present. A lateral X-ray view might be helpful in detecting anterior pneumothorax.

Clinical Presentation

Infants with a small pneumothorax may be asymptomatic. Depending on the severity of the air leaks, the onset of symptoms may be rapid or gradual. Rapid onset usually occurs with either a large or a tension pneumothorax. With a large pneumothorax, infants usually present

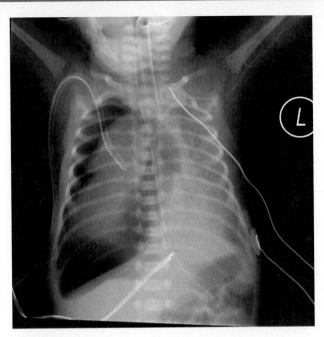

FIGURE 14-11 Radiologic image showing a pneumothorax. The pneumothorax is seen as a dense dark area with absent lung markings.

Case courtesy of Dr Angela Byrne, Radiopaedia.org, rID: 7589

with signs of respiratory distress, including tachypnea, grunting, pallor, retractions, and cyanosis. On physical exam, there will be chest asymmetry with enlargement of the affected side, decreased breath sounds on the affected side, and a shift of the point of maximal cardiac impulse away from the affected side.[85,89]

Hypotension, bradycardia, and hypoxemia occur with large pneumothorax secondary to increased intrathoracic pressure, decreased venous return, and decreased cardiac output.[85,88] Due to the loss of lung volume on the affected side, ventilation/perfusion mismatch occurs with pneumothoraces. Arterial blood gas analysis reveals acidosis, hypercarbia, and hypoxemia.[85,88]

There are several complications associated with pulmonary air leaks. In the immediate phase following the occurrence of the pneumothorax, there is a decrease in the lung compliance, compression atelectasis, and hypoxemia.[89] As a consequence of hypoxemia, the infant may develop hypoxemia-induced pulmonary arterial vasoconstriction, vasospasm, and pulmonary hypertension. The excessive intrathoracic pressure that develops during tension pneumothorax can result in a decrease of cardiac output and profound hypotension. Pulmonary interstitial emphysema may also be a complication to pneumothoraces. Additionally, complications may arise from the treatment of pneumothorax. In particular, infants will be at risk for developing bronchopulmonary dysplasia. When chest tube placement is needed, the complications may include bruising of the diaphragm and mediastinal structures, perforation of the lung with possible hemorrhage, cardiac tamponade, and phrenic nerve injury.[90]

Treatment

Small pneumothoraces in spontaneously breathing infants will typically resolve in 1 to 2 days. These infants should be monitored closely, and oxygen supplementation should be provided as needed to maintain adequate saturation; however, the rate of resolution of spontaneous pneumothoraces is not improved with oxygen supplementation.[91] In mechanically ventilated infants, ventilator settings should be adjusted to avoid alveolar distention and to minimize mean airway pressure by reducing peak inspiratory and alveolar pressures, positive end-expiratory pressure, and inspiratory time.

For symptomatic infants who are not mechanically ventilated, **thoracentesis** may be the only intervention needed to treat pneumothorax and should be considered as a temporizing measure in infants who require ventilation.[91] Thoracentesis involves aspiration of accumulated air with a syringe attached to a 23- or 25-gauge scalp vein needle or an 18- to 20-gauge angiocatheter.

Pneumothorax that develops in a mechanically ventilated infant is best treated with chest tube placement and underwater seal for drainage with continuous suction at a pressure of 10 to 15 cmH$_2$O. Appropriate positioning of the chest tube and resolution of the pneumothorax are assessed by chest radiographs. Resolution of pneumothorax usually occurs in 2 to 3 days.

Pneumomediastinum

Pneumomediastinum is also a pulmonary air leak. This type of air leak occurs when alveolar rupture causes an accumulation of air in the mediastinal space.

Diagnosis

Pneumomediastinum is usually suspected on the routine newborn examination when heart sounds are distant. The diagnosis is made based on a chest radiograph. Pneumomediastinum is most reliably seen on a left anterior oblique view, in which minimal air in the mediastinum surrounds the thymus and lifts it from the cardiac shadow, resulting in the characteristic spinnaker sail sign (**Figure 14-12**), which derives its name from its visual resemblance to the headsail of a boat. This radiologic finding occurs with a spontaneous anterior pneumomediastinum and usually resolves without specific treatment.

Clinical Presentation

Most cases of pneumomediastinum are asymptomatic. Clinically significant pneumomediastinum may result in tachycardia, tachypnea, and cyanosis.

Pneumomediastinum is associated with a range of complications, including lung collapse, subcutaneous emphysema, and pneumopericardium.[92] **Figure 14-13** shows radiologic evidence of subcutaneous emphysema, in which air is present in the subcutaneous tissues of the chest and neck in a small child with a pneumomediastinum.

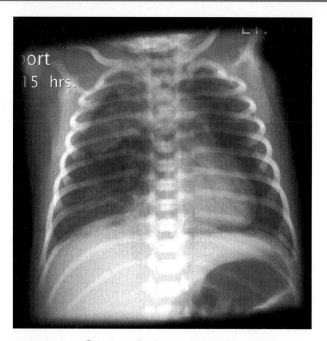

FIGURE 14-12 Pneumomediastinum seen on a chest radiograph. In this image, air is in the mediastinum and surrounds the thymus, lifting it from the cardiac shadow. The pattern of air is the characteristic spinnaker sail sign.
Courtesy of A. Prof Frank Gaillard, Radiopaedia.org, rID: 6353.

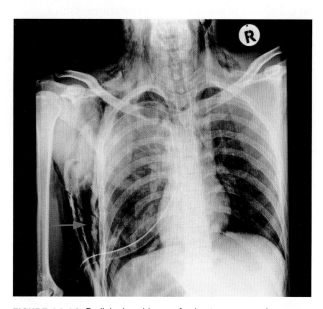

FIGURE 14-13 Radiologic evidence of subcutaneous emphysema extending from the neck to the chest in an adolescent with a pneumomediastinum.
© Sopone/Shutterstock.

In severe cases, so much air is built up in the chest that it compresses the heart and the great blood vessels, causing hemodynamic compromises and cardiac dysfunction.[87]

Treatment

Pneumomediastinum does not require a specific treatment, as it usually resolves spontaneously within a few days. However, adequate monitoring of the infant should be maintained for early recognition and intervention should cardiopulmonary compromise or other air leaks, such as a pneumothorax, develop. If a tension pneumomediastinum is suspected, infants should be treated emergently with ultrasound-guided percutaneous drainage of the tension pneumomediastinum.[93]

Disorders of the Pleura

Disorders of the pleura can occur from many different sources. Pleural disorders may manifest from illness, injury, or medication or reactions to medications. Treatment depends on the type and severity of the condition affecting the pleural space.

Pleural Effusion

The normal pleural space contains approximately 1 mL of fluid. Any abnormal collection of fluid in the pleural space is considered a **pleural effusion** (Figure 14-14). It is the most common manifestation of pleural disease, with approximately 1.5 million pleural effusions diagnosed in the United States each year. They are generally classified as either a transudate or an exudate, and classification is based on the mechanism of fluid formation and pleural fluid chemistry.[94] **Transudate** results from an imbalance in oncotic and hydrostatic pressures, whereas exudates are the result of inflammation of the pleura or decreased lymphatic drainage. In some cases, the pleural fluid may have a combination of transudative and exudative characteristics. Pleural effusion is an

TABLE 14-6
Common Causes of Pleural Effusion in Infants and Children

Cause	Frequency of Occurrence
Pneumonia (parapneumonic effusion)	50–70%
Renal disease	9%
Trauma	7%
Viral disease	7%
Malignancy	5–10%
Congenital heart disease	5–11%
Other (liver failure, sickle cell anemia, meningitis)	3%

indicator of an underlying disease that may be caused by pulmonary or nonpulmonary conditions.

Etiology

Pleural effusions result from disruption of the balance between hydrostatic and oncotic forces in the visceral and parietal pleurae and lymphatic drainage. Several etiologies cause pleural effusions (Table 14-6).

Transudates are due to an imbalance in hydrostatic and oncotic forces in the chest. Major causes of transudative pleural effusion include congenital heart disease, congestive heart failure, hepatic cirrhosis, peritoneal dialysis, nephrotic syndrome, and pulmonary embolus. However, transudates can also be caused by the movement of fluid from peritoneal spaces or by iatrogenic infusion into the pleural space from misplaced or migrated central venous catheters or nasogastric feeding tubes. In clinical practice, transudates are often multifactorial, with renal failure plus cardiac failure plus poor nutritional status being a common trilogy.[94,95]

Exudates arise from pleural or lung inflammation, impaired lymphatic drainage of the pleural space, transdiaphragmatic movement of inflammatory fluid from the peritoneal space, altered permeability of pleural membranes, and increased capillary wall permeability or vascular disruption.[95] Exudates often require more extensive evaluation and treatment than transudates.

Pathophysiology

The regulated fluid balance in the pleural space is disrupted when local or systemic disorders occur. Alterations of local factors include leaky capillaries from inflammation due to infection, infarction, or tumor while alterations of systemic factors can be caused by an elevated pulmonary capillary pressure with heart failure, excess ascites with cirrhosis, or low oncotic pressure due to hypoalbuminemia.[96] When the accumulated fluid is rich in protein

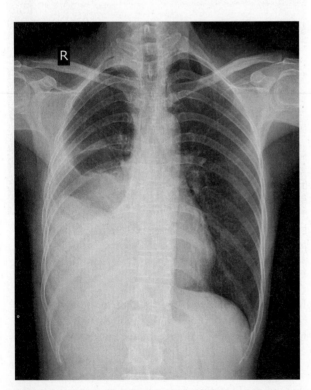

FIGURE 14-14 Posteroanterior chest X-ray (left) and computed tomography scan (right) showing a pleural effusion in the right hemithorax.
© Jarva Jar/Shutterstock.

and lactic dehydrogenase (LDH), it is called exudate; if it is low in protein and LDH, it is called a transudate.

Diagnosis

Auscultation and percussion are valuable initial assessment tools when a pleural effusion is suspected. However, imaging tests are essential for definitive diagnosis. On chest radiograph, a pleural effusion appears as a white space blunting the costophrenic angle at the base of the lung (Figure 14-14). Fluid aspiration by thoracentesis is required to differentiate between a transudate and an exudate. Differentiation between transudates and exudates is based on the chemical characteristics of the accumulated fluid (**Table 14-7**).

Clinical Presentation

The clinical manifestations of pleural effusion are variable and often are related to the underlying disease process. Dyspnea is a common symptom. Cough may be present and is often mild and nonproductive. Pleuritic chest pain commonly occurs and may be mild or severe. This pain is typically described as localized sharp or stabbing pain; however, pain can be felt in the ipsilateral shoulder or upper abdomen. Other symptoms associated with pleural effusion may be present as a reflection of the primary underlying disease process, such as lower extremity edema in congestive heart failure, or cutaneous changes and ascites in liver disease.[97]

Children may be asymptomatic if the effusion is small. However, with significant pleural effusions, findings may include diminished or inaudible breath sounds, dullness to percussion, decreased tactile fremitus, asymmetrical chest expansion, diminished expansion on the side of the effusion, and mediastinal shift away from the effusion in severe cases.[97]

The pleural effusion formation causes flattening or inversion of the diaphragm, mechanical dissociation of the visceral and parietal pleurae, and a restrictive ventilatory defect.[97] Increased peak airway and peak alveolar pressures may be seen in infants with pleural effusion who are intubated and mechanically ventilated. These increases in pressures will predispose the infant to ventilator-induced lung injuries. Significant pleural effusions can also lead to hypoxemia that will necessitate the use of excessive concentrations of inspired oxygen and place the

infants at further risk for complications, such as bronchopulmonary dysplasia and retinopathy of prematurity.

Treatment

Respiratory symptoms and complications resulting from pleural effusion are best treated with drainage of the pleural effusion to relieve symptoms. Subsequent management of pleural effusion, whether transudative or exudative, should be focused on treating the underlying medical disorder. Discontinuation of some medications that are known to cause pleural effusions, such as procainamide, hydralazine, quinidine, nitrofurantoin, dantrolene, methysergide, procarbazine, and methotrexate, might be needed if the medical condition of the patient allows.

Immediate and urgent drainage of parapneumonic effusions that are frankly purulent, with a pH less than 7.0 to 7.1 and bacteria on Gram stain or culture, is needed to prevent rapid coagulation and formation of fibrous peels that might require surgical decortication.[98] Parapneumonic effusions that are not of the nature just described will improve clinically within 1 week with the appropriate antibiotic treatment. Parapneumonic effusions that cannot be drained adequately by needle or small-bore catheters may require surgical intervention.

In unusual cases, surgery might be required to close diaphragmatic defects to prevent recurrent accumulation of pleural effusions in patients with ascites and to ligate the thoracic duct to prevent re-accumulation of effusions.[98] **Pleurodesis** by insufflating talc directly onto the pleural surface using video-assisted thoracoscopy can be employed to sclerose the pleural space and prevent recurrence of pleural effusion. However, the use of talc can produce fever, chest pain, nausea, and possibly acute lung injury. Decortication is usually required for trapped lungs to remove the thick, inelastic pleural peel that restricts ventilation and produces progressive or refractory dyspnea.

Therapeutic thoracentesis with a catheter rather than a needle is used to remove larger amounts of pleural fluid to alleviate dyspnea and to prevent ongoing inflammation and fibrosis in parapneumonic effusions. This procedure is indicated when mediastinal shift is away from the pleural effusion. Only moderate amounts of pleural fluid should be removed to prevent reexpansion pulmonary edema. Large amounts of pleural fluid can be removed if pleural pressure is monitored by pleural manometry and is maintained above -20 cmH$_2$O.[99]

Complicated parapneumonic effusions require drainage by tube thoracostomy. Small-bore tubes, size 7 to 14 French, inserted at the bedside or under radiographic guidance have been demonstrated to provide adequate drainage.[100]

Chylothorax

Chylothorax, also known as chylopleura, refers to the presence of chyle in the pleural space secondary to

---

TABLE 14-7

Chemical Composition of Transudate versus Exudate

Type of Effusion	Pleural Liquid Concentration		Pleural/Serum Concentration Ratio		
	Protein	LDH	Protein	LDH	pH level
Transudate	<3 g/dL	<2/3	<0.5	<0.6	>7.45
Exudate	>3 g/dL	>2/3	>0.5	>0.6	<7.3

leakage from the thoracic duct. Chylothorax can be caused by trauma to the neck or thorax or by an obstruction of the thoracic duct.[101]

Etiology

Causes of chylothorax are either traumatic or nontraumatic. Malignancies account for more than 50% of the nontraumatic cases; lymphoma is the most common cause of malignant etiologies, with non-Hodgkin lymphoma being more likely than Hodgkin lymphoma. Other nonmalignant etiologies are classified into idiopathic, congenital, and miscellaneous. Congenital chylothorax is the leading cause of pleural effusion in neonates.[101] Miscellaneous causes include cirrhosis, tuberculosis, sarcoidosis, amyloidosis, and filariasis.[101]

Surgical trauma is the leading cause of chylothorax. Cardiothoracic surgery has been associated with 69% to 85% of cases of chylothorax in children.[102] Nonsurgical trauma, usually penetrating trauma, is the second leading cause of chylothorax, accounting for approximately 25% of cases.[103]

Pathophysiology

Chylous fluid leaking from the thoracic duct accumulates in the pleural cavity, usually on the right side, and causes acute or chronic alterations in the pulmonary mechanics. Considerable amounts of fat and lymphocytes may be lost due to the leakage of chyle from the thoracic duct. Eosinophils are also present in a higher proportion than in circulating blood. If left untreated, chylothorax can lead to significant nutritional and immunologic pathology. Protein loss in the drained lymphatic fluid can lead to hypoalbunemia, nutritional compromise, and metabolic complications. The chyle appears to have a bacteriostatic property, which accounts for the rare occurrence of infection complicating chylothorax.[101]

Chylothorax in children falls under two categories: congenital and acquired. Congenital chylothorax can represent a significant management challenge: A higher proportion of children with congenital chylothorax fail conservative therapy than those with acquired causes.[103] The majority of acquired cases in infants and children are secondary to traumatic injuries. Direct traumatic injuries to the thoracic duct, as well as thrombosis of the superior vena cava, account for the majority of acquired chylothorax cases.[104]

Diagnosis

Chyle is often suspected only after a thoracentesis. The confirmation of chylothorax is based on pleural fluid analysis and imaging techniques. Pleural fluid analysis for the diagnosis of chylothorax involves the analysis of fluid collected by thoracentesis for cell count and differential, pH, triglycerides, glucose, cholesterol, LDH, total protein, cytology, and microbiologic smear and culture. Triglyceride levels greater than 110 mg/dL

lead to a high suspicion of chylothorax; conversely, if the level is less than 50 mg/dL, chylothorax is unlikely. When triglyceride levels are between 50 and 110 mg/dL, lipoprotein analysis should be performed. Chylomicrons in the fluid establish the diagnosis of chylothorax.[101] Cell counts reveal a predominance of lymphocytes, usually greater than 80% of the total nucleated cell count. Lactic dehydrogenase in chyle is typically low and remains in the transudative range in chylous pleural fluid.[97] Chylous fluid usually has a pH range of 7.40 to 7.80.[101]

Another useful test is the ingestion of lipophilic dye or radio-labeled triglyceride (131I-triolein). Presence of the dye color in the fluid within 1 hour or detection of high radioactivity in the pleural fluid after 48 hours confirms the presence of chylothorax.[101] Lymphangiography may be helpful in defining the site of chyle leak or obstruction or penetrating trauma in spontaneous chylothorax and in lymphangiomatous malformations. Lymphangiography has also demonstrated a therapeutic role in assisting occlusion of the postoperatively damaged lymphatic vessel. This may occur from an inflammatory granulomatous reaction by the lipiodol dye during extravasation.

Once a chylothorax has been diagnosed, imaging techniques are used to identify the site and cause of chyle leakage. Demonstration of chyle leakage by direct visualization or lymphangiography has been the gold standard for the diagnosis of a chylothorax. Conventional chest radiography can identify the side of the chest with the effusion (**Figure 14-15**) but is not helpful in determining the etiology of the chylothorax. Chest computed tomography (CT) of the thorax and abdomen is typically needed to identify the site of thoracic duct rupture. When the site of chyle leakage remains uncertain after chest CT, lymphangiography or lymphoscintigraphy may be helpful.[101]

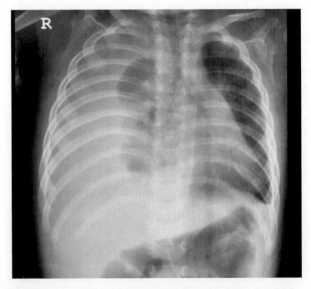

FIGURE 14-15 Chest radiography identifying an effusion due to chyle, or a chylothorax.

Courtesy of Dr. Mohammad Ashkan Moslehi, Radiopaedia.org, rID: 19158.

Clinical Presentation

Most children with a chylothorax remain asymptomatic. Children with a significant amount of chyle accumulation in the pleural space present with dyspnea and tachypnea. Chest pain and fever are uncommon because chyle is not irritating to the pleural surface. Findings on physical examination are nonspecific and include decreased breath sounds and shifting dullness. Traumatic chylothorax usually develops within 2 to 10 days postinjury while in nontraumatic chylothorax, the onset of symptoms is more insidious.[103,104] Spontaneous chylothorax may rarely present as a sudden neck mass.[105] The severity of symptoms is related to the rate of accumulation of chyle and to the size of the pleural effusion.

Due to the loss of chyle, which is rich in fats, proteins, electrolytes, bicarbonate, lymphocytes, and fat-soluble vitamins, some serious complications of chylothorax may occur in patients, such as malnutrition, weakness, dehydration, metabolic acidosis, and compromised immunologic status. Hypoalbuminemia and lymphopenia with prolonged loss of chyle increase the risk of systemic bacterial and viral infections.[101,103]

Treatment

Treatment of chylothorax should be directed at the underlying cause. The thoracic duct leak closes spontaneously in nearly 50% of patients, but surgical management often is pursued after failure of conservative therapies.[105,106]

The placement of a chest tube and continuous drainage of fluid from the pleural space is the initial or conservative management approach.[105,106] This normalizes pleural pressure and reexpands the partially collapsed lungs. Because up to 3L of chyle may drain daily, large amounts of fluid, electrolytes, fat, protein, and lymphocytes may be lost, leading to severe nutritional depletion and an immunodeficient state. Replacements of fluids, electrolytes, protein, fat, and lymphocytes are essential when large amounts of chyle are drained. If drainage from the pleural space does not decrease and remains unchanged, parenteral alimentation should be started.[105,107] Radiotherapy to the mediastinum to resolve the tumor mass in patients with lymphoma is helpful, as the chylothorax in these patients is secondary to lymphoma.[105,106] Somatostatin, a peptide hormone that regulates the endocrine system, or octreotide, a cyclic octapeptide administered at 3.5 to 12 mcg/kg/hour, have shown some success in treating pediatrics with postoperative and iatrogenic chylothorax.[105,106]

Surgical intervention in chylothorax should be considered when the following conditions exist: (1) average daily loss exceeds 1L to 1.5L per year of age in children for a 5-day period, (2) chyle flow has not diminished over 14 days, (3) nutritional complications appear imminent, or (4) accumulation of chyle is continuous despite chest tube drainage.[101]

Thoracic duct ligation is the standard surgical intervention.[106,108] Most recently, video-assisted thoracic surgery and fluoroscopic percutaneous embolization have provided an effective and potentially less invasive approach to chylothorax.[108] A pleuroperitoneal shunt can be successful for refractory chylothorax but is associated with blood loss requiring transfusion.[109] Talc pleurodesis is often used for malignant chylothorax.[110]

Hemothorax

The presence of blood in the pleural space is known as **hemothorax** (**Figure 14-16**). The source of blood may be the chest wall, lung parenchyma, heart, or great vessels secondary mainly to a blunt trauma, iatrogenic causes,[111] or a spontaneous occurrence.[112]

Etiology

Penetrating injuries of the lung, heart, great vessels, or chest wall are the most common causes of a hemothorax. This type of trauma may be accidental, deliberate, or iatrogenic in origin.[113,114] Blunt chest trauma results in hemothorax when a laceration of internal vessels occurs[113,114] while central venous catheter and thoracotomy tube placement are primary iatrogenic causes.[104,114] Other nontraumatic or spontaneous causes of hemothorax are listed in **Table 14-8**.

Pathophysiology

The development of a hemothorax is manifested mainly by hemodynamic and respiratory physiologic responses. The degree of hemodynamic response is determined by the amount and rapidity of blood loss. Early recognition of signs and symptoms of significant blood loss and poor perfusion is essential to patient outcome.[114] Normal respiratory movement of air to the lung may be hampered by the space-occupying effect of a significant

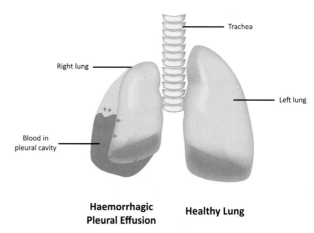

FIGURE 14-16 Illustration of a hemothorax.
© joshya/Shutterstock.

TABLE 14-8
Causes of Nontraumatic or Spontaneous Hemothorax

Hemorrhagic disease of the newborn (e.g., vitamin K deficiency, Henoch-Schönlein purpura, beta thalassemia/hemoglobin E disease)
Primary or metastatic neoplasia
Congenital cystic adenomatoid formation
Type IV Ehlers-Danlos syndrome
Von Recklinghausen disease
Blood dyscrasias
Pulmonary embolism with infarction
Torn pleural adhesions in association with spontaneous pneumothorax
Bullous emphysema
Necrotizing infections
Tuberculosis
Pulmonary arteriovenous fistulae
Hereditary hemorrhagic telangiectasia
Thoracic aortic aneurysm or aneurysm of the internal mammary artery
Intralobar and extralobar sequestration
Abdominal pathology (e.g., ancreatic pseudocyst, splenic artery aneurysm, or hemoperitoneum)

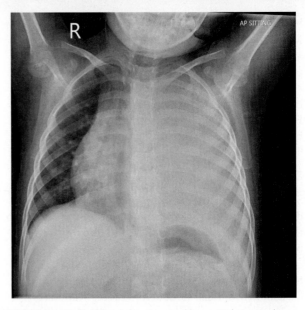

FIGURE 14-17 Right hemothorax caused by a gunshot wound to the chest.

Courtesy of Dr. Henry Knipe, Radiopaedia.org, rID: 41474.

accumulation of blood within the pleural space. In trauma cases, derangements of ventilation and oxygenation variables may result, especially if associated with injuries to the chest wall.[114]

Late physiologic sequelae of unresolved hemothorax include empyema and fibrothorax. If undetected or improperly treated, empyema can lead to bacteremia and septic shock. Fibrothorax traps the lung in position and prevents it from full expansion, causing persistent atelectasis of portions of the lung and reduction in pulmonary function.[114]

Diagnosis

A chest radiograph, preferably in the upright position, is the primary diagnostic tool in the detection of hemothorax. In blunt trauma cases, hemothorax is frequently associated with other chest injuries visible on the chest radiograph, such as rib fractures, pneumothorax, or a widening of the superior mediastinum (**Figure 14-17**). However, additional studies with ultrasonography and CT may be needed for identification and quantification of a hemothorax.[114] Ultrasonography plays a complementary role in specific cases where the chest X-ray findings of hemothorax are equivocal. Bedside echocardiography can provide immediate and accurate information regarding the pericardium and possible presence of serious cardiac injury and pericardial effusion.[114] CT is a highly accurate diagnostic study for pleural fluid or blood and is particularly helpful in localizing collections of blood[114] that may not be evident on the initial chest radiograph.

Measurement of the hematocrit of pleural fluid is virtually never needed in a patient with a traumatic hemothorax; however, it is necessary for the analysis of a bloody effusion from a nontraumatic cause. A hemothorax is present when the hematocrit of the pleural fluid is at least 50% that of the peripheral blood.[114]

Clinical Presentation

Symptoms and findings associated with hemothorax in trauma vary widely, depending on the amount and rapidity of bleeding, the existence and severity of underlying pulmonary disease, and the nature and degree of associated injuries. Chest pain, dyspnea, tachypnea, and shallow breathing are common symptoms.[114] In severe cases, hypoxemia may be present. Diminished ipsilateral breath sounds and dull percussion are noted. With substantial blood loss, hypotension and tachycardia are present.[114] Although hemothorax is associated with chest wall injuries, bony fractures of the chest wall are not necessarily present in infants and children with hemothorax.

Hemodynamic manifestations associated with massive hemothorax are those of hemorrhagic shock. Depending on the amount and rate of bleeding, symptoms can range from mild to severe derangements in hemodynamic variables.[114]

Delayed hemothorax can occur at some interval after blunt chest trauma. In such cases, the initial evaluation reveals findings of rib fractures without any evidence of hemothorax. However, hours to days later, a hemothorax is seen. The mechanism is believed to be either rupture of a trauma-associated chest wall hematoma into the pleural space or displacement of rib fracture edges with eventual disruption of intercostal vessels during respiratory movement or coughing.

Lysis of red blood cells and the increase in the protein concentration of the pleural fluid will lead to an increase in the osmotic pressure within the pleural cavity. This favors transudation of fluid into the pleural space and the progression of small asymptomatic hemothorax into a large and symptomatic bloody pleural effusion.

In nontraumatic hemothorax, symptoms and clinical findings are variable, depending on the underlying pathology. Hemothorax due to acute hemorrhage from structures within the chest, such as arteriovenous malformation, can produce profound hemodynamic changes and symptoms of shock. Occult hemorrhage is most commonly related to metastatic disease or complications of anticoagulation. In such cases, bleeding into the pleural cavity occurs slowly, resulting in subtle or absent changes in hemodynamics. When the effusion is large enough to produce symptoms, dyspnea is usually the most prominent complaint. Signs of anemia may also be present. Other findings include dullness to percussion and decreased breath sounds over the area of the hemothorax.

After full drainage and evacuation of the hemothorax, reexpansion pulmonary edema may occur. A hemothorax that is not fully drained will lead to clotted hemothorax, which may become infected, and empyema can develop. Even if it remains uninfected, clotted hemothorax will progress to a fibrothorax secondary to fibrin deposition. This can lead to lung entrapment, persistent atelectasis, and impaired pulmonary function.[114]

Treatment

Initial treatment of hemothorax is directed toward cardiopulmonary stabilization and evacuation of the pleural blood collection. A hemothorax must be effectively managed to prevent complications, such as fibrothorax and empyema.

Tube thoracostomy drainage is the primary mode of treatment for hemothorax, and as many as 70% to 80% of patients who sustain traumatic hemothorax are successfully treated by tube thoracostomy drainage and require no further therapy.[113,114] However, this procedure is relatively contraindicated when significant pleural adhesions are present. Drainage of hemothorax in a patient with a coagulopathy should be performed with great care; normalization of coagulation function should be initiated before drainage of the hemothorax, if possible. If drainage is incomplete as visualized on the postthoracostomy chest radiograph, placement of a second drainage tube should be considered.

Video-assisted thoracoscopic surgery has been used as an alternative treatment to tube thoracostomy. It permits direct removal of the clot and precise placement of the chest tubes, and it is associated with fewer postoperative complications and shorter hospital stays.[113,114]

Thoracotomy is the procedure of choice for surgical exploration of the chest for massive hemothorax, persistent bleeding, late management of retained clot, drainage of empyema, or decortication.[113,114] During the surgical exploration, the source of bleeding is controlled and the hemothorax is evacuated.

Postoperative ventilator management should progress according to the individual status of the patient. When no other significant injury or disease process is present, weaning and extubation may be quick. In more critically ill patients, such as those with severe chest wall injuries or those requiring massive transfusion, ventilator management might be more challenging and must be tailored to the condition of the patient.

Case Study 1

A 3-month-old female presents with a 4-day history of cough, rhinorrhea, congestion, and fevers. Today her mother noticed she was breathing faster and looked like she was having difficulty breathing. She has been taking less formula than normal. Her 3-year-old sister had a cold last week. On physical exam her temperature is 39.0°C, heart rate is 150 beats per minute, respiratory rate is 70 breaths per minute, and blood pressure is 90/50 mm Hg. Her oxygen saturation is 90%. She appears alert but agitated and is tachypneic and coughing with nasal congestion with a lot of secretions. She has significant work of breathing, with subcostal and intercostal retractions. On auscultation of her lungs, breath sounds are decreased and wheezing is heard on both inspiration and expiration. A prolonged expiratory phase is also noted. The wheezing has a "wet" quality to it. Sputum culture was sent at this time, patient is RSV+.

1. You are requested to assess the child. What respiratory treatment considerations would you recommend at this time?

The patient is admitted to the inpatient floor, where she received oxygen therapy by heated high-flow nasal cannula at an FiO₂ of 0.36. The patient required Q1 to Q2 hours suctioning for thick secretions. An IV was placed for decreased feeds and dehydration. The patient was weaned from heated high flow nasal cannula therapy to room air. Feeds improved, and she was discharged 2 days later.

2. What are specific diagnostic tests for confirming RSV infection?

3. When would you consider using palivizumab?

Case Study 2

An 18-month-old male presented to the emergency department with a chief complaint of cough. He had a two day history of rhinorrhea; fever; a hoarse cry; a progressively worsening, harsh, "barky" cough; and a whistling sound when he breathes. He has been drinking, but his appetite is diminished. His past medical history is unremarkable. His 5-year-old brother also has cold symptoms. Physical exam includes heart rate at 138 beats per minute, respiratory rate at 38 breaths per minute, blood pressure of 90/63 mm Hg, and oxygen saturation of 95% on room air. He is awake and alert, in moderate respiratory distress, and with subcostal and intercostal retractions. Work of breathing increases with nasal flaring when he gets upset. He has a dry, barking cough and a hoarse cry. He has some clear mucus rhinorrhea but no nasal flaring. His pharynx is slightly injected. He has good aeration bilaterally upon auscultation and has inspiratory stridor at rest. No wheezing or rhonchi are noted. His extremities are warm and pink with good perfusion, capillary refill <2 seconds.

1. **How would you classify this patient according to the Westley croup severity scale?**

2. **You are called to the room to do an assessment. What respiratory treatment considerations would you recommend at this time?**

He is treated with nebulized racemic epinephrine; his coughing subsides and his stridor resolves. A lateral neck X-ray was also completed at this time, which reveals no prevertebral soft tissue widening or evidence of epiglottitis. The subglottic region is mildly narrowed. He is treated with oral dexamethasone. He is discharged home after 1 hour of monitoring, and his parents were instructed to treat him with humidified mist therapy.

3. **What is the most common cause of laryngotracheobronchitis?**

References

1. Teshome G, Gattu R, Brown R. Acute bronchiolitis. *Pediatr Clin North Am.* 2013;60(5):1019-1034.

2. Nicolai A, Ferrara M, Schiavariello C, et al. Viral bronchiolitis in children: a common condition with few therapeutic options. *Early Hum Dev.* 2013;89(Suppl 3):S7-S11.

3. Pickles RJ, DeVincenzo JP. Respiratory syncytial virus (RSV) and its propensity for causing bronchiolitis. *J Pathol.* 2015;235(2):266-276.

4. Greenough A, Cox S, Alexander J, et al. Health care utilisation of infants with chronic lung disease, related to hospitalisation for RSV infection. *Arch Dis Child.* 2001;85(6):463-468.

5. Homaira N, Oei JL, Mallitt KA, et al. High burden of RSV hospitalization in very young children: a data linkage study. *Epidemiol Infect.* 2015;2:1-10.

6. McNamara PS, Flanagan BF, Smyth RL, Hart CA. Impact of human metapneumovirus and respiratory syncytial virus co-infection in severe bronchiolitis. *Pediatr Pulmonol.* 2007;42(8):740-743.

7. Semple MG, Cowell A, Dove W, et al. Dual infection of infants by human metapneumovirus and human respiratory syncytial virus is strongly associated with severe bronchiolitis. *J Infect Dis.* 2005;191(3):382-386.

8. Sieminska A, Kuziemski K. Respiratory bronchiolitis-interstitial lung disease. *Orphanet J Rare Dis.* 2014;9:106. doi:10.1186/s13023-014-0106-8.

9. Hasegawa K, Mansbach JM, Camargo CA Jr. Infectious pathogens and bronchiolitis outcomes. *Expert Rev Anti Infect Ther.* 2014; 12(7):817-828.

10. Piedimonte G. Origins of reactive airways disease in early life: do viral infections play a role? *Acta Paediatr Suppl.* 2002;91(437):6-11.

11. Borchers AT, Chang C, Gershwin ME, Gershwin LJ. Respiratory syncytial virus—a comprehensive review. *Clin Rev Allergy Immunol.* 2013;45(3):331-379.

12. Husain S, Singh N. Bronchiolitis obliterans and lung transplantation: evidence for an infectious etiology. *Semin Respir Infect.* 2002; 17(4):310-314.

13. Mustafa G. Bronchiolitis: the recent evidence. *J Ayub Med Coll Abbottabad.* 2014;26(4):602-610.

14. Mailaparambil B, Grychtol R, Heinzmann A. Respiratory syncytial virus bronchiolitis and asthma-insights from recent studies and implications for therapy. *Inflamm Allergy Drug Targets.* 2009;8(3):202-207.

15. Ravaglia C, Poletti V. Recent advances in the management of acute bronchiolitis. *F1000Prime Rep.* 2014;6:103-111.

16. Ralston S, Hill V. Incidence of apnea in infants hospitalized with respiratory syncytial virus bronchiolitis: a systematic review. *J Pediatr.* 2009;155(5):728-733.

17. Anderson LJ. Respiratory syncytial virus vaccines for otitis media. *Vaccine.* 2000;19(Suppl 1):S59-S65.

18. Menchise A. Myocarditis in the setting of RSV bronchiolitis. *Fetal Pediatr Pathol.* 2011;30(1):64-68.

19. Piastra M, Caresta E, Tempera A, Langer A, Zorzi G, Pulitano S. Sharing features of uncommon respiratory syncytial virus complications in infants. *Pediatr Emerg Care.* 2006;22(8):574-578.

20. Hasegawa K, Mansbach JM, Camargo CA Jr. Infectious pathogens and bronchiolitis outcomes. *Expert Rev Anti Infect Ther.* 2014;12(7):817-828.

21. Piippo-Savolainen E, Korppi M. Wheezy babies—wheezy adults? Review on long-term outcome until adulthood after early childhood wheezing. *Acta Paediatr.* 2008;97(1):5-11.

22. Sweetman LL, Ng YT, Butler IJ, Bodensteiner JB. Neurologic complications associated with respiratory syncytial virus. *Pediatr Neurol.* 2005;32(5):307-310.

23. American Academy of Pediatrics Subcommittee on Diagnosis and Management of Bronchiolitis. Diagnosis and management of bronchiolitis. *Pediatrics.* 2006;118(4):1774-1793.

24. Ralston SL, Lieberthal AS, Meissner HC, et al. Clinical Practice Guideline: The diagnosis, management, and prevention of bronchiolitis. *Pediatrics.* 2014;134(5):e1474-e1502.

25. Ralston S, Garber M, Narang S, et al. Decreasing unnecessary utilization in acute bronchiolitis care: results from the value in inpatient pediatrics network. *J Hosp Med.* 2013;8(1):25-30.

26. Johnson LW, Robles J, Hudgins A, Osburn S, Martin D, Thompson A. Management of bronchiolitis in the emergency department: impact

of evidence-based guidelines? *Pediatrics.* 2013;131(Suppl 1): S103-S109.

27. Florin TA, Byczkowski T, Ruddy RM, Zorc JJ, Test M, Shah SS. Variation in the management of infants hospitalized for bronchiolitis persists after the 2006 American Academy of Pediatrics bronchiolitis guidelines. *J Pediatr.* 2014;165(4):786-792.

28. Iwane MK, Chaves SS, Szilagyi PG, et al. Disparities between black and white children in hospitalizations associated with acute respiratory illness and laboratory-confirmed influenza and respiratory syncytial virus in 3 US counties—2002-2009. *Am J Epidemiol.* 2013;177(7):656-665.

29. Centers for Disease Control and Prevention. Respiratory syncytial virus circulation in the United States, July 2012–June 2014. *MMWR.* 2014;62:141-144.

30. Gomez RS, Guisle-Marsollier I, Bohmwald K, Bueno SM, Kalergis AM. Respiratory syncytial virus: pathology, therapeutic drugs and prophylaxis. *Immunol Lett.* 2014;162(1 Pt A):237-247.

31. Luo G, Nkoy FL, Gesteland PH, Glasgow TS, Stone BL. A systematic review of predictive modeling for bronchiolitis. *Int J Med Inform.* 2014;83(10):691-714.

32. Nokso-Koivisto J, Marom T, Chonmaitree T. Importance of viruses in acute otitis media. *Curr Opin Pediatr.* 2015;27(1):110-115.

33. Oray-Schrom P, Phoenix C, St Martin D, Amoateng-Adjepong Y. Sepsis workup in febrile infants 0-90 days of age with respiratory syncytial virus infection. *Pediatr Emerg Care.* 2003;19(5): 314-319.

34. Pickles RJ, DeVincenzo JP. Respiratory syncytial virus (RSV) and its propensity for causing bronchiolitis. *J Pathol.* 2015;235(2):266-276.

35. Somech R, Spirer Z. Uncommon presentation of some common pediatric diseases. *Adv Pediatr.* 2003;50:269-304.

36. Williams JV. The clinical presentation and outcomes of children infected with newly identified respiratory tract viruses. *Infect Dis Clin North Am.* 2005;19(3):569-584.

37. Díez-Domingo J, Pérez-Yarza EG, Melero JA, et al. Social, economic, and health impact of the respiratory syncytial virus: a systematic search. *BMC Infect Dis.* 2014;14:544-558.

38. Lin JA, Madikians A. From bronchiolitis guideline to practice: a critical care perspective. *World J Crit Care Med.* 2015;4(3):152-158.

39. American Academy of Pediatrics Committee on Infectious Diseases; American Academy of Pediatrics Bronchiolitis Guidelines Committee. Updated guidance for palivizumab prophylaxis among infants and young children at increased risk of hospitalization for respiratory syncytial virus infection. *Pediatrics.* 2014;134(2):e620-e638.

40. Engelhardt OG, Fodor E. Functional association between viral and cellular transcription during influenza virus infection. *Rev Med Virol.* 2006;16(5):329-345.

41. Matsuzaki Y, Abiko C, Mizuta K, et al. A nationwide epidemic of influenza C virus infection in Japan in 2004. *J Clin Microbiol.* 2007;45(3):783-788.

42. Gubareva LV, Kaiser L, Hayden FG. Influenza virus neuraminidase inhibitors. *Lancet.* 2000;355(9206):827-835.

43. Wu G, Yan SM. Mutation trend of hemagglutinin of influenza A virus: a review from a computational mutation viewpoint. *Acta Pharmacol Sin.* 2006;27(5):513-526.

44. Bouvier NM. Animal models for influenza virus transmission studies: a historical perspective. *Curr Opin Virol.* 2015;13:101-108.

45. Bell D, Nicoll A, Fukuda K, et al. Non-pharmaceutical interventions for pandemic influenza, national and community measures. *Emerg Infect Dis.* 2006;12(1):88-94.

46. Dwyer DE, Smith DW, Catton MG, Barr IG. Laboratory diagnosis of human seasonal and pandemic influenza virus infection. *Med J Aust.* 2006;185(Suppl 10):S48-S53.

47. Williams LO, Kupka NJ, Schmaltz SP, Barrett S, Uyeki TM, Jernigan DB. Rapid influenza diagnostic test use and antiviral prescriptions in outpatient settings pre- and post-2009 H1N1 pandemic. *J Clin Virol.* 2014;60(1):27-33.

48. Liu PY, Wang LC, Lin YH, Tsai CA, Shi ZY. Outbreak of influenza A and B among military recruits: evidence from viral culture and polymerase chain reaction. *J Microbiol Immunol Infect.* 2009; 42(2):114-121.

49. Jung YJ, Kwon HJ, Huh HJ, Ki CS, Lee NY, Kim JW. Comparison of the AdvanSure real-time RT-PCR and Seeplex RV12 ACE assay for the detection of respiratory virus. *Journal of Viral Methods.* 2015;224:42-46.

50. van Vugt SF, Broekhuizen BD, Zuithoff NP, et al. Validity of a clinical model to predict influenza in patients presenting with symptoms of lower respiratory tract infection in primary care. *Fam Pract.* 2015;32(4):408-414.

51. Flannery B, Clippard J, Zimmerman RK, et al. Early estimates of seasonal influenza vaccine effectiveness—United States, January 2015. *MMWR Morb Mortal Wkly Rep.* 2015;64(1):10-15.

52. Influenza vaccination coverage among pregnant women—United States, 2012-13 influenza season. *MMWR Morb Mortal Wkly Rep.* 2013;62(38):787-792.

53. Interim adjusted estimates of seasonal influenza vaccine effectiveness—United States, February 2013. *MMWR Morb Mortal Wkly Rep.* 2013;62(7):119-123.

54. Gensheimer KF, Meltzer MI, Postema AS, Strikas RA. Influenza pandemic preparedness. *Emerg Infect Dis.* 2003;9(12):1645-1648.

55. Fiore AE, Fry A, Shay D, et al. Antiviral agents for the treatment and chemoprophylaxis of influenza—recommendations of the Advisory Committee on Immunization Practices (ACIP). *MMWR Recomm Rep.* 2011;60(1):1-24.

56. Adisasmito W, Chan PK, Lee N, et al. Effectiveness of antiviral treatment in human influenza A(H5N1) infections: analysis of a Global Patient Registry. *J Infect Dis.* 2010;202(8):1154-1160.

57. Chamni S, De-Eknamkul W. Recent progress and challenges in the discovery of new neuraminidase inhibitors. *Expert Opin Ther Pat.* 2013;23(4):409-423.

58. Lee V, Yap J, Cook AR, et al. Effectiveness of public health measures in mitigating pandemic influenza spread: a prospective sero-epidemiological cohort study. *J Infect Dis.* 2010;202(9): 1319-1326.

59. Bjornson CL, Johnson DW. Croup in children. *CMAJ.* 2013;185(15): 1317-1323.

60. Zoorob R, Sidani M, Murray J. Croup: an overview. *Am Fam Physician.* 2011;83(9):1067-1073.

61. Worrall G. Croup. *Can Fam Physician.* 2008;54(4):573-574.

62. Rajapaksa S, Starr M. Croup-assessment and management. *Aust Fam Physician.* 2010;39(5):280-282.

63. Bjornson CL, Johnson DW. Croup. *Lancet.* 2008;371(9609):329-339.

64. Petrocheilou A, Tanou K, Kalampouka E, Malakasioti G, Giannios C, Kaditis AG. Viral croup: diagnosis and a treatment algorithm. *Pediatr Pulmonol.* 2014;49(5):421-429.

65. Hoa M, Kingsley EL, Coticchia JM. Correlating the clinical course of recurrent croup with endoscopic findings: a retrospective observational study. *Ann Otol Rhinol Laryngol.* 2008;117(6):464-469.

66. Khemani RG, Schneider JB, Morzov R, Markovitz B, Newth CJ. Pediatric upper airway obstruction: interobserver variability is the road to perdition. *J Crit Care.* 2013;28(4):490-497.

67. Everard ML. Acute bronchiolitis and croup. *Pediatr Clin North Am.* 2009;56(1):119-133.

68. Tibballs J, Watson T. Symptoms and signs differentiating croup and epiglottitis. *J Paediatr Child Health.* 2011;47(3):77-82.

69. Mazza D, Wilkinson F, Turner T, Harris C; Health for Kids Guideline Development Group. Evidence based guideline for the management of croup. *Aust Fam Physician.* 2008;37(6 Spec No):14-20.

70. Bjornson C, Russell KF, Vandermeer B, Durec T, Klassen TP, Johnson DW. Nebulized epinephrine for croup in children. *Cochrane Database Syst Rev.* 2011;CD006619.

71. Russell K, Wiebe N, Saenz A, et al. Glucocorticoids for croup. *Cochrane Database Syst Rev.* 2004;CD001955.

72. Scolnik D, Coates AL, Stephens D, Da Silva Z, Lavine E, Schuh S. Controlled delivery of high vs low humidity vs mist therapy for croup in emergency departments: a randomized controlled trial. *JAMA.* 2006;295(11):1274-1280.

73. Beckmann KR, Brueggemann WM Jr. Heliox treatment of severe croup. *Am J Emerg Med.* 2000;18(6):735-736.

74. Weber JE, Chudnofsky CR, Younger JG, et al. A randomized comparison of helium-oxygen mixture (Heliox) and racemic epinephrine for the treatment of moderate to severe croup. *Pediatrics.* 2001;107(6):E96.

75. Rizk HG, Nassar M, Rohayem Z, Rassi SJ. Hypoplastic epiglottis in a non-syndromic child: a rare anomaly with serious consequences. *Int J Pediatr Otorhinolaryngol.* 2010;74(8):952-955.

76. Wallenborn PA III, Postma DS. Radiation recall supraglottitis. A hazard in head and neck chemotherapy. *Arch Otolaryngol.* 1984;110(9):614-617.

77. Katori H, Tsukuda M. Acute epiglottitis: analysis of factors associated with airway intervention. *J Laryngol Otol.* 2005;119(12):967-972.

78. Loftis L. Acute infectious upper airway obstructions in children. *Semin Pediatr Infect Dis.* 2006;17(1):5-10.

79. Sobol SE, Zapata S. Epiglottitis and croup. *Otolaryngol Clin North Am.* 2008;41(3):551-566.

80. Rotta AT, Wiryawan B. Respiratory emergencies in children. *Respir Care.* 2003;48(3):248-258.

81. Jenkins IA, Saunders M. Infections of the airway. *Paediatr Anaesth.* 2009;19(Suppl 1):118-130.

82. Chandradeva K, Palin C, Ghosh SM, Pinches SC. Percutaneous transtracheal jet ventilation as a guide to tracheal intubation in severe upper airway obstruction from supraglottic oedema. *Br J Anaesth.* 2005;94(5):683-686.

83. Alter SJ. Spontaneous pneumothorax in infants: a 10-year review. *Pediatr Emerg Care.* 1997;13(6):401-403.

84. Johnson NN, Toledo A, Endom EE. Pneumothorax, pneumomediastinum, and pulmonary embolism. *Pediatr Clin North Am.* 2010;57(6):1357-1383.

85. Giuliani S, Franklin A, Pierce J, Ford H, Grikscheit TC. Massive subcutaneous emphysema, pneumomediastinum, and pneumopericardium in children. *J Pediatr Surg.* 2010;45(3):647-649.

86. Pauzé DR, Pauzé DK. Emergency management of blunt chest trauma in children: an evidence-based approach. *Pediatr Emerg Med Pract.* 2013;10(11):1-22.

87. Takada K, Matsumoto S, Hiramatsu T, et al. Spontaneous pneumomediastinum: an algorithm for diagnosis and management. *Ther Adv Respir Dis.* 2009;3(6):301-307.

88. Dotson K, Johnson LH. Pediatric spontaneous pneumothorax. *Pediatr Emerg Care.* 2012;28(7):715-720.

89. da Silva PS, de Aguiar VE, Fonseca MC. Iatrogenic pneumothorax in mechanically ventilated children: incidence, risk factors and other outcomes. *Heart Lung.* 2015;4(3):238-242.

90. Ogunleye EO. Principles of chest tube insertion. *Nig Q J Hosp Med.* 2012;22(1):65-68.

91. Baumann MH. Management of spontaneous pneumothorax. *Clin Chest Med.* 2006;27(2):369-381.

92. Cullen ML. Pulmonary and respiratory complications of pediatric trauma. *Respir Care Clin N Am.* 2001;7(1):59-77.

93. Sogut O, Cevik M, Boleken ME, Kaya H, Dokuzoglu MA. Pneumomediastinum and subcutaneous emphysema due to blunt neck injury: a case report and review of the literature. *J Pak Med Assoc.* 2011;61(7):702-704.

94. Segura RM. Useful clinical biological markers in diagnosis of pleural effusions in children. *Paediatr Respir Rev.* 2004;5(Suppl A):S205-S212.

95. Prais D, Kuzmenko E, Amir J, Harel L. Association of hypoalbuminemia with the presence and size of pleural effusion in children with pneumonia. *Pediatrics.* 2008;121(3):e533-e538.

96. Givan DC, Eigen H. Common pleural effusions in children. *Clin Chest Med.* 1998;19(2):363-371.

97. Beers SL, Abramo TJ. Pleural effusions. *Pediatr Emerg Care.* 2007;23(5):330-334.

98. Paraskakis E, Vergadi E, Chatzimichael A, Bouros D. Current evidence for the management of paediatric parapneumonic effusions. *Curr Med Res Opin.* 2012;28(7):1179-1192.

99. Feller-Kopman D, Parker MJ, Schwartzstein RM. Assessment of pleural pressure in the evaluation of pleural effusions. *Chest.* 2009;135(1):201-209.

100. Cafarotti S, Dall'Armi V, Cusumano G, et al. Small-bore wire-guided chest drains: safety, tolerability, and effectiveness in pneumothorax, malignant effusions, and pleural empyema. *J Thorac Cardiovasc Surg.* 2011;141(3):683-687.

101. Talwar A, Lee H. A contemporary review of chylothorax. *Indian J Chest Dis Allied Sci.* 2008;50(4):343-351.

102. Milonakis M, Chatzis AC, Giannopoulos NM, et al. Etiology and management of chylothorax following pediatric heart surgery. *J Card Surg.* 2009;24(4):369-373.

103. Tutor JD. Chylothorax in infants and children. *Pediatrics.* 2014;133(4):722-733.

104. Achildi O, Smith BP, Grewal H. Thoracoscopic ligation of the thoracic duct in a child with spontaneous chylothorax. *J Laparoendosc Adv Surg Tech A.* 2006;16(5):546-549.

105. Soto-Martinez M, Massie J. Chylothorax: diagnosis and management in children. *Paediatr Respir Rev.* 2009;10(4):199-207.

106. Suddaby EC, Schiller S. Management of chylothorax in children. *Pediatr Nurs.* 2004;30(4):290-295.

107. Lopez-Gutierrez JC, Tovar JA. Chylothorax and chylous ascites: management and pitfalls. *Semin Pediatr Surg.* 2014;23(5):298-302.

108. Nadolski G, Itkin M. Thoracic duct embolization for the management of chylothoraces. *Curr Opin Pulm Med.* 2013;19(4):380-386.

109. Shiraga K, Terui K, Ishihara K, et al. Pleuroperitoneal shunt for refractory chylothorax accompanied with a mediastinal lymphangioma: a case report. *Ann Thorac Cardiovasc Surg.* 2014;20:654-658.

110. Banjer AH, Siddiqui MA, Al-Fattani MO, Nigme BA. Malignant chylothorax treated by talc pleurodesis: a case report and review of the literature. *Ann Saudi Med.* 1998;18(6):550-552.

111. Karavis MY, Argyra E, Segredos V, Yiallouroy A, Giokas G, Theodosopoulos T. Acupuncture-induced haemothorax: a rare iatrogenic complication of acupuncture. *Acupunct Med.* 2015;33(3):237-241.

112. Patrini D, Panagiotopoulos N, Pararajasingham J, Gvinianidze L, Iqbal Y, Lawrence DR. Etiology and management of spontaneous haemothorax. *J Thorac Dis.* 2015;7(3):520-526.

113. Choi PM, Farmakis S, Desmarais TJ, Keller MS. Management and outcomes of traumatic hemothorax in children. *J Emerg Trauma Shock.* 2015;8(2):83-87.

114. Broderick SR. Hemothorax: etiology, diagnosis, and management. *Thorac Surg Clin.* 2013;23(1):89-96.

15

Chronic Respiratory Disorders of the Child

Tim Opt'Holt

Lisa Johnson

Teresa A. Volsko

© Anna Rucak/ShutterStock, Inc.

OUTLINE

OBJECTIVES

1. Describe the pathophysiology of asthma.
2. List the tests used to diagnose asthma.
3. Explain the therapies used in the step-wise approach to the treatment of asthma.
4. Discuss the importance of an asthma action plan.
5. Differentiate among SABAs, LABAs, and ICSs.
6. Discuss the essential elements of asthma treatment across the continuum of care.
7. List the complications associated with poor asthma control.
8. Describe the pathophysiology of cystic fibrosis (CF).
9. List the tests used to diagnose CF.
10. Explain the therapies used in the daily treatment of CF.
11. List the four pillars of CF care.
12. Discuss how an acute exacerbation is identified and treated.
13. List the complications associated with CF.

KEY TERMS

airway clearance
  therapy (ACT)
allergic bronchopulmonary
  aspergillosis (APBA)
asthma
asthma action plan
bronchoprovocation
  challenge test
cepacia syndrome
cystic fibrosis
  transmembrane
  conductance
  regulator (CFTR)
cystic fibrosis (CF)
distal intestinal obstruction
  syndrome (DIOS)

forced expiratory volume
  in 1 second (FEV$_1$)
inhaled corticosteroids
  (ICSs)
ivacaftor
long-acting beta2-agonists
  (LABAs)
lung clearance index (LCI)
massive hemoptysis
meconium ileus
minor hemoptysis
peak flow meter
short-acting beta2-agonists
  (SABAs)
steatorrhea
sweat chloride test

Introduction

Asthma and cystic fibrosis are two chronic diseases that require the use of respiratory modalities to maintain health and prevent acute exacerbations or flare-ups of the disease process. Clinicians play an important role in helping the child and family understand their disease process, their therapeutic regimen, and how to recognize the need to contact their healthcare provider for additional intervention or escalation of care.

Asthma

Asthma is one of the most common and serious chronic diseases in childhood. According to the Centers for Disease Control and Prevention (CDC) National Health Interview Survey conducted in 2012, over 10 million children in the United States younger than age 18 years have been diagnosed with asthma.[1] The Environmental Protection Agency (EPA) ranked asthma as third for the cause of hospitalization among children younger than the age of 15 and noted, on average, that 1 out of every 10 school-aged children has an asthma diagnosis. Asthma accounts for over 10.5 million school days missed per year.[2]

Asthma also accounts for significant morbidity and mortality. Asthma was the cause for 479,300 hospitalizations, 1.9 million emergency department visits, and 8.9 million doctor visits in 2009.[3] Data from the CDC's Asthma's Impact on the Nation factsheets reveal that about nine people die from asthma each day.[3] The economic cost for asthma in the United States is $56 billion each year, with the average yearly cost to care for a child with asthma at $1,039.[3]

Etiology

The National Institutes of Health (NIH) National Asthma Education and Prevention Program (NAEPP) Guidelines for the Diagnosis and Management of Asthma Expert Panel Report 3 (EPR-3) define **asthma** as follows:

> A chronic inflammatory disorder of the airways in which many cells and cellular elements play a role: in particular, mast cells, eosinophils, neutrophils (especially in sudden onset, fatal exacerbations, occupational asthma, and patients who smoke), T lymphocytes, macrophages, and epithelial cells. In susceptible individuals, this inflammation causes recurrent episodes of coughing (particularly at night or early in the morning), wheezing, breathlessness, and chest tightness. These episodes are usually associated with widespread but variable airflow obstruction that is often reversible either spontaneously or with treatment.[4]

These guidelines continue to characterize this complex disorder by stating that, if left untreated, the interaction between the inflammation in the airway causes variable and recurring symptoms, airflow obstruction, bronchial hyperresponsiveness, and ongoing underlying inflammation.[4] **Figure 15-1** illustrates how the airways react to certain stimuli—smooth muscles that wrap around the airways tighten, the airway wall becomes inflamed, and thick mucus is produced.

The exact cause of asthma is not known, and there is no cure. However, asthma can be managed very well with medication and by controlling environmental factors, such as allergens and irritants. Researchers continue to explore the inflammatory process in hopes of finding a cause and cure for this disease. The EPR-3 guidelines describe the development of asthma as a relationship between host factors (genetic and environmental exposures) that occurs during the development of the immune system early in life.[4]

Pathophysiology

Although the cause may not be known, the bronchi appear to be hyperreactive to stimuli, increasing the production of immunoglobulin E (IgE), mast cell degranulation, and release of inflammatory mediators. Due to this response in the airway, the lung tissue swells, causing the airways to be overly reactive. Mucus production increases, adding to the constriction of the airways. Inflammation, if left untreated, can cause permanent structural changes, also known as airway remodeling. It is important to note that airway remodeling can be prevented or minimized with proper asthma management.

Diagnosis

A detailed medical history and physical examination are important to the diagnosis of asthma. For the child older than 1 year of age who presents with their first episode of wheezing, a family history of asthma or allergies may be suggestive of a diagnosis of asthma.

Past Medical and History of Present Illness

The medical history should ascertain the factors contributing to the abrupt episode of wheezing, shortness of breath, chest discomfort, and/or nocturnal awakenings for dyspnea. It is important for the clinical team to identify the factors or stimuli that trigger the acute asthma exacerbation, such as exposure to changes in weather (cold, heat), emotions (crying, laughing), animal dander (cat, dog, horse), or environmental exposures (pollen, smoke).

An account of the frequency of symptoms and the number of physician office visits, emergency department visits, hospitalizations, and intensive care unit (ICU) admissions for asthma are important for identifying the severity risk for and control of this chronic condition. This history should also include quality of life determinants, such as the number of missed school- and/or workdays associated with asthma exacerbations.

Diagnostic Testing

Spirometry is essential for the diagnosis and management of asthma in children older than 5 years of age. The forced vital capacity (FVC), **forced expiratory**

Pathology of Asthma

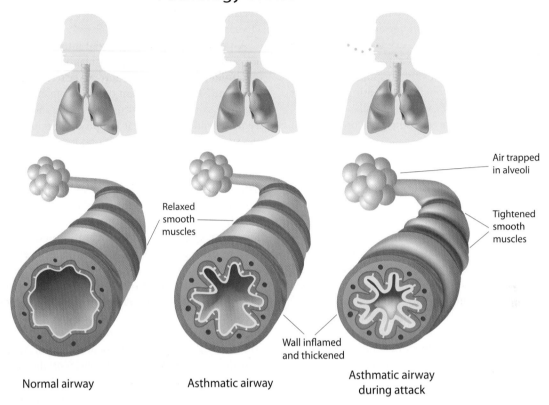

Air trapped
in alveoli

Relaxed
smooth
muscles

Tightened
smooth
muscles

Wall inflamed
and thickened

Normal airway   Asthmatic airway   Asthmatic airway
during attack

FIGURE 15-1 In the asthmatic airway, the airway wall thickens, smooth muscle spasms, and there is an increase in mucus production.
© Alila Medical Media/Shutterstock.

volume in 1 second (FEV$_1$), and ratio of forced expiratory volume in 1 second to forced vital capacity (FEV$_1$/FVC%) are most commonly used.

Typically, when the child is not having an exacerbation of asthma and is free of asthma exacerbation symptoms, the FEV$_1$/FVC should be within the normal range, which is ranked by age.

The FEV$_1$ measures small-airway obstruction. Typically, spirometry is performed before and after bronchodilator administration to determine the presence of airway obstruction and the response to bronchodilator therapy. An FEV$_1$ is measured prior to a bronchodilator treatment and again 15 minutes after bronchodilator administration to determine reversibility of airway obstruction. Reversibility, or an indicator of airway responsiveness to bronchodilator administration, is defined as an increase in FEV$_1$ and FVC of 12%.[5] Airway response to bronchodilator treatment is a key feature of asthma. Spirometry is patient effort dependent. It is important for the clinician who performs the test to be trained in coaching children on the proper way to perform the maneuver in order to obtain a satisfactory test.

Additional diagnostic testing, such as a bronchoprovocation challenge; chest radiograph; allergy testing; and sputum, blood, or urine testing, may be needed to differentiate asthma from other childhood diseases, especially if the child is too young to perform spirometry

or is not responding to bronchodilator therapy. It is important to remember that bronchoprovocation challenge and/or allergy testing are never conducted when the child is symptomatic or experiencing an acute exacerbation of asthma. The **bronchoprovocation challenge test** is more commonly used in the adult population, but it has been used in older children. The test is performed in a clinic setting using either methacholine or mannitol. Following baseline spirometric testing, the child repeatedly inhales a dose of methacholine by aerosol mist or dry powder in increasing concentrations until hyperreactivity of the small airways is noted. Spirometry is performed after each dose to evaluate response, or a reduction in FEV$_1$. A 20% reduction of FEV$_1$ is considered a positive test.[6,7] A short-acting bronchodilator is administered to reverse the effects of the methacholine. Mannitol challenge testing is a new method used for assessment of asthma and is reported to be especially helpful with diagnosing exercise-induced asthma. Prefilled mannitol capsules in escalating doses are administered by a dry powder inhaler device. Spirometry testing is performed 60 seconds after each dose, watching for a 15% fall in FEV$_1$ value.[8]

Exercise tolerance tests may be performed to diagnose exercise-induced asthma. A variety of forms of exercise, including bicycle ergometry and running on a treadmill or free running, have been used. The child is monitored during the exercise interval, which lasts approximately 5 to 8 minutes. Exercise may be graded, or the intensity elevated, in order to increase the child's heart rate to 85% of predicted for age and gender. Spirometry is performed prior to exercising and in between each exercise interval. A decline in FEV_1 of 15% or greater is indicative of a positive response.[9] However, when compared to bronchoprovocation challenge using pharmacologic agents, exercise challenge is less sensitive and may be a poorer predictor of bronchial hyperresponsiveness.[9,10]

A chest radiograph has little value in the diagnosis of asthma. Typically the chest radiograph is normal, but it may be helpful to exclude other diagnoses. Allergy testing may be performed to check for sensitivities to common allergens that cause bronchial reactivity. When identified, education about avoidance of allergens is often beneficial for preventing future asthma exacerbations. Sputum, blood, or urine testing can also assist with diagnosing allergic sensitivities, elevated IgE levels, and other comorbid conditions.

A combination of a positive family history, the intermittent presence of typical asthma symptoms, spirometry indicating reversible obstruction, and ruling out of asthma mimics are instrumental in the diagnosis of asthma.

Classifying Asthma Severity

Once a diagnosis of asthma has been made, classifying and assessing asthma severity by using evidence-based national guidelines will assist with creating a treatment plan to achieve asthma control. The EPR-3 guidelines divide recommendations for asthma assessment and treatment into three age ranges: 0 to 4 years, 5 to 11 years, and 12 years and older.

Asthma severity is categorized into two domains—impairment and risk—and four classifications: intermittent, mild persistent, moderate persistent, and severe persistent. The impairment domain concentrates on symptoms and lung function.[4] Knowing the current frequency and intensity of symptoms and lung function measurements can assist with obtaining an appropriate treatment plan. The risk domain is a predictor of future asthma exacerbations. Medical history, along with past visits to the emergency department, hospitalizations, unscheduled clinic visits, and oral corticosteroid use, for asthma exacerbations play a big part in assessing the risk factor. Other predictors include monitoring for reduction in lung growth and medication side effects from the treatment plan.

The four classifications of asthma are based on frequency of daytime and nighttime symptoms, frequency of reliever/rescue medication usage, interference with normal activity, lung function measurements, and oral corticosteroid usage. Recommendations for medical providers on how to initiate a treatment plan and to adjust the treatment plan by the patient's response to therapy are presented in **Table 15-1**, which provides an example of an asthma severity table for children 4 years of age or younger.[4] The National Asthma Guidelines provide tables for children within each of the three aforementioned age ranges.

TABLE 15-1
An Example of Classifying Asthma Severity for Children 4 Years of Age or Younger

Components of Severity		Classification of Asthma Severity 0–4 Years of Age			
		Intermittent	Persistent		
			Mild	Moderate	Severe
Impairment	Symptoms	≤2 days/week	>2 days/week, but not daily	Daily	Throughout the day
	Nighttime awakenings	0	1–2 times/month	3–4 times/month	>1 time/week
	SABA for symptoms	≤2 days/week	>2 days/week, but not daily	Daily	Several times per day
	Interference with normal activity	None	Minor limitation	Some limitation	Extremely limited
Risk	Exacerbations requiring oral systemic corticosteroids	0–1/year	>2 exacerbations in 6 months requiring oral systemic corticosteroids or 4 wheezing episodes/1 year lasting >1 day AND risk factors for persistent asthma		
			Consider severity and interval since last exacerbation. Frequency and severity may fluctuate over time.		

SABA = short-acting beta2-agonist

Data from National Asthma Education and Prevention Program Expert Panel Report 3. Guidelines for the diagnosis and management of asthma. National Heart Lung and Blood Institute, National Institutes of Health: U.S. Department of Health and Human Services; 2007 Aug 28. Report no. 07-4051. Full Report.

Clinical Presentation

The physical examination of the child is very important. The combination of a detailed history and physical examination are helpful in differentiating asthma from other childhood diseases, such as bronchiolitis, and foreign body obstruction. Children experiencing an acute exacerbation of asthma will have varying degrees of respiratory distress, depending on the severity of airway constriction, inflammation, and obstruction. **Table 15-2** provides a list of common symptoms associated with an acute exacerbation of asthma. The physical examination of a child who has asthma, but who is not currently experiencing an acute exacerbation of asthma, is generally normal.

Management

There are four key components for achieving and then controlling asthma: (1) assess and monitor asthma severity and control, (2) partner with patients and families to educate them on their asthma plan of care, (3) control environmental factors and comorbid conditions that trigger asthma exacerbations, and (4) prescribe appropriate medications for treatment of asthma.

Assess and Monitor Asthma Severity and Control

The NAEPP's EPR-3 recommends a step-wise approach to asthma treatment based on an assessment of the child's severity and control.[4] These guidelines serve as a

standardized tool based on the best available evidence. Treatment depends on collaboration between the family and the clinical team to identify and minimize asthma exacerbation triggers, formulation of a plan that establishes management goals to improve asthma control, and enhanced patient and family satisfaction with their asthma care. Asthma care, including pharmacologic intervention, escalates, described in the guidelines as "step up," during an acute exacerbation, when asthma symptoms worsen or when the child's asthma is not well controlled. Treatment deescalates or is "stepped down" when asthma is controlled.

Step-Wise Approach

A child with poorly controlled asthma will have symptoms that frequently interfere with age-appropriate activity and require short-acting beta2-agonists (SABAs) for symptom relief several times per day. **Table 15-3** outlines the classification for asthma control for children 4 years of age and younger. Pharmacologic management depends on the child's asthma severity and level of control. **Table 15-4** outlines the step-wise approach to care for children 4 years of age or younger with intermittent or persistent asthma. A comprehensive home asthma management plan should include trigger identification and a strategy for trigger avoidance, the use of quick-relief medications to relieve symptoms of an acute exacerbation, and, depending on the severity of asthma, the use of long-term controller medications.

It is important to assess a patient's adherence to therapy, investigate environmental changes that may trigger an asthma exacerbation, rule out comorbid conditions, and assess the child's ability to properly administer medication, such as observing inhaler technique to ensure proper administration, before stepping up or escalating therapy. It is equally important for the primary care team to decrease pharmacologic therapy when the child's asthma control improves and sustains that improvement for least 3 months.

Educate Children and Their Families/Caregivers

Education is a key element of asthma home management. Children and their families must be able to differentiate controller medications from those used for quick relief and understand the plan of care for maintaining health and addressing asthma symptoms. NAEPP recommends that asthma education be provided and reinforced by the healthcare team during every opportunity with the patient. Asthma self-management education is a partnership among the child, their parents or caregivers, and the interdisciplinary healthcare team. Asthma education should include information on how to control asthma symptoms or to maintain health and prevent asthma exacerbations. The use of open-ended communication allows the child and family to have an

---

TABLE 15-2
Common Symptoms Associated with an Acute Exacerbation of Asthma

Upper airway inflammation • Nasal secretions • Swelling of the nasal mucosa • Nasal polyps
Wheezing • Wheezing on exhalation • Bilateral wheezing
Retractions
Hyperexpansion of the thorax
Changes in the skin • Atopic dermatitis • Eczema • Allergic shiners (dark circles under the eyes)
Accessory muscle use
Cough
Shortness of breath
Tachypnea
Pulses paradoxis

TABLE 15-3
Matrix Used to Assess Asthma Control for Children 4 Years of Age or Younger

Components of Control		Classification of Asthma Control 0–4 Years		
		Well Controlled	Not Well Controlled	Very Poorly Controlled
Impairment	Symptoms	≤2 days/week	>2 days/week	Throughout the day
	Nighttime awakenings	≤1 night/month	>1 night/month	>1 night/week
	Interference with normal activity	None	Some limitation	Extremely limited
	SABA use for symptoms	≤2 days/week	>2 days/week	Several times per day
Risk	Exacerbations requiring oral systemic corticosteroids	0–1/year	2–3/year	>3/year
	Treatment-related adverse effects	Medication side effects can vary in intensity from none to very troublesome and worrisome. The level of intensity does not correlate to specific levels of control but should be considered in the overall assessment of risk.		
Recommended action for treatment		*Maintain current treatment. *Regular follow-up every 1–6 months. *Consider step down if well controlled for at least 3 months.	*Step up (1 step). *Reevaluate in 2–6 weeks. *If no clear benefit in 4–6 weeks, consider alternative diagnoses or adjusting therapy. *For side effects, consider alternative treatment options.	*Consider short course of oral systemic corticosteroids. *Step up (1–2 steps). *Reevaluate in 2 weeks. *If no clear benefit in 4–6 weeks, consider alternative diagnoses or adjusting therapy. *For side effects, consider alternative treatment options.

NOTE: Before step up in therapy, review adherence to medications, inhaler technique, and environmental control. If alternative treatment option was used in a step, discontinue it and use preferred treatment for that step.

SABA = short-acting beta2-agonist

*2007 NIH/NHLBI Asthma Guidelines

Data from National Asthma Education and Prevention Program Expert Panel Report 3. Guidelines for the diagnosis and management of asthma. National Heart Lung and Blood Institute, National Institutes of Health: U.S. Department of Health and Human Services; 2007 Aug 28. Report no. 07-4051. Full Report.

active role in preparing and using their asthma plan of care or asthma treatment plan. Emergency phone numbers are listed on the plan in case urgent medical attention is needed. Giving the families some scenarios during education will provide them with the opportunity to see how to respond and allow them to ask questions.

Peak Flow Monitoring

Measurement of peak expiratory flow is an effective way to monitor airflow during forced expiration. Peak flow monitoring is not as sensitive as the FEV_1 to changes in the diameter of the small airways. However, it does provide an objective indicator of lung function, especially in patients with persistent asthma and/or those who are not adept at perceiving the frequency or severity of asthma symptoms. Peak flow monitoring and symptom monitoring are considered appropriate ways of determining the action plan for asthma management.

A **peak flow meter** is used to measure how much air can move out of the airway with a momentary blast of exhalation. Peak flow helps the patient monitor airway changes so that they can take their reliever medication quickly according to their asthma action plan.

The meter is marked by a provider using either a predicted value from a nomogram or after determining the child's personal best. To obtain a personal best value, three peak flow measurements should be performed every day in the morning and evening for a 2- to 3-week period when the child's asthma is well controlled. The highest value among the three measurements is the personal best. Instructions for peak flow use are found in **Figure 15-2**.

The patient is instructed to keep a diary of the readings and concurrent symptoms and triggers so that the provider can guide the child and family on the appropriate actions to take. Using the meter on a regular basis can provide more information about a patient's asthma severity and control. Because effort and technique play an important role for obtaining accurate readings, children should be observed and coached on correct use of the peak flow meter on a daily basis.

TABLE 15-4
An Example of a Step-Wise Approach for the Management of Children 4 Years of Age and Younger with Intermittent and Persistent Asthma

Intermittent Asthma	Persistent Asthma: Daily Medication					
	Consult with asthma specialist if step 3 care or higher is required.					
	Consider consultation at step 2.					
					Step 6	Step up if needed
				Step 5	Preferred:	(First, check adherence, inhaler technique, environmental control)
			Step 4	Preferred:		
		Step 3	Preferred:		High dose ICS + either LABA or montelukast	**Assess Control**
	Step 2	Preferred:		High-dose ICS + either LABA or montelukast	Oral systemic corticosteroids	
Step 1	Preferred:		Medium-dose ICS + either LABA or montelukast			Step down if possible
Preferred:		Medium-dose ICS				
	Low-dose ICS					Asthma is well controlled for at least 3 months
SABA PRN						
	Alternative: Cromolyn or montelukast					

Patient Education and Environmental Control at Each Step

Quick-Relief Medications for All Patients:
*SABA as needed for symptoms. Intensity of treatment depends on severity of symptoms.
*With viral respiratory infection: SABA q 4–6 hours up to 24 hours (longer with physician consult). Consider short course of oral systemic corticosteroids if exacerbation is severe or patient has history of previous severe exacerbations.
*Caution: Frequent use of SABA may indicate the need to step up treatment.

ICS = inhaled corticosteroid; LABA = long-acting beta2-agonist; SABA = short-acting beta2-agonist

Note: Studies on children 0–4 years of age are limited. Step 2 preferred therapy is based on Evidence A.

All other recommendations are based on expert opinion and extrapolation from studies in older children.

*2007 NIH/NHLBI Asthma Guidelines

Data from National Asthma Education and Prevention Program Expert Panel Report 3. Guidelines for the diagnosis and management of asthma. National Heart Lung and Blood Institute, National Institutes of Health: U.S. Department of Health and Human Services; 2007 Aug 28. Report no. 07-4051. Full Report.

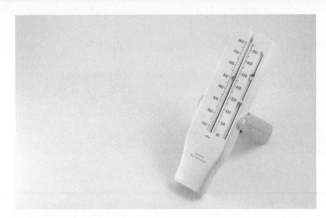

FIGURE 15-2 A peak flow meter with the green, yellow, and red zones marked. The zone markings correspond to the plan of care outlined on the child's asthma action plan.
© Rob Byron/Shutterstock.

Asthma Action Plan

The written **asthma action plan** (Figure 15-3) uses peak flow and symptom monitoring to determine the actions a child and family need to take in response to changes in the child's symptoms. Children with asthma should have home and school treatment plans to ensure consistent care. Coaches and school nurses should have a copy of the child's asthma action plan and should be able to perform peak flow monitoring and administer medications. Asthma action plans are often based on the colors of a traffic light: green, yellow, and red. Use of these colors provides a visual indication of the severity of symptoms during an acute exacerbation, with green signifying symptoms that are the least severe and red indicating the most severe. The asthma action plan illustrated in Figure 15-3 provides instructions for the type and dose of medication to administer, when to escalate care, and who to call for help for each of the three colored zones.

The green zone means "go" and indicates that the child's asthma is controlled. The child may be symptom-free or intermittently experiencing mild symptoms. Daily controller medications are administered as indicated in this section of the plan, and type and dose of reliever medication prior to exercise, or when intermittently symptomatic, are outlined. Peak flow for the green zone is typically >80% of the child's personal best.

Patients in the yellow zone have had an exposure to triggers and experience an increase in frequency and severity of symptoms. Symptoms include cough, which may worsen at night or with exercise; wheezing; chest tightness; itchy, runny nose; and/or itchy, sore throat. The peak flow rate in this zone is lower than that in the green zone, ranging from 50% to 80% of the child's personal best. The yellow zone means to slow down and take caution. The instructions in this section concentrate on using prescribed quick-relief medications as well as when to contact the physician or healthcare provider. The yellow zone also provides instructions

for stepping up care, which includes increasing the frequency and/or dose of the quick-reliever medication. Medications, such as a course of oral corticosteroids, may be initiated if the prescribed quick-reliever medication is ineffective (usually within 24 hours) in alleviating symptoms.

The red zone denotes that the child's symptoms are severe and peak flow is <50% of their personal best. Red zone or late-warning signs include refractory shortness of breath, nasal flaring, retractions, grunting, difficulty walking or talking, and/or cyanosis of the lips or fingernails. Action should be taken immediately if the child reaches this zone. Reliever medication is given in this zone at a faster pace, and the patient/caregiver must proceed to the emergency department or call 911 immediately. Recognizing the signs of an asthma episode early and taking immediate action are important. Early treatment can keep an asthma episode from becoming worse.

Other components of asthma education that can be discussed by the healthcare provider are basic asthma facts, what asthma is, the purpose of medications, how to use any devices prescribed, asthma triggers, how to avoid triggers, and the importance of scheduled asthma checkups. Education can be overwhelming to children and their families, so reviewing the components of asthma education during well-child primary care visits or throughout the length of the emergency department visit or hospitalization is helpful. Tailor the education to the age and literacy level of the child and family. It is also important to be mindful of the child/family's cultural background. If English is not the family's native language, interpretive services may be required to explain the elements of care and to provide education in a manner in which the child and family will best understand.

Control Environmental Triggers and Comorbid Conditions

Identifying and reducing exposures to allergens and irritants have been shown to reduce asthma exacerbations. **Table 15-5** lists the broad categories the NAEPP identifies as contributing factors for asthma exacerbations and provides some examples of the conditions and/or tangible items for each of the factors.[4] Education on trigger identification and limiting exposure to the irritants, allergens, and other factors contributing to asthma exacerbations is a key component of asthma control.[11] The literature reports that severe or difficult-to-treat asthma in children and adolescents is characterized by high frequencies of comorbid allergic diseases, allergen sensitization, and high IgE levels.[12] These children may benefit from allergy skin testing to identify the indoor, outdoor, and seasonal allergen triggers.[13] Identifying the precipitants and predictors of asthma exacerbations can be used to construct an

Asthma Action Plan

Name: _____ DOB:_____

Doctor: _____ Date:_____

Phone for Doctor or Clinic: _____

Predicted/Personal Best Peak Flow Reading:_____

Asthma Triggers
Try to stay away from or control these things:

□ Exercise	□ Smoke, strong odors or spray
□ Mold	□ Colds/Respiratory infections
□ Chalk dust/dust	□ Carpet
□ Pollen	□ Change in temperature
□ Animals	□ Dust mites
□ Tobacco smoke	□ Cockroaches
□ Food _____	□ Other _____

1. Green – Go

- Breathing is good.
- No cough or wheeze.
- Can work and play.

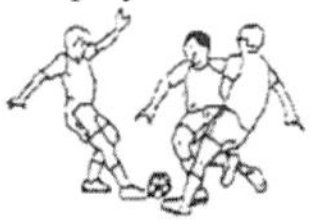

Or Peak Flow _____ to _____ (80-100%)

Use these controller medicines *every day* to keep you in the green zone:

Medicine: How much to take: When to take it: □ Home □ School

_____

_____

_____

5-15 minutes before very active exercise, use □ Albuterol _____ puffs.

2. Yellow – Caution

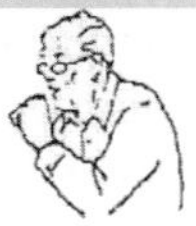

Coughing 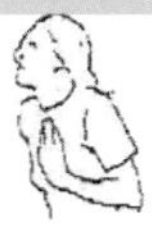   Wheezing

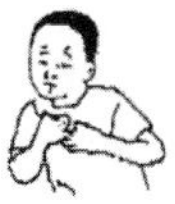

Tight Chest 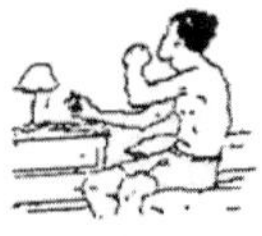   Wakes up at night

Or Peak Flow _____ to _____ (50-80%)

Keep using controller green zone medicines everyday.

Add these medicines to keep an asthma attack from getting bad:

Medicine	How much to take	When to take it
Albuterol or _____	□ 2 puffs by inhaler □ 4 puffs by inhaler □ with spacer, if available □ by nebulizer	□ May repeat every 20 min up to 3 doses in first hour, if needed

If symptoms *DO NOT* improve after first hour of treatment, then go to *red zone.*

If symptoms *DO* improve after first hour of treatment, then continue:

| Albuterol or _____ | □ 2 puffs by inhaler □ 4 puffs by inhaler □ with spacer, if available □ by nebulizer | □ Every 4 - 8 hours for _____ days |

_____, ____times a day for _____days □ Home □ School
(oral corticosteroid)   (how much)

Call your doctor if still having some symptoms for more than 24 hours!

3. Red – Stop – Danger

- Medicine is not helping.
- Breathing is hard and fast.
- Nose opens wide.
- Can't walk.
- Ribs show.
- Can't talk well.

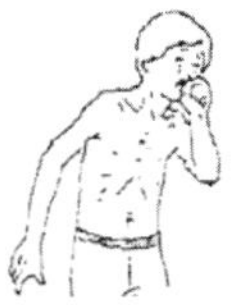

Or Peak Flow _____ (Less than 50%)

Call your doctor and/or parent/guardian *NOW!*
Take these medicines until you talk with a doctor or parent/guardian:

Medicine:	How much to take:	When to take it:
Albuterol or _____	□ 2 puffs by inhaler □ 4 puffs by inhaler □ with spacer, if available □ by nebulizer	□ May repeat every 20 minutes until you get help

_____, ____times a day for _____days □ Home □ School
(oral corticosteroid)   (how much)

Call 911 for severe symptoms, if symptoms don't improve, or you can't reach your doctor and/or parent/guardian.

Physician Signature _____   Date_____   Phone_____

WHITE – PATIENT   YELLOW – CHART   PINK – SCHOOL

Provided by Community Care of N.C., N.C. Asthma Program, and Asthma Alliance of N.C.   10/08

FIGURE 15-3 An example of an asthma action plan, outlining the symptoms and peak flow measurements that correspond to each of the zones (green, yellow, and red) and the treatment plan.

Asthma Action Plan sample courtesy of Asthma Alliance of North Carolina. www.communitycarenc.org/media/tool-resource-files/nc-asthma-action-plan-nc-dhhsdpi-english.pdf

effective, individualized asthma management approach and educational plan for the child and family.[14]

Counseling the patient on how to modify or eliminate exposure to allergens may not always be a simple step. Some patients may be sensitive or emotionally attached to an animal in their home. Therefore, the family may not be willing to remove the animal from the home and be averse to discussing this subject. Education, in this case, would focus on minimizing the child's exposure to the allergen rather than removing the

TABLE 15-5

Categories and Examples of Conditions or Factors That May Trigger an Acute Exacerbation of Asthma

Inhaled Allergens	Occupational Factors	Irritants	Comorbid Conditions	Other
• Animal dander • House dust mites • Cockroach allergen • Indoor mold • Pollen	• Chemicals • Dust • Cleaners • Grain/flour dust	• Environmental tobacco smoke • Indoor/outdoor • Air pollution • Wood fires • Strong fumes (e.g., paint, perfumes, scented candles/ soaps/lotions) • Glues • Insect sprays	• Allergic bronchopulmonary aspergillosis • Rhinitis/sinusitis • Obesity • Obstructive sleep apnea • Stress, depression, and psychosocial factors	• Medication and food • sensitivities • Airway infections • Sulfite sensitivity • Female hormones • Weather changes

Data from National Asthma Education and Prevention Program Expert Panel Report 3. Guidelines for the diagnosis and management of asthma. National Heart Lung and Blood Institute, National Institutes of Health: U.S. Department of Health and Human Services; 2007 Aug 28. Report no. 07-4051. Full Report.

allergen from the home. Education would then focus on keeping the pet out of the child's bedroom, grooming the pet regularly, and home cleaning tips on removing dander and fur from flooring and furniture.

There are many inhalant allergens, such as house dust mites, cockroaches, and mold, that a child may be exposed to in their home environment, school, childcare facility, or work. Parents may even bring a trigger from their place of employment home on their clothing and expose the child. Therefore, trigger identification and control needs to be broad-based and encompass all the touchpoints the child and family encounter.

Irritants can cause asthma to get worse and to interfere with asthma control if not addressed. The literature reports a link between increased asthma symptoms, poor asthma control, and increased morbidity and mortality among children exposed to environmental tobacco smoke.[15] The educational and self-management plan should incorporate information on avoiding secondhand smoke exposure as well as smoking cessation counseling resources.

Air quality can make breathing difficult on days when pollen counts are high, nitric oxide levels are elevated, or ozone levels are increased. Educating children and their families on the resources available to alert them to the air quality in their area is helpful. Some television and radio stations and newspapers report air quality data and provide environmental alerts. Smartphone apps are also available that provide air quality alerts, making it convenient for families to plan activities that will minimize environmental triggers.

Other indoor irritants include strong fumes from cleaning products, gas stoves or appliances that are not vented properly, wood-burning stoves or fireplaces, perfumes, colognes, paints, glues, insect sprays, or other aerosol sprays. It is also important to educate the child and family on the methods to avoid these triggers and the benefits of trigger avoidance in achieving

asthma control to decrease or prevent future asthma exacerbations.

Diagnosing and treating comorbid conditions can also improve asthma control. Extreme weather changes (hot and cold) can cause an attack. Helpful techniques for teaching a child how to protect their airway, including wearing a scarf, cupping their hands over their mouth and nose, or using their coat collar, can be very beneficial when going outside on cold days. Encouraging families to comply with seasonal flu vaccines to minimize upper respiratory infections like flu or colds and lower respiratory infections like pneumonia and bronchitis is also helpful and one of the key elements of preventive care.[16]

Prescribe Pharmacologic Asthma Treatment

Medications used to treat asthma can be divided into two categories: quick relief and controller. Quick-relief medications are also called rescue medications. They are used during an acute exacerbation to treat bronchospasm and airway constriction by relaxing bronchial smooth muscles. Controller medications are used to maintain health. These medications help prevent acute exacerbations of asthma by relaxing bronchial smooth muscles or by decreasing airway inflammation. Typically the controller medications used to relax bronchial smooth muscles have a longer duration to onset and a longer half-life.

Quick Relievers

Quick-relief medications, also known as **short-acting beta2-agonists (SABAs)**, are prescribed for all patients who have asthma to treat bronchoconstriction and bronchospasm during an acute exacerbation. The onset of action is rapid, or within 3 to 5 minutes following administration, and the effects last for 4 to 6 hours.

Quick-relief medications should not be used on a regular basis. Children who are symptomatic and require the use of quick-relief medications more than twice weekly is a sign that asthma is poorly controlled. The clinical team should then review the child's asthma plan of care and, depending on the asthma severity, add controller medications. Changes to the plan of care should be discussed with the family, and patient/family education should be provided. An exception to routine use would be the prophylactic use of SABAs 10 to 15 minutes prior to exercise or physical activities for children diagnosed with exercise-induced bronchospasm to prevent shortness of breath, coughing, and other symptoms during their physical activity.

The most common side effects are tremor, restlessness, headache, and tachycardia. Common SABA and manufacturer recommendations for initial dosing are listed in **Table 15-6**. Children with asthma should be instructed on the importance of keeping the SABA readily available. The child and family should be instructed on how to follow the asthma action plan and to properly use the quick-relief medication.

Children whose symptoms are not relieved by albuterol require combination therapy with other quick-relief medications, such as corticosteroids and/ or ipratropium bromide (Atrovent). Oral systemic corticosteroids are used in conjunction with SABAs during a moderate to severe asthma exacerbation to assist with quick relief for the patient. Ipratropium is not generally used to treat asthma, but it may be used to treat asthma exacerbations in combination with a short-acting bronchodilator to provide a synergetic effect. This treatment regimen typically occurs in the emergency department.

Controller Medications

Controller medications are prescribed for daily use and recommended for patients who have persistent asthma. Different classes of controller medications are available: corticosteroids, leukotriene modifiers, **long-acting beta2-agonists (LABAs)**, and theophylline. Combination therapy, such as a corticosteroid and a LABA, may also be prescribed. The most common and most effective controller medications are the **inhaled corticosteroids (ICSs)**. Table 15-7 lists common

TABLE 15-6
Formulations of Quick-Relief Medications

Medication Name	Dosing	Delivery Device
AccuNeb (albuterol for nebulization)	Children 2–12 years of age: 0.63 mg albuterol/3 mL administered by nebulization	Nebulizer
	Children 6–12 years of age with more severe asthma (baseline FEV_1 less than 60% predicted), weight >40 kg, or children 11–12 years of age: 1.25 mg albuterol/3 mL	
Albuterol 0.083%	2.5 mg albuterol/3 mL	Nebulizer
Albuterol 0.5%	Children 2–12 years of age: Initial dosing should be based on body weight (01.–0.5 mg/kg per dose), with subsequent dosing titrated to achieve the desired clinical response. Dosing should not exceed 2.5 mg three to four times daily by nebulization.	Nebulizer
	Adults and children 12 years of age and older: 2.5 mg of albuterol administered three to four times daily by nebulization.	
ProAir (albuterol sulfate) HFA	90 mcg per inhalation. Dosing for adults and children 4 years of age and older is two inhalations.	MDI
Proventil (albuterol sulfate) HFA	90 mcg per inhalation. Dosing for adults and children 4 years of age and older is two inhalations.	MDI
Ventolin (albuterol sulfate) HFA	90 mcg per inhalation. Dosing for adults and children 4 years of age and older is two inhalations.	MDI
Xopenex (levalbuterol) HFA	45 mcg per inhalation. Dosing for adults and children 4 years of age and older is two inhalations.	MDI
Xopenex nebulized (levalbuterol)	Children 6–11 years of age: 0.31 mg	Nebulizer
	Children ≥12 years of age: 0.63 mg, 1.25 mg	

MDI = metered dose inhaler

TABLE 15-7
A List of Inhaled Controller Medications

Medication Name	Class	Strengths	Low Dose			Medium Dose			High Dose		
			Child 0–4 Years of Age	Child 5–11 Years of Age	Child ≥12 Years of Age and Adults	Child 0–4 Years of Age	Child 5–11 Years of Age	Child ≥12 Years of Age and Adults	Child 0–4 Years of Age	Child 5–11 Years of Age	Child ≥12 Years of Age and Adults
Aerospan (flunisolide) HFA	ICS	80 mcg per inhalation	NA	160 mcg	320 mcg	NA	160–320 mcg	>320–640 mcg	NA	320 mcg	>640 mcg
Alvesco (ciclesonide) HFA	ICS	80 or 160 mcg per inhalation	NA	80–160 mcg	160–320 mcg	NA	160–320 mcg	>320–640 mcg	NA	320 mcg	>640 mcg
Arnuity Ellipta (fluticasone furoate)	ICS	100 or 200 mcg per inhalation	NA	NA	100 mcg	NA	NA	100–200 mcg	NA	NA	200 mcg
Asmanex (mometasone) DPI	ICS	110 or 220 mcg per actuation	NA	110 mcg	110–220 mcg	NA	220–440 mcg	>220–440 mcg	NA	>440 mcg	>440 mcg
Flovent (fluticasone) DPI	ICS	50, 100, or 250 mcg per dose	NA	100–200 mcg	100–300 mcg	NA	>200–400 mcg	>300–500 mcg	NA	>400 mcg	>500 mcg
Flovent (fluticasone) HFA	ICS	44, 110, or 220 mcg per actuation	88–176 mcg	88–176 mcg	88–264 mcg	>176–352 mcg	>176–352 mcg	264–440 mcg	>352 mcg	>352 mcg	>440 mcg
Pulmicort (budesonide) DPI Flexhaler	ICS	90 or 180 mcg per dose	NA	180–360 mcg	180–540 mcg	NA	360–720 mcg	540–1080 mcg	NA	>720 mcg	>1080 mcg
Pulmicort (budesonide) Respules	ICS	0.25, 0.5, or 1.0 mg per unit dose	0.25–0.5 mg	0.5 mg	NA	>.05–1.0 mg	1.0 mg	NA	>1.0 mg	2.0 mg	NA
QVAR (beclomethasone) HFA	ICS	40 or 80 mcg per actuation	NA	80–160 mcg	80–240 mcg	NA	>160–320 mcg	>240–480 mcg	NA	>320 mcg	>480 mcg

Drug	Class	Strengths available										
Advair (fluticasone and salmeterol) DPI	ICS and LABA	100/50, 250/50, or 500/50 mcg per inhalation	NA	100/50 1 puff bid	NA	100/50 1 puff bid	NA	100/50 1 puff bid	250/50 1 puff bid	NA	100/50 1 puff bid	250/50–500/50 1 puff bid
Advair (fluticasone and salmeterol) HFA	ICS and LABA	45/21, 115/21, or 230/21 mcg per inhalation	NA	NA	NA	45/21 2 puffs bid	NA	NA	115/21 2 puffs bid	NA	NA	230/21 2 puffs bid
Dulera (mometasone and formoterol)	ICS and LABA	100/5 or 200/5 mcg per inhalation	NA	NA	NA	100/5 2 puffs bid	NA	NA	200/5 2 puffs bid	NA	NA	200/5 2 puffs bid
Symbicort (budesonide and formoterol) HFA	ICS and LABA	80/4.5 or 160/4.5 mcg per inhalation	NA	NA	NA	80/4.5 2 puffs bid	NA	NA	160/4.5 2 puffs bid	NA	NA	160/4.5 2 puffs bid
Serevent (salmeterol) DPI	LABA	50 mcg per dose	NA	50 mcg 1 puff bid	NA	50 mcg 1 puff bid	NA	50 mcg 1 puff bid	50 mcg 1 puff bid	NA	50 mcg 1 puff bid	50 mcg 1 puff bid
Foradil (formoterol) DPI	LABA	12 mcg per inhalation	NA	12 mcg 1 puff bid	NA	12 mcg 1 puff bid	NA	12 mcg 1 puff bid	12 mcg 1 puff bid	NA	12 mcg 1 puff bid	12 mcg 1 puff bid

corticosteroids and corticosteroid/LABA formulations used for asthma control, along with the drug's strength and dosage. ICSs generally cause mild side effects, such as throat and mouth irritation, hoarseness, and oral yeast infections (thrush).[17] Children should be instructed to use a spacer device when administering the ICS by metered dose inhaler (MDI) and to rinse their mouth after using the medication to prevent oral yeast infections. Long-term use of these medications in children has shown a slight growth delay, but studies have found no evidence that children fail to reach their full height potential.[18] Oral systemic corticosteroids, such as prednisone and methylprednisolone, may be used for asthma treatment but are associated with more side effects than inhaled corticosteroids. A 5- to 7-day course of oral prednisone during asthma exacerbations effectively relieves inflammation, but long-term use is generally not recommended.

Leukotrienes are chemical mediators of inflammation, produced by airway mast cells. Mast cells degranulate during an acute exacerbation and release leukotrienes, which cause bronchial smooth muscle contraction, mucus production, and eosinophil migration from the blood to the bronchi. Leukotriene receptor antagonists block leukotrienes from interacting with their receptor sites. They are most effective for children with allergic asthma and nasal allergies. Three leukotriene modifiers are commercially available: zafirlikast (Accolate, not recommended for children younger than 5 years), zileuton (Zyflo, not recommended for children), and montelukast (Singulair). Only montelukast is

available for children as a chewable tablet (4 and 5 mg) and as oral granules (4 mg, to be mixed with food or liquid; see **Table 15-8**).

LABAs are inhaled medications that have a slightly longer onset of action but provide bronchodilation for a longer duration of time (e.g., 12 hours). Salmeterol (Serevent) and formoterol (Foradil) are the most commonly prescribed LABAs for the treatment of moderate to severe asthma. LABAs are not to be used as monotherapy; rather, this medication is combined with ICSs to relax airways and reduce inflammation. Common formulations include fluticasone and salmeterol (Advair Diskus or MDI), budesonide and formoterol (Symbicort MDI), and mometasone and formoterol (Dulera MDI; see Table 15-7).

Theophylline is a methylxanthine that is used for relief and prevention of bronchoconstriction. Although used more routinely in the treatment of chronic obstructive pulmonary disease, theophylline is recommended only as an alternative to the recommended drugs for asthma due to its difficult management. Theophylline is more commonly seen in children hospitalized with a severe asthma exacerbation that is refractory to conventional emergency care. In the acute care setting, the use of theophylline IV in combination with SABA and steroid therapy was associated with a shorter hospital length of stay, improved steroid responsiveness, and reduced duration of oxygen use in children hospitalized with status asthmaticus.[19] Common trade names include Theo-24 and Elixophyllin. The therapeutic window for this medication is narrow; therefore,

TABLE 15-8
Noninhaled Controller Medications Used in the Treatment of Asthma

Medication Name	Class	Dose
Methylprednisolone, prednisolone, prednisone	Oral systemic corticosteroid	0–11 years: short course "burst" 1–2 mg/kg/day, maximum 60 mg/day, for 3–10 days
		≥12 years: short course "burst" 40–60 mg/day as single dose or two divided doses for 5–10 days
Montelukast sodium (Singulair)	Leukotriene modifier	12–23 mos: 4 mg sprinkles with 1 spoonful of CAIR (carrots, applesauce, ice cream, or rice); 1–5 years: 4 mg chewable tablet
		6–14 years: 5 mg chewable tablet
		>15 years: 10 mg tablet
Zafirlukast (Accolate)	Leukotriene modifier	7–11 years: 10 mg bid; >12 years: 20 mg bid
Zileuton (Zyflo) Zileuton CR (Zyflo-extended release)	Leukotriene modifier	12 years or older: Immediate release: 600 mg orally four times per day; Extended release:1200 mg orally twice a day (within one hour after morning and evening meals); Max dose 2400 mg
Omalizumab (Anti IgE)	Immunomodulator	≥12 years: 150–375 mg SC q 2–4 weeks, depending on body weight and pretreatment serum IgE level
Theophylline	Methylxanthine	Maintenance dose: 42 days to 18 days starting dose 20 mg/kg/day orally; Alternate dosing [(0.2 cage in weeks + 5)] x kg = 24 hour oral dose in mg; 1–8 years: 20–24 mg/kg/day; 9–11 yrs: 16 mg/kg/day; 12–15 yrs: 13 mg/kg/day; 16 yrs or older: 10 mg/kg/day; Do not exceed 900 mg/day

routine or regularly scheduled theophylline blood levels are needed to make sure the correct dose is being prescribed. Possible side effects include insomnia, gastroesophageal reflux, nausea, and arrhythmia.

Omalizumab is a recombinant humanized anti-IgE monoclonal antibody approved in the United States for moderate to severe persistent allergic asthma (severe persistent asthma in the European Union) that is uncontrolled despite treatment with ICSs and LABAs.[20] NAEPP recommends consideration of omalizumab (Xolair) for patients 12 years and older with moderate to severe persistent asthma when asthma is not well controlled, who have a documented allergy to at least one perennial allergen, and IgE levels are in the range of 30 to 700 units.[5]

Management of an Acute Exacerbation

Asthma action plans are very helpful for patients to know how to recognize and respond to worsening asthma and when to seek medical care. However, when a child's symptoms cannot be controlled by treatment outlined on the asthma action plan, or they become worse, emergency treatment is warranted.

Emergency Department Treatment

The emergency department (ED) serves as an important access point for children experiencing asthma exacerbations. For some families, the ED visit may be the only source for care because many families lack a medical home or primary care provider. ED visits for acute exacerbations of asthma are on the rise, many of which can be potentially preventable and/or contribute to an increased risk for fatal asthma.[21] Thus, the interaction the medical team has with the patient and family in the ED is crucial.

Urgent asthma care requires early identification and classification of the exacerbation severity and the prompt involvement of the interdisciplinary team. Early identification, accurate assessment of the severity of airway obstruction, and response to therapy are fundamental to the treatment of patients experiencing acute asthma symptoms in the ED setting. Asthma severity scoring tools are often used to objectively rate or classify the severity of the exacerbation. The use of a scoring tool reduces variability in rating the severity of the asthma exacerbation and, when coupled with a care path or asthma treatment protocol, can improve timeliness of care, reduce variation in practice, and improve adherence to evidence-based care.[22,23] There are several asthma scoring tools available for use. **Figure 15-4** provides an example of one asthma scoring tool, the pediatric asthma score. This tool uses a simple rating system to identify the severity of the acute exacerbation. Higher scores signify a greater deviation from normal, indicating a severe asthma exacerbation. In this example, the scoring tool was modified from its original form to describe dyspnea and respiratory rate in greater detail, with descriptions appropriate for different age ranges.

Treatment in the emergency department focuses on relieving bronchospasm, reducing airway inflammation, and preventing respiratory failure. As with the treatment of an acute exacerbation in the home management of an asthma exacerbation, administration of

	1	2	3
Respiratory rate 1–3 years 4–5 years 6–12 years >12 years	≤34 ≤30 ≤26 ≤23	35–39 31–35 27–31 24–27	≥40 ≥36 ≥31 ≥28
Oxygen Requirement	>95% on room air	90–95% on room air	<90% on room air or requiring any amount of O$_2$
Retractions	None of intercostal	Intercostal and substernal OR nasal flaring (infants)	Intercostal, substernal, and supraclavicular OR nasal flaring and head bobbing (infants)
Dyspnea 1–4 years	Normal feeding, vocalization, and play	Decreased appetite, coughing after play, hyperactivity	Stops eating or drinking, stops playing, OR drowsy and confused and/or grunting
Dyspnea >5 years	Counts to ≥10 in one breath OR speaks in complete sentences	Counts to 4–6 in one breath OR speaks in partial sentences	Counts to ≤3 in one breath OR speaks in single-word grunts
Auscultation	Normal breath sounds and end-expiratory wheezes	Expiratory wheezing	Inspiratory and expiratory wheezing to diminished breath sounds
Total PAS	Mild 5–7	Moderate 8–11	Severe ≥12

FIGURE 15-4 An example of an asthma scoring tool, the modified pediatric asthma score.

a quick-relief medication or beta2-agonists is first-line therapy. Initial treatment of a child experiencing a mild exacerbation of asthma consists of a single short-acting beta2-agonist by nebulizer or MDI. Those presenting with a moderate to severe exacerbation require care escalation, which includes additional beta2-agonist treatments, typically three treatments spaced 15 minutes apart; the addition of inhaled ipratropium bromide; and administration of systemic corticosteroids.[4]

Medications that also may be initiated in the ED as second-line therapy include continuous nebulization of beta2-agonists and a dose of intravenous magnesium sulfate.[24,25] Additional therapy that is administered for those patients refractory to first- and second-line therapies or who present with a life-threatening exacerbation includes heliox and noninvasive positive pressure ventilation.[26]

Children who respond to ED treatment and are discharged home require asthma education and an asthma action plan outlining the medications to continue, new medications to begin, and when to follow up with the primary care provider. The goal of asthma education in this setting is to provide the child and family with an asthma management foundation from which the primary care team can build upon. The literature reports that children with one asthma-related ED visit are more likely to experience a subsequent ED visit within 1 year.[27] Children more likely to return with an asthma exacerbation within 1 week of discharge from the ED for asthma-related symptoms include those meeting any of the following criteria:

- Younger than 2 years of age
- Categorized with persistent asthma
- On government-assisted insurance
- Reporting a poor quality of life due to asthma symptoms
- An increased use of healthcare resources in the preceding 12 months for asthma[28]

Children and families who receive asthma education and demonstrate an understanding of the plan for controlling asthma and who can recognize an acute exacerbation, how to treat symptoms according to the asthma action plan of care, and have a scheduled follow-up visit with a primary care physician are less likely to revisit the ED for an asthma-related illness.[29]

Management in the Hospital

Children requiring hospitalization are those who have a poor response to therapy within the first few hours of treatment (2–4) in the ED or who have a repeat visit within 24 hours of discharge home from the ED. Those with poor access to medical care, or previous hospital admission requiring treatment in the ICU or ventilatory assistance, may also require hospitalization. In the latter case, the decision to admit the child for additional acute

TABLE 15-9

Complications Associated with Ventilatory Support of the Child with Status Asthmaticus

Air trapping
ARDS
Auto-PEEP
Death
Hypotension
Pulmonary air leaks (pneumothorax, pneumomediastimum)

ARDS = acute respiratory distress syndrome; PEEP = positive end-expiratory pressure

care depends on a combination of the child's response to therapy and the family's understanding of the asthma care plan and demonstrated ability to administer medications and follow the post-ED discharge plan of care.

Children who are refractory to first- and second-line therapy and demonstrate respiratory muscle fatigue are at high risk for respiratory failure. Elective intubation and ventilatory support may be required to stabilize the child and prevent cardiorespiratory arrest. Low tidal volume or lung protective strategies are essential to minimize complications associated with mechanical ventilatory support. Table 15-9 provides a list of complications associated with mechanically ventilating a child with asthma who is refractory to medical treatment. Providing sufficient time to exhale, or a sufficient expiratory time, will avoid worsening air trapping and increasing resistance through the narrowed conducting airways. First- and second-line therapies are continued. Sedation may be required and is dependent on the peak ventilating pressures and hemodynamic, acid–base, and oxygenation status.

Children discharged home also require asthma education and an asthma action plan outlining the medications to continue, new medications to begin, and when to follow up with the primary care provider. During the acute care stay, the clinical team has an opportunity to work with the child and family to reinforce asthma education. The child and/or family should demonstrate the ability to distinguish the controller from quick-relief medications as well as the ability to administer the medication properly.

Complications

Missed school and work time and a reduced ability to lead a healthy, active lifestyle are associated with poor asthma control. Respiratory failure secondary to an exacerbation that is refractory to treatment may occur. More than one asthma hospital admission, three ED visits, or five physician visits for asthma exacerbation–related symptoms is associated with an increased risk of mortality. Complications associated with mechanical ventilatory support of asthma patients with respiratory failure include pneumothorax, hypotension, and acute respiratory distress syndrome.

Outcomes

The development of evidence-based guidelines facilitates better management of children with asthma. Partnering with patients and families to improve adherence to the asthma plan of care improves asthma control and quality of life.

Cystic Fibrosis

Cystic fibrosis (CF) is a life-limiting autosomal recessive disorder affecting approximately 80,000 individuals worldwide. Scientific progress in the understanding of the pathophysiology of CF and advancements in clinical treatment have improved the median predicted survival rate and quality of life for those affected by this disease.

Etiology

CF is caused by a single gene defect on chromosome 7. Those with the gene defect may be unaffected by the disease and carry the mutated gene, or they may be affected and have the genetic condition. Persons who carry a single mutated **cystic fibrosis transmembrane conductance regulator (CFTR)** gene along with a normal CFTR allele are termed *carriers*. Carriers have few or no symptoms attributable to CF, but their children may be affected: Each child conceived from two CF carriers has a 25% chance of being affected with CF, a 50% chance of being a CF carrier, and a 25% chance of not having a gene defect (**Figure 15-5**). Since the discovery of the CFTR gene in 1989, more than 1800 individual mutations have been identified.[30] The most common mutation is F508del, which accounts for 66% of CF alleles reported worldwide.[30] Approximately half of all persons with CF are homozygous for this mutation or have an F508del/F508del mutation.[30] The prevalence of individual mutations varies, with the F508del mutation being more common in those who are Caucasian.[31]

Mutations in the CFTR gene have been categorized into groups that reflect the mechanism for decrease or loss of CFTR function. The groups, in which the mutations may permit the production of adequate CFTR levels, result in less severe manifestations of the disease. Current research in CF is investigating specific CFTR defects and determining ways to treat it.

Pathophysiology

CFTR is a chloride channel expressed in the apical membrane of epithelial cells lining the lung, pancreas, gut, sweat duct, reproductive tract, kidney, liver, and submucosal glands. CFTR regulates several ion

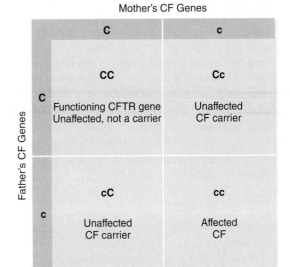

FIGURE 15-5 Children born to parents who carry one CF mutated gene have a 25% chance of being born with two gene mutations (cc) and having CF, a 50% chance of becoming a carrier for this disease (Cc), and a 25% chance of having no gene mutation (CC).

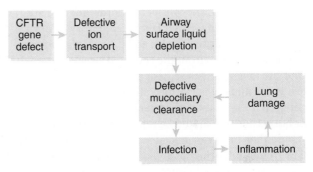

FIGURE 15-6 The sequelae of events that contribute to lung damage and the decline in lung function.

conductance pathways, including epithelial sodium, chloride, and potassium channels, as well as bicarbonate transport.[32] Loss of a normally functioning CFTR can have a profound impact on water and electrolyte transport across the epithelium. Pulmonary impact may include a reduction in intact mucin (mucus) in the CF airway, leaving the airway more vulnerable to chronic bacterial infection and airway inflammation (**Figure 15-6**). The sequelae of mucus retention, chronic bacterial infection, and airway obstruction contribute to lung damage, which can be quantified by the measurable reduction in lung function.

Diagnosis

The diagnosis of CF is based on the combination of one or more typical phenotypic features and evidence of CFTR malfunction. The phenotypic findings can be present on physical exam or through diagnostic testing, such as chest radiography and pulmonary function testing or laboratory evaluation.

Newborn Screening

There are several tests available to detect abnormalities in the CFTR. In the United States, all newborns are screened for CF. As with all newborn screening, within the first few days of life blood is taken for analysis from the baby's heel. Although not used in all states, the ImmunoReactive Trypsinogen (IRT) screens for CF in the newborn. In those states in which the IRT is not used, genetic screening is performed. Genetic screening or a sweat chloride test is commonly performed when the IRT screen is positive or high.

Sweat Chloride Testing

Evidence of CFTR dysfunction is typically provided by a **sweat chloride test**, which can be performed in children older than 6 months. A minimum of 75 mg of sweat over a 30-minute interval must be collected to perform the analysis. A chloride concentration of more than 60 mmol/L on two or more occasions is suggestive of CF. Sweat chloride values may be elevated (i.e., between 60–80 mmol/L) in non-CF-related diseases, such as atopic dermitis and anorexia nervosa. Values between 40 and 60 mmol/L are considered borderline and are more suggestive of CF in infants. Laboratory errors are common with this technique, and even a small amount of water vapor loss from the collected sweat can concentrate ions and cause a false-positive test result. If the test is not initially performed at a Cystic Fibrosis Foundation (CFF)–accredited center, a subsequent positive or borderline test should be repeated. The repeat test should then be performed at a center accredited by the CFF to minimize the possibility that inaccurate results from variations in laboratory testing will result.

Genetic Testing

CFTR mutational analysis is used to identify CF alleles, and genetic testing is used as a complement to IRT and sweat testing. The identification of two disease-causing CFTR mutations is highly specific for the diagnosis of CF. CFTR mutation analysis lacks sensitivity and usually screens for only 32 to 70 common mutations. Although mutation analysis does detect up to 95% of CF alleles, it does not identify all the known mutations capable of causing CF. A family history of CF should also be sought in support of a clinical CF diagnosis.

Clinical Presentation

There is a broad range of clinical features that may present with CF. These include pulmonary and extrapulmonary manifestations. Clinical manifestations depend on a combination of genetic (modifier genes) and environmental factors. There are, for example, individuals with CF whose CFTR mutation is associated with pancreatic sufficiency and mild pulmonary impairment. A summary of the common manifestations associated with CF can be found in **Table 15-10**.

TABLE 15-10
Common Phenotypic Features of CF

Pulmonary	Chronic sinopulmonary disease
	Nasal polyps and chronic sinus (but not middle ear) involvement
	Chronic cough, especially with sputum expectoration
	Persistent infection with typical cystic fibrosis pathogens (e.g., *Staphylococcus aureus*, *Pseudomonas aeruginosa*, *Burkholderia cepacia*, atypical *Mycobacteria*)
	Persistent chest radiographic abnormality (e.g., bronchiectasis, hyperinflation, atelectasis)
	Airway obstruction pattern on pulmonary function testing
	Digital clubbing
Gastrointestinal	Intestinal: Meconium ileus, rectal prolapse, distal intestinal obstruction syndrome
	Pancreatic: Pancreatic insufficiency, recurrent pancreatitis
	Hepatic: Focal biliary cirrhosis
	Nutritional: Malnutrition, hypoproteinemia, fat-soluble vitamin deficiency
Electrolyte and metabolic	Salt loss syndrome
	Acute salt depletion, especially with water loss, such as during exercise in heat
	Chronic metabolic alkalosis
Reproductive	Male urogenital abnormality
	Obstructive azoospermia resulting from congenital bilateral absence of the vas deferens

Extrapulmonary Manifestations

There are several manifestations of CF that affect other organs within the body. The frequency and severity with which children are affected with extrapulmonary manifestations depends on a combination of the genetic mutation and environmental factors.

Gastrointestinal

Meconium ileus occurs in approximately 18% of all newborns with CF.[33] A **meconium ileus** is an intestinal obstruction that results from the impaction of thick, tenacious meconium in the distal small bowel of a newborn. A barium enema is used to identify the site of the obstruction.[33] Depending on the severity, the obstruction may be cleared with enema-guided radiography or may require surgical intervention.

Intestinal obstruction may also occur after the newborn period. Typically, the obstruction occurs in the distal or terminal ileum and is associated with the passage of large amounts of food that are not completely digested into the small bowel. Patients with **distal intestinal obstruction syndrome (DIOS)** present with a myriad of symptoms, including right lower quadrant pain, anorexia, nausea, vomiting, and occasionally fever.[34] DIOS is typically associated with poor adherence to pancreatic enzyme therapy but can occur with enzyme intolerance, especially in small children.

Pancreatic

Pancreatic insufficiency is present from birth in a majority of patients with CF.[35] Destruction of acinar pancreatic tissue, pancreatic ductular obstruction, and pancreatic enzyme deficiency result in maldigestion of fats and proteins. Stools are foul smelling, bulky, and have an oily appearance. If uncorrected, malabsorption results in failure to gain weight and stunting of linear growth. Exocrine pancreatic enzyme supplements are required to address malabsorption and minimize the **steatorrhea.** Because fat is malabsorbed, the diet for those with CF concentrates on high-energy, high-calorie foods that are lower in fat.

Children with CF may present with signs and symptoms of vitamin deficiency, including fatigue, muscle aches and weakness, pale or yellowish skin color, and tingling of extremities. Impaired absorption of fat-soluble vitamins causes the deficiency. Prophylactic supplementation of vitamins A, D, E, and K can prevent this from occurring.

Gradual loss of insulin production may occur as the child grows into adulthood. Because children with CF are living longer, the propensity for comorbidities, such as CF-related diabetes, increases. In the United States, among those older than 18 years of age, the prevalence of CF-related diabetes requiring chronic insulin therapy ranges from 15% to 30%.[36] Clinical manifestations of CF-related diabetes include failure to gain or maintain weight despite nutritional intervention, poor growth, and unexplained decline in lung function.[36] Typically caloric restriction is not required, as obesity and CF are a rare combination. A high-calorie diet, consisting of 40% fat, and insulin therapy are used as primary management strategies.

Reproductive Tract

Male infertility is nearly universal, with more than 98% of cases resulting from an obstruction of the vas deferens.[37] During physical examination, the clinician may not be able to palpate the vas deferens. Consequently, the volume of ejaculate is one-third to one-half the normal volume and does not contain spermatozoa. Sperm are developed in the testes and can be harvested by micro-aspiration as a component of family planning.

Very few women, only 20%, experience infertility issues.[38] Reproductive issues vary and include anovulation and changes in the cervical mucus that impair implantation. Pregnancy in women with CF may have a negative impact on lung function and contribute to an increased risk of CF comorbid conditions as well as the risk of death. Women with CF must consider the impact pregnancy will have on their health as well as the health of their unborn child when considering conceiving.

Sweat Glands

Reduced sodium chloride absorption in the sweat duct is a common clinical feature and the reason sweat chloride is elevated in individuals with CF.[39] This reduction in sodium chloride reabsorption may predispose those with CF to salt depletion. Vomiting, diarrhea, or exercise/play can easily cause salt/volume loss in young children with CF. These children will present with lethargy, anorexia, and hypochloremic acidosis. Increased salt intake is encouraged when there is an increased risk for salt loss (i.e., during viral illness where vomiting and diarrhea present or during activities in which the child will sweat).

Pulmonary Manifestations

Children with cystic fibrosis have pulmonary manifestations. Because there is no known cure, respiratory therapy is aimed at minimizing the frequency and severity of acute exacerbations and reducing the rate of decline in lung function.

Upper Respiratory Tract

Chronic rhino-sinusitis and opacification of paranasal sinuses are common to nearly all individuals with CF, although some will appear relatively asymptomatic.[40] Commonly reported symptoms include anosmia, headache, facial pain, nasal obstruction, chronic congestion, and nasal discharge. Nasal endoscopy typically reveals mucosal edema, purulent discharge, and nasal polyposis. Upon visual inspection, the bridge of the nose may be widened. Imaging by computed tomography (CT) demonstrates sinus hypoplasia or aplasia with generalized opacification. The type of bacteria associated with sinus disease varies with age and is similar to that isolated from the individual's lower respiratory tract.

The therapeutic goal for CF-related sinusitis is to ameliorate symptoms. Treatment includes the use of hypertonic saline, topical and systemic steroids, and antibiotics. Endoscopic sinus surgery is considered when medical management fails to alleviate symptoms. Following endoscopic procedures, medical management is very important because sinus symptoms and nasal polyps often reoccur.

Lower Respiratory Tract

Newborns with CF, identified by newborn screening, appear to have normal lung function, implying normal intrauterine lung development.[41] Clinical symptoms or evidence of increased airway resistance and gas trapping often develop very early in life. However, in a minority of patients with CFTR mutations associated with milder pulmonary involvement, the clinical symptoms associated with lower respiratory tract manifestations may not be apparent until adulthood.

There is a triad of pulmonary manifestations that occur in the lung: Those affected with CF have an increased number of goblet cells and submucosal gland hypertrophy, contributing to increased production of airway secretions that are dehydrated and viscid.

A cough that becomes persistent and productive of purulent sputum over time is the hallmark symptom. During an acute exacerbation, individuals with CF present with increased cough, sputum, fatigue, anorexia, weight loss, and decreased lung function. Exacerbations negatively impact clinical stability. During an exacerbation, more intensive therapy is required. The therapeutic goals in the treatment of an acute exacerbation are to alleviate symptoms and to restore lost lung function through the use of antibiotics, nutritional support, and airway clearance maneuvers. As the child grow and develops, exacerbations become more frequent, and depending on the bacteria causing the exacerbation, the individual with CF may be less responsive to these interventions and thus at risk for respiratory failure.

Management

In the past decade, a paradigm shift in the medical management of CF has occurred. The focus was predominately reactive, concentrating efforts on alleviating symptoms and correcting pulmonary and extrapulmonary organ dysfunction. Currently there is a shift in focus to preventive care, including delaying the onset of the initial and minimizing subsequent pulmonary infections and preserving lung function.

There are four key pillars of CF care: prompt identification and treatment of pulmonary infections, suppression of airway inflammation, relief of airway obstruction, and attention to nutritional status and nutritional support.[42]

Standard Respiratory Therapy

Treatment of CF lung disease can be categorized as therapies used to prevent deterioration of lung function and those used to treat acute exacerbations. Although therapies are being developed that are aimed at the correction of either the gene defect or the ion transport abnormalities that characterize CF epithelia, currently available therapies either promote the physical removal of airway secretions or reduce airway infection and inflammation. A successful outcome of this research is

ivacaftor (Kalydeco), the first available CFTR modulator therapy drug that targets the underlying cause of CF. Ivacaftor is an oral medication that was approved for use in 2012 for people with CF 6 years of age and older with the CFTR gene mutation G551D, which is a Class III mutation. This medication is classified as a "potentiator" because it improves (*potentiates*) the function of the CFTR protein on the cell surface by allowing Cl absorption in the sweat gland, decreasing sweat Cl concentration. Patients on this medication show marked improvement in lung function and weight gain, which are strong predictors of life expectancy in CF. However, only 4% of people with CF have the G551D mutation. Further research is aimed at determining the effectiveness other CFTR modulator therapies that may treat the other 96% of the CF population.

Identification and Treatment of a Pulmonary Exacerbation

Prompt identification and treatment of pulmonary infections are essential components of CF care. Pulmonary exacerbations are associated with inflammation and impaired mucociliary clearance, which contributes to worsening airway obstruction, a decline in lung function, and a profound negative impact on perceived quality of life.

Identification of a Pulmonary Exacerbation

Sputum culture and sensitivity identify the infectious agent and antimicrobial agents that are most effective. Over time, the organisms that a patient with CF is colonized or infected with may change, or multiple organisms may be present. Obtaining a sputum culture and sensitivity when an acute exacerbation is suspected is an important part of the treatment plan.

The respiratory tract of newborns often becomes infected with typical CF pathogens early in life. *Staphylococcus aureus* and *Haemophilus influenzae* are often the first organisms detected. *H. influenzae*, however, rarely persists beyond childhood while *S. aureus* may not persist after its initial isolation during childhood or may be isolated for the first time during the adult years.[43] The prevalence of *S. aureus* is nearly 50% in newly diagnosed children and peaks in school-age children (6–10 years) to just over 55%, then gradually decreases to 33% during adulthood. Methicillin-resistant *S. aureus* (MRSA) strains are becoming increasingly more prevalent in persons with CF. Infection with MRSA is associated with more rapid decline in pulmonary function, more frequent exacerbations than infection with *Pseudomonas aeruginosa*, and decreased survival.[44,45]

The airways of CF patients have a propensity to become persistently infected with otherwise uncommon gram-negative pathogens. These form bacterial biofilms in the airway, making eradication particularly difficult. *P. aeruginosa* is the most common and clinically significant pathogen colonizing and infecting the airways of those with CF. The prevalence ranges from about 25% during the first year of life to nearly 80% in adulthood.[44,45] With the progression of lung disease, *P. aeruginosa*, particularly the mucoid and biofilm form, is often the only organism recovered from sputum and may be present with different antibiotic sensitivity patterns. Efforts focus on avoiding or delaying the onset of infection with this organism, as it is a predictor of worsening lung function and survival.[45]

Burkholderia cepacia complex is highly transmissible organism and is difficult to treat because it is often resistant to antimicrobial therapy. Although the precise pathogen and host factors are unknown, a subset of patients will have **cepacia syndrome**,[46] characterized by fever and sepsis after initial infection and a precipitous and often fatal decompensation in their clinical condition. Strong evidence exists that person-to-person spread of *B. cepacia* complex occurs; therefore, stringent infection control measures are now advocated for outpatient and hospitalized care.

Fungi and molds, such as *Aspergillus*, are frequently cultured from the respiratory secretions of CF patients. Although much less common, **allergic bronchopulmonary aspergillosis (APBA)** may occur. The diagnosis of ABPA is based on five clinical features: new infiltrates, wheezing, increased cough, expectoration of brown plugs, and/or an unexplained deterioration in lung function. Immunologic sensitivity to *Aspergillus* or other fungi, including elevated titers of *Aspergillus* precipitating antibodies and high total IgE levels above 500 IU, should also prompt consideration of this diagnosis. Therapy includes systemic corticosteroids and antifungal medications.

Clinically, during an acute exacerbation, the child will have malaise, lack of appetite, increased cough, and sputum production and will complain of increasing dyspnea. Fever may also be present. In addition to clinical findings, radiography and pulmonary function studies are of value in quantifying the severity of the disease, detecting an acute exacerbation, and monitoring the response to therapy.

Early in the course of this disease, chest radiographs are normal and have little diagnostic value. In children, hyperinflation, followed by increased interstitial markings, may be the first radiographic findings. As the disease progresses, these increased interstitial markings develop into the typical findings of cystic bronchiectasis. The right upper lobe is more frequently and severely affected than the left, although the rationale is not quite clear. Despite high densities of bacteria in airways, findings consistent with bacterial pneumonia are not generally seen, even during an acute exacerbation. Airway obstruction from retained secretions commonly manifests radiologically as segmental or subsegmental atelectasis and lobar collapse. Chest radiography is also useful for the detection of complications of CF lung disease, which include lobar collapse and pneumothorax.

High-resolution CT scans of the chest may also be useful to detect early pathologic changes, such as bronchiectasis, that are not visible on routine chest radiograph early in the course of the disease. Chest CT is of value during the evaluation of a patient with chronic cough and sputum production who is not otherwise known to have bronchiectasis. More recently, magnetic resonance imaging (MRI) has emerged as an alternative, radiation-free imaging technique for quantitative assessment of CF lung disease. In addition to structural lung damage, chest MRI enables noninvasive assessment of abnormalities in lung perfusion and ventilation characteristically associated with mucus plugging in CF lung disease.[47]

Pulmonary function testing is a reliable method used to quantify the severity of CF lung disease. It is also an objective means to detect a decline or deterioration in the child's clinical status, necessitating more intensive therapy. Pulmonary function testing is also used to measure the response to therapy. Effective therapeutic interventions will manifest as improved lung function (i.e., lung function returns to or near to the pre-exacerbation baseline) or a plateau, demonstrating that lung function is no longer declining as a result of the acute exacerbation.

Initially, obstruction of small airways is detected. This is indicated by reduced flow at low lung volumes (e.g., FEF25–75%) and gas trapping with an increase in the ratio of residual volume to total lung capacity (RV/TLC).[48] As the disease progresses, pulmonary function tests demonstrate progressive reduction in FEV_1, followed by decreased functional vital capacity (FVC). The FEV_1 is the accepted indicator of disability and is somewhat predictive of length of survival.[49] An FEV_1 of about 30% of predicted often is used as one of the factors taken into consideration for lung transplant evaluation.[49]

Lung clearance index (LCI) is a more sensitive test, especially in the early stages of CF, when lung pathology is more difficult to detect. LCI is also easier for younger patients to perform.[50] LCI is measured by performing an inert gas washout using a low concentration of an inert gas.

Treatment of an Acute Exacerbation of CF Lung Disease

Treatment of CF lung disease focuses on therapies aimed at preventing deterioration of lung function and those used to treat acute exacerbations. Inhaled medications, including a proteolytic, an antibiotic, and **airway clearance therapy (ACT)**, are essential components of routine care. However, when the child with CF has an acute exacerbation, airway clearance therapy is intensified. Therefore, the frequency with which a child's routine ACT regimen is performed may be increased (i.e., a child performing high-frequency chest wall compressions twice daily at home may require this therapy to be performed three to four times per day during an acute exacerbation). Another form of ACT may also be added (i.e., the addition of oscillatory positive expiratory pressure therapy to the ACT regimen of a child who performs high-frequency chest wall compression as routine home therapy). ACT in combination with nutrition, antibiotic, and anti-inflammatory therapy provide optimal care during an acute exacerbation by

treating infection, reducing airway inflammation, and mobilizing and clearing retained secretions. CF airway secretions are difficult to clear because of their lower viscosity and higher tenacity. Table 15-11 provides a list of inhaled medications frequently used to reduce airway resistance, enhance secretion mobilization, and treat infection. The aforementioned therapies are also important in daily maintenance care to prevent secretion retention, progressive airway obstruction, and inflammation. In addition to inhaled medications, performing ACT promotes the expectoration of airway secretions. ACT is a cornerstone of CF care that has several therapeutic modalities available for use, including postural drainage and clapping, oscillatory positive expiratory pressure (OPEP) devices, high-frequency chest wall compression, and breathing techniques. No one technique is superior, but it is important to incorporate patient preference into the decision-making process; age and other factors will influence airway clearance technique selection (Table 15-12). Patients and families should be included as informed consumers when a decision regarding the type of ACT to be incorporated into the child's plan of care is made. Patients and, in the case of very small children, families are more likely to be adherent to therapy when their preferences are taken into consideration. By identifying clinical characteristics associated with the risk for airway obstruction, malnutrition, and decline in lung function, clinicians may be better equipped to promptly recognize and treat pulmonary exacerbations, which can ultimately improve their patient's long-term prognosis. Respiratory therapists play a key role in the treatment of patients with pulmonary

TABLE 15-11
Inhaled Medications Used During Daily or Routine Care as Well as in the Treatment of an Acute Exacerbation of CF

Inhaled Agent	Rationale
Dornase alfa	Decreases secretion tenacity by degrading DNA polymers
Bronchodilator (beta-adrenergic agonist)	May protect against bronchospasm induced by expectorants and/or antibiotics No proven effect on airway clearance
Hypertonic saline or mannitol	May improve airway surface fluid hydration, increase mucin secretion, and increase cough effectiveness
Antibiotic (TOBI, Cayston)	Treat pulmonary bacterial infection

TABLE 15-12
Common Airway Clearance Techniques for Patients with CF

Technique	Age Considerations	Ability to Be Used Concurrently with Aerosol Therapy	Other Factors for Consideration
Postural drainage and clapping	No age limitations	When patient is positioned upright	Time/labor intensive Positions may need modification
Active cycle of breathing	Begin at 3–4 years Coaching until ~10 years	Yes	Takes time to learn May be difficult to perform during an exacerbation or with severe lung disease
Autogenic drainage	Begin at ~10–12 years of age	No	May be difficult to perform during an exacerbation or with severe lung disease Takes concentration
Oscillatory positive expiratory pressure	Children and adults	With some devices, such as the Acapella and AerobiKa	Difficult to determine the pressure delivered to the patient
High-frequency chest wall compression	>2–3 years of age	Yes	Precaution needs to be taken with indwelling catheters and chest tubes
Exercise	Children and adults	No	Bronchospasm oxygen desaturation

manifestations of CF. Respiratory therapists not only are essential in providing direct care but also are instrumental in ensuring that patients and families properly perform inhaled medication and airway clearance therapies. As an integral member of the interdisciplinary team, respiratory therapists should continually evaluate ACT for therapeutic effectiveness and recommend changes to the plan of care as needed.

Although the prompt treatment of airway obstruction, infection, and inflammation are key components of care for CF patients, complicated treatment regimens and lengthy treatment times contribute to nonadherence. Optimal management may be hindered by other patient-related factors, such as depression, lack of disease-related education aimed at performing airway clearance therapies properly, and limited understanding of medication/therapy regimens to promote self-care. Adverse effects of therapy, such as toxicity, unpalatable taste, and drug interactions; inconvenience of medication delivery systems and airway clearance modalities; and lack of clinician time dedicated to patient/family education, are factors that contribute to nonadherence to the prescribed plans of care. Technologic advances in antimicrobial therapy and inhaled delivery systems bring the promise of improved tolerance, reduced treatment times, and enhanced adherence to recommended care.

Nutritional Support

Attention to nutritional status and focus on nutritional support are two of the pillars of CF care. There is an interrelationship between lung function and nutritional status. Progressive lung disease further increases calorie requirements by the increase in the child's work of breathing. The basic tenets of nutritional repletion in CF include the use of pancreatic enzyme replacement therapy and following a high-calorie, high-protein, unrestricted diet. Children who receive aggressive nutritional support with adequate pancreatic replacement management should have both normal growth and lung function preservation. During an acute exacerbation, increasing calorie intake is necessary to combat the higher energy expenditure due to the increased work of breathing. Routine assessment of the child's nutritional status includes anthropometric parameters and, as the child matures, an annual assessment of body composition, bone density, glucose tolerance, and various biochemical and micronutrient levels.

Complications

Hemoptysis, pneumothorax, and respiratory failure are major pulmonary complications that tend to occur in association with more severe lung disease. In the adult CF population, major hemoptysis and pneumothorax each occurs in about 1% of patients annually.

Hemoptysis in CF may range from minor blood streaking of the sputum, requiring little intervention, to massive bleeding (more than 240 mL in 24 hours). **Minor hemoptysis** is common and usually self-limited, although it may indicate an exacerbation of lung disease. **Massive hemoptysis** most commonly comes from the bronchial artery circulation, which is at systemic arterial pressure. The new occurrence of any amount of bleeding may signal the presence of an increased infection or inflammation and the need for intensified treatment. It is important to identify the cause of a minor amount of hemoptysis to determine if intensified treatment with antibiotics is really necessary. Medications, such as nonsteroidal inflammatory agents, aspirin, or penicillin, can cause a new occurrence of bleeding. Vitamin K deficiency may also contribute to new onset of bleeding.

Hemoptysis greater than 240 mL in 24 hours from bronchiectatic airways occurs in approximately 5% of patients[51] and may lead to airway obstruction and asphyxiation. Hypotension, anemia, and chemical pneumonitis may result from massive hemoptysis. Bronchial artery embolization may be required to control bleeding and to minimize the propensity for adversely impacting the unaffected lung. Hemoptysis that persists for several days (such as 100 mL/day for 3 days) also should be considered a major bleeding event. This type of bleeding may be a precursor to massive bleeding, and these children require hospitalization and treatment with antibiotics based on their recent sputum culture results. Airway clearance is temporarily withheld, and patients are encouraged to suppress vigorous cough efforts. Bed rest may also be used to lessen the likelihood of further bleeding. However, suspending ACT, coughing, and mobility should not be continued for prolonged periods in patients with advanced lung disease, as these patients will most likely suffer further complications from inadequate airway clearance.

Spontaneous pneumothorax is typically caused by rupture of subpleural air cysts. Pneumothorax occurs in approximately 16% to 20% of patients but is more common in those reaching adulthood.[52] Most patients complain of a sudden increase in dyspnea or chest discomfort. However, some may be asymptomatic. The presence of a newly detected pneumothorax requires hospitalization, irrespective of whether chest tube insertion is initially planned. Asymptomatic pneumothoraces that occupy less than 20% of the hemithorax may not require treatment, but clinical monitoring is needed to assess progression.[52] Larger pneumothoraces leading to symptoms should be treated with a chest tube. The chest tube may be removed once the pneumothorax has resolved.

Most patients who suffer massive hemoptysis or pneumothorax can be treated successfully. However, respiratory failure, as the result of progressive airway obstruction and destruction, typically results in death.

Hypoxemic and hypercapnic respiratory failure occurs in the late stages of CF.[52] Treatment of hypoxemia may improve both the quality and the duration of life. Ventilation/perfusion mismatch and hypoxemia occur as infection and inflammation progress and airway obstruction and parenchymal destruction worsen. Increased partial pressure of carbon dioxide, intrapulmonary shunt, reduced mixed venous saturation resulting from increased oxygen consumption, malnutrition, and weakness also contribute to hypoxemia.[52]

The use of noninvasive mechanical ventilation (NIV) has been used to alleviate respiratory muscle fatigue in CF patients with severe end-stage lung disease. NIV may be used alone or in conjunction with long-term oxygen therapy. The literature reports that NIV can improve nocturnal ventilation, oxygenation, sleep quality, and functional capacity.[53,54] The initial goal of treating hypoxemic respiratory failure is to correct reversible processes. This includes treating airway infection, clearing retained secretions, improving nutrition, and medically managing other complications that occur. Supplemental oxygen may be needed to maintain an SpO_2 of greater than or equal to 90%. Even when daytime oxygen saturation is adequate, hypoxemia during sleep or exercise may occur. Assessment of nocturnal oxygen saturation is important in those with severe lung disease or an FEV_1 ≤30% of predicted. Low resting oxygen saturations can contribute to cor pulmonale.

Outcomes

Cystic fibrosis is a life-limiting disease. Treatment at an approved CF center and adherence to the therapeutic plan of care can increase longevity and quality of life. Lung transplantation is an accepted therapy for end-stage CF lung disease, but there are often long waiting times before organ availability, with waiting times exceeding 2 years at some centers. Those with an FEV_1 of less than 30% of predicted; hypercapnia (PCO_2 ≥45 mm Hg); the presence of an accelerated clinical decline, characterized by more frequent exacerbations that respond incompletely to aggressive therapy; recurrent pneumothoraces; massive hemoptysis; or pan-resistant organisms should receive prompt consideration for a lung transplantation referral.[55] CF lung transplant recipients have good outcomes after lung transplantation, and quality of life is dramatically improved. However, those with CF are still prone to the common complications germane to all lung transplant recipients, including primary graft dysfunction, acute and chronic rejection, infections, malignancies, and renal failure.

Case Study 1

A 7-year-old female weighing 26 kg presents to the emergency department with an asthma exacerbation. Her mother reports she has had an upper respiratory tract infection for the last 2 days and has been using her albuterol inhaler more frequently. Today she has received treatments every 2 to 3 hours but still complains of shortness of breath and has frequent coughing. She reports taking her controller medication, Flovent 44 mcg 2 puffs bid as prescribed. Her mother states that the patient uses her controller medication every day. Your assessment reveals the following: an alert yet anxious 7-year-old, sitting on the edge of the bed leaning forward. She has moderate intercostal retractions. You ask her to tell you her name and favorite activity at school, but she must stop and take a breath after four words. At this time, vitals are as follows: heart rate of 140 beats per minute, respiratory rate of 42 breaths per minute, SpO_2 at 93% on room air, blood pressure of 90/60 mm Hg, temperature of 37.5°C. Upon auscultation, breath sounds are diminished with very faint expiratory wheezes throughout all lung fields.

1. **You are called to the room. What is your recommendation at this time?**

Your reassessment after an hour reveals the following: heart rate of 156 beats per minute, respiratory rate of 36 breaths per minute, SpO_2 at 95% on room air. Mild intercostal retractions persist. Breath sounds reveal increased expiratory wheezes throughout all lung fields. The patient status has improved after an additional hour of observation (heart rate of 140 beats per minute, respiratory rate of 28 breaths per minute, SpO_2 at 98%, blood pressure of 88/60 mm Hg). Intercostal retractions are no longer present. Breath sounds show improved air entry throughout all lung fields, and few expiratory wheezes persist. The patient is discharged home with follow up with her primary care physician in 2 days.

2. **What key components are necessary for improving this patient's asthma control?**

3. **Are there other recommendations that you might make for this patient at this time?**

Case Study 2

A 9-month-old child presents with a history of poor growth and a chronic cough. He was postterm (41 weeks' gestation), born to a 30-year-old gravida 1 para 1 mother with an uncomplicated pregnancy. Soon after birth, he developed respiratory distress and was admitted to the neonatal intensive care unit, where he was mechanically ventilated for 2 days and discharged after a week. He was initially breastfed, but due to frequent vomiting and loose bowel movements, he was changed to formula feeding. Despite trials of different types of formula, he continued with bloating, diarrhea, and failure to thrive (weight <5th percentile). He developed a daily cough and some respiratory difficulty. At 6 months of age, he was again hospitalized for respiratory distress. He continued to have loose, large, greasy, foul-smelling stools and failure to thrive. A sweat test and genetic testing were recommended. At this time the patient is alert and in no distress, heart rate is 120 beats per minute, respiratory rate is 40 breaths per minute, blood pressure is 85/65 mm Hg, temperature is 37.5°C, and oxygen saturation is 96% on room air. He continues to be small for his age. Heart regular. Lungs with good aeration and mild wheezing and rales. Color and perfusion are good. Sweat test revealed weight 120 mcg; 105 mmol/L. Cystic fibrosis mutation analysis from the genetic testing was positive for one copy of Delta F508 and one copy of R1066C.

1. **What will be the key pillar of care for the patient newly diagnosed with CF?**

2. **What is the most common pathogen present in patients with CF?**

3. **This patient is in the <5th percentile for weight. What therapeutic intervention should be implemented?**

References

1. Bloom B, Jones LI, Freeman G. Summary health statistics for U.S. children: National Health Interview Survey, 2012. National Center for Health Statistics. *Vital Health Stat.* 2013;258:1-81.

2. United States Environmental Protection Agency. Asthma facts, March 2013. http://www.epa.gov/asthma/pdfs/asthma_fact_sheet_en.pdf. Accessed August 15, 2015.

3. Centers for Disease Control and Prevention. Asthma's impact on the nation. Data from the CDC National Asthma Control Program. Atlanta, GA: US Department of Health and Human Services, CDC: 2011. Available at http://www.cdc.gov/asthma/impacts_nation/asthmafactsheet.pdf. Accessed September 1, 2015.

4. National Asthma Education and Prevention Program Expert Panel Report 3. *Guidelines for the Diagnosis and Management of Asthma.* National Heart Lung and Blood Institute, National Institutes of Health: U.S. Department of Health and Human Services; 2007 Aug 28. Report no.: NIH Publication No.07-4051. Full Report.

5. Miller MR, Hankinson J, Brusasco V, et al. Standardisation of spirometry. *Eur Respir J.* 2005;26(2):319-338.

6. Sverrild A, Porsbjerg C, Thomsen SF, Backer V. Airway hyper-responsiveness to mannitol and methacholine and exhaled nitric oxide: a random-sample population study. *J Allergy Clin Immunol.* 2010;126(5):952-958.

7. Cockcroft DW, Davis BE. Diagnostic and therapeutic value of airway challenges in asthma. *Curr Allergy Asthma Rep.* 2009;9(3):247-253.

8. Anderson SD. Provocative challenges to help diagnose and monitor asthma: exercise, methacholine, adenosine, and mannitol. *Curr Opin Pulm Med.* 2008;14(1):39-45.

9. Zaczeniuk M, Woicka-Kolejwa K, Stelmach W, Podlecka D, Jerzyńska J, Stelmach I. Methacholine challenge testing is superior to the exercise challenge for detecting asthma in children. *Ann Allergy Asthma Immunol.* 2015;115(6):481-484.

10. Anderson SD, Charlton B, Weiler JM, et al. Comparison of mannitol and methacholine to predict exercise-induced bronchoconstriction and a clinical diagnosis of asthma. *Respir Res.* 2009;10:4.

11. Liccardi G, Cazzola M, D'Amato M, D'Amato G. Pets and cockroaches: two increasing causes of respiratory allergy in indoor environments. Characteristics of airways sensitization and prevention strategies. *Respir Med.* 2000;94(11):1109-1118.

12. Haselkorn T, Szefler SJ, Simons FE, et al. Allergy, total serum immunoglobulin E, and airflow in children and adolescents in TENOR. *Pediatr Allergy Immunol.* 2010;21(8):1157-1165.

13. Sicherer SH, Wood RA; American Academy of Pediatrics Section on Allergy and Immunology. Allergy testing in childhood: using allergen-specific IgE tests. *Pediatrics.* 2012;129(1):193-197.

14. Cook J, Saglani S. Pathogenesis and prevention strategies of severe asthma exacerbations in children. *Curr Opin Pulm Med.* 2016;22(1):25-31.

15. Wang Z, May SM, Charoenlap S, et al. Effects of secondhand smoke exposure on asthma morbidity and health care utilization in children: a systematic review and meta-analysis. *Ann Allergy Asthma Immunol.* 2015;115(5):396-401.

16. Murphy EV. Improving influenza vaccination coverage in the pediatric asthma population: the case for combined methodologies. *Yale J Biol Med.* 2014;87(4):439-446.

17. Spantideas N, Drosou E, Bougea A, Assimakopoulos D. Inhaled corticosteroids and voice problems. What is new? *J Voice.* 2016;S0892-1997(16)30266-1.

18. Hossny E, Rosario N, Lee BW, et al. The use of inhaled corticosteroids in pediatric asthma: update. *World Allergy Organ J.* 2016;9:26.

19. Eid NS, O'Hagan A, Bickel S, Morton R, Jacobson S, Myers JA. Anti-inflammatory dosing of theophylline in the treatment of status asthmaticus in children. *J Asthma Allergy.* 2016;9:183-189.

20. Milgrom H, Berger W, Nayak A, et al. Treatment of childhood asthma with anti-immunoglobulin E antibody (omalizumab). *Pediatrics.* 2001;108(2):E36.

21. Nath JB, Hsia RY. Children's emergency department use for asthma, 2001-2010. *Acad Pediatr.* 2015;15(2):225-230.

22. Zemek R, Plint A, Osmond MH, et al. Triage nurse initiation of corticosteroids in pediatric asthma is associated with improved emergency department efficiency. *Pediatrics.* 2012;129(4):671-680.

23. Ducharme FM, Chalut D, Plotnick L, et al. The Pediatric Respiratory Assessment Measure: a valid clinical score for assessing acute asthma severity from toddlers to teenagers. *J Pediatr*. 2008;152(4):476-480.

24. Torres S, Sticco N, Bosch JJ, et al. Effectiveness of magnesium sulfate as initial treatment of acute severe asthma in children, conducted in a tertiary-level university hospital: a randomized, controlled trial. *Arch Argent Pediatr*. 2012;110(4):291-296.

25. Phumeetham S, Bahk TJ, Abd-Allah S, Mathur M. Effect of high-dose continuous albuterol nebulization on clinical variables in children with status asthmaticus. *Pediatr Crit Care Med*. 2015;16(2):e41-e46.

26. Basnet S, Mander G, Andoh J, Klaska H, Verhulst S, Koirala J. Safety, efficacy, and tolerability of early initiation of noninvasive positive pressure ventilation in pediatric patients admitted with status asthmaticus: a pilot study. *Pediatr Crit Care Med*. 2012;13(4):393-398.

27. Walsh-Kelly CM, Kelly KJ, Drendel AL, Grabowski L, Kuhn EM. Emergency department revisits for pediatric acute asthma exacerbations: association of factors identified in an emergency department asthma tracking system. *Pediatr Emerg Care*. 2008;24(8):505-510.

28. Tolomeo C, Savrin C, Heinzer M, Bazzy-Asaad A. Predictors of asthma-related pediatric emergency department visits and hospitalizations. *J Asthma*. 2009;46(8):829-834.

29. Guttmann A, Zagorski B, Austin PC, et al. Effectiveness of emergency department asthma management strategies on return visits in children: a population-based study. *Pediatrics*. 2007;120(6):e1402-e1410.

30. Cystic Fibrosis Foundation. *Patient Registry Annual Data Report for 2014*. Bethesda, MD: Cystic Fibrosis Foundation; 2015.

31. Giorgi G, Casarin A, Trevisson E, et al. Validation of CFTR intronic variants identified during cystic fibrosis population screening by a minigene splicing assay. *Clin Chem Lab Med*. 2015;53(11):1719-1723.

32. Cotton CU, Stutts MJ, Knowles MR, Gatzy JT, Boucher RC. Abnormal apical cell membrane in cystic fibrosis respiratory epithelium. An in vitro electrophysiologic analysis. *J Clin Invest*. 1987;79(1):80-85.

33. Dupuis A, Keenan K, Ooi CY, et al. Prevalence of meconium ileus marks the severity of mutations of the cystic fibrosis transmembrane conductance regulator (CFTR) gene. *Genet Med*. 2016;18(4):333-340.

34. Taege L, Shepherd B. The pathologic findings of distal intestinal obstruction syndrome, a commonly occurring but rarely described complication of cystic fibrosis. *Pathology*. 2016;48(Suppl 1):S82-S83.

35. Assis DN, Freedman SD. Gastrointestinal disorders in cystic fibrosis. *Clin Chest Med*. 2016;37(1):109-118.

36. Brennan AL, Beynon J. Clinical updates in cystic fibrosis-related diabetes. *Semin Respir Crit Care Med*. 2015;36(2):236-250.

37. Chotirmall SH, Mann AK, Branagan P, et al. Male fertility in cystic fibrosis. *Ir Med J*. 2009;102(7):204-206.

38. Sueblinvong V, Whittaker LA. Fertility and pregnancy: common concerns of the aging cystic fibrosis population. *Clin Chest Med*. 2007;28(2):433-443.

39. Nussbaum E, Boat TF, Wood RE, et al. Cystic fibrosis with acute hypoelectrolytemia and metabolic alkalosis in infancy. *Am J Dis Child*. 1979;133(9):965-966.

40. Chang EH. New insights into the pathogenesis of cystic fibrosis sinusitis. *Int Forum Allergy Rhinol*. 2014;4(2):132-137.

41. Chow C, Landau L, Taussig L. Bronchial mucus glands in the newborn with cystic fibrosis. *Eur J Pediatr*. 1982;139(4):240-243.

42. Cohen-Cymberknoh M, Shoseyov D, Kerem E. Managing cystic fibrosis: strategies that increase life expectancy and improve quality of life. *Am J Respir Crit Care Med*. 2011;183(11):1463-1471.

43. Janhsen WK, Arnold C, Hentschel J, et al. Colonization of CF patients' upper airways with *S. aureus* contributes more decisively to upper airway inflammation than *P. aeruginosa*. *Med Microbiol Immunol*. 2016;205(5):485-500.

44. Dasenbrook EC, Merlo CA, Diener-West M, Lechtzin N, Boyle MP. Persistent methicillin-resistant *Staphylococcus aureus* and rate of FEV_1 decline in cystic fibrosis. *Am J Resp Crit Care Med*. 2008;178(8):814-821.

45. Vanderhelst E, De Meirleir L, Verbanck S, Piérard D, Vincken W, Malfroot A. Prevalence and impact on FEV_1 decline of chronic methicillin-resistant *Staphylococcus aureus* (MRSA) colonization in patients with cystic fibrosis. A single-center, case control study of 165 patients. *J Cyst Fibros*. 2012;11(1):2-7.

46. Lynch JP. Burkholderia cepacia complex: impact on the cystic fibrosis lung lesion. *Semin Respir Crit Care Med*. 2009;30(5):596-610.

47. Mall MA, Stahl M, Graeber SY, Sommerburg O, Kauczor HU, Wielpütz MO. Early detection and sensitive monitoring of CF lung disease: prospects of improved and safer imaging. *Pediatr Pulmonol*. 2016;51(S44):S49-S60.

48. Bakker EM, Borsboom GJ, van der Wiel-Kooij EC, Caudri D, Rosenfeld M, Tiddens HA. Small airway involvement in cystic fibrosis lung disease: routine spirometry as an early and sensitive marker. *Pediatr Pulmonol*. 2013;48(11):1081-1088.

49. Harun SN, Wainwright C, Klein K, Hennig S. A systematic review of studies examining the rate of lung function decline in patients with cystic fibrosis. *Paediatr Respir Rev*. 2016;20:55-66.

50. Stahl M, Wielpütz MO, Graeber SY, et al. Comparison of lung clearance index and magnetic resonance imaging for assessment of lung disease in children with cystic fibrosis. *Am J Respir Crit Care Med*. 2017;195(3):349-350.

51. Flume PA, Yankaskas JR, Ebeling M, Hulsey T, Clark LL. Massive hemoptysis in cystic fibrosis. *Chest*. 2005;128(2):729-738.

52. Flume PA. Pulmonary complications of cystic fibrosis. *Respir Care*. 2009;54(5):618-627.

53. Lima CA, Andrade Ade F, Campos SL, et al. Effects of noninvasive ventilation on treadmill 6-min walk distance and regional chest wall volumes in cystic fibrosis: randomized controlled trial. *Respir Med*. 2014;108(10):1460-1468.

54. Katz ES. Cystic fibrosis and sleep. *Clin Chest Med*. 2014;35(3):495-504.

55. Hadjiliadis D. Special considerations for patients with cystic fibrosis undergoing lung transplantation. *Chest*. 2007;131(4):1224-1231.

16

Pediatric Neurodisability Disorders

Robert H. Warren

Farrah D. Jones

© Anna Rubak/ShutterStock, Inc.

OUTLINE

OBJECTIVES

1. Explain the pathophysiology of neurodisability disorders affecting the infant and child.
2. Identify the clinical symptoms of neurodisability disorders affecting the infant and child.
3. Discuss the diagnosis of neurodisability disorders affecting the infant and child.
4. Define the pulmonary composite for the infant and child with neurodisability disorders.
5. Identify the pulmonary composite factors and the particular role each plays in airway secretion overload and pulmonary dysfunction.
6. Discuss how airway secretion overload can progress to chronic lung disease.
7. Explain the approach to physical assessment of the infant and child with a neurodisability disorder.
8. Describe the effects of chronic bacterial colonization on the pulmonary stability of the infant and child with a neurodisability disorder.
9. Develop a respiratory management plan for the infant and child with a neurodisability disorder and pulmonary compromise.
10. Understand the role of airway clearance in the respiratory management plan of the infant and child with a neurodisability disorder and pulmonary compromise.
11. Discuss the importance of education and skills validation for the caregiver of the infant and child with a neurodisability disorder and pulmonary compromise.
12. Recognize the psychological characteristics of the caregiver of the infant and child with a neurodisability disorder.

KEY TERMS

airway secretion overload
bacterial colonization
cerebral palsy (CP)
Guillain-Barré
  syndrome (GBS)
mitochondrial disorders
muscular dystrophy (MD)
myasthenia gravis
neurodisability disorders
ptosis

pulmonary composite
skills validation
spina bifida
spinal muscular
  atrophy (SMA)
stertor
stridor
transverse myelitis
traumatic brain injury

Introduction

Pediatric patients with a primary neurodisability who have secondary pulmonary complications represent a population consisting of both congenital and acquired etiologies for their primary diagnosis. Ongoing pulmonary assessment is critical in stabilizing chronic pulmonary disease and preventing irreversible pulmonary dysfunction that often presents in these patients.

Neurodisability Disorders

Congenital **neurodisability disorders** as well as acquired conditions, such as **traumatic brain injury**, make up a challenging list of diagnoses. **Table 16-1** lists congenital neurodisability disorders while **Table 16-2** lists neurodisability disorders that are acquired.

Although many of the primary neurodisability disorders are relatively rare, **Table 16-3** lists those seen commonly in the pediatric population. To develop an appropriate respiratory management plan, one should be readily familiar with the disorder's etiology, how it

TABLE 16-1
Congenital Neurodisability Disorders

Bethlehem myopathy
Cerebellar atrophy
Cervicothoracic syringomyelia/syrinx
CHARGE syndrome
Cockayne syndrome
Congenital hypomyelination syndrome
Congenital scoliosis
CFC syndrome
Down syndrome
Fredericks ataxia
Jacho-Levin syndrome
Metachromatic leukodystrophy
Muscular dystrophy
Myotonic dystrophy
Neiman pick
Neuronal migration disorder
Partial complex IV mitochondrial disease
Pompe disease
Soto syndrome
Spina bifida
Spinal muscular atrophy, types I and II
Thoracic dystrophy
Undiagnosed mitochondrial disorder
Undiagnosed neurodegenerative disorder
X-linked myotubular myopathy

TABLE 16-2
Acquired Neurodisability Disorders

Complications of prematurity
Term newborns with neurologic insults at birth
Traumatic brain injury
Spinal cord injury
Kernicterus

TABLE 16-3
Common Pediatric Neurodisability Disorders

Muscular dystrophy (MD)
Spinal muscular atrophy (SMA)
Cerebral palsy (CP)
Spina bifida
Guillain-Barré syndrome
Myasthenia gravis
Transverse myelitis

TABLE 16-4
Most Common Types of Muscular Dystrophy

Duchenne
Myotonic
Becker
Congenital
Limb-girdle
Facioscapulohumeral
Oculopharyngeal
Distal
Emery-Dreifuss

is identified, and the primary symptoms that would be expected to be seen.

Muscular Dystrophies

The muscular dystrophies are a group of genetic disorders that are characterized by progressive muscular degeneration and weakness. There are more than 30 forms of **muscular dystrophy (MD)**. This weakness is usually due to abnormalities in muscle proteins caused by genetic mutations. Diagnosis can be made through history and physical exam, genetic testing, or muscle biopsy. **Table 16-4** lists the most common types of muscular dystrophy; Duchenne muscular dystrophy is seen most often and is one of the most severe forms. Several muscular dystrophies can affect the muscles of the respiratory system, causing difficulty with swallowing, ineffective cough, and respiratory failure.[1]

Spinal Muscular Atrophy

Spinal muscular atrophy (SMA) is a group of hereditary diseases that progressively cause muscle weakness and wasting of muscle (atrophy). They are the second most common autosomal-recessive inherited disorders (cystic fibrosis being the most common). The disorders are caused by a mutation in a gene known as the survival motor neuron gene 1 (SMN1). The abnormal gene causes motor neurons in the spinal cord to degenerate and die.[2] This can be offset by a neighboring SMN2 gene that is similar in function. As shown in **Table 16-5**, there are four types of SMA: types I, II, III, and IV. Prognosis depends upon the type, with type I (also known as Werdnig-Hoffman disease) being the most severe form,

TABLE 16-5
Types of Spinal Muscular Atrophy

Type	Usual Onset	Description
I	Birth to 6 months	Severe weakness; often fatal
II	6 months to 2 years	Unable to walk; may have respiratory symptoms
III	18 months to adolescence	Mildest form in children; may need wheelchair
IV	Early adulthood	Rarely occurs; mild motor impairment

followed in decreasing severity by II, III, and IV. The type is determined by the age at onset of symptoms and by the copies of SMN2 gene that are present. Definitive diagnosis is made through genetic testing. Respiratory symptoms can include a weak cry and cough, swallowing and feeding difficulty, abdominal breathing, and respiratory failure.[3] Death is most often due to respiratory complications.

Cerebral Palsy

The term **cerebral palsy (CP)** refers to a group of non-progressive neurodisability disorders that appear in infancy or early childhood and permanently affect body movement and muscle coordination. It is caused by brain injury or abnormal development of the brain. The majority of cases of cerebral palsy are congenital, although a small number of children have cerebral palsy as the result of brain damage in the first few months or years of life. The most common causes of acquired CP are brain infections, such as bacterial meningitis or viral encephalitis, and head injury as a result of a motor vehicle crash, fall, or child abuse.[4] There is no definitive diagnostic test for CP. If a child does not meet developmental milestones, the presence of characteristic symptoms and the use of testing to rule out other neurodisabilities can be used to diagnose CP. Respiratory symptoms associated with CP can range from impaired airway clearance to respiratory failure requiring mechanical ventilation.

Spina Bifida

Spina bifida is a disorder involving incomplete development of the brain, spinal cord, and/or their protective coverings. This occurs during the first month of pregnancy, when the fetal spine fails to close properly. The result is permanent nerve damage with varying degrees of paralysis of the lower limbs.[5] Research indicates that inadequate maternal intake of folic acid during pregnancy is the major cause of spina bifida. Diagnosis is usually made prenatally by ultrasound or amniocentesis and postnatally with radiologic studies. Respiratory

symptoms are restrictive in nature and caused by scoliosis or other spinal malformations.

Guillain-Barré Syndrome

Guillain-Barré syndrome (GBS) is a rare disorder in which the body's immune system attacks the nerves. Tingling and weakness in the legs are usually the first symptoms. Over the course of hours, days, or weeks, symptoms can spread to the upper body and increase in intensity. Complaints often include dyspnea, dysphagia, and slurred speech, and progression may lead to muscle paralysis with respiratory failure.[6] The exact cause of GBS is unknown, but it usually follows a viral or bacterial infection of the respiratory or gastrointestinal systems. In rare cases, surgery and vaccinations have triggered GBS. Diagnosis is made through a history and physical exam. A nerve conduction velocity test can help in diagnosis, with signals traveling slower along the nerves affected by GBS. A spinal tap showing an elevated protein level in the cerebrospinal fluid strongly supports the diagnosis. Respiratory symptoms are related to respiratory muscle weakness and can sometimes require mechanical ventilation.

Myasthenia Gravis

Myasthenia gravis is a chronic autoimmune neuromuscular disease that causes varying degrees of muscle weakness. In **myasthenia gravis**, the body's own antibodies block, alter, or destroy acetylcholine receptors, which in turn disrupts the transmission of nerve impulses to the muscles.[7] The most commonly affected muscles are those that control the eyes, face, speech, and swallowing. Diagnosis is made through a neurologic exam and patient history. Early symptoms include drooping of one or both eyelids (**ptosis**), double vision (diplopia), dysphagia, and slurred speech. Muscle weakness can spread from the face and neck to the arms, hands, and legs. In rare cases it may progress to involve the muscles of the respiratory system and lead to respiratory failure and the need for mechanical ventilation. Muscle weakness that increases during periods of activity and improves after periods of rest is a key characteristic of myasthenia gravis. Although patients may go into remission, there is no known cure for this disorder.

Transverse Myelitis

Transverse myelitis is a neurodisability disorder caused by inflammation of an area across the spinal cord, resulting in damage to the myelin that covers nerve cells. Researchers are uncertain of the causes of transverse myelitis, but it is believed to result from viral infections or abnormal immune responses.[8] Some cases have occurred following vaccinations. Diagnosis is provided through a medical history and neurologic examination. Symptoms usually develop within hours and become worse within a few days. The most common early symptom is sudden pain, usually in the lower back. Other symptoms associated with transverse myelitis are muscle weakness in the limbs, sensory disturbances (numbness, tingling, coldness, or burning) in the legs or feet and toes, fatigue, and bladder and bowel dysfunction. Respiratory symptoms include muscle weakness or paralysis and may range from impaired airway clearance to respiratory failure.

Mitochondrial Disorders

Mitochondrial disorders are a group of neuromuscular diseases that occur when there is damage to the mitochondria in the cells. Enzymes within the mitochondria change nutrients into cellular energy; mitochondrial failure leads to death of the cells and ultimately organ failure. These disorders can be caused by genetic mutation or may be acquired following the adverse effects from drugs or infections.[9] Diagnosis is made from the clinical picture obtained through a neurologic exam and the medical history. The symptoms of mitochondrial disorders may include muscle weakness or exercise intolerance, heart failure or rhythm disturbances, dementia, movement disorders, stroke-like episodes, deafness, blindness, droopy eyelids, limited mobility of the eyes, vomiting, and seizures. Muscle biopsy and genetic testing can also be used to confirm the diagnosis. Respiratory symptoms are a result of muscle weakness or abnormalities in the brain leading to respiratory control issues.

The Pulmonary Composite

Faced with such a large, heterogeneous group of primary neurologic diagnoses, it becomes a challenge for the healthcare professional to evaluate and manage the secondary pulmonary complications. However, a careful examination of this patient population reveals similarities of physical abnormalities and pulmonary symptoms. This allows for the development of individualized respiratory care management plans.

Careful historical assessment can identify a set of etiologic factors that come into play on a routine basis in this population, each contributing to the production or retention of secretions, regardless of the primary neurologic diagnosis. The pulmonary symptoms can be relegated to this set of factors—to be defined as the **pulmonary composite**—applicable to all neurodisability patients with pulmonary complications. The number of specific primary neurologic diagnoses in the pediatric age group that have the potential to have secondary pulmonary complications is extensive.

Airway Secretion Overload

A broad etiologic concept is that, regardless of the neurologic diagnosis, the primary finding in these patients is related to the presence of excessive airway secretions. The introduction, production, and retention of

TABLE 16-6
Pulmonary Composite

Pulmonary Composite Factors	Effect on Secretion Accumulation
Drooling	Introduction
Gastroesophageal reflux	Introduction
Dysphagia	Introduction
Seizure	Introduction
Recurrent respiratory illness	Production
Hypotonia	Production/retention
Hypopneic breathing pattern	Production/retention
Spasticity	Production/retention
State of ambulation	Production/retention

secretions creates a clinical picture that can be referred to as **airway secretion overload**. Airway secretions naturally occur in the airway and are responsible for maintaining normal airway function. When disease states result in excessive secretion accumulation, the stage is set for the beginning of chronic pulmonary dysfunction, which over time may progress to respiratory failure and the need for mechanical ventilator support.

A major key to successful respiratory care management of the patient with neurodisability is to identify the factors that make up the pulmonary composite in each individual patient and to address each factor so as to minimize its impact on the total airway secretion overload status of the patient. **Table 16-6** lists the pulmonary composite factors and the particular role each plays in airway secretion overload and pulmonary dysfunction.

Chronic Lung Disease

A major beginning point in the progression of excessive airway secretions to chronic lung disease is the presence of an ineffective cough. This is one of the most commonly seen factors in the pulmonary composite regardless of the primary diagnosis. An ineffective cough, which is most closely linked to hypotonia and the ambulatory status of the patient, sets the stage for secretion retention.

Secretions also commonly invade the airway overtly due to aspiration from dysphagia and gastroesophageal reflux. Over time, chronic secretion retention results in airway hyposensitivity as irritant fiber receptors cease to respond to both the volume and the irritant effect of airway secretions. Secretion retention also leads to airway inflammation, resulting in mucosal gland proliferation and hypertrophy, as the mucous glands react to the inflammatory response. Finally, retained secretions

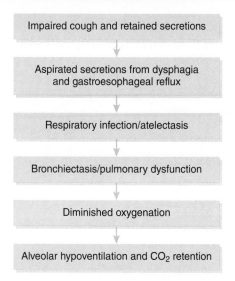

FIGURE 16-1 Evolution of chronic lung disease in children with neurodisability disorders.

become a perfect milieu for chronic bacterial infection, producing more inflammation and more airway secretion production. As seen in **Figure 16-1**, the result is a vicious cycle leading to airway and parenchymal destruction. The end result is hypoxia and chronic hypoventilation with CO_2 retention. This progressive sequence of events forms the basis for the selection of medications and therapy devices that should be included in a patient's individualized respiratory care plan. An effective management plan would reduce the impact of airway secretion production and accumulation. This leads to an increase in pulmonary stability and a decrease in the degree of progression and the severity of chronic pulmonary dysfunction. Reducing the specific effect of each factor in the pulmonary composite may delay the progression of chronic lung disease, in some cases for years.

Patient Assessment

The pulmonary composite can be used as a guide in the clinical assessment of the patient during pulmonary clinic visits. These periodic visits are needed to update the patient's pulmonary history and to obtain a physical assessment. Laboratory data may be obtained on a regular basis as well as on a semi-urgent basis should the patient present to the clinic visit in an unstable condition. The approach to the patient in the clinic setting should be outlined in an organized fashion.

Patient History

It is important to inquire as to the presence or absence of each pulmonary composite factor as well as the relative degree of activity of the factor. For example, if seizure activity has been significantly increased since the last clinical assessment, then there may be an increase

in the total sum of airway secretions and thus an increase in pulmonary symptoms. If ambulation has been decreased significantly for whatever reason, then an increase in potential accumulation of secretions is possible. This process of reasoning can be followed through for each factor in the composite.

Physical Examination

Physical assessment begins with making an initial overview observation of the patient in totality prior to the use of palpation, percussion, or by examination using the stethoscope. Much can be gained by observing components of the composite factor, such as spasticity, seizure activity, and drooling. Audible airway sounds can denote an increase in airway secretions, which may be accompanied by increased respiratory rates if not mild respiratory distress.

A "hands-on" approach is used to evaluate tracheal positioning, assess for extremity edema, and examine the nail beds for clubbing. Palpation of the chest can determine asymmetry and diaphragm movement as well as identify the location of the point of maximal impulse of the heart. Abdominal palpation can identify any liver or spleen enlargement, which may indicate chronic obstructive pulmonary changes due to an increase in lung volume and airway disease.

Audible noises heard on auscultation of the respiratory system include **stridor**, **stertor**, and the noises produced as turbulent airflow passes around, under, and above fixed secretions in the large airways. It is incumbent upon the respiratory care practitioner to become an expert in the use of the stethoscope. The need for expertise in auscultation is necessary for routine physical examination, to assess efficacy of respiratory therapy treatments, and to be able to identify acute pulmonary changes when the patient is in respiratory distress.

Pulmonary Function

Obtaining objective pulmonary function data is a major challenge in the neurodisability patient. Routine spirometry, which is the most commonly used laboratory parameter to identify both restrictive and obstructive pulmonary dysfunction, especially as it is performed over time, is unfortunately rarely applicable to this patient population due to the neurologic and cognitive deficits caused by the patient's primary disease process. Pulmonary function data that can be of benefit include measurement of the resting tidal volume to evaluate the presence or absence of hypopnea and the use of end-tidal CO_2 measurement to document hypoventilation. Because a significant factor in the pulmonary composite is chronic aspiration, the presence of dead space ventilation due to the acquired airway disease produced by aspiration makes the end-tidal CO_2 value unreliable and may underestimate CO_2 elevation due to pulmonary insufficiency. For that reason, it is important to correlate on a periodic basis the end-tidal CO_2 with the CO_2 assessment from blood gas analysis. As long as the correlation between end-tidal CO_2 and blood gas analysis is stable, end-tidal CO_2 monitoring may be considered reliable. This is seen when the patient is evaluated in a steady clinical state. The unreliability of end-tidal CO_2 monitoring is found most often when assessing a patient during an acute respiratory illness; therefore, clinical judgement is required to decide when end-tidal CO_2 measurements are valid data in assessment.

Radiography

The chest radiograph of a patient with a primary neurologic diagnosis who has secondary pulmonary complications must be evaluated carefully. The chest radiograph is used primarily when an acute respiratory illness is present. Where there is a history of recurrent respiratory illness, and especially when factors related to aspiration are present, the chest radiograph will usually become abnormal over time and demonstrate chronic changes of atelectasis that remain even when the patient is stable. This becomes problematic if serial chest radiographs obtained over the years are not available during an acute illness. This is because chronic changes on the chest radiograph can easily be misinterpreted as acute changes when the patient presents with other acute symptoms of fever or respiratory distress. An improper diagnosis of pneumonia may be made and unnecessary hospitalizations and medical treatment undertaken when the proper diagnosis is, for example, a simple viral respiratory illness.

When there are significant upper respiratory symptoms, especially mucopurulent nasal discharge with associated fever and tenderness and swelling over the area of the maxillary sinuses, there may be an indication to obtain a single Water's view of the maxillary sinuses. When acute sinus disease is present, the medical management required is more intensive, as has been documented in the patient with cystic fibrosis.[10]

Assessment of Bacterial Colonization

Chronic **bacterial colonization** is considered to be that condition in which bacteria are identified in the airway even though the patient is otherwise stable and free of acute respiratory illness. Secretions that accumulate in the airways provide a perfect environment for bacterial invasion and chronic bacteria residence. Over time, multiple organisms can take up residence in the airway and remain there for years. Etiologic factors, primarily viral disease, such as the common cold, will cause exponential growth of the bacteria that are chronically present in the airway, producing symptoms of cough, congestion, and fever. When the acute illness is resolved, the bacterial colony count in the airway is reduced, acute symptoms disappear, and the bacteria return to a status of colonization.

TABLE 16-7
Organisms Commonly Found in Patients with Neurodisability

Pseudomonas aeruginosa
Stenotrophomonas maltophilia
Serratia marcescens
Moraxella catarrhalis
Methicillin-resistant Staphylococcus aureus (MRSA)
Methicillin-sensitive Staphylococcus aureus (MSSA)
Haemophilus influenzae
Group B streptococcus
Streptococcus pneumonia
Acinetobacter baumanii
Acinetobacter calcoacetuis
Serratia liquificacins
Haemophilus parainfluenzae

Bacterial colonization is present in the airway of the patient with neurodisability. This was demonstrated in a recent study that looked at 92 patients who had undergone tracheostomy placement due to upper airway obstruction related to their neurodisability.[11] Specific etiologic factors of the intermittent upper airway obstruction included severe hypotonia with inability to maintain an open airway, inability to clear secretions leading to respiratory distress, and multiple recurrent acute respiratory illnesses. **Table 16-7** lists the multiple organisms identified in subjects within this particular study.

The presence of chronic bacterial colonization may result in recurrent acute infection, mucus plugging, and atelectasis, leading ultimately to bronchiectasis and chronic pulmonary insufficiency, and is a significant factor in the progression of chronic lung disease and respiratory failure. An important component in the management of the acute respiratory illness is an initial aggressive increase in respiratory therapy using medications and devices to clear airway mucus. This is more important in the resolution and stabilization of the acute illness than antibiotic therapy, although antibiotic therapy must always be a consideration.[12] This further makes an important case for obtaining periodic respiratory cultures to monitor the organisms present, to determine when new organisms appear, and especially to see the antibiotic sensitivities to the bacteria. It is somewhat controversial that a culture taken while a patient is in a stable clinical state at a routine clinic visit can be used to direct antibiotic therapy in an acute illness.[13] It should be appreciated that the relationship exists between chronic bacterial colonization and changes in airway inflammation.[14–16]

Respiratory Management Plan

Individualization of the respiratory management plan is the key to care of the neurodisability patient. Management includes the following three areas: inhaled medications, airway clearance techniques, and ventilatory support. The plan should be created to address the patient's clinical presentation of pulmonary symptoms. It should also be uniquely tailored not only in the selection of the specific medication but also to the method of delivery, patient interface, frequency of therapy, and ability of the caregiver to perform the therapy.

Medication Selection

Bronchodilators, anti-inflammatories, mucolytics, and antibiotics are all inhaled medications that may be incorporated into the respiratory management plan for the neurodisability patient.[17] Bronchodilators are used to relieve acute bronchospasm, facilitate secretion removal, prevent bronchospasm due to irritation caused by mucolytics, and possibly promote ciliary function. Albuterol and ipratropium bromide are the most common bronchodilators used in the neurodisability patient population. Anti-inflammatories reduce airway swelling and inflammation. As previously stated, airway inflammation leads to increased secretion production, so the addition of an anti-inflammatory to the respiratory management plan can help to interrupt this cycle of chronic secretion production. Mucolytics are very effective in facilitating airway clearance by thinning thick, retained secretions that have the potential to lead to mucus-plugging and atelectasis. Most mucolytics can be very irritating to the airway, causing bronchospasm, so they should always be given in conjunction with a bronchodilator. Inhaled antibiotics are used to treat acute bacterial pulmonary infections. **Table 16-8** lists medications that are commonly administered as an aerosol to infants and children with neurodisability disorders and pulmonary compromise.

After selecting the appropriate medications based on the clinical picture, the appropriate delivery method must be chosen. Medications may be delivered using nebulization devices or metered dose inhalers (MDIs). A holding chamber should always be used to deliver MDI medications to the spontaneously breathing patient. Available in mouthpiece, face mask, and tracheostomy tube options, the mouthpiece chambers are not typically used in the neurodisability population because the patient is unable to produce a good seal around the mouthpiece. For those patients with shallow breathing patterns, a nonvalved holding chamber is used in conjunction with a self-inflating resuscitation bag to deliver MDI medications with hyperinflation.[17] However, there are no data to substantiate the idea that patients with shallow breathing patterns and reduced inspiratory flow rates benefit from hyperinflation techniques. Nebulized medications, with or without hyperinflation with a resuscitation bag, are delivered using an aerosol face mask or a connection to the tracheostomy tube.

When a patient requires more than one inhaled medication, as so many neurodisability patients with pulmonary complications do, the order in which each medication is given should be carefully considered. The rule to follow is "bronchodilator—mucolytic—anti-inflammatory—antibiotic." Bronchodilators are given first to dilate the airways and to aid in secretion removal. Mucolytics are delivered next to thin the secretions, making for easier clearance. After secretions have been cleared, the anti-inflammatory medication is introduced, followed by any inhaled antibiotics.

Airway Clearance Therapy

Because airway secretion overload is a major component of the pulmonary picture in neurodisability patients, airway clearance is an essential part of the respiratory management plan. Airway clearance techniques are used to both mobilize and remove secretions from the airways. The use of traditional forms of positive expiratory pressure (PEP) or vibratory PEP therapy are typically unsuccessful in the neurodisability patient due to the need for patient cooperation. Chest physiotherapy (CPT) with postural drainage is an effective method of airway clearance and is typically the first choice because it requires minimal equipment. However, CPT is highly dependent upon the technique of the person performing the therapy as well as the patient's ability to tolerate it. It is often more effective in infants and smaller patients because it is easier for the caregiver to correctly position the child. High-frequency chest wall oscillation with a therapy vest does not require patient cooperation and is much less labor intensive for the caregiver; however, the vibration created can trigger or increase the frequency of seizures for some neurodisability patients. For patients with in-dwelling ports or gastrostomy tubes, special padding can be used to prevent the vest from irritating those sites. Intra-pulmonary percussive ventilation is a very effective means of airway clearance

TABLE 16-8
Inhaled Aerosol Medications Common to Patients with Neurodisability and Pulmonary Compromise

Bronchodilators	Anti-Inflammatories	Mucolytics	Antibiotics
Albuterol (Proventil) Levalbuterol (Xopenex) Ipratropium bromide (Atrovent)	Fluticasone (Flovent) Budesonide (Pulmicort)	Dornase alpha (Pulmozyme) Acetylcysteine (Mucomyst) Sodium bicarbonate Hypertonic saline	Tobramycin (TOBI) Ceftazidime (Fortaz)

in patients with tracheostomies. Treatment can be delivered using a mask interface to patients without a tracheostomy, but effectiveness may be reduced and it can also be difficult for caregivers to perform.

Once secretions have been mobilized, they must be removed from the airway. This process must be facilitated in patients who have an ineffective cough due to muscle weakness, as there are reported cases of patients receiving secretion mobilization therapy without facilitated secretion removal that resulted in respiratory distress.[18] The manually assisted cough is a technique in which the caregiver uses their hands to physically apply pressure underneath the diaphragm to increase the expiratory flow during a cough. This technique can be effective but requires patient cooperation and can be affected by the caregiver's limitations. The cough assist device is another technique used to remove secretions. This device facilitates a cough by delivering positive pressure during inspiration to increase the size of the breath and then immediately creating negative pressure to increase the expiratory force. The cough assist device can be applied with a face mask or directly to a tracheostomy tube. This is a valuable therapy for the neurodisability patient, not only for secretion removal but also for lung expansion. Patients using a mask may have difficulty adjusting to the mask and/or positive pressure, so mask and/or pressure desensitization may be necessary to help improve patient tolerance.

Frequency of Therapy

The final step in developing the respiratory management plan is determining the frequency of selected medications and airway clearance. Frequency of therapy is determined by patient symptoms and their response to the management plan. Some patients may require medication and airway clearance therapy only as needed during acute illnesses while others may require it four times daily to maintain clinical stability. The frequency of therapy should be adjusted in response to changes in the patient's clinical picture.

Mechanical Ventilation

Regardless of the degree of expertise of respiratory care management provided by the caregiver, there will always be a certain number of patients who progress to the need for evaluation of mechanical ventilator support. The need for ventilation is predicted through diagnosis, assessment of the pulmonary composite, and trends in diagnostic and clinical presentation information. Specific neurologic diagnoses lend themselves to clinical patterns with the potential for pulmonary insufficiency. For example, chronic respiratory failure is generally anticipated in those diagnoses with progressive muscle weakness, such as the muscular dystrophies and spinal muscular atrophies, and is often within predictable time frames.

Specific diagnostic information and clinical symptoms are used to determine the need to initiate mechanical ventilation. Daytime hypercapnia ($PaCO_2$ greater than 45 torr) and nocturnal hypoventilation (SpO_2 less than 88% for 5 consecutive minutes) are established indications for the initiation of ventilator support. Patient symptoms, including fatigue, respiratory accessory muscle use, tachypnea, and dyspnea, as well as recurrent pulmonary exacerbations requiring frequent hospital admissions, are all common indicators of the need for mechanical ventilation.[19]

If proper management of the patient and proper consultation with the caregivers has been carried out over time, the decisions made at this point regarding whether to proceed with mechanical ventilator support will be easier and made with less anxiety and emotional upheaval within the family. The interim step of providing ventilator support only at night, for example, is becoming more acceptable to the family. This is especially true with the developing expertise in the use of noninvasive mechanical ventilation techniques; thus, there are several points in time along the pathway leading to respiratory failure where caregivers may decide on partial ventilator management strategies, such as nighttime mechanical ventilation only. Use of noninvasive interfaces can avoid and delay the question of tracheostomy tube placement. This allows more time for caregivers to develop their thoughts and to be more confident of the decisions they ultimately make. Unfortunately, there are times when pulmonary events are sudden and require fairly quick decisions regarding comprehensive ventilator support. Because of this possibility, it is even more important that consultations between the caregivers and the healthcare team be carried out early and often so as to better prepare families for the decision making required in such acute circumstances.

If routine clinic appointments are part of the management plan, the healthcare team will acquire a clinical database over time that will allow some degree of prediction as to the speed and severity of progressive pulmonary dysfunction. This can be used to provide information and recommendations to the family regarding pulmonary deterioration and again allow for decision making to be a much more deliberate and thought-out process, especially regarding the institution of mechanical ventilator support.

Caring for the Caregiver

Due to the labor-intensive respiratory care management required in many patients with a neurodisability, this chapter would be incomplete without consideration of the caregivers. The primary caregiver of the child with a neurodisabilty can generally be characterized, with respect to medical training, as a lay person who is required usually on a daily basis to utilize medical

Respiratory Care Management

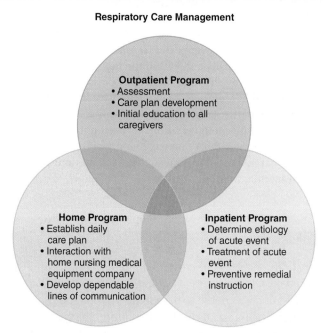

FIGURE 16-2 Respiratory care management programs for patients with neurodisability.

equipment, administer multiple medications, and determine the frequency and intensity of respiratory therapy based on their child's respiratory symptoms. It is incumbent on the caregiver to be knowledgeable about devices and medications as well as to be competent in clinical assessment.

Figure 16-2 demonstrates the three areas of activity where the respiratory management plan is used for the child with a neurodisability and pulmonary compromise. The caregiver is involved in all three. At home, the caregiver is predominantly the active deliverer of the respiratory management plan. In the outpatient setting, the caregiver can demonstrate knowledge and expertise that they provide for the patient at home. During a hospitalization, the caregiver works with the inpatient team to understand the "breakdown" that occurred in the home setting and resulted in the need for hospitalization. It may not be a breakdown due to lack of proper care but instead the development of an acute respiratory illness that prevents the child from maintaining clinical stability at home.

Caregiver Education

When pulmonary symptoms appear and the need for respiratory management is determined, the caregiver should receive instruction in delivering medications and use of the airway clearance devices. Education may begin during the child's hospitalization or initiated during a clinic visit. This may be further augmented by instruction from the home medical equipment company staff, primarily on the devices the company is providing. Although initial instruction, especially if received in a hospital setting, may be comprehensive, the follow-up

encounters during routine pulmonary clinic visits are usually relatively brief and focused on specific problems. Furthermore, home medical equipment company protocols are quite varied and often without any standardization of instruction.

Caregiver Skills Validation

Because caregivers must remain skilled in the daily respiratory management that their child may require, many medical facilities who care for these patients and follow them on an outpatient basis are now utilizing annual or semi-annual skills validation for the caregivers.[20–22] **Skills validation** is a well-known concept in the medical profession and is an important tool used to document ongoing competency. Caregivers are informed that the skills validation will be performed at an upcoming clinic visit and are instructed to bring their home equipment with them. During the visit, they are asked to set up the equipment and to perform therapy as they do at home. If any deficiencies are identified during the skills validation session, remedial education can be provided at that time.

Psychological Characteristics of Caregivers

Although daily respiratory therapies can often take up the greater part of the day, especially in the patient with significant chronic pulmonary disease, the caregiver also has responsibility in most cases for all activities of daily living. This includes providing for enteral nutrition and managing multiple medications for the nonpulmonary problems, including, for example, seizures, spasticity, and drooling. The question of how the caregivers sustain themselves over time, often for decades, with this heavy workload is important. This is especially true if the caregiver is having difficulty keeping up with the multiple tasks and responsibilities and therefore has the potential for serious psychological and physical health issues themselves.

A study conducted in 2009 was designed to psychologically characterize caregivers and to identify the characteristics that allowed them to carry out the daily tasks of providing for their child over time while maintaining their own physical and mental health.[23] The study group consisted of 62 caregivers who underwent a battery of tests to determine their psychological makeup. The result was the separation of the caregivers into three specific groups based on the results of the psychological testing. The Resilient group were those described as having high tendencies toward extroversion and low trends toward neuroticism. They were, as a group, open, conscientious, and agreeable in nature. The Undercontrollers exhibited neuroticism to a fairly high degree and as a group tended to have a decrease in characteristics of conscientiousness and agreeableness. The third group, the Overcontrollers, demonstrated high levels of neurotic tendencies and tended to be introverted. Overall, the Resilient group's test results demonstrated less anxiety and generally good mental health. A final conclusion of the study was to further investigate ways to improve the psychological health of both the Undercontroller and the Overcontroller subjects who had the potential to have more difficulty in being long-term caregivers.

Conclusion

The pediatric patient with a primary neurodisability who has secondary pulmonary complications is a major challenge for the respiratory care practitioner. Chronic pulmonary symptoms must be stabilized to reduce the frequency of acute events and to provide overall stability, both clinically and within the home. Providing optimum airway clearance on a daily basis is time consuming and in many cases labor intensive. It becomes a large piece of the daily activities not only for the patient but also for the caregivers. For this reason it is imperative that the respiratory management plan be one that can be carried out in the most effective and time-efficient manner possible.

Case Study 1

A 5-month-old girl is admitted to a university hospital because of severe hypotonia. Her medical history included being born at 37 weeks' gestational age with a birth weight of 2000 g. Apgar scores were 7 at 1 minute and 9 at 5 minutes. Although she had intrauterine growth retardation, no specific abnormality was observed, and there was no history of neurologic disease in either parent's family. Physical exam revealed that she could not control her head. She babbled, looked alert, showed social smiling, and could contact her eyes with her mother's eyes, but her posture was severely hypotonic. Deep tendon reflexes were absent. Upper extremity power was grade 3 and lower extremity power was grade 2. Tongue fasciculation was observed. One week later she developed respiratory distress and was noted to have frequent aspiration. She had a bell-shaped chest and weak cry. She was intubated and mechanical ventilation was initiated. Over the next 3 weeks, she was gradually weaned to noninvasive ventilation. She was eventually discharged home requiring noninvasive ventilation at night and secretion clearance modalities as part of her daily therapy.

1. **How is a definitive diagnosis of SMA obtained?**

2. **What landmark observation on a chest radiograph is indicative of SMA?**

3. **What specific airway clearance modalities would be appropriate for this infant?**

Case Study 2

A 5-year-old previously healthy boy presents to the emergency department with a 4-day history of hoarseness and sore throat, nonproductive cough, decreased oral intake, decreased activity, and joint pain. Five days prior, he had reported pain in all extremities, including both arms and legs. Upon admission, he reported worsening, diffuse pain throughout his body and he refused to walk. Upon physical examination he was found to be alert and afebrile with a mild tachycardia. He had generalized weakness and diffuse pain still. He was admitted to the general pediatrics floor with a diagnosis of a viral infection with myalgia and dehydration. After day 3 of his hospital stay, he exhibited poor head control, reduced truncal strength, and progressive weakness of his arms and legs. Due to progressive respiratory failure, he was intubated. At this time a neurology consultation was obtained, revealing an alert patient with bilateral facial weakness and symmetrically flaccid limbs. Deep tendon reflexes were absent, and there was no Babinski sign. In the intensive care unit, he developed mild dysautonomia, including intermittent tachycardia and hypertension that self-resolved without intervention. A spinal tap and electromyography confirmed the clinical diagnosis of Guillain-Barré syndrome, and he was treated with 2 g/kg of intravenous immunoglobulin over the next 2 days. He was discharged home after 4 weeks in a rehabilitation unit.

1. **What is Guillain-Barré syndrome?**

2. **What is the typical progression of weakness in Guillain-Barré syndrome?**

3. **How can a diagnosis of Guillain-Barré syndrome be confirmed?**

References

1. Emery AEH. The muscular dystrophies. *Lancet.* 2002;359(9307):687-695.
2. Prior TW. ACMG Practice Guidelines: Carrier screening for spinal muscular atrophy. *Genet Med.* 2008;10(11):840-842.
3. Wang CH, Finkel RS, Bertini ES, et al. Consensus statement for standard of care in spinal muscular atrophy. *J Child Neurol.* 2007; 22(8):1027-1049.
4. MacLennan AH, Thompson SC, Gecz J. Cerebral palsy: causes, pathways, and the role of genetic variants. *Am J Obstet Gynecol.* 2015;213(6):779-788.
5. Liptak GS, Dosa NP. Myelomeningocele. *Pediatr Rev.* 2010;31(11): 443-450.
6. Rosen BA. Guillain-Barré syndrome. *Pediatr Rev.* 2012; 33(4):164-171.
7. Peragallo JH. Pediatric myasthenia gravis. *Semin Pediatr Neurol.* 2017;24(2):116-121.
8. Absoud M, Greenberg BM, Lim M, et al. Pediatric transverse myelitis. *Neurology.* 2016;87(Suppl 2):S46-S52.
9. Ching-Shiang C, Hsiu-Fen L, Chi-Ren T, et al. Clinical manifestations in children with mitochondrial diseases. *Pediatr Neurol.* 2010;43(3):183-189.
10. Illing EA, Woodworth BA. Management of the upper airway in cystic fibrosis. *Curr Opin Pulm Med.* 2014;20(6):623-631.
11. McCaleb R, Warren RH, Willis D, Maples HD, Bai S, O'Brien CE. Description of respiratory microbiology of children with long-term tracheostomies. *Respir Care.* 2016;61(4):447-452.
12. Rusakow L, Guarin M, Wegner CB, Rice TB, Mischler EH. Suspected respiratory tract infection in the tracheostomized child. *Chest.* 1998;113(6):1549-1554.
13. Cline JM, Woods CR, Ervin SE, Rubin BK, Kirse DJ. Surveillance tracheal aspirate cultures do not reliably predict bacteria cultured at the time of an acute respiratory infection in children with tracheostomy tubes. *Chest.* 2012;141(3):625-631.
14. Chalmers JD, Smith MP, McHugh BJ, Doherty C, Govan JR, Hill AT. Short- and long-term antibiotic treatment reduces airway and systemic inflammation in non-cystic fibrosis bronchiectasis. *Am J Respir Crit Care Med.* 2012;186(7):657-665.
15. Finney LJ, Ritchie A, Pollard E, Johnston SL, Mallia P. Lower airway colonization and inflammatory response in COPD: a focus on Haemophilus influenza. *Int J Chron Obstruct Pulmon Dis.* 2014; 9:1119-1132.
16. Tufvesson E, Bjermer L, Ekberg M. Patients with chronic obstructive pulmonary disease and chronically colonized with Haemophilus influenza during stable disease phase have increased airway inflammation. *Int J Chron Obstruct Pulmon Dis.* 2015;10: 881-889.
17. Warren RH, Willis D. Airway secretions in pediatric patients with neurodisability. http://respiratory-care-sleep-medicine.advanceweb .com/Features/Articles/Airway-Secretions-Pediatric-Neurodisability .aspx. January 25, 2011. Accessed November 9, 2015.
18. Willis LD, Warren RH. Acute hypoxemia in a child with neurologic impairment associated with high-frequency chest-wall compression. *Respir Care.* 2007;52(8):1027-1029.
19. Hill NS. Ventilator management for neuromuscular disease. *Semin Respir Crit Care Med.* 2002;23(3):293-305.
20. Gilabert S, Rubinsztajn R. Optimization of respiratory management at home by the family. Presented at: 14th International Conference on Home Mechanical Ventilation; March 2015; Lyon, France.
21. Syed F, Snow N, Daniels C, et al. Knowledge and skills retention of caregivers of children receiving long-term invasive mechanical ventilation at home. Presented at: 14th International Conference on Home Mechanical Ventilation; March 2015; Lyon, France.
22. Keating JM, Wakeman R, Halley G. An education programme to support caregivers to children requiring long term invasive ventilation. Presented at: 14th International Conference on Home Mechanical Ventilation; March 2015; Lyon, France.
23. Blucker RT, Elliott TR, Warren RH, Warren AM. Psychological adjustment of family caregivers of children who have severe neurodisabilities that require chronic respiratory management. *Fam Syst Health.* 2011;29(3):215-231.

17

Sleep-Disordered Breathing in Infants and Children

Gulnur Com

Iris A. Perez

Thomas G. Keens

OUTLINE

OBJECTIVES

1. Recognize the spectrum of sleep-disordered breathing in children.
2. Discuss the components of polysomnography and a child-friendly laboratory.
3. Explain the pathophysiology of pediatric sleep-disordered breathing.
4. Differentiate among obstructive sleep apnea, central sleep apnea, and upper airway resistance syndrome.
5. List the risk factors of obstructive sleep apnea.
6. Recognize the clinical presentation of a child with sleep-disordered breathing.
7. Describe the diagnostic tests used to evaluate pediatric sleep-disordered breathing.
8. Learn the indications, complications, and outcomes of adenotonsillectomy in children.
9. Discuss the indications of positive airway pressure therapy for sleep-disordered breathing and how to achieve successful treatment.
10. Describe the clinical presentation of congenital central hypoventilation syndrome.
11. Explain the treatment options for congenital central hypoventilation syndrome.
12. Describe the role diaphragm pacing has in treatment of congenital central hypoventilation syndrome.

KEY TERMS

adenotonsillar hypertrophy
adenotonsillectomy (AT)
adherence programs
apnea
central sleep apnea
congenital central
  hypoventilation
  syndrome (CCHS)
diaphragm pacing
Epworth Sleepiness
  Scale (ESS)
esophageal manometry
excessive daytime
  sleepiness (EDS)
negative pressure
  ventilation
noninvasive positive pressure
  ventilation (NPPV)

non-rapid eye
  movement (NREM)
obstructive sleep
  apnea (OSA)
periodic breathing
polysomnography (PSG)
positive airway pressure
rapid eye movement (REM)
respiratory inductance
  plethysmography
sleep architecture
sleep-disordered breathing
sleep hygiene
titration study
upper airway resistance
  syndrome

Introduction

Sleep occupies a major portion of infant and childhood years, and poor sleep is one of the most common complaints brought up by parents during a health maintenance visit. Sleep-related problems, such as poor sleep hygiene, insufficient sleep, and nighttime awakenings, are quite common from infancy through adolescence. Although approximately 25% to 40% of children experience some type of sleep problems, sleep disorders that meet diagnostic criteria of International Classification of Sleep Disorders are less common.[1] Sleep disorders, such as hypersomnia syndromes and narcolepsy, periodic limb movement disorder, restless leg syndrome, circadian rhythm disorders, and obstructive sleep apnea (OSA), are frequently considered adult sleep disorders, yet they often originate in childhood. Clinical manifestations of sleep disorders in a child can be vastly different from those seen in an adult. Although many adults with sleep disorders experience daytime somnolence, mood disorders, and academic performance deficit due to poor sleep quality/quantity, children experience behavioral problems, such as hyperactivity, impaired social functioning, and irritability.[2] The impact of insufficient sleep on the developing brain of a child can present as learning problems, memory deficit, and decreased executive functions. Overactivity, opposition, poor impulse control, depression, risk-taking behavior, and noncompliance are well known consequences of OSA in adolescents.[1-3] Finally, sleep problems/disorders in children have a major impact on the family.

Evaluation of Pediatric Sleep Disorders

Obtaining a physical examination, medical history, and sleep history are essential in the evaluation of pediatric sleep disorders. Patients are then referred to a sleep lab for polysomnography and possibly other sleep studies.

History

Evaluation of sleep disorders begins with obtaining a detailed medical history. Questions to investigate routine sleep practice, also called **sleep hygiene**, include evening routine, time to go to bed, bedtime behavior, sleep environment, nocturnal and morning behavior, and daytime functioning. In older children, well-established sleep questionnaires can be used to assess daytime sleepiness. One such questionnaire, the **Epworth Sleepiness Scale (ESS)**, asks caregivers to rate how often their child will doze off or fall asleep in different situations, such as watching television, doing homework, and riding in a car. The American Academy of Pediatrics (AAP) recommends that during routine health maintenance visits, caregivers of children be asked about sleep-related symptoms, especially snoring.[4] The BEARS is a simple screening algorithm developed to assess sleep-related disorders in the primary care setting. This tool asks questions regarding sleep problems in five different domains, each represented by a letter:

- **B**edtime problems
- **E**xcessive daytime sleepiness
- **A**wakenings during the night
- **R**egularity and duration of sleep
- **S**noring[2]

Any child who snores on most nights should undergo diagnostic evaluation. Other potential symptoms of sleep-disordered breathing should be investigated in children with attention-deficit/hyperactivity disorder (ADHD), behavioral problems, or poor school performance.[4]

Polysomnography

Polysomnography (PSG) is the most commonly used test for the evaluation and diagnosis of sleep disorders. **Table 17-1** lists the multiple physiologic variables related to sleep and wakefulness that can be simultaneously recorded with PSG. Other tests used for the evaluation of pediatric sleep disorders include the multiple sleep latency test (MSLT) for the assessment of daytime sleepiness and diagnosis of narcolepsy, actigraphy to assess periodic limb movements and circadian rhythm disorders as well as insomnia, and sleep questionnaires to assess daytime sleepiness.

Overnight PSG is indicated for the assessment of sleep disorders in a variety of conditions seen in children. Recommendations regarding the use of PSG in pediatric patients were addressed by the American Academy of Sleep Medicine (AASM) Task Force in 2011.[5] **Table 17-2** lists these indications.

Components of Polysomnography

In 2007, the AASM published a manual for scoring sleep that recommended that PSG include specific components. An electroencephalogram (EEG), electrooculogram (EOG), and electromyelogram (EMG) are needed to determine sleep staging, characterize sleep architecture, and score arousals during sleep.[5] Sleep state is staged as **non-rapid eye movement (NREM)** and **rapid eye movement (REM)** sleep. **Sleep architecture** is characterized by several measures, which include sleep time, sleep efficiency, sleep onset latency, awake time after sleep onset, and percentage of sleep time spent in NREM stage and in REM sleep.

The AASM recommends using an oronasal thermal sensor to detect complete airflow cessation, or **apnea**, and a nasal air pressure transducer to detect hypopnea.[6] **Respiratory inductance plethysmography** is used to determine respiratory movements or effort and is an alternative signal for identifying apnea. Although it is not a standard measure in adults, end-tidal CO_2 monitoring is used to identify hypoventilation and is an alternative signal choice for identifying apnea.[6,7] Limb electrodes are placed to detect periodic limb movements, which may

TABLE 17-1
Physiologic Variables Obtained during a Polysomnography Recording[5]

Physiologic Variable	Purpose of the Measurement	Interpretation/ Reporting
EEG/EOG/ EMG	Stage sleep; detect seizure activities and arousals	Percentage of REM and non-REM sleep; arousal index; total sleep time; wake time; sleep onset latency; REM latency
Airflow/ nasal airway pressure	Detect apnea, hypopnea, RERA	AHI REM RDI index
ETCO$_2$	Detect apnea; monitor CO$_2$ levels	ETCO$_2$ trend; % time while ETCO$_2$ >50 torr
Chest and abdominal belts	Detect central apnea, obstructive apnea	AHI Thoraco-abdominal asynchrony
Pulse oximetry	Detect hypoxemia, desaturations; titrate oxygen	Percent time spent while SpO$_2$ measured below certain levels; ODI
ECG	Detect cardiac arrhythmia, decelerations	Heart rate range; rhythm abnormalities
Body position	Determine association between body position and respiratory events	Supine AHI
Video recording	Stage sleep; detect seizure activities and parasomnias	

EEG = electroencephalogram; EOG = electrooculogram;
EMG = electromyoclogram; REM = rapid eye movement;
RERA = respiratory effort related arousal; AHI = apnea hypopnea index;
RDI = respiratory disturbance index; ETCO$_2$ = end-tidal carbon dioxide;
ODI = oxygen desaturation index; ECG = electrocardiogram

Data from Aurora RN, Zak RS, Karippot A, et al. Practice Parameters for the respiratory indications for polysomnography in children. *SLEEP*. 2011; 34(3); 379-388.

TABLE 17-2
Indications of PSG in Children (AASM Consensus Statement, 2011)[4]

Diagnosis of OSA
Initial titration of positive airway pressure (PAP) therapy
Assessment of chronic positive airway pressure therapy
Diagnosis of congenital central hypoventilation syndrome (CCHS)
Prior to and following adenotonsillectomy to diagnose OSA and assess for residual symptoms
Diagnosis of obesity hypoventilation syndrome
Assessment of obstructive and restrictive pathophysiology in neuromuscular conditions
Supplemental oxygen titration in children with chronic hypoxemia or respiratory insufficiency
Prior to tracheostomy decannulation
Periodic evaluation of noninvasive and invasive ventilation with ventilator settings adjustment
Evaluation of daytime sleepiness
Determine presence and severity of periodic limb movement
Evaluation of infants who have experienced an apparent life-threatening event

Data from Marcus CL, Brooks LJ, Ward SD, et al. Diagnosis and management of childhood obstructive sleep apnea syndrome. *Pediatrics*. 2012; 130:e714-755.

There are many routines a sleep laboratory can adapt to meet the needs of the families, ease the burden on the children and technologists, and improve the diagnostic quality of the polysomnogram.[8,9] Schedule the child and parent for a tour of the sleep lab prior to the study. This visit can prepare the child for what will occur and ease anxiety during the study.[8] Allow the child to sit on the parent's lap during the hookup and explain each step in a child-friendly and developmentally appropriate manner, as shown in **Figure 17-2**.

Obstructive Sleep Apnea

The American Thoracic Society defines **obstructive sleep apnea (OSA)** as a disorder of breathing during sleep characterized by prolonged partial upper airway obstruction and/or intermittent complete obstruction during sleep that disrupts alveolar gas exchange and normal sleep patterns.[8]

Snoring is the most common symptom of **sleep-disordered breathing** and has a prevalence of 3% to 12% in preschool children.[4,8] Because OSA is common and frequently underdiagnosed, the AAP recommends that all children be screened by history for snoring.[4] The spectrum of OSA includes primary (habitual) snoring, upper airway resistance syndrome (UARS), obstructive hypoventilation, and intermittent obstruction of the upper airway.[6] Primary snoring refers to children who snore regularly or at least 3 or more nights per week and do not have gas exchange abnormalities, sleep disruption, or daytime symptoms.[10,11]

OSA is conservatively estimated to affect 1% to 3% of the pediatric population; therefore, not every child with snoring will be diagnosed with OSA.[4,7,11] Obstructive hypoventilation is a pattern of persistent partial upper

be cause for sleep disturbances. An electrocardiogram (ECG) to detect cardiac rate and rhythm abnormalities and a pulse oximeter to monitor oxygen saturation are standard physiologic parameters of PSG. Additionally, snoring, body position monitoring, and video recordings are essential to PSG. **Figure 17-1** is representative of the monitoring that occurs during PSG.

Polysomnography in a Child-Friendly Laboratory

In pediatric patients, especially toddlers and preschoolers, performing PSG can be challenging. Children may be frightened and uncooperative with the attachment of probes and electrodes. They may also have difficulty sleeping in a strange environment.[8] Children with neurodisability and autistic features and those with sensorial issues are of particular challenge.

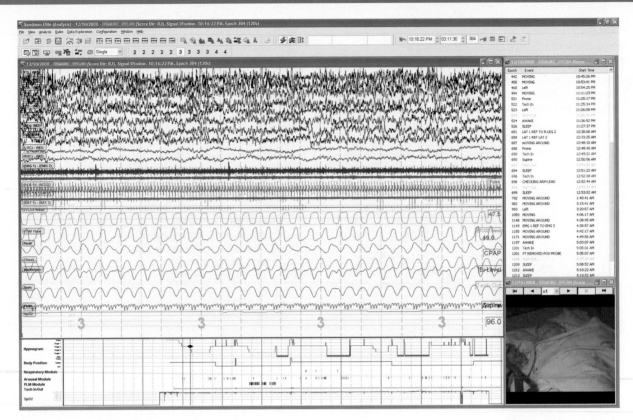

FIGURE 17-1 Example of a normal polysomnogram.
Courtesy of Natus Medical Incorporated.

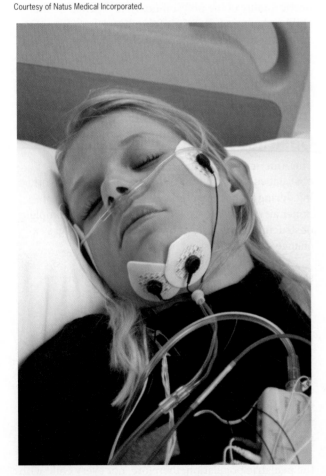

FIGURE 17-2 A child prepared for overnight polysomnography.
© BSIP SA/Alamy Stock Photo.

airway obstruction associated with gas exchange abnormalities, including CO_2 retention.

Etiology and Pathophysiology

The etiology of OSA is complex. It is well known that childhood OSA is not simply a problem with enlarged tonsils and adenoids. Studies have demonstrated that children with OSA have narrower upper airways compared with controls.[11] However, the basic underlying pathology of OSA involves not only anatomical narrowing but also increased upper airway collapsibility (i.e., hypotonia); abnormal neural control of the upper airway muscles; and other genetic, hormonal, and metabolic factors.[7,11] The upper airway collapsibility and neuromuscular compensation are major determinants of airway patency, as evidenced by observations showing that OSA predominantly occurs in REM sleep, when the upper airway muscle tone is at the lowest level.[7,8,10,11] It has been shown that in children with OSA, the upper airway is more collapsible compared with control subjects not only during sleep but also during wakefulness.[11] In healthy subjects, the transition to sleep state results in changes within the respiratory system to accommodate a decreased metabolic rate. This includes a decrease in tidal volume and minute ventilation accompanied by reduced upper airway dilator muscle activity and decreased airway caliber. The result is a mildly increasing $PaCO_2$ and decreasing PaO_2. This normal phenomenon is magnified in patients with OSA.[10,11]

Risk Factors

Enlarged tonsils and adenoids are the most common causes of upper airway narrowing in otherwise healthy children with OSA. Hypertrophied nasal turbinates, swollen nasal mucosa, a large uvula, and a crowded soft palate can also cause narrowing of the upper airway passage. The size and location of the adenotonsillar tissue are influenced by genetic factors, infection, and inflammation. Although an oral exam may reveal large tonsils, there is no clear linear correlation of increased size of tonsils and adenoids with a greater severity of OSA.[4,10] The prevalence of OSA is significantly increased in children with craniofacial syndromes and dysmorphic facial features, such as the midfacial hypoplasia seen in children with Down syndrome and the small and recessed mandible associated with Pierre-Robin sequence.[4,10] Children with neuromuscular disorders tend to have a loss in upper airway muscle tone and a high prevalence of OSA. Obesity has been shown to be an independent risk factor for OSA, with the reported OSA prevalence in obese children at around 37% to 66%.[12] Conditions associated with narrowing of the upper airway due to deposition of complex carbohydrates in the airway or those conditions affecting the neural control or collapsibility of the airway have a high prevalence of OSA; these include mucopolysaccharidoses, Prader-Willi syndrome, meningomyelocele, and Chiari malformations. Male gender, a family history of OSA, asthma, and a history of prematurity are other factors found to be associated with OSA.[10] **Table 17-3** summarizes the risk factors associated with a high prevalence of OSA.[4]

Clinical Presentation

Children with OSA classically present with snoring that worsens during upper respiratory infections. Dysphagia may occur in young children with significant tonsil enlargement. Infants may present with stridor that worsens during feeding or with activity. Stridor may also indicate the existence of laryngomalacia, vocal cord abnormalities, and subglottic stenosis.[10] During sleep,

TABLE 17-3
Risk Factors for Obstructive Sleep Apnea

Adenotonsillar hypertrophy
Obesity
Craniofacial anomalies (e.g., recessed chin, micrognathia, midface hypoplasia)
Genetic syndromes (e.g., Down syndrome, achondroplasia, Treacher Collins syndrome)
Prader-Willi syndrome
Cerebral palsy
Neuromuscular disorders
Meningomyelocele
Achondroplasia
Mucopolysacchariodosis
Family history of obstructive sleep apnea
Sickle cell disease
Asthma/allergy

some children may experience increased respiratory effort, episodes of pauses in breathing or apnea, mouth breathing, gasping for air following an obstructive event, restless sleep, enuresis, and profuse sweating.[4,7] Daytime signs and symptoms associated with OSA may include mouth breathing and hyponasal speech. Affected children are often difficult to awaken or may complain of a headache in the morning. In patients with OSA, subjective **excessive daytime sleepiness (EDS)** is a more common symptom in adults than in young children. However, the incidence of EDS is higher in adolescents and obese children.[2,11]

Caregivers and clinicians should question daytime napping and complaints of sleepiness as well as falling asleep in school, on short car rides, or on the school bus. Problems with attention and hyperactivity; irritable mood; learning difficulties; and oppositional behaviors, including impulsivity, rebelliousness, and aggression can be associated with OSA in children.[3,4,11] Children may experience worsening school performance and declining grades. Multiple studies have demonstrated an association between OSA and cognitive functioning, including reduced psychomotor efficiency, poor memory recall, and lower scores on standardized academic tests.[13-17] Reports of improvement in behavior and cognition following treatment of OSA support a causal relationship between neurobehavioral consequences and OSA and the belief that timely treatment will lead to reversibility of such deficits in children with OSA.[13]

Diagnosis

Studies that evaluated the use of history alone for the diagnosis of OSA have found poor sensitivity and specificity.[18] Although children with OSA are more likely to have such symptoms as witnessed apnea, cyanosis, and labored breathing, no questionnaire has positive and negative predictive values that are high enough to warrant use as a primary diagnostic tool.[10] However, questionnaires can be used as a screening tool, such that a negative score would be unlikely to miss a diagnosis of OSA, but a positive score would be unlikely to accurately diagnose a particular child with certainty.[4]

Physical examination of a child with suspected OSA includes assessment of growth and careful inspection of the head and neck for craniofacial abnormalities, including midfacial hypoplasia; retrognathia; micrognathia; macroglossia; and narrow, high-arched palate. Typical presentation of hypertrophic adenoids, or adenoid facies, is a long, open-mouthed face with hyponasal speech. The nasal passages should be inspected for nasal septum deviation, masses, inflammation, and polyps. Pale nasal mucosa and swollen inferior turbinates suggest nasal allergies. The oropharynx is examined for the shape of the hard and soft palate and to assess the size of the tonsils, soft palate, and uvula. Tonsil grading is typically on a scale of 0 to 4, with 0 having surgically absent tonsils and 4 having tonsils that are touching each other. Otolaryngologists use nasopharyngoscopy to visualize the nasal passages, nasopharynx, oropharynx, hypopharynx, and larynx. This office-based procedure is particularly useful to assess the size of the adenoids.[10]

Overnight Polysomnography

According to the AAP, PSG is indicated for the diagnosis of OSA in children.[4] Overnight PSG performed in a laboratory is considered the gold standard for diagnosis of OSA because it provides an objective, quantitative evaluation of disturbances in respiratory and sleep patterns.[7] PSG identifies children with severe OSA and those who are at risk for the complications of untreated OSA. It also detects children who are at risk for postoperative complications following upper airway surgery and would, therefore, benefit from inpatient observation postoperatively.[4,10] Finally, PSG helps identify children who are at high risk for persistence of OSA following

upper airway surgery. A nap study, which is a shortened PSG, is not recommended for the evaluation of OSA in children.[4] Table 17-4 lists what is typically included in a PSG report. Figure 17-3 is an example of a PSG recording with obstructive apneas, desaturation, and arousals.

Other Tests for the Diagnosis of Obstructive Sleep Apnea

Home sleep testing or portable monitoring has been used increasingly in adults; however, it is not the standard of care in the pediatric population.[4] Overnight continuous pulse oximetry recording alone is insufficient for the diagnosis of OSA due to poor sensitivity and specificity, although positive predictive value of pulse oximetry is as high as 97%.[10] With the universal availability of smartphones, video recordings obtained by parents and presented to physicians have become common practice. Studies correlating video recording systems to PSG have been encouraging. Diagnosing OSA using home audio recordings in addition to a clinical evaluation revealed a sensitivity of 71% to 92% and a specificity of 29% to 80%.[19] Children with a PSG diagnosis of severe OSA should undergo testing that includes an ECG and an echocardiogram to evaluate cardiac function and anatomy and to assess pulmonary arterial pressures. Lateral soft tissue imaging of the head and neck is a useful tool for the evaluation of adenoids and the upper airway passage. CT imaging of craniofacial structure is helpful in planning therapy for high-risk children with a diagnosis

TABLE 17-4
Components of a Polysomnography Report

Description of sleep architecture
Number and duration of apneas
Number and duration of hypopneas
Apnea hypopnea index (AHI)
Relationship among AHI, body positions, and sleep stages
Oxygen desaturations
End-tidal CO_2 measurements

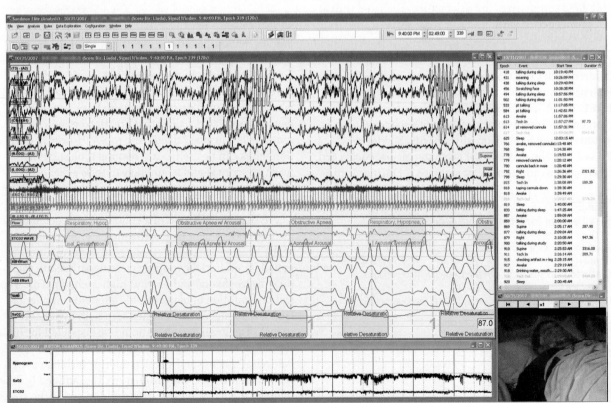

FIGURE 17-3 Polysomnography demonstrating flow limitations associated with arousals and desaturations during obstructive events.
Courtesy of Natus Medical Incorporated.

of OSA related to anatomic abnormalities.[10] Sleep endoscopy, or drug-induced sleep endoscopy, is a relatively new tool to study the airway dynamically in a sleeping patient with OSA. Sleep endoscopy can help the surgeon identify the location of an obstruction and tailor the operative procedure to the patient's specific condition.[20]

Management

Treatment options for pediatric patients with OSA are still evolving. The degree of OSA often determines the treatment. Although management of mild OSA may consist only of medication, such as inhaled nasal corticosteroids, moderate to severe OSA will most likely include surgical intervention and/or positive airway pressure therapy.

Surgical Intervention

Adenotonsillar hypertrophy is the most common cause of OSA, and **adenotonsillectomy (AT)** continues to be the primary treatment of this condition in children.[4] AT is mostly associated with a low complication rate. Minor complications include postoperative pain and poor oral intake; more severe complications include bleeding, swallowing difficulty, anesthetic complications, respiratory compromise due to worsening of the upper airway obstruction, pulmonary edema, oxygen desaturation, oropharyngeal stenosis, velopharyngeal insufficiency, and aspiration, especially in children with poor oro-motor skills.[4,10] Although AT can be safely performed in the vast majority of children as an outpatient procedure, there are some children who will require postoperative observations. Factors that may increase the risk of postoperative complications include age younger than 3 years, severe OSA, the presence of cardiac complications, and obesity. **Table 17-5** summarizes the risk factors for postoperative complications following AT.[4,10]

AT improves not only OSA symptoms but also sleep quality and homeostasis.[4,10,21] Additionally, AT improves daytime behavior, academic performance, neurocognitive functioning, and quality of life.[13–17,21] Although AT is the primary treatment of OSA in children, the outcomes of AT may not be as favorable as expected,

---

TABLE 17-5
Risk Factors for Postoperative Complications Following Adenotonsillectomy

Younger than 3 years of age
Severe obstructive sleep apnea
Morbid obesity
Neuromuscular disease
Pulmonary hypertension
Down syndrome
Craniofacial anomalies
Asthma
Sickle cell disease
Failure to thrive
History of respiratory compromise or anesthesia complications
Congenital heart disease

---

particularly when OSA is severe and/or when obesity is present.[22–28] Reports from studies of the efficacy and outcome of AT in pediatric OSA have demonstrated large variability in the frequency of residual OSA after AT, ranging from 19% to 73%.[3,28] Children with severe OSA, asthma, age older than 7 years, and obesity are at risk for persistent (residual) OSA after AT.[4,21–28] Therefore, postoperative PSG is recommended in 6 to 8 weeks following surgery for those with risk factors for residual OSA.[10] Postoperative symptoms, such as snoring and witnessed apnea, correlate well with persistence of OSA following AT. Therefore, patients with mild to moderate OSA who have complete resolution of signs and symptoms require follow-up clinically. A repeat PSG is performed if their symptoms persist or reemerge.[4,10]

Infants and children with craniofacial abnormalities and severe OSA can benefit from skeletal advancement procedures to prevent tracheostomy or to facilitate tracheostomy decannulation.[10] Two procedures performed with satisfactory results in children include mandibular distraction osteogenesis and rapid maxillary expansion. Few reports have investigated the efficacy of airway surgeries other than AT for the treatment of OSA in children.[28–30] Combined surgeries of AT, turbinectomy and/or septoplasty, tongue-hyoid advancement, uvulopalatoplasty, conventional mandibular advancement, distraction osteogenesis of the mandible, and tongue reduction in children with neurodisability showed a significant improvement of OSA following surgery.[30] A retrospective study of a group of severely obese children with OSA who underwent AT and uvulopharyngopalatoplasty (UPPP) suggested that adding UPPP to AT may be beneficial in selected pediatric cases.[28] Although the majority of children with laryngomalacia may be managed expectantly, infants who have laryngomalacia that results in OSA and/or feeding difficulties can be managed with a supraglottoplasty.[10] Patients with severe OSA who are refractory to surgical and PAP therapy may need a tracheostomy to bypass the obstructive airway.

Positive Airway Pressure

Positive airway pressure is the second-line treatment for pediatric patients who do not improve following AT or when surgery is not possible or indicated. It is often indicated for children with OSA related to obesity, craniofacial anomalies, and neuromuscular disorders.[10,31] The current standard of practice includes performing a PAP **titration study** in the sleep laboratory. During the study, the PAP is adjusted or titrated to find the optimal pressure that will prevent upper airway obstruction. Education about PAP therapy should be provided prior to a titration study.

Evidence-based guidelines that recommend when to use continuous positive airway pressure (CPAP) and when to use bilevel ventilation are limited. It is common practice to switch the treatment from CPAP to bilevel therapy when high pressures are needed to relieve upper airway obstruction and/or the patient cannot tolerate high pressures during the PAP titration study. Additionally, bilevel therapy is the treatment of choice for OSA with hypoventilation, with coexisting muscle weakness, or with extreme obesity that results in obesity hypoventilation syndrome.[31]

Patient comfort is the most important concern in selecting the PAP interface. The headgear should be snug, but not tight, with special attention paid to prevent skin breakdown over the nasal bridge and forehead.[10] Use of a mask can result in nasal dryness or congestion, epistaxis, eye irritation, skin compromise, and gastric distention. These issues must be addressed and regular follow-ups scheduled to investigate interface-related problems. Changes in the craniofacial structures of a growing child will affect the airway anatomy and neuromuscular function, which will in turn impact PAP pressures. For this reason, expert opinions recommend periodic re-titration studies for children treated with PAP.[31]

Although PAP therapy is safe and effective in children, extensive behavioral conditioning is needed to achieve satisfactory adherence.[32] Treatment of OSA with PAP is complicated initially by patient difficulty in adjusting to the PAP interface and air pressure and later by poor long-term adherence.[32–38] This is especially true in the pediatric population. Data from adult studies indicate that 5% to 50% of patients discontinue PAP therapy in the first week of treatment, with a long-term adherence rate ranging from 17% to 71%.[36] In children, PAP adherence varies, depending on the population studied, definitions used to measure adherence, and the technique used for assessing adherence.[32] Reports have shown that adolescents and African American adults and children are less likely to maintain use of PAP therapy.[34–38] It has also been reported that within 2 years of PAP therapy initiation, as many as 86% of children are lost to follow-up of their clinic appointments.[28]

PAP **adherence programs** have been developed to improve adherence with PAP in the inpatient and outpatient settings. These programs attempt to build a positive, supportive relationship with patients and families by implementing behavioral interventions and desensitization protocols that will facilitate PAP introduction and maintain long-term adherence.[32] Education of patients and caregivers regarding the medical necessity of PAP and addressing barriers causing poor adherence have been found to improve adherence to PAP treatment in adults with OSA.[39] In a recent study, the addition of a respiratory therapist to the sleep disorders clinic staff improved PAP adherence in children and adolescents with OSA.[39]

Additional Therapy

There are increasing data on the efficacy of anti-inflammatory therapies, including intranasal corticosteroids and the leukotriene receptor antagonist montelukast in the management of mild OSA.[40–42]

Intranasal steroids may be helpful if adenoid hypertrophy is the predominant cause of mild OSA in children. Although intranasal steroids have not been found to impact tonsil size, there has been a significant decrease in adenoid size and in symptom scores in patients receiving montelukast.[10] For patients with hypoxemia who are waiting for definitive therapy or those who have no other treatment options, supplemental oxygen may be administered.[10] When used during sleep, oral appliances function to enlarge the upper airway by positioning the mandible and tongue forward. Although frequently used in the adult population with snoring or mild to moderate OSA, there are insufficient data in children with regard to treatment with oral appliances.[4,10] Weight loss and lifestyle intervention can be effective treatments for mild OSA in obese children.[43,44]

Complications and Outcomes

Studies suggest that childhood OSA may be associated with cardiovascular morbidity.[4,41] In patients with severe OSA, intermittent hypoxemia associated with respiratory events during sleep may have a potential role in increased pulmonary arterial pressures. Studies have also shown that cardiac changes occur in the presence of OSA, with an effect on both ventricles.[7,10,41] Arousal from sleep is a protective mechanism that reestablishes breathing, but frequent arousals may cause sleep fragmentation and sympathetic activation that in turn may result in high systolic blood pressure.[4,41] Although the current data on OSA and markers of systemic inflammation in children are limited and contradictory, there are recent studies indicating that OSA can induce local and systemic inflammation.[42,45]

The more serious potential consequence of intermittent hypoxemia is the behavioral and cognitive adverse effect of this phenomenon on the developing brains of children.[13–17] Childhood OSA has been associated with cognitive deficits that include general intelligence as well as processing level.[4] Sleep fragmentation is commonly seen in adults but is much less frequent in children. Multiple studies support a causal relationship between nighttime sleep fragmentation and daytime neurobehavioral dysfunction.[4] Behavioral consequences of untreated OSA include hyperactivity, attention deficit, ADHD symptoms, depression, aggression, and abnormal social behaviors.[13–17] Studies examining changes in behavior and/or cognition after surgical treatment of OSA showed posttreatment improvement of behavior, quality of life, hyperactivity, ADHD, and impulsivity. These results suggest that early diagnosis and treatment of pediatric OSA may improve a child's long-term cognition and academic performance.[4,10,13,21]

Upper Airway Resistance Syndrome

Similar to OSA, patients with **upper airway resistance syndrome** present with complaints of EDS, tiredness, and frequent awakenings during sleep. However, unlike OSA, the patient does not have apnea, hypopnea, or gas exchange abnormalities.[6,46] UARS was initially identified by Guilleminault when he described 25 pediatric patients with symptoms of snoring, daytime sleepiness, and behavioral problems. When compared to healthy controls, the PSG variables of this patient group showed significantly larger swings in the esophageal pressures (Pes) during sleep.[47,48] They also demonstrated intermittent tachypnea, arrhythmias, and snoring. However, none of them had significant oxyhemoglobin desaturation or met the criteria for OSA. Following tonsillectomy and/or adenoidectomy, all PSG variables, as well as clinical sleepiness, were improved in these children with UARS.[47,48]

Pathophysiology and Clinical Presentation

UARS is characterized by intermittently high negative airway pressures during inspiration that lead to arousals and sleep fragmentation. It is also associated with increased upper airway collapsibility during sleep.[46] Children with UARS arouse with less respiratory effort than do children with OSA or primary snoring. Studies indicate that the levels of negative intra-thoracic pressures generated are the primary physiologic change inducing arousal. Although children with UARS typically have frequent snoring, restlessness during sleep, and sweating, they also may present with daytime sleepiness or fatigue. Other characteristics include decreased appetite, poor school performance, and behavioral problems.[10,47] The true prevalence of UARS is unknown, and studies suggest that significant neurocognitive abnormalities may occur even in children with primary snoring.[10]

Diagnosis

PSG is the only tool to identify patients with UARS. The original case series of patients with UARS were detected by implementing **esophageal manometry** to routine PSG. These patients displayed repetitive increased upper airway resistance that was defined by high negative inspiratory Pes occurring concomitant with decreased oro-nasal airflow without frank apnea or oxygen desaturation.[46]

There is no standard clinical diagnosis of UARS, and routine PSG testing does not include Pes measurement. Therefore, the diagnosis of UARS is made based on the clinical symptoms and PSG findings showing arousals without frank respiratory events. A patient who presents with daytime sleepiness and has an increased arousal index during PSG should raise suspicion of UARS.[46]

Management

Treatment of UARS is similar to OSA, with the first-line treatment being surgical intervention with AT. Daytime sleepiness has been shown to improve after AT.[47] Similarly, PAP therapy improved objective sleepiness measured by MSLT testing in adults with UARS.[46]

Central Sleep Apnea

Central sleep apnea refers to a heterogeneous group of sleep disorders in which respiratory effort is diminished or absent in an intermittent fashion during sleep.[49] In children, physiologic central apneas are common during normal sleep, occurring mostly during sleep-wake transition. Up to 40% of healthy children have been found to exhibit central apnea.[49] Another type of physiologic central apnea occurs following an arousal or after a sigh.[50] These central apneas are usually brief and do not cause significant oxygen desaturation unless cardiopulmonary systems are compromised. The International Classification of Sleep Disorders describes several different entities of central sleep apnea:

- Primary central sleep apnea
- Cheyne-Stokes breathing-central sleep apnea pattern
- High-altitude periodic breathing
- Central sleep apnea due to medical conditions other than Cheyne-Stokes
- Central sleep apnea due to drugs or substances
- Primary sleep apnea of infancy[51]

Common conditions associated with central apnea in children are summarized in **Table 17-6**.

Periodic breathing may occur frequently in premature infants or in children who reside at high altitude and is occasionally seen in older children with central nervous system abnormalities. The polysomnographic definition of **periodic breathing** refers to a sequence of three or more consecutive respiratory pauses lasting 3 or more seconds, with 20 seconds or less of normal respiration between pauses.[6] In preterm infants, periodic breathing is common, with an incidence of 7% in babies born at 34 to 35 weeks' gestation, 54% at 30 to 31 weeks' gestation, and nearly all infants born at less than 29 weeks' gestation.[51] **Figure 17-4** shows periodic breathing captured by an apnea monitor.

TABLE 17-6
Conditions Associated with Central Apnea in Children

High altitude
Narcotic use
Primary central apnea
Apnea of prematurity
Primary sleep apnea of infancy
Hypothyroidism
Multiple system atrophy (Shy-Dragger syndrome)
Familial dysautonomia
Postpolio syndrome
Medullary respiratory center damage due to tumor, infarction, or infection
Arnold-Chiari malformation type I and type III
Cervical cordotomy
Muscular dystrophy
Prader-Willi syndrome
Idiopathic cardiomyopathy

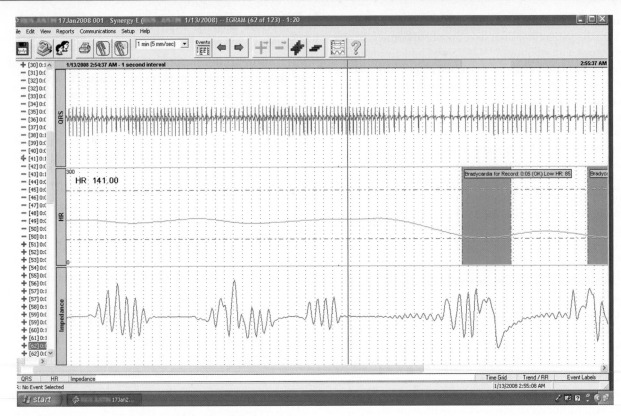

FIGURE 17-4 A periodic breathing episode captured with a home apnea monitor.
Courtesy of Circadiance.

Etiology and Pathophysiology

One must have an appreciation of normal respiratory control mechanisms to understand the underlying pathophysiology of central sleep apnea. Control of breathing begins with the central respiratory drive and operates as a negative feedback loop.[52] The respiratory center in the brainstem establishes the basic rhythm of breathing with inputs from peripheral feedback components, including the upper airway, lungs, and peripheral arterial chemoreceptors. The rate and depth of respiration are also modified by peripheral and central chemoreceptors located in the brain, aortic arch, and carotid arteries. The arterial chemoreceptors in the carotid body contain specialized oxygen-sensing cells that can perceive acute changes in arterial oxygen tension and initiate a quick response.[53] Peripheral chemoreceptors are also sensitive to changes in pH and CO_2 tension as well as to temperature, glucose, and osmolality.[52,53] During wakefulness, signals from cortical areas of the brain affect respiration with a mechanism named behavioral control. For example, while a person is awake, the frequency and depth of respiration can be increased and the breath voluntarily held. During sleep, behavioral control is lost and chemical control is the major mechanism

regulating ventilation, with the $PaCO_2$ being the major stimulus for ventilation.[53] Indeed, during sleep, all individuals are susceptible to breathing cessation should the $PaCO_2$ fall below a critical threshold known as the apnea threshold.

Central sleep apnea is most often seen during NREM sleep, when behavioral influence is the lowest.[49] Normal sleep is characterized by a slightly decreased PaO_2, increased $PaCO_2$, and higher $PaCO_2$ apneic threshold. Reduction of $PaCO_2$ below the $PaCO_2$ set point can result in central apneas. Central apneic events commonly occur during sleep-wake transition, when the $PaCO_2$ set point is being adjusted and there is instability of ventilation control.[49–54] Once stable sleep is reached, healthy children should not have more than one central apnea per hour of sleep.[55]

Fetal response to anoxia and hypercapnia are different from those of the adult. While adults respond to anoxia and hypercapnia with an immediate increase in ventilation, the fetus responds to hypoxia by decreasing breathing activity.[52,54] Maturation of respiration is incomplete at birth, and both term and preterm neonates initially respond to hypoxia like the fetus, with hypoventilation and apnea. However, they gradually develop an increase in hypoxic sensitivity over the first weeks of life. When hypoxic sensitivity is mature, the infant is less likely to become apneic to respond to a hypoxic stimulus. Apnea of prematurity occurs predominantly during active, REM sleep and is uncommon during quiet sleep.[52,54]

Clinical Presentation

Parental observations of respiratory pauses during sleep with or without color changes is the most common presentation of central apnea in children. Older children who complain of insomnia may be unable to maintain sleep due to several awakenings during the night. These may include a gasp for air and a choking sensation. Headaches upon awakening are common in patients with severe alteration of blood gases during sleep.[49]

Diagnosis

In adults, the PSG definition of central apnea refers to the cessation of airflow greater than 90% for 10 seconds or longer without any respiratory effort. In children, central apnea should last 20 seconds or longer, or an event should last for at least two missed breaths and be associated with arousal, an awakening, or ≥3% arterial oxygen desaturation.[6] Central apneas are most prevalent in the transition from wake to sleep and when patients sleep in the supine position. The central events may be associated with variable degrees of hypoxemia depending on the cardiorespiratory reserves of the child. Cheyne-Stokes breathing is described as a 10- to 60-second episode of hyperventilation following the central apnea, with a gradual decrease in tidal volume leading to the cessation of airflow.[51] This type of breathing is seen in adults and is associated with congestive heart failure.

In the healthy population, a central apnea index greater than 1 is considered abnormal; however, the true cutoff level of central apnea that may indicate central nervous system abnormalities is unknown.[55] Chiari malformation (CM) is characterized by herniation of a portion of the cerebellum through the foramen magnum and is associated with a high prevalence of sleep-disordered breathing.[56] Due to the association between central sleep apnea and CM, several publications have recommended obtaining magnetic resonance imaging (MRI) in children with central apnea to rule out any brainstem pathology.[57] Conversely, it does seem prudent to consider screening CM patients for sleep disordered breathing. By using a cutoff level of a central apnea index >5/hour, one study found that the most common identifiable risk factor for central apnea was a neurologic disorder. This study confirmed that any child with a central apnea index of 5 and higher warrants full clinical assessment, including neuro-imaging.[57]

Management

There are no clear guidelines available on when or whether to treat central sleep apnea in the absence of symptoms. In adults, up to 20% of central sleep apnea cases resolve spontaneously.[49] Therefore, if the patient is not symptomatic and experiences central sleep apnea during sleep-wake transition without significant oxygen desaturation, observation may be the only appropriate action. Studies have shown that both central and obstructive apnea events improved following decompression surgery in children with Chiari I malformation.[56]

PAP is the second line of treatment for children with central apnea associated with gas-exchange abnormalities. Any patient with central sleep apnea and significant hypoxemia who cannot tolerate PAP treatment is a potential candidate for a trial with supplemental oxygen.[10]

Complications and Outcomes

The major complications of central apnea are related to the cardiovascular effects, including hypertension and cardiac arrhythmias. Untreated central apnea in patients with CM may result in tonsillar herniation and catastrophic outcomes.[56] Periodic breathing resolves on its own with altitude change and the maturation of the brain. Home cardiorespiratory monitoring with an apnea monitor may be necessary for patients with apnea of prematurity.

Congenital Central Hypoventilation Syndrome

Congenital central hypoventilation syndrome (CCHS), also known as Ondine's curse, is a rare genetic disorder characterized by severe alveolar hypoventilation and autonomic nervous system dysfunction.[58–60] It is due to a mutation in the PHOX2B gene that is essential in the migration of neural crest cells and the development of the autonomic nervous system.[61,62] All CCHS patients have abnormal ventilation both awake and asleep, but hypoventilation is always worse during sleep.[58,60,63,64] Alveolar hypoventilation is worse during NREM sleep than during REM sleep.[65] Affected patients have absent or negligible ventilatory sensitivity to hypercapnia and hypoxemia; therefore, all CCHS patients require ventilatory support throughout life.[58,60,64,66]

Epidemiology

The incidence of CCHS is not well known, but it is estimated in France as 1 in 200,000 live births and 1 in 148,000 live births in Japan.[67,68] The majority of CCHS cases involve PHOX2B mutations that are inherited in an autosomal dominant pattern.[60,69] Although most CCHS patients do not have parents with CCHS, thus they presumably had a spontaneous PHOX2B mutation, CCHS males and females have a 50% chance of passing CCHS on to their children in each pregnancy.[60]

Clinical Presentation

The clinical presentation of CCHS varies depending on the severity of the disorder and the PHOX2B gene mutation.[60,68] Most CCHS patients present with apnea, cyanosis, or hypoventilation in the newborn period and require assisted ventilation. When intubated, some infants cannot be extubated or cannot be weaned from mechanical ventilation. Many CCHS infants do not breathe at all during the first few months of life but may mature to a pattern of adequate breathing during wakefulness while apnea or hypoventilation persists during sleep. This apparent improvement is due to normal maturation of the respiratory system and does not represent a change in the basic disorder.[60,66,70] Others present at a later age with cyanosis, edema, an apparent life-threatening event, or signs of right heart failure.[60,70,71] Finally, some patients present in older childhood or adulthood as an adverse reaction to general anesthesia, pneumonia, or other stress.[72–74] Thus, any child or adult with a delay in waking or achieving adequate ventilation following general anesthesia or who is unable to be extubated after appropriate treatment of pneumonia should be suspected of CCHS and a PHOX2B gene mutation study performed.

In general, CCHS patients who are otherwise clinically healthy usually breathe well enough while awake that they require ventilatory support only during sleep. However, often dependent upon the gene mutation, there are those who hypoventilate so severely during wakefulness that they require full-time ventilatory support.[60,75]

CCHS is a generalized disorder of the autonomic nervous system, and it affects more than just control of breathing. Associated abnormalities include Hirschsprung's disease, neural crest tumors, life-threatening arrhythmias, ophthalmologic abnormalities, and abnormal glucose metabolism.[70,76–90]

Diagnosis

The diagnosis of CCHS is suspected when patients present with hypoventilation that is worse during sleep but is not caused by lung disease, ventilatory muscle weakness, or obvious neurologic disorders. It is confirmed by testing for mutations in the PHOX2B gene. Identification of the specific PHOX2B mutation aids in predicting the severity of ventilatory control, the risk of associated complications, and other adverse consequences.[60]

While waiting for genetic test results, the following tests should be performed to rule out other causes of hypoventilation:

- MRI and/or CT scans of the brain and the brainstem to rule out gross anatomic lesions
- Metabolic screen and neurologic evaluation
- PSG with appropriately collected respiratory data to establish the presence of hypoventilation and sleep-related breathing disorder

- Daytime blood gas analysis during wakefulness to document daytime hypoventilation
- Chest radiograph
- Fluoroscopy of the diaphragms
- Echocardiogram[60]

Management

The goal in the treatment of CCHS is to ensure adequate ventilation when the patient is unable to achieve adequate gas exchange through spontaneous breathing. CCHS patients generally have minimal lung disease, so they have many options for ventilatory support:

- Tracheostomy and positive pressure ventilation
- **Noninvasive positive pressure ventilation (NPPV)**
- Negative pressure ventilation
- Diaphragm pacing

Oxygen administration alone is inadequate because although it improves oxygenation and relieves cyanosis, hypoventilation persists.[60]

Tracheostomy and Positive Pressure Ventilation

Infants with CCHS are often very unstable during the first year of life, with minor respiratory infections causing complete apnea during both sleep and wakefulness. Therefore, mechanical ventilation with a tracheostomy in place is initially recommended for all CCHS infants.[60] Ventilator settings are adjusted to achieve an end-tidal $PaCO_2$ between 30 and 35 mm Hg while maintaining the SpO_2 at greater than 94%. Patients ventilated in this manner tend to have more reserve for acute respiratory infections or changes in pulmonary mechanics and are less likely to develop pulmonary hypertension. The pressure control with assist control mode is used to achieve these targets. A relatively smaller tracheostomy tube is recommended because it is less likely to cause tracheomalacia. A smaller tracheostomy tube also allows a large expiratory leak so that a child's voice may continue to be heard.[91]

Noninvasive Positive Pressure Ventilation

Modes of ventilation for older children who are stable and require support only during sleep include NPPV, bilevel positive airway pressure, or average volume assured pressure support ventilation. A nasal or face mask is used for the interface.[60,92] Although there are reports of younger children ventilated solely with NPPV, the American Thoracic Society recommends noninvasive ventilation in the older, stable patients.[60,93–95] Because CCHS patients do not increase their respiratory rate or tidal breaths with hypoxemia or hypercapnia, only the spontaneous-timed or timed modes guarantee breath delivery. The difference between the inspired positive airway pressure and the expired positive airway pressure is used to provide an optimal tidal volume. Long-term use of NPPV with a nasal mask interface can be associated with midface hypoplasia.[95] Therefore, patients must be monitored for development of midface hypoplasia and dental malocclusion.

Negative Pressure Ventilation

Negative pressure ventilators include the chest shell, wrap, or tank. To generate ventilation, these ventilators apply a negative pressure to the outside of the chest and abdomen during inspiration.[95,96] Airway occlusion may occur with **negative pressure ventilation** because there is no synchronous activation of the upper airway muscles that normally occurs during spontaneous breathing. Rarely used in the pediatric population today, these ventilators are not portable and have largely been replaced by NPPV.

Diaphragm Pacing

Diaphragm pacing is an attractive treatment option for CCHS patients. It provides daytime ventilatory support for those who are 24-hour ventilator dependent, allowing for mobility and independence from the ventilator during the day. It can be the sole source of ventilation, permitting tracheal decannulation for those patients who are ventilator dependent only during sleep.[60,66,75]

As opposed to a conventional mechanical ventilator, diaphragm pacing uses the child's own diaphragm as the respiratory pump. As seen in **Figure 17-5**, a diaphragm pacer system involves four components:

- Electrodes that are surgically implanted on the phrenic nerves
- Receivers that are surgically implanted on the abdomen or chest bilaterally
- External antennae that are placed over the receivers
- An external battery-operated portable transmitter

The external transmitter generates electrical energy similar to radio frequency via an external antenna that is placed over the receiver. The receiver converts the energy to electrical current that is then conducted to the phrenic nerve, stimulating the diaphragm to contract.

Diaphragm pacing uses the diaphragm as the ventilator. Therefore, patients who are candidates for pacing must have normal diaphragm function, an intact phrenic nerve, and little or no lung disease. Obesity is a contraindication to successful diaphragm pacing as a high amount of adipose tissue increases the distance between the antenna and receiver of the diaphragm pacer. This results in increased variability in the signal received by the receiver.[75,97]

Diaphragm pacers are surgically implanted on the phrenic nerves using a thoracoscopic approach.[98,99] The pacers are tested intraoperatively, so neuromuscular blocking agents are not given for the surgery.

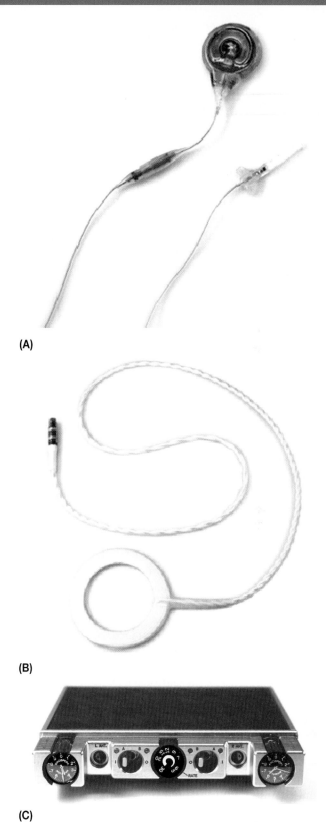

(A)

(B)

(C)

FIGURE 17-5 Components of a diaphragm pacer system. (**A**) Electrodes and receivers are surgically implanted on the phrenic nerves and on the abdomen or chest. (**B**) An external antenna is placed over a receiver. (**C**) The external battery-operated portable transmitter generates electrical energy via the antennae that are over the receivers.

Courtesy of Avery Biomedical Devices, Inc.

The diaphragm pacers are not used right away; instead, patients are returned to positive pressure ventilation with a tracheostomy for 6 to 8 weeks to allow time for healing. To initiate pacing, patients are readmitted to the hospital, where the settings are established and adjusted. Pacing begins at 1 to 1½ hours per night. To train the diaphragm and prevent fatigue, time on the pacers is gradually increased by 30 to 60 minutes each week.[75,97,98] This has been found to be necessary even with those patients who breathe spontaneously while awake. The probable reason is that the phrenic nerve electrode stimulates those fibers that happen to touch the electrode by chance, which are not the same fibers that are stimulated during spontaneous breathing. Another theory is that the electrical impulse profile of the diaphragm pacers is different from the natural phrenic nerve impulses. In either case, this necessitates training the diaphragm to accept longer periods of pacing without fatigue. In general, it takes 2 to 3 months to establish full pacing during sleep. Once on full pacing, if a patient with a tracheostomy does well for 3 months, then decannulation is considered.[75] Diaphragm pacing for more than 14 hours a day is not recommended because of the risk of diaphragm fatigue. When a patient requires ventilator support for 24 hours a day, then a backup form of ventilation should be available to use during part of the day.[91]

On the night of pacing initiation, the pacers are started by turning on both sides, whether the patient is awake or asleep, as the goal is to begin training the diaphragm. Mechanical ventilation is not applied while the patient is on diaphragm pacing. The patient is monitored using continuous pulse oximetry and an end-tidal CO_2 monitor. If the SpO_2 falls below 95% and/or the end-tidal CO_2 rises above 40 torr, then the pacers are adjusted by slightly increasing the tidal volume settings. If the patient experiences shoulder pain with a pacer breath, the tidal volume is set too high. After 90 minutes, the pacing is discontinued, and for the remainder of the night the patient is ventilated using the home ventilator at the usual settings. If there is a fall in the SpO_2, increase in the end-tidal CO_2, or decrease in diaphragmatic contraction before the 90-minute period has elapsed, then diaphragm fatigue is occurring. At this point, the pacing is stopped and home ventilation is resumed.

When considering decannulation of a patient who is ventilator dependent only during sleep, the patient should undergo full laryngoscopy and bronchoscopy to ensure a patent airway. An overnight PSG with the tracheostomy tube capped is performed to assess readiness for decannulation. During the sleep study, diaphragm pacer settings are also adjusted to achieve optimal gas exchange and relieve OSAs, if present. If the patient has adequate oxygenation and ventilation while using diaphragm pacers with the tracheostomy tube capped, then decannulation is scheduled. Following decannulation, the patient is observed for 1 to 2 nights in the hospital.[75]

Pulse oximetry and end-tidal CO_2 monitors are crucial in monitoring patients with CCHS at home and in the hospital. Alarm thresholds are set well below the desired goals to decrease nuisance alarms and to provide the caregivers adequate time to respond to potential emergencies. Apnea/bradycardia monitoring alone is not adequate, as many patients hypoventilate but are not apneic. Furthermore, for those children ventilated by diaphragm pacing, the pacer artifacts may falsely elevate the heart rate.[60]

Patients with CCHS are likely to be more sensitive to respiratory depressant effects of inhalational anesthetics, narcotics, and benzodiazepines. When these patients receive sedation medications, they must receive ventilator support and be monitored continuously with a pulse oximeter and end-tidal CO_2 monitor. Because of their abnormal responses to hypoxia and hypercapnia, if these patients have any unexplained problem, such as seizure or lethargy, they should be stabilized by hyperventilation with 100% oxygen until the source of the problem can be identified. In children with CCHS, hypoventilation should be considered the source of the problem until proven otherwise. A brief period of hyperventilation will not be harmful but may be lifesaving.[91]

To assess ventilator status and to adjust ventilator settings, patients should undergo at least yearly PSG. An annual echocardiogram is also recommended to evaluate for pulmonary hypertension. If a patient develops progressive pulmonary hypertension and cor pulmonale, until proven otherwise it must be assumed to be the result of inadequate ventilator settings, and ventilator support should be adjusted accordingly.[60]

Complications and Outcomes

CCHS is a lifelong disorder, with patients requiring ventilatory support for life. The reported overall mortality rate ranges between 8% and 38%, with most deaths occurring before 2 years of age.[67,70,99] Cause of death varies but is linked to tracheostomy and ventilator dependence.[67] Many children survive to adolescence and adulthood. Complications of CCHS include cardiac failure and hypoxic seizures, but these improve with correction of ventilatory support.[100,101] Development of neurocognitive deficiencies has been attributed to inadequate ventilation.[100,102,103] To confer the best outcome, early recognition and initiation of optimal ventilatory support are crucial in preventing the negative sequelae associated with hypoxia.

Case Study 1

A previously healthy 10-year-old boy presents to his pediatrician's office for his annual checkup. His parents are concerned about his quality of sleep. They report that he snores during sleep, takes naps during the day, and has difficulty concentrating in school. After a thorough sleep history, it is determined that he often plays on his iPad just before sleep each night and that his father uses a CPAP machine at home during sleep. On physical exam, he has a BMI greater than the 95th percentile, and his tonsils are enlarged with a rating of 2+ on the Brodsky scale. The remainder of the examination is unremarkable, and he is otherwise considered healthy. After recommending healthy weight programs and the elimination of electronic screen-time before sleep, the next steps in diagnosis and treatment are discussed. It is decided that he is

at significant risk for OSA and is a likely candidate for adenotonsillectomy. He is scheduled for an overnight polysomnography test and a referral is made for consultation with an ENT specialist. Following examination by the ENT specialist and interpretation of the sleep study results, he undergoes an adenotonsillectomy. Subsequently there is improvement in OSA symptoms, and no further treatment is indicated.

1. **What are common causes of obstructive sleep apnea in children?**
2. **What recommendations does the American Academy of Pediatrics give for the management of OSA in children?**
3. **What is considered the gold standard for the diagnosis of OSA in children?**

Case Study 2

Following an uncomplicated vaginal delivery, a 39-week 3550 g male infant was born to a gravida 3 para 3 mother. The Apgar score was 8 at 1 minute and 10 at 5 minutes. At 6 hours of age, the infant was transferred to the neonatal intensive care unit of a children's hospital because of intermittent episodes of cyanosis. Antibiotics were given after a complete septic workup was completed. None of the cultures showed evidence of bacteria. Because of frequent apnea and oxygen desaturation with CO_2 retention, the infant was intubated; saturation was maintained well when he was awake, but while asleep he had cyanosis and was entirely dependent on the ventilator with no respiratory effort noted. There were no remarkable findings on chest radiography, CT scan, electrocardiogram, echocardiogram, and neurologic examinations. The infant failed multiple attempts at extubation after developing severe hypoxia and hypercapnia. A permanent tracheostomy was performed for long-term ventilator

support after rigid bronchoscopy ruled out any airway abnormality. Congenital central hypoventilation syndrome (CCHS) was suspected because of cyanosis occurring only during sleep and dysregulation of the body temperature. Genetic studies were performed, and CCHS was diagnosed from mutation in the PHOX2B gene. At 6 months of age, the infant remained ventilator dependent with a tracheostomy 24 hours a day. He was discharged home with developmental milestones, including gross motor, fine motor, and social interaction, normal for a 6-month-old infant.

1. **Describe the severity and clinical presentation of congenital central hypoventilation syndrome (CCHS) in the newborn period.**
2. **What disorders might be considered in the differential diagnosis of CCHS?**
3. **What options are available for the treatment of CCHS in an infant?**

References

1. Meltzer LJ, Plaufcan MR, Thomas JH, Mindell JA. Sleep problems and sleep disorders in pediatric primary care: treatment recommendations, persistence, and health. *J Clin Sleep Med.* 2014;10:421-426.
2. Mindel JA, Owens JA. *A Clinical Guide to Pediatric Sleep: Diagnosis and Management of Sleep Problems.* Philadelphia, PA: Lippincott Williams & Wilkins; 2003.
3. Ivanenko A, Crabtree VM, Gozal D. Sleep and depression in children and adolescents. *Sleep Med Rev.* 2005;9:115-129.
4. Marcus CL, Brooks LJ, Ward SD, et al. American Academy of Pediatrics. Diagnosis and management of childhood obstructive sleep apnea syndrome. *Pediatrics.* 2012;130:e714-e755.
5. Aurora RN, Zak RS, Karippot A, et al. Parameters for the respiratory indications for polysomnography in children. *SLEEP.* 2011;34:379-388.
6. Iber C. *The AASM Manual for the Scoring of Sleep and Associated Events: Rules, Terminology and Technical Specifications.* Westchester, FL: American Academy of Sleep Medicine; 2007.
7. Jambhekar S, Carroll JL. Diagnosis of pediatric obstructive sleep disordered breathing: beyond the gold standard. *Expert Rev Respir Med.* 2008;2:791-809.

8. Beck SE, Marcus CL. Pediatric polysomnography. *Sleep Med Clin.* 2009;4:393-406.

9. Zaremba EK, Barkey ME, Mesa C, Sanniti K, Rosen CL. Making polysomnography more "child friendly": a family-centered care approach. *J Clin Sleep Med.* 2005;1:189-198.

10. Sheldon SH, Ferber R, Kryger MH, Gozal D. *Principles and Practice of Pediatric Sleep Medicine.* Philadelphia, PA: Elsevier Saunders; 2014.

11. Katz ES, D'Ambrosio CM. Pathophysiology of pediatric obstructive sleep apnea. *Proc Am Thorac Soc.* 2008;5:253-262.

12. Redline S, Tishler PV, Schluchter M, et al. Risk factors for sleep-disordered breathing in children: associations with obesity, race, and respiratory problems. *Am J Respir Crit Care Med.* 1999;159:1527-1532.

13. Gozal D, Kheirandish-Gozal L. Neurocognitive and behavioral morbidity in children with sleep disorders. *Curr Opin Pulm Med.* 2007;13:505-509.

14. Chervin RD, Archbold KH, Dillon JE, et al. Inattention, hyperactivity, and symptoms of sleep-disordered breathing. *Pediatrics.* 2002;109:449-456.

15. Gozal D. Sleep-disordered breathing and school performance in children. *Pediatrics.* 1998;102:616-620.

16. Bass JL, Corwin M, Gozal D, et al. The effect of chronic or intermittent hypoxia on cognition in childhood: a review of the evidence. *Pediatrics.* 2004;114:805-816.

17. Chervin RD, Dillon JE, Archbold KH, Ruzicka DL. Conduct problems and symptoms of sleep disorders in children. *J Am Acad Child Adolesc Psychiatry.* 2003;42:201-208.

18. Carroll JL, McColley SA, Marcus CL, et al. Inability of clinical history to distinguish primary snoring from obstructive sleep apnea syndrome in children. *Chest.* 1995;108:610-618.

19. Sivan Y, Kornecki A, Schonfeld T. Screening obstructive sleep apnoea syndrome by home videotape recording in children. *Eur Respir J.* 1996;9:2127-2131.

20. Golbin D, Musgrave B, Succar E, Yaremchuk K. Clinical analysis of drug-induced sleep endoscopy for the OSA patient. *Laryngoscope.* 2016;126(1).doi:10.1002/lary.25516.

21. Marcus CL, Moore RH, Rosen CL, et al. Childhood Adenotonsillectomy Trial (CHAT). A randomized trial of adenotonsillectomy for childhood sleep apnea. *N Engl J Med.* 2013;368:2366-2376.

22. Bhattacharjee R, Kheirandish-Gozal L, Spruyt K, et al. Adenotonsillectomy outcomes in treatment of obstructive sleep apnea in children: a multicenter retrospective study. *Am J Respir Crit Care Med.* 2010;182:676-683.

23. Mitchell RB, Kelly J. Outcomes of adenotonsillectomy for obstructive sleep apnea in obese and normal-weight children. *Otolaryngol Head Neck Surg.* 2007;137:43-48.

24. Tauman R, Gulliver TE, Krishna J, et al. Persistence of obstructive sleep apnea syndrome in children after adenotonsillectomy. *J Pediatr.* 2006;149:803-808.

25. Brietzke SE, Gallagher D. The effectiveness of tonsillectomy and adenoidectomy in the treatment of pediatric obstructive sleep apnea/hypopnea syndrome: a meta-analysis. *Otolaryngol Head Neck Surg.* 2006;134:979-984.

26. Mitchell RB. Adenotonsillectomy for obstructive sleep apnea in children: outcome evaluated by pre-and postoperative polysomnography. *Laryngoscope.* 2007;117:1844-1854.

27. Guilleminault C, Li K, Quo S, Inouye RN. A prospective study on the surgical outcomes of children with sleep-disordered breathing. *Sleep.* 2004;27:95-100.

28. Com G, Carroll JL, Tang X, et al. Characteristics and surgical and clinical outcomes of severely obese children with obstructive sleep apnea. *J Clin Sleep Med.* 2015;11:467-474.

29. Hartzell LD, Guillory RM, Munson PD, et al. Tongue base suspension in children with cerebral palsy and obstructive sleep apnea. *Int J Pediatr Otorhinolaryngol.* 2013;77:534-537.

30. Cohen SR, Lefaivre JF, Burstein FD, et al. Surgical treatment of obstructive sleep apnea in neurologically compromised patients. *Plast Reconstr Surg.* 1997;99:638-646.

31. Kushida CA, Chediak A, Berry RB, et al. Clinical guidelines for the manual titration of positive airway pressure in patients with obstructive sleep apnea. Positive Airway Pressure Titration Task Force; American Academy of Sleep Medicine. *J Clin Sleep Med.* 2008;4:157-171.

32. Harford KL, Jambhekar S, Com G, et al. Behaviorally based adherence program for pediatric patients treated with positive airway pressure. *Clin Child Psychol Psychiatry.* 2013;18:151-163.

33. Marcus CL, Rosen G, Ward SL, et al. Adherence to and effectiveness of positive airway pressure therapy in children with obstructive sleep apnea. *Pediatrics.* 2006;117:e442-e451.

34. O'Donnell AR, Bjornson CL, Bohn SG, Kirk VG. Compliance rates in children using noninvasive continuous positive airway pressure. *Sleep.* 2006;29:651-658.

35. Uong EC, Epperson M, Bathon SA, Jeffe DB. Adherence to nasal positive airway pressure therapy among school-aged children and adolescents with obstructive sleep apnea syndrome. *Pediatrics.* 2007;120:e1203-e1211.

36. Weaver TE. Adherence to positive airway pressure therapy. *Curr Opin Pulm Med.* 2006;12:409-413.

37. Sawyer AM, Gooneratne NS, Marcus CL, et al. A systematic review of CPAP adherence across age groups: clinical and empiric insights for developing CPAP adherence interventions. *Sleep Med Rev.* 2011;6:343-356.

38. Beebe DW, Byars KC. Adolescents with obstructive sleep apnea adhere poorly to positive airway pressure (PAP), but PAP users show improved attention and school performance. *PLoS One.* 2011; 6:e16924.

39. Jambhekar SK, Com G, Tang X, et al. Role of a respiratory therapist in improving adherence to positive airway pressure treatment in a pediatric sleep apnea clinic. *Respir Care.* 2013;58:2038-2044.

40. Goldbart AD, Goldman JL, Veling MC, Gozal D. Leukotriene modifier therapy for mild sleep-disordered breathing in children. *Am J Respir Crit Care Med.* 2005;172:364-370.

41. Gozal D, Kheirandish-Gozal L. Cardiovascular morbidity in obstructive sleep apnea: oxidative stress, inflammation, and much more. *Am J Respir Crit Care Med.* 2008;177:369-375.

42. Gozal D, Crabtree VM, Sans Capdevila O, et al. C-reactive protein, obstructive sleep apnea, and cognitive dysfunction in school-aged children. *Am J Respir Crit Care Med.* 2007;176:188-193.

43. Verhulst SL, Franckx H, Van Gaal L, De Backer W, Desager K. The effect of weight loss on sleep-disordered breathing in obese teenagers. *Obesity (Silver Spring).* 2009;17(6):1178-1183.

44. Kalra M, Inge T, Garcia V, et al. Obstructive sleep apnea in extremely overweight adolescents undergoing bariatric surgery. *Obes Res.* 2005;13:1175-1179.

45. Gozal D, Serpero LD, Kheirandish-Gozal L, et al. Sleep measures and morning plasma TNF-alpha levels in children with sleep-disordered breathing. *Sleep.* 2010;33:319-325.

46. Exar EN, Collop NA. The upper airway resistance syndrome. *Chest.* 1999;115:1127-1139.

47. Guilleminault C, Stoohs R, Clerk A, et al. From obstructive sleep apnea syndrome to upper airway resistance syndrome: consistency of daytime sleepiness. *Sleep.* 1992;15(Suppl 6):S13-S16.

48. Guilleminault C, Stoohs R, Clerk A, et al. A cause of daytime sleepiness: the upper airway resistance syndrome. *Chest.* 1993;104:781-787.

49. Becker K. Central sleep apnea syndromes treatment & management. https://emedicine.medscape.com/article/304967-treatment. Accessed November 30, 2015.

50. Fukumizu M, Kohyama J. Central respiratory pauses, sighs, and gross body movements during sleep in children. *Physiol Behav.* 2004;82(4):721-726.

51. American Academy of Sleep Medicine. *International Classification of Sleep Disorders: Diagnostic and Coding Manual.* 2nd ed. Westchester, NY: American Academy of Sleep Medicine; 2005.

52. Stokowski LA. A primer on apnea of prematurity. *Adv Neonatal Care.* 2005;5:155-170.

53. Carroll JL, Agarwal A. Development of ventilatory control in infants. *Paediatr Respir Rev.* 2010;11:199-207.

54. Paul K, Melichar J, Miletín J, Dittrichová J. Differential diagnosis of apneas in preterm infants. *Eur J Pediatr.* 2009;168:195-201.

55. Traeger N, Schultz B, Pollock AN, et al. Polysomnographic values in children 2-9 years old: additional data and review of the literature. *Pediatr Pulmonol.* 2005;40:22-30.

56. Tran K, Hukins CA. Obstructive and central sleep apnea in Arnold-Chiari malformation: resolution following surgical decompression. *Sleep Breath.* 2011;15:611-613.

57. Kritzinger FE, Al-Saleh S, Narang I. Descriptive analysis of central sleep apnea in childhood at a single center. *Pediatr Pulmonol.* 2011;46:1023-1030.

58. Mellins RB, Balfour HH, Turino GM, Winters RW. Failure of automatic control of ventilation (Ondine's curse). Report of an infant born with this syndrome and review of the literature. *Medicine.* 1970;49:487-504.

59. Weese-Mayer DE, Rand CM, Berry-Kravis EM, et al. Congenital central hypoventilation syndrome from past to future: model for translational and transitional autonomic medicine. *Pediatr Pulmonol.* 2009;44:521-535.

60. Weese-Mayer DE, Berry-Kravis EM, Ceccherini I, et al. An official ATS clinical policy statement: congenital central hypoventilation syndrome: genetic basis, diagnosis, and management. *Am J Respir Crit Care Med.* 2010;181:626-644.

61. Amiel J, Laudier B, Attié-Bitach T, et al. Polyalanine expansion and frameshift mutations of the paired-like homeobox gene PHOX2B in congenital central hypoventilation syndrome. *Nat Genet.* 2003;33:459-461.

62. Weese-Mayer DE, Berry-Kravis EM, Zhou L, et al. Idiopathic congenital central hypoventilation syndrome: analysis of genes pertinent to early autonomic nervous system embryologic development and identification of mutations in PHOX2b. *Am J Med Genet.* 2003;123A:267-278.

63. Paton JY, Swaminathan S, Sargent CW, et al. (1993). Ventilatory response to exercise in children with congenital central hypoventilation syndrome. *Am Rev Respir Dis.* 1993;147:1185-1191.

64. Paton JY, Swaminathan S, Sargent CW, Keens TG. Hypoxic and hypercapnic ventilatory responses in awake children with congenital central hypoventilation syndrome. *Am Rev Respir Dis.* 1989;140:368-372.

65. Fleming PJ, Cade D, Bryan MH, Bryan AC. Congenital central hypoventilation and sleep state. *Pediatrics.* 1980;66:425-448.

66. Chen ML, Keens TG. Congenital central hypoventilation syndrome: not just another rare disorder. *Paediatr Respir Rev.* 2004;5: 182-189.

67. Trang H, Dehan M, Beaufils F, et al. The French Congenital Central Hypoventilation Syndrome Registry: general data, phenotype, and genotype. *Chest.* 2005;127:72-79.

68. Shimokaze T, Sasaki A, Meguro T, et al. Genotype-phenotype relationship in Japanese patients with congenital central hypoventilation syndrome. *J Hum Genet.* 2015;60:473-477.

69. Sritippayawan S, Hamutcu R, Kun SS, et al. Mother-daughter transmission of congenital central hypoventilation syndrome. *Am J Respir Crit Care Med.* 2002;166:367-369.

70. Weese-Mayer DE, Silvestri JM, Menzies LJ, Morrow-Kenny AS, Hunt CE, Hauptman SA. Congenital central hypoventilation syndrome: diagnosis, management, and long-term outcome in thirty-two children. *J Pediatr.* 1992;120:381-387.

71. Fine-Goulden MR, Manna S, Durward A. Cor pulmonale due to congenital central hypoventilation syndrome presenting in adolescence. *Pediatr Crit Care Med.* 2009;10:e41-e42.

72. Barratt S, Kendrick AH, Buchanan F, Whittle AT. Central hypoventilation with PHOX2B expansion mutation presenting in adulthood. *Thorax.* 2007;62:919-920.

73. Little R. A 2-year old with no ventilator requirement but who cannot be extubated. *Semin Pediatr Neurol.* 2008;15:157-159.

74. Mahfouz AKM, Rashid M, Khan MS, Reddy P. Late onset congenital central hypoventilation syndrome after exposure to general anesthesia. *Can J Anaesth.* 2011;58:1105-1109.

75. Diep B, Wang A, Kun S, et al. Diaphragm pacing without tracheostomy in congenital central hypoventilation syndrome patients. *Respiration.* 2015;89:534-538.

76. Vanderlaan M, Holbrook CR, Wang M, et al. Epidemiologic survey of 196 patients with congenital central hypoventilation syndrome. *Pediatr Pulmonol.* 2004;37:217-229.

77. Low KJ, Turnbull AR, Smith KR, et al. A case of congenital central hypoventilation syndrome in a three-generation family with non-polyalanine repeat PHOX2B mutation. *Pediatr Pulmonol.* 2014;49:e140-e143.

78. Swaminathan S, Gilsanz V, Atkinson J, Keens TG. Congenital central hypoventilation syndrome associated with multiple ganglioneuromas. *Chest.* 1989;96:423-424.

79. Gronli JO, Santucci BA, Leurgans SE, et al. Congenital central hypoventilation syndrome: PHOX2B genotype determines risk for sudden death. *Pediatr Pulmonol.* 2008;43:77-86.

80. Movahed MR, Jalili M, Kiciman N. Cardiovascular abnormalities and arrhythmias in patients with Ondine's curse (congenital central hypoventilation) syndrome. *Pacing Clin Electrophysiol.* 2005;28:1226-1230.

81. Silvestri JM, Hanna BD, Volgman AS, et al. Cardiac rhythm disturbances among children with idiopathic congenital central hypoventilation syndrome. *Pediatr Pulmonol.* 2000;29:351-358.

82. Woo MS, Woo MA, Gozal D, et al. Heart rate variability in congenital central hypoventilation syndrome. *Pediatr Res.* 1992;31:291-296.

83. Basu AP, Bellis P, Whittaker RG, et al. Teaching neuroimages: alternating ptosis and Marcus Gunn jaw-winking phenomenon with PHOX2B mutation. *Neurology.* 2012;79:e153.

84. Bucci MP, Kapoula Z, Yang Q, et al. Saccades, vergence and combined eye movements in a young subject with congenital central hypoventilation syndrome (CCHS). *Strabismus.* 2003;11: 95-107.

85. Goldberg DS, Ludwig IH. Congenital central hypoventilation syndrome: ocular findings in 37 children. *J Pediatr Ophthalmol Strabismus.* 1996;33:175-180.

86. Michel G, Villega F, Desprez P, et al. Ondine's curse and rare oculomotor abnormalities: a case report. *J Fr Ophtalmol.* 2006;29:422-425.

87. Farina MI, Scarani R, Po' C, et al. Congenital central hypoventilation syndrome and hypoglycaemia. *Acta Paediatr.* 2012;101: e92-e96.

88. Gelwane G, Trang H, Carel JC, et al. Intermittent hyperglycemia due to autonomic nervous system dysfunction: a new feature in patients with congenital central hypoventilation syndrome. *J Pediatr.* 2013;162:171-176.

89. Hennewig U, Hadzik B, Vogel M, et al. Congenital central hypoventilation syndrome with hyperinsulinism in a preterm infant. *J Hum Genet.* 2008;53:573-577.

90. Marics G, Amiel J, Vatai B, et al. Autonomic dysfunction of glucose homoeostasis in congenital central hypoventilation syndrome. *Acta Paediatr.* 2013;102:e178-e180.

91. Perez IA, Keens TG, Ward SL. Central hypoventilation syndrome. In: Kheirandish-Gozal L, Gozal D, eds. *Sleep Disordered Breathing in Children.* New York, NY: Springer; 2012:391-408.

92. Vagiakis E, Koutsourelakis I, Perraki E, et al. Average volume-assured pressure support in a 16-year-old girl with congenital central hypoventilation syndrome. *J Clin Sleep Med.* 2010;6:609-612.

93. Kam K, Bjornson C, Mitchell I. Congenital central hypoventilation syndrome; safety of early transition to non-invasive ventilation. *Pediatr Pulmonol.* 2014;49:410-413.

94. Migliori C, Cavazza A, Motta M, et al. Early use of nasal-BiPAP in two infants with congenital central hypoventilation syndrome. *Acta Paediatr.* 2003;92:823-826.

95. Tibballs J, Henning RD. Noninvasive ventilatory strategies in the management of a newborn infant and three children with

congenital central hypoventilation syndrome. *Pediatr Pulmonol.* 2003;36:544-548.

96. Hartmann H, Jawad MH, Noyes J, et al. Negative extrathoracic pressure ventilation in central hypoventilation syndrome. *Arch Dis Child.* 1994;70:418-423.

97. Chen ML, Tablizo MA, Kun S, Keens TG. Diaphragm pacers as a treatment for congenital central hypoventilation syndrome. *Expert Rev Med Devices.* 2005;2:577-585.

98. Nicholson KJ, Nosanov LB, Bowen KA, et al. Thoracoscopic placement of phrenic nerve pacers for diaphragm pacing in congenital central hypoventilation syndrome. *J Pediatr Surg.* 2015;50:78-81.

99. Shaul DB, Danielson PD, McComb JG, Keens TG. Thoracoscopic placement of phrenic nerve electrodes for diaphragmatic pacing in children. *J Pediatr Surg.* 2002;37:974-978.

100. Marcus CL, Jansen MT, Poulsen MK, et al. Medical and psychosocial outcome of children with congenital central hypoventilation syndrome. *J Pediatr.* 1991;119:888-895.

101. Oren J, Kelly DH, Shannon DC. Long-term follow-up of children with congenital central hypoventilation syndrome. *Pediatrics.* 1987;80:375-380.

102. Charnay AJ, Antisdel-Lomaglio JE, Zelko FA, et al. Congenital central hypoventilation syndrome: neurocognition already reduced in preschool-age children. *Chest.* 2016;149:809-815.

103. Zelko FA, Nelson MN, Leurgans SE, et al. Congenital central hypoventilation syndrome: neurocognitive functioning in school age children. *Pediatr Pulmonol.* 2010;45:92-98.

18

Childhood Disorders Requiring Respiratory Care

Joyce Baker
Jamie L. Sahli
Katherine R. Ward
Kimberly L. DiMaria

OUTLINE

OBJECTIVES

1. Identify common childhood disorders impacting respiratory care.
2. Describe the underlying etiology and pathophysiology of each childhood disorder.
3. Recognize clinical presentations and diagnosis of each childhood disorder.
4. Determine the best way to manage each childhood disorder.
5. Recognize complications and define processes for the best outcomes for each childhood disorder.

KEY TERMS

antepartum
cricothyrotomy
Cushing's triad
cytokines
encephalopathy
extracorporeal membrane
  oxygenation (ECMO)
exudative phase
fibroproliferative phase
flail chest
focal bronchiectasis
fluoroscopy
Glasgow Coma Scale (GCS)
granulomas

intrapartum
lactate
meninges
nonaccidental trauma (NAT)
noncardiogenic
  pulmonary edema
noncommunicable
pulmonary vascular
  resistance
rigid bronchoscopy
surface tension
systemic vascular
  resistance (SVR)

Introduction

Respiratory disorders are one of the most common causes of morbidity and mortality in children. Many disorders have respiratory involvement as a complication of the disease process. Understanding the etiology and pathophysiology of common childhood diseases that impact the respiratory system provides insight into the need for respiratory intervention.

Acute Respiratory Distress Syndrome

First recognized in 1967, acute respiratory distress syndrome (ARDS) was previously termed *adult* respiratory distress syndrome or simply respiratory distress syndrome (RDS). The name was changed in 1994 by the American-European Consensus Conference to recognize that this condition also affects children.[1] ARDS is defined as acute, **noncardiogenic pulmonary edema** with bilateral pulmonary infiltrates on chest X-ray (CXR) and a PaO_2 to FiO_2 ratio of <200 (**Table 18-1**).[2]

Etiology

ARDS results from lung injury that damages the alveolar capillary membrane, impairing the ability to maintain lung fluid balance. As a result, fluid leaks from the capillary bed into the alveolar space. ARDS is classified as primary or secondary. Although lung injury can result from a variety of causes, classification of ARDS depends on how lung injury occurs. Primary ARDS is caused by conditions that injure the alveolar capillary membrane and disrupt this protective lung barrier. Exposure to noxious gases, such as chlorine; aspiration of gastric contents; pneumonia; and pulmonary contusions caused by chest trauma are among the conditions that cause primary ARDS (**Table 18-2**). Infection, specifically pneumonia,[3] is the most common cause of primary ARDS in pediatrics. Secondary ARDS occurs as a result of a complication of an injury or illness that indirectly causes lung injury. A severe reaction to a blood transfusion, sepsis, and pancreatitis are a few examples of conditions that cause secondary ARDS (Table 18-2).[2]

These conditions cause systemic inflammation, which results in the release of proinflammatory mediators and neutrophils into the alveoli. This inflammatory cascade of events affects the integrity of the alveolar capillary membrane, causing fluid leakage into the alveolar space.

Pathophysiology

Regardless of the inciting cause of the lung injury, all cases of ARDS typically advance through a series of three phases: acute or exudative, fibroproliferative, and chronic or recovery (**Table 18-3**). Progression through each phase is often recognized using clinical, radiographic, and histopathologic features.[2] Infants and smaller children are at higher risk of complications

TABLE 18-2
Etiology of Acute Respiratory Distress Syndrome

Direct Lung Injury	Indirect Lung Injury
Pneumonia	Sepsis
Aspiration	Shock
Pulmonary contusion	Burns
Fat or air embolism	Pancreatitis
Submersion injury	Cardiac bypass surgery
Inhalational injury	Transfusion-related lung injury
Reperfusion injury	Drug overdose or toxic ingestion

TABLE 18-3
Phases of Acute Respiratory Distress Syndrome: Characteristics and Pathophysiology

Acute/Exudative	Fibroproliferative	Chronic/Recovery
4–7 days	7–21 days	>21 days
Interstitial and alveolar edema	Chronic inflammation	Removal of edema
• Disruption of gas exchange • Arterial hypoxemia • Late arterial hypercarbia	Fibrosis	Proliferation of type II cells
Loss of surfactant	Loss of alveolar architecture	Differentiation into type I cells
Decreased lung compliance		Endothelial progenitor influx
Acute inflammation		Resolution of inflammation
		Remodeling of fibrotic areas

TABLE 18-1
Acute Respiratory Distress Syndrome Diagnostic Criteria

Acute onset
Bilateral infiltrates
PaO_2/FiO_2 <200
Noncardiogenic origin: • Pulmonary artery wedge pressure <18 mm Hg • No clinical evidence of left atrial hypertension

given their smaller airways, increased airway resistance, and lower functional residual capacity.[3]

In a healthy lung, two separate barriers form the alveolar capillary membrane: the capillary endothelium and the alveolar epithelium, which are separated by the interstitium.[4] The alveolar epithelium is composed of type I and II cells, covering 90% and 10%, respectively, of the surface. The main function of this interface is gas exchange. After oxygen is inhaled, it is diffused through the thin wall of the alveolar epithelium into the capillaries before being transported to the tissues. Carbon dioxide from tissue metabolism is carried back to the lung through venous circulation and easily diffuses from the capillaries through thin alveolar walls before being exhaled. In order to maintain functional gas exchange, alveoli must remain appropriately expanded. The LaPlace equation illustrates the direct relationship between surface tension (T) and the pressure (P) required for maintaining an open spherical structure with a certain radius (r):[2]

$$P = 2T/r$$

Surface tension within the alveoli is drastically reduced by surfactant, which is manufactured by type II cells lining the walls of the alveoli. Surfactant significantly reduces the pressure required to open the alveoli or to maintain alveolar expansion. The presence of tight junctions within the epithelium protects the alveolus from vascular fluid entry. Fluid movement from the capillaries into the interstitium is normally controlled by a delicate balance of hydrostatic and oncotic pressures. This balance prevents vascular fluid from entering the alveolar air space and allows it to be removed by the lymphatic system and returned back into the systemic circulation.[5]

Acute/Exudative Phase

The first phase is known as the **exudative phase**, which is characterized by disrupted fluid balance following injury to the alveolar–capillary barrier. Damage to the tight junctions of the alveolar epithelium allows edema or fluid into the alveolar air space, impairing gas exchange.[5] During this phase, patients first present with arterial hypoxemia, followed by arterial hypercarbia.

As damage occurs to the alveolar epithelium, type II epithelial cells are also damaged and surfactant production inhibited. The loss of surfactant, which maintains alveolar surface tension, causes alveolar and small airway collapse during expiration. The pressure required to open a collapsed alveolus, despite the radius, increases proportionally and reduces pulmonary compliance, or makes the lungs stiffer and more difficult to ventilate.[2] Damage to the alveolar epithelium also leads to an acute inflammatory response and to the release of a variety of proinflammatory **cytokines**, including tumor necrosis factor alpha, interleukin (IL)-6, IL-8, and IL-10. IL-8,

specifically, is a neutrophil chemoattractant, which causes a neutrophil influx and subsequent release of cytokines that cause more lung injury. No single cytokine has been identified as the main contributor of overall inflammation or ultimate damage; rather, it is the balance of proinflammatory and anti-inflammatory cytokines that determines extent and duration of injury.[5] Some patients move through the acute/exudative phase and then have a rapid recovery with complete resolution. Other patients move from this initial phase into the fibroproliferative phase, a second, more-damaging phase.

Fibroproliferative Phase

The second phase, called the **fibroproliferative phase**, is characterized by continued inflammatory response, fibrosis, and scarring of the alveolar–capillary unit.[2] Scarring and fibrosis result from a maladaptive repair response to the initial injury. During this phase, mesenchymal cells and fibroblasts deposit various collagen types and fibronectin, which disrupt and potentially obliterate alveolar architecture and disrupt alveolar function. Patients who progress into this phase have an increased risk of death from ARDS.[5]

Chronic/Recovery Phase

The final phase of ARDS is the chronic/recovery phase. This phase involves recovery or resolution of all the disruptions present in the previous phases: repair of capillary endothelium, repair of alveolar epithelium, removal of alveolar edema, removal of inflammatory cells, and remodeling of fibrotic tissue. As alveolar and interstitial fluids are removed, the alveolar epithelium repair begins. The alveolar epithelium is repaired by remodeling or the action of type II cells, which proliferate along the damaged walls and differentiate as needed into type I cells. Capillary endothelial recovery is less well understood but likely follows migration of progenitor cells to the area of injury. In some patients, the fibrosis may be too extensive to repair, leaving chronically scarred and poorly functioning alveoli unable to return to their previous functional state (Table 18-3).[5]

Diagnosis

The diagnosis of ARDS is made by a combination of CXR and arterial blood gas (ABG) information. Fluid or edema in the alveolar spaces is seen as bilateral infiltrates on CXR (**Figure 18-1**) while ABGs are needed to determine the level of hypoxemia. Patients with ARDS have a low PaO_2 while receiving oxygen at an FiO2 ≥0.50. The $PaO_2/FiO2$ is used to quantify the degree of oxygenation impairment. A $PaO_2/FiO2$ ratio <200 is seen with ARDS. The PaO_2 also provides the ability to calculate the oxygenation index (OI), which may guide management decisions. It is important to determine if

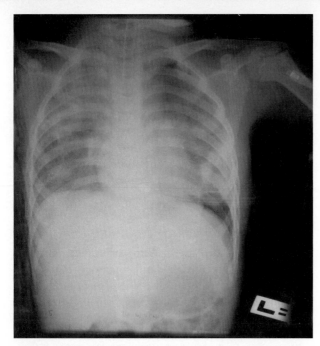

FIGURE 18-1 Chest radiograph of an intubated child with bilateral infiltrates.

© Santibhavank P/Shutterstock.

hypoxemia is caused by a cardiac or pulmonary problem. The patient history can be helpful in determining if the patient currently has or had a cardiac condition, and an echocardiogram is often used to rule out a cardiac cause for the oxygenation problem.

Blood tests, such as a complete blood count (CBC), can help identify the presence of infection, a cause of ARDS. Although a very high or low white blood cell (WBC) count can signal an infection, further testing is needed to identify the specific organism and to guide treatment. A bronchoalveolar lavage can be used to obtain a sputum culture and to evaluate the extent of neutrophil activation within the lung.

Clinical Presentation

The patient will present with tachypnea and a labored breathing pattern. By definition, hypoxemia will be present. Auscultatory findings include areas of diminished breath sounds and adventitious breath sounds, including rales or crackles indicating edema.

Other signs and symptoms relate directly to the etiologies of ARDS. For example, if bacterial pneumonia is the cause of ARDS, the patient may be febrile and have an elevated WBC count. A thorough history and physical examination are essential and will help delineate potential causes and complicating factors.

Treatment

It is important to identify the etiology to effectively manage the disease course.[3]

Initially, supplemental oxygen is needed to address hypoxemia. However, nasal cannula or simple face mask is generally not sufficient to correct the oxygen defect. Noninvasive ventilation (NIV) in the form of continuous positive airway pressure or bilevel positive airway pressure can be utilized and may reduce intubation rates if used early in the course of the disease.[6] However, intubation will be necessary in children whose PaO_2/FiO_2 does not respond to NIV or whose disease state is severe.

A "lung protective" strategy should be used with NIV and invasive ventilation. The Pediatric Acute Lung Injury Consensus Conference Group recommends ventilatory strategies that avoid overdistention and minimize the cyclic opening and closing of alveoli to reduce the risk for further lung injury. Therefore, the goal is to reduce mean airway pressure (MAP) below 30 mm Hg. This can best be achieved with low tidal volumes (V_T) in the physiologic range of 5 to 8 mL/kg ideal body weight for patients with a better respiratory system and V_T of 3 to 6 mL/kg predicted body weight for patients with poor respiratory compliance.[7] Peak end-expiratory pressure (PEEP) above atmospheric is needed to prevent alveolar collapse at end inspiration and to improve oxygenation. Hemodynamic stability, oxygenation, and respiratory system compliance should be closely monitored during PEEP titration.[7] The literature supports maintaining an SpO_2 of 88% to 92%.[7] Unless contraindicated, permissive hypercapnia, allowing a less than normal blood pH, will help prevent high lung pressures.[8] High-frequency oscillatory ventilation (HFOV) may be considered as an alternative for patients who fail to improve with conventional ventilation. Close monitoring of oxygenation, hemodynamic stability, and acid–base balance are essential when setting and adjusting MAP and oscillatory rate. There are cases where **extracorporeal membrane oxygenation (ECMO)** is required. Calculating the OI helps determine what degree of escalation may be necessary. OI is calculated as follows:

$$OI = ((FiO_2 \times MAP))/(PaO_2)$$

With an OI >20, HFOV should be considered; for an OI ≥40, ECMO should be considered.[9]

Prone positioning is an early intervention that improved oxygenation and reduced ventilator-associated injury in adult trials but not in pediatrics.[3] The literature suggests that early use in ARDS may reduce both short- and long-term mortality.[10]

Conservative fluid management is another intervention that has shown benefit in adult studies. One of the hallmarks of the disease is excess fluid; therefore, administering a limited amount of additional fluids—only enough to maintain appropriate hydration—is indicated.[11]

There are many interventions that may or have been used that do not improve overall outcome, including the use of surfactant to reduce alveolar surface tension and help maintain expansion,[12] inhaled nitric oxide,[13] and corticosteroids.[14] The use of these interventions is not supported in pediatrics.

Mortality rates may be as high as 40% to 60%. Often, mortality is related to the presence of multiorgan dysfunction rather than the primary respiratory disease. Indicators of poor outcomes, therefore, include other organ dysfunction and extremities of age. Interestingly, OIs do not accurately predict outcome. Despite the significant acute injury to the lung, most survivors do recover normal pulmonary function within about a year after illness.[5]

Systemic Inflammatory Response Syndrome and Sepsis

Sepsis and septic shock typically result from a severe infection caused by bacteria, viruses, fungi or parasites, and/or toxins produced by these organisms.[15] Septic shock is one of the leading causes of morbidity and mortality in children[16] Research has played a major role in helping the medical community gain a better understanding of the pathophysiology and preventive strategies to improve clinical outcomes.[16]

Etiology

Sepsis is an inflammatory response triggered by infection that can range from mild symptoms to severe organ dysfunction and death. Because of the spectrum of clinical presentation, standardized definitions of systemic inflammatory response syndrome (SIRS), sepsis, severe sepsis, and septic shock have been created to better describe this disease process.

According to the 2012 Surviving Sepsis Campaign, sepsis is defined as "the presence (probable or documented) of infection together with systemic manifestations of infection."[17] The infection can be bacterial, viral, or fungal and can originate in the blood, lungs, urinary tract, brain, skin, bone, or soft tissue.

Gram-positive bacteria, *Staphylococcus* specifically, are the most common cause of pediatric sepsis.[18] Gram-negative bacteria, such as *Escherichia coli*, *Klebsiella*, *Pseudomonas*, *Serratia*, and *Enterobacter*, are less commonly the cause of sepsis, but gram-negative sepsis is typically more severe and carries an increased mortality rate.[19]

Sepsis remains a significant health problem worldwide. In the United States, sepsis causes more than 75,000 hospital admissions and 10,000 deaths among the pediatric population.[18]

Pathophysiology

The initial inflammatory response of SIRS can be triggered by an infectious or noninfectious cause. Once activated, the immune system responds by producing both inflammatory and anti-inflammatory cytokines. Persistent infection and release of toxins from bacteria cause excessive release of proinflammatory cytokines. The overproduction of inflammatory cytokines causes an imbalance between the pro- and anti-inflammatory responses, therefore causing widespread inflammation that can lead to sepsis, severe sepsis, and septic shock.[20]

Pediatric patients with sepsis often display signs of profound volume depletion.[19] Typically, these patients present with a low cardiac output (CO) and elevated **systemic vascular resistance (SVR)**, or "cold shock." However, CO and SVR will fluctuate throughout the course of illness, necessitating changes to vasopressor therapy. Because of the decreased CO, oxygen delivery to tissues is decreased. As SIRS progresses to sepsis and septic shock, tissue hypoxia worsens, which further compromises perfusion.

Diagnosis

There is no clinical test to determine if a patient has sepsis. Instead, there are well-described criteria that, when met, place a patient along a continuum ranging from SIRS to septic shock. Pediatric-specific criteria for SIRS, sepsis, severe sepsis, and septic shock were adapted from the adult sepsis criteria (**Table 18-4**). Mortality rates are significantly improved when sepsis is diagnosed and treatment is initiated quickly. Therefore, it is essential that clinicians are familiar with sepsis criteria and have a high level of suspicion for sepsis if a pediatric patient presents with fever or hypothermia in the presence of hypoperfusion (delayed capillary refill time, decreased urine output, and altered mental status).

TABLE 18-4
SIRS Criteria for Younger Than 18 Years

SIRS Criteria*
Temperature >38°C (100.4°F) or <36°C (96.8°F)
Heart rate >90 beats/min
Respiratory rate >20 breaths/min or $PaCO_2$ <32 mm Hg
WBC >12,000/mm³, <4,000/mm³, or >10% bands
Sepsis Criteria (SIRS plus infection)
Suspected or present infection
Severe Sepsis Criteria
Lactic acidosis
Blood pressure <90 mm Hg or drop >40 mm Hg from baseline
Septic Shock
Hypotension, despite adequate fluid resuscitation
* ≥2 meets SIRS definition

To meet SIRS criteria, a patient must have either hypothermia/hyperthermia or leukocytosis/leukopenia in addition to tachycardia or tachypnea. Sepsis is defined as "SIRS in the presences of, or as a result of suspected or proven infection."[21,22] Cultures from blood, respiratory secretions, cerebrospinal fluid (CSF), urine, and wound or tissue may show evidence of infection, although a negative culture does not rule out sepsis. A patient with sepsis will also typically display elevated inflammatory markers, including C-reactive protein, sedimentation rate, and procalcitonin. Severe sepsis occurs when a patient meets SIRS criteria and also has evidence of either cardiovascular instability and/or ARDS in addition to pulmonary, renal, neurologic, hepatic, or hematologic dysfunction. Septic shock is defined as sepsis accompanied by cardiovascular dysfunction.[22]

Clinical Presentation

A septic patient displays evidence of compromised perfusion and temperature instability (fever or hypothermia). In warm shock, patients present with brisk or flashy capillary refill time, wide pulse pressure, flushed appearance, and bounding pulses. In comparison, patients in cold shock will demonstrate the effects of vasoconstriction, which include weak pulses, delayed capillary refill time (>2 seconds), cool extremities, and mottling. A fever is the most common evidence of temperature instability and one of the criteria for SIRS and sepsis, although some patients will present with lower than normal core body temperatures. Tachycardia is a hallmark sign of SIRS and is a pediatric patient's method of compensating for decreased CO. Hypotension in pediatric patients is a late sign because an infant or child with decreased CO will compensate until they are severely ill, at which time profound hypotension will occur.

Signs of decreased end-organ perfusion, such as altered level of consciousness, decreased urine output, tachypnea, elevated blood **lactate**, and hypoxia, are later signs of distress and place the patient in the severe sepsis or septic shock categories. Altered mental status in a pediatric patient can manifest as irritability, inconsolability, confusion, or lethargy.

Treatment

A landmark study by Rivers et al.[23] reported that early goal-directed therapy significantly reduced mortality among adult patients with sepsis. Since that time, SIRS and sepsis management have become guideline driven, with specific and time-sensitive goals to quickly identify sepsis and initiate therapy to improve perfusion and oxygen delivery while identifying and treating the underlying cause of infection.

Initial management includes administration of high-flow oxygen to achieve and maintain an oxygen saturation of 94% and intravenous or intraosseous access and fluid resuscitation. An oxygen mask, high-flow nasal cannula, or noninvasive positive pressure therapy may be used to stabilize the patient's oxygenation status. The device used depends on the patient's degree of hypoxemia and ability to tolerate the device. Fluid resuscitation with isotonic crystalloid IV fluids, normal saline, or Lactated Ringer's are administered in 20 mL/kg aliquots.[23] Patient assessment is essential during fluid resuscitation. The patient should be reassessed after each bolus for response to therapy, increased perfusion, fluid overload, crackles, hepatomegaly, and hypoxemia.

Additional diagnostic testing includes blood, urine, sputum, and CSF cultures to determine the causative agents, ideally prior to the initiation of broad-spectrum antibiotic therapy, and to guide antimicrobial therapy.[24] However, obtaining cultures should not interfere with the goal of administering broad-spectrum antibiotic therapy within 1 hour of recognition of signs and symptoms of sepsis. A complete metabolic panel, complete blood count, blood gas, and lactate level are also helpful in assessing acid–base balance and electrolyte status. Hypoglycemia and hypocalcemia should be corrected if present.

If perfusion does not improve after the initial fluid resuscitation, fluid-refractory shock should be considered and vasoactive medications, such as dopamine, epinephrine, or norepinephrine, initiated. Epinephrine is recommended as the first-line treatment for cold shock and norepinephrine as the first-line treatment for warm shock. Central venous access should be considered for the safer delivery of vasoactive medications. Prior to placement of the central venous catheter, vasoactive medications can be administered peripherally. After initial stabilization, treatment should continue in the intensive care unit (ICU), where the patient's ventilatory and hemodynamic status can be closely monitored.

Intubation and mechanical ventilation should be considered for patients whose hemodynamic status does not improve after fluid resuscitation and initiation of inotropic support. As approximately 40% of CO is used to support the respiratory muscles, mechanical ventilatory support can be used to offset some of this demand.[25] Mechanical ventilation will decrease left ventricular afterload, which is beneficial for patients with cold shock and high SVR.

Prior to intubation or central venous catheter placement, sedation with ketamine is recommended.[26] Etomidate may cause adrenal suppression, preventing endogenous stress response during critical illness, and is therefore contraindicated in sepsis.

Patients with compromised perfusion after 1 hour of fluid resuscitation and vasoactive support are categorized as catecholamine-resistant shock and require prompt administration of hydrocortisone.

Management at this time is focused on maintaining an age-appropriate blood pressure, specifically targeting a MAP of 55 mm Hg for an infant and 65 mm Hg for a child. Central venous pressure (CVP) should be monitored and therapy directed at maintaining a normal CVP, or a CVP between 5 and 10 cm H_2O. Mixed venous saturations, or SvO_2, should also be monitored and therapy targeted at maintaining SvO_2 >70% obtained with a pulmonary artery catheter or venous blood gas.[26]

ECMO should be considered for shock persisting after fluid resuscitation, vasoactive support, and initiation of steroids. Prior to the initiation of ECMO, the patient should be evaluated for the presence of a pericardial effusion and/or pneumothorax.

Despite recent advancements in sepsis guidelines, sepsis and septic shock remain a leading cause of death. The hospital mortality rate for pediatric patients with severe sepsis is 10%.[27] Approximately 68% of pediatric patients with septic shock who require ECMO survive.[28]

Shock

Shock is a syndrome of decreased perfusion and inadequate oxygen delivery to the tissues that could result in single or multiorgan failure.[29] Shock is categorized into three different stages: compensated, uncompensated, and irreversible. Blood pressure and CO are within normal limits with compensated shock. However, as a compensatory mechanism for decreased tissue perfusion, tachycardia is present. Cardiac output is low and hypotension present with uncompensated shock. Irreversible shock involves damage to the brain and heart.[30] There are four types of shock. Depending on the type of shock, the etiology, clinical presentation, and management will vary.

Etiology

Primary types of shock include hypovolemic, disruptive, cardiogenic, and obstructive (Table 18-5). Cellular hypoperfusion occurs with all four types of shock.

Hypovolemic shock is the most common cause of shock in infants and children.[29] It occurs when there is insufficient intravascular fluid volume due to hemorrhage, vomiting, diarrhea, dehydration, diabetes insipidus, burns, movement of fluid from intravascular space as in third spacing, or osmotic diuresis.

Distributive shock is characterized by a maldistribution of blood flow, caused by profound vasodilation and venodilation. Dilation of the vascular bed, regardless of the cause, produces the effect of relative hypovolemia and the organs perceive perfusion is inadequate. The most common cause of disruptive shock is an anaphylactic reaction from exposure to an allergen. The most common allergens causing anaphylactic shock in children are foods, medications, and insect stings.[31] Neurogenic shock, a type of distributive shock, results from loss of vascular tone and usually follows an injury to the brain or spinal cord.

Cardiogenic shock is caused by a severe myocardial dysfunction that compromises CO. It can be systolic or diastolic in nature. Common causes of cardiogenic shock in pediatric patients are cardiomyopathy, cardiac tamponade, arrhythmias, congenital heart disease, and myocarditis.

Obstructive shock is caused by a physical obstruction to adequate cardiac output. Examples include pulmonary embolism, tension pneumothorax, congenital heart defects, such as critical aortic stenosis, and cardiac tamponade.

TABLE 18-5
Comparison of the Types of Shock

Type of Shock	Pathophysiology	Signs and Symptoms	Causes
Hypovolemic (volume loss)	Decreased CO Increased SVR	Hypotension Tachycardia Hypoxia Low red blood cell count and hematocrit Prolonged capillary refill Low urine output	Trauma Hemorrhage (internal or external) Severe dehydration Severe vomiting Severe diarrhea
Disruptive (inadequate perfusion)	Increase CO Decreased SVR	Severe hypovolemia and vascular collapse Decreased contractility and dysrhythmias Hypoxia Capillary leaking	Anaphylaxis Sepsis Drug overdose Brain or spinal cord injury
Cardiogenic (pump failure)	Decreased CO Normal or increased SVR	Hypotension Tachycardia Blood pressure <90 mm Hg or <40 mm Hg less than baseline Fluid volume not affected Pulmonary congestion	Cardiac arrest Ventricular dysrhythmias Cardiac tamponade Congenital heart disease Myocarditis
Obstructive	Decreased CO Increased SVR	Paradoxical pulse Muffled heart sounds Sudden onset of shortness of breath Hypoxia	Cardiac tamponade Pulmonary embolus Tension pneumothorax Congenital heart defects

Pathophysiology

Regardless of the etiology of shock, the common feature is an imbalance between the supply of oxygen and nutrients and the cellular demand. When the supply cannot meet the demand, cellular hypoperfusion and anaerobic metabolism occur. When cells use anaerobic metabolism to produce energy, lactic acid is produced.

Hypovolemic shock occurs when there is volume loss, either intravascular, extravascular, or both. Decreased circulating volume causes decreased preload and subsequently decreased CO. In hypovolemic shock, the relative size of the blood vessels does not change; instead, there is insufficient volume to adequately fill the space.

Unlike hypovolemic shock, a patient with distributive shock does not sustain blood volume loss. Instead, there is a maldistribution of blood flow. Disruptive shock is caused by dilation of veins and arteries, leading to hypoperfusion of organs. Anaphylactic shock is an example of a type of distributive shock. When anaphylaxis occurs, there is a release of inflammatory mediators in response to an allergen. The inflammatory mediators cause vasodilation and vascular permeability, exacerbating symptoms that include, but are not limited to, angioedema, itching, and bronchospasm. Hypotension, tachycardia, and decreased CO also occur. Septic shock is another example of distributive shock. Septic shock occurs as an immune response to an infectious trigger resulting in excessive release of inflammatory cytokines, which cause low CO and hypoxia.[32] Neurogenic shock transpires from a spinal cord or brain injury that significantly limits the body's ability to regulate the sympathetic nervous system. As such, no system is available to oppose a parasympathetic response, and hypotension, bradycardia, and occasionally hypothermia ensue.

Cardiogenic shock occurs as a result of myocardial dysfunction leading to decreased CO. The weakened myocardium is unable to fully eject blood volume during systole, resulting in high end-diastolic volumes in both the right and the left ventricle and congestion in the pulmonary veins, which results in pulmonary edema, hypoxia, and increased work of breathing.

Diagnosis

There is no one diagnostic test to determine the presence of shock. Typically a diagnosis is made by careful examination of vital signs, capillary refill, and level of consciousness. Blood tests, radiographic assessments, echocardiogram of the heart, assessment of adequate systemic blood flow, and patient history collectively assist in determining the diagnosis and determinant of the cause.

Capillary refill assessment is an easy, rapid, noninvasive method to assess perfusion. Capillary refill can be assessed at the nail bed or on a fleshy part of the skin (forearm, thigh, etc.) by applying light pressure to the area, then releasing the pressure. When the pressure is released, there is initial noted blanching of skin. Perfusion is normal if the blanched area returns to a pink color in less than 2 seconds.[33] A normal capillary refill is predictive of superior vena cava oxygen saturations of greater than or equal to 70%.[33] Inadequate or delayed tissue perfusion is present when there is a greater than 3-second delay in the blanching returning to a normal or pink color.

Clinical Presentation

Regardless of the etiology of shock, patients will present with evidence of decreased systemic perfusion, tachycardia, tachypnea, decreased urine output, a change in mental status, and elevated lactate. Hypotension is a late and ominous sign of shock. For pediatric patients, a decrease in the systolic blood pressure can be the last vital sign to show evidence of shock. In compensated shock, a patient presents with decreased tissue perfusion, but blood pressure is within normal limits. This phase can last for a few minutes to hours depending on the etiology of the shock. A pediatric patient can be severely ill and still present with a normal blood pressure. Uncompensated shock occurs when inadequate perfusion and hypotension are present (Table 18-6). Patients with hypovolemic shock typically have a metabolic acidosis and compensate by increasing their respiratory rate. Therefore, tachypnea is a common presenting symptom of hypovolemic shock. Other symptoms of hypovolemic shock include tachycardia, weak pulses, delayed capillary refill time, cool extremities, mottling, decreased urine output, and changes in level of consciousness.

Distributive shock presentation will vary depending on the etiology. Disruptive shock can occur with an anaphylactic, or severe allergic, reaction; sepsis; drug overdose; or spinal cord injury. Patients with anaphylaxis can present with hives, itching, stridor, wheezing, laryngeal edema, tachycardia, and hypotension. If not recognized and treated, anaphylactic shock can lead to cardiopulmonary collapse and death. Signs of

TABLE 18-6
Systolic Blood Pressure Abnormalities Associated with Decompensated Shock

Age	Systolic Blood Pressure (SBP)
Neonate	<60 mm Hg
Infant	<70 mm Hg
Child (1–10 years)	<70 mm Hg + (2 × age in years)
Child (>10 years)	<90 mm Hg

septic shock include fever or hypothermia, tachycardia, tachypnea, and hypoxemia. Depending on the cause, the WBC count may be elevated or low. Patients with cold shock will have cool and pale extremities with weak pulses. Patients with warm shock will have a brisk capillary refill and bounding pulses. Neurogenic shock may occur in patients who have sustained a spinal cord injury. Signs of neurogenic shock include profound hypotension with a wide pulse pressure accompanied by a normal heart rate or bradycardia.

Pulmonary venous congestion and subsequent pulmonary edema often occur with cardiogenic shock. As a result, patients will have increased work of breathing. Decreased cardiac output with this type of shock is manifested as weak pulses, cool extremities, and delayed capillary refill time, in addition to the other signs of increased end-organ dysfunction. If the myocardial dysfunction is severe enough, patients will display signs of congestive heart failure, which include jugular venous distention, hepatomegaly, and crackles.

Obstructive shock presents similarly to hypovolemic shock. As the severity of this type of shock worsens, patients will begin to display subtle signs of venous congestion, such as increased work of breathing, jugular venous distention, muffled heart sounds, and narrow pulse pressure, which are not consistent with hypovolemia.

Treatment

Management strategies vary and depend on the type of shock affecting the child. However, therapy is targeted at improving perfusion while treating the underlying cause. There are three primary goals of therapy in the first hours following clinical presentation: maintain oxygenation, ventilation, and achieve normal perfusion. Ongoing assessment and adjustments to interventions are necessary until the child has stabilized. Fluid resuscitation can be crucial to reversing hypovolemic and disruptive shock; however, patients with cardiogenic shock may worsen with additional fluid resuscitation. Venous access is an essential first step to fluid resuscitation. When the care team is unable to place an intravenous catheter peripherally, a central venous catheter or intraosseous catheter (IO) may be used. An isotonic crystalloid solution, such as normal saline or Lactated Ringer's, is used for fluid resuscitation. A fluid bolus of 20 mL/kg of isotonic crystalloid solution is administered by an IO or IV push over a 5-minute period.

The amount of fluid administered is determined by clinical assessment of urine output, blood pressure, capillary refill, and laboratory values. The fluid bolus can be repeated a second or third time if needed. After the third fluid bolus, if blood loss or hemorrhage is suspected, administration of packed red blood cells at 10 to 15 mL/kg or whole blood at 20 mL/kg should be considered.

Pharmacologic support includes inotropics, vasopressors, and alpha-adrenergic agonists to improve peripheral perfusion. In septic shock, antibiotics are administered. Adjunctive medications, such as diphenhydramine, ranitidine, methylprednisolone, and inhaled bronchodilators, may be used to treat trigger symptoms in anaphylaxis.

Organ dysfunction during or after shock is common, typically with the kidneys, blood coagulation, lungs, liver, and gastrointestinal system being the most affected. If shock is not recognized and corrected in the early stages, then profound hypotension, cardiac arrest, and possibly death can occur.

Meningitis

Meningitis is an inflammation of the **meninges**, or the three connective tissue layers that protect the brain and spinal cord, caused by an infection. The meninges contain CSF and support the blood vessels that run throughout the central nervous system. Cerebral edema and elevated intracranial pressures for an extended period of time cause neurologic damage.

Etiology

Meningitis can occur in children of any age. The brain parenchyma and blood vessels may also be inflamed, resulting in endothelial cell injury, vessel stenosis, and secondary ischemia.[30] According to the Centers for Disease Control and Prevention, infants, unvaccinated children, those living in close quarters (dormitory rooms, community housing, etc.), immunocompromised children, and those traveling abroad are at increased risk.[34]

Pathophysiology

There are several different organisms that can cause meningitis, and in some cases meningitis can develop secondary to an illness or medication. Viral meningitis is the most common cause of meningitis in the United States and is far less serious than bacterial meningitis.[34] Viral meningitis presents with flu-like symptoms and can often remain undiagnosed. Common viruses contributing to meningitis include enterovirus, influenza, herpesvirus, and arboviruses. It can also occur with or following the measles or mumps.

Ear and sinus infections, skull fractures, or surgical sites provide a mode of entry for bacteria to enter the bloodstream or meninges. Bacteria that cause meningitis vary by age group (**Table 18-7**) and include *Streptococcus pneumoniae* (pneumococcus), *Neisseria meningitidis* (meningococcus), *Haemophilus influenzae* (*Haemophilus*), *Escherichia coli* (*E. coli*), and *Listeria monocytogenes* (*Listeria*). Meningococcus is the leading cause of bacterial meningitis and is spread through the exchange of respiratory secretions. Fungal meningitis is typically caused by a fungus called *Cryptococcus* and affects children with immune deficiencies. Fungal and bacterial meningitis is life threatening if left untreated. Meningitis can also result from noninfectious causes, such as chemical reactions, drug allergies, some types of cancer, and inflammatory diseases.[34]

TABLE 18-7
Types of Bacteria Commonly Causing Meningitis by Age Group

Age Group	Primary Organism Causing Meningitis
Newborns	Group B *streptococcus* *Escherichia coli* *Listeria monocytogenes*
Infants and children	*Streptococcus pneumoniae* *Neisseria meningitides* *Haemophilus influenzae* type b
Adolescents and young adults	*Neisseria meningitides* *Streptococcus pneumoniae*
Older adults	*Streptococcus pneumoniae* *Neisseria meningitides* *Listeria monocytogenes*

Data from Meningitis. Centers for Disease Control and Prevention. www.cdc.gov/meningitis/bacterial.html. Updated April 1, 2014. Accessed August 27, 2015.

Diagnosis

The diagnosis is based on a combination of medical history, physical examination, and diagnostic tests, including blood cultures and/or CSF cultures obtained by lumbar puncture. Definitive diagnosis and treatment are based on the organism grown in the CSF. Levels of glucose and protein in the CSF are able to help determine if meningitis is viral or bacterial.[35,36]

Clinical Presentation

Meningitis symptoms vary depending on the age of the patient, cause of the infection, and acuteness of the illness. There are three acuity phases; acute, subacute (1–7 days), and chronic (>7 days). Symptoms may appear acutely (<24 hours) or subacutely (1–7 days) following a cold, diarrhea, and/or vomiting. Primary symptoms of meningitis include a triad of nuchal rigidity (neck stiffness), photophobia (intolerance of bright light), and headache. However, patients may also present with lethargy, irritability, skin rashes, vomiting, and even seizures (**Figure 18-2**). Infants with meningitis commonly present with extreme irritability, lethargy, fever, poor feeding, or bulging fontanelles. Viral meningitis may be mild enough where it may go undiagnosed and resolve within 7 to 10 days, even without treatment.

Meningitis

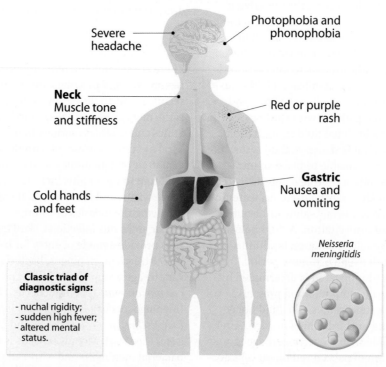

FIGURE 18-2 Signs and symptoms of meningitis.
© Designua/Shutterstock.

Treatment

Treatment includes supportive care and antimicrobial therapy. Broad-spectrum antibiotic therapy is often started until culture and sensitivity results identify the causative organism. Once the organism causing meningitis is identified, antimicrobial (antifungal, antiviral, antibiotic) therapy may be changed to match the sensitivity of the organism. In severe cases, patients may require fluid resuscitation, anticonvulsants, vasopressors, and mechanical ventilation. Corticosteroids may be administered to reduce cerebral edema and seizure activity. Noninfectious causes of meningitis, such as an allergic reaction, cancer, or autoimmune disease, may also be treated with corticosteroids. In some cases, no treatment is required because the condition can resolve on its own.

The complications of meningitis can be severe. Delay in treatment increases the risk for long-term seizures, hearing loss, learning disabilities, gait problems, brain damage, and kidney failure.

The incidence of meningitis has decreased in the past two decades.[37,38] Vaccinations for *H. influenzae*, *S. pneumoniae*, and *N. meningitides* help to reduce the incidence.[34] Bacterial meningitis, however, is associated with a high mortality rate.

Hypoxic Ischemic Encephalopathy

Hypoxic ischemic **encephalopathy** (HIE) occurs when there is inadequate oxygen delivery to the brain. It is one of the major causes of acute mortality in infants and chronic neurologic disabilities (cerebral palsy, learning disorders, and epilepsy) in survivors.[39]

Etiology

HIE is typically observed in fetuses and newborn infants who have experienced interrupted umbilical cord–blood flow during the **antepartum** or **intrapartum** period. Interruption of blood flow may result from a variety of conditions, including a prolapsed cord with cord compression, placental abruption, or placental insufficiency. HIE is also associated with prolonged traumatic events where there is suspicion of inadequate oxygenation and ventilation. Despite earlier recognition and advances in perinatal monitoring, HIE remains a serious condition that causes significant mortality and long-term morbidity in newborns. Maternal factors that increase the risk of HIE in infants include maternal diabetes, pregnancy-induced hypertension, heart or renal disease, and administration of anesthetics or analgesics. Infant risk factors include premature birth, multiple births, intrauterine growth retardation, fetal anomalies, and presence of thick meconium at birth. Traumatic HIE in infants and children is not common and often can be secondary from near drowning, strangling, choking, suffocation, cardiac arrest, head trauma, or carbon monoxide poisoning.[39]

Pathophysiology

The brain requires and consumes oxygen to provide the energy necessary to maintain systemic physicochemical activity. In adults, the brain represents up to 2% of total body weight and accounts for 20% of the resting total body oxygen consumption.[40] However, in infants and children, the brain represents up to 10% of total body weight, with as much as 50% of total body oxygen consumption, for the first decade of life.[41,42] HIE occurs as a result of prolonged (5 minutes or longer) systemic hypoxemia and normal or reduced cerebral blood flow. The body's response to prolonged systemic hypoxemia is to increase cerebral blood flow through an increase in epinephrine and redistribution of CO to shift blood flow to the essential organs, such as the brain, kidneys, and liver. Hypoxemia that occurs for five minutes or longer can result in long-term neurologic effects or brain death.

Diagnosis

Diagnosis of HIE is based on maternal history; overview of the incident prior to the hypoxic insult; and physical examination, including neurologic assessments, laboratory tests, and diagnostic procedures. Diagnostic procedures, including head ultrasound, computed tomography (CT) scan, electroencephalogram (EEG), and magnetic resonance imaging (MRI), can help to determine the area of the brain affected and the quality of brain activity. HIE guidelines from the American Academy of Pediatrics and the American College of Obstetrics and Gynecology require all the clinical presentations shown in **Table 18-8** to be present for a formal diagnosis of acute neurologic injury in a newborn.[43]

Clinical Presentation

Initially, the acute response to hypoxia is tachypnea, tachycardia, and hypertension. As hypoxia continues, symptoms change to bradycardia, hypotension, agonal respirations, or apnea that eventually results in HIE. Chronic signs and symptoms of HIE will vary depending upon the age of the child and the severity of the insult (**Table 18-9**).

TABLE 18-8
Clinical Presentation of Acute Neurologic Injury

Profound metabolic or mixed acidemia (pH <7)
Persistence of an Apgar score of 0–3 for longer than 5 minutes
Neonatal neurologic sequelae (e.g., seizures, coma, hypotonia)
Multiple organ involvement (e.g., kidney, lungs, liver, heart, intestines)

TABLE 18-9
Chronic Symptoms Associated with Hypoxic Ischemic Encephalopathy

	Mild	Moderate	Severe
Infant	• Duration <24 hours with hyperalertness • Uninhibited Moro and stretch reflexes • Sympathetic effects • Normal EEG • Slight increase in muscle tone • Poor feeding • Excessive crying or sleepiness	• Lethargy • Sluggish grasping or sucking reflexes • Seizures • Periods of apnea • Decreased spontaneous movements with or without seizures	• Seizures • No response to physical stimulation • Irregular respirations • Hypotonia • No reflexes (cough, gag, sucking) • Disturbances in ocular motion and/or dilated pupils • Bulging fontanelle • Irregularities in heart rate and blood pressure • Stupor • Flaccidity • Suppressed brainstem and autonomic functions • EEG with isopotential areas or with infrequent periodic discharges
Infant and child	• Obeys or has localized motor function • Disoriented and confused at times • Spontaneous eye opening	• Withdrawal or abnormal flexion to pain • Incomprehensible speech • Eye opening to pain	• Abnormal extension • No response to pain or stimulation • No reflexes (cough, gag, sucking) • Disturbances in ocular motion and/or dilated pupils • Irregularities in heart rate and blood pressure

Data from Zanelli SA, Kaugman DA. Hypoxic-ischemic encephalopathy clinical presentation. *Medscape*. http://emedicine.medscape.com/article/973501-overview#a5. Updated: January 16, 2015. Accessed August 29, 2015; Battin M. Newborn services clinical guideline: Neonatal encephalopathy. www.adhb.govt.nz/newborn/Guidelines/Neurology/NE.htm. Accessed August 31, 2015; and Lane Medical Library: Stanford Medical. Neurological assessment. http://lane.stanford.edu/portals/cvicu/HCP_Neuro_Tab_4/Neuro_Assessment.pdf. Accessed August 29, 2015.

Treatment

Clinical management varies and is dependent on the age of the child and the time period from insult. Prevention of HIE of the newborn begins before or during delivery. Antepartum support includes maintaining adequate maternal blood pressure and oxygenation and positioning of the mother to support adequate placental blood flow.[44] It is also important for the prenatal team to be aware of the risk factors associated with maternal conditions. Intrapartum interventions include minimizing trauma to the infant during delivery, suctioning mouth and nares immediately at delivery, maintaining adequate oxygenation and ventilation, and temperature and glucose regulation.[45] If the newborn requires cardiopulmonary resuscitation, respiratory and cardiac support should be provided according to the Neonatal Resuscitation Guidelines established by the American Heart Association and the American Academy of Pediatrics. Postacute care of a newborn with suspected HIE includes intentional hypothermia (33–36.5°C) through head or whole-body cooling for over a period of 48 to 72 hours.[46] The literature reports that therapeutic hypothermia significantly reduces the risk of mortality in this population.[47]

Initial evaluation for infants or children presenting with traumatic injury and suspected hypoxia includes airway patency, ventilation and oxygenation requirements, circulation status, and stabilization of cervical spine. Emergent surgical intervention and monitoring of intracranial pressures may be necessary. A mortality rate of approximately 20% is associated with an elevated intracranial pressure.[48] Following the initial stabilization, a thorough history should be obtained and a head-to-toe assessment completed.

HIE remains one of the most serious birth complications and is associated with long-term neurologic complications in survivors.[46] Long-term complications include cerebral palsy, severe visual deficits, severe motor or sensory loss, cognitive delay, fine or gross motor dysfunction, hearing loss, cognitive dysfunction, and learning disabilities.[47,49] Chronic management of HIE includes seizure control and supportive care for neurologic development.

HIE occurs in 1 to 3 per 1000 live full-term births.[50] In the postnatal period, the mortality rate is 15% to 20%, and the morbidity rate for severe and permanent neuropsychologic deficits is 25%.[51] Therapeutic hypothermia significantly reduces the risk of mortality.[47] Approximately 3000 children die from posttraumatic asphyxia or HIE each year.[52] Very little data are available reporting the long-term disabilities associated with HIE in children.[52]

Unintentional Injuries

Unintentional injuries are the leading cause of disability and death in children older than 1 year of age. Children are more vulnerable to unintentional injuries because they are smaller in size, have slower development and reflexes, are naturally curious, and are inexperienced to risk. Unintentional injuries include foreign body aspiration, poisoning, near drowning, and trauma. This type of injury has a predictable course and is preventable when proper precautions are taken to protect and direct children.

Foreign Body Aspiration

Foreign body aspiration occurs when a solid or semisolid object becomes lodged in the larynx or trachea. Objects large enough to cause a near-complete obstruction of the upper airway cause asphyxia that may result in death or anoxic brain injury. Lesser degrees of obstruction beyond the carina are less fatal and may result in injury, with less serious harm.

Etiology

Foreign body aspiration is the fourth leading cause of nonfatal injury in children 1 to 4 years of age.[53] Infants and toddlers explore their surroundings through seeing, touching, hearing, smelling, and tasting, which predisposes them to a greater risk of placing objects in their mouth.[54] Children also lack molar teeth, decreasing their ability to sufficiently chew food, and they also tend to talk, laugh, and run while chewing. Aspiration of a foreign object is rarely observed and only recognized after onset of respiratory symptoms. The size, composition, and location of the item aspirated will determine the respiratory system response. Raisins, hot dogs, seeds, nuts, and small toys or parts of toys are among the most commonly aspirated objects.[54]

Pathophysiology

Foreign objects lodged in the upper airway, supraglottis, or esophagus may compress the airway, causing respiratory distress, laryngospasm, or acute asphyxiation. More than 22% of foreign body aspirations occur in the larynx and trachea.[55] A majority of objects, or 55%, that pass the carina lodge in the right mainstem bronchus, 18% lodge in the left mainstem bronchus, and slightly over 1% in both bronchi.[55]

Diagnosis

Many parents are unaware or do not remember an incident that resulted in the foreign body aspiration, particularly if the incident occurred 5 or more days prior to the onset of symptoms.[56] Fifty percent of cases are not detected within the first 24 hours and one-quarter of cases are undetected for more than 1 month.[57] Children with foreign body aspiration of the upper airway present with a more acute onset of symptoms, including a sudden onset of choking, coughing, shortness of breath, and unilateral wheezing.

Although a chest X-ray is typically ordered to confirm the diagnosis in children with a suspected foreign body aspiration of the lower airway, radiologic findings are normal in 30% of patients with early diagnosis (<24 hours) because the object may not be radiolucent and initial airway inflammation has not yet occurred.[57] Children with a late diagnosis (>24 hours) may present with fever, coughing, unilateral wheezing, and shortness of breath. In 50% of patients with a late diagnosis, radiologic findings showed atelectasis or consolidation.[57,58] Right-sided foreign body aspirations tend to be more quickly diagnosed than left-sided or esophageal aspirations (**Figure 18-3**). **Fluoroscopy** and CT scanning may be helpful when the chest radiograph is normal.[59] When radiographic studies are inconclusive or fail to identify a foreign object in the airway when there is high suspicion, a bronchoscopy should be performed.[59] The combination of symptoms, radiologic findings, and bronchoscopy help formally diagnose foreign body aspiration (Figure 18-3).

Clinical Presentation

A child with a foreign body aspiration causing total or near-total occlusion of the upper airway will present with severe respiratory distress. The episode typically begins with a sudden episode of choking. The child may clutch their neck, a universal sign for choking. Often with a complete or near-complete upper airway obstruction, no breath sounds are heard during inspiration. Within the first 24 hours of aspiration of a foreign body into the lower airway, children will present with unilateral wheezing, cough, stridor, respiratory distress, cyanosis, and/or voice changes.[59] When aspiration of a foreign body occurred more than 24 hours before the onset of symptoms, children present with fever,

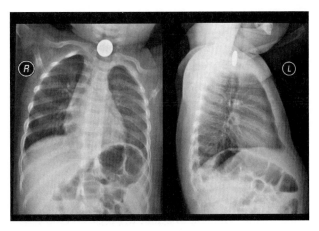

FIGURE 18-3 Radiologic image of a foreign body aspiration. The foreign body is lodged in the child's esophagus.
© Hong xia/Shutterstock.

persistent or recurrent cough, wheezing, persistent or recurrent pneumonia or atelectasis, lung abscess, **focal bronchiectasis**, or hemoptysis.[59]

Treatment

Treatment depends upon the child's clinical presentation and the location of the object in the airway. A complete obstruction of the upper airway requires immediate and emergent action with the intent to dislodge the object from the airway and to reestablish ventilation. If the object is visible, attempts to remove it should be made. It is not appropriate to blindly probe or sweep the mouth or upper airway because of the risk of pushing the object lower into the airway and/or changing the object's position in the airway and worsening the obstruction. In some cases, there is a need to perform an emergent **cricothyrotomy** to prevent death or anoxic event. Children who present with suspected partial obstruction without clinical compromise should be encouraged to cough and to use their body's natural reflexes to remove the object. A controlled flexible bronchoscopy or laryngoscopy should be performed in children who are unable to effectively cough and expectorate the aspirated foreign body. **Rigid bronchoscopy** should be used to immediately remove a foreign body in children presenting with partial obstruction and clinical compromise.[60,61] Inhaled corticosteroids, bronchodilators, and chest physiotherapy with postural drainage are ineffective and should not be used to remove the object. If the obstruction occurred more than 24 hours before onset of symptoms, and sputum cultures confirm bacterial infection, antibiotics may be prescribed. Systemic corticoid steroids, such as prednisolone or prenisone, are useful when significant airway edema is observed or if granulation tissue is present.[59]

Complications increase as time elapses between the initial aspiration event to diagnosis and removal. Complications include atelectasis, lung abscess, hemoptysis, focal bronchiectasis, or HIE if prolonged airway blockage occurs.[58]

Foreign body aspiration is one of the top five causes of death in children ages 1 to 4 years.[60] If the object is successfully removed easily and quickly, lung pathology resolves within 1 week.[61] Resolution of radiographic changes occurs more slowly when objects are difficult to remove or when airway inflammation and/or **granulomas** are present.[61]

Blunt Trauma

Trauma is an injury to the body caused from any external source. It is the leading cause of death in children in the United States.[62,63] The mortality rate for trauma is higher than all communicable diseases, including influenza, and **noncommunicable** diseases, including leukemia.[64] Approximately 15,000 pediatric deaths occur annually from trauma in the United States. Males are twice as likely as females to die from trauma, and children in southern states have the highest incidence of trauma death.[61] Inflicted trauma, or violence, has been the leading cause of death among African American male adolescents for more than a decade.[65]

Nonfatal trauma was the source of an estimated 9 million emergency department visits and approximately 3 million trauma-related hospital stays, resulting in approximately $32 billion in medical and lost-work costs.[63,65] **Nonaccidental trauma (NAT)** may be due to abuse or self-harm. Accidental and nonaccidental trauma impose a significant physical, psychological, emotional, and financial burden on children and their families.

Etiology

Mechanisms of injury for blunt trauma may vary and include motor vehicle crashes (MVCs), falls, pedestrian injuries (pedestrian or bicyclist struck by a moving vehicle), striking objects, blasts, and NAT or child abuse.[63]

Motor vehicle crashes are a leading cause of death in children, accounting for more than 800 deaths and 180,000 injuries per year.[66] MVCs are the most expensive trauma-related cause in the United States, as children are more likely to sustain severe injury requiring longer hospital stays and increased medical costs as compared to adults.[67] Trauma injuries are exacerbated by children not properly restrained as recommended, especially in rollover crashes, the most severe type of MVC.[68]

NAT is the general term used to describe physical child abuse. Federal guidelines define child abuse as follows:

> Any recent act or failure to act on the part of a parent or caretaker which results in death, serious physical or emotional harm, sexual abuse or exploitation; or an act or failure to act, which presents an imminent risk of serious harm.[69]

Pediatric abusive head trauma, also known as shaken baby syndrome, is a form of child abuse defined as an injury to the skull or intracranial contents of a child younger than 5 years due to inflicted blunt impact or violent shaking. Incidence peaks in the second month of birth as parents are unprepared for the demands of crying babies.[70]

Of the 679,000 cases of child abuse reported in 2013, 18% suffered from physical trauma.[69] It is assumed that the number of victims is higher but not always reported to the state authorities. Of those cases, the majority of victims were younger than 3 years of age. Although biological mothers were the most likely perpetrators, physical abuse can occur with males and females, and the perpetrators may not always be the biological parents.[69]

Prevalent risk factors for child abuse include financial hardship or the need to use public assistance programs, such as Medicaid, social security, supplemental nutrition programs, or public housing services, to meet the family's minimum needs.[69] Children with physical and/or emotional disabilities have an increased risk for NAT.

Pathophysiology

Blunt trauma damages surrounding tissue and blood vessels near the area of impact without breaking the skin. The specific pathophysiology depends on the mechanism of injury and the affected area(s). Head and chest injuries typically lead to severe complications.[71,72]

Blunt trauma to the head causes an accumulation of blood within the cranium, termed intracranial hemorrhage.[73] Victims of NAT are more likely to suffer from intracranial hemorrhage as compared to children with accidental injuries.[71] Abusive head trauma also results in retinal hemorrhages, which are caused by the violent repeated movement of the brain and ocular vessels against the skull. The repeated shaking causes shearing in the tissues, blood leakage and accumulation, and retinal tearing.[70] Intracranial and retinal hemorrhages cause intracranial pressure (ICP) to rise, which increases the risk for brain herniation and subsequent multiorgan failure.[74]

Blunt trauma to the chest may cause a pulmonary contusion. Compared to adults, children have more elastic cartilage and increased chest wall compliance. This physiologic difference predisposes the lungs to injury when blunt chest trauma occurs. Pulmonary contusions often occur from shearing forces of the lung parenchyma and vessels as the lungs strike the rib cage.[72] Contusion or bruising of the lung tissue leads to hemorrhage, inflammation, and increased capillary permeability, which in turn lead to ventilation/perfusion mismatch, edema, hypoxia, and hypercarbia.[75] Pneumothorax and hemothorax commonly accompany pulmonary contusion.

Severe hemorrhage, regardless of area of impact or damage, leads to a decrease in blood volume, blood pressure, and organ perfusion. The cascade of low tissue perfusion can lead to multiorgan failure, which is the primary cause of death in trauma patients.[76]

Diagnosis

Children involved in a traumatic event require a variety of imaging studies. Chest radiographs are helpful for identifying rib fractures, airway damage, pulmonary contusion, and pneumothorax. Children suspected as being victims of abuse require a complete skeletal radiograph to look for current and old fractures. The presence of old fractures or spiral fractures on a skeletal series are commonly seen with physical abuse (**Figure 18-4**).

Patients with altered mental status and mechanism of injury suspicious for head trauma warrant head CT to identify hemorrhage and tissue damage.[77] MRI provides greater detail and may be used to assess the extent of tissue damage. Ultrasound imaging may be used to identify internal bleeding, especially in the abdomen and chest. ABG sampling is useful in evaluating acid–base and oxygenation status. Electrocardiograms identify any arrhythmias as a result of blunt trauma to the heart, hypovolemia, hypoxemia, and/or electrolyte or acid–base imbalances.

Clinical Presentation

Dependent on condition, mechanism of injury, and number of body areas involved, patients may present with hypotension, tachycardia, tachypnea, hypoxia, respiratory distress, cyanosis, and apnea. Inspection reveals external tissue damage, such as abrasions, bleeding, or petechiae. Palpation is used to identify tenderness, swelling, or pain at the site(s) of impact. Auscultation may reveal diminished breath sounds over an area of contusion or pneumothorax.

Neurologically, the patient may present with an altered mental status. The **Glasgow Coma Scale (GCS)** is a numeric scoring system used to evaluate patient alertness following head injury. The scale ranges from 3 to 15 and is shown in **Table 18-10**. A lower score indicates a decreased level of consciousness and more severe head trauma; a score of 8 or less indicates that the patient will likely be in a coma and that the outcome is poor.[78,79]

Treatment

Trauma protocols according to the American Heart Association life support guidelines should be implemented upon the patient's arrival to the emergency department. Typically, the interdisciplinary team responding to the trauma is led by a physician or advanced provider experienced in pediatric trauma.[81] A detailed record of the assessment and treatment of the trauma patient should be transcribed in the electronic health record.

Assessment of the patient's airway, breathing, and circulation is essential. Children with a patent airway and hypoxemia require supplemental oxygen. Intubation may be necessary to establish a patent airway and to prevent or address hypoxia. A pediatric nonrebreathing mask may be used at an oxygen flowrate that keeps the bag partially inflated during inspiration, usually 10 to 15 L/minute, quickly to deliver higher concentrations of oxygen. A heated high-flow nasal cannula (HFNC) may also be used and can deliver precise oxygen concentrations. Theoretically, the flow provided by an HFNC washes out dead space and maximizes pulmonary gas exchange.[82] NIV may be initiated to reduce the work of breathing in children with intact airway reflexes in respiratory distress.

Intubation and mechanical ventilatory support are required for children who present with respiratory failure and are unable to protect their airway.[83] Lung protective strategies should be used for initial ventilator settings and ongoing ventilator management. An open

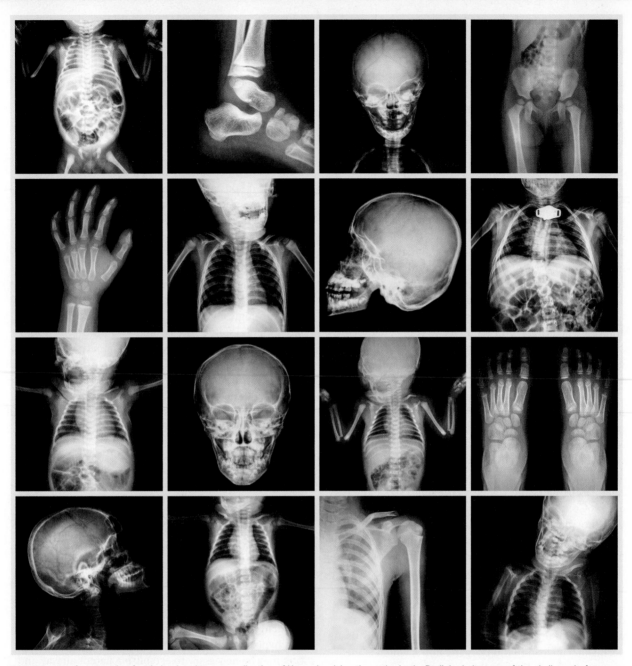

FIGURE 18-4 An example of a skeletal series, or a collection of X-rays involving the entire body. Radiologic images of the skull, neck, face, spine, shoulder, thorax, abdomen, and extremities are shown.
© Puwadol Jaturawutthichai/Shutterstock.

lung strategy, low tidal volumes (6–8 mL/kg), and high PEEP levels (8–14 cm H_2O), should be used to prevent volutrauma and barotrauma, which contribute to an inflammatory response of the compromised lung.[84]

Modes of ventilation that increase mean airway pressure to improve oxygenation, such as airway pressure release ventilation and nonconventional ventilation, including high-frequency ventilation, as well as inhaled nitric oxide, neuromuscular blockers, and prone positioning, may be used if moderate to severe ARDS persists.[7] Pediatric patients are more commonly monitored with pulse oximetry rather than with invasive blood gases; therefore, SpO_2/FiO_2 (S/F) ratios are frequently used. An S/F ratio of less than 270 corresponds to a PaO_2/FiO_2 (P/F) ratio less than 300 torr (mild ARDS).[7] Recommended guidelines prefer OI to be used to monitor oxygenation if the pediatric patient is intubated, but P/F or S/F ratios may be used when the patient is receiving support with noninvasive or HFNC.[7]

Mechanical ventilation has the potential to increase ICP, as positive pressure ventilation increases intrathoracic pressure and can decrease cerebral venous return. Permissive hypercapnia should not be used as a ventilation strategy with mechanically ventilated patients with respiratory distress syndrome and traumatic brain injury. Rather, in this subset of patients, $PaCO_2$ should

TABLE 18-10
Behaviors and Responses Evaluated through the Glasgow Coma Scale[76,80]

Behavior	Response	Score
Eye opening	Spontaneous	4
	Verbal command	3
	Open to pain	2
	Not opening	1
Verbal	Oriented	5
	Consolable but confused	4
	Inconsistent, inconsolable	3
	Inconsolable, agitated	2
	No response	1
Motor	Obeys commands	6
	Localizes pain	5
	Withdraws from pain	4
	Flexes from pain	3
	Extends from pain	2
	No motor response	1

Note: A score is assigned to each of the behaviors depending on the child's response.

Data from Kaplan JL, Porter RS. *Merck Manual of Diagnosis and Therapy.* 19th ed. Whitehouse Station, NJ: Merck Sharp & Dohme; 2011; and Hess D, MacIntyre N, Galvin W, Mishoe S. *Respiratory Care Principles and Practice.* 3rd ed. Burlington, MA: Jones & Bartlett Learning; 2016.

be maintained within the range of 35 to 45 mm Hg.[85] An elevated CO_2 will dilate the cerebral blood vessels and increase blood flow to the brain, which can cause a rise in ICP. ECMO may be required for trauma patients whose pulmonary gas exchange cannot be stabilized or maintained with mechanical ventilation. The National Trauma Bank reports that approximately 154 pediatric trauma patients required the use of ECMO in a current 4-year period.[86] ECMO supports both ventilation and perfusion (venoarterial) or oxygenation and ventilation only (venovenous).[80] Head injury and ARDS are the primary reasons that trauma patients require ECMO support.[86]

The use of blood product transfusion, mainly packed red blood cells (PRBCs), may also be necessary for trauma patients. PRBC transfusion is required in patients who have hemodynamic instability from severe hemorrhage. Although it may be a lifesaving therapy, there are complications associated with PRBCs, such as transfusion-related lung injury.[87] Patients who required transfusion of PRBCs have significantly worse clinical outcomes as compared to patients who did not.

Vessel rupture, tracheobronchial tears, cardiac tamponade, cardiac arrhythmias, cervical spine injuries, abdominal and diaphragm injuries, and fractured bones are possible complications of trauma. Patients who present with injuries to multiple areas of the body have poorer outcomes.[88] The mortality rate for children with multiple trauma, including those with chest trauma, is approximately 34% to 37%.[89] Multiple-trauma patients also have longer ventilator usage periods. The literature reports that 56% of children with multiple trauma required intubation for at least 24 hours.[79] More than half, 55%, of patients required ECMO and survived.[86] Mortality rates are lower among children treated at designated pediatric trauma centers.[90] Long-term closed-head injury may occur as the ultimate and most serious complication. Abuse accounts for more than 95% of all closed-head injury during the first year of life and 85% of all injuries before the second birthday.[91,92]

Public education is the primary focus of childhood trauma prevention. Education and public awareness campaigns focus on two primary areas: proper use of car seats or automotive restraints and prevention of child abuse. Studies show that properly restrained children are at a significantly lower risk of sustaining serious or fatal injury. *Healthy People 2020*, an evidence-based report published by the U.S. Department of Health and Human Services, reported that children are not always restrained in the proper type of seat and positioned in the correct manner. According to the *Healthy People 2010* report, only 86% of infants younger than 1 year were properly secured in rear-facing car seats, only 72% of children aged 1 to 3 years were secured in front-facing car seats, and a staggering 42% of children aged 4 to 7 years were observed in high-backed booster seats.[93] Seatbelts were only observed in 78% of children between 8 and 12 years of age.[93] Considering the devastation caused by MVCs, especially to unrestrained or improperly restrained passengers, it is imperative to continue with public health campaigns around proper use of automotive restraints.

Prevention of child abuse is a matter of public policy. At a minimum, each state has a local child protective services department that investigates abuse allegations. Teachers, daycare providers, or healthcare providers have an obligation to report suspected abuse. Funding for prevention strategies is provided by the federal government and directed toward community-based programs to strengthen and support families and to keep children in a healthier environment. Federal money is also allocated to assist with the financial burden of foster care and with the adoption of children who are no longer safe in their current home when abuse has taken place.[69]

Penetrating Trauma

Penetrating trauma can occur from accidental or nonaccidental causes. The surgical and medical management of the child and outcome depends on the mechanism and severity of the injury.

Etiology

Penetrating trauma causes organ tissue damage by external objects that have broken through the skin's surface. Penetrating trauma may be caused by glass or fragments of the vehicle during a motor vehicle crash, such weapons as knives, bullets, or blasts, or any other types of sharp objects that pierce the body.[80]

Pathophysiology

Flail chest is most commonly associated with high-impact thoracic blunt trauma and results from severe anteroposterior compression found in MVCs, blasts, or penetrating trauma.[94] It is defined as a fracture of two or more contiguous ribs in two or more places.[95] The segment of fractured ribs creates a paradoxical breathing pattern, moving inward with inspiration and outward with expiration (**Figure 18-5**). Pain associated with the flail segment leads to splinting, hypoventilation, and suppressed cough effort. As a result, atelectasis and mucus accumulation from poor airway clearance occurs. Pulmonary contusion, pneumothorax, and/or hemothorax commonly accompany flail chest and contribute to respiratory failure.[75,96,97]

External hemorrhage occurs when major organs or blood vessels are ruptured or pierced by penetrating trauma. Blood loss leads to hypoperfusion, shock, and subsequent multiorgan failure.

Clinical Presentation

The clinical presentation in penetrating trauma is similar to blunt trauma. The type and severity of signs and symptoms depend on the extent of the injury. Hypotension, tachycardia, tachypnea, hypoxia, respiratory distress, cyanosis, and apnea may be present. Auscultation may reveal diminished breath sounds over an area of fracture, contusion, or hemopneumothorax. Altered mental status may accompany a head injury.

Treatment

Management of flail chest is generally supportive. Pain control, fluid management, and aggressive airway clearance are shown to have the best outcomes for flail chest. Intubation and mechanical ventilation may be required when pulmonary contusion, pneumothorax, and/or hemothorax are present. Surgical fixation of the chest wall may be necessary when extensive rib fractures are present. Cables, wires, or fragment plates may be used to secure the ribs. Titanium plates have shown promise in reconstructing the ribs and in securing the chest wall. Respiratory failure may occur and is typically attributed to an accompanying pulmonary contusion rather than to the flail segment.[75,96] When the flail segment is associated with penetrating trauma, holding pressure on the site of external bleeding is appropriate to minimize blood loss. IV fluid is rapidly given (20 mL/kg) to replace fluid volume and prevent shock.

Complications of penetrating injury include pneumonia, ARDS, sepsis, shock, and abdominal and vessel injury; the most serious complication is long-term closed-head injury.[75,96,97]

Poisoning

Poisoning is the exposure to a substance that results in toxicity.[76] Children younger than 4 years have the highest

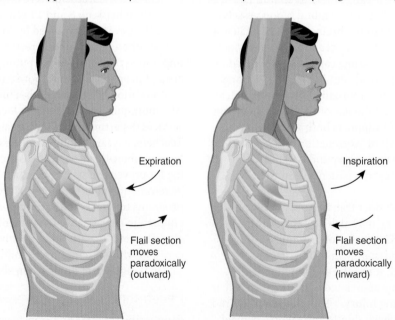

FIGURE 18-5 Schematic of a flail chest. The flail segment moves inward during inspiration and outward during exhalation.

rates of poisoning.[63] According to the Centers for Disease Control and Prevention, poisoning represents 5% of the accidental injury deaths among children.[61] Males are twice as likely as females to die from poisoning.[63]

Etiology

The poisoning can be either accidental or nonaccidental. Younger children are naturally curious, and they tend to taste or eat a majority of things they come in contact with. Poisoning from household chemicals or accidental ingestion of medication is a serious concern. In older children, such as adolescents, suicide is the third leading cause of death, and a large percentage of the suicides are from poisoning. White adolescent males have a higher incidence of suicide, whereas adolescent females have a higher rate of ingestion as the method of attempted suicide. Poisoning in this population can occur from ingestion of solids or liquids or inhalation of gases, such as carbon monoxide.[98]

Pathophysiology

Ingested toxins cause direct and indirect organ damage. When orally ingested, toxins may damage the tissue of the gastrointestinal tract and when metabolized can cause acute liver failure.[76]

Inhalation of gases disrupts tissue oxygenation and leads to hypoxia. Carbon monoxide competitively binds to hemoglobin to form carboxyhemoglobin, a nonfunctional type of hemoglobin that causes anemic hypoxia. Cyanide gas blocks the tissue-binding sites for oxygen, leading to histotoxic hypoxia. Neither gas will interfere with the partial pressure of oxygen in the arterial blood; instead, the oxygen-carrying capacity of RBCs and delivery of oxygen to the tissues are impaired. Depending on the agent, gas inhalation poisoning can be difficult to diagnose. Other toxic gases commonly associated with poisoning include phosgene, nitrogen oxides, and hydrogen chloride.[98]

Diagnosis

Diagnosis of poisoning can be difficult as there are a number of chemicals that have similar clinical presentations. A detailed recent history is a valuable diagnostic tool. If the patient is unable to offer a history, family members or friends should be asked to provide details of the circumstances that led them to seek medical care. Physical assessment includes obtaining vital signs; evaluation of pupil size and reactivity, skin color, and motor activity; and checking for skin marks and the presence of odors. Toxicology tests, CXR, electrocardiogram, and a blood co-oximetry test may be used to identify the causative agent.[99]

Clinical Presentation

Clinical symptoms depend on the substance and amount of toxicity produced by the substance ingested or inhaled. **Table 18-11** summarizes common toxins, presenting symptoms, and management.

Treatment

The primary step in management of a patient suspected of poisoning is to maintain a stable, patent airway and adequate tissue perfusion. Once the patient is stable from a cardiopulmonary standpoint, a care plan may be established. Gastric lavage, activated charcoal, bowel irrigation, and continuous renal replacement therapy may

TABLE 18-11
Common Poisons, Their Accompanying Clinical Presentation, and Management[76,98–100]

Substance	Clinical Presentation	Management
Carbon monoxide	Lethargy Headache Coma	High-dose oxygen
Cyanide gas	Lethargy Headache	Oxygen Amyl nitrite, hydroxocobalamin, sodium nitrite IV
Opioids	Lethargy Pinpoint pupils Respiratory depression	Naloxone
Ethylene glycol (antifreeze)	Altered mental status (inebriation)	Gastric aspiration
Ethanol (alcohol)	Altered mental status (inebriation)	Supportive, IV fluids
Hydrocarbons (lamp oil, gasoline)	Respiratory distress	Surfactant
Acetaminophen	Nonspecific	Acetylcysteine (Mucomyst) orally or via nasogastric tube
Antihistamine	Altered mental status Flushed skin Tachycardia Dilated pupils	Activated charcoal
Stimulants	Alertness Agitation Tachycardia Hypertension Dilated pupils	Sedatives

Data from Kaplan JL, Porter RS. *Merck Manual of Diagnosis and Therapy.* 19th ed. Whitehouse Station, NJ: Merck Sharp & Dohme; 2011; Shepherd G, Klein-Schwartz W. Accidental and suicidal adolescent poisoning deaths in the United States, 1979–1994. *Arch Pediatr Adolesc Med.* 1998;152:1181-1185; Dale DC, ed. *Infectious Diseases: The Clincian's Guide to Diagnosis, Treatment, and Prevention.* New York, NY: WebMD; 2003.; and Mastropietro C, Valentine K. Early administration of intratracheal surfactant (calfactant) after hydrocarbon aspiration. *Pediatrics.* 2011;127(6):e1600-e1604. doi:10.1542/peds.2010-3229.

be used for ingestions.[99] High-dose oxygen is the treatment of choice for carbon monoxide poisoning; hyperbaric oxygen, which increases the atmospheric pressure up to three atmospheres, has also been used with mixed reviews regarding efficacy.

Complications and outcomes depend on the substance and the amount ingested or inhaled. At high levels of toxicity, respiratory failure, liver failure, seizures, coma, or death may occur. At low levels, hypotension or hypertension may occur and require care in the ICU and a prolonged hospital stay.

Near Drowning

Near or unintentional drowning is ranked fifth among the leading causes of unintentional injury death in the United States.[101] One in five children younger than 14 years of age dies from near drowning.[102] Children aged 1 to 4 years and adolescents aged 15 to 19 years are at highest risk and have the highest mortality rate.[102,103] Adolescent males have increased risk-taking behaviors and are approximately four times more likely than females to have submersion injuries.[103]

Etiology

Drowning is defined as "the process of experiencing respiratory impairment from submersion/immersion in a liquid" and is classified as either fatal or nonfatal.[104] Such terms as wet, dry, passive, active, or secondary are no longer used to describe the injury.[104] Drowning can occur in lakes; oceans; rivers; swimming pools; open wells; bathtubs; or, for a small child, in only a few inches of water, such as a bucket, puddle, toilet, or other areas of shallow water. Worldwide, drowning is a leading cause of death among infants, children, and adolescents.[105] Pre-schoolers, 5 years of age or younger, are more likely to drown in bathtubs and pools as compared to teenagers, who are more likely to sustain submersion injury in open water, such as a lake or river.[106] Other risk factors that increase the likelihood of this type of injury include alcohol use and having an underlying seizure disorder:[107,108] Epilepsy increases an individual's risk of drowning by nearly 20% as compared to those without a seizure disorder.[109] A majority, approximately 80%, of drownings are preventable. Such actions as adult supervision while children are bathing or playing in or around water, fencing around pools, teaching children how to swim, responsible alcohol consumption during aquatic events, and lifeguard supervision are effective deterents.[110]

Pathophysiology

Once the victim is submerged and they no longer have access to oxygen in the atmosphere, hypoxia ensues. The typical drowning sequence starts with an immediate struggle as the victim's airway moves below the surface of the water. This progresses to a period where the victim may become motionless as they hold their breath and attempt to clear their nasopharynx by swallowing the water. Breath holding continues until the drive to breathe is too strong to resist and the victim inhales the fluid medium into their lungs and triggers a reflex cough or laryngospasm. The lack of access to oxygen and the fluid aspiration that occurs during a drowning event contribute to the development of hypoxia. Loss of consciousness immediately follows.[105,111] The drowning process, from submersion or immersion to loss of consciousness, lasts only a few minutes. If the victim is not rescued and the hypoxia reversed, death will occur.

Hypoxia affects every organ system and causes a spectrum of damage depending on the duration of the injury. Victims who are rescued quickly and sustain a brief hypoxic episode may have minimal consequences. Victims of a prolonged submersion often suffer cardiac arrest and irreversible brain damage.

Near-drowning victims require mechanical ventilatory support. The fluid aspirated into the lungs causes surfactant washout and increased permeability of the alveolar–capillary membrane. Surfactant-deficient alveoli are prone to collapse and atelectasis occurs. The increased permeability of the alveolar–capillary membrane causes noncardiogenic pulmonary edema and subsequent decreased gas exchange. ARDS occurs and is characterized by decreased lung compliance, ventilation/perfusion mismatch, hypercarbia, hypoxia, and respiratory acidosis.[105,111,112] Cerebral hypoxia causes global brain injury in the form of HIE, the extent of which is determined by the duration of hypoxia. Lack of oxygen to the neurons in the brain leads to cell damage and death. Cytotoxic cerebral edema develops, which, if severe enough, can cause increased ICP and decreased cerebral blood flow. Cerebral hypoxia and its effects are the primary cause of morbidity and mortality for drowning victims.

The hypoxia and sympathetic response causes the heart rate, **pulmonary vascular resistance**, and systemic vascular resistance to increase. As a result, myocardial work and oxygen consumption are increased. This stress response occurs as the body becomes progressively more hypoxemic, which will further compromise myocardial contractility and function. Victims are initially tachycardic and hypertensive but will become bradycardic and hypotensive as hypoxia worsens. Pulseless electrical activity typically precedes cardiac arrest.[110]

Diagnosis

Diagnosis of a submersion or immersion injury can be made with bystander-reported history. Drownings can be intentional or unintentional; therefore, it is essential to consider NAT, suicide, or homicide as the etiology of the submersion or immersion event.

Clinical Presentation

There is a broad spectrum of symptoms of a drowning injury, depending primarily on the length of submersion. A victim of a brief submersion may be asymptomatic, whereas a victim who sustained a prolonged submersion may present in cardiopulmonary arrest.

Neurologic manifestations of HIE can present as confusion, disorientation, seizures, altered mental status, evidence of intracranial hypertension, such as **Cushing's triad**, or coma. Respiratory manifestations include tachypnea, hypoxia, wheezing, increased work of breathing, pulmonary edema, crackles, blood-tinged secretions, and respiratory failure. Cardiac manifestations range from tachycardia, bradycardia, hypotension, and possible arrhythmias to cardiac arrest. Patients typically present with a mixed respiratory and metabolic acidosis.

Treatment

Victims who are rescued quickly have a brief period of hypoxia and may require few interventions. Alternatively, victims of a prolonged submersion may develop cardiac arrest and require cardiopulmonary resuscitation (CPR), intubation, and ventilatory support. The primary goals of management of a drowning victim are restoration of oxygenation and prevention of further hypoxia.

After the victim is rescued from the water, basic CPR should be initiated. Begin chest compressions if a pulse is not detected and rescue breathing if the child is apneic. Cervical spine immobilization should be implemented for suspected head or neck injury, such as a diving accident or a fall into water.

As with any trauma, management is initially focused on airway, breathing, and circulation, followed by a secondary survey to evaluate for further trauma. Not every drowning victim will require a hospital admission. A majority of victims are promptly rescued, aspirate only a small amount of water, and have a brief episode of hypoxia. These patients will likely be asymptomatic and will not require hospitalization.

Mild hypoxia can be managed with supplemental oxygen. Mechanical ventilation is required for patients with insufficient respiratory effort or profound oxygenation and ventilation defects. Circulation may be supported by fluid boluses and vasoactive medications. A nasogastric tube should be placed for gastric decompression as the victim likely swallowed water during the event, increasing the high risk for aspiration, especially if bag-mask ventilation is required. Arterial blood gases are useful in quantifying the severity of the ventilation and oxygenation defects.

Hospital management focuses on reversing hypoxia, preventing secondary injury, and supportive care. Ventilator management for drowning victims should follow ARDS or "open lung" strategies. Permissive hypercapnia is contraindicated for patients with cerebral insult and concern for intracranial hypertension because high CO_2 can worsen an elevated ICP. Additionally, steroids, bronchodilators, and prophylactic antibiotics are not included as standard management.[111] Antibiotic therapy should be considered when fever, persistent or new infiltrates on chest X-ray, organisms are identified on culture and sensitivity results from a tracheal aspirate, or leukocytosis develops.[105]

Neuroprotective strategies, such as maintaining $PaCO_2$ between 35 and 45 mm Hg, normothermia, normoglycemia, and avoiding hypotension, are essential for preventing secondary injury to the brain. Additionally, the head of the patient's bed should be elevated and their head kept in the midline position to enhance venous drainage. Clinical seizures should be treated with an antiepileptic agent.

Arrhythmias or cardiac arrest should be managed according to the Pediatric Advanced Life Support algorithm using CPR, defibrillation, and pharmacologic agents specific to the arrhythmia noted on the cardiac monitor. ECMO may be required when supplemental oxygen, mechanical ventilation, and vasoactive support fail to correct hypoxemia and disturbances in acid–base balance.

The length of submersion and duration of hypoxia are the most significant contributing factors to the victim's outcome.[113]

Case Study 1

A 23-month-old, 15.4 kg male child presented to the emergency department (ED) through triage with his mother. The mother stated that she noticed he had a fever that morning and he had not been eating well since the previous night. She indicated that her son vomited green fluid once that morning and was complaining that his stomach hurt. Once in the treatment room, the mother denied any past medical issues.

There were no known complications at birth, and she denied any drug use during pregnancy. The patient had no known allergies and was up to date on his required childhood immunizations but had not received a flu vaccination. Initial vital signs were as follows: heart rate 190 beats per minute, respiratory rate 40 breaths per minute, blood pressure 100/50 mm Hg, temperature 39.2°C, oxygen saturation 98% on room

(continues)

Case Study 1 (continued)

air, capillary refill less than 2 seconds. The child appeared toxic as evidenced by his poor response to interaction and listlessness. Upon further examination, the patient's skin was dry, dusky, and appeared ashen. He was unable to follow objects with his gaze, and his pupils were dilated with sluggish response to light. He did not produce tears. Lung sounds were clear and equal bilaterally, and no respiratory distress was noted. The patient's pulse was rapid, regular, and bounding. The complete blood cell count reported a white blood cell count of 4.5 x 103/mcL, with zero neutrophils both segmented and absolute. His hemoglobin was 12.0 g/dL, his hematocrit was 39%, and he had an elevated lymphocyte count of 89%. A rapid influenza screen was positive for influenza A.

1. **What is your initial impression of this patient?**

The vital signs were stable for the next 15 minutes, then he vomited bilious fluid and his heart rate decreased to less than 60 beats per minute while his blood pressure became undetectable and his breathing was agonal. CPR was begun, the patient was placed on a monitor/defibrillator with pediatric pads, and a size 4.0 endotracheal tube was placed by the ED physician. After 3 minutes, the patient's heart rate and blood pressure were normalized, and the patient was transferred to the ICU.

2. **What is the diagnosis?**

3. **What is your recommended treatment plan?**

Case Study 2

You have just arrived for your 7AM shift on a cold February morning when an unresponsive 21-month-old girl is brought in by emergency medical services. On arrival to the ED, she is noted to be lethargic and flaccid. She is immediately placed on a cardiorespiratory monitor and the following vital signs are obtained: heart rate 160 beats per minute, respiratory rate 36 breaths per minute, blood pressure 85/58 mm Hg, temperature 37.8°C, oxygen saturation 100% on facemask oxygen. On physical examination, she has sluggish opening of her eyes to voice. She moans and localizes to pain, and her skin is pale. She is not apneic or cyanotic. Other than her altered level of consciousness, the rest of her physical examination is normal. She is managing her airway appropriately. Emergency medical services reports that they checked her serum glucose and it was normal. Her mother arrives 20 minutes later and states that the child was

previously healthy, and she was in her normal state of health when she placed her in the crib at bedtime. The mother says she went to check on her daughter this morning when she did not wake at her normal time and found her unresponsive. She has not had any fevers, upper respiratory symptoms, diarrhea, or rashes. There is no history of trauma, and the child has been in the care of her mother. The mother also stated that she needed to use a space heater because the weather has been so cold out. She also stated that she has not been feeling well, with headache and nausea upon waking this morning.

1. **Based on your assessment, what diagnosis would you suspect?**

2. **What key lab value would identify differential diagnosis?**

3. **What is the main treatment for this patient?**

References

1. Bernard G, Artigas A, Brigham K, et al. The American-European Consensus Conference on ARDS. Definitions, mechanisms, relevant outcomes, and clinical trial coordination. *Am J Respir Crit Care Med*. 1994;149(3):818-824.

2. Ventre K, Arnold J. Acute lung injury and acute respiratory distress syndrome. In: Helfaer M, Nichols D, eds. *Rogers' Handbook of Pediatric Intensive Care*. 4th ed. Philadelphia, PA: Wolters Kluwer; 2009:201-207.

3. Randolph A. Management of acute lung injury and acute respiratory distress syndrome in children. *Crit Care Med*. 2009;37(8):2448-2454.

4. Ware M, Matthay M. The acute respiratory distress syndrome. *N Engl J Med*. 2000;342(18):1334-1349.

5. Ware L. Pathophysiology of acute lung injury and the acute respiratory distress syndrome. *Semin Respir Crit Care Med*. 2006;27(4): 337-349.

6. Piastra M, De Luca D, Pietrini et al. Noninvasive pressure-support ventilation in immunocompromised children with ARDS: a feasibility study. *Intensive Care Med*. 2009;35(8):1420-1427.

7. Rimensberger PC, Cheifetz IM. Ventilatory support in children with pediatric acute respiratory distress syndrome. Proceedings from the Pediatric Acute Ling Injury Consensus Conference. *Pediatr Crit Care Med*. 2015;16(5):S51-S60.

8. Ventilation with lower tidal volumes as compared with traditional tidal volumes for acute lung injury and the acute respiratory distress syndrome. The Acute Respiratory Distress Syndrome Network. *N Engl J Med.* 2000;342:1301-1308.

9. Ferguson N, Cook D, Gordon G, et al. High-frequency oscillation in early acute respiratory distress syndrome. *N Engl J Med.* 2013;368:795-805.

10. Guérin C, Reignier J, Richard JC, et al. Prone positioning in severe acute respiratory distress syndrome. *N Engl J Med.* 2013;368:2159-2168.

11. Wiedemann H, Wheeler A, Bernard G, et al. Comparison of two fluid-management strategies in acute lung injury. *N Engl J Med.* 2006;354:2564-2575.

12. Duffett M, Choong K, Ng V, et al. Surfactant therapy for acute respiratory failure in children: a systematic review and meta-analysis. *Crit Care.* 2007;11:R66.

13. Adhikar N, Burns K, Friedrich J, et al. Effect of nitric oxide on oxygenation and mortality in acute lung injury: systematic review and meta-analysis. *BMJ.* 2007;334:779.

14. Peter J, John P, Graham P, et al. Corticosteroids in the prevention and treatment of acute respiratory distress syndrome (ARDS) in adults: meta-analysis. *BMJ.* 2008;336:1006-1009.

15. Santhanam S. Pediatric sepsis. Medscape Website. http://emedicine.medscape.com/article/972559-overview. Updated September 29, 2015. Accessed October 12, 2015.

16. Zehava NL. The history of sepsis management over the last 30 years. *Clin Pediatr Emerg Med.* 2014;15(2):116-119.

17. Dellinger RP, Levy MM, Rhodes A, et al. Surviving sepsis campaign. *Crit Care Med.* 2013;41(2):580-637.

18. Hartman ME, Linde-Zwirble WT, Angus DC, Watson RS. Trends in the epidemiology of pediatric severe sepsis. *Pediatr Crit Care Med.* 2013;14(7):686-693.

19. Simmons ML, Durham SH, Carter CW. Pharmacological management of pediatric patients with sepsis. *AACN Adv Crit Care.* 2012;23(4):437-448; quiz 449-450.

20. Sagy M, Al-Qaqaa Y, Kim P. Definitions and pathophysiology of sepsis. *Curr Probl Pediatr Adolesc Health Care.* 2013;43(10):260-263. doi:10.1016/j.cppeds.2013.10.001.

21. Goldstein B, Giroir B, Randolph A. International pediatric sepsis consensus conference: definitions for sepsis and organ dysfunction in pediatrics. *Pediatr Criti Care Med.* 2005;6(1):2-8.

22. Kaplan LJ. Systemic inflammatory response syndrome. Medscape Website. http://emedicine.medscape.com/article/168943-overview. Updated March 30, 2015. Accessed October 12, 2015.

23. Rivers E, Nguyen B, Havstad S, et al. Early goal-directed therapy in the treatment of severe sepsis and septic shock. *N Engl J Med.* 2001;345(19):1368-1377.

24. Kumar A, Roberts D, Wood KE, et al. Duration of hypotension before initiation of effective antimicrobial therapy is the critical determinant of survival in human septic shock. *Crit Care Med.* 2006;34(6):1589-1596.

25. Zawistowski CA. The management of sepsis. *Curr Probl Pediar and Adol Health Care.* 2013;43(10):285-291.

26. Brierley J, Carcillo JA, Choong K, et al. Clinical practice parameters for hemodynamic support of pediatric and neonatal septic shock: 2007 update from the American College of Critical Care Medicine. *Crit Care Med.* 2009;37(2):666-688.

27. Watson RS, Carcillo JA, Linde-Zwirble WT, Clermont G, Lidicker J, Angus DC. The epidemiology of severe sepsis in children in the United States. *Am J Respir Crit Care Med.* 2003;167(5):695-701.

28. Skinner SC, Iocono JA, Ballard HO, et al. Improved survival in venovenous vs venoarterial extracorporeal membrane oxygenation for pediatric noncardiac sepsis patients: a study of the Extracorporeal Life Support Organization registry. *J Pediatr Surg.* 2012;47(1):63-67.

29. Pasman EA. Shock in pediatrics. Medscape Website. http://emedicine.medscape.com/article/1833578-overview. Updated March 30, 2015. Accessed October 12, 2015.

30. Hay WW Jr, Hayward AR, Levin MJ, Sondheimer JM. In: Hay WW, Hayward AR, Levin MJ, Sondheimer JM, eds. *Current Pediatric Diagnosis & Treatment.* (15th ed.). New York, NY: Lange Medical Books/McGraw-Hill; 1999:680-681.

31. Lieberman P, Camargo CA, Bohlke K, et al. Epidemiology of anaphylaxis: findings of the American College of Allergy, Asthma and Immunology Epidemiology of Anaphylaxis Working Group. *Ann Allergy Asthma Immunol.* 2006;97(5):596-602.

32. Sagy M, Al-Qaqaa Y, Kim P. Definitions and pathophysiology of sepsis. *Curr Probl Pediar Adolesc Health Care.* 2013;43(10):260-263.

33. Raimer PL, Han YY, Weber MS, Annich GM, Custer JR. A normal capillary refill time of $\leq$ 2 seconds is associated with superior vena cava oxygen saturations of $\geq$ 70%. *J Pediatr.* 2011;158(6):968-972.

34. Meningitis. Centers for Disease Control and Prevention Website. http://www.cdc.gov/meningitis/bacterial.html. Updated April 1, 2014. Accessed August 27, 2015.

35. Spanos A, Harrell FE Jr, Durack DT. Differential diagnosis of acute meningitis: an analysis of the predictive value of initial observations. *JAMA.* 1989;262:2700-2707.

36. Bonsu BK, Harper MB. Differentiating acute bacterial meningitis from acute viral meningitis among children with cerebrospinal fluid pleocytosis: a multivariable regression model. *Pediatr Infect Dis J.* 2004;23:511-517.

37. Nigrovic LE, Fine AM, Monuteaux MC, Shah, SS, Neuman MI. Trends in the management of viral meningitis at United States children's hospitals. *Pediatrics.* 2013;131(4):670-676. doi:10.1542/peds.2012-3077.

38. Thigpen MC, Whitney CG, Messonnier NE, et al. Bacterial meningitis in the United States, 1998–2007. *N Engl J Med.* 2011;364(21):2016-2025. doi:10.1056/NEJMoa1005384.

39. Kriel RL, Krach LE, Luxenber MG, Jones-Saete C, Sanchez J. Outcome of severe anoxic/ischemic brain injury in children. *Neurology.* 1994;10(3):207-212.

40. Clarke DD, Sokoloff L. Regulation of cerebral metabolic rate. In: Siegel GJ, Agranoff BW, Albers RW, et al., eds. *Basic Neurochemistry: Molecular, Cellular and Medical Aspects.* 6th ed. Philadelphia, PA: Lippincott-Raven; 1999.

41. Kennedy C, Sokoloff L. An adaptation of the nitrous oxide method to the study of the cerebral circulation in children; normal values for cerebral blood flow and cerebral metabolic rate in childhood. *J. Clin. Invest.* 1957;36:1130-1137.

42. Grande CF. Energy metabolism of the brain in children. *An Esp Pediatr.* 1979;12(3):235-244.

43. Zanelli SA, Kaugman DA. Hypoxic-ischemic encephalopathy clinical presentation. Medscape Website. http://emedicine.medscape.com/article/973501-overview#a5. Updated January 16, 2015. Accessed August 29, 2015.

44. Battin M. Newborn services clinical guideline: neonatal encephalopathy. http://www.adhb.govt.nz/newborn/Guidelines/Neurology/NE.htm. Accessed August 31, 2015.

45. Lane Medical Library: Stanford Medical. Neurological assessment. http://lane.stanford.edu/portals/cvicu/HCP_Neuro_Tab_4/Neuro_Assessment.pdf. Accessed August 29, 2015.

46. Allen KA, Brandon DH. Hypoxic ischemic encephalopathy: pathophysiology and experimental treatments. *Newborn Infant Nurs Rev.* 2011;11(3):125-133. doi:10.1053/j.nainr.2011.07.004.

47. Shah PS. Review hypothermia: a systematic review and meta-analysis of clinical trials. *Semin Fetal Neonatal Med.* 2010;15(5):238-246.

48. Fakhry SM, Trask AL, Waller MA, Watts DD. Management of brain-injured patients by an evidence-based medicine protocol improves outcomes and decreases hospital charges. *J Trauma.* 2004;56(3):492-499; discussion 499-500.

49. Ray M. *Hypoxia Ischemic Encephalopathy. Treatment and Prognosis in Pediatrics.* 1st ed. Kathmandu, Nepal: Jaypee Brothers Medical Publishers; 2013.

50. Graham EM, Ruis KA, Hartman AL, Northington FJ, Fox HE. A systematic review of the role of intrapartum hypoxia-ischemia in the causation of neonatal encephalopathy. *Am J Obstet Gynecol.* 2008;199(6):587-595.

51. Vannucci RC, Perlman JM. Interventions for perinatal hypoxic-ischemic encephalopathy. *Pediatrics.* 1997;100(6):1004-1014.

52. Centers for Disease Control and Prevention. Traumatic brain injury in the United States: assessing outcomes in children. http://www.cdc.gov/traumaticbraininjury/assessing_outcomes_in_children.html#2. Accessed August 31, 2015.

53. National Center for Injury Prevention and Control, Centers for Disease Control and Prevention. WISQARS, 2010. http://webappa.cdc.gov/cgi-bin/broker.exe. Accessed August 23, 2015.

54. Centers for Disease Control and Prevention. Protect the ones you love: child injuries are preventable, 2012. http://www.cdc.gov/safechild/NAP/background.html. Accessed August 23, 2015.

55. Saki N, Nikakhlagh S, Rahim F, Abshirini H. Foreign body aspirations in infancy: a 20-year experience. *Int J Med Sci.* 2009;6(6):322-328. doi:10.7150/ijms.6.322.

56. Bittencourt PF, Camargos PA, Scheinmann P, de Blic J. Foreign body aspiration: clinical, radiological findings and factors associated with its late removal. *Int J Pediatr Otorhinolaryngol.* 2006;70(5):879-884.

57. Wiseman NE. The diagnosis of foreign body aspiration in childhood. *J Pediatr.* 1984;19(5):531-535.

58. Karakoç F, Karadağ B, Akbenlioğlu C, et al. Foreign body aspiration: what is the outcome? *Pediatr Pulm.* 2002;34(1):30-36. doi:10.1002/ppul.10094.

59. Concepcion E, Bye MR. Pediatric airway foreign body. Medscape Website. http://emedicine.medscape.com/article/1001253-overview#a5. Accessed October 14, 2015.

60. Warshawsky ME. Foreign body aspiration treatment & management. Medscape Website. http://emedicine.medscape.com/article/298940-treatment. Updated November 20, 2013. Accessed August 23, 2015.

61. Chung MK, Jeong HS, Ahn KM, et al. Pulmonary recovery after rigid bronchoscopic retrieval of airway foreign body. *Laryngoscope.* 2007;117(2):303-307.

62. National Center for Injury Prevention and Control, Centers for Disease Control and Prevention. WISQARS, 2013. http://webappa.cdc.gov/cgi-bin/broker.exe. Accessed August 23, 2015.

63. Borse NN, Gilchrist J, Dellinger AM, Rudd RA, Ballesteros MF, Sleet DA. *CDC Childhood Injury Report: Patterns of Unintentional Injuries among 0–19 Year Olds in the United States, 2000–2006.* Atlanta, GA: Centers for Disease Control and Prevention, National Center for Injury Prevention and Control; 2008.

64. Ten leading causes of death and injury. Centers for Disease Control and Prevention Website. http://www.cdc.gov/injury/wisqars/leadingcauses.html. Updated March 31, 2015. Accessed August 23, 2015.

65. Cunningham RM, Carter PM, Ranney M, et al. Violent reinjury and mortality among youth seeking emergency department care for assault-related injury: a 2-year prospective cohort study. *JAMA Pediatr.* 2015;169(1):63-70. doi:10.1001/jamapediatrics.2014.1900.

66. A national action plan for child injury prevention. Centers for Disease Control and Prevention Website. http://www.cdc.gov/safechild/NAP/. Updated June 17, 2015. Accessed August 15, 2015.

67. Gardner R, Smith G, Chany A, Fernandez S, McKenzie L. Factors associated with hospital length of stay and hospital charges of motor vehicle crash-related. *Arch Pediatr Adolesc Med.* 2007;161(9):889-895. doi:10.1001/archpedi.161.9.889.

68. Refaat H. *National Highway Traffic Safety Administration. Children Injured in Motor Vehicle Traffic Crashes.* Published by U.S. Department of Transportation, National Highway Traffic Safety Administration. May 2010. http://www-nrd.nhtsa.dot.gov/Pubs/811325.pdf. Accessed August 15, 2015.

69. U.S. Department of Health and Human Services, Administration for Children and Families, Administration on Children, Youth and Families, Children's Bureau. *Child Maltreatment 2013.* http://www.acf.hhs.gov/programs/cb/research-data-technology/statistics-research/child-maltreatment. Accessed August 15, 2015.

70. Shiau T, Levin A. Retinal hemorrhages in children: the role of intracranial pressure. *Arch. Pediatr Adoles Med.* 2012;166(7):623-628. doi:10:1001/archpediatrics.2016.46.

71. DiScala C, Sege R, Li G, Reece R. Child abuse and unintentional injuries: a 10 year retrospective. *Arch Pediatr Adolesc Med.* 2000;154:16-22.

72. Sharma O, Oswanski M, Stringfellow K, Raj S. Pediatric blunt trauma: a retrospective analysis in a level I trauma center. *Am Surg.* 2006;72:538-543.

73. Lo W, Lee J, Rusin J, Perkins E, Roach ES. Intracranial hemorrhage in children: an evolving spectrum. *Arch Neurol.* 2008;65 (12):1629-1633.

74. Bennett T, Riva-Cambrin J, Keenan H, Korgenski EK, Bratton S. Variation in intracranial pressure monitoring and outcomes in pediatric traumatic brain injury. *Arch Pediatr Adolesc Med.* 2012;166(7):641-647.

75. Vana G, Neubauer D, Luchette, F. Contemporary management of flail chest. *Am Surg.* 2014;80:527-535.

76. Kaplan JL, Porter RS. *Merck Manual of Diagnosis and Therapy.* 19th ed. Whitehouse Station, NJ: Merck Sharp & Dohme; 2011.

77. Rozzelle CJ, Aarabi B, Dhall SS, et al. Management of pediatric cervical spine and spinal cord injuries. In: Guidelines for the management of acute cervical spine and spinal cord injuries. *Neurosurgery.* 2013;72(2):205-226.

78. Nigrovic L, Lee L, Hoyle J, et al. Prevalence of clinically important traumatic brain injuries in children with minor blunt head trauma and isolated severe injury mechanism. *Arch Pediatr Adolesc Med.* 2012;166(4):356-361. doi:101001/archpediatrics.2011.1156.

79. Lichenstein R, Glass T, Quayle K, et al. Presentations and outcomes of children with intraventricular hemorrhages after blunt head trauma. *Arch Pediatr Adolesc Med.* 2012;166(8);725-731. doi:10.1001/archpediatrics.2011.1919.

80. Hess D, MacIntyre N, Galvin W, Mishoe S. *Respiratory Care Principles and Practice.* 3rd ed. Burlington, MA: Jones & Bartlett Learning; 2016.

81. American Heart Association. *Advanced Cardiovascular Life Support Provider Manual.* Dallas, TX: American Heart Association; 2011.

82. Mayfield S, Jauncey-Cooke J, Hough, J, Schilbler A, Gibbons K, Bogossian F. High-flow nasal cannula therapy for respiratory support in children. *Cochrane Database Syst Rev.* 2014;3:CD009850. doi:10.1002/14651858.CD009850.pub2.

83. Frat J, Thille A, Mercat, et al. High-flow oxygen through nasal cannula in acute hypoxemic respiratory failure. *N Engl J Med.* 2015;372(23):2185-2196.

84. National Institutes of Health, ARDS Network. Ventilation with lower tidal volumes as compared with traditional tidal volumes for acute lung injury and the acute respiratory distress syndrome. *N Engl J Med.* 2000;342:1301-1308.

85. Khemani RG, Markovitz BP, Curley MAQ. Characteristics of children intubated and mechanically ventilated in 16 PICUs. *Chest.* 2009;136(3):765-771. doi:10.1378/chest.09-0207.

86. Bembea M, Almuqati R, Haider A, Haur E. Extracorporeal membrane oxygenation use in trauma patients: a report from the national trauma bank. *Pediatr Crit Care Med.* 2014;15(4).

87. Hassan N, DeCou J, Reischman D, et al. RBC transfusions in children requiring intensive care admission after traumatic injury. *Pediatr Crit Care Med.* 2014;15(7):306-313. doi:10.1097/PCC.0000000000000192.

88. Mohn-Brown EL, Burke KM, Eby L. *Medical-Surgical Nursing Care.* 4th ed. Upper Saddle River, NJ: Pearson Education; 2016.

89. Haxhija Q, Nores H, Schober P, Hollwarth M. Lung contusion-lacerations after blunt trauma in children. *Pediatr Surg Int.* 2004;20:412-414. doi:10.1007/s00383-004-1165-z.

90. Odetola F, Mann C, Hansen K, Patrick S, Bratton S. Source of admission and outcomes for critically injured children in the mountain states. *Arch Pediatr Adolesc Med.* 2010;164(3):277-282.

91. Sills M, Libby A, Orton H. Prehospital and in-hospital mortality: a comparison of intentional and unintentional traumatic brain injuries in Colorado children. *Arch Pediatr Adolesc Med.* 2005;159:665-670.

92. Reece R, Sege R. Childhood head injuries: accidental or inflicted? *Arch Pediatr Adolesc Med.* 2000;154:11-15.

93. U.S. Department of Health and Human Services. *Healthy People 2020*. https://www.healthypeople.gov/.

94. Wanek S, Mayberry JC. Blunt thoracic trauma: flail chest, pulmonary contusion and blast injury. *Crit Care Clin*. 2004;20(1):71-81.

95. Battle CE, Evans PA. Predictors of mortality in patients with flail chest: a systemic review. *Emerg Med J*. 2015;32(12):961-965.

96. Cannon R, Smith J, Franklin G, Harbrecht B, Miller F, Richardson J. Flail chest injury: are we making any progress? *Am Surg*. 2012;78(4):398-402.

97. Trinkle JK, Richardson JD, Franz JL, et al. Management of flail chest without mechanical ventilation. *Ann Thorac Surg*. 1975;19:355-363.

98. Shepherd G, Klein-Schwartz W. Accidental and suicidal adolescent poisoning deaths in the United States, 1979–1994. *Arch Pediatr Adolesc Med*. 1998;152:1181-1185.

99. Dale DC, ed. *Infectious Diseases: The Clincian's Guide to Diagnosis, Treatment, and Prevention*. New York, NY: WebMD; 2003.

100. Mastropietro C, Valentine K. Early administration of intratracheal surfactant (calfactant) after hydrocarbon aspiration. *Pediatrics*. 2011;127(6):e1600-e1604. doi:10.1542/peds.2010-3229.

101. Web-based injury statistics query and reporting system (WISQARS). Centers for Disease Control and Prevention, National Center for Injury Prevention and Control Website. http://www.cdc.gov/injury/wisqars. Accessed October 5, 2015.

102. Laosee OC, Gilchrist J, Rudd R. Drowning 2005–2009. *MMWR*. 2012;61(19):344-347.

103. Cantwell GP. Drowning. Medscape Website. http://emedicine.medscape.com/article/772753-overview. Updated September 25, 2015. Accessed October 14, 2015.

104. Van Beeck EF, Branche CM, Szpilman D, Modell JH, Bierens JJLM. A new definition of drowning: towards documentation and prevention of a global public health problem. *Bull World Health Organ*. 2005;83(11):853-856.

105. Moon RE, Long RJ. Drowning and near-drowning. *Emer Med*. 2002;14(4):377-386.

106. Quan L, Gore EJ, Wentz K, Allen J, Novack AH. Ten-year study of pediatric drownings and near-drownings in King County, Washington: lessons in injury prevention. *Pediatrics*. 1989;83(6):1035-1040.

107. American Academy of Pediatrics Committee on Injury, Violence, and Poison Prevention. Prevention of drowning. *Pediatrics*. 2010;126(1):178-185. http://doi.org/10.1542/peds.2010-1264.

108. Peden MM. World report on child injury prevention. World Health Organization. Published 2008. http://www.who.int/violence_injury_prevention/child/injury/world_report/en/. Accessed August 154, 2015.

109. Bell GS, Gaitatzis A, Bell CL, Johnson AL, Sander JW. Drowning in people with epilepsy: how great is the risk? *Neurology*. 2008;71(8):578-582.

110. Bierens JJLM, Knape JTA, Gelissen HPMM. Drowning. *Curr Opin Crit Care*. 2002;8(6):578-586.

111. Szpilman D, Bierens JJLM, Handley AJ, Orlowski JP. Drowning. *N Eng J Med*. 2012;366(22):2102-2110. http://doi.org/10.1056/NEJMra1013317.

112. Lord SR, Davis PR. Drowning, near drowning and immersion syndrome. *J Royal Army Med Corps*. 2005;151(4):250-255.

113. Suominen P, Baillie C, Korpela R, Rautanen S, Ranta S, Olkkola KT. Impact of age, submersion time and water temperature on outcome in near-drowning. *Resuscitation*. 2002;52(3):247-254.

19
Cardiopulmonary Monitoring

Kellianne Flemming
Teresa A. Volsko

OUTLINE

OBJECTIVES

1. Explain the uses and limitations of noninvasive cardiorespiratory monitoring in infants and children.
2. Describe the rationale for assessing pre- and postductal oxygen saturations.
3. Differentiate between mainstream and sidestream capnometers.
4. Describe the value of capnometry as an adjunct to cardiorespiratory monitoring in mechanically ventilated infants and children.
5. List the factors or conditions that can limit the accuracy of transcutaneous O_2 and CO_2 monitoring.
6. List the techniques used to reduce false alarms and to improve the accuracy of monitoring by impedance pneumography.
7. Describe the clinical conditions in which near infrared spectroscopy may be used in lieu of pulse oximetry.
8. Describe the procedure for percutaneous arterial blood sampling.
9. List the sampling sites commonly used to perform an arterial puncture.
10. List the sites used for capillary blood gas sampling.
11. List the indications for arterial and capillary blood gas sampling.
12. Describe the importance of caring for arterial and capillary blood gas samples prior to analysis.
13. List the sites used for artery cannulation in infants and children.
14. Calculate mean blood pressure.
15. Describe the uses for inline blood gas monitoring.
16. Explain the methods used for central venous catheter insertion.
17. List the indications for central venous and pulmonary artery catheter insertion.
18. List the normal values for hemodynamic parameters.
19. Describe the hemodynamic values that can be derived from pulmonary artery catheter monitoring.

KEY TERMS

arterial blood gas analysis
arterial catheters
capillary blood gas
capnography
capnometry
central venous catheter
cut-down procedure
Dunn formula
impedance pneumography
mean blood pressure (MAP)
modified Allen's test
near infrared
    spectroscopy (NIRS)
peripheral artery catheter
peripherally inserted
    central catheter (PICC)
photoplethysmography
pulmonary artery catheters
pulse contour analysis
pulse oximetry
spectrophotometry
transcutaneous carbon
    dioxide tension ($PtcCO_2$)
transcutaneous oxygen
    tension ($PtcO_2$)
transilluminating light
umbilical artery
    catheter (UAC)
umbilical venous
    catheter (UVC)

Introduction

Cardiopulmonary monitoring is used to evaluate and quickly identify conditions requiring therapeutic intervention. Monitoring involves the interpretation of numeric values and waveforms associated with various noninvasive and invasive monitoring devices. Noninvasive monitoring of oxygenation and ventilation status is important to the care of critically ill children. Noninvasive monitoring of oxygen saturation, transcutaneous oxygen and carbon dioxide tensions, as well as end-tidal carbon dioxide, minimize the need for repeated blood gas analysis. This in turn reduces blood loss, which is extremely important in fragile, very low birthweight, or premature infants. This chapter will describe the operational concepts, patient application, indications for use, limitations and hazards, waveform analysis, and factors affecting accuracy of noninvasive and invasive devices used to monitor the cardiorespiratory status of infants and children.

Noninvasive Monitoring

Monitoring oxygenation and adequacy of gas exchange is an important component of care for children receiving some form of respiratory support. There are a variety of noninvasive monitors available for use. It is essential for the clinician to understand the factors associated with the use of noninvasive monitors. This section will review the types of noninvasive monitors commonly used to evaluate an infant's and child's response to therapeutic intervention.

Pulse Oximetry

Pulse oximetry is widely used to noninvasively monitor oxygenation status and to provide objective data to guide care. These devices are relatively inexpensive and routinely used across the continuum of care, such as in the neonatal and pediatric intensive care units, in outpatient clinics, and in extended care and homecare settings. Pulse oximetry provides continuous, instantaneous monitoring of heart rate and hemoglobin oxygen saturation, reported as SpO_2.

Operational Concepts

These devices determine SpO_2 using **spectrophotometry** and photoplethysmography.[1,2] Spectrophotometry is based on the Beer-Lambert law, which states that every substance has its own pattern of light absorption. Pulse oximeters use two light wavelengths (red and infrared) in the spectrophotometric analysis. SpO_2 values reflect the amount of light absorbed as the two wavelengths pass through a vascularized site and will vary depending on the presence or amount of oxygenated blood. Oxygenated blood absorbs less red light (600–750 nm) and more infrared light (850–1000 nm) than deoxygenated blood. **Photoplethysmography** uses light to analyze variations in volume changes in tissue during pulsatile blood flow to distinguish between arterial and venous blood flow. Although pulse oximetry correlates closely to arterial blood's oxygen saturation, it should never be misinterpreted as an actual arterial blood oxygen saturation (SaO_2) and should be correlated with an arterial blood gas.[3,4]

Patient Application

The pulse oximeter consists of a sensor, commonly referred to as a probe; a processor; and a display unit. The probe has two sides. One side contains independent LED light sources, one red and the other infrared. The opposite side houses the photodetector. The light sources and photodetector must be lined up over a perfused area, such as the nail bed or area of tissue that allows the light sources to pass through (**Figure 19-1**). The detected wavelengths of light create signals that are sent to a microprocessor for amplification, resulting in the pulsatile waveform display and corresponding SpO_2.[3] **Figure 19-2** shows the different types of probes used with a pulse oximeter in infants and children.

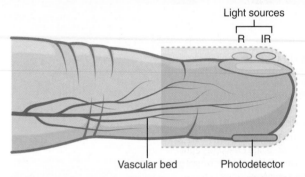

FIGURE 19-1 An example of the pulse oximeter sensor. This illustration demonstrates the correct alignment of the photo detectors.

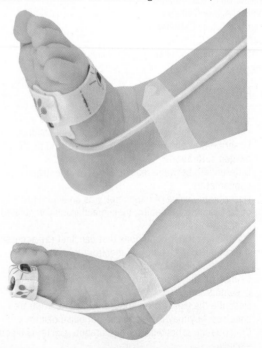

FIGURE 19-2 Pulse oximeter probes can be wrapped around a digit on the hand or foot or positioned on the wrist, hand, or foot.
Courtesy of Nonin.

Clinical Considerations in Neonates

Prior to the use of pulse oximetry, it was common for the clinical team to assess an infant's color in order to determine if tissue oxygenation was adequate. However, this practice has fallen out of favor and is not routinely used because color is a poor indicator of tissue oxygenation. The literature reports that wide variations in SpO_2, from 10% to 100%, were observed in infants perceived to be pink.[5,6]

Shortly after birth, as newborns transition to extrauterine life, pulse oximetry is beneficial in guiding oxygen management. Current recommendations in the literature are to achieve a target SpO_2 range of 85% to 90% at 3 minutes of life.[6] Sensors can be applied and a monitored value obtained in as quickly as 15 seconds, achieving reliable SpO_2 readings within the first minute of life.[6] After transition to extrauterine life is complete, it is expected that full-term infants maintain an SpO_2 range of 93% to 100%.[7]

Some infants need further care in the neonatal intensive care unit (NICU) for respiratory insufficiency due to respiratory distress syndrome (RDS), meconium aspiration, or congenital anomalies, such as diaphragmatic hernia or congenital heart defects. In the NICU, oxygen saturation monitoring by pulse oximetry is a standard of care and is often reported as the fifth vital sign. Oximetry is especially valuable in the care of infants with congenital heart defects to ensure that saturations remain in the prescribed range appropriate for the defect. Recently, pulse oximetry has been recommended (and mandated in some states) for newborn screening of congenital heart disease (CHD). Screening is recommended to take place between 24 and 48 hours of life and consists of placing a sensor on the right hand or arm and either foot to determine if there are pre- and postductal differences in SpO_2. If pre- and postductal saturations are less than 95% when measured in a quiet newborn, or if there is greater than a 3% difference in pre- and postductal saturations, the test is reported as "positive." Infants with positive results require a complete cardiac evaluation to determine the type, presence, and severity of the CHD.[8,9]

When first initiating the use of oximetry in preterm infants, sensors were commonly placed on the mid- or forefoot. Studies have shown that the fastest and most reliable SpO_2 readings have been measured using the right hand because this extremity has a higher blood pressure, is well perfused, and represents the preductal oxygenation status during the first several minutes of life.[10,11] There are many factors that affect the accuracy of pulse oximetry in the neonate that clinicians should be aware of, as they can contribute to inaccurate readings. Vernix, poor perfusion, tissue edema, bright ambient light, poor skin integrity, and acrocyanosis reduce measurement accuracy.[12,13] Practitioners caring for patients with continuous oximetry must be aware that sensors have been associated with light burns at the probe or sensor site and hospital-acquired pressure ulcers. Preterm infants are most at risk, due to the reduced integrity (thin and fragile) of their skin. Therefore, the location of the sensor should be routinely rotated as specified by organizational or hospital policy.

Clinical Considerations in the Pediatric Patient

Pulse oximetry also varies throughout the day in children. Saturations are lowest in the morning and highest in the late afternoon. Studies have shown that altitude affects oxygenation and contributes to variations in SpO_2, with mean values ranging from 97% to 99% in healthy children at sea level and lower readings (i.e., 93–95%) at higher elevations.[14]

Pulse oximetry is a standard of care in children. Oxygen saturations are typically monitored when disease processes, such as asthma, pneumonia, and bronchiolitis, contribute to ventilation/perfusion mismatch. Pulse oximetry is not a reliable indicator of ventilation. Hypoxemia may occur in the presence of laryngeal or tracheal obstruction, vocal cord dysfunction, or foreign body aspiration, but it is a secondary outcome due to hypoventilation.

Limitations

Most pulse oximeters are unable to distinguish between hemoglobin that is saturated with oxygen with that saturated with carbon monoxide because oxygen and carbon monoxide have similar light absorption qualities.[15] It is important to recognize the limitations of the pulse oximeter that is in use. Assuming that all pulse oximeters can differentiate between carboxyhemoglobin saturation and oxygen saturation can be a safety concern. Pulse oximeters without the specific technology to differentiate between oxygen and carbon monoxide will display an SpO_2 of 100% for hemoglobin that is fully saturated, whether it is saturated with oxygen or carbon monoxide. Therefore, patients suspected of carbon monoxide inhalation should have a blood gas analysis by hemoximetry to verify tissue oxygenation.

Fetal hemoglobin and hemoglobin S, commonly found in patients with sickle cell anemia, do not affect the reliability of pulse oximetry. However, practitioners should be aware that the measured SpO_2 may not accurately reflect tissue oxygenation due to cardiac output and shifts in the oxygen dissociation curve.[1,2]

Sensor positioning plays an important role in ensuring that the values displayed on the oximeter are accurate. Similar to placement in infants, sensors used with children are most commonly placed on the fingers and toes or around the hands and feet. When perfusion is poor, placing the sensor centrally, such as on the earlobe, may improve the accuracy of the SpO_2 reading. Reluctant sensors are useful for patients with extremity or digit deformities, those with active seizures, and/or patients with burns. Accuracy can also be affected by motion artifact, bright ambient light, skin pigmentation, colored nail polish, and intravenous dyes.[16,17]

Capnometry and Capnography

Capnometry and capnography are noninvasive measurements of the partial pressure of CO_2 at the end of a tidal breath and reflect a patient's ventilation metabolism, circulation, and ventilation status.[18]

Operational Concepts

Capnometry is a digital, numeric measurement of CO_2 at the end of a tidal breath while **capnography** is the graphical representation of ventilation. Most capnographs have the ability to display a breath-to-breath waveform in addition to a trend graph of end-tidal CO_2 values over time. End-tidal CO_2 monitoring devices differ in capabilities, with some having only capnometry capabilities and others having the ability to display the numeric value simultaneously with the capnograph.

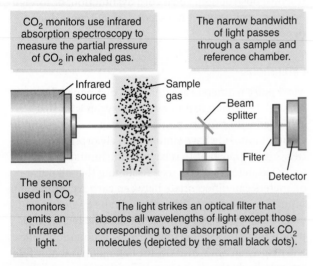

CO$_2$ monitors use infrared absorption spectroscopy to measure the partial pressure of CO$_2$ in exhaled gas.

The narrow bandwidth of light passes through a sample and reference chamber.

Infrared source — Sample gas — Beam splitter — Filter — Detector

The sensor used in CO$_2$ monitors emits an infrared light.

The light strikes an optical filter that absorbs all wavelengths of light except those corresponding to the absorption of peak CO$_2$ molecules (depicted by the small black dots).

FIGURE 19-3 An illustration of CO_2 gas analysis by an end-tidal CO_2 monitor.

There are two types of devices capable of monitoring the partial pressure of CO_2 at the end of a tidal volume breath ($pETCO_2$). Mainstream CO_2 monitoring devices use a small infrared sensor consisting of an optical bench and a cuvette or sample cell to measure the amount of CO_2 molecules within the gas flow pathway through infrared light absorption. As the infrared light passes through a sample chamber, a lens focuses any unabsorbed infrared light to the photodetector. Because carbon dioxide absorbs infrared light, the more infrared light that arrives at the detector, the lower the content of CO_2 in the exhaled gas and vice versa (**Figure 19-3**).[19] Sidestream employs the same analysis theory, but rather than measuring CO_2 molecule content directly in the flow of the gas path, a sampling port is placed inline with the flow of gas from the patient. Gas sampled or withdrawn from the flow of gas from intubated and spontaneously breathing, nonintubated patients is analyzed at a remote monitor.[20]

Patient Application

Mainstream sampling is typically used with infants and children who are intubated. The cuvette used to measure $pETCO_2$ adds weight to the patient-ventilator circuit and may make positioning and kangaroo care challenging, especially when used with low birthweight infants, whose tracheal tubes are small and thin (i.e., 2.0–3.5 mm inner diameter).[21] **Figure 19-4** illustrates the configuration of mainstream sampling inline with a ventilator circuit.

Unlike mainstream sampling, sidestream analyzers sample exhaled gas by pulling exhaled gas from the circuit. A special cannula, shown in **Figure 19-5**, enables the sidestream analyzer to be used with spontaneously breathing patients.[22] A sample port facilitates its use with intubated and mechanically ventilated infants and children. As this type of monitor withdraws gas from the patient-ventilator circuit, devices with a high sampling rate may cause auto-triggering and reduce tidal volume delivery in neonates and small children, resulting in hypercapnia.[23]

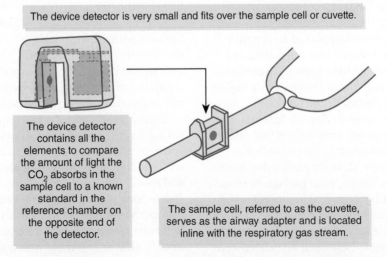

The device detector is very small and fits over the sample cell or cuvette.

The device detector contains all the elements to compare the amount of light the CO$_2$ absorbs in the sample cell to a known standard in the reference chamber on the opposite end of the detector.

The sample cell, referred to as the cuvette, serves as the airway adapter and is located inline with the respiratory gas stream.

FIGURE 19-4 An illustration of a mainstream capnograph used to sample CO_2 inline with a ventilator circuit.

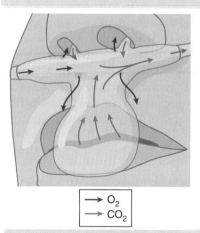

In addition to collecting expired CO_2, these delivery devices also administer oxygen.

→ O_2
→ CO_2

Notice that within the cannula, there are separate ports or routes for O_2 delivery and CO_2 collection or aspiration.

FIGURE 19-5 An illustration of a cannula used to sample CO_2 with a sidestream monitoring device.

TABLE 19-1
Characteristics of Adaptors Used with Mainstream and Sidestream CO_2 Capnographs and Capnometers

	Dead Space (cc)	Flow Resistance (cm H$_2$O)

Mainstream
  Adult/pediatric
  Infant
	5–8
	<1
		<0.3 at 30 L/min
		<1.3 at 10 L/min

Sidestream
  Adult/pediatric
  Infant
	<5
	<1
		N/A

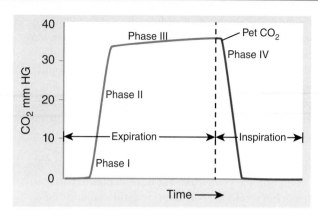

FIGURE 19-6 An illustration of the four phases of a normal capnograph: Phase I, the beginning of exhalation; Phase II, the expiratory upstroke; Phase III, the plateau; and Phase IV, the downstroke or beginning of inspiration.

TABLE 19-2
Uses for End-Tidal CO_2 Monitoring

Dislodged endotracheal tube (ETT)
ETT obstruction
Patient-ventilator disconnection
Noninvasive monitoring of ventilation and detection of respiratory depression (i.e., during procedural sedation, with patient-controlled analgesia, postoperatively)
Effectiveness of cardiopulmonary resuscitation
Determining return of spontaneous circulation
Differentiating esophageal from tracheal intubation
Identification of hypo- and hyperventilation
Identification of bronchoconstriction

Both mainstream and sidestream capnography add some dead space to the circuit, which can impede ventilation in the neonatal population. Current technology allows adaptors to be lightweight and to have minimal dead space and resistance to flow (**Table 19-1**). Although manufacturer-specific, infant sensors are typically used in pediatric patients who are younger than 1 year or weigh less than 10 kg.

Waveform Analysis

Capnography is a useful tool. The shape of the waveform can be used to identify ventilation, airway, and patient-ventilator circuit issues, such as airway obstruction, circuit disconnection, circuit leak, bronchospasm, accidental extubation, and hypo- or hyperventilation. There are four distinct phases of a normal capnograph, which are shown in **Figure 19-6**. Phase I represents anatomic dead space and the beginning of expiration, which form the baseline of the capnograph. Phase II

represents the beginning of exhalation, where there is a mixture of anatomic dead space and alveolar gas. There is an upstroke of the capnograph during this phase. Phase III is the alveolar plateau, reflecting alveolar emptying. The numeric value for end-tidal CO_2 is captured at the end of this plateau. Phase IV appears as an expiratory downstroke signaling the beginning of inspiration. A normal waveform should begin and end at baseline with a plateau that is not sloped.

Anomalies in the shape and size of the waveform can signal changes in the patient's ventilatory status, problems with the integrity of the patient-ventilator circuit, airway obstruction, or a malpositioned tracheal tube.

Clinical Considerations

End-tidal CO_2 monitoring is a noninvasive technology that can be used along the continuum of care. Uses for end-tidal CO_2 gas monitoring are found in **Table 19-2**. Continuous waveform capnography is useful in verifying tracheal placement of an endotracheal tube following intubation and during transport as a tool to guide ventilator management, diagnostically to identify airway abnormalities, and as an adjunct to monitor cardiopulmonary integrity and the effectiveness of chest compressions during resuscitation.[24] **Table 19-3** provides examples of capnographs that identify a clinical or equipment issue.

End-tidal CO_2 monitoring by nasal cannula in spontaneously breathing patients is also beneficial for evaluating the ventilatory status of pediatric patients receiving moderate conscious sedation and during postoperative care.[25] This technology has also proven to be reliable in monitoring seizure disorder patients to evaluate the patient's need for mechanical ventilation.[26] Capnometry is the standard of care for the ventilated patient in the pediatric ICU and during interfacility transport. Following intubation, capnography provides a faster, more reliable distinction between tracheal and esophageal intubation when compared to colorimetric CO_2 detectors.[27]

Capnometry and capnography monitoring are valuables tools during resuscitation. During cardiac arrest, pETCO2 often abruptly falls to very low levels at the onset of a cardiac arrest, increases after the onset of effective cardiopulmonary resuscitation, and returns to normal levels at the return of spontaneous circulation.[28]

Hazards/Complications

Added weight to the ETT and ventilator circuit of neonates and small children may increase the risk for ETT malposition. Sidestream devices that require larger samples of gas for analysis can cause hypoventilation in children with small tidal volumes.

Limitations

There are no absolute contraindications for the use of capnography in spontaneously breathing or mechanically ventilated infants and children. Its use with uncuffed ETTs may lower pETCO2 readings and provide an erratic capnograph pattern and pETCO2 value due to variable leaks. The pETCO2 values may also not to correlate with the $PaCO_2$ due to gas leaking around the ETT.

Transcutaneous Monitoring

Transcutaneous monitoring (TCM) is a noninvasive method of measuring carbon dioxide and oxygen tension across the skin. Although SpO_2 provides a more global perspective regarding oxygenation, **transcutaneous oxygen tension (PtcO2)** provides an estimation of oxygenation at the tissue level. Although these measurements may not always be equal to arterial values for O_2 and CO_2, there are reports of good agreement between transcutaneous PaO_2/$PaCO_2$ measurements and corresponding arterial values (mean bias 0.3 and 0.4, respectively) in very low birthweight infants.

It is important to note that $PtcO_2$ may not be reflective of PaO_2.[29] TCMs are useful for monitoring changes in CO_2 when nonconventional ventilation (i.e., high-frequency oscillation and jet ventilation) are used. Originally designed for use in the neonate, the technology has advanced to make transcutaneous O_2 and CO_2 useful tools in the hospitalized pediatric patient. Transcutaneous CO_2 and O_2 monitoring have demonstrated value in evaluating cardiac performance and tissue perfusion and in guiding the care of severely injured pediatric patients.[30]

Operational Concepts

TCMs use a heated sensor, placed on the surface of the skin, to measure O_2 and CO_2 tensions. Heat warms the skin to approximately 40°C to 43°C and dilates the capillary bed, which increases gas solubility and allows O_2 and CO_2 to diffuse more readily from the capillary lumen to the sensor. The heat applied to the surface area of the skin causes an increase in metabolic rate by approximately 4% to 5% for every degree Celsius, causing an increase in CO_2 production at the site. Transcutaneous monitors use a servo-controlled thermistor to regulate the temperature of the heating element in the sensor, which lightly adheres to the skin. The temperature used depends on the age of the patient and the skin thickness. Compared to an older child, lower temperatures are required to heat the skin of a neonate and to increase the arterial blood supply to the dermal capillary bed beneath the sensor.

Most sensors are combined and have the ability to measure CO_2 and O_2. A miniaturized Severinghaus electrode is used to electrochemically calculate $PaCO_2$ diffusing across the sensor's membrane. CO_2 reacts with the electrolyte solution in the electrode to form bicarbonate and hydrogen ions. The hydrogen ions produced have a linear relationship to the amount of CO_2 diffusing across the membrane and a voltage change between two cells in the sensor, which measures the change and converts it and display a **transcutaneous carbon dioxide tension (PtcCO2)** reading in mm Hg on the monitor.

A miniaturized polarographic Clark electrode, contained within the sensor, measures transcutaneous PaO_2. Similar to the Clark electrodes contained within blood gas analyzers, a platinum or gold cathode surrounding a silver anode is housed in an electrolyte chamber. A semipermeable membrane covers the chamber, allowing gases to diffuse from the surface of the skin. Heat used to facilitate vasodilation also enhances the diffusion of O_2 across the skin's surface to the sensor. Oxygen penetrating the sensor's membrane creates a current as it comes in contact with the cathode, generating an electrical current. The current produced is directly proportional to the concentration of oxygen against the outer membrane's surface. The monitor measures this current's voltage, and then converts and displays it as mm Hg.

TABLE 19-3
Examples of Capnographs That Identify a Clinical or Equipment Issue

Waveform Description	Representative Waveform	Potential Clinical or Equipment-Related Causes
Baseline increases with each breath		Inadequate inspiratory flow, causing the patient to rebreathe CO_2 Air trapping Malfunctioning CO_2 absorber (anesthesia machine)

End-tidal CO_2 is rising		Hypoventilation caused by:
		  Sedation
		  Worsening clincial condition (worsening compliance, yielding lower tidal volume delivery during pressure control ventilation)
		  Patient-controlled pain medication administration
		  Increase in metabolic rate (such as a rapid rise in body temperature)

End-tidal CO_2 is decreasing		Hyperventilation
Erratic waveform		Variable leak from a malfunctioning pilot balloon on a cuffed ETT or a capnograph from an uncuffed ETT Partially obstructed ETT Hypoventilation in a spontaneously breathing child following surgery, with procedural sedation or pain management
Cleft noted during Phase III		A dip or a cleft in Phase III of the waveform represents the patient initiating a breath. This can occur when the effects of a paralytic agent are wearing off. A patient with an inspiratory effort that is weak and a trigger sensitivity that is not set sensitive enough for the patient to trigger a mechanical breath
Absent Phase III		Airway obstruction or bronchospasm

Some monitors incorporate the ability to monitor SpO_2 through the use of an ear sensor. This sensor incorporates technology identical to pulse oximetry explained earlier.

Patient Application

A small adhesive disc is used to secure the sensor, commonly referred to as a probe, to the skin. It is important for the sensor to be flush with the skin; therefore, sensors are typically placed centrally, on the chest or abdomen with infants and chest or forehead with children.[31] Avoid applying the probe to a bony area, like the sternum or scapula, as these areas do not have sufficient underlying tissue to allow for CO_2 diffusion.

Depending on the skin thickness of the patient and the temperature used to heat the skin, the probe is removed every 3 to 4 hours and the site is changed. Localized erythema may be present at the site when the sensor is initially removed and should dissipate shortly. It is important to follow manufacturer's recommendations for use, which include setting the temperature according to patient type (neonate, infant, child, adolescent, etc.), sensor location, and the maximum time a sensor can be left in one location.

Transcutaneous monitors do require some maintenance. The CO_2 sensor requires routine calibrations when the monitor is in use to verify proper electrode response. Although manufacturer-specific, a two-point calibration, using 5% and 10% CO_2 gas, is required every 24 hours when continuous CO_2 monitoring is used. A one-point calibration is typically performed every 4 hours when the monitor is used. A variance of ± 2 mm Hg for the one-point calibration and ± 4 mm Hg for the two-point calibration signify proper sensor function. During calibration, a CO_2 value falling outside of the variance limits indicates a need to troubleshoot the problem.

The oxygen sensor requires a two-step calibration process as well. First, a zero calibration is performed, either by exposing the sensor membrane to a special solution or by electronically performing this procedure through the monitoring device. A high-point calibration is then performed by exposing the sensor to ambient air (with an oxygen concentration of 20.9%). Some monitors have preset the values for barometric pressure while others require manual adjustment. A reference chart is typically provided if manual adjustment is required.

The sensor also requires routine changes in the electrolyte solution and outer covering or membrane. Routine membrane maintenance is typically performed weekly.

Clinical Considerations

Transcutaneous monitoring is valuable as a trending tool. Uses include monitoring patients at risk for hypoventilation, during conscious sedation or patient-controlled analgesia, evaluating the need for ventilatory support, and with ventilator management.[32]

Indications

Transcutaneous O_2 and CO_2 monitoring provide continuous trending of ventilation and oxygenation status, reducing the need for serial blood gas sampling. This type of monitoring is especially useful for noninvasively evaluating the ventilatory status of a patient receiving high-frequency oscillatory ventilation and jet ventilation, where $pETCO_2$ monitoring is not an option. It is especially useful in patients who do not have an indwelling arterial catheter and require arterial puncture to evaluate oxygenation and ventilatory status. The ability to also monitor SpO_2 provides the clinician with a reliable method of noninvasively monitoring oxygenation and ventilation status.[33]

Hazards/Complications

There are no absolute contraindications for transcutaneous monitoring. Alternative monitoring devices should be considered in patients with skin integrity concerns, such as burns or Stevens-Johnson syndrome. Thermal injury is a hazard of transcutaneous monitoring. In patients where continuous monitoring is indicated, sensors should be relocated every 4 hours or as dictated by institutional policy. Great care should be used in placing and relocating sensors on neonates and populations with skin integrity concerns.[13]

Conditions Adversely Affecting Accuracy

TCM may not accurately estimate the PaO_2 and should not be used as the only assessment for oxygenation. $PtcPO_2$ changes are useful in detecting changes in tissue perfusion[34] and in guiding therapy for necrotizing enterocolitis.[35]

Device-related limitations include the amount of time it takes to perform routine maintenance (i.e., membrane and electrolyte solution changes) and sensor calibration, as well as the time it takes for the sensor to equilibrate, once it is affixed to the skin, before displaying a result. Clinical limitations are primarily based on skin integrity. Operator errors create opportunities for inaccurate display of $PtcCO_2$ and $PtcO_2$ values. **Table 19-4** outlines the operator error and clinical conditions contributing to inaccurate $PtcCO_2$ and $PtcO_2$ results. Therefore, upon initial use, when possible, it is important to validate the transcutaneous measurements with an arterial blood gas. This validation will reveal the gap between transcutaneous and arterial measures and provide the respiratory care practitioner with additional information on which to base clinical and troubleshooting decisions should changes in values occur during monitoring.

Nonphysiologic factors may also affect $PtcCO_2$ and $PtcO_2$ measurements. These factors include ambient-air

TABLE 19-4

Factors Contributing to Inaccurate Assessment of Transcutaneous O_2 and CO_2

Clinical Condition or Contributing Factor	Result
Hyperoxemia (PaO_2 >100 mm Hg)	Increased $PtcCO_2$
Poor perfusion	Decreased $PtcCO_2$
Use of vasoactive agents	Decreased $PtcCO_2$
Improper sensor placement or application	Increased or decreased $PtcCO_2$
Subcutaneous edema	Decreased $PtcCO_2$
Increased capillary blood flow due to activity	Increased $PtcCO_2$
Sensor placed on extremities with decreased perfusion	Decreased $PtcCO_2$

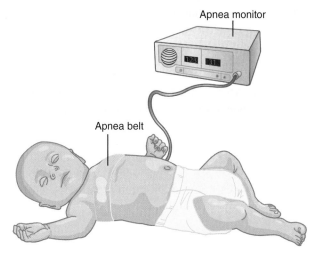

FIGURE 19-7 An illustration of the soft belt used to hold the electrodes securely against the chest wall during home infant apnea monitoring.

temperature, humidity, barometric pressure, membrane thickness, rate of O_2 and CO_2 diffusion across electrolyte solution contained within the electrode, and the polarization voltage across the electrode.

Impedance Pneumography

Impedance pneumography is a noninvasive method to monitor changes in the breathing activity of infants and children. Electrodes are placed on the infant's or child's chest wall and are typically held in place by a soft wrap. The electrodes are attached to a monitor by leads and a cable, similar in appearance to those used for electrocardiogram monitoring.

Operational Concepts

The monitors using electrical impedance pass safe, low-amplitude, high-frequency current through the chest through two electrodes placed on the chest. Small changes in the electrical impedance between the two electrodes are detected as the chest wall expands and contracts with breathing. The electrical signal or impedance changes are reflective of the volume of gas entering and exiting the lungs.[36] Depending on the type of monitor used, a waveform may be displayed as the modulated signal, which represents tidal breathing and the respiratory rate.

This technology has been incorporated into equipment used for diagnostic testing, mechanical ventilators, and infant home apnea monitors. Apnea is measured indirectly and signaled when there is an absence of chest wall movement. To differentiate between central and obstructive apnea, diagnostic monitoring systems incorporate impedance pneumography with a nasal thermistor, proximal airway sensor, and/or infrared CO_2 sensor.

Home apnea monitors use this technology and are designed to detect breathing pattern and heart rate changes and to alert the caregivers of those changes. The same electrodes used to monitor voltage variations during thoracic movement also monitor the electrical activity of the heart and determine heart rate. Thresholds for apnea and high and low heart rate alerts are preset per protocol or physician order.

Patient Application

Because the technology is incorporated into mechanical ventilators, diagnostic equipment, and home apnea monitors, impedance pneumography is indicated for patients requiring monitoring of the rate and depth of respirations across the continuum of care. Depending on the type of monitor used, the electrodes can be nondisposable pads that can be placed on the skin and secured with a soft wrap belt (**Figure 19-7**). Disposable electrodes with adhesive backs, which adhere to the skin, may also be used. Electrode position is important to ensure the accuracy of the impedance signal. The electrodes should not be placed in close proximity. Placing one electrode on the right side and the other on the left side of the chest is optimal, as this placement technique will minimize false alerts for apnea or low tidal volume due to inadvertent small changes in the impedance signal caused when electrodes are placed too closely together. Correct placement area extends from the nipple line to the axilla. Avoid placing the electrodes too close to the bottom of the ribcage, near the abdomen. The monitor will detect interference at this point, which will reduce the accuracy of the impedance signal. Placing the electrodes in the axillary pit may cause skin irritation, especially if nondisposable electrodes and a wrap belt are used.

It is important to keep the skin under the electrodes free from oils or lotions, which can interfere with the impedance signal. Washing the skin with mild soap and water prior to the application of the electrodes is helpful. Rotating the electrode site often can prevent skin irritation or breakdown. Special consideration should be taken in patients with skin integrity concerns.

The disposable or reusable electrodes are connected to the monitoring system by lead wires, which plug into a cable attached to the monitoring device. Monitors used for diagnostic testing or home apnea monitoring can discern between equipment problems, such as a loose or disconnected lead wire, and a physiologic event. The apnea delay time, as well as alarm limits for high and low heart rate and respiratory rate, are adjustable for home apnea monitors.

Clinical Considerations

Although the technology for impedance pneumography has improved throughout the years, there remain issues with accurately differentiating respiratory impedance from cardiac artifact. Placing the electrodes in the proper position is helpful in reducing false alarms on apnea monitors and in obtaining accurate data for tidal volume and respiratory rate evaluation on diagnostic equipment employing this technology.

Apnea delay time and high and low alarm limits for respiratory and heart rates require a physician's order for home apnea monitoring. The settings may change over the monitoring period based upon the number and type of events the infant is experiencing.

Conditions Adversely Affecting Accuracy

Limitations for impedance pneumography can be divided into two categories: patient factors and technology issues. Changes in the infant's position, especially side lying, can position the electrodes closer together. If nondisposable electrodes are used, the side-lying position can cause gaps in the belt, loosening the belt and the electrode placement against the chest, and so impedance signals are not accurately captured. This results in false apnea, or low respiratory rate, alarms on home apnea monitors, and reduces both low tidal volumes and respiratory rate on diagnostic equipment and mechanical ventilators using this technology.

Impedance pneumography cannot accurately distinguish between cardiac oscillation and respiratory impedance signals. This may result in an inaccurate interpretation of respiratory rate. Placing the electrodes in the proper position may minimize, but does not completely correct, this limitation. Because this technology does not directly measure airflow, impedance pneumography cannot directly distinguish a central from an obstructive or mixed apnea. Additionally, for home monitoring equipment, the technology is less sophisticated than that employed in diagnostic equipment or mechanical ventilators. Therefore, it is important to note that although a respiratory rate is displayed, the monitor does not evaluate the effectiveness of ventilation.

Near Infrared Spectroscopy

Near infrared spectroscopy (NIRS) is a noninvasive tool that provides real-time continuous monitoring of regional tissue oxyhemoglobin saturation (rSO_2).

Operational Concepts

Much like the pulse oximetry technology discussed previously, NIRS uses the Beer-Lambert law to determine the absorption of NIR light by oxyhemoglobin, which translates to tissue oxygenation. NIRS is most commonly used in infants and children who have undergone cardiac surgery or who are critically ill and at risk for low cardiac output syndrome.[37,38]

Patient Application

Common locations for placement of the sensors are the forehead and the abdomen or low back at T-10 to L-2. Because the skull is easily penetrated by near infrared light, sensors placed on the forehead provide a real-time assessment of regional cortical oxygenation[39,40] (**Figure 19-8**).

Clinical Considerations

An acceptable range of rSO_2 is 55% to 80%. Absolute values less than 50% or a decrease in baseline rSO_2 by 20% indicate a need for intervention. Patients with rSO_2 less than 45% or a decrease from baseline of 25% have shown less favorable neurologic outcomes than those who remained within the defined acceptable rSO_2 range.[40]

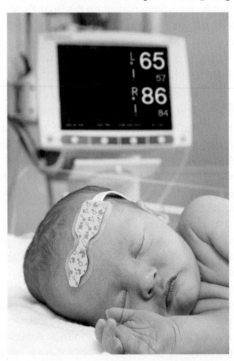

FIGURE 19-8 A near infrared spectroscopy monitoring of an infant. The sensor is small and placed on the infant's forehead, which provides immediate assessment of regional cortical oxygenation.

Sensors placed on the abdomen or low back, often referred to as renal NIRS, are reflective of tissue oxygenation of the kidneys. Renal NIRS has been effective in providing accurate, real-time analysis of tissue oxygenation due to the kidneys' superficial location and the pediatric patient's thin skin and minimal subcutaneous fat layer. Because infants and children are at risk for end-organ failure, especially renal failure, following cardiac surgery, trending renal NIRS has become a standard practice in many pediatric ICUs.

NIRS has also been quickly adopted as a noninvasive monitoring tool to measure cerebral oxygenation during and after pediatric cardiac surgery, in patients supported by extracorporeal membrane oxygenation, and in critically ill patients at risk for decreased end-organ perfusion. NIRS monitoring is useful for trending patient oxygenation as well as reflecting acute changes, which alert practitioners to a possible acute decompensation of the patient's cardiopulmonary or hemodynamic status.

Hazards/Complications

Improved light technology reduces but does not eliminate the potential for the NIRS sensors to cause thermal burns. As with any device that adheres to the skin, special care should be taken when applying and removing sensors, as skin tears are a possible iatrogenic injury. This is especially important when applying the sensor to infants and children who are known to have compromised skin integrity.

Conditions Adversely Affecting Accuracy

There are several factors and/or conditions that limit the accuracy with which NIRS monitors and displays rSO_2 values. Skin pigmentation and jaundice are among the most common factors limiting the monitor's accuracy. Sensor placement may also adversely affect accuracy. Patients with severe tissue edema or sensors placed in areas with large amounts of adipose tissue can display inaccurate rSO_2 values. Additionally, sensors placed over tissue with underlying muscle may cause inaccurate readings because myoglobin will contribute to the measurement. Oxygen has a high affinity to myoglobin, which will result in an overestimation of tissue oxygenation. The effect myoglobin causes is similar to that with carboxyhemoglobin and pulse oximetry; the monitoring system is unable to effectively differentiate a myoglobin signal from a hemoglobin signal. It is important to note that the sensors are single-patient use, which can be expensive. Studies to further investigate the cost/benefit analysis are needed.

Invasive Monitoring

Invasive monitors require vascular access to evaluate oxygenation status, adequacy of gas exchange, and acid–base balance. Invasive monitors may also be used to assess intrapulmonary shunt, differences in arterial-venous oxygen content, and oxygen consumption.

Arterial Blood Gas Analysis

Arterial blood gas analysis provides a reliable evaluation of oxygenation, gas exchange, and acid–base balance[41] and is often used in diagnostic evaluation and to assess the child's response to therapeutic interventions.[42] **Table 19-5** outlines the approximate normal blood gas ranges for arterial blood.

Arterial Sampling Procedure

Arterial sampling may be performed as needed by a percutaneous puncture or by cannulation of a peripheral artery. Adherence to the process steps for obtaining an arterial sample is essential to minimize procedural complications and to obtain a quality sample of blood for analysis.

Sampling Sites for the Neonate and Child

There are several potential access sites to perform an arterial puncture or for cannulation and securement

TABLE 19-5
Normal Blood Gas Ranges for Arterial Blood, Stratified by Age

	Preterm Infant	Newborn Term Infant	Term Infant to Toddler	Children
Age range	<39 weeks' gestational age	40 weeks' gestational age	40 weeks' gestational age to 2 years of age	>2 years of age
pH	≥7.20–7.24	7.30–7.40	7.30–7.40	7.35–7.45
$PaCO_2$ (mm Hg)	45–55	30–40	30–40	35–45
PaO_2 (mm Hg)	45–65	60–90	80–100	80–100
HCO_3 (mEq/L)	15–18	20–22	20–22	22–24

of an arterial line. The umbilical artery provides a reliable route for continuous monitoring of arterial blood for blood gas analysis and blood pressure monitoring as well as an access site for intravenous fluid administration.[43] Reliable vascular access can quickly and painlessly occur immediately after birth in high-risk newborns and often avoids the painful skin punctures needed for other forms of vascular access, such as peripherally inserted central catheters and surgically inserted central venous catheters. Closed-loop blood analysis devices can be used to analyze arterial blood for blood gas and chemistry monitoring without the risk of blood loss. Typically, closed loop blood gas monitors automatically withdraw 1.5 mL of blood from the indwelling catheter, perform the required analysis (i.e., blood gas, electrolytes, hemoglobin), and reinfuse the blood used for analysis. Closed-loop analysis devices can be used with umbilical or peripheral arterial catheters.

Cannulation for arterial catheter placement can be performed in a variety of locations in children. The radial artery has adequate collateral circulation to an extremity that can be easily accessed and manipulated during the insertion procedure. The nerves and veins in the wrist area are not directly adjacent to the radial artery, minimizing risk of injury or inadvertent venous cannulation. The femoral artery is less commonly used in children because of its close proximity to the femoral nerve and vein. Cannulation here can be also challenging in children because of the artery's nearness to the hip joint. Generally, use of the femoral artery is reserved for emergent access.

The radial and femoral arteries may also be used as an arterial puncture site. Similar to rationale for their use with arterial catheter insertion, the radial artery is preferred, and the femoral artery is reserved for access by highly skilled clinicians in emergency situations. The brachial artery is also less commonly used for arterial puncture. Similar to the femoral artery, it is more difficult to palpate, does not have collateral circulation, and is the main feed for a large distal circulatory network. A list and description of common arterial puncture sites are found in **Table 19-6**.

Arterial Puncture

There are instances when the need for arterial blood gas analysis is infrequent. In these instances, a percutaneous arterial puncture is obtained. Obtaining an arterial blood gas sample percutaneously requires skill and is more challenging than performing an arterial puncture in an adult. Depending on the child's age, it may be difficult to get the child to cooperate and remain still during the procedure, so two care providers should be used so that one can assist with stabilizing the extremity used for the procedure.

It is important to recognize that an arterial puncture is a painful procedure and can cause a stress response in infants and children. Analgesic agents, such as a topical anesthetic cream, a lidocaine injection at the site, or a short-acting oral analgesic agent, may be used for pain control during the procedure. The type of agent used depends on the age of the patient, hemodynamic stability, and type and duration of the procedure. Parental support during the procedure may be helpful in calming and providing comfort to a young child.

The use of a **transilluminating light** or devices that use near infrared light may be helpful in identifying the vessel selected for access.[44,45]

Prior to performing the arterial puncture, a **modified Allen's test** is used to verify the presence or absence of collateral circulation. A passive method for

TABLE 19-6
A Comparison of Arterial Sites That May Be Used for Peripheral Arterial Puncture of Infants and Children

Artery	Good Collateral Circulation at Site	Ease of Access
Temporal	Yes	An option for premature infants. Artery has two branches, which are larger than the radial artery and are relatively superficial.
Axillary	No	A skilled clinician is required.
Radial	Yes	Extremity can be easily accessed and manipulated.
Ulnar	Yes	Not as easily accessed as the radial artery. Artery runs adjacent to the ulnar nerve.
Brachial	No	Not as easily accessed as the radial artery.
Femoral	No	A skilled clinician is required.
Posterior tibial	Yes	Extremity can be easily accessed and manipulated.
Dorsalis pedis	Yes	Extremity can be easily accessed and manipulated.

performing the Allen's test may be used when the child is unable to follow commands. A second caregiver or parent may provide assistance when performing the passive method. To perform the passive method, elevate or gently squeeze the child's hand while the radial and ulnar arteries are occluded.

Regardless of the technique used, the color of the palm of the infant's or child's hand will change from blanched to pink within 5 seconds of releasing the ulnar artery when collateral circulation is adequate.

Table 19-7 outlines the steps used in preparing for and performing a percutaneous arterial puncture.

Care of Puncture Site

Prior to performing the procedure, it is important to cleanse the site with an antiseptic wipe. Alcohol and povidone-iodine wipes are commonly included in arterial blood gas kits.

Prior to the puncture, it is important to observe the selected puncture site for contusions, swelling, or breakdown.

TABLE 19-7
The Preparation and Procedural Steps for Performing a Percutaneous Arterial Puncture

Phase	Procedure Steps

Preparing for the procedure	1. Perform hand hygiene.
	2. Introduce yourself to the patient and family and explain the procedure.
	3. Adhere to standard precautions, including the use of hand hygiene before donning gloves and protective garments.
	4. Select the sample site by palpating a pulse.
	5. Perform a modified Allen's test (if applicable; i.e., for radial puncture).
	6. Cleanse the site with an antiseptic swab, allowing the area to air dry before proceeding.
	7. While the cleaned area dries, prepare a clean field and assemble the blood gas equipment for use.
	  a. Preheprinized 1.0-mL syringe with 25-gauge preheprinized needle or 25-gauge butterfly needle infusion kit
	  b. Sterile gauze pad
	  c. Needle capping protection device (varies by manufacturer)
	  d. Patient label
	8. Cleanse gloves with an antiseptic wipe and palpate the site selected for specimen collection.
	9. Communicate to the patient and family that the procedure will begin.

Collecting the specimen	10. While palpating the arterial pulse, gently position the butterfly needle, or needle and syringe, on the skin (against blood flow) with the bevel up at a 45-degree angle.
	11. Advance the needle gently into the artery.
	12. Observe the hub of the needle for a flash of blood, which indicates arterial access.
	  a. If no flash occurs, gently withdraw the needle, while continuing to palpate the pulse, until the hub can be seen at the skin's surface.
	  b. Continue to observe the hub for the blood flash.
	  c. If no flash is seen, palpate the pulse, redirect the needle, and gently advance into the artery.
	  d. Connect the butterfly needle to the syringe and gently aspirate until the sample is obtained.
	13. Once the sample is obtained, withdraw the needle and hold firm pressure on the puncture site for at least 5 minutes with the sterile gauze pad.
	  a. Pressure should be held for a longer period of time in patients with coagulopathy or those receiving anticoagulation therapy.

Preparing the sample for analysis	14. While simultaneously holding pressure to the puncture site, remove any air bubbles from the syringe and protect and remove the needle, using the manufacturer-provided safety shield. 15. Cap the syringe. 16. Gently rotate the sample to mix the blood and heparin. This can be accomplished by rolling the capped syringe between the index finger and the thumb. 17. Apply the patient label to the sample.

Care of the sampling site and postprocedure infection control measures	18. Observe the puncture site.
	  a. If bleeding is noted, continue to hold pressure, assessing the site every few minutes.
	  b. Note any changes to the puncture site, such as new onset of bruising, swelling, blanching, etc.
	  c. Document the procedure in the patient's medical record.
	19. Doff protective garments and perform hand hygiene.

Transporting the sample for analysis and documenting care	20. Document the procedure in the electronic health record:
	  a. Puncture site
	  b. Quality of blood obtained
	  c. How the patient tolerated the procedure
	21. Transport the sample for analysis using standard precautions.

Following the procedure, hold pressure to the puncture site for a minimum of 5 minutes. Patients with coagulopathy or those receiving anticoagulation therapy will most likely require the site to be held for a longer period of time. If the site requires pressure for longer than 10 minutes, arrange for another healthcare provider to transport the sample for analysis.

Once the bleeding has stopped, inspect the puncture site for changes in the condition of the skin. Always document skin abnormalities noted prior to and/or after the procedure, as well as any complications, in the electronic health record.

Care of Sample

After obtaining the sample, air bubbles should be immediately removed. It is essential to follow manufacturer instructions for safe capping of the needle. Needle shields are provided with arterial blood gas kits and although the designs may differ, the shields allow for the needle to be safely capped using one hand, minimizing the risk of an accidental needle stick to the healthcare provider. Butterfly needles generally do not have needle shields and thus should be carefully removed from the syringe by twisting at the hub.

Once the needle is safely removed and the syringe capped, mix the sample to blend the heparin and the blood. Gently rolling the syringe between the index finger and thumb can easily accomplish this. The sample should be labeled immediately and transported within 10 to 15 minutes of collection to ensure accurate results. Samples that are not analyzed within 15 minutes will metabolize and may yield inaccurate results.

Clinical Considerations

Arterial blood gas puncture is an invasive procedure. There is pain and, for some children, anxiety associated with this procedure. Care should be taken to evaluate the frequency with which blood gas results are needed to guide care. Communicating that need to the interprofessional team and incorporating it into the patient plan of care is a better practice. Frequent need for blood gas results may require an indwelling arterial catheter to minimize the number of punctures an infant or child will need to endure.

Indications

The analysis of arterial blood provides a reliable assessment of oxygenation, ventilation, and acid–base balance.[41] Arterial blood gas results are used as a diagnostic tool as well as to guide care by assessing the child's response to therapy.[42] The indications for arterial blood gas analysis are outlined in **Table 19-8**.

Hazards/Complications

The most common complication associated with an arterial puncture is bruising or hematoma formation

---

TABLE 19-8
Indications for Arterial Blood Gas Analysis

To evaluate:
Acid–base balance
Ventilation effectiveness
Oxygenation
Hemoglobin concentrations and oxygen-carrying capacity
Differential diagnoses

To quantify:
Degree of intrapulmonary shunting
Cardiopulmonary response to therapeutic interventions

To identify:
Dyshemoglobinemia, such as carboxyhemoglobin, methemoglobin, and fetal hemoglobin*

To monitor:
Therapeutic responses to invasive and noninvasive medical interventions
Disease severity and progression

*Arterial blood gas analysis by hemoximetry is necessary to identify dyshemoglobinemia.

---

at the site. This is commonly seen with coagulopathy issues or when pressure is not held long enough to stop all bleeding. Pain is also associated with this invasive procedure as well as inadvertent contact of the needle to surrounding nerves or bone (more common with attempts to access the radial and brachial arteries).[46] Thromboses, arterial spasm, nerve palsy, pseudoaneurysm, and arteriovenous fistula are also complications.[47] Infection can also occur. The use of proper technique, including standard precautions, maintaining a clean field while preparing for the procedure, and using sterile gauze to hold pressure on the site following sample collection, will minimize the risk for infection.

Damage to the artery targeted for access may impair circulation to the extremity. To minimize this risk, it is essential to ensure that collateral circulation is present prior to performing the procedure.

Contraindications/Limitations

Arterial puncture should not be performed at a site with compromised collateral circulation, where skin integrity is compromised (skin tears or breakdown are present), or a surgical shunt. Extremities where there is evidence of peripheral vascular disease or where infection is present should also be avoided.

Conditions Adversely Affecting Accuracy

The quality of the sample can be adversely affected by collection technique or the manner in which the sample is handled following specimen collection. During collection, the needle may enter a vein, causing a flash of blood in the hub, with lack of blood flow into the syringe. Venous blood can affect the validity of test results by raising the $PaCO_2$ and reducing the PaO_2.

After collecting the sample, it is essential to ensure that air bubbles larger than 5% of the sample are removed from the syringe. Contamination of the blood gas sample with air will lower the $PaCO_2$ and elevate the PaO_2. Improper mixing of the anticoagulant within the syringe may cause the specimen to clot, requiring the sample to be redrawn. Pre-analytical errors can occur when there is a delay in analyzing the specimen. The blood will metabolize in the syringe when there is a delay of greater than 15 minutes for a sample that remains at room temperature or greater than 60 minutes for a sample that is collected and stored at 4°C.

Capillary Blood Gas Analysis

Capillary blood gas sampling is a useful alternative for assessing acid–base balance and ventilation in infants and children. Blood obtained from a capillary blood gas sample correlates well with the pH, $PaCO_2$, HCO_3, and base excess (BE) obtained from an arterial sample and provides a less invasive sampling method.[48] Compared to values obtained from an arterial sample, the PaO_2 does not correlate well and is lower than the PaO_2 obtained from an artery, although it does correlate well with the PaO_2 obtained from venous blood.[49]

Capillary Sampling Procedure and Sampling Sites for the Neonate and Child

The quality of the sample depends on the site preparation and the sampling technique. In order to obtain a capillary sample that will best reflect that of arterial blood, the site must be properly prepared by warming the puncture area. Warming the area will increase circulation to the arterioles in the extremity selected for use.

A capillary blood gas sample can be obtained from the foot, finger, or earlobe.[50] The posterolateral aspect of the foot provides a safe site for capillary blood gas sampling. This area is just anterior to the heel of the foot, which reduces the risk for inadvertent puncture of the bone, which is prominent on the back of the heel, or the posterior tibia artery, which runs along the medial aspect of the foot.

The fleshy surface of the fingers or toes, known as the palmar, also provides a safe site for capillary sampling in infants and children. These areas should be avoided in preterm infants because there is a higher risk of causing trauma to the nerve endings of the developing neonate.

The earlobe provides another site for capillary blood gas sampling in children. Earlobe sampling provides a slightly more accurate reflection of arterial CO_2 and PaO_2 as compared to capillary samples drawn from the fingers, toes, or foot.[50] **Figure 19-9** illustrates the recommended sites for capillary blood collection as well as the techniques used to stabilize the area or extremity from which the sample will be drawn.

It is important to evaluate the site prior to specimen collection. The area should be free from trauma (bruising), edema, infection, or skin breakdown. **Table 19-9** outlines the procedure for obtaining a capillary blood gas sample for analysis.

Care of Puncture Site

Assessing the site of any percutaneous blood sampling is important. Always observe the potential site for contusions, swelling, or skin breakdown. Following the procedure, hold pressure to the collection area for a minimum of 5 minutes. Patients with coagulopathy or those receiving anticoagulation therapy will most likely require the site to be held for a longer period of time. If the site requires pressure for longer than 10 minutes, arrange for another healthcare provider to transport the sample for analysis.

Once the bleeding has stopped, inspect the puncture site for changes in the condition of the skin. Always document skin abnormalities noted prior to and/or after the procedure as well as any complications in the electronic health record. An adhesive bandage may be used to cover the site once the bleeding has stopped and the site has been inspected. Weigh the risk for bandaging the site, especially if fingers or toes were used for the procedure. Bandages may cause a choking risk for toddlers or small children who may put their digit in their mouth.[51]

Care of Sample

After obtaining the sample, the labeled capillary tube should be immediately taken to the laboratory for analysis. Because the capillary tubes are fragile, it is not advisable to use a pneumatically powered transport tube system to send the sample for analysis.

There may be occasions when the sample cannot be analyzed promptly after collection. In this instance, the sample will need to be mixed within the heparinized capillary tube and sealed. To mix the sample and prevent clotting, gently cap the ends of the capillary tube and roll the tube between the fingers and the palm, as shown in **Figure 19-10A**. Mixing can also be accomplished by inserting a metal filing, also known as a flea, into one end of the capillary tube. Seal both ends of the tube by gently inserting rubber caps. (The caps and mixing fleas are provided with capillary tube kits.) Mix the sample by running a small magnet horizontally along the side of the capillary tube, as shown in **Figure 19-10B**. When a mixing flea is used, the flea must be removed before the sample is analyzed. To remove the flea, uncap one end and run the magnet horizontally in one direction along the sample from the capped end to the open end. This will move the flea to the open end of the tube, where it can be easily removed.

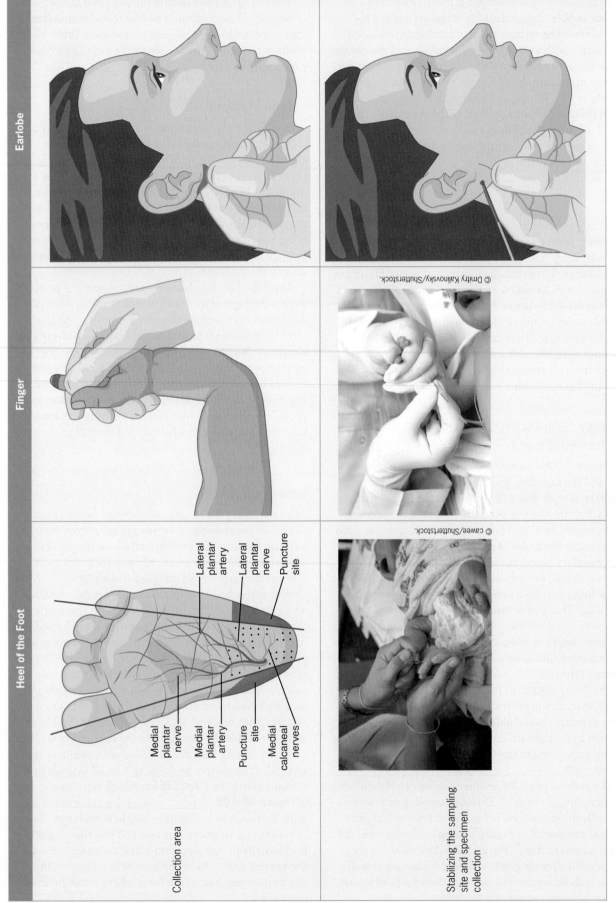

Earlobe

Finger

© Dmitry Kalinovsky/Shutterstock.

Heel of the Foot

Lateral plantar artery

Lateral plantar nerve

Puncture site

Medial plantar nerve

Medial plantar artery

Puncture site

Medial calcaneal nerves

Collection area

© cawee/Shutterstock.

Stabilizing the sampling site and specimen collection

FIGURE 19-9 An illustration of the sites used for capillary blood gas sampling. The area shaded in red highlights the recommended area to collect the sample.

TABLE 19-9
The Preparation and Procedural Steps for Performing a Capillary Blood Gas Puncture

Preparing for the procedure	1. Perform hand hygiene.
	2. Introduce yourself to the patient and family and explain the procedure.
	3. Adhere to standard precautions, including the use of hand hygiene before donning gloves and protective garments.
	4. Select the collection site.
	5. Warm the area using a wet cloth pre-warmed to approximately 42°C or a commercially available warming pack.
	  a. Apply the cloth or pack to the area. Allow the area to warm for 5–10 minutes before removing the warming cloth or pack.
	  b. To avoid burning the skin, do not to use cloths that exceed the recommended temperature.
	  c. A dry cloth or tape can be used to hold the warming cloth or pack, respectively, in place.
	6. Assess for the need for pain control.
	  a. Obtain an order for a topical anesthetic cream if needed.
	7. Remove the warming cloth or pack.
	  a. Cleanse the site with an antiseptic wipe and dry with a sterile gauze pad to minimize hemolyzing the blood.
	  b. Apply anesthetic cream to the puncture site prior to collecting the specimen as needed.
	8. Immobilize the area selected for the procedure by:
	  a. Holding the patient's digit with your thumb and forefinger for a finger stick
	  b. Grasping the earlobe
	  c. Grasping the foot and positioning the thumb along the arch of the foot and the forefinger, wrapped around the upper portion of the heel (in a C shape)

Collecting the specimen	9. Position the lancet on the skin. Lancets vary in size and include those with a safety feature, which will automatically pierce and withdraw the blade into a housing.
	  a. Do not direct the lancet over bone.
	  b. Lancets that automatically trigger, when actuated, will pierce the skin at a depth of 1–2 mm.
	  c. To manually pierce the skin, quickly and gently pierce the skin with a smooth continuous motion, at a depth of 1–2 mm. Superficially puncturing the skin may require a second stick to produce a free flow of blood sufficient enough to fill the capillary tube.
	  d. To minimize the chances of slicing or digging into the infant's or child's skin, avoid puncturing the skin multiple times or using a twisting motion to pierce the skin.
	10. Maintain moderate pressure on the heel or fingertip while slightly releasing the pressure the thumb is placing on the infant's heel or fingertip. This will allow blood to flow more freely from the site.
	  a. To avoid hemolyzing the blood, do not squeeze or massage the collection site.
	11. Wipe the first drop of blood from the site with a sterile gauze pad. This will reduce contaminating the sample with intrastitial, intracellular, and/or lymphatic fluid.
	12. Holding the capillary tube horizontal to the puncture site, with the opening angled downward, place the tip of the capillary tube into the drop of blood.
	  a. Do not hold the tip of the capillary tube against the puncture site.
	  b. Keep the opening of the capillary tube in constant contact with the blood droplets until the blood fills the capillary tube. The amount of blood collected depends on the size of the capillary tube, which typically ranges from 40–125 µL.
	  c. Do not expose the capillary tip to air between droplet collections.
	  d. Do not scrape the skin's surface to collect the sample, as this will increase the likelihood of introducing air into the sample.
	13. After collecting the sample, hold pressure on the puncture site with a sterile gauze pad.
	  a. Hold pressure for approximately 5 minutes or until bleeding stops.
	  b. Pressure should be held for a longer period of time for children with coagulopathy or those receiving anticoagulation therapy.
	14. Apply the patient label to the sample.

Care of the sampling site and postprocedure infection control measures	15. Observe the puncture site.
	  a. If bleeding is noted, continue to hold pressure, assessing the site every few minutes.
	  b. Note any changes to the puncture site, such as new onset of bruising, swelling, blanching, etc.
	  c. Document the procedure in the patient medical record.
	16. Doff protective garments and perform hand hygiene.

Transporting the sample for analysis and documenting care	17. Document the procedure in the electronic health record:
	  a. Puncture site
	  b. Quality of blood obtained
	  c. How the patient tolerated the procedure
	18. Transport the sample for analysis using standard precautions.

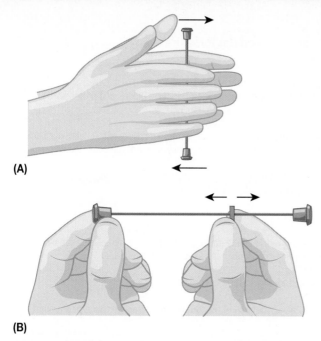

(A)

(B)

FIGURE 19-10 Mixing a capillary sample by (A) gently rolling the sample between the fingers and the palm or (B) inserting a metal filing, or flea, and using a magnet to move the filing within the blood sample.

Clinical Considerations

Capillary sampling should be performed only when there is a documented need for intermittent assessment of an infant's or child's acid–base balance. This form of blood gas sampling is not recommended when frequent assessment is required or when the need for an arterial assessment of oxygenation and ventilation exists.

The integrity of a capillary sample is important. A poor-quality sample can impair effective medical management and contribute to poor patient outcomes. Factors that can contribute to a poor-quality sample include contamination of the sample with air and lymphatic fluid, insufficient sample, or clots in the capillary tube. During transition to extrauterine life, peripheral perfusion is poor; therefore, capillary punctures should not be performed in newborn infants younger than 24 hours of age.

Indications

Capillary blood gas sampling provides an invasive alternative to arterial blood gas sampling when blood gases are of value to the management of the infant or child, including monitoring the severity and/or progression of disease status as well as evaluating a patient's response to therapeutic intervention. Capillary blood gas sampling is less invasive than percutaneous arterial blood gas sampling and is often used when access to arterial blood is not available. Capillary blood gas results are helpful when assessing the accuracy of non-invasive monitoring, such as transcutaneous and end-tidal values for CO_2 and SpO_2 trends.

Hazards/Complications

Although this procedure is less invasive than a percutaneous arterial puncture, complications may occur, especially if variations in the procedure occur. Use of a warming cloth that is heated to temperatures above 42°C increases the likelihood of causing thermal injury to the skin. Puncturing the skin in an area that is outside of the recommended collection site, such as the posterior medial aspect of the heel, can lacerate the tibial artery. Lancing the posterior curvature of the heel can injure bone and cause osteomyelitis and/or calcification. The risk for nerve damage is increased as well when a lancet is used in areas of the heel, fingers, or toes that are not recommended. As with any invasive procedure, the risk of infection and bleeding exists. Hematoma is a common finding when pressure is not held on the site until all bleeding stops.

Disadvantages/Limitations

Preparation of the puncture site is a crucial step in the sampling procedure. A site that is not properly warmed will yield capillary pH and CO_2 values that correlate poorly with arterial values. Warming is necessary to arterialize the sample. Variability in capillary O_2 values precludes its use for adequately assessing oxygenation status.

Conditions Adversely Affecting Accuracy

There are several clinical conditions that can affect the quality of the sample and accuracy with which the blood obtained reflects the infant's or child's acid–base balance. Conditions that reduce cardiac output and contribute to peripheral blood pooling, such as cor pulmonale, hypotension, hypothermia, hypovolemia, and shock, may elevate $PaCO_2$ values.

The gap between arterial and arterialized capillary oxygen tensions will narrow in the presence of hypoxemia. Children with congenital cardiac disease require special consideration as well. Consideration should be given to the type of cardiac disorder affecting the child as well as the therapeutic interventions (e.g., surgical repair, medications) the child received.

Umbilical Artery Catheter

Arterial catheters are useful when frequent sampling of arterial blood is required for the management of a critically ill infant or child. Arterial catheters also provide continuous blood pressure monitoring, which is useful with infants and children who are not hemodynamically stable.

Placement

After birth, the umbilical stump provides access to the umbilical artery, making access and cannulation easier, as compared to peripheral artery cannulation.

Cannulating the umbilical artery shortly after birth is preferable because these vessels will spasm as arterial tensions rise, reducing the ease with which they can be accessed.[52]

An umbilicus contains two arteries and a vein. The hands of a clock are often used to describe the position of the umbilical vessels. While standing at the foot of the newborn, the two arteries are located at the 5 and 7 o'clock positions, as seen in **Figure 19-11**.

Cannulation of the umbilical artery is a surgical procedure, requiring the use of aseptic technique. There are two positions for a properly placed umbilical artery catheter: high and low. Historically, a measure of shoulder to umbilicus length, also known as the **Dunn formula**, was used to determine initial catheter placement.[52] A chart or nomogram was then used to determine the depth with which the catheter was initially advanced and anchored into place. The literature reports that this method often overestimates insertion length, especially in very low birthweight babies.[52,53] The use of a weight-based formula to determine initial insertion depth—insertional length (cm) = (4 x birth weight [kg]) + 7—resulted in significantly fewer malpositioned umbilical artery catheters.[54,55]

The tip of the **umbilical artery catheter (UAC)** overlies the 6th to 8th thoracic vertebrae in the high-lying position and the 3rd to 4th lumbar vertebrae in the low-lying position. Once the high or low position is determined and the distance for catheter insertion is calculated, the sterile catheter is gently inserted and advanced through the artery, using a rotating motion. Blood will flow freely through the catheter when it is patent and unobstructed. Once in position, using

aseptic technique, the catheter is connected to a fluid-pressure transducer system and the transducer is calibrated. The transducer should be positioned at the level of the right atrium.

Sutures are generally used to secure the umbilical catheter into the artery through the umbilical skin, and then tied around the umbilical stump. Tape can be used to stabilize the catheter by tethering it to the infant's abdomen. A chest and abdominal radiograph is used to confirm UAC position.

Clinical Considerations

Historically, the selection of the high or low position for UAC placement has been the subject of much debate. Currently, there are no evidence-based recommendations for the optimal position. The literature does report, however, a lower incidence of clinical vascular complications, such as arterial vasospasm and lower extremity blanching, with high-lying umbilical artery catheters.[56,57] Most physicians and practitioners inserting UACs use the position favored at the institution granting their medical privileges.

Indications

UACs are commonly used for blood sampling and invasive monitoring of blood pressure. A UAC provides painless, quick, and reliable vascular access immediately after birth in high-risk newborns and avoids the painful skin punctures needed for a peripherally placed arterial catheter.

Direct measurement of systolic, diastolic, and mean blood pressure are useful in determining the hemodynamic status of critically ill patients. **Mean blood pressure (MAP)** represents the force with which the left ventricle must pump, providing an assessment of left ventricular afterload. The MAP is calculated and displayed on the monitor when an indwelling arterial catheter is in place. MAP can be calculated by using the systolic and diastolic pressures obtained by noninvasive blood pressure monitoring through the following formula:

$$MAP = [(2 \times \text{diastolic blood pressure}) + (\text{systolic blood pressure})] / 3$$

Monitoring pulse pressure, or the difference between systolic and diastolic blood pressure, is helpful in determining volume status and determining the efficacy of fluid resuscitation. A narrowing or decreasing pulse pressure may indicate hypovolemia. During fluid resuscitation, increasing pulse pressure will occur with the restoration of a normal volume status.

Arterial access, through an indwelling catheter, provides a connection to an inline blood gas monitor. This closed system allows for continuous monitoring of blood gases, electrolytes, and hemoglobin by sampling a small amount, approximately 1.5 mL, of blood. After the

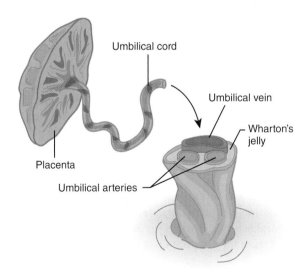

FIGURE 19-11 An illustration of the positions of the umbilical arteries and vein in the stump of the umbilical cord following birth. The arteries are smaller in size and located at the 5 and 7 o'clock positions. The vein is larger, more oblong shaped, and found near the 12 o'clock position.

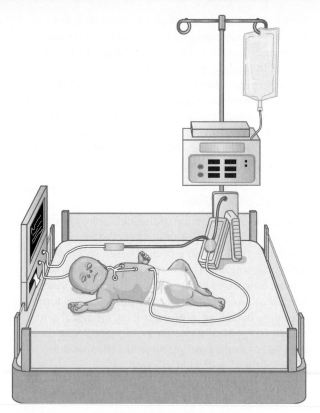

FIGURE 19-12 An illustration of the configuration and use of an inline continuous blood gas monitor.

blood crosses the microelectrochemical sensor for analysis, the patient is reinfused with 1.0 mL of the blood used for analysis, minimizing blood loss. **Figure 19-12** provides an illustration of the ViaMedical inline blood gas monitor (International Biomedical, Austin TX).

Hazards/Complications

Incorrect placement of the UAC increases the risk for catheter-associated complications, such as increased risk for thromboses of the lower extremities, bowel, and kidneys and bleeding and circulation disturbances.[58] Adjusting the catheter position and drifting from aseptic technique during line care increases infant handling and infection risk.[58]

Disadvantages/Limitations

Distal hypoperfusion may follow arterial cannulation. Therefore, it is important for the infant's pelvic area and feet to be visible at all times, facilitating assessment of adequate circulation. The risks and benefits of cannulation should be weighed prior to catheter placement.

Conditions Adversely Affecting Accuracy

Catheter malposition increases the likelihood for complications, some of which may be life threatening. The

accuracy of invasive blood pressure monitoring may be adversely affected by transducer position. It is essential for the transducer to be free of blood and maintained at the level of the right atrium. Monitoring arterial pressure waveforms is helpful in determining the quality of the signal and precision of the systolic, diastolic, and mean pressures displayed on the monitor. A dampened signal denotes the need to calibrate the transducer. Treatment based on erroneous blood pressure readings contributes to poor patient outcomes.

Peripheral Artery Catheter

Peripherally inserted arterial lines are useful when frequent sampling of arterial blood is required for the management of a critically ill child and where cannulation of the umbilical artery is not a viable option. Similar to a UAC, a **peripheral artery catheter** also provides continuous blood pressure monitoring.

Placement in an Infant or Child

Cannulation of the artery can be accomplished by percutaneous puncture or by making a small surgical incision in the skin to allow direct access to the vessel, also known as the cut-down method. The radial artery is the most commonly used site. However, the dorsalis pedis and posterior tibial arteries provide viable options if cannulation of the radial artery cannot be accomplished. Arterial catheters range in size from 10 to 22 gauge for children and 22 to 24 gauge for newborns and infants. The literature reports the benefits of using ultrasound to guide peripheral arterial line placement. The use of ultrasound guidance for the placement of radial arterial catheters reduces the time and number of attempts required for cannulation, especially among less experienced practitioners.[59]

Clinical Considerations

Prior to cannulation, it is important to assess the collateral circulation of the extremity selected for potential use by performing a modified Allen's test. This invasive procedure is not without risk for complications. The risks and benefits of peripherally cannulating the artery, especially when performed in infants and very small children, should be weighed prior to performing the procedure.

There is an increased risk of complications with cannulation of the brachial, femoral, and superficial temporal arteries. These sites are not considered as first choices for percutaneous or surgical access of the artery.

Indications

The indications for a peripherally inserted arterial catheter mirror those of UACs. The arterial lines are commonly used for blood sampling and invasive monitoring of blood pressure. As with a UAC, an inline continuous closed-loop blood gas monitor may be used.

Hazards/Complications

The insertion of a peripheral artery catheter carries a risk for catheter-associated infections. To minimize the risk for infection, adherence to aseptic technique and catheter-related bloodstream infection bundles is essential.[60] Bleeding and thrombosis are also complications associated with indwelling arterial catheters. The risk of thrombosis increases proportionally with the size and duration of catheter placement. Children younger than 5 years of age carry a higher risk for complications and should be closely monitored for signs of thrombosis.[61]

Disadvantages/Limitations

Insertion of peripheral artery catheters can be challenging and is associated with a low first-attempt success rate, especially when less experienced practitioners perform the procedure.[61] Repeated attempts for vascular access are associated with a higher complication rate and can delay patient care.[61]

Conditions Adversely Affecting Accuracy

Conditions that adversely affect the accuracy of invasive blood pressure measurements or blood gas results mirror those associated with the use of a UAC. Catheter malposition will increase the likelihood for circulatory impairment of the extremity distal to the catheter tip. The accuracy of invasive blood pressure monitoring may be adversely affected by transducer position. Poor patient outcomes may occur when treatment is based on erroneous blood gas or pressure readings.

Central Venous Catheter

There are several types of central venous access. The types of access devices differ with indications for use. The frequency of catheter use, availability of access sites, and expected duration of therapy should be considered when selecting the type of venous access device to place. Although a topical anesthetic is frequently used before accessing a central vein, sedation and analgesia are necessary for pain control.[62]

Placement in a Neonate or Child

A **central venous catheter** may be placed percutaneously or through surgical cannulation, known as the cut-down method. The **cut-down procedure** is typically used to access the internal and external jugular and common facial, brachial, femoral, and saphenous veins. This method requires expertise to minimize the propensity for surgical complications, including bleeding, vessel perforation, and nerve and/or muscle damage.[63]

The internal and external jugular, brachial, and saphenous veins may also be accessed percutaneously. The subclavian vein is also a commonly accessed vessel by percutaneous cannulation. A flush line, pressure transducer, and pressure-monitoring device are required for invasive monitoring of right atrial pressures. The pressure waveform provides guidance for the depth of insertion.[63] Similar to the placement of arterial lines, radiographic confirmation of line position is required following placement.[63]

Clinical Considerations

The **umbilical venous catheter (UVC)** is most commonly used in critically ill newborn infants. Cannulation of the umbilical vein provides easy access and preserves the integrity of the small-caliber peripheral veins, especially in preterm infants.

Another option for central access in infants and children is a **peripherally inserted central catheter (PICC)**. A PICC is generally threaded percutaneously through a superficial vein and can be used to administer vasoactive medications and parenteral nutrition.

Indications

Central venous catheters provide a direct route for fluid, medication, and nutritional support to the central circulation. Assessing a central vein is preferable when antibiotic or chemotherapeutic medication delivery is irritating to the peripheral veins (causes a burning sensation or vasospasm), in children with limited or difficult peripheral access, and those requiring frequent blood collection.[64]

Central venous catheters can be used to monitor hemodynamic status by measuring central venous and right atrial pressures, which are helpful in managing fluid administration.

Central access through the internal and external jugular, brachial, femoral, subclavian, and saphenous veins provides a route for infusing larger volumes of fluid as well as for monitoring right atrial pressures.[64] Monitoring right atrial pressures is helpful in assessing tricuspid valve performance, intravascular volume, and myocardial function. Pressure trends are useful for guiding therapy, especially fluid balance. Normal values for right atrial pressures range from 2 to 7 cm H_2O but vary with changes in intrapleural and thoracic pressure. **Table 19-10** outlines the clinical conditions associated with variances in central venous pressures.

Hazards/Complications

Studies comparing complications from central venous access devices identified that most occur with PICCs

TABLE 19-10
Common Conditions Associated with Changes in Central Venous Pressure

	Increased Central Venous Pressure	Decreased Central Venous Pressure
Clinical condition	Hypervolemia	Severe dehydration
	Increased systemic vasoconstriction	Hemorrhage
	Left ventricular failure	Profound vasodilation
	Tricuspid stenosis	Shock
	Tricuspid regurgitation	Hypovolemia
	Increased pulmonary vascular resistance	
	Cardiac tamponade	

(51%) and fewer (1.6%) with UVCs.[65] As with any indwelling catheter, the risk for catheter-associated bloodstream infection exists.[65]

During insertion, pneumothorax can occur.[65] Dysrhythmias are often associated with catheter malposition and occur in response to right ventricular irritation by the catheter tip. There is also the risk for thromboembolism and migration of the emboli to the pulmonary vasculature, especially when the catheter is in place for a prolonged period of time.[63]

Disadvantages/Limitations

The caliber of the central line may limit its use. The lumen of a PICC line can be extremely small, especially when the use is for a preterm or low birthweight infant. The small lumen often makes these lines unsuitable for blood sampling or hemodynamic monitoring. Because of the risks of infection, PICCs are used for intermediate duration of therapy, extending from 1 to 6 months.[66]

Conditions Adversely Affecting Accuracy

Catheter migration and subsequent malposition will affect pressure readings. Right atrial pressures are also affected by changes in thoracic and intrapleural pressure. Caution should be used when basing decisions on trends that include values obtained during mechanical ventilatory support.

Pulmonary Artery Catheter

Pulmonary artery catheters, also known as Swan Ganz catheters, provide direct monitoring of pulmonary and intracardiac pressures and measurement of mixed venous oxygen tensions and cardiac output. Left arterial pressure estimations can be obtained by performing a pulmonary artery wedge pressure.

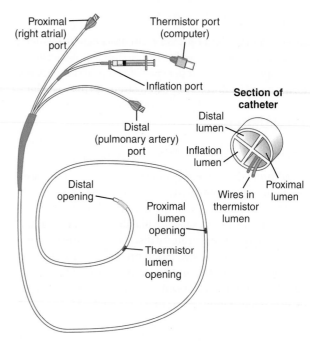

FIGURE 19-13 An illustration of a pulmonary artery catheter.

Placement in a Neonate or Child

Preparation for insertion is essential. The child is typically placed in a Trendelenburg position to enhance neck vein filling, which facilitates catheter float through the tricuspid valve into the right ventricle. This position also used to prevent air emboli. The conventional pulmonary artery catheter has four ports (**Figure 19-13**). Prior to insertion, the catheter is primed with an intravenous flush solution. The integrity of the balloon is also assessed by injecting air into the balloon lumen and verifying that the balloon, located on the catheter's distal tip, inflates and remains inflated until manually deflated by removing air from the balloon lumen.

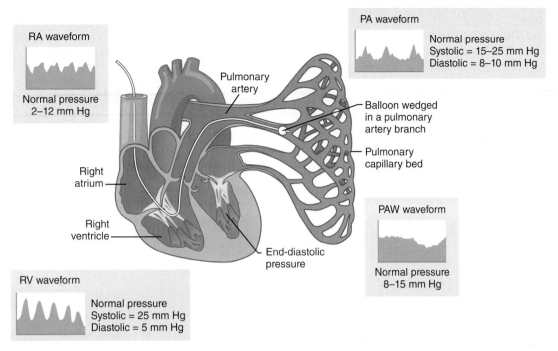

FIGURE 19-14 Waveforms from the various locations of a pulmonary artery catheter.

Cannulation of a large vessel is required. This can be accomplished surgically, by a cut-down technique, or through percutaneous insertion. The left subclavian or right internal jugular vein is frequently used because the predesigned curvature of the catheter allows for ease of access, even in the most unfavorable conditions, such as a pulmonary hypertensive crisis. The femoral artery may also be used; however, access to the pulmonary artery is more difficult with this approach because of the torturous path the catheter must travel. Fluoroscopy-guided insertion may be helpful when congenital anomalous venous connections are suspected.[67] The balloon is inflated after insertion of the distal portion of the catheter. The air-filled balloon helps the catheter flow through the major vessels and right chamber of the heart to the pulmonary artery. The location of the catheter is confirmed by observing the pressure waveforms on the cardiac monitor (**Figure 19-14**).

Clinical Considerations

The use of pulmonary catheters in critically ill infants and young children is much less frequent than in critically ill teens and adults. The risk of complications is much higher in infants and young children, which must be weighed against the monitoring benefits. The pressures and normal ranges for their respective values obtained from pulmonary artery catheterization are found in **Table 19-11**. Fluid balance, intrapleural pressure, and cardiac function can cause variations in pulmonary

TABLE 19-11
Normal Range Values for Pressures Obtained from Pulmonary Artery Catheterization

Monitored Pressure	Range (mm Hg)
Mean right atrial	2–7
Pulmonary artery systolic	15–30
Pulmonary artery diastolic	5–15
Mean pulmonary artery	10–20
Pulmonary capillary wedge	5–15

artery and capillary wedge pressures. **Table 19-12** outlines the clinical conditions that can cause alterations in pulmonary artery pressures. Pulmonary capillary wedge pressures will be increased with intravascular fluid overload and left ventricular failure.

Pressure and cardiac output measurements can be used to derive several hemodynamic parameters. **Pulse contour analysis** is a minimally invasive technique that uses pressure measurements obtained from a pulmonary artery or central venous catheter to continuously calculate cardiac output. Stroke volume and cardiac index can be accurately derived from variations in the arterial pressure waveform during mechanical ventilation.[68] **Figure 19-15** illustrates how stroke volume and cardiac output can be derived from the arterial pressure waveform. A central venous

TABLE 19-12
Conditions That Will Cause Pulmonary Artery Pressure to Vary from Normal

Conditions Causing Pressures to Increase	Conditions Causing Pressures to Decrease
Increased pulmonary vascular resistance Mitral stenosis Left ventricular failure Hypervolemia/intravascular fluid overload Pulmonary edema Increase in pulmonary blood flow (i.e., congenital heart defects with a left-to-right shunt)	Hypovolemia pulmonary vasodilation

TABLE 19-13
Calculated Parameters Used to Construct a Hemodynamic Profile and Values Within the Normal Range

Hemodynamic Parameter	Range of Normal Values
Cardiac index	3.5–4.5 L/min/m^2
Stroke volume	50–80 mL/heartbeat
Stroke volume index	30–65 mL/heartbeat/m^2
Systemic vascular resistance	11–18 mm Hg/L/min
Pulmonary vascular resistance	1.5–3.0 mm Hg/L/min
Shunt fraction	<5%

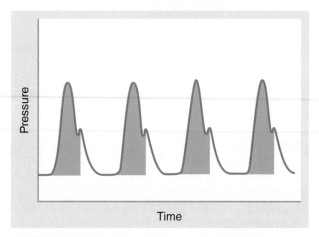

FIGURE 19-15 An illustration of the use of pulse count analysis to derive stroke volume and cardiac output. Stroke volume is reflected by the red-colored area under the systolic part of the pressure curve of one heartbeat. Cardiac output is calculated beat to beat and is the product of stroke volume and heart rate (stroke volume x heart rate).

catheter may be used in lieu of a pulmonary artery catheter when pulse contour analysis is used, making it an attractive alternative for infants and children.

Values obtained from pulmonary artery pressure monitoring can be used to calculate parameters that will provide a comprehensive hemodynamic profile. The parameters and normal range values are found in **Table 19-13**.

Indications

Pulmonary artery catheters measure hemodynamic parameters and are used to measure cardiac output, evaluate cardiomyopathy and intravascular volume, and determine shock state. The presence and severity of valvular heart disease and pulmonary hypertension can also be assessed.

Hazards/Complications

Complications can occur during the insertion of a pulmonary artery catheter or while the catheter is indwelling. Bleeding, pneumothorax, arrhythmias, and perforation of the right atria and ventricle can occur during catheter insertion. Overinflation of the balloon can contribute to balloon rupture and subsequent air emboli or, if the balloon remains intact, cause structural damage to the pulmonary artery. To minimize the potential for pulmonary infarction, care should be taken to avoid positioning the catheter in the wedge position for prolonged periods of time.

Complications associated with an indwelling catheter include catheter-associated bloodstream infections and thrombosis.

Disadvantages/Limitations

The skill required for insertion and complications associated with insertion limit the utility in infants and small children.

Conditions Adversely Affecting Accuracy

Variations in pulmonary capillary wedge pressure may occur during mechanical ventilatory support. Pulmonary capillary wedge pressure reflects the pressures on the left side of the heart, which are obtained when blood flow is absent on the pulmonary capillary bed. Change in intrapulmonary pressure will affect pulmonary capillary wedge pressures. As intrapulmonary pressures rise, more pressure is transmitted to adjacent cardiovascular structures. The use of positive end-expiratory pressure (PEEP) will elevate pulmonary capillary wedge pressure. It is important to follow trends and to interpret values cautiously when changes in PEEP and pulmonary compliance occur.

Case Study 1

A 16-year-old girl with a history of poorly controlled asthma presents to the emergency department with worsening shortness of breath. She is in severe respiratory distress despite receiving albuterol every 2 hours at home. She is placed on a cardiopulmonary monitor and a pulse oximeter. Vitals signs are as follows: heart rate 120 beats per minute, respiratory rate 30 breaths per minute, blood pressure 125/90 mm Hg, temperature 37.5°C, oxygen saturation 86% on room air. You are asked to initiate continuous albuterol at 15 mg/hr and to obtain a blood gas. After obtaining the arterial blood gas supplies, you enter the room, introduce yourself to the patient, and describe the procedure to her.

Prior to performing the radial artery puncture, you perform the modified Allen's test. The color of the palm changed from blanched to pink in <5 seconds.

You proceed with the procedure, obtain a sample for analysis, and apply pressure to the puncture site until bleeding has stopped. The blood gas is analyzed with a point-of-care blood gas machine. The arterial blood gas test indicates a pH of 7.54, CO_2 of 26 mm Hg, PaO_2 of 60 mm Hg, bicarbonate level of 22 mEq/L, base excess of 0.8 meq/L and Pa. A chemistry panel demonstrates a sodium level of 138 mEq/L and chloride level of 103 mEq/L. The physician asks you to interpret the arterial blood gas and to make recommendations for care.

1. **Was collateral circulation adequate prior to performing the arterial sample.**

2. **If the patient was unable to follow your direction for the modified Allen's test, describe how you would assess collateral circulation.**

3. **What is your interpretation of this arterial blood gas?**

4. **What other recommendations would you make at this time?**

Case Study 2

A 6-week-old infant presents to the emergency department with complaints of color changes with a choking and coughing episode. The mother reported that the child had a bluish discoloration of his face with the episode. Upon presentation, the infant appeared alert and in no distress. Vital signs are as follows: heart rate 122 beats per minute, respiratory rate 30 breaths per minute, blood pressure 90/54 mm Hg, SpO_2 100% on room air. The patient was triaged and placed on a cardiorespiratory monitor.

The infant's mother stated that the event occurred about 10 minutes after she had finished breastfeeding and had placed him on his back in his crib. She said that she had heard him making choking and gurgling sounds and had gone back to his room to check on him, where she noticed that his face had turned bluish purple. She further noted that when she picked her son up, he was limp and did not seem to be breathing. She immediately shouted for her husband while she "blew air into his mouth." After about 10 seconds, she said her infant responded and seemed to be back to his normal self.

A chest radiograph was ordered and results were unremarkable. The infant was admitted to pediatric services for overnight evaluation with impedance pneumography with pH by an esophageal monitoring catheter. The patient had no further apneic episodes during admission but did have reflux after most feeds. No further interventions were required during the hospital stay, and the infant was discharged home the following day after parental education on home management of infantile gastroesophageal reflux disease.

1. **What does impedance pneumography monitor?**

2. **Could this type of monitoring be performed with a home device?**

3. **What are the limitations to using an impedance pneumography monitor on the patient in this case study?**

References

1. Salyer JW. Neonatal and pediatric pulse oximetry. *Respir Care.* 2003;48(4):386-396; discussion 397-398.
2. Sinex JE. Pulse oximetry: principles and limitations. *Am J Emerg Med.* 1999;17(1):59-67.
3. Bell C, Luther MA, Nicholson JJ, Fox CJ, Hirsh JL. Effect of probe design on accuracy and reliability of pulse oximetry in pediatric patients. *J Clin Anesth.* 1999;11(4):323-327.
4. Sahni R. Continuous noninvasive monitoring in the neonatal ICU. *Curr Opin Pediatr.* 2017;29(2):141-148. doi:10.1097/MOP.0000000000000459.
5. O'Donnell CP, Kamlin CO, Davis PG, Carlin JB, Morley CJ. Clinical assessment of infant colour at delivery. *Arch Dis Child Fetal Neonatal Ed.* 2007;92:F465-F467.
6. Dawson JA, Davis PG, O'Donnell CP, Kamlin CO, Morley CJ. Pulse oximetry for monitoring infants in the delivery room: a review. *Arch Dis Child Fetal Neonatal Ed.* 2007;92(1):F4-F7.

7. Toth B, Becker A, Seelbach-Göbel B. Oxygen saturation in healthy newborn infants immediately after birth measured by pulse oximetry. *Arch Gynecol Obstet*. 2002;266(2):105-107.

8. de Wahl-Granelli A, Wennergren M, Sandberg K, et al. Impact of pulse oximetry screening on the detection of duct dependent congenital heart disease: a Swedish prospective screening study in 39,821 newborns. *BMJ*. 2009;338:a3037.

9. Reich JD, Miller S, Brogdon B, et al. The use of pulse oximetry to detect congenital heart disease. *J Pediatr*. 2003;142(3):221-222.

10. Meier-Stauss P, Bucher HU, Hürlimann R, König V, Huch R. Pulse oximetry used for documenting oxygen saturation and right-to-left shunting immediately after birth. *Eur J Pediatr*. 1990;149(12):851-855.

11. Mariani G, Dik PB, Ezquer A, et al. Pre-ductal and post-ductal O₂ saturation in healthy term neonates after birth. *J Pediatr*. 2007;150(4):418-421.

12. Das J, Aggarwal A, Aggarwal NK. Pulse oximeter accuracy and precision at five different sensor locations in infants and children with cyanotic heart disease. *Indian J Anaesth*. 2010;54(6):531-534.

13. Griksaitis MJ, Scrimgeour GE, Pappachan JV, Baldock AJ. Accuracy of the Masimo SET LNCS neo peripheral pulse oximeter in cyanotic congenital heart disease. *Cardiol Young*. 2016;26(6):1183-1186.

14. Shrestha S, Shrestha S, Shrestha L, Bhandary N. Oxygen saturation of hemoglobin in healthy children of 2–14 years at high altitude in Nepal. *Kathmandu Univ Med J*. 2012;10(37):40-43.

15. Nilson D, Partridge R, Suner S, Jay G. Noninvasive carboxyhemoglobin monitoring: screening emergency medical services patients for carbon monoxide exposure. *Prehosp Disaster Med*. 2010;25(3):253-256.

16. Ralston AC, Webb RK, Runciman WB. Potential errors in pulse oximetry. III: effects of interferences, dyes, dyshaemoglobins and other pigments. *Anaesthesia*. 1991;46(4):291-295.

17. Hinkelbein J, Genzwuerker HV, Sogl R, Fiedler F. Effect of nail polish on oxygen saturation determined by pulse oximetry in critically ill patients. *Resuscitation*. 2007;72(1):82-91.

18. Siobal MS. Monitoring exhaled carbon dioxide. *Respir Care*. 2016;61(10):1397-1416.

19. Hess D. Capnometry and capnography: technical aspects, physiologic aspects, and clinical applications. *Respir Care*. 1990;35(6):557-573.

20. Casati A, Gallioli G, Scandroglio M, Passaretta R, Borghi B, Torri G. Accuracy of end-tidal carbon dioxide monitoring using the NBP-75 microstream capnometer. A study in intubated ventilated and spontaneously breathing nonintubated patients. *Eur J Anaesthesiol*. 2000;17(10):622-626.

21. Bhat YR, Abhishek N. Mainstream end-tidal carbon dioxide monitoring in ventilated neonates. *Singapore Med J*. 2008;49(3):199-203.

22. Tobias JD, Flanagan JFK, Wheeler TJ, Garrett JS, Burney C. Noninvasive monitoring of end-tidal CO₂ via nasal cannulas in spontaneously breathing children during the perioperative period. *Crit Care Med*. 1994;22(11):1805-1808.

23. Friesen RH, Alswang M. End-tidal PCO₂ monitoring via nasal cannulae in pediatric patients: accuracy and sources of error. *J Clin Monit*. 1996;12(2):155-159.

24. Bhende MS. End-tidal carbon dioxide monitoring in pediatrics—clinical applications. *J Postgrad Med*. 2001;47(3):215-218.

25. Hart LS, Berns SD, Houck CS, Boenning DA. The value of end-tidal CO₂ monitoring when comparing three methods of procedural sedation for children undergoing painful procedures in the emergency department. *Pediatr Emerg Care*. 1997;13:189-193.

26. Abramo TJ, Wiebe RA, Scott S, Goto CS, McIntire DD. Noninvasive capnometry monitoring for respiratory status during pediatric seizures. *Crit Care Med*. 1997;25(7):1242-1246.

27. Bhende MS. Capnography in the paediatric emergency department. *Peds Emerg Care*. 1999;15:64-69.

28. Hatlestad D. Capnography as a predictor of the return of spontaneous circulation. *Emerg Med Serv*. 2004;33(8):75-80.

29. Sandberg KL, Brynjarsson H, Hjalmarson O. Transcutaneous blood gas monitoring during neonatal intensive care. *Acta Paediatr*. 2011;100(5):676-679.

30. Martin M, Brown C, Bayard D, et al. Continuous noninvasive monitoring of cardiac performance and tissue perfusion in pediatric trauma patients. *J Pediatr Surg*. 2005;40(12):1957-1963.

31. Restrepo RD, Hirst KR, Wittnebel L, Wettstein R. AARC clinical practice guideline: transcutaneous monitoring of carbon dioxide and oxygen: 2012. *Respir Care*. 2012;57(11):1955-1962.

32. Tobias JD. Transcutaneous carbon dioxide monitoring in infants and children. *Paediatr Anaesth*. 2009;19(5):434-444.

33. Bernet V, Döll C, Cannizzaro V, Ersch J, Frey B, Weiss M. Longtime performance and reliability of two different PtcCO₂ and SpO₂ sensors in neonates. *Paediatr Anaesth*. 2008;18(9):872-877.

34. Rithalia SV, George RJ, Tinker J. Continuous tissue pH and transcutaneous PO₂ measurement as an index of tissue perfusion in critically ill patients. *Resuscitation*. 1981;9(1):67-74.

35. Buntain WL, Conner E, Emrico J, Cassady G. Transcutaneous oxygen (tcPO2) measurements as an aid to fluid therapy in necrotizing enterocolitis. *J Pediatr Surg*. 1979;14(6):728-732.

36. Malmberg LP, Seppä VP, Kotaniemi-Syrjänen A, et al. Measurement of tidal breathing flows in infants using impedance pneumography. *Eur Respir J*. 2017;49(2):1600926.

37. Tsang R, Checchia P, Bronicki RA. Hemodynamic monitoring in the acute management of pediatric heart failure. *Curr Cardiol Rev*. 2016;12(2):112-116.

38. Hampton DA, Schreiber MA. Near infrared spectroscopy: clinical and research uses. *Transfusion*. 2013;53(Suppl 1):52S-58S.

39. Scheeren TW, Schober P, Schwarte LA. Monitoring tissue oxygenation by near infrared spectroscopy (NIRS): background and current applications. *J Clin Monit Comput*. 2012;26(4):279-287.

40. Ghanayem NS, Hoffman GM. Near infrared spectroscopy as a hemodynamic monitor in critical illness. *Pediatr Crit Care Med*. 2016;17(8 Suppl 1):S201-S206.

41. Breen PH. Arterial blood gas and pH analysis. Clinical approach and interpretation. *Anesthesiol Clin North Am*. 2001;19(4):885-906.

42. Davis MD, Walsh BK, Sittig SE, Restrepo RD. AARC clinical practice guideline: blood gas analysis and hemoximetry: 2013. *Respir Care*. 2013;58(10):1694-1703.

43. Nash P. Umbilical catheters, placement, and complication management. *J Infus Nurs*. 2006;29(6):346-352.

44. de Graaff JC, Cuper NJ, Mungra RA, Vlaardingerbroek K, Numan SC, Kalkman CJ. Near-infrared light to aid peripheral intravenous cannulation in children: a cluster randomised clinical trial of three devices. *Anaesthesia*. 2013;68(8):835-845.

45. Cuper NJ, Klaessens JH, Jaspers JE, et al. The use of near-infrared light for safe and effective visualization of subsurface blood vessels to facilitate blood withdrawal in children. *Med Eng Phys*. 2013;35(4):433-440.

46. Matheson L, Stephenson M, Huber B. Reducing pain associated with arterial punctures for blood gas analysis. *Pain Manag Nurs*. 2014;15(3):619-624.

47. Dogan OF, Demircin M, Ucar I, Duman U, Yilmaz M, Boke E. Iatrogenic brachial and femoral artery complications following venipuncture in children. *Heart Surg Forum*. 2006;9(4):E675-E680.

48. Escalante-Kanashire R, Tantalean-Da-Fiebo J. Capillary blood gases in a pediatric intensive care unit. *Crit Care Med*. 2000;28(1):224-226.

49. Yidizdas D, Yapicioglu H, Yilmaz HL, Sertdemir Y. Correlation of simultaneously obtained capillary, venous and arterial blood gases of patients in a pediatric intensive care unit. *Arch Dis Child*. 2004;89(2):176-180.

50. Zavorsky GS, Cao J, Mayo NE, Gabbay R, Murias JM. Arterial verses capillary blood gases: a meta-analysis. *Respir Physiol Neurobiol*. 2007;155(3):268-279.

51. Committee on Injury, Violence, and Poison Prevention. Prevention of choking among children. *Pediatrics*. 2010;125(3):601-607.

52. Prince AM. Tips for successful umbilical artery catheterization. *J Ark Med Soc*. 2007;103(7):181-183.

53. Lopriore E, Verheij GH, Walther FJ. Measurement of the 'shoulder-umbilical' distance for insertion of umbilical catheters in newborn babies: questionnaire study. *Neonatology*. 2008;94(1):35-37.

54. Wright IM, Owers M, Wagner M. The umbilical arterial catheter: a formula for improved positioning in the very low birth weight infant. *Pediatr Crit Care Med.* 2008;9(5):498-501.

55. Min SR, Lee HS. Comparison of Wright's formula and the Dunn method for measuring the umbilical arterial catheter insertion length. *Pediatr Neonatol.* 2015;56(2):120-125.

56. Marshall M. Radiographic assessment of umbilical venous and arterial catheter tip location. *Neonatal Netw.* 2014;33(4):208-216.

57. Barrington KJ. Umbilical artery catheters in the newborn: effects of position of the catheter tip. *Cochrane Database Syst Rev.* 2000;(2):CD000505.

58. Hermansen MC, Hermansen MG. Intravascular catheter complications in the neonatal intensive care unit. *Clin Perinatol.* 2005;32(1):141-156.

59. Kantor DB, Su E, Milliren CE, Conlon TW. Ultrasound guidance and other determinants of successful peripheral artery catheterization in critically ill children. *Pediatr Crit Care Med.* 2016;17(12):1124-1130.

60. Düzkaya DS, Sahiner NC, Uysal G, Yakut T, Çitak A. Chlorhexidine-impregnated dressings and prevention of catheter-associated bloodstream infections in a pediatric intensive care unit. *Crit Care Nurse.* 2016;36(6):e1-e7.

61. Scheer B, Perel A, Pfeiffer UJ. Clinical review: complications and risk factors of peripheral arterial catheters used for haemodynamic monitoring in anaesthesia and intensive care medicine. *Crit Care.* 2002;6(3):199-204.

62. Mickler PA. Neonatal and pediatric perspectives in PICC placement. *J Infus Nurs.* 2008;31(5):282-285.

63. Ullman AJ, Marsh N, Mihala G, Cooke M, Rickard CM. Complications of central venous access devices: a systematic review. *Pediatrics.* 2015;136(5):e1331-e1344.

64. Barczykowska E, Szwed-Kolinska M, Wrobel-Bania A, Slusarz R. The use of central venous lines in the treatment of chronically ill children. *Adv Clin Exp Med.* 2014;23(6):1001-1009.

65. Taylor JE, McDonald SJ, Earnest A, et al. A quality improvement initiative to reduce central line infection in neonates using checklists. *Eur J Pediatr.* 2017;176(5):639-646.

66. Chesshyre E, Goff Z, Bowen A, Carapetis J. The prevention, diagnosis and management of central venous line infections in children. *J Infect.* 2015;71(Suppl 1):S59-S75.

67. Tripathi M, Kumar N, Singh PK. Pulmonary artery catheter insertion in a patient of dextrocardia with anomalous venous connections. *Indian J Med Sci.* 2004;58(8):353-356.

68. Hadian M, Kim HK, Severyn DA, Pinsky MR. Cross-comparison of cardiac output trending accuracy of LiDCO, PiCCO, FloTrac and pulmonary artery catheters. *Crit Care.* 2010;14(6):R212.

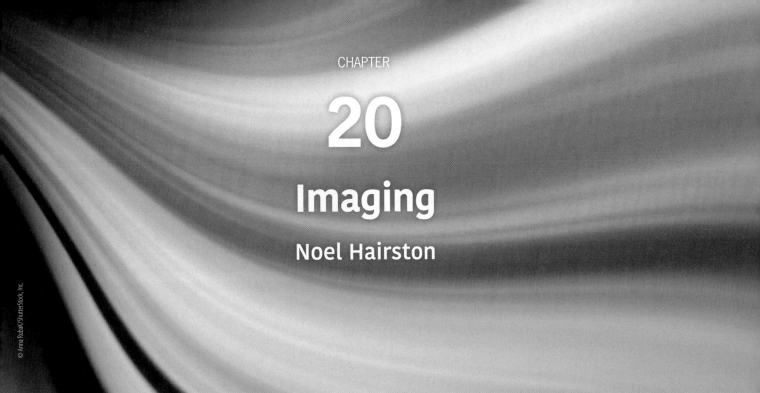

CHAPTER

20
Imaging

Noel Hairston

OUTLINE

Introduction
Anteroposterior and Posteroanterior Views
Chest Radiography
  Lateral Decubitus
  Oblique
  Neck
  Examination of Anatomical Structures
  Lines/Drains and Tubes
Computerized Tomography
Magnetic Resonance Imaging
References

OBJECTIVES

1. List the indications for chest radiography.
2. Explain the concerns associated with radiation exposure in pediatric patients.
3. Describe how to evaluate the technical quality of chest radiography.
4. Explain the importance of patient and head positioning during chest radiography.
5. List the indications for frontal and lateral neck radiography.
6. Differentiate between the church steeple and thumb-like signs.
7. Differentiate among lateral decubitus, oblique, anteroposterior, and posteroranterior views.
8. Describe the common radiologic abnormalities seen in the airway, pleura, and lung parenchyma.
9. Explain proper radiologic position of common lines and drains, such as peripherally inserted central catheter, umbilical artery catheter, umbilical venous catheter, and nasogastric tube.
10. List the contraindications of magnetic resonance imaging.

KEY TERMS

anteroposterior (AP)
computerized tomography scan
lateral decubitus
magnetic resonance imaging
oblique
peripherally inserted central catheter (PICC)
posteroanterior (PA)
radiolucent
umbilical artery catheter (UAC)
umbilical venous catheter (UVC)

331

Introduction

Radiography has advanced tremendously over the years. Historically, when a chest radiograph was obtained, a film was used, which required manual development. After the image processing, the film was hand delivered to a physician for review and interpretation. This process was quite lengthy and much different from the process we currently use. Today, radiographic images are obtained and ready for interpretation almost instantaneously. Portable machines obtain radiographic images at the point of care, such as the patient's bedside. Typically, portable radiologic imaging occurs when transport to a central radiology department is not optimal. Portable machines are common in neonatal and pediatric intensive care units, especially when intubated patients require imaging. The radiologist or attending physician has the ability to review the images electronically and even to have a specialist review and interpret the reading from a separate location, expediting care. Radiographs are viewed digitally and most frequently use a Picture Archiving and Communication System (PACS) monitor, a monitor on the portable unit, or with a radiologist in the radiology department.[1] In addition to streamlining workflow, digital imaging systems, such as PACS, allow radiograph images to link to the electronic health record, which ties the image to the patient's clinical data and minimizes the propensity for lost or missing films.[2] The use of digital images allows the user to adjust the quality of the image, reducing the need to repeat radiographs because films were over- or underexposed.[3]

Radiographic assessment of the chest is critical in determining accurate diagnosis and proper treatment. A respiratory care practitioner is able to visualize anatomy; assess airway patency; evaluate abnormalities; and assess and verify the position of lines, drains, and tubes. Pediatric radiation exposure is a particular concern because infants and children are more radiosensitive than adults. Infants and children also have a longer span of time for any detrimental effects of radiation exposure, such as cancer, to manifest, and the use of equipment and exposure settings designed for adults may result in excessive radiation exposure if used on pediatrics.[4,5] Where there is a need for imaging, the as low as reasonably achievable (ALARA) principle should always be followed.[6]

Normal anatomy is distinguishable by the amount of the X-ray beam that is absorbed. For instance, bone and metallic hardware (orthopedic hardware, etc.) appear white because the higher absorption rate of radiation results in less to expose the film. In contrast, air has little absorption; the lungs, for example, appear black on the radiograph.

Anteroposterior and Posteroanterior Views

Anteroposterior (AP) and **posteroanterior (PA)** views are differentiated by the position of the patient in relationship to the radiation source. In the AP view, the patient

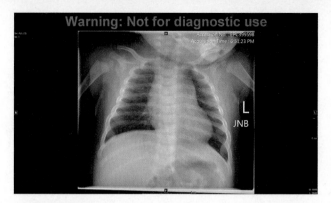

FIGURE 20-1 AP view of a neonate demonstrating a lordotic appearance due to lack of thoracic curvature.
Courtesy of Akron Children's Hospital.

lies on their back and the radiographic beam enters from front to back. The PA view is the opposite—the patient either is in a prone position or is standing, and the radiographic beam enters from back to front.

Neonatal AP chest radiographs (CXRs) tend to have a lordotic appearance because of the lack of thoracic curvature that develops with age. It is important to consider this distortion when reviewing the image. The image of the chest is obtained during the inspiratory phase for neonates and infants receiving ventilatory support. Occasionally, the provider requests an inspiratory pause during the CXR. The inspiratory hold enables the image to capture the lungs fully inflated for a better evaluation (**Figure 20-1**).

Chest Radiography

Chest radiography has been used as a diagnostic tool for more than a century. Chest radiographs provide clinicians with images that allow for examination of the heart, lungs, and thorax; identify presence and/or progression of pathology; and assess the position of lines, drains, and tubes.

Lateral Decubitus

The **lateral decubitus** position evaluates the presence of air or fluid in the pleural space. Positioning is important to obtain an image that can reveal air or fluid that is abnormally in the pleura. When the clinician is evaluating for air in the pleural space or for a pneumothorax, the patient lies with the affected side of the thorax facing up or away from the bed or cart.[7] Clinicians prefer this view because AP CXRs have poor sensitivity for occult pneumothoraces.[8] Positioning the patient with the affected side down helps to evaluate for a pleural effusion or the presence of fluid in the pleural space.[9] Frequently, clinicians request this view to determine the presence of a foreign body aspiration.[10] Air trapping during expiration in a confined or isolated area is suggestive of a complete bronchial obstruction. Normally, the lung loses volume during expiration. However, when a foreign body lodges in the airway and completely obstructs the airway, air is unable to escape from that area, and the affected portion of the lung will remain

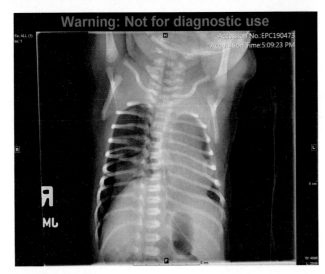

FIGURE 20-2 Lordotic radiographic view showing the presence of free air in the pleural space. The arms and chin are raised to minimize interference.
Courtesy of Akron Children's Hospital.

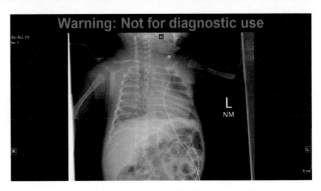

FIGURE 20-3 An oblique image, in which there is a 45-degree rotation of the chest for better evaluation of the airway and lung fields.
Courtesy of Akron Children's Hospital.

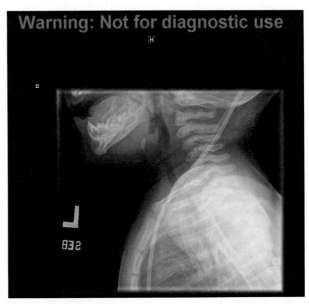

FIGURE 20-4 Lateral neck radiograph demonstrating the steeple sign commonly associated with croup.
Courtesy of Akron Children's Hospital.

inflated. Proper positioning is critical for a good image. Arms and chin must be raised and remain out of range of the image. Elevating the neonate or infant on a radiolucent sponge prevents the chest from sinking into the cart pad. When the body sinks into the cart pad, artifact lines superimpose over the lateral lung field, obscuring the image. Additionally, fluid in the pleural cavity will also obscure an image. Because fluid sinks to the lowest level, there is potential for the fluid to superimpose with the cart pad, which will obscure the image (**Figure 20-2**).

Oblique

The **oblique** position gains an additional perspective of the lungs. The oblique rotation will place the anatomic structures in a different position to provide further evaluation of areas previously superimposed on the AP/PA image. This position also elongates the ribs to allow for better determination of a fracture. This is especially helpful when evaluating an infant or a child for fractures due to abuse or nonaccidental trauma.[11] As with all radiographs, proper position is critical. An oblique image, if evaluating the lung field, requires a 45-degree rotation of the chest, whereas an oblique for the heart requires a 60-degree rotation. If the rotation is not accurate, distortion and magnification of anatomic structures can occur (**Figure 20-3**).

Neck

The thoracic trachea and mainstem bronchi are prominent on routine CXRs. Soft tissue neck films are useful and further evaluate the extrathoracic airway. These views may show a mass effect resulting from retropharyngeal abscess or reveal distortion related to a foreign object. The adenoids are located posterior to the nasopharynx on the lateral neck radiograph. The lateral neck radiograph allows for visualization of the palatine

tonsils, located between the oropharynx and nasopharynx. Enlargement of these two structures is a leading cause of sleep-related apnea as well as airway obstruction related to swelling from acute infection.[12]

Croup is the most common cause of upper airway obstruction in children between 6 months and 3 years of age.[13] Most cases are viral in nature and cause stridor with a barking cough. Frontal and lateral neck radiographs may demonstrate subglottic narrowing below the vocal chords with loss of the normal shouldering and overdistention of the hypopharynx, resulting in the church steeple appearance (**Figure 20-4**).[14]

It is important to evaluate a child presenting with stridor for a foreign body aspiration. Children, especially toddlers, often put food or toys in their mouths. However, they often do not chew the food well enough to allow it easy passage into the esophagus. The larger pieces of food, commonly a peanut, piece of candy, or hot dog, are aspirated rather than swallowed and obstruct the trachea or bronchus. Additionally, a coin or small toy ingested into the esophagus may cause compression of the trachea (**Figure 20-5**). A history of choking typically

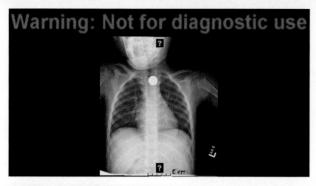
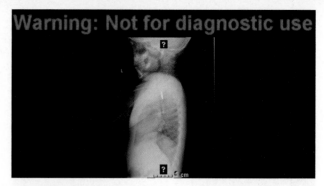

FIGURE 20-5 Radiologic images showing a coin lodged in the esophagus.
Courtesy of Akron Children's Hospital.

prompts the evaluation for aspiration or ingestion of a foreign object. A lateral neck view, as well as views of the chest and abdomen, are helpful in locating the object.

Radiation exposure is always a concern, and the need for imaging should be evaluated. Although no parent wants their child subjected to the hazards associated with radiation exposure, a radiograph is often critical to diagnose respiratory and cardiac-related problems. Proper selection of the technique and patient position are critical to the evaluation of the radiologic image of the neck and chest. Obtaining the right type of view with little to no interference will minimize the need to repeat the imaging study. Improper positioning may also result in a misinterpretation of the image. For example, chest rotation can cause image distortion, show improper tube or line placement, and result in a missed diagnosis.

Examination of Anatomical Structures

Many structures of the chest are readily visible on a chest radiograph. These include bony structures such as the ribs, clavicles, sternum, and spine in addition to the lungs, trachea, hila, diaphragm, lung fissures, heart, aorta, and esophagus. Other important structures, such as the phrenic nerve, are not visible for evaluation. Anatomical structures such as the pleura are only clearly visible when an abnormality exists.

Chest and Neck

When viewing a chest radiograph, it is important to be able to identify the anatomic structures of the thorax, pleura, hilar region, lung fields, heart and vasculature, and the soft tissues. The clavicular heads meet just above the mediastinum, at the first thoracic vertebra (T1), to form the thoracic inlet. The trachea descends vertically between the clavicular heads and appears as a radiolucent structure positioned over the spine. In neonates, the trachea may not align perfectly with the spine because of the lack of thoracic curvature. The trachea bifurcates at the carina into the right and left mainstem bronchi at the 6th thoracic vertebrae (T6) in children and the 4th thoracic vertebra (T4) in neonates. The ribs should be symmetrical. A normal rib cage has 12 pairs of ribs. Children with congenital anomalies of the chest, such as Jarcho-Levin

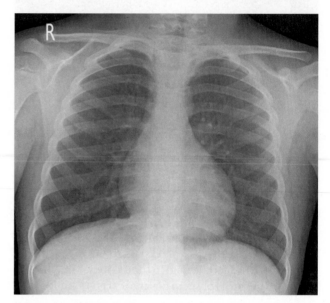

FIGURE 20-6 CXR showing normal anatomic structures.
Case courtesy of Dr. Jeremy Jones, Radiopaedia.org, rID: 41667.

syndrome, may have a crab-shaped chest and fused ribs.[15] Children with skeletal dysplasia may have asymmetrical and/or short ribs.[16] Intercostal spaces are evenly spaced. Widened intercostal spaces and flattened diaphragms are associated with hyperinflation. Narrowed intercostal spaces signify decreased lung volumes, which are often seen with atelectasis. The right hemidiaphragm is typically slightly higher than the left. The liver rests below the right and the stomach below the left hemidiaphragms. Because the lungs are filled with air and normally do not contain fluid or blood, they appear **radiolucent**.

The heart and vasculature are located in the center of the chest, in the mediastinal area. A CXR does not present the heart in detail. However, the shape and size can be examined on a CXR. **Figure 20-6** shows the normal anatomic structures in an older child. **Figure 20-7** identifies the structures typically seen on a lateral view of the neck. This view allows for evaluation of the cervical spine, oropharynx, and upper airway.

Lines/Drains and Tubes

A CXR also determines placement of internal lines and tubes. The accuracy of placement is extremely

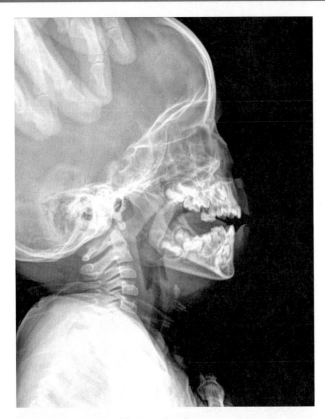

FIGURE 20-7 A view of the lateral neck.
© Xray Computer/Shutterstock.

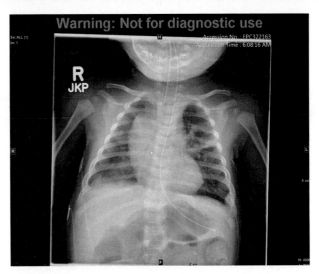

FIGURE 20-8 An AP view of an intubated infant. The tip of the ETT is just below the thoracic inlet. A nasogastric tube is seen in the stomach.
Courtesy of Akron Children's Hospital.

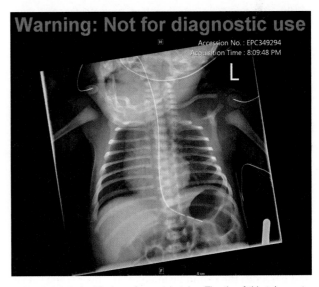

FIGURE 20-9 An AP view of a gastric tube. The tip of this tube rests in the stomach, below the left hemidiaphragm.
Courtesy of Akron Children's Hospital.

important for proper patient monitoring, treatment, and care. As previously discussed, positioning of the patient is crucial in determining placement. Small variations, such as flexion or extension of the patient's neck, may result in a need to repeat the image and subject the child unnecessarily to additional radiation exposure.

Tracheal Tubes

The endotracheal tube (ETT) should reside below the thoracic inlet and above the carina (level of T4 on a neonate and T6 in children). Because the distance between the thoracic inlet and the carina is minimal in a neonate, migration of the tube within a few millimeters can position the ETT shallowly and at risk for unplanned extubation or too deeply in the trachea and at risk for an endobronchial intubation (**Figure 20-8**). Keep head rotation to a minimum because the ETT tip can move superiorly and inferiorly, making it difficult to determine the actual position. The tracheal length in a child is shorter compared to an adult. Small changes in head position can malposition the ETT. Head extension can move the ETT superiorly; depending on the initial position of the ETT, this may place the tip of the tube above the thoracic inlet or even in the esophagus. Head flexion can cause the ETT to migrate deeply into the trachea and position the tip at the carina or within a mainstem bronchus. Endobronchial intubations most frequently occur in the right mainstem bronchus. If undetected, an ETT positioned in the right main bronchus results in hyperinflation of the right lung and collapse

of the contralateral lung. The AP/PA frontal view is the primary choice to evaluate the distance from the ETT to the carina.

Gastric Tubes (NG/OG)

Gastric tubes should follow a vertical path along the midline of the chest. The tip should rest in the stomach, below the left hemidiaphragm (**Figure 20-9**). This tube should not coil in the chest or follow along the trachea and bronchus.

Central Lines: Peripherally Inserted Central Catheter

A **peripherally inserted central catheter (PICC)** line, inserted through a peripheral vein, rests in the thoracic

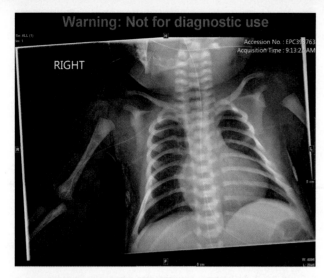

FIGURE 20-10 An AP view of a PICC line confirming placement following insertion.
Courtesy of Akron Children's Hospital.

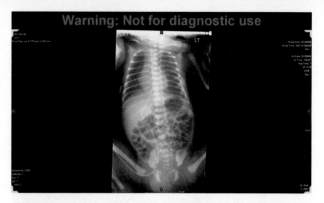

FIGURE 20-11 AP projection demonstrating correct UVC line placement.
Courtesy of Akron Children's Hospital.

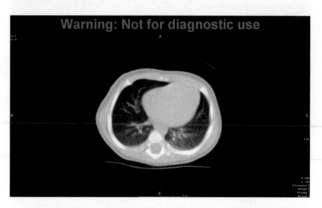

FIGURE 20-12 CT of the chest, showing the heart, lungs, and vertebrae.
Courtesy of Akron Children's Hospital.

portion of the vena cava or right atrium of the heart (**Figure 20-10**). A PICC allows concentrated solutions to be delivered with less risk of complications.

Possible complications associated with PICC insertion include pneumothorax, hemothorax, hematoma, and/or infection. Although there are risks, a PICC provides an alternative for pediatric patients needing frequent labs, small injections, or recurring intravenous medication.

Umbilical Vessel Catheters and Vein and Artery Catheters

The **umbilical venous catheter (UVC)** and **umbilical artery catheter (UAC)** are specific to newborn infants or neonates. This is because as the infant ages, the umbilical cord dries up and falls off. If not cannulated, the umbilical vein closes soon, fewer than 7 days after birth, and becomes the round ligament of the liver. The UVC is useful for exchange transfusions; for monitoring central venous pressure; and for the infusion of fluids, including emergency vascular access for the administration of fluids, blood products, or medications. The umbilical vein is found with the two umbilical arteries in the cord stump and travels to the inferior vena cava (IVC) by the left portal vein and ductus venosus. The ductus venosus begins at the left portal vein and enters the IVC closely related to the hepatic veins. The correct position of the tip of the UVC is at or close to the inferior cavoatrial junction (**Figure 20-11**). Misplacement can occur among other places, in normal anatomy, at the level of the left portal vein and at the level of the hepatic veins.

UAC uses include monitoring blood pressure and obtaining arterial samples for blood gas, electrolyte, and lactate analysis. The UAC is passed through either one of the two umbilical arteries and descends to the iliac artery before ascending to the aorta. Appropriate placement of the tip is in either a low (L3–L4) or high (T6–T10) position.

This avoids the tip being associated with the origin of major aortic vessels.

Computerized Tomography

A **computerized tomography scan** (CT) generates and records many X-ray images as the detector moves around the patient's body. A computer reconstructs all the individual images into cross-sectional images or "slices" of internal organs and tissues. A CT exam involves a higher radiation dose than conventional radiography because many individual X-ray projections are used to construct the CT image.

CT evaluates internal organs, bones, soft tissues, and blood vessels (**Figure 20-12**). It often helps diagnose chest pain or evaluates for injury after trauma. CT is the modality of choice for distinguishing cellulitis from an abscess, which will appear as a walled-off fluid collection needing surgical drainage. Diagnostic needle aspiration of a lung abscess depends on accessibility of the abscess and sufficient size for proper collection for diagnosis. It is often performed with CT guidance.

CT offers much more diagnostic information than a CXR but at a much higher radiation dose. The U.S. Food and Drug Administration states that "the probability for absorbed x rays to induce cancer or heritable mutations leading to genetically associated diseases in offspring is thought to be very small for radiation doses of the magnitude that are associated with CT procedures."[17] High doses of radiation can lead to tissue changes, such as skin reddening, cataracts, and hair loss.[18] Pediatric radiation exposure is highly regulated and monitored to prevent such occurrences.

CT, although delivering useful information, can be difficult to obtain. CT imaging necessitates the patient to lie extremely still, which often requires sedation or general anesthesia to obtain adequate images.

Magnetic Resonance Imaging

Magnetic resonance imaging (MRI) uses a combination of magnetism, radio waves, and computer processing to create detailed anatomic images (**Figure 20-13**). Unlike imaging techniques generated with ionizing radiation, with MRI there is no exposure to radiation.

MRI is the imaging modality of choice in a vast array of pediatric conditions, particularly in neurologic, musculoskeletal, and some cardiovascular diseases. Advantages of MRI include excellent image quality, superior soft tissue contrast, and lack of ionizing radiation.

With radiation safety becoming more prevalent, the need for imaging without ionizing radiation is in high demand. Although MRI is safer in regard to radiation exposure, it has some risks as well. A person may *not* have an MRI if the following contraindications exist:

- Metallic fragments and clips (such as aneurysm clips) can shift or heat up due to the magnetic field.
- Magnetically activated implanted devices, such as cardiac pacemakers, insulin pumps,

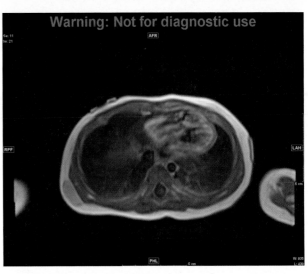

FIGURE 20-13 MRI of the thorax, showing the heart, lung, and spine.

Courtesy of Akron Children's Hospital.

neurostimulators, and cochlear implants, may be deprogrammed.
- Metal hardware (such as orthopedic rods) may heat up or cause artifacts in the image. Titanium has become widely accepted due to its MRI compatibility.

One of the biggest challenges in MRI is patient cooperation. Limiting patient motion is particularly demanding due to MRI's long scan times. Swaddling is a technique used in the hospital settings to soothe infants. The technique requires that an infant be fed just prior to an exam, then swaddled, avoiding the need for sedation/anesthesia.

Case Study 1

A previously healthy 5-year-old boy weighing 21 kg is brought to an urgent care center for difficulty breathing. Three days prior he had a runny nose, cough, and low-grade fevers up to 38.3°C. He continued to take liquids well, but his solid intake has decreased. His mother reported this morning his temperature was 39.4°C, and he was breathing fast and working hard to breathe. He is not taking medications other than acetaminophen. His immunizations are up to date for his age. He does not have a history of choking or vomiting. Upon initial assessment, vital signs: temperature 40°C, heart rate 128 beats per minute, respiratory rate 38 breaths per minute, blood pressure 90/70 mm Hg, oxygen saturation 88% on room air. He is awake and alert and in moderate distress. His nasal mucosa is erythematous with yellowish discharge. His mucous membranes are dry. Subcostal and intercostal retractions are present, oxygen saturation at this time is

89% on room air. Breaths sounds reveal decreased air entry over right lower lobe with crackles; no wheezes are noted. There is dullness to percussion at the right base and increased vocal fremitus over the right base.

1. **What will you recommend for next steps at this time?**

The patient was placed on 2 L/minute nasal cannula, labs were drawn, and a chest X-ray ordered. Oxygen saturation increased to 95%. Results from a complete blood count revealed the following: white blood cell count 21,000, 75% segs, 10% bands, 12% lymphs, 3% monos, 1% eos, hemoglobin 12.4, and platelet count 250,000. Chest radiograph reveals infiltrates in the right lower lobe.

2. **Based on the clinical findings, what diagnosis would you suspect?**

Case Study 2

A 6-year-old male presented to his pediatrician with a 1-week history of cough and shortness of breath, but no fever, as reported by the mother. The boy has no previous history of illness or asthma. Clinically the child was in moderate respiratory distress and has oxygen saturations in the mid 80s. The pediatrician immediately called 911, and the patient was transported to the emergency department. On admission his vitals were as follows: heart rate 130 beats per minute, respiratory rate 36 breaths per minute, blood pressure 100/80 mm Hg, temperature 38.0°C, oxygen saturation 94% on 4 L/minute nasal cannula. There was a shift of the mediastinum to the right and stony dullness to percussion on the left, indicative of a left-sided pleural effusion. Breath sounds were diminished on the left side, and no wheezing was noted. Anterior and lateral chest X-rays were ordered to rule out a foreign body. Imaging confirmed no foreign body was present, a left-sided pleural effusion and a widened superior mediastinum were noted. The pleural effusion was evacuated and sent to the lab. The widened superior mediastinum became more apparent on the repeat chest x-ray. A CT was ordered, which confirmed the presence of a large superior mediastinal mass. Cytology of the effusion revealed atypical lymphocytes suggestive of a malignancy. The child's white cell count was normal, with no atypical lymphocytes on the smear. The superior mediastinal mass was biopsied by the cardiothoracic surgery team, and a bone marrow aspirate and trephine (BMAT) was performed at the same time. The BMAT was not suggestive of malignancy. Histology of the mass itself revealed a T-cell lymphoblastic lymphoma.

1. Can definitive diagnosis of a mediastinal mass be made via chest X-ray?

2. Why did the patient receive a subsequent CT scan after a chest X-ray confirmed a widened superior mediastinum?

3. What other diagnostic approach could be used to confirm the presence of a tumor?

References

1. Al-Hajeri M, Clarke M. Future trends in Picture Archiving and Communication System (PACS). *Conf Proc IEEE Eng Med Biol Soc.* 2015:6844-6847.

2. Beird LC. How to satisfy both clinical and information technology goals in designing a successful picture archiving and communication system. *J Digit Imag.* 2000;113(2 Suppl 1):10-12.

3. Bedel V, Zdanowicz M. PACS strategy for imaging centers. *Radiol Manage.* 2004;26(5):24-29.

4. Scaife ER, Rollins MD. Managing radiation risk in the evaluation of the pediatric trauma patient. *Semin Pediatr Surg.* 2010;19(4):252-256.

5. Kharbanda AB, Flood A, Blumberg K, Kreykes NS. Analysis of radiation exposure among pediatric trauma patients at national trauma centers. *J Trauma Acute Care Surg.* 2013;74(3):907-911.

6. McGiff TJ, Danforth RA, Herschaft EE. Maintaining radiation exposures as low as reasonably achievable (ALARA) for dental personnel operating portable hand-held x-ray equipment. *Health Phys.* 2012;103(2 Suppl 2):S179-S185.

7. Beres RA, Goodman LR. Pneumothorax: detection with upright versus decubitus radiography. *Radiology.* 1993;186(1):19-22.

8. Matsumoto S, Kishikawa M, Hayakawa K, Narumi A, Matsunami K, Kitano M. A method to detect occult pneumothorax with chest radiography. *Ann Emerg Med.* 2011;57(4):378-381.

9. Kocijancic I. Diagnostic imaging of small amounts of pleural fluid: pleural effusion vs. physiologic pleural fluid. *Coll Antropol.* 2007;31(4):1195-1199.

10. Assefa D, Amin N, Stringel G, Dozor AJ. Use of decubitus radiographs in the diagnosis of foreign body aspiration in young children. *Pediatr Emerg Care.* 2007;23(3):154-157.

11. Marine MB, Corea D, Steenburg SD, et al. Is the new ACR-SPR practice guideline for addition of oblique views of the ribs to the skeletal survey for child abuse justified? *Am J Roentgenol.* 2014;202(4):868-871.

12. Tagaya M, Nakata S, Yasuma F, et al. Relationship between adenoid size and severity of obstructive sleep apnea in preschool children. *Int J Pediatr Otorhinolaryngol.* 2012;76(12):1827-1830.

13. Hammer J. Acquired upper airway obstruction. *Paediatr Respir Rev.* 2004;5(1):25-33.

14. Darras KE, Roston AT, Yewchuk LK. Imaging acute airway obstruction in infants and children. *Radiographics.* 2015;35(7):2064-2079.

15. Martinez Santos JL, Dmytriw AA, Fermin S. Neurosurgical management of a large meningocele in Jarcho-Levin syndrome: clinical and radiological pearls. *BMJ Case Rep.* 2015. doi:10.1136/bcr-2015-210240.

16. Toru HS, Nur BG, Sanhal CY, et al. Perinatal diagnostic approach to fetal skeletal dysplasias: six years experience of a tertiary center. *Fetal Pediatr Pathol.* 2015;34(5):287-306.

17. Frush DP. Pediatric CT: practical approach to diminish the radiation dose. *Pediatr Radiol.* 2002;32(10):714-717.

18. Brenner D, Elliston C, Hall E, Berdon W. Estimated risks of radiation-induced fatal cancer from pediatric CT. *Am J Roentgenol.* 2001;176(2):289-296.

Pulmonary Function Testing in the Pediatric Population

M. Barbara Howard

OUTLINE

OBJECTIVES

1. Recognize the age divisions for pediatric pulmonary function testing.
2. Discuss ways to communicate with children, prior to and during testing, that will assist in obtaining reliable data.
3. Explain the two methods of obtaining a height measurement in children.
4. List the components that can be obtained during standard spirometry.
5. Understand the criteria for acceptable and repeatable tests specific to the pediatric population.
6. Discuss the relationship between predicted values and actual measurements.
7. Given an observed measurement value and a predicted value, calculate the percent predicted.
8. Describe the technique used to obtain pre- and post-bronchodilator measurements.
9. Discuss the role that pre- and post-bronchodilator testing has in identifying obstructive disorders.
10. Distinguish between obstructive and restrictive patterns indicated through spirometry measurements.
11. Explain the insight gained through comparing and trending test results.
12. Appreciate the challenges faced when interpreting spirometry and obtaining reliable data in the pediatric population.

13. Compare the three techniques used to obtain lung volume measurements.
14. Explain the ATS protocol criteria for a methacholine challenge.
15. List the pediatric disorders that may be identified through exercise testing.
16. Describe the performance of exercise testing in children.
17. List the two modalities used in performing exercise testing in children.
18. Discuss the value of the cough peak flow measurement.
19. Explain the method used to measure DL_{CO} and the modifications that may be made when testing children.
20. List the lung measurements that can be collected through infant pulmonary function testing.
21. Describe the single-breath measurement of nitric oxide in children and its significance.
22. Explain the method of multiple breath washout and its role in assessing distribution of ventilation.
23. Discuss the role of bedside pulmonary function testing and the measurements that can be obtained.

KEY TERMS

bedside pulmonary function testing
bicycle ergometer
body plethysmography
bronchoprovocation
compliance
cough peak flow (CPF)
diffusing capacity (DL_{CO})
eucapnic voluntary hyperpnea (EVH)
exercise-induced bronchospasm (EIB)
expiratory reserve volume (ERV)
FEV_1/FVC ratio
flow-volume loop
forced expiratory flow rate over the midportion of exhalation ($FEF_{25-75\%}$)
forced expiratory volume in 1 second (FEV_1)
forced vital capacity (FVC)
functional residual capacity (FRC)
helium dilution
impulse oscillometry (IOS)
infant pulmonary function test (IPFT)
inspiratory capacity (IC)
lung clearance index (LCI)
mannitol challenge

maximal expiratory pressure (MEP)
maximal inspiratory pressure (MIP)
methacholine challenge
minute ventilation
multiple breath washout (MBW)
nitric oxide (NO)
nitrogen washout
percent predicted
pre- and post-bronchodilator testing
provocation dose (PD_{20})
pulmonary function testing
raised volume rapid thoracoabdominal compression technique (RV/RTC)
residual volume (RV)
respiratory resistance (Rint)
specific airway conductance (sGaw)
specific airway resistance (sRaw)
spirometry
thoracic gas volume (TGV)
tidal volume (Vt)
total lung capacity (TLC)
vocal cord dysfunction (VCD)

Introduction

Respiratory disorders account for most hospitalizations and are a leading cause of morbidity and mortality in children. **Pulmonary function testing** is an integral part of assessing and monitoring respiratory status and diagnosing pediatric respiratory diseases. Testing is most

TABLE 21-1

Age Divisions for Pediatric Pulmonary Function Testing

Division	Age
Infants and toddlers	Younger than 3 years of age
Preschool age	3–6 years of age
School age	6–10 years of age

often indicated in children who present with chronic symptoms of coughing or wheezing. It is used to diagnose and monitor diseases, including asthma, cystic fibrosis, and disorders that impact lung function, such as muscular dystrophy or pectus excavatum. Age breaks for pulmonary function testing in pediatrics are listed in **Table 21-1**. Children older than 10 years of age have the same guidelines as adults.

As our focus intensifies to a better understanding of pediatric pulmonary physiology and the need for early intervention, testing in younger children has gained significant interest. However, standard pulmonary function testing is effort dependent, and obtaining these tests in the pediatric population presents unique challenges. There are specific considerations and adjustments to be made to obtain accurate pulmonary function measurements in children.

Infants and toddlers are unable to follow specific instructions and to adequately execute the maneuvers necessary for the performance of standard pulmonary function tests. Therefore, the focus of this chapter will be on testing in children older than 3 years of age. It will address the following:

- Challenges of testing the pediatric patient
- Challenges in obtaining reliable data in this population
- Guidelines, tips, and tools to assist in obtaining reliable data
- Testing options for patients who are unable to be tested in a laboratory setting
- Efforts, both from clinical and research perspectives, at obtaining pulmonary function measurements in children younger than 6 years of age

Preparing a Child for Testing

Most of the preparations for performing standard pulmonary function testing in the pediatric population take place before patients are brought to the lab. An experienced pulmonary technologist with the ability to connect with, engage, and motivate children is essential. Although there are limitations, children as young as 4 years of age can attempt and sometimes perform testing maneuvers. By 5 years of age, most children can perform spirometry with good technique and repeatability, although this may require practice and more than one visit or training session.

Communication

Children are fearful of the unknown, and it takes time and patience to gain their confidence. First and foremost, they need to be informed and reassured that there is no pain associated with these tests. Such comments as "There are no needles" and "Nothing hurts" are helpful. An anxious or nervous child does not process the directions or perform well. Anxious parents often arrive for testing with anxious children. An explanation of the tests prior to the appointment can help allay any fears or concerns the child and/or parent may have.

A kid-friendly testing area relaxes patients, making them comfortable and better able to understand what is expected during the test. Wall murals, posters, and equipment decorated with stickers are easy ways to accomplish this. Talking directly to children in a way they can understand helps establish a connection that can make them more receptive to listening. Repeating directions and asking children if they understand or have any questions empowers them, as they feel part of the process.

Incentives and Directions

Breathing is a very abstract concept that children are not able to envision; therefore, it is important to relate it to something they have done or seen, like blowing out candles or blowing bubbles. Using a pinwheel is helpful in showing children that something happens if you blow fast and long. Technology not only has given us better ways to measure the lower flow rates and smaller volumes that children have but also has provided us with incentive computer screens. These screens are complete with everything from blowing leaves off trees to dragons blowing fire, which helps to motivate children in the same way video games do. Simple strategies like being demonstrative and changing the intonation of your voice help maintain the child's attention to directions. It is equally important for the technologist to pay attention to how the child is responding to coaching techniques and to make appropriate changes when necessary. No two children are alike and they do not learn in the same way—what works for one child may not work for another.

Variables That Can Affect Testing

How the child feels on the day of the test can dramatically affect the outcome of the testing session. Being overtired, anxious, uncomfortable, or in pain, or something as common as needing to use the restroom, are all variables that can affect the success of the testing session. In general, early morning is best for younger children as they are less likely to be tired or easily distracted. When a child is hospitalized or chronically ill, it is important to address as many variables as possible prior to testing, such as not scheduling a session immediately after a blood draw or when the child has emesis. This is especially important when testing is being conducted at the bedside. A child's first reaction when unfamiliar equipment is brought into the hospital room is to question if it is going to cause pain. Introducing yourself to the child and explaining what will be done before bringing the equipment into the room may help alleviate anxiety.

Involving Parents

Keeping the focus on the child while being flexible and recognizing situations where exceptions should be made can provide better outcomes. This is especially important when testing very timid or fearful children. The technologist should appreciate parental concerns and address them while also taking into consideration the child's willingness or needs. Although having more than one person other than the child and technologist in the room may cause the child's attention to be easily diverted, allowing parents to stay in the room during testing can at times be helpful and not a distraction. If the parent wishes to be present or the child is too anxious or refuses to be tested alone, it is recommended that the parent sit behind the technologist so that the technologist has the child's full attention. In some situations, it may be helpful to have the child sit on a parent's lap and touch the equipment to help allay fears and to make the child more comfortable. Demonstrating the tests on a parent can be just the right icebreaker to relax children enough to try the test on their own.

Ending a Testing Session

It is important that the technologist recognize when a session should end, as repeated efforts may frustrate the child and prove counterproductive for future visits. Informing the parents that these tests require maximal, repeatable efforts that may take more than one session is also important so that the child and/or parent does not see the session as a failure. The goal should be to make as much positive progress in a testing session as possible so that future sessions will be more productive, especially with preschool children. Providing praise and a positive attitude during testing, and giving incentive prizes, such as a pinwheel that was used for demonstration, can set the groundwork for the best cooperation and outcomes from children when attempting these tests.

Equipment Used for Testing

The most common pulmonary function test performed in both children and adults is **spirometry**. This testing can occur in a variety of locations: in physician offices, dedicated diagnostic laboratories, and even at the patient's bedside. Spirometry can be performed using a handheld device that the child blows into. Testing for lung volumes and airway resistance can be done using a body plethysmograph.

Whether using a handheld device or a body plethysmograph, the equipment should meet or exceed the equipment performance standards set by the American Thoracic Society (ATS). Daily calibration and a level of quality assurance, depending on the sophistication of the equipment, should be in place to ensure accurate, consistent performance of the equipment.[1] It is best to use smaller or tapered mouthpieces and cushioned or padded nose clips that are "kid comfortable" while still able to maintain a seal. A calibrated stadiometer is used to obtain the height at each testing session, as lung function is directly correlated to height, age, sex, and race. The measurement is done with the shoes removed and the child standing straight and looking forward. Measuring the arm span may be used in children who are unable to stand for a height measurement.[2] When this is done, it should be noted in the comment section of the report.

Standard Spirometry Measurements

Accurate spirometry measurements require that patients completely fill their lungs to **total lung capacity (TLC)** and then blow that air out as fast and long as possible to **residual volume (RV)**. This effort provides various volume and flow measurements, with the most common or standard measurements as follows:

- **Forced vital capacity (FVC)**
- **Forced expiratory volume in 1 second (FEV$_1$)**
- **FEV$_1$/FVC ratio**
- **Forced expiratory flow rate over the midportion of exhalation (FEF$_{25-75\%}$)**

Maximal Expiratory Measurements

The FVC represents how large the lungs are and is measured in liters. The FEV$_1$, also measured in liters, is reflective of flow in the large or central airways in adults; however, in children, this measurement also reflects flow in the medium to small airways because their lungs are smaller and empty more quickly. At a more sophisticated level, measured flow can be plotted on a Y axis and volume on the X axis, providing inspiratory and expiratory flow-volume loops. The shape of flow-volume loops in young children is initially convex and then linearizes over time due to the elastic properties of the growing lung. As shown in **Figure 21-1**, curvature or concavity of the loop provides additional information concerning the presence of obstruction in children.[3]

The FEF$_{25-75\%}$ measurement represents flow rate measured over the midportion of a maximal exhalation. This measurement is accurate only if the patient consistently blows to RV and produces multiple repeatable

measurements. Children often tighten or tense their upper airway when executing FVC maneuvers. This may also occur prior to suppressing a cough or during coughing, as often occurs in patients with cystic fibrosis who have copious secretions. This can be subtle and difficult to detect, or grossly obvious, as with glottis closure, as seen in **Figure 21-2.** Measurements of FEF$_{25-75\%}$

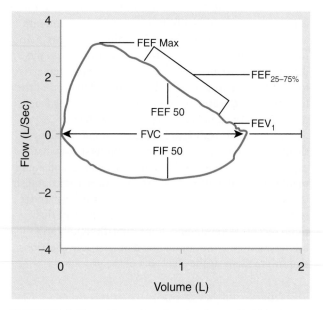

FIGURE 21-1 Normal flow-volume loop in a 6-year-old child.

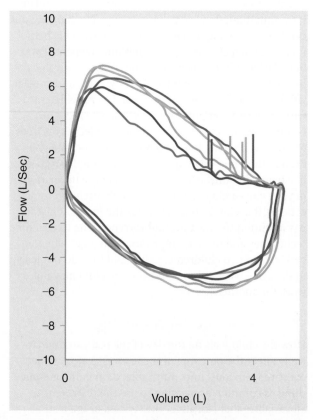

FIGURE 21-2 Flow-volume loop demonstrating upper airway tension in a patient coughing during testing.

from efforts that have evidence of upper airway tension or glottis closure are not accurate. In diagnostic laboratories with experienced technologists, the variability in the $FEF_{25-75\%}$ is significantly less. This has also become evident in multicenter research studies where efforts have increased over the past 10 to 15 years to standardize the performance and accuracy of spirometry, especially in the pediatric population.[4,5]

Maximal Inspiratory Measurements

Maximal inspiratory measurements can provide information regarding extrathoracic obstruction. For this maneuver, the patient is instructed to blow out to RV and then to inhale maximally to TLC. Children tend to exhale maximally and then terminate the breath instead of following exhalation with a maximal inspiration. Therefore, these efforts should be measured after the child has consistently been able to perform maximal exhalations. The descending limb or curve of the flow-volume loop provides information on instantaneous flows during inspiration. The maximum inspiratory flow at 50% of FVC ($FIF_{50\%}$) and the ratio of maximum expiratory to inspiratory flow at 50% of FVC ($FEF_{50\%}/FIF_{50\%}$) are helpful in identifying intrathoracic versus extrathoracic airflow limitation. Because the opening of the vocal cords should be approximately the same at both 50% of the forced expiratory capacity and 50% of the maximal inspiratory capacity, the ratio should not be greater than 1.0. A ratio of greater than 1.0 suggests an extrathoracic obstruction, as seen in patients with tracheomalacia, subglottic stenosis, or growths in the upper airway. Patients with evidence of **vocal cord dysfunction (VCD)** show significant variability in their maximal inspiratory loops. As shown in **Figure 21-3**, there is evidence of truncating, blunting, and flattening as they try to maximally inspire through adducted vocal cords.[6]

Acceptable and Repeatable Tests

As described earlier, there are three phases to performing spirometry correctly, the first being an inhalation that completely fills the lungs. This is followed by blasting or blowing the air out as fast as possible and then exhaling completely until no more air can be exhaled. To ensure accuracy and repeatability, the patient needs to perform the spirometry with proper technique at least three times. In adults with proper coaching, this can be achieved in three to eight attempts. This usually takes longer in children; therefore, it is important to allocate more time in obtaining these measurements.

Table 21-2 lists additional criteria for acceptable and repeatable tests, including those specific to the pediatric population. The ATS guidelines for accurate testing state that during the FVC maneuver, adults should blow at least 6 seconds or until a plateau of less than 25 mL/second is reached. In children younger than

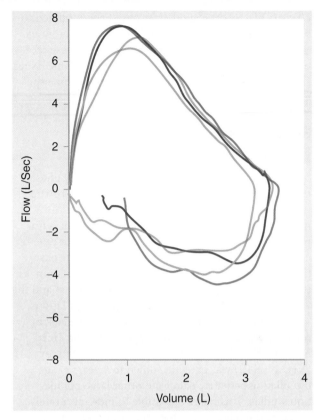

FIGURE 21-3 Maximal inspiratory loops demonstrating variability, as is seen in vocal cord dysfunction.

TABLE 21-2
Criteria for Acceptable and Repeatable Tests

Start of Test
- School age: Extrapolated volume of less than 150 mL OR 5% of the FVC*
- Preschool age: Extrapolated volume of less than 80 mL OR 12.5% of the FVC*

*The greater value is used.

Free from Artifacts (for all ages)
- Cough, especially in first second
- Glottis closure or hesitation
- Leak around the mouth
- Premature termination
- Submaximal effort

End of Test
- School age: Volume-time curve demonstrates a plateau in volume less than 25 mL/sec for at least 1 second
- Preschool age: Not defined

Repeatability
- School age
  - Three acceptable maneuvers
  - Two largest efforts of FVC and FEV_1 are within 150 mL or within 100 mL if the FVC is less than 1000 mL
- Preschool age
  - Two acceptable maneuvers
  - Second-highest FVC and FEV_1 are within 100 mL or 10% of the highest value, whichever is greatest

10 years of age, these guidelines have been modified to blowing greater than 3 seconds because smaller lungs empty more quickly. It is important to view these recommendations with the understanding that some issues still need clarification for better standardization, especially in preschool children.[1,7]

Reference Sets and Predicted Values

Spirometry measurements from the expiratory phase can identify various disease patterns, such as obstruction, restriction, or a combination. To evaluate the measurements obtained and what they mean, it is important to compare them to predicted values or reference equations from similar populations. In the past this has been a challenge in the pediatric population, as there were limited studies performed in children and the values were derived from relatively small populations.

Two efforts have been made to address the lack of reference values across a broad age range. The Third National Health and Nutrition Examination Survey (NHANES III) was extended down to 4 years of age by collating pediatric data from other large population studies. This made it possible to more accurately describe the relationship between spirometric measurements and height and age within the pediatric population. Published in 2007 and referred to as "Reference Ranges for Spirometry across All Ages", these reference equations provide a seamless transition from preschool through adolescence and into adulthood.[8] In 2012, the Global Lung Initiative (GLI), a task force of the European Respiratory Society, published a report providing normal spirometry values. These values were the result of a study based on over 97,000 records from healthy males and females across five continents. It led to equations for predicted values and age-appropriate lower limits of normal for spirometric indices in patients aged 3 to 95 years.[9] Other reference equations are available. Laboratory equipment often comes with multiple reference sets available to the user. It is important to choose the reference set that is most appropriate for the population being tested and the technology being used. Use of reference equations that extrapolate values for young children from data on older children should not be used, as linear relationship in school- and preschool-age children is not the same as that in older children and adults.[4]

Spirometry is generally expressed as **percent predicted**, where observed is the absolute measurement and predicted is from the reference equation that incorporates sex, age, height, and race.

$$\text{Percent Predicted} = (\text{Observed Value} \div \text{Predicted Value}) \times 100$$

To avoid incorrectly flagging results as abnormal, age-specific cutoffs should be used for the lower limits of normal in children. It is important to look at both percent predicted values and absolute values when comparing or trending results in children, as there is an age-related natural change in lung function over time.

Interpreting Spirometry Data

Once appropriate reference equations have been selected and predicted normal values calculated, the process to evaluate spirometry results is established. Baseline values that are greater than 80% of the predicted values are, by definition, within normal limits. Based on the percent predicted values, we can begin to identify and quantify patterns of disease presence or change that may have occurred. **Table 21-3** compares obstructive and restrictive lung patterns. Monitoring the efficacy of therapies, interventions (such as hospitalization), and research drugs is done through comparing and trending spirometry data.

Obstructive and Restrictive Disorders

Significant decreases from predicted values in the FEV_1, FEV_1/FVC ratio, and/or $FEF_{25-75\%}$ indicate a baseline obstruction. To evaluate if the obstruction is reversible, four puffs of albuterol are administered using a metered dose inhaler (MDI) and holding chamber.[1] Most children who can perform spirometry consistently have no problem using an MDI with a holding chamber. However, if the child is having trouble holding a breath following a puff of albuterol, then nebulized albuterol would be an alternative; some laboratories routinely nebulize albuterol in place of an MDI. Spirometry testing is repeated 15 to 20 minutes after the administration of albuterol and results are compared to pre-bronchodilator baseline measurements. **Pre- and post-bronchodilator testing** provides information regarding airway hyperresponsiveness or airway reactivity, as seen in asthma. The technologist should be confident that baseline efforts are maximal and repeatable before administering a bronchodilator so that any improvements due to training and/or effort are not misinterpreted. Sometimes this may just require a little more time, allowing the child a comfort break or deferring to another testing session.

Even though children may present with clinical symptoms of airway obstruction disorders, they often

TABLE 21-3
Spirometry and Disease Patterns

Spirometry Test	Obstructive	Restrictive	Mixed
FVC	normal or ↓	↓	↓
FEV_1	↓	↓	↓
FEV_1/FVC	↓	normal or ↑	↓

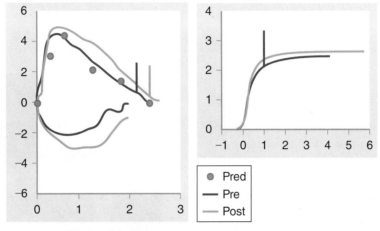

Spirometry	Pre-Bronch			Post-Bronch		
	Pred	Actual	% Pred	Actual	% Pred	% Chng
FVC (L)	2.35	2.45	104	2.63	111	+7
FEV$_1$ (L)	2.05	2.12	103	2.39	116	+12
FEV$_1$/FVC (%)	87	87	99	91	104	+4
FEF 25% (L/sec)	4.46	4.24	95	4.85	108	+14
FEF 75% (L/sec)	1.43	1.11	77	1.88	131	+69
FEF 25–75% (L/sec)	2.42	2.23	92	3.34	137	+49
FEF Max (L/sec)	3.09	4.51	145	4.89	158	+8

- ● Pred
- — Pre
- — Post

FIGURE 21-4 Spirometry pre- and post-bronchodilator showing significant response to bronchodilator.

have spirometry values that are within normal limits or even above normal. In many of these cases, test results following albuterol inhalation show a significant improvement in FEV$_1$ (>10%) or FEF$_{25-75\%}$ (>25%), which is indicative of airway reactivity or hyperresponsiveness. This is demonstrated in **Figure 21-4**.

Accurate FEF$_{25-75\%}$ measurements are helpful in following young children with cystic fibrosis when the disease is more confined to the periphery of their lungs.[10] Children with asthma can have borderline or no significant response noted in their FEV$_1$ (<10%) yet have a significant response in their FEF$_{25-75\%}$ (>25%) postalbuterol. These data are helpful in identifying and monitoring progression of asthma and the efficacy of medications.[11]

Spirometry data can also indicate a restrictive disorder. Restrictive patterns may be seen in children with interstitial lung disease, pulmonary fibrosis secondary to chemotherapy or radiation, scoliosis, obesity, and neuromuscular diseases, such as muscular dystrophy or amyotrophic lateral sclerosis (ALS). A reduction or a borderline reduction in FVC and an FEV$_1$ with a normal or increased FEV$_1$/FVC ratio is indicative of but not definitive for a restrictive process.

Trending Results

Trending percent predicted values over time gives insight into the progression of chronic diseases, such as cystic fibrosis and muscular dystrophy. In children with

asthma, spirometry can be used to assess the severity of the disease and how well it is controlled, evaluate the response to medications, and help in determining changes in the treatment plan. **Table 21-4** demonstrates how monitoring spirometry values can indicate progression of a disease. When comparing or trending results to previous visits in young children, it is important to realize that from one visit to the next there can be some variability in the child's performance. There may also be a lack of reproducibility due to a training affect or other contributing factors.

Interpretation Challenges

Interpretation of spirometry in the pediatric population can be challenging. An important component of interpretation is the technologist's comments on how well the tests were performed and if they met ATS guidelines. During spirometry testing, the goal should be to meet or exceed the ATS recommendations; however, when this is not possible, data obtained may still be useful for lung function evaluation. An example is when a child consistently takes a full breath in but maximally blows out for only 2 seconds without a plateau. In this case, the FEV$_1$ would not be affected and may be helpful in assessing lung function, but the FVC, FEV$_1$/FVC ratio, and FEF$_{25-75\%}$ would not be accurate measurements. Another example is the child who produces one effort that is technically acceptable but is unable to produce another good-quality effort during

TABLE 21-4
Trended Data in a Patient with Cystic Fibrosis Showing a Progressive Decline in Lung Function

Visit Date Pre	FVC L	FVC % Predicted	FEV_I L	FEV_I % Predicted	FEF 25–75% L/Sec
9/3/2013 13:13:55	1.61	125	1.40	122	1.46
12/3/2013 14:19:37	1.59	123	1.45	125	2.03
3/11/2014 13:06:05	1.57	117	1.38	115	1.76
6/17/2014 13:22:02	1.53	111	1.40	114	2.02
9/23/2014 13:03:12	1.41	97	1.24	96	1.57

the testing session. The information obtained, including documentation about lack of repeatability, may be helpful in assessing the child. This is a case in which post-albuterol testing should be deferred until repeatable baseline tests are obtained. Trending or comparing future tests to these types of measurements is not advised.

Preschoolers often do not exhale for more than 1 second, and recent studies have investigated the clinical usefulness of $FEV_{0.5}$ and $FEV_{0.75}$ in this age group. It was concluded that more research was needed to assess the utility and clinical applicability of these measurements. In this age group, all data obtained (not just selected data) should be available or accessible for review and interpretation.[4]

Beyond Spirometry: Lung Volumes and Airway Resistance

Measurement of lung volumes, or more specifically **functional residual capacity (FRC)** and TLC, can identify a restrictive pattern. The volume of the lung can be determined with one of three techniques: (1) **helium dilution**, (2) **nitrogen washout**, and (3) body plethysmography. Lung volume measurements by gas dilution or washout pose similar problems in children as they do in adults. Both methods measure lung volumes in communication with the mouth. In patients with airway obstruction and gas trapped in the lung, these methods often underestimate the actual lung volume. Both testing methods require a tight seal around the mouth and nose while the patient breathes a dry gas for several minutes. This requirement, along with a wait time between tests for the lung to equilibrate, make the testing process longer and more challenging in children.

Unlike helium dilution and nitrogen washout, **body plethysmography**, also known as a body box, measures all the gas within the lung. As shown in **Figure 21-5**, body plethysmographs are designed for the patient to sit inside the chamber while breathing through a mouthpiece with a nose clip in place.

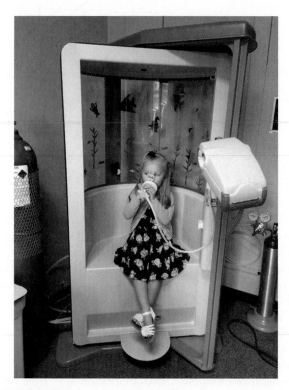

FIGURE 21-5 A 4-year-old child performing spirometry in a body plethysmograph.

The patient breathes normally until a stable tidal volume is observed, at which point a shutter occludes at the mouth. When the shutter opens, the patient is instructed to take a deep breath in followed by a complete exhalation, which gives a vital capacity (VC). Exhalation should be maximal but not forced or blasted out like the FVC. The VC is then divided into the subdivisions of **inspiratory capacity (IC)** and **expiratory reserve volume (ERV)**. **Figure 21-6** is an example of reduced lung volume measurements indicating restriction. The body plethysmograph method provides multiple **thoracic gas volume (TGV)** measurements in a short period with minimal patient effort. For these reasons, it is the preferred method for measuring lung volumes in children and adults. When FRC

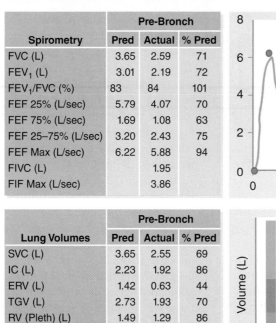

Spirometry	Pre-Bronch		
	Pred	Actual	% Pred
FVC (L)	3.65	2.59	71
FEV$_1$ (L)	3.01	2.19	72
FEV$_1$/FVC (%)	83	84	101
FEF 25% (L/sec)	5.79	4.07	70
FEF 75% (L/sec)	1.69	1.08	63
FEF 25–75% (L/sec)	3.20	2.43	75
FEF Max (L/sec)	6.22	5.88	94
FIVC (L)		1.95	
FIF Max (L/sec)		3.86	

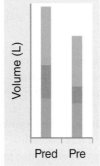

Lung Volumes	Pre-Bronch		
	Pred	Actual	% Pred
SVC (L)	3.65	2.55	69
IC (L)	2.23	1.92	86
ERV (L)	1.42	0.63	44
TGV (L)	2.73	1.93	70
RV (Pleth) (L)	1.49	1.29	86
TLC (Pleth) (L)	4.96	3.85	77
RV/TLC (Pleth) (%)	30	34	112
Trapped Gas (L)			

FIGURE 21-6 Spirometry and lung volumes showing a restrictive pattern.

or TGV measurements are combined with a measured VC, IC, and ERV, we also obtain indirect measurements of RV, TLC, and RV/TLC ratio, which are instrumental in further differentiating obstruction from restriction.[12]

Bronchoprovocation and Exercise Testing

As important as it is to identify disease and progression of disease, it is equally important not to misinterpret what is normal. Baseline spirometry is only as sensitive as the predicted values chosen. For example, when baseline spirometry is within normal limits and there is a borderline or no significant response to a bronchodilator, yet clinical symptoms persist, a **bronchoprovocation** test may be indicated. This test assesses bronchial hyperresponsiveness (BHR) or airway hyperresponsiveness (AHR). Depending upon the presentation of symptoms, a **methacholine challenge** or an exercise-induced bronchospasm test can be helpful in further assessing the patient.[13]

Methacholine Challenge

The ATS protocol criteria for a methacholine challenge are the same for children as adults.[14] Baseline spirometry is performed; the patient is then given increasing doses of methacholine. After each dose, spirometry is performed to document any changes in FEV$_1$. A drop of 20% or greater from baseline, called the **provocation dose (PD$_{20}$)**, is considered significant, and the degree of hyperresponsiveness is related to the cumulative dose of methacholine when this drop occurred. There are also abridged protocols for performing methacholine challenges where doses are skipped. Although this has been proven useful in decreasing the test time in adults, it is important to be cautious in using the abridged protocol with children, especially the young child, as they have smaller airways and flow rates can significantly drop more quickly.[15] It is also recommended to perform pre- and post-bronchodilator testing using albuterol prior to a methacholine challenge so as not to do unwarranted testing. This also ensures that the child is able to perform repeatable spirometry in a timely fashion, as the methacholine challenge is time specific.

Exercise Testing

Children who have dyspnea with exertion or exercise are often identified when they start school or become involved in organized sports and activities. This may be because, prior to engaging in these activities, they may have self-limited their activity when they felt short of breath. Also, parents may have nothing to compare their child's activity level to. Whatever the reason, dyspnea in children can prevent them from wanting to engage in exercise or limit their ability to excel in an activity they enjoy. Exercise testing in children is helpful in identifying **exercise-induced bronchospasm (EIB)**, VCD, cardiac anomalies, and their level of fitness. It can

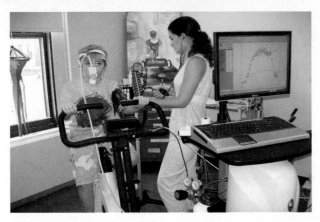

FIGURE 21-7 A 10-year-old child undergoing exercise testing using a bicycle ergometer.

also be used to evaluate patients with chest deformities, such as pectus excavatum and pectus carinatum. A **bicycle ergometer**, as seen in **Figure 21-7**, is the preferred modality to use in children as they are more familiar with bicycles than treadmills. It is easier to monitor oxygen saturation, blood pressure, and electrocardiogram with fewer artifacts from motion. There is also less chance of the child falling, should they become dizzy or ill. It is the preference of the laboratory as to whether a cycle ergometer or treadmill is used.

It is important to familiarize the child with the treadmill and bicycle ergometer and how they work prior to testing. To perform an EIB test and to meet ATS protocol criteria, the patient must be able to quickly increase their heart rate to 90% of the predicted maximum rate, with a corresponding increase in minute ventilation of $17.5 \times FEV_1$ or greater, and to maintain a steady state for 4 to 6 minutes.[16] Additionally, the child must be able to consistently perform maximal, repeatable spirometry measurements within a reasonable time. This is because postexercise spirometry testing is also time sensitive. It requires FVC maneuvers every 5 to 10 minutes, up to 30 minutes postexercise, to document any significant decreases in FEV_1, $FEF_{25-75\%}$, or **specific airway conductance (sGaw)**.

VCD affects children and young adults with an average age of onset of 14.5 years. It has been reported more frequently in females than males (2:1) with or without a history of respiratory problems.[17] Laryngoscopy performed while the patient is exercising visualizes the movement of the vocal cords and any abnormalities that may be present. Monitoring inspiratory curves for variability and flow limitation before, during, and after exercise and noting any clinical symptoms, such as abrupt onset of stridor, are helpful but not as definitive as laryngoscopy. These methods are, however, less invasive and better tolerated by children.

The level of fitness, or lack thereof, is often the cause of dyspnea in children, especially in those with a high body mass index. The protocol of choice to evaluate the level of fitness is an incremental or ramp protocol to evaluate cardiorespiratory response. This would also be the protocol to use to evaluate the effect that chest wall anomalies, such as pectus excavatum and pectus carinatum, may have on the cardiorespiratory system.[18] There has been discussion over the years as to the best way to evaluate dyspnea in children: to differentiate the level of fitness or to use an EIB protocol. Although it may be convenient to attempt to achieve both assessments with one testing session, this requires two different protocols. The first is a progressive increase in work while the EIB protocol is an abrupt increase of work and steady state. The progressive protocol may condition the airways and prevent an EIB response while the EIB protocol does not give a true reflection of cardiopulmonary adaptation to exercise. Additionally, the patient usually does not reach and maintain target ventilations necessary to elicit bronchospasm when performing a progressive or incremental test. Therefore, best practice guidelines would dictate that in such patients, especially those with a cardiac concern, a progressive protocol test be performed first and then an EIB protocol only if necessary.

Considerations, challenges, and limitations of exercise testing in children would include the child's ability to perform spirometry in a timely fashion and their ability to pedal or run to a predetermined heart rate and/or ventilation, and the technologist's ability to motivate and coach the child to accomplish this. Exercise equipment used for testing in the pediatric population may need to be modified to accommodate the smaller stature of younger children. Safety considerations include having appropriate resuscitation equipment immediately available and Pediatric Advanced Life Support (PALS)–trained and –certified staff. An identified physician should be either in the room or able to quickly respond if necessary.[19]

Mannitol Challenge

In general, children as young as 7 years of age can perform an exercise test; however, some children, and some adults, cannot achieve and/or maintain the recommended target heart rate and ventilation to evaluate EIB. Optional testing to assess bronchial hyperresponsiveness for these individuals includes the **mannitol challenge** and the **eucapnic voluntary hyperpnea (EVH)** tests, which also act indirectly to elicit bronchoconstriction. The mannitol challenge requires the patient to inhale increasing doses of mannitol, a naturally occurring sugar alcohol, which is administered as a dry powder through an inhaler device. Each inhalation is followed by measurements of the FEV_1. There must be a 15% fall in the FEV_1 from baseline or a 10% fall between two consecutive doses to be considered a positive test.[20]

Eucapnic Voluntary Hyperpnea Testing

EVH testing involves the patient breathing at a high level of ventilation ($35 \times FEV_1$) with replacement of the exhaled CO_2. This is accomplished by inhaling a dry gas containing 4.9% CO_2, 21% O_2, and balanced N_2 at room temperature for 6 minutes. FEV_1 is measured at 1, 3, 5, 7, and 10 minutes after the challenge. A fall from baseline in the FEV_1 of 15% or more defines an abnormal response.[21] Patients must still be able to perform maximal repeatable spirometry in a reasonable amount of time, as these are also time-sensitive tests.

Specialized Tests

Children with neuromuscular disease, such as Duchenne muscular dystrophy (DMD) and spinal muscular atrophy, present with a restrictive pattern as their disease progresses. Due to muscle weakness and fatigue, these patients lose the ability to fully inhale or exhale, cough effectively, or ventilate sufficiently for normal gas exchange. It is important to monitor the progression of their disease so that supportive interventions, such as bilevel positive airway pressure, therapy with a cough-assist device, or continuous mechanical ventilation, are made available when needed. The current standard of care for DMD is routine assessment of pulmonary function. This assessment should include oxyhemoglobin saturation by pulse oximetry, spirometric measurements of FVC, FEV_1, maximal mid-expiratory flow rate, maximum inspiratory and expiratory pressures, and cough peak flow.[22,23]

Maximal Inspiratory and Expiratory Pressures

Maximal inspiratory pressure (MIP) and **maximal expiratory pressure (MEP)** are measured when the patient inspires or expires maximally against an occlusion for 1 to 3 seconds. These measurements can be obtained using handheld devices, within a body plethysmograph, or interfaced with a laptop. Smaller mouthpieces that are flanged should be used to help maintain a good seal around the mouth and prevent leaks. The measured pressure is recorded in cm H_2O. MIP primarily measures inspiratory muscle strength; a reduced MIP measurement may indicate a need for ventilatory support. MEP measures the accessory muscles and elastic recoil of the lungs. A low or reduced MEP indicates a loss of force to cough effectively. An MEP greater than 60 cm H_2O suggests difficulty in clearing secretions and the need for a cough-assist device. MIP and MEP measurements require at least three maximal efforts within 10% or 10 cm H_2O. The maximal value should be reported.[24] The limited studies of maximal inspiratory and expiratory pressures in children show relatively large variability.[25]

Cough Peak Flow

Cough peak flow (CPF) measures the velocity of air as a patient coughs into a flow measuring device, such as a peak flow meter. This measurement represents the effectiveness of a patient's cough for clearing secretions.

A reduced value may indicate the need for a cough-assist device. The measurement is obtained by holding a mask firmly against the child's face as the child is coached to cough as hard as possible. Coughing is something children are familiar with doing and can relate to; however, to get maximal results, a maximal inspiration is required prior to the cough. This may take practice. Similar to a peak flow measurement, CPF is measured in L/second or L/minute. Measurements of less than 270 L/minute would suggest use of a cough-assist device.[22]

Cough peak flow, as well as MIP and MEP, can frighten children as they attempt to breathe against an occlusion or have a mask held firmly against their face. Allowing the child to hold the device and having a parent demonstrate the procedure may be helpful. Calm reassurance and taking breaks between efforts so that the child does not become fatigued can usually provide better results.

Diffusing Capacity

Patients with restrictive and/or obstructive lung disease may also have a reduction in the available surface area that maintains normal gas exchange within the lungs. Diseases in children that may produce this are interstitial lung disease and pulmonary fibrosis secondary to chemotherapy or radiation. It may also be seen in immunologic disorders, such as scleroderma and systemic lupus erythematosus.

The **diffusing capacity (DL_{CO})** is a test that indirectly measures gas transport at the alveolar level. The most common method used to measure DLco is the single breath or breath hold technique ($DL_{CO}sb$). This requires a sequence of maneuvers where the patient blows out to RV and then rapidly inspires a very low concentration of 0.3% carbon monoxide to TLC. This is followed by a 10-second breath hold and then a rapid exhalation. Typically, the initial 750 mL of anatomical dead space in the exhalant is flushed or discarded and the remainder is collected and analyzed as the alveolar sample. The change in inhaled to exhaled carbon monoxide is attributed to diffusion across the alveolar capillary bed.

There are many inherent variables affecting the results, such as hemoglobin, volume of inspiration, length of breath, time to TLC, and added driving pressures, such as those seen in a Valsalva maneuver. The ATS guidelines for adults are the same for children.[26] This maneuver is very difficult for small children and even older children and may require more than one session before obtaining accurate repeatable results.

A recent hemoglobin measurement is needed to correct the actual DL_{CO} measurement for an accurate measurement of diffusion, as hemoglobin directly affects the transfer and pickup of carbon monoxide by the blood. If a recent hemoglobin is not available, it is recommended that this be done after testing is complete and that the child is not made aware of this possibility, as it can produce significant anxiety that can affect the testing session. There is currently available a pulse oximetry system that has the option to noninvasively measure multiple additional blood constituents and physiologic parameters, including total hemoglobin, methemoglobin, and carboxyhemoglobin. In children with normal hemoglobin and mild anemia, there was a positive correlation between this indirect measurement and a direct measurement. However, more studies are necessary in children with moderate and severe anemia.[27]

Considerations and modifications when performing DL_{CO} testing in children with lung volumes less than 1.5 L would include the ability to reduce the dead space washout (<750 mL) on the system so that there is a sufficient alveolar sample for analysis. The demand valve mechanism that allows the flow of tracer gas must be easily triggered or opened by the child's inspiration. Until recently there were limited reference equations in children, making it more difficult to interpret these tests in the pediatric population.[28]

Infant and Toddler Pulmonary Function Testing

The importance of understanding how infant and toddler lungs function, grow, and present with disease has gained increasing interest over the past four decades. Early diagnosis and treatment has been shown to slow the progression and to reduce the mortality of various diseases in children with such disorders as bronchopulmonary dysplasia and cystic fibrosis.[29,30] Children younger than 3 years of age cannot execute and perform the standard pulmonary function tests thus far discussed. Therefore, the focus in this age group has shifted to tests that require sedation or minimal patient cooperation in infants, toddlers, and preschoolers. Many efforts at accomplishing this have been met with a multitude of challenges and obstacles over the years. As far back as the 1970s, efforts were being made to study and measure passive respiratory mechanics in infants.

Equipment Used

Through collaborative and cooperative efforts worldwide supported by research funding and the commitment of private industries, there have been systems that measure pulmonary function in infants commercially available since the 1990s. The system or Plexiglas body plethysmograph, similar to the one used in older children and adults, is a pressure-variable chamber that provides measurements of lung volumes, capacities, and flows, as well as compliance and resistance, as seen in **Figure 21-8**.

Obtaining Measurements

Infants as young as 17 weeks and up to approximately 3.5 years of age can be tested using these systems. An

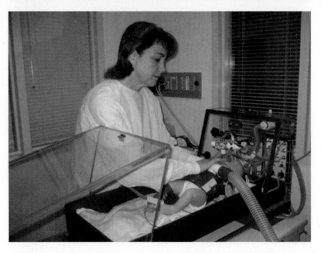

FIGURE 21-8 An infant undergoing pulmonary function testing with a body plethysmograph.

infant pulmonary function test (IPFT) gathers measurements similar to those obtained during spirometry and plethysmography in older children and adults. However, these tests require the infant to be sleep-deprived and sedated during testing. The flow and volume measurements collected are adjusted for the lower lung volumes and flows in infants. Equipment should be calibrated with a smaller 1-L syringe to ensure accuracy.[31]

As the infant breathes for several efforts against a closed-mouth valve within the sealed chamber, a pneumotach and transducers measure the resulting changes in box and mouth pressure. These changes are then applied to the inverse relationship of volume and pressure, as expressed by Boyle's law, to calculate the FRC.

To obtain measurements similar to FVC, often referred to as **raised volume rapid thoracoabdominal compression technique (RV/RTC)**, the infant's inspiratory effort is augmented by 30 cm H_2O positive pressure applied to the breathing circuit. This pressure is applied to the face mask at the beginning of two to five successive, spontaneous inspirations until a pause occurs at end expiration. This is also referred to as activating the Hering-Breuer reflex. Pressure is then applied to an inflatable bladder that is secured in place over the infant's chest with a hugger vest. This forces the air out of the lungs and is measured and displayed as an expiratory flow-volume curve.[32] Pre- and post-bronchodilator testing can also be performed if the child remains asleep.

Challenges

Although infant pulmonary function testing requires no patient cooperation, it is not without challenges. The testing process requires highly trained and dedicated staff and the use of sophisticated equipment, and it is very time consuming, taking approximately 2 to 4 hours to obtain measurements. A great deal has been learned about infant pulmonary physiology with IPFT. However, because this testing cannot be done quickly or easily, it does not provide the lung function monitoring that is needed routinely to manage patient care. Sedating an infant or toddler poses risks that require continuous monitoring throughout testing by staff trained and certified in PALS.[33] Reference values are available but limited.[34]

Children between the ages of 3 and 6 years, also referred to as preschoolers, present the most challenge when attempting to measure lung function. Efforts in this age group have also focused on minimal cooperation, such as breathing normally through a mouthpiece with nose clips or through a mask, which in and of itself is not an easy feat in a conscious preschooler. Some examples of tests that require minimal effort would include tidal volume measurements, various methods that measure airway resistance, measurement of indirect biomarkers, and multiple breath washout tests.

Flow-Volume Loops

A **flow-volume loop** can also be measured during tidal volume breathing. The highest flow generated during a tidal volume breath normally occurs within the initial third of the expiration. These loops look similar to and can mimic standard FVC loops with characteristic shapes. Concavity of the expiratory curve with a normal volume may indicate an obstructive process. Decreased volumes but with normal flow on the expiratory curve may indicate a restrictive process. Flow limitation on the inspiratory curve by flattening is characteristic of a variable extrathoracic obstruction. If this flattening is also evident on the expiratory portion of the loop, it may reflect a fixed obstruction.[4] Measuring tidal volume loops pre- and post-bronchodilator inhalation has provided evidence of reactivity.[35]

Airway Resistance

Airway resistance contributes to how easily air flows in and out of the lungs. This measurement during tidal breathing is reflective of airway caliber. Increased airway resistance contributes to airflow limitation and is associated with an obstructive pattern, as seen in asthma. Other methods to measure airway resistance in the preschooler include a modified procedure for measurement of **specific airway resistance (sRaw)** using whole-body plethysmography, the interrupter technique for measurement of **respiratory resistance (Rint)**, and **impulse oscillometry (IOS)**.[36]

Measurement of sRaw requires the child to be seated in the body plethysmograph with the door closed. A mouthpiece with a nose clip in place is used to breathe through a pneumotach. During tidal volume breathing, flow is measured by the pneumotach and the change in pressure is measured by pressure transducers in the plethysmograph. The sRaw is calculated from the change in volume divided by the change in flow. An advantage of this measurement in children is that sRaw is independent of height and gender, which facilitates the interpretation of measurements over time.[37] However, the equipment used for these measurements is not portable. It also requires the child to sit totally enclosed in a plethysmograph and to tolerate a mouthpiece and nose clip while breathing.

The interrupter technique for measuring Rint is a noninvasive method for determining airway resistance in children. This handheld device is comprised of a flowmeter, a pressure measurement device, and a flow interruption system. As the child breathes normally through a mouthpiece with a nose clip in place, flow is intermittently occluded. To calculate resistance, mouth pressure recorded immediately after the occlusion is related to the mouth pressure recorded before the occlusion.[38] Measurement of Rint is performed during normal tidal volume breathing, making it a feasible test in the preschool-age group. Reference values have been published, but there is still a need for standardization of methods used between laboratories.[4]

Measurement through IOS is another way to noninvasively determine airway resistance in the preschooler. For this test, the child breathes through a pneumotach with a mouthpiece and nose clip in place. Downstream from the pneumotach is a miniature loudspeaker that produces forced oscillations generated by soundwaves with a range of frequencies into the airway. Flow and pressure are measured at the mouth. The resultant pressures and flows at the mouth in response to the oscillations are measured. The pressure oscillations generated by the soundwaves are either referred to as respiratory resistance (Rrs), which are in phase with the airflow, of which airway resistance is the most significant, or respiratory reactance (Xrs), which are those out of phase with the airflow and are determined by the elastic and inertial properties of the respiratory system. The data collected from these signals represent total respiratory system resistance and contain contributions from both the lung and the chest wall. IOS has been shown to be well suited to studies in children or in adults who cannot perform spirometry, such as those with neuromuscular disease. Reference values are limited as they are derived from different populations, devices, and techniques.[39]

Nitric Oxide Measurement

Measurement of **nitric oxide (NO)**, a substance normally found in exhaled air, can be useful in monitoring airway inflammation, such as that present in asthma and cystic fibrosis. Significantly higher levels of NO are present when there is tissue inflammation. Therefore, measurement of exhaled NO has been considered an index or indicator of airway inflammation in asthma. There are several commercially available systems that make this measurement by single or multiple breaths. The single breath method involves the child taking a deep breath to TLC and immediately exhaling at a rate of approximately 50 mL/second into a device. Many systems come with graphics that help the child exhale at or around this rate. Results of this test are based on a mean of two to three values and are expressed in parts per billion (ppb). Various studies have looked at the usefulness of these measurements as indirect biomarkers when asthma is present, controlled, or not controlled by inhaled corticosteroids.[40]

Multiple Breath Washout

Multiple breath washout (MBW) is a method that has gained considerable interest in identifying lung disease in children with cystic fibrosis and is thought to be more sensitive than spirometry in accomplishing this. MBW is used to measure FRC and to assess distribution of ventilation. When this process is affected by disease, it becomes less efficient and results in nonuniformity of ventilation distribution across the lungs. This is often referred to as ventilation inhomogeneity. **Lung clearance index (LCI)** is the cumulative expired volume needed to clear a tracer gas from the lungs divided by the FRC. It is a means to measure ventilation inhomogeneity. This can be done with a variety of tracer gases, but nitrogen, a resident gas, is most commonly used.

During MBW, the child uses a flanged mouthpiece with a nose clip or mask to breathe nitrogen through a pneumotach until a stable baseline tidal volume is established. At end exhalation the child begins breathing 100% oxygen and is coached to breathe normally until the resident nitrogen is washed out to 1/40th of the initial concentration. This is referred to as the washout phase. Leaks in the system, especially around the child's mouth or nose, allow entrainment of nitrogen and provide erroneous results. Time between tests is required for the wash-in phase, which allows for the reequilibration of oxygen and nitrogen in the lungs.[41] Because of the challenges and inherent variables in obtaining these tests, especially in preschoolers, it is recommended that they be performed by trained and nationally certified technologists.

The tests that have been discussed for measuring lung function in infants and preschoolers are options that are feasible in young children who cannot perform standard spirometry. Although technically the child does not have to perform or execute maneuvers, they still must be able to understand what is going to occur and what is expected of them. They must also be capable of relaxing and breathing normally. This requires time, patience, and a technologist familiar with techniques used to relax and reduce anxiety in children. Additionally more research is needed to standardize methods and techniques, establish predicted values, and evaluate usefulness in the clinical setting.

Bedside Pulmonary Function Testing

Advances in technology have made it possible to bring many of the standard pulmonary function tests performed in the laboratory to the patient's bedside. This is an important option in evaluating critically ill patients in the intensive care unit as well as patients in isolation and those who are unable to go to the laboratory.

Equipment Used

Equipment or devices used for **bedside pulmonary function testing** range from hand spirometers to state-of-the-art ventilators to complete mobile PFT labs. In the intensive care unit, bedside pulmonary function measurements and respiratory mechanics play a major role in weaning patients from mechanical ventilation.[42] They are also used to monitor a patient's response to pharmacologic and therapeutic interventions.[43]

State-of-the-art ventilators can provide diagnostic measurements while monitoring the patient. These systems measure flows and pressures from which calculated values, such as compliance and resistance, can be displayed or reported in various relationships, including flow-volume and pressure-volume loops. Pressure, flow, and volume measurements can be displayed continuously, providing a dynamic representation of the patient's respiratory status. Conditions under which the patient is breathing must be considered when reviewing the results. These include the mode of ventilation, amount of ventilator support, and presence of spontaneous breathing.

Bedside Measurements

Tidal volume (Vt) is the basic unit of respiration and is measured in milliliters. It is correlated to body weight and is reported in milliliters per kilogram (mL/kg). Respiratory rate or frequency is the number of breaths a minute and is one of the first indicators that the child is in distress. Time spent in the inspiratory and expiratory phases of the tidal volume are referred as T_I and T_E, respectively. They are also expressed as a ratio (T_I/T_E) or as a fraction of total time (T_I/total). Typically, expiratory time will be greater than inspiratory time as it is the passive phase of respiration. If the inspiratory time is longer than the expiratory time, then the patient may be experiencing air trapping. **Minute ventilation**, which is a product of respiratory rate and tidal volume, is expressed as liters per minute or liters per minute per kilogram (L/min/kg). This measurement is an important guide in weaning a patient from a ventilator.[44]

Compliance is defined as the change in volume divided by the change in pressure and is used to describe the elastic properties of the respiratory system. It is reflective of how easily the lungs fill and empty. Compliance can be measured statically (static or specific compliance) or dynamically (dynamic compliance). A difference in compliance occurs throughout the lung, making it a more useful measurement when measured at a known lung volume. Dynamic compliance is measured during tidal volume breathing and is affected by resistance. If graphic displays of tidal volume show a return to 0 at end inspiratory and expiratory, it is assumed that pressures have equalized within the lung. Pressure-volume loops graphically display a relation between tidal volume (vertical axis) and pressure (horizontal axis). If this relationship were linear, it would result in a straight line. By drawing a line through the loop at the end points of the tidal breath, the resulting slope of the line is proportional to compliance—the more vertical the line, the more compliant the lung, meaning less pressure is needed for the tidal volume, as seen in **Figure 21-9**.[45] Compliance is decreased in such diseases as bronchopulmonary dysplasia and respiratory distress syndrome of the newborn.

Airway resistance is defined as the change in flow divided by the change in pressure. Resistance measurements have been used to assess the severity of infant respiratory diseases and the efficacy of bronchodilator therapy.[46]

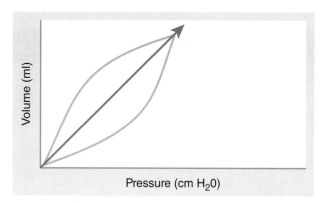

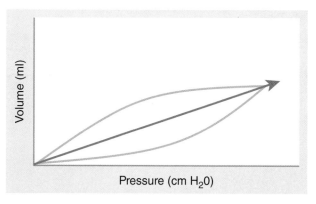

FIGURE 21-9 Pressure-volume loops of compliance.

Mobile Testing

Commercially available mobile PFT systems provide many of the same measurements we have previously discussed, including spirometry, lung volumes by washout technique, tidal volume loops, resistance measurements, compliance by passive occlusion, DL_{CO}, and exercise testing, at the bedside. This option provides the advantage of testing the patient in the comfort and privacy of their room. For patients in isolation or at risk for nosocomial infections, such as immunosuppressed patients and patients with cystic fibrosis, it provides an option for least exposure. Additionally, performing bedside PFTs also addresses many of the issues of the changing landscape of health care, such as readily available results for patient management and care and providing additional testing options for increased productivity and decreased wait time.

Considerations and Limitations

Bedside pulmonary function testing is covered under the same guidelines, standards, and protocols that are used in the laboratory, including calibration, quality control, infection control, and competency of the staff performing these tests. Additionally, considerations and limitations discussed in performing these tests in the pediatric population must be considered. Often, when equipment becomes easier to use and more readily available, standards and guidelines may be compromised.

Considerations of and limitations to performing tests at the bedside would include the patient's status and ability to perform the tests. For example, some children are too sick to perform spirometry or to cooperate enough to just breathe quietly. As previously stated, bringing equipment into a child's room can cause anxiety. Meeting with the child and parent prior to testing and using a booklet in a storybook format that describes the testing is helpful. Using a stuffed animal to demonstrate the test and then giving that animal as a prize is often just the right incentive. Flexibility, patience, and timing are very important in performing bedside pulmonary function tests in children.

Summary

Pulmonary function testing in the pediatric population assists in identifying, grading, and monitoring various disease states. Special attention is given to the integral role the skilled technologist has in getting the child to perform the maneuvers necessary for measurements of standard pulmonary function tests. Techniques, modifications, and considerations for performing various tests in children are critical in obtaining usable data. Pulmonary function measurements are needed in infants and preschoolers for early diagnosis and intervention.

Case Study 1

An 8-year-old male is referred to a pediatric pulmonologist for evaluation because of continued cough and wheezing and the need for oral steroids four times in the past year. His medical history includes being born prematurely at 27 weeks' gestation, remaining hospitalized for 5 months after birth with a diagnosis of bronchopulmonary dysplasia, and requiring supplemental oxygen for the first 10 months of life. Over the past 8 years, he has had frequent ED visits with more than 2 hospitalizations per year for viral-induced cough and wheeze. His symptoms have been managed with the following:

- Leukotriene inhibitor taken daily
- Combination corticosteroid and long-acting bronchodilator inhalations twice per day
- Albuterol inhalations as needed

The pulmonologist ordered pulmonary function tests that included spirometry with lung volumes, pre- and post-bronchodilator, and DLco. He was able to perform spirometry that met ATS criteria. However, his DLco measurements could not be obtained after multiple attempts. On the day of the test, his mother stated that he was taking all the medications just listed, but he had not used albuterol for several weeks and had no symptoms. The spirometry test results were as follows:

- Decreased FVC
- Decreased FEV_1
- Normal FEV_1/FVC ratio
- Decreased TLC
- Decreased $FEF_{25-75\%}$
- Increased RV/TLC ratio

Post-bronchodilator measurements revealed a 15% increase in the FEV_1, significant improvement in the $FEF_{25-75\%}$, and a reduction in the RV/TLC ratio.

1. **These test results indicate which of the following disease patterns: restrictive, obstructive, or mixed?**

2. **How would you interpret the results of the pre- and post-bronchodilator testing?**

3. **What do the test results tell you about the efficacy of the current medication regimen?**

Case Study 2

A 13-year-old girl presents to the pulmonary function laboratory for exercise-induced bronchospasm (EIB) testing. She had been well until the start of soccer season 2 months ago. Twice while running she became short of breath and "thought she was going to pass out". During a recent soccer game, she became severely dyspneic and was taken to the local emergency department (ED). By the time she reached the ED, she was not wheezing or coughing and her dyspnea had resolved. She was discharged and referred to her local pediatrician for follow-up, where she was prescribed an albuterol inhaler to use 20 minutes prior to exercise. Over the past 2 weeks, she has had 2 more episodes of dyspnea during games and states that "the albuterol didn't help" and that her throat hurts and it is difficult to breathe in or catch her breath.

EIB testing was performed on the cycle ergometer. She had no coughing or wheezing; however, at end-exercise she experienced significant stridor and respiratory distress. Her blood pressure increased from a baseline of 108/76 to 156/75 prior to termination of the test. Baseline pulmonary function results showed a normal FVC, FEV_1, and $FEF_{25-75\%}$. Post-exercise measurements showed no significant changer from baseline. After interpretation of the test results, a diagnosis of vocal cord dysfunction was made.

1. **Based on the test results, did this patient have a positive EIB test?**

2. **What is the classic presentation of a patient with vocal cord dysfunction?**

3. **How is a definitive diagnosis of vocal cord dysfunction made, and how is it managed?**

References

1. Miller MR, Hankinson J, Brusasco V, et al. Standardisation of spirometry. *Eur Respir J.* 2005;26(2):319-338.
2. Torres LA, Martinez FE, Manço JC. Correlation between standing height, sitting height, and arm span as an index of pulmonary function in 6–10-year-old children. *Pediatr Pulmonol.* 2003;36(3):202-208.
3. Nève V, Matran R, Baquet G, et al. Quantification of shape of flow-volume loop of healthy preschool children and preschool children with wheezing disorders. *Pediatr Pulmonol.* 2012;47(9):884-894.
4. Beydon N, Davis SD, Lombardi E, et al. An official American Thoracic Society/European Respiratory Society statement: pulmonary function testing in preschool children. *Am J Respir Crit Care Med.* 2007;175(12):1304-1345.
5. Rao DR, Gaffin JM, Baxi SN, Sheehan WJ, Hoffman EB, Phipatanakul W. The utility of forced expiratory flow between 25% and 75% of vital capacity in predicting childhood asthma morbidity and severity. *J Asthma.* 2012;49(6):586-592.
6. Bakker E, Volpi S, Salonini E, et al. Improved treatment response to dornase alfa in cystic fibrosis patients using controlled inhalation. *Eur Respir J.* 2011;38(6):1328-1335.
7. Pellegrino R, Viegi G, Brusasco V, et al. Interpretative strategies for lung function tests. *Eur Respir J.* 2005;26(5):948-968.
8. Stanojevic S, Wade A, Stocks J, et al. Reference ranges for spirometry across all ages: a new approach. *Am J Respir Crit Care Med.* 2008;177(3):253-260.
9. Quanjer PH, Stanojevic S, Cole TJ, et al. Multi-ethnic reference values for spirometry for the 3–95-yr age range: the global lung function 2012 equations. *Eur Respir J.* 2012;40(6):1324-1343.
10. Seed L, Wilson D, Coates AL. Children should not be treated like little adults in the PFT lab. *Respir Care.* 2012;57(1):61-74.
11. Marseglia GL, Cirillo I, Vizzaccaro A, et al. Role of forced expiratory flow at 25–75% as an early marker of small airways impairment in subjects with allergic rhinitis. *Allergy Asthma Proc.* 2007;28(1):74-78.
12. Flesch JD, Dine CJ. Lung volumes: measurement, clinical use, and coding. *Chest.* 2012;142(2):506-510.
13. Joos G, O'Connor B. Indirect airway challenges. *Eur Respir J.* 2003;21(6):1050-1068.
14. Crapo R, Casaburi R, Coates A, et al. Guidelines for methacholine and exercise challenge testing-1999. This official statement of the American Thoracic Society was adopted by the ATS Board of Directors, July 1999. *Am J Respir Crit Care Med.* 2000;161(1):309.
15. Le Souëf PN, Sears MR, Sherrill D. The effect of size and age of subject on airway responsiveness in children. *Am J Respir Crit Care Med.* 1995;152(2):576-579.
16. Parsons JP, Hallstrand TS, Mastronarde JG, et al. An official American Thoracic Society clinical practice guideline: exercise-induced bronchoconstriction. *Am J Respir Crit Care Med.* 2013;187(9):1016-1027.
17. Ibrahim WH, Gheriani HA, Almohamed AA, Raza T. Paradoxical vocal cord motion disorder: past, present and future. *Postgrad Med J.* 2007;83(977):164-172.
18. Jaroszewski D, Notrica D, McMahon L, Steidley DE, Deschamps C. Current management of pectus excavatum: a review and update of therapy and treatment recommendations. *J Am Board Fam Med.* 2010;23(2):230-239.
19. Paridon SM, Alpert BS, Boas SR, et al. Clinical stress testing in the pediatric age group: a statement from the American Heart Association Council on Cardiovascular Disease in the Young, Committee on Atherosclerosis, Hypertension, and Obesity in Youth. *Circulation.* 2006;113(15):1905-1920.
20. Kersten ET, Driessen JM, van der Berg JD, Thio BJ. Mannitol and exercise challenge tests in asthmatic children. *Pediatric Pulmon.* 2009;44(7):655-661.
21. Brummel NE, Mastronarde JG, Rittinger D, Philips G, Parsons JP. The clinical utility of eucapnic voluntary hyperventilation testing for the diagnosis of exercise-induced bronchospasm. *J Asthma.* 2009;46(7):683-686.
22. Finder J, Birnkrant D, Carl J, et al. Respiratory care of the patient with Duchenne muscular dystrophy: ATS consensus statement. *Am J Respir Crit Care Med.* 2004;170(4):456-465.
23. Birnkrant DJ, Bushby K, Amin RS, et al. The respiratory management of patients with Duchenne muscular dystrophy: a DMD Care Considerations Working Group specialty article. *Pediatric Pulmonol.* 2010;45(8):739-748.
24. ATS/ERS statement on respiratory muscle testing. *Am J Respir Crit Care Med.* 2002;166(4):518-624.
25. Tomalak W, Pogorzelski A, Prusak J. Normal values for maximal static inspiratory and expiratory pressures in healthy children. *Pediatric Pulmonol.* 2002;34(1):42-46.
26. Macintyre N, Crapo R, Viegi G, et al. Standardisation of the single-breath determination of carbon monoxide uptake in the lung. *Eur Respir J.* 2005;26(4):720-735.
27. Patino M, Schultz L, Hossain M, et al. Trending and accuracy of noninvasive hemoglobin monitoring in pediatric perioperative patients. *Anesth Analg.* 2014;119(4):920-925.
28. Kim YJ, Christoph K, Yu Z, Eigen H, Tepper RS. Pulmonary diffusing capacity in healthy African-American and Caucasian children. *Pediatr Pulmonol.* 2015;51(1):84-88.
29. Filbrun AG, Popova AP, Linn MJ, McIntosh NA, Hershenson MB. Longitudinal measures of lung function in infants with bronchopulmonary dysplasia. *Pediatr Pulmonol.* 2011;46(4):369-375.
30. Stocks J, Lum S. Applications and future directions of infant pulmonary function testing. *Prog Respir Res.* 2005:78-91.
31. Lesnick BL, Davis SD. Infant pulmonary function testing: overview of technology and practical considerations—new current procedural terminology codes effective 2010. *Chest.* 2011;139(5):1197-1202.
32. Sly PD, Tepper R, Henschen M, Gappa M, Stocks J. Tidal forced expirations. ERS/ATS Task Force on Standards for Infant Respiratory Function Testing. European Respiratory Society/American Thoracic Society. *Eur Respir J.* 2000;16(4):741-748.
33. AARC Clinical Practice Guideline. Infant/toddler pulmonary function tests. *Respir Care.* 1995;40(7):761-768.
34. Jones M, Castile R, Davis S, et al. Forced expiratory flows and volumes in infants: normative data and lung growth. *Am J Respir Crit Care Med.* 2000;161(2):353-359.
35. Carlsen K, Carlsen KL. Tidal breathing analysis and response to salbutamol in awake young children with and without asthma. *Eur Respir J.* 1994;7(12):2154-2159.
36. Kaminsky DA. What does airway resistance tell us about lung function? *Respir Care.* 2012;57(1):85-99.
37. Bisgaard H, Nielsen KG. Plethysmographic measurements of specific airway resistance in young children. *Chest.* 2005;128(1):355-362.
38. Child F. The measurement of airways resistance using the interrupter technique (Rint). *Paediatr Respir Rev.* 2005;6(4):273-277.
39. Davis SD. Neonatal and pediatric respiratory diagnostics. *Respir Care.* 2003;48(4):367-385.
40. Taylor D, Pijnenburg M, Smith A, Jongste J. Exhaled nitric oxide measurements: clinical application and interpretation. *Thorax.* 2006;61(9):817-827.
41. Subbarao P, Stanojevic S, Brown M, et al. Lung clearance index as an outcome measure for clinical trials in young children with cystic fibrosis. A pilot study using inhaled hypertonic saline. *Am J Respir Crit Care Med.* 2013;188(4):456-460.
42. Grinnan DC, Truwit JD. Clinical review: respiratory mechanics in spontaneous and assisted ventilation. *Crit Care.* 2005;9(5):472-484.
43. Nikischin W, Brendel-Müller K, Viemann M, Oppermann H, Schaub J. Improvement in respiratory compliance after surfactant therapy evaluated by a new method. *Pediatr Pulmonol.* 2000;29(4):276-283.
44. Bhutani VK, Sivieri EM. Clinical use of pulmonary mechanics and waveform graphics. *Clin Perinatol.* 2001;28(3):487-503.
45. Harris RS. Pressure-volume curves of the respiratory system. *Respir Care.* 2005;50(1):78-99.
46. Allen J, Baryishay E, Bryan A, et al. Respiratory mechanics in infants: physiological evaluation in health and disease. *Am Rev Respir Dis.* 1993;147(2):474-496.

22

Airway Management

Stephen Stayer
Laura Ryan
Lee Evey

OUTLINE

OBJECTIVES

1. Discuss the indications, hazards, complications, and contraindications of upper and lower airway devices.
2. Describe the technique used to insert a laryngeal mask airway (LMA).
3. Explain the calculation used to select endotracheal tube (ETT) size.
4. List the equipment essential to the preparation for endotracheal intubation.
5. Explain the different techniques used to intubate the trachea.
6. Describe the methods used to confirm tracheal ETT placement.
7. Discuss the clinical considerations for evaluating tracheostomy tube size.
8. List the indications, contraindications, and hazards of suctioning.
9. List suction pressures.
10. Differentiate between deep and shallow suctioning.
11. Describe how suction catheter size is selected.

KEY TERMS

decannulation
endotracheal tube
laryngeal mask airway (LMA)
Murphy eye
nasopharyngeal airway

oropharyngeal airway
rima glottides
suctioning
supraglottic airway (SGA)
tracheostomy tube

Introduction

Establishing and maintaining airway patency is crucial to the care of infants and children. It is essential to recognize not only the signs of airway compromise but also the need to secure an airway in those with respiratory distress and/or pending respiratory failure. Clinicians need to be familiar with the indications, proper uses, and limitations of airway management equipment to minimize the propensity for harm during care.

Upper Airway Devices

Upper airway obstruction describes partial or complete obstruction of gas flow through the oro- or nasopharyngeal airway, past the base of the tongue. It impedes spontaneous ventilation or effective bag-mask ventilation. It is most commonly encountered among patients with obesity, those with a decreased level of consciousness due to relaxation of airway musculature, or those with certain anatomic findings, such as a small mandible or large tongue.

Upper airway devices do not provide lower airway protection. Rather, they are designed to relieve upper airway obstruction (i.e., oro- or nasopharyngeal airways) or to provide a conduit to the lower airway (supraglottic airway devices, laryngeal mask airway) and a temporary means to provide assisted ventilation.

Oropharyngeal Airways

An **oropharyngeal airway** is a rigid, c-shaped device that is inserted through the mouth to provide a clear passage of airflow past the obstruction of the tongue and upper airway tissue to the level of the supraglottic area. Some styles of oropharyngeal airways have a hollow center, allowing for suctioning of the airway and the passage of airflow through the lumen of the device (**Figure 22-1**).

An oropharyngeal airway is indicated when spontaneous ventilation is partially or fully obstructed or mask ventilation is inadequate despite optimal facemask

position, mask fit, and mask seal. When correctly positioned, the oropharyngeal airway displaces the tongue forward, away from the palate and the posterior wall of the pharynx. The distal portion rests just above the larynx. Oropharyngeal airways are manufactured in several different sizes, and choosing the correct size is imperative because an airway that is either too short or too long could exacerbate airway obstruction. The correct size for an oropharyngeal airway can be determined by measuring the device against the patient's face. The appropriately sized oropharyngeal airway should extend from the level of the patient's teeth (or alveolar ridge) to the angle of the mandible (**Figure 22-2**).

An oropharyngeal airway is inserted through the mouth. The use of a tongue depressor can facilitate insertion. The clinician holds the mouth open with the nondominant hand. If a tongue depressor is used, it is held by the dominant hand to depress the tongue. The nondominant hand holds the airway with the concavity facing rostrally and inserts it into the mouth. Once the distal end of the airway passes the upper teeth, the device is rotated 180 degrees and simultaneously advanced along the surface of the tongue. The clinician should be careful not to abrade the palate or other oropharyngeal structures during insertion. Spontaneous ventilation should immediately improve with proper positioning of the oral airway. Should the patient require ventilatory assistance, mask ventilation can again be implemented or resumed and air movement evaluated. The device does not need to be secured and can remain in place until either the patient's breathing improves or a more definitive airway, such as an endotracheal tube, is inserted. To remove the oropharyngeal airway, gently pull in a slightly caudal direction to allow the oropharyngeal airway to follow the natural course of the patient's airway.

Oropharyngeal airways are useful adjuncts to mask ventilation in the case of upper airway obstruction or in the sedated patient breathing spontaneously. However, they are not well tolerated in awake patients

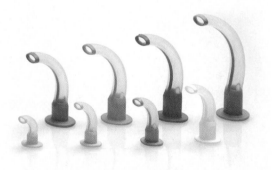

FIGURE 22-1 The Guedel airway has a hollow center that allows air to flow through and provides a path to facilitate suctioning.

Courtesy of Intersurgical Ltd/Wikimedia Commons.

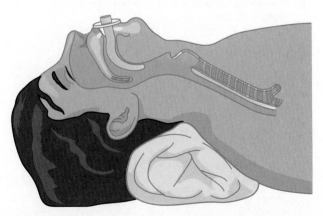

FIGURE 22-2 An illustration of a properly placed oral airway, which extends from the patient's teeth to the angle of the mandible.

and can induce coughing, gagging, and choking. Their use should be reserved for deeply sedated or anesthetized patients.

Nasopharyngeal Airways

The **nasopharyngeal airway** is a device designed to maintain or improve upper airway patency by creating a conduit from the tip of the nose to the hypopharynx. This device often bypasses an upper airway obstruction. Unlike the oropharyngeal airway, the nasopharyngeal airway is a soft, flexible tube. The proximal end of the device, or flange, is flared to prevent it from advancing in the nasopharynx, and some nasopharyngeal airways are adjustable to ideally position the length of the airway (**Figure 22-3**). When properly placed, the distal aperture should rest just superior to the epiglottis (**Figure 22-4**). The nasopharyngeal airway is better tolerated than the oropharyngeal airway and can be used in either awake or asleep patients.

The nasopharyngeal airway is indicated to treat upper airway obstruction, either in an awake patient exhibiting signs of respiratory distress or in an unconscious patient to facilitate effective mask ventilation. A spectrum of different sizes is available. The correct size should extend from the naris to the meatus of the ear. Typically the nasopharyngeal airway will be 2 to 4 cm longer than the appropriate oropharyngeal airway in a given patient.

Lubricate the nasopharyngeal airway prior to insertion to allow smooth passage through the nasopharynx.

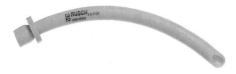

FIGURE 22-3 An adjustable nasopharyngeal airway. The circle portion just below the flange can be moved along the body of the airway to adjust its length.

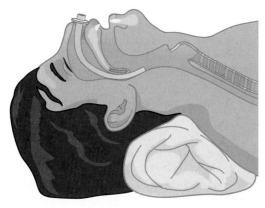

FIGURE 22-4 In a properly inserted nasopharyngeal airway, the flange rests at the nares and the distal end rests superior to the epiglottis.

A vasoconstrictor, such as oxymetazoline, can be sprayed into the nose to reduce the risk of epistaxis. Initial insertion should be aimed directly posterior along the floor of the nasal passage. Attempting to insert the nasopharyngeal airway in a superior direction should be avoided because this could cause injury to the nasal turbinates. The device is smoothly advanced until the flange rests against the naris. If resistance is encountered, attempt to turn the device while applying gentle pressure, and if resistance continues, the nasopharyngeal airway should be removed and insertion attempted in the opposite naris, as exerting force could produce a nose bleed. Securing the nasopharyngeal airway is rarely necessary, but in the presence of a tenuous airway, such as postsurgery or with facial trauma, the device may be secured in place with sutures or tape.

Typically, a nasopharyngeal airway is much better tolerated compared to the oropharyngeal airway. Although oropharyngeal airway use is essentially limited to the unconscious patient with absent airway reflexes, the nasopharyngeal airway is often well tolerated in awake patients.

Although nasopharyngeal airways are an excellent adjunct for effective ventilation, they are not suitable in all patients. Due to the risk of epistaxis, nasopharyngeal airways should be avoided in patients with impaired coagulation from either pharmacologic anticoagulation or a pathologic bleeding disorder. Nasopharyngeal airways are contraindicated in head trauma or facial trauma because, if the facial bones or basilar skull are compromised (broken), there is a potentially fatal risk of passing the nasopharyngeal airway through the cribiform plate into the brain.

Supraglottic Airway Devices

A **supraglottic airway (SGA)** provides an unobstructed airway from the mouth to the suprglottic area and a 15-mm connector to provide positive pressure ventilation. There are a number of different SGAs available for use.

Laryngeal Mask Airway

One of the first to be developed, the mostly widely used SGA is the **laryngeal mask airway (LMA)** developed by Dr. Archie Brain in 1981. The LMA was originally designed as an alternative to facemask ventilation for delivering anesthesia when endotracheal intubation was impossible. Currently, there are many different types of SGAs, and their clinical application has broadened to include a role in anesthesia, resuscitation, and intensive care.

The original LMA developed is a reusable silicone device that can be autoclaved and reused up to 40 times, and it is still commercially available. Several manufacturers produce disposable versions that are typically made of polyvinyl chloride. The LMA is a

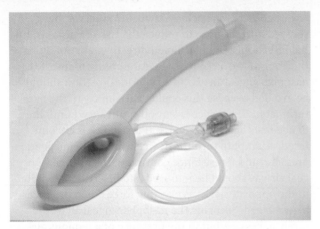

FIGURE 22-5 A laryngeal mask airway is available in a variety of sizes to facilitate insertion in very small or larger children.
© Michael Pervak/Shutterstock.

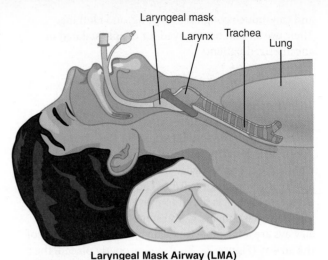

Laryngeal Mask Airway (LMA)

FIGURE 22-6 An illustration of a laryngeal mask airway properly positioned in the airway.

small, elliptically shaped mask designed to fit in the hypopharynx and to provide a conduit that bypasses the upper airway and allows positive pressure ventilation. The rim of the mask is an inflatable cuff, which is connected to a pilot tube and balloon through which the cuff is inflated and intracuff pressure can be monitored (**Figure 22-5**). There is an anterior aperture that, when correctly positioned, will overlie the laryngeal inlet. On the posterior surface of the mask, a ventilating tube extends from the central aperture to the mouth, with a standard 15-mm adapter allowing connection to a breathing circuit. Properly positioned, the distal aperture opens to the laryngeal inlet, and the tip of the cuff rests in the proximal esophagus posterior to the cricoid cartilage (**Figure 22-6**). Upon inflation of the cuff, a seal is created within the hypopharynx, allowing for positive pressure ventilation.

The LMA is available in sizes ranging from infant to adult, and correct size is usually determined by the patient's weight. The manufacturer recommends choosing the largest size that fits in the oral cavity, then inflating the cuff to the minimum pressure that will allow ventilation using up to 20 cm H_2O of pressure to the airway without significant air leak.

Prior to insertion of the LMA, the patient is placed in the sniffing position. The cuff of the LMA is fully deflated, ensuring that the posterior surface of the mask is smooth and wrinkle-free (although some recommend having a slight amount of air in the cuff). The tip of the LMA should be deflected backward, away from the aperture, encouraging the LMA to slide posterior to the epiglottis without pushing it over the glottic opening. The posterior (pharyngeal) surface should be lubricated to facilitate smooth insertion. Using the nondominant hand at the patient's occiput to extend the head, the LMA is held in the dominant hand like a pencil, with the index finger at the junction of the mask and barrel. The LMA is inserted into the mouth and advanced against the hard palate toward the larynx until resistance is felt. The hand is then removed and the cuff

inflated to an intracuff pressure of less than 60 cm H_2O. The LMA can be secured with tape.

Laryngeal masks and other SGAs are poorly tolerated in awake or lightly anesthetized patients. Insertion in a patient who has an intact gag reflex can result in coughing, laryngospasm, gagging, and emesis. Contraction of the pharyngeal and laryngeal musculature prevents optimal positioning of the LMA. The LMA partially protects the airway from pharyngeal secretions but does not protect the patient from aspiration of gastric contents. The cuff need not be deflated prior to removal, as the inflated cuff may aid in extraction of oropharyngeal secretions.

After becoming commercially available in the United Kingdom in 1988 and the United States in 1991, the LMA gained wide acceptance for its role in anesthesia practice and airway management. Over the first 3 years of clinical availability, the LMA replaced the endotracheal tube (ETT) as the airway management technique in >40% of routine general anesthesia.[1] With widespread use, numerous other SGAs were introduced, with design modifications aimed to provide more dependable positive pressure ventilation. Design modifications included disposability to minimize the potential for cross-contamination, an integrated bite block, and features to reduce the risk of pulmonary aspiration of gastric contents. Several SGAs were invented that had the ability to accommodate decompression of the stomach by passing a suction or nasogastric tube. Modifications were made to facilitate intubation through the lumen of some SGAs.[2]

There are several advantages to using an LMA compared to endotracheal intubation. Insertion of an LMA is simple and easy to learn and has a high success rate, even among inexperienced operators. Insertion is typically faster and does not require a laryngoscope. Insertion is also accomplished with a lighter level of anesthesia, and no muscle relaxation is necessary. There are fewer changes in hemodynamics or intracranial and intraocular pressure compared to tracheal intubation and extubation.[3–7] There is decreased laryngeal trauma associated with LMA use versus tracheal intubation.[8] When used for administration of general anesthesia, there is a lower incidence of postoperative sore throat when using the LMA.[9] Compared to facemask ventilation, the LMA is easier to learn and use and provides a better seal in bearded patients or those with abnormal facial anatomy.[10] The LMA protects the airway from secretions and may reduce the risk of facial nerve injury and eye trauma.[11]

Esophageal-Tracheal Combitube

The Esophageal-Tracheal Combitube (Covidien-Nellcor, Boulder, CO) is another laryngeal airway that has proven especially useful in the prehospital setting or other emergency situations because it is inserted blindly and ventilation can be established whether the device enters the trachea or the esophagus. Unfortunately, the Combitube can only be used in the adult population, as no pediatric sizes are available.

King Laryngeal Tube

The Laryngeal Tube (LT; King Systems, Noblesville, IN) is an SGA that is easy to insert and designed to minimize airway trauma. There are several variations of the design in the LT family, and all are composed of a slightly curved tube with a larger proximal pharyngeal cuff and a smaller distal esophageal cuff (**Figure 22-7**). Both are low-pressure, high-volume cuffs served by a common inflation line, designed to equalize pressures between the two cuffs. A ventilating lumen exists between the two cuffs to allow air movement through the larynx. It is available in both disposable and reusable models, and modifications exist to allow suction through the distal tip and a ventilating lumen that will accept a flexible bronchoscope or tube exchanger for tracheal intubation. It is available in pediatric sizes for children as small as 12 kg and 35 inches tall.

Both cuffs are deflated and lubricated prior to insertion. With the head in neutral or sniffing position, the LT is inserted in the midline of the mouth. It is advanced along the hard palate in a caudal direction until resistance is felt. The cuffs are inflated to a pressure no greater than 60 cm H_2O. Position is confirmed by auscultating breath sounds and detecting CO_2 on capnometry.

Clinical Application/Indications of Laryngeal Airways

Although the LMA was originally designed for administration of anesthesia, the use of laryngeal airways has expanded to play an important role in many avenues of airway management. The most critical new role for SGAs is to rescue the airway when traditional attempts to oxygenate or ventilate the patient fail. In the American Society of Anesthesiologists' Difficult Airway

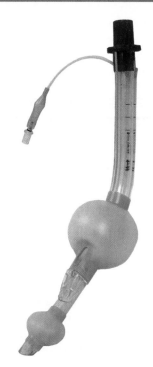

FIGURE 22-7 An example of a laryngeal tube (King LTS).
Courtesy of King Systems.

Algorithm, the LMA is recommended for patients in whom initial intubation attempts fail and facemask ventilation is inadequate.[12] In an observational study, the LMA provided rescue ventilation in 94% of patients in whom tracheal intubation and mask ventilation were impossible.[13,14] In the pediatric population, the LMA has been shown to prevent significant desaturation in patients with difficult airways.[15,16]

SGAs also serve as an aide to tracheal intubation. This technique is particularly useful in patients with a known difficult airway or those who have had a rescue laryngeal airway placed for emergency ventilation and oxygenation. A key advantage is the ability to continue ventilation through the device during the intubation. Several different modifications were made to early SGAs to provide a conduit for either blind or fiberoptic intubation. In the perfectly positioned LMA, where the ventilating aperture lies against the glottic inlet, blind tracheal intubation is possible. However, in children it is common to have the epiglottis fold inside the mask of the LMA yet not produce airway obstruction. Therefore, in children we recommend inserting a fiberoptic bronchoscope through the LMA where a complete view of the glottis is possible in the majority of patients,[15,17] making fiberoptic-guided techniques for intubation a safer option than blind intubation techniques.

Airway management of children is a significant challenge in the emergency prehospital setting. Often, personnel lack advanced airway management expertise, some standard supplies are not available, and physical conditions are suboptimal. Optimal patient preparation is impossible. Although tracheal intubation is the gold standard for securing the airway, it is often difficult and occasionally impossible in the prehospital setting. Because of their ease of insertion and ability to provide reliable ventilation better than bag-mask ventilation, SGAs have come to play a prominent role in prehospital airway management. They can also be inserted without mobilization of the cervical spine, which is advantageous in trauma patients. Tracheal intubation is also a challenge during a cardiopulmonary resuscitation and often requires cessation of chest compressions. There is a high incidence of failed intubations, unrecognized esophageal intubation, and unrecognized dislodgement of the tracheal tube. For these reasons, the use of an SGA device has been recognized as an acceptable method of airway management during cardiopulmonary resuscitation.[16,18]

Complications

Although they have proven to be a safe and effective adjunct to airway management, a significant failure rate exists with the use of SGAs. The majority of devices report a failure rate of 0% to 5%.[19] Ventilatory failure most likely results from a malpositioned device, which can partially or completely obstruct the airway.[20] This may be exacerbated by an improperly sized device. Torque from the ventilator circuit can induce mechanical kinking or twisting of the ventilation shaft and compromised ventilation, especially in smaller devices for pediatric patients.

Pulmonary aspiration of gastric contents remains a rare but potential risk associated with SGA use. The incidence of pulmonary aspiration with LMA use is between 0.85 and 2/10,000 patients.[20–22] There is *no* increased risk of aspiration with positive pressure ventilation through an LMA compared to an ETT.[23] Most correctly positioned laryngeal airway devices have a high esophageal seal pressure ($>$50–60 cm H_2O),[19] inhibiting esophageal insufflation, but the LMA is associated with a reduced lower esophageal sphincter tone compared to facemask ventilation.[22,24] Newer designs of SGAs have aimed to reduce the risk of pulmonary aspiration, incorporating gastric vents to decompress the stomach. Factors that likely increase the risk of aspiration include improper positioning of the device and excessive peak airway pressures. Cadaver studies have demonstrated esophageal insufflation with airway pressures $>$20 cm H_2O through various SGA devices, including those with modifications to reduce the risk of aspiration.[23] For this reason, airway pressures should be maintained at $<$20 cm H_2O whenever possible. Despite these findings, the use of an SGA should still be considered in an emergency situation, even for patients at increased risk for aspiration.

Airway injury can occur with SGA use, most likely related to improper positioning of the device or excessive cuff pressure. Postoperative sore throat is common after SGA use, and tongue congestion or edema can occur if the SGA is improperly positioned or holds high intracuff pressure.[25] Avulsion of the frenulum of the tongue can occur if the tongue is caught by the mask during insertion. If intracuff pressure exceeds the pressure of the pharyngeal mucosa, local tissue necrosis and resulting edema can occur. Compression injuries to pharyngeal nerves have been reported, including the lingual, hypoglossal, and recurrent laryngeal nerves.[26] In order to minimize the risk of airway injury, cuffs should be inflated to a pressure no greater than 60 cm H_2O. Package inserts of some devices recommend a maximum volume of air to be inflated as well. Use of a manometer attached to the pilot balloon can confirm an appropriate cuff pressure.

Contraindications

The routine use of SGAs should be avoided in patients who have an increased risk of pulmonary aspiration, such as those with active gastroesophageal reflux, intestinal obstruction, hiatal hernia, pregnancy, recent trauma, or intoxication. Because peak airway pressures are limited when ventilating through an SGA, they are best avoided in patients with low pulmonary compliance. SGAs should not be used in the presence of pharyngeal pathology, such as pharyngeal abscess or obstruction. In an emergency situation, however, providing oxygenation and ventilation is of utmost importance and the use of an SGA should be considered, even in the presence of these risk factors.

Limitations

Although they play a prominent role in airway management, SGAs are not considered a definitive airway and should be exchanged for a tracheal tube in patients who have continued need for ventilatory support. They may not provide adequate ventilation in patients with lung pathology requiring high inspiratory pressures. There also exists a low but identified risk for pulmonary aspiration of gastric contents.

Lower Airway Devices

Lower airway devices provide a definitive method for securing an airway, removing airway secretions, and providing the lower airway with aspiration protection. Lower airway devices can be inserted through the nares or mouth (i.e., endotracheal tubes) or permanently placed surgically or percutaneously (tracheostomy tube).

Endotracheal Tubes

The most definitive method of securing the airway is endotracheal intubation, whether to provide positive pressure ventilation, effective suctioning of lower airway material, or protection from pulmonary aspiration.

Description

Polyvinylchloride (PVC) is the most commonly used material to produce an **endotracheal tube**. The tubes are designed with a gentle curve, making it easier to pass around the tongue without the need for a stylet. If a more acute curve in the ETT is required, a stylet can be inserted within the lumen of the ETT and used to alter the shape or curve of the tube. It is important to ensure that the more rigid tip of the stylet is not advanced beyond the tip of the ETT, which may injure glottic or subglottic structures. The tip of the ETT has a 45-degree bevel that makes it easier to pass between the vertical vocal cords. If the ETT is advanced beyond the carina, it will most often pass into the right mainstem bronchus because the bevel contacts the carina and displaces the ETT to the right. If left mainstem intubation is desired, the ETT can be turned 180 degrees so that the bevel will direct the ETT to the left. Most ETTs have a **Murphy eye**, an additional orifice on the side of the ETT at the distal tip (**Figure 22-8**). The Murphy eye will allow bilateral lung ventilation when the tip of the ETT sits close to the carina; gas is able to pass to one lung out of the distal orifice of the ETT and to the other lung through the Murphy eye. Lastly, many manufacturers place markings on the ETT indicating the proper depth of insertion when aligning these markings with the vocal cords.

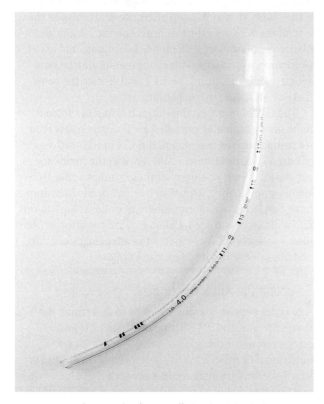

FIGURE 22-8 An example of an uncuffed endotracheal tube.
© poolsarp/Shutterstock.

Indications

Tracheal intubation is most commonly indicated to provide positive pressure ventilation to treat respiratory failure. An ETT is sometimes placed to bypass an obstruction between the mouth or nose and the mid-trachea. Other indications include facilitating airway suctioning when a cough and less invasive suctioning are ineffective or for airway protection (**Table 22-1**). A child who does not have protective airway reflexes, most commonly from anesthetics or poisoning, and who is also at risk for emesis is at increased risk of aspiration pneumonitis. Rarely, tracheal intubation is used to isolate one lung—for example, during thoracic surgery. Specialized ETTs and bronchial blockers are used in these situations. Many times, tracheal intubation is indicated for surgery under general anesthesia. General anesthesia can be administered without an ETT, but intubation is most commonly used for major surgical procedures and for laparoscopic and thoracoscopic procedures where spontaneous ventilation is compromised. Endotracheal intubation is frequently indicated for airway surgery, and in children the most common airway procedures are adenoidectomy and tonsillectomy.

Hazards/Complications

Caution should be used when tracheal intubation with positive pressure ventilation is used to bypass an airway obstruction because of the risk of intrathoracic airway collapse. Therefore, tracheal intubation is contraindicated for patients with airway collapse from a mediastinal mass.

The timing of intubation is also important. As tracheal intubation is most commonly performed for respiratory failure or general anesthesia, failure to intubate in a timely manner may rapidly lead to patient injury or death. Backup systems should always be in place to care for patients with unanticipated difficult intubation. During the procedure, there is a risk of stress hormone release, leading to systemic hypertension, pulmonary hypertension, tachycardia, and increased intracranial pressure. A vagal response during laryngoscopy and ETT placement may cause bradycardia or even asystole.

TABLE 22-1
Indications for Endotracheal Intubation

Provide positive pressure ventilation from respiratory failure
Bypass supraglottic, glottic, and subglottic airway obstruction
Airway suctioning
Airway protection from gastric aspiration
Lung isolation
Surgery with general anesthesia

Although not a direct complication of tracheal intubation, ventilator-associated pneumonia is a common source of morbidity among intubated and ventilated intensive care unit (ICU) patients.

Postintubation croup (also referred to as postextubation croup) occurs in 0.1% to 1% of children.[27,28] Factors associated with increased risk of croup include an ETT with an outer diameter (OD) that is too large for the child's airway, no leak at >25 cm H_2O pressure or resistance at the time of insertion, repeated attempts at intubation, traumatic intubation, patient age between 1 and 4 years, coughing while intubated with an ETT, and previous history of croup.

Ninety percent of acquired subglottic stenoses are the result of tracheal intubation, particularly prolonged intubation.[29,30] However, preterm neonates less commonly develop subglottic stenosis because the immature cricoid cartilage is thought to be less susceptible to ischemic injury.[30,31] An ischemic injury occurs secondary to pressure exerted from the ETT on the lateral wall of the trachea, producing mucosal ulcerations and necrosis. Granulation tissue forms within these ulcerations, ultimately resulting in a narrowed airway from scar tissue.[32,33]

Types of Tubes

Most standard ETTs are made of PVC. There are recent advances in ETT design for infants and children. For example, some ETTs are manufactured from softer polyurethane and have a cuff that is high volume, low pressure, similar to cuffed ETTs used for older children and adults. The cuff may be positioned more distally on the tube to facilitate insertion below the cricoid cartilage. The Murphy eye is eliminated because of thin ETTs with a distal cuff placement. Other specialized tubes are designed for specific surgical procedures (**Table 22-2**).

Cuffed versus Uncuffed

Traditionally, uncuffed endotracheal tubes were used in children younger than 8 years because a seal can be made between the wall of the ETT and the tracheal mucosa at the level of the cricoid cartilage.[32] The complete ring of the cricoid cartilage was thought to be the narrowest portion of the pediatric airway. More recent evidence has shown the narrowest portion of the airway to be the **rima glottides** (the level of the vocal cords),[33,34] and the cricoid cartilage is not circular but rather more elliptical in shape. An ETT that makes a good seal at the level of the cricoid exerts more pressure on the lateral mucosa than mucosa in the anterior-posterior dimension.[34] For this reason, some manufacturers of cuffed ETTs have the cuff positioned below the level of the cricoid cartilage.

Small changes in the internal diameter of an ETT more significantly affect airway resistance when ETTs

TABLE 22-2
Types and Uses of Specialized ETTs

Type of ETT	Use
Metal tubes	Laser surgery on the airway. Metal is used because PVC is flammable.
Double lumen tubes	Facilitates single (unilateral) lung ventilation
Bronchial blockers built into the ETT or used in conjunction with standard ETTs	Facilitates single (unilateral) lung ventilation
Specialized curved ETTs designed by Ring, Adaire, and Elwyn (RAE)	Oral RAE tubes are used for cleft palate and adenotonsillectomy surgery. Nasal RAE tubes are used for dental procedures.

have a small internal diameter (ID). Assuming the gas flow is laminar, the change in resistance between a 7.5- and a 7.0-mm ETT is 24%. However, the change in resistance between a 3.5- and a 3.0-mm ETT is close to 50%.[35] Therefore, it is recommended to decrease the size of the ETT by 0.5 mm ID when using a cuffed tube. Cuffed tubes are now standardly used for pediatric patients for anesthesia and intensive care, yet controversy remains regarding the use of cuffed tubes during infancy.[36] One significant advantage of a cuffed ETT is the ability to maintain an adequate seal between the wall of the ETT and the tracheal mucosa.[37] Modern pediatric ventilators will effectively coordinate and assist ventilation in patients with spontaneous efforts; however, an air leak around the ETT will reduce the sensitivity or eliminate this capability.

The risk of injury to the subglottic mucosa from a tight-fitting cuffed or uncuffed ETT exists. A few studies comparing the use of cuffed ETTs in ICU settings in children have not found a difference in the incidence of subglottic injury; however, all these studies suffer from small sample size.[38] Studies in the anesthesia literature have significantly larger numbers of patients and do not find a difference in the incidence of stridor after intubation.[39–42] **Table 22-3** compares the advantages of cuffed and uncuffed tubes in infants and children.

Selecting the Appropriate Size

Age is the primary parameter used to determine the correct size of an ETT. The head and neck typically grow even when there is growth reduction due to nutritional or other causes; therefore, weight-based or length-based formulas are less accurate.[43,44] One of the most commonly used formulas dates back to a publication from 1957:[45]

Age (years) + 4/16 (age 2 and older)

TABLE 22-3
Comparison of the Advantages of Cuffed and Uncuffed Tubes in Infants and Children

	Cuffed ETT	Uncuffed ETT
Advantages	Accurate ventilator sensing of spontaneous effort	Less airway resistance to gas flow
	Less need for multiple laryngoscopies to size the best-fitting tube	
	Better protection against aspiration	
Disadvantages	Greater ETT resistance to gas flow	Poor seal will lead to poor coordination with modern ventilators

TABLE 22-4
SOAPPIM Mnemonic for Endotracheal Intubation

S	Suction
O	Oxygen source
A	Airway(s)
P	Pharmacy (pharmaceutical agents)
P	Personnel
I	Intravenous access
M	Noninvasive monitors (heart rate, blood pressure, oxygen saturation, and CO_2 detection)

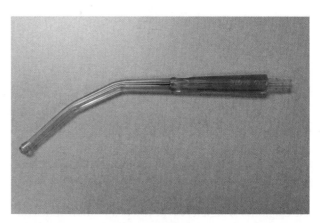

FIGURE 22-9 An example of a yankauer-style suction used for larger children.

ETT Insertion

ETTs can be inserted using digital technique (by feel), blind technique (usually nasal intubation), direct laryngoscopy, video laryngoscopy, a lighted video stylet, or fiberoptic laryngoscopy. Standard equipment should be routinely prepared and checked before proceeding with intubation. One mnemonic used as a checklist memory aid is SOAPPIM (Table 22-4). A large-bore, multi-orifice suction is required to remove secretions or vomitus that may obstruct the view of the larynx. In larger children and adults, the yankauer-style suction is typically preferred (Figure 22-9). Although smaller, pediatric yankauer suction is available, but the device may still be too large for a neonate infant and a flexible suction may be used instead. Typically, a 14 Fr catheter that provides continuous suction is preferred because this will not be used to suction the trachea and functions more like a yankauer-style suction.

In addition to the appropriately sized ETT, a tube 0.5 mm smaller should be readily available. The smaller tube can be used when the clinician performing the intubation is unable to pass the appropriate-size tube due to airway edema or anomaly. Appropriately sized oral airways should also be prepared for immediate use. Sedatives and analgesics should be prepared, along with muscle relaxants if indicated. IV access is helpful for pre-intubation medication and/or emergency drug administration. Patients who are hypovolemic may develop significant hypotension from the conversion of spontaneous ventilation, with associated negative intrathoracic pressure, to positive pressure ventilation. Volume administration of a balanced salt solution is frequently indicated.

Technically skilled personnel should be performing tracheal intubation; the care team should be aware of immediate patient needs during the procedure and be prepared to assist with bag-mask ventilation, administration of additional medications, and monitoring of the patient's vital signs as the laryngoscopist is focused on the technical task. Also, because failure to intubate can rapidly lead to patient harm, a backup plan to call for additional skilled assistance should be considered.

Direct Laryngoscopy (DL)

Anatomic differences between children and adults require a difference in intubating techniques.[46–50] The Miller (straight) blade is commonly used to expose the glottis because of these anatomic differences. The infant larynx is positioned more superiorly, at the level of the second cervical vertebral body as opposed to the fourth, as seen with older children and adults. This position gives the larynx a more anterior appearance

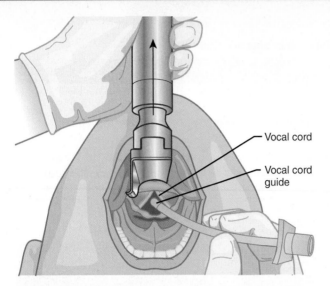

FIGURE 22-10 Illustrated view of the glottis during intubation with a Miller blade.

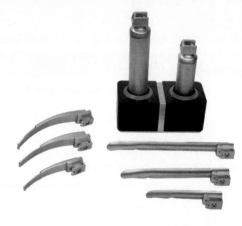

FIGURE 22-11 Handles of laryngoscopes (small and large), as well as two styles of blades: Macintosh blades (left) and Miller blades (right).

© Terayut Janjaranuphab/Shutterstock.

when performing laryngoscopy. A curved blade (Macintosh) can displace the larynx even more anteriorly, worsening visualization of the glottic opening. Also, the epiglottis in a child is more omega shaped and hangs over the glottic opening compared to the adult, where the epiglottis is parallel to the trachea.[51] Many times the laryngoscopist must lift the epiglottis to obtain a good view of the glottic opening (**Figure 22-10**). The Miller blade is designed to easily lift the epiglottis without producing trauma. Many other laryngoscope blade designs exist; however, the Miller and Macintosh blades are the most commonly used (**Figure 22-11**).

The laryngoscope blade is inserted slightly to the right side of the mouth and advanced under constant vision along the surface of the tongue as the tip of the blade is placed in the vallecula. The tongue is then displaced to the left as the laryngoscope blade is moved more to the midline, exposing the glottic opening. If the epiglottis is still covering the glottic opening, it can be lifted with the tip of the blade (Figure 22-10). The laryngoscope blade should *not* be used as a fulcrum with pressure applied to the teeth or alveolar ridge. If the laryngoscope blade is blindly advanced deep into the mouth, the tip of the blade typically advances into the esophagus. The blade can then be withdrawn until the epiglottis falls and subsequently advanced into the vallecular. This technique should be avoided because there is a greater risk of laryngeal trauma when the tip of the blade scrapes the arytenoids and aryepiglottic folds.

The goal of laryngoscopy for tracheal intubation is to optimally align the oral, pharyngeal, and tracheal axes. In older children and adults, this generally requires placing a folded towel or blanket under the head. Because of the large occiput in smaller children and infants, simple head extension will accomplish this alignment. It is common for the inexperienced

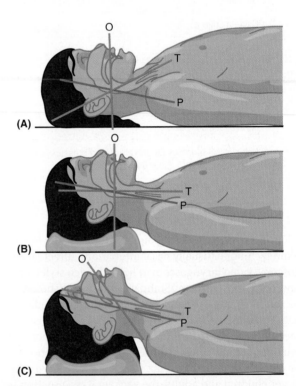

FIGURE 22-12 The three planes: oral (O), pharyngeal (P), and tracheal (T). Head position affects alignment of the three planes and visualization of the vocal cords. (**A**) Lack of alignment when the head is held in a neutral position. (**B**) The use of a head roll begins to move the larynx more anteriorly. (**C**) Simple head extension aligns the three planes in smaller children; head extension with a head roll (pictured) can be used to align the three plans in the older child.

laryngoscopist to place a roll under the shoulders of infants and children. Even though this may improve the laryngeal view, especially when the laryngoscopist is seated, this extreme neck extension position typically misaligns the oral, pharyngeal, and tracheal axes, making intubation more difficult and placing the larynx very anterior in appearance (**Figure 22-12**).[52–54]

Videolaryngoscopy

Improvements of small video cameras and optical lenses have led to the development of a wide variety of videolaryngoscopes. These scopes enhance the ability to visualize the larynx of children who are difficult to intubate. All these tools require practice to acquire appropriate expertise. They should be used periodically for routine laryngoscopy in order to maintain practice and familiarity with the differences in technique required to master these tools. Compared to standard direct laryngoscopy, videolaryngoscopy typically requires more time to intubate, and blood or secretions in the airway limit the utility of these devices.[55–59] The glidescope is one of the most popular devices available. The blade has an accentuated curvature with a high-resolution camera at the tip of the blade, and it has an incorporated anti-fog system. A variety of blade sizes are available, from neonatal to adult. Because of the extreme curvature of the laryngoscope blade, the ETT requires a stylet that should be molded to the shape of the blade. The blade is inserted in the center of the mouth and the tongue is not swept to the side. Once the ETT is positioned at the laryngeal inlet, the stylet is withdrawn, allowing the ETT to pass into the trachea. When a poor view is encountered, it is most commonly due to wrong blade size, excess head extension, and/or failure to lift the blade. Similar to standard direct laryngoscopy, the best view of the larynx is obtained from a straight lift of the blade rather than from rocking the blade back against the incisors where the tip of the blade is forced more anteriorly.

Fiberoptic Intubation

The fiberoptic bronchoscope is one of the most versatile tools used to intubate children with a difficult airway. This tool does not require neck extension and is useful when the neck is fused or should not be manipulated. It can be used with a sedated, spontaneously breathing patient, improving safety over the use of anesthetics and muscle relaxants. It can also be used in combination with the LMA. Once the LMA is successfully inserted, the fiberoptic bronchoscope can be passed through the LMA, where it typically exits above the laryngeal inlet. In children, the epiglottis frequently folds within the mask portion of the LMA. This positioning of the epiglottis generally does not interfere with LMA function; however, visualization of the larynx using fiberoptic bronchoscopy is more difficult, and blind insertion of the ETT through the LMA will traumatize laryngeal structures.

Confirming the Tube Position

The routine use of capnography provides rapid and reliable evidence of tracheal intubation. A true capnographic display is more reliable than the colorimetric devices because the waveform has better diagnostic properties. The colormetric devices display a color change, typically from purple to yellow, when carbon dioxide (CO_2) is detected. Bag-mask ventilation often causes some CO_2 to enter the stomach, and a slight color change is sometimes seen with esophageal intubation. This color change will quickly disappear. A capnographic display will demonstrate a low value of CO_2 in this setting that also disappears with ventilation. CO_2 detection may produce false-negative results (the patient is properly intubated, yet there is no CO_2 detected) during full cardiac arrest. If there is no pulmonary blood flow, there will be no CO_2 delivered to the alveoli. Capnography can be used to determine the effectiveness of cardiopulmonary resuscitation (CPR), as a higher CO_2 number indicates adequate pulmonary blood flow and therefore better cardiac output.[60–62]

Other markers of tracheal intubation are less reliable than CO_2 detection; these include bilateral auscultation of breath sounds, auscultation over the abdomen, fog in the ETT, symmetric chest rise, and the absence of gastric insufflation. Because breath sounds in children are transmitted, it is best to listen for breath sounds in the axilla and apices to determine if there is endobronchial intubation; listening over the anterior chest is less reliable. Likewise, gastric ventilation can often be heard over the chest and can fool the examiner. The gold standard for determining optimal positioning of the ETT is plain chest radiography, which should be obtained as soon as possible after tracheal intubation, unless very short-term intubation is planned.

Securing the Tube

Traditionally, tape has been used to secure ETTs, and this remains the most common method of securing ETTs placed for anesthesia (**Figure 22-13**). There are several commercially available securing systems that minimize movement of the ETT yet allow access to the mouth for oral care. Most of these devices adhere to the face, but some also are secured behind the neck.

For neonatal patients, one of the most popular devices is the Neobar (Neotech, Valencia, CA; **Figure 22-14**). The Neobar is available in several sizes, and using the best-fit bar is key to success. Oral care is easier, and it is also easier to avoid skin injury using this securement device; however, there may be a higher risk of self-extubation. One small retrospective study reported that the Neobar was more likely to position the ETT high compared to standard tape, which may increase the risk for unplanned extubation.[63]

It is important to properly insert the ETT in mid-trachea of neonatal patients. The term neonate has a 5-cm distance from vocal cords to carina.[64] Therefore, placing the ETT in the mid-trachea and securing the ETT with minimal movement is key to avoiding endobronchial intubation or unanticipated extubation. Head flexion or extension will move the tip of the ETT, even when well secured. There are several formulas the clinician can use to predict the depth of insertion (Table 22-5). It is important to note that the formulas have not been prospectively validated.[65]

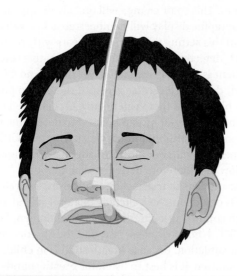

FIGURE 22-13 Securing an ETT with tape in which a Y slit is made in the tape. One end affixes to the upper lip, and the other is used to wrap around the ETT to hold it in place.

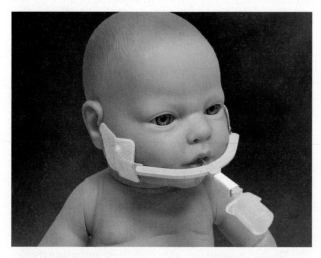

FIGURE 22-14 The Neobar, a commercially available ETT holder.
Courtesy of Neotech Products.

Cuff Pressure Monitoring

Cuff pressures that exceed 25 mm Hg will produce mucosal ischemia that may heal with scar tissue, producing subglottic stenosis. Therefore, cuff pressure should be checked and monitored a few times per day.

Extubation

All equipment and personnel needed for intubation should also be available at the time of extubation, in case there is a need for immediate reintubation. Prior to extubation, the ETT should be cleared of secretions and the oropharynx suctioned. One of two techniques is commonly used. The first technique is to insert a suction catheter beyond the tip of the ETT and to apply suction while removing both the suction catheter and the ETT. This is thought to suction secretions from the airway as the ETT is removed. More commonly, one large positive pressure breath is administered as the ETT is removed to ensure that the first phase of respiration without the ETT is exhalation. This way, any residual secretions will not be pulled into the airway.

Unplanned Extubation

Translaryngeal, standard ETTs are inherently unstable. Patient movement or traction of the ETT or ventilator circuit can lead to unplanned extubation. ICUs that care for intubated patients must have immediate access to intubation tools and personnel. In the event of an unplanned intubation, bedside personnel must be skilled in bag-mask ventilation to temporize and maintain ventilation and oxygenation while gathering equipment and personnel. Patients who are known to be difficult to intubate should have a bedside sign or indicator to avoid delay in contacting an expert in intubation, such as an anesthesiologist or otolaryngologist.

Tracheal Abnormalities

A smaller-size ETT should be used for patients with known tracheal stenosis. Review available records from previous intubations to determine the best size ETT to use, and if intubation records are not available, multiple smaller-size ETT should be available from 0.5 mm smaller ID to 2 mm smaller.

TABLE 22-5
Formulas for Predicting the Depth of ETT Insertion, Stratified by Age

Insertion Depth (cm)	<1 year of age	>1 year of age
Nasotracheal	$\left[\dfrac{weight}{2}\right] + 9$	$\left[\dfrac{age}{2}\right] + 15$
Orotracheal	$\left[\dfrac{weight}{2}\right] + 8$	$\left[\dfrac{age}{2}\right] + 13$

Patients with trachemalacia typically can be intubated with a normal-size tube for age, although some authors suggest using an ETT that is 0.5 mm smaller than predicted so as not to place excess pressure on the tracheal mucosa.

Granulomas form in the airway from prior airway injury and reduce the diameter of the trachea. To prevent further injury, use an ETT that is 0.5 mm smaller than predicted.

Tracheostomy Tubes

A **tracheostomy tube** provides a stable airway for many infants and children requiring airway and chronic respiratory support. A tracheostomy tube is inserted into an artificial opening, known as a stoma, in the trachea. Although a tracheostomy tube can be inserted percutaneously, most infants and small children require it to be placed surgically. After surgery, the tracheostomy tube is sutured in place to prevent movement or inadvertent removal until the stoma has had time to heal. In most cases, the stoma will heal in approximately 7 days, at which time the sutures are removed; the tracheostomy tube is replaced or exchanged for another tube of the same size and type, and it is secured with ties.

Indications

Some of the most common indications for a tracheostomy in children are listed in **Table 22-6.**

There are many types of tracheostomy tubes, including cuffed or uncuffed, fenestrated or unfenestrated, single cannula or a tube with an inner cannula (**Figure 22-15**). There are also a variety of types of neck flanges to choose from. The child's age, medical condition, structure of neck and face, presence of airway anomalies, and need for ventilatory assistance affect the tracheostomy tube type, length, and flange design used.[66]

A tracheostomy should not limit a child's activities. Prior to performing a tracheostomy, consideration should be given to the child's medical needs and degree of disability.

TABLE 22-6
Common Indications for Tracheostomy

• Laryngomalacia
• Need for prolonged mechanical ventilation
• Control of airway secretion
• Upper airway obstruction
• Central hypoventilation syndrome
• Airway trauma
• Tracheomalacia

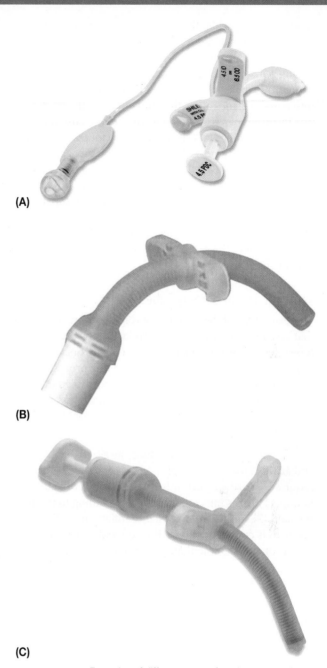

FIGURE 22-15 Examples of different types of tracheostomy tubes: (**A**) cuffed, (**B**) uncuffed, and (**C**) extended length.

(**A**) ©2018 Medtronic. All rights reserved. Used with the permission of Medtronic; (**B**) and (**C**) Courtesy of Smiths Medical.

Hazards/Complications

Complications associated with tracheostomy can occur during or shortly after the surgical procedure or as a consequence of long-term use. Bleeding can occur at the stoma or within the airway. Depending on the length of the tube and the presence of airway anomalies, the distal tip of the tube can rub against the tracheal wall, causing irritation or abrasion. When this occurs, the patient may have blood-tinged, or blood-streaked, secretions. As with any artificial airway, there is the potential for accidental removal, or decannulation. Clinicians should avoid placing undue tension on the proximal end of the tube, especially when the patient is receiving mechanical ventilation. Should decannulation occur before the stoma is healed, there is a risk of creating a false track during reinsertion. A false track occurs when the tracheotomy tube is inserted through the stoma and passed into a tissue plane rather than the lumen of the trachea. The insertion of a tracheostomy tube into a false track is an airway emergency. It is imperative for the clinician to immediately remove the tracheostomy tube; provide ventilation if needed, with the stoma occluded; and prepare to reestablish a patent airway. If direct laryngoscopy can be performed, the child should be orally intubated.

Granulation or scar tissue can form in the airway or at the stoma. Infection in the trachea or lower airway can also occur. The presence of blood or secretions can occlude the airway.

Types of Tracheostomy Tubes

There are many different types of tracheostomy tubes that can be used for infants and children. The type of tube selected for use depends on several factors. The two most common used in the decision making process are the purpose for the airway (airway anomaly, need for long term mechanical ventilation) and the child's age.

Cuffed Tubes

Cuffed tracheostomy tubes reduce the risk of aspiration and are also used when high ventilation pressures are required. There are currently three methods of cuff inflation: (1) Air is injected into the pilot tubing to inflate the cuff, (2) sterile water is used to inflate the cuff, and (3) foam is contained within the cuff and, when the pilot tube is opened, ambient air pressure inflates the cuff.

Uncuffed Tubes

Children who do not require high airway pressures or who are not at risk for aspiration most commonly receive an uncuffed tracheostomy tube. Uncuffed tubes do not exert pressure on the tracheal mucosa, thereby reducing the risk of mucosal injury, the development of granulation tissue, and scarring.

Jackson Silver

Metal tubes are sometimes used in special circumstances, such as after laryngeal reconstruction surgery. Most metal tubes have an inner cannula that reduces the inner diameter of the tube, and the inner cannula can be easily removed for cleaning.

Procedure for Tracheostomy Tube Change

Cleaning the stoma and changing the tracheostomy tube is an essential component of care.[67] Parents are taught how to perform tracheostomy care in the home for those children transitioning from the acute care to the long-term or homecare setting. **Table 22-7** outlines the technique used to care for a tracheostomy tube.

TABLE 22-7

Procedure for Performing Stoma Care and Changing a Tracheostomy Tube

- Gather supplies and have suction readily available.
- Use clean technique—hand washing with the use of nonsterile gloves.
- Place child in a comfortable position.
- Suction the tracheostomy tube prior to changing.
- Prepare the new tube by completely inserting obturator and applying a water-soluble lubricant.
- Hold on to the current tube hub while unfastening the ties.
- Remove the old tube.
- Insert the new tube on inspiration.
- Remove obturator.
- Fasten with tracheostomy tube ties or commercial tube holder.

During daily stoma care, the site should be inspected for redness, irritation, bleeding, or increased secretions. Secretion removal or suctioning is important to the care of infants and children with an artificial airway. Suctioning can be accomplished in two ways. The suction catheter can be inserted into the proximal end or hub of the tracheostomy tube and suction applied to clear secretions that have been coughed into the hub. This method is often used when the patient has a strong cough and does not have difficulty mobilizing and/or expelling secretions. The goal is to clear secretions from the hub and to prevent reentry of mobilized secretions into the airway.

Suctioning can also be performed similar to the procedure performed for intubated patients. The suction catheter can be advanced the length of, but not extending beyond the distal end or tip of, the tracheostomy tube and suction applied as the catheter is withdrawn. Prior to suctioning, the suction depth is calculated to ensure that the catheter does not extend beyond the distal tip of the tube. The use of premarked catheters is strongly recommended to ensure insertion to the correct depth, at the tip of the tracheostomy tube. This will reduce the risk of epithelial damage to the tracheal mucosa.[69] Suction pressures, for pediatric patients, are typically limited to 80 to 100 mm Hg.

Securing the Tracheostomy Tube

There are three common methods of securing the tracheostomy tube: (1) twill ties, (2) a commercially manufactured securement device, and (3) a stainless steel beaded chain. Twill ties are low cost and readily available. Twill ties are disposed of after each use or when the ties are changed during stoma care. Commercially manufactured securing devices are made of a soft material that adheres with Velcro. This type of securement device can be washed and reused. A stainless steel beaded chain is not commonly used. As with the commercially manufactured device, the steel beaded chain also can be easily washed and reused.

The tracheostomy tube is held securely to avoid slippage of the tube in the trachea and evenly to avoid pulling on the stoma. The ties are tightened to allow one finger to easily slide beneath the tie.[68]

Confirming Tube Position

A tracheostomy tube is placed as a surgical procedure, most commonly performed under general anesthesia. During placement, the anesthesiologist confirms bilateral breath sounds, and if the length of the tube is questionable, the surgeon may perform a bronchoscopic evaluation to ensure that the tube is in good position and that the shaft is an appropriate length. A CXR can be used to confirm proper tube placement as well.

Speaking/Phonation Devices

When a tracheostomy is considered, better practices recommend referral to a speech pathologist to facilitate a communication and feeding plan. Prior to trialing a speaking valve, the child must be medically stable. Evaluation of the tracheostomy size is also important. The tracheal cannula diameter must not exceed two-thirds of the tracheal lumen, unless a fenestrated tube is used. Should this diameter exceed two-thirds of the tracheal lumen, there is a risk that airflow around the tracheostomy tube will be obstructed or limited. In this case, expired gas will fail to effectively pass through the vocal cords, making phonation difficult. Children with cuffed tracheostomy tubes must be evaluated for the risk of aspiration and their ability to tolerate a deflated cuff. Cuff deflation and the sensation of air through the vocal cords may alarm some children. The communication plan should include a process to prepare and support the child and parent/caregiver(s) through this experience.

Patients with significant medical complications who are unable to tolerate a speaking valve can use language boards, electronic communication devices, or sign language.

Decannulation

Typically, an endoscopic evaluation of the airway is performed to evaluate anatomic structure and vocal cord function prior to elective **decannulation**, or removal of the tracheostomy tube. Patients who tolerate tracheostomy tube capping for 24 to 48 hours are candidates for decannulation. After decannulation, the stoma typically spontaneously closes within hours or days. For those whose stoma remains partially or fully open, a surgical closure is necessary.

Clinical Considerations

Patients with tracheostomy tubes require follow-up by an otolaryngologist to evaluate airway patency, airway function, and the development of granulation tissue around the stoma or within the airway. Evaluating the size of the tracheostomy tube with growth is often necessary. This ensures correct placement of the distal tip in the trachea and minimizes the resistive work of breathing associated with the tube's diameter. If the tracheostomy tube is alleviating an airway obstruction, such as a stenosis, evaluating the tracheostomy tube size is crucial with growth to minimize inadvertent airway compromise due to insufficient tracheostomy tube length.

Unplanned Decannulation

In some instances, an unplanned decannulation can be life threatening, especially for the child receiving mechanical ventilatory support. A spare tracheostomy tube of the same size and a tube one size smaller should always be readily available for immediate insertion. If the clinician is unable to reinsert the same size tube, a smaller one should be attempted. Orotracheal intubation by direct laryngoscopy should be performed in most patients whose tracheosomy tube cannot be reinserted.

Patient/Family Education

The goal of education is to ensure that the caregivers are confident and have demonstrated ability in caring for their child with a tracheostomy tube before transition to the home.

Homecare teaching commonly begins before the tracheostomy is placed and continues throughout the hospitalization. Training is multifaceted and inclusive of all aspects of care, from activities of daily living to operation and basic equipment troubleshooting. Typically, more than one direct caregiver is trained. Training includes didactic instruction and demonstration (Table 22-8). The parent(s) and/or direct caregiver(s) return demonstrations and are assessed on their ability

---

TABLE 22-8

Content Areas Included in a Teaching Plan for a Child Transitioning from Hospital to Home with a Tracheostomy

- Routine tracheostomy tube change
- Suctioning
- Manual ventilation
- Ventilator training if patient requires mechanical ventilation
- Use and storage of oxygen if patient requires supplemental oxygen
- Use of a heat and moisture exchanger
- Use of a speaking valve
- Prevention of unplanned decannulation and reinsertion of tracheostomy tube following an unplanned decannulation
- CPR
- Use of a specialized airway bag to keep all necessary supplies (extra tracheostomy tube, ties, suction catheters, etc.) organized
- Use of and basic mechanical ventilator troubleshooting

TABLE 22-9
Equipment Needed to Perform Tracheal Suctioning

- Adjustable vacuum source
- Sterile suction catheters with thumb regulation port
- Sterile gloves
- Eye protection
- Mask and gown
- Oxygen delivery system (bag-valve mask or ventilator if closed suction technique is performed)

TABLE 22-10
Potential Complications Associated with Suctioning a Tracheostomy Tube

Decrease in dynamic lung compliance
Atelectasis
Hypoxemia
Tissue trauma to the tracheal or bronchial mucosa
Pulmonary hemorrhage from mucosal trauma
Interruption of mechanical ventilation
Bronchoconstriction/bronchospasm
Microbial colonization of lower airways
Systemic hypertension
Pulmonary hypertension
Hypotension
Increased intracranial pressure
Bradycardia or other arrhythmias, including cardiac arrest

to provide care safely in the home. Some hospitals require the parent/caregiver to perform 12 to 24 hours of continuous care in a homelike setting with clinical staff in close proximity and available to answer questions or intervene if necessary.

If the child requires mechanical ventilation, the local emergency medical system (EMS) and power companies should be notified of the address of the technology-dependent child. In the event of a natural disaster or medical emergency, the appropriate local agencies and personnel are then made aware that a child requiring electrical power for life-support systems is in a residence.

Suctioning

Suctioning involves the manual removal of secretions from a patient's airway and is commonly performed in patients with an artificial airway. Retained secretions can produce respiratory distress, increased work of breathing, a decrease in oxygen saturation, hypercapnia, and atelectasis and can lead to pulmonary infection. Other reasons for suctioning include coarse breath sounds or "noisy" breathing, the inability to cough up secretions, new areas of atelectasis noted on a CXR, visible secretions in the patient's airway, or clinical deterioration. More subtle indications that suggest the need for suctioning include changes in the patient's ventilator settings, such as an increase in peak inspiratory pressure when set in volume control ventilation, or a decrease in tidal volume during pressure control ventilation.[69,70] Suctioning involves applying negative pressure from a vacuum source through a collection tube. Collection tubes can either be flexible suction catheters or rigid devices with a suction tip on the end, such as a yankauer-style device. The equipment needed for suctioning is listed in **Table 22-9**.

Hazards/Complications

Suctioning is not always a benign procedure. Suctioning is *never* contraindicated when it is needed or an indication exists. Potential associated complications of open and/or closed suctioning are found in **Table 22-10**.

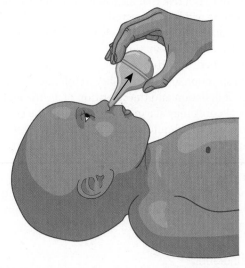

FIGURE 22-16 An illustration of nasal suctioning with a bulb syringe. The arrow illustrates the flow of nasal secretions once the squeezed bulb reinflates.

Bulb Suctioning

Bulb suctioning is typically reserved for infants and small children and is defined as the act of removing secretions from a patient's nasal passage using a bulb device (**Figure 22-16**). To use bulb suction, you squeeze the air out of the bulb, gently insert it into the infant's nostril, and release the bulb, creating a vacuum as the bulb reinflates. This action will pull mucus out of the infant's nostril.

Nasotracheal Suctioning

Nasotracheal suctioning (NTS) is intended to remove accumulated saliva, pulmonary secretions, blood, vomitus, and other foreign material from the trachea and nasopharynx that cannot be removed naturally by the patient.[71] NTS is performed by inserting a flexible catheter into the patient's nasal passages and pharynx in order to remove secretions. Secretion clearance is accomplished by applying negative pressure, at the recommended vacuum pressure, to a flexible catheter.[72,73]

To facilitate passing the suction catheter into the airway, position the patient in the sniffing position, or with the head slightly extended (Figure 22-12). Gently insert the catheter through the nostril, directing it toward the septum and floor of the nasal cavity. Negative pressure should not be applied during catheter insertion. If resistance is felt, twirl the catheter (roll it gently between your index finger and thumb) and then advance. The patient may cough as the catheter enters the posterior larynx.

Indications

NTS is indicated to maintain a patent airway and to remove secretions in patients who have difficulty expectorating mobilized secretions. Indications for the need of NTS mirror those for suctioning associated with an artificial airway. The patient may have secretions visible in the airway (secretions bubbling from the nares or mouth), coarse breath sounds or "gurgling" may be heard on auscultation, or the patient may exhibit signs of increased work of breathing or complain that they feel their secretions did not clear with coughing.

The only absolute contraindications for NTS are in patients diagnosed with epiglottitis or croup. Relative contraindications include occluded nasal passages; nasal bleeding; head, neck, or facial trauma; bleeding disorder/coagulopathy; irritable/reactive airway; and following tracheal reconstruction surgery.[71,74]

NTS is a blind procedure and is not without risks or complications. Inserting the catheter into the oropharynx or esophagus may cause the patient to gag and vomit, increasing the risk for aspiration. Repositioning the patient and/or catheter is appropriate at this time. Always be ready to suction the oropharynx if needed. Special consideration should be made for patients who have recently eaten or who have gastric tube feedings. The determination to suction should be done in close coordination with the nurse caring for the patient. Hazards or complications are listed in **Table 22-11**.[71]

Suctioning and Artificial Airway

Suctioning is the most common procedure performed in the ICU for patients with an artificial airway.[73]

TABLE 22-11
Hazards/Complications Associated with Nasotracheal Suctioning

Mechanical trauma (nose bleeding)
Hypoxia/hypoxemia
Bradycardia, other arrhythmias, or cardiac arrest
Hypotension/hypertension
Respiratory arrest
Paroxysmal coughing
Gagging/vomiting
Laryngospasm
Bronchoconstriction/bronchospasm
Infection
Atelectasis
Increased intracranial pressure
Pneumothorax

TABLE 22-12
Recommended Vacuum Pressures Used for Suctioning the Airway

Population	Pressure (mm Hg)
Neonates	60–80
Infants	80–100
Children	100–120
Adults	100–150

The presence of an artificial airway, such as an ETT, impairs the cough reflex and increases mucus production, thereby producing the need for suctioning. The ideal suction procedure should be painless, safe, effective, and free of associated adverse events. In order to optimize safety, the provider should consider the patient's lung compliance, the vacuum pressure used for the suctioning procedure, the size of the suction catheter, and the time taken to pass the catheter and collect secretions.

Use of correct suction catheter size and vacuum pressure are essential. Vacuum pressures vary by age and are listed in **Table 22-12**. The use of smaller catheters at lower vacuum pressures leads to ineffective secretion clearance.

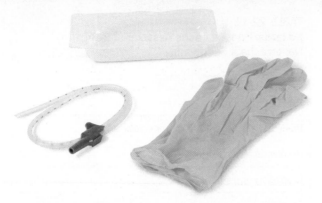

FIGURE 22-17 An example of an open suction kit. The kit contains sterile gloves, a suction catheter, and a container to hold sterile water to flush the secretions from the catheter.
© Medline Industries, Inc. 2018

Hazards/Complications

Although suctioning is a routine procedure performed in the ICU on a daily basis, as with NTS, it is not without complications. Careful adherence to the procedure is the best way to avoid potential hazards or complications, such as oxygen desaturation, bronchospasm, nosocomial infection, pain, anxiety, dyspnea, tachycardia, and increased intracranial pressure.

The routine use of normal saline lavage prior to suctioning may be associated with adverse events and can actually increase the risk of nosocomial pneumonia by dislodging bacteria from the tracheal walls.

Desired Outcomes

Clinical outcomes associated with suctioning include an improvement in breath sounds, improvement in arterial blood gases or oxygen saturation, decrease in airway resistance with a concomitant decrease in peak inspiratory pressure, and increase in tidal volume delivery during pressure ventilation.[69]

Suctioning Techniques

Suctioning may be done with the child disconnected from ventilatory support (also know as the open procedure) or while the child remains connected to the patient-ventilator circuit (closed procedure). Although differences in the open and closed suction procedures differ, the indications, risks, and complications are similar.

Open

The open suction procedure requires the patient to be disconnected from ventilator support to insert a suction catheter into the ETT to remove secretions. In the hospital setting, sterile technique is used. A clean technique is often used in the homecare setting to suction patients with a tracheostomy who may or may not require mechanical ventilation. This procedure may pose an increased risk of exposing the patient to environmental contamination if proper technique is

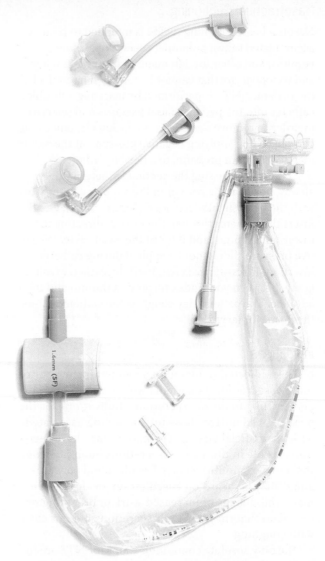

FIGURE 22-18 An example of a closed suction system.
Used with permission from Avanos Medical.

not maintained.[75–77] Suction catheters are available in a variety of designs, with most including a thumb port to apply suction and distal side suction ports to decrease mucosal damage caused by applying vacuum at a single end port (**Figure 22-17**). Suction catheters are sized in French units for the external circumference and are typically 22 inches long.[69] It is important to select the appropriate-size catheter to prevent atelectasis or hypoxemia when negative pressure is applied.

Closed

The closed suction technique involves attaching a sterile suction system inline in the patient's ventilator circuit (**Figure 22-18**). Use of a closed suction system maintains ventilation and oxygen delivery during the suction procedure. The literature reports that the use of closed suction results in fewer procedure-associated oxygen desaturations.[76]

Catheter Size Selection

It is recommended to use smaller catheters whenever possible. The negative pressure that is transmitted to the airways is determined by a combination of the catheter size as well as the vacuum pressure. Large catheter sizes and increased vacuum pressures are associated with increased negative tracheal pressures during endotracheal suctioning.[72] Therefore, it is recommended to use smaller catheter sizes whenever possible for suctioning an artificial airway.

Measuring the Size of Suction Catheters

To estimate the proper size of a suction catheter for endotracheal suctioning, first multiply the tube's inner diameter by 2, then use the next smallest size catheter. For example, if the patient has a size 5.0 ETT: 2 x 5 = 10, and the next smallest size is an 8.[75]

Suction Depth

Many studies address the difference between deep suction procedures and shallow suction procedures. A deep suction procedure is described as the catheter being passed into the ETT until a cough or gag reflex is obtained while a shallow suction procedure is described as the catheter being passed into the ETT so that the catheter goes to the tip of the ETT but does not extend beyond the length of the tube.[77] When deep suctioning was compared to shallow suctioning in neonatal patients, there was no significant difference in oxygen saturations or heart rate; therefore, there appears to be no added cardiovascular risk to a neonatal patient from deep suctioning.[77] However, shallow suctioning is recommended to prevent trauma to the tracheal mucosa.[77]

Case Study 1

A 5-year-old boy presented to the emergency department with signs of acute airway obstruction and stridor. The signs and symptoms had begun the day before, with a respiratory infection, and had quickly progressed. His mother reported that the child ate peanuts as well. On arrival, the boy was restless and agitated, with dyspnea and tachypnea. He was sitting in a tripod position, and audible inspiratory stridor in the head-up position was noted. Cyanosis was present and his oxygen saturation by pulse oximetry was 85%. His vital signs upon admission were as follows: temperature 37.8ºC, blood pressure 90/60 mm Hg, heart rate 160 beats per minute, respiratory rate 38 breaths per minute. The chest examination revealed decreased aeration bilaterally, transmitted sounds from the upper airway, and wheezing and whispery sounds.

Systemic corticosteroids and 100% oxygen by face mask were given immediately. The physician asks you to prepare for intubation to assure an airway is secured.

1. **What size and type of ETT will you prepare for this patient?**

2. **What mnemonic is used as a checklist memory aid for equipment essential for endotracheal intubation?**

   The child was successfully intubated and transferred to the ICU.

3. **Is there another method the physician may have chosen because of the upper airway obstruction and associated risks?**

Case Study 2

A 10-month-old girl was transported to the emergency department by paramedics. She has a history of fever and had a seizure at home. On arrival, the patient was not actively seizing, but she was apenic with an oxygen saturation of 75%. You position the head, open the airway, and, using the EC-clamp technique, you provide oxygen by a bag-valve-mask resuscitator. You suction the airway to remove oral secretions. At this time, the physician takes over manual ventilation and asks you to prepare for intubation. He would like an oral airway, with appropriate ETT size, stylet, and

laryngoscope handle and blades. Using SOAPPIM, you prepare for intubation.

1. **What size ETT, oral airway, stylet, and laryngoscope blades will you prepare for this patient?**

   The patient is intubated without any adverse intubation-associated events.

2. **How do you confirm endotracheal tube placement in the pediatric patient?**

3. **What other intubation device could have been used for this patient?**

References

1. Hagberg C. *Benumof and Hagberg's Airway Mangement*. 3rd ed. Philadelphia, PA: Elsevier; 2012.

2. Hernandez MR, Klock PA, Ovassapian A. Evolution of the extraglottic airway: a review of its history, applications, and practical tips for success. *Anesth Analg*. 2012;114(2):349-365.

3. Wilson IG, Fell D, Robinson SL, Smith G. Cardiovascular responses to insertion of the laryngeal mask. *Anaesthesia*. 1992;47(4):300-302.

4. Braude N, Clements EA, Hodges UM, Andrews BP. The pressor response and laryngeal mask insertion. A comparison with tracheal intubation. *Anaesthesia*. 1989;44(7):551-554.

5. Agrawal G, Agarwal M, Taneja S. A randomized comparative study of intraocular pressure and hemodynamic changes on insertion of proseal laryngeal mask airway and conventional tracheal intubation in pediatric patients. *J Anaesthesiol Clin Pharmacol*. 2012;28(3):326-329.

6. Ismail SA, Bisher NA, Kandil HW, Mowafi HA, Atawia HA. Intraocular pressure and haemodynamic responses to insertion of the i-gel, laryngeal mask airway or endotracheal tube. *Eur J Anaesthesiol*. 2011;28(6):443-448.

7. Igboko JO, Desalu I, Akinsola FB, Kushimo OT. Intraocular pressure changes in a Nigerian population—effects of tracheal tube and laryngeal mask airway insertion and removal. *Niger Postgrad Med J*. 2009;16(2):99-104.

8. Tanaka A, Isono S, Ishikawa T, Sato J, Nishino T. Laryngeal resistance before and after minor surgery: endotracheal tube versus laryngeal mask airway. *Anesthesiology*. 2003;99:252-258.

9. Brimacombe J. The advantages of the LMA over the tracheal tube or facemask: a meta-analysis. *Can J Anaesth*. 1995;42(11):1017-1023.

10. Parmet JL, Colonna-Romano P, Horrow JC, Miller F, Gonzales J, Rosenberg H. The laryngeal mask airway reliably provides rescue ventilation in cases of unanticipated difficult tracheal intubation along with difficult mask ventilation. *Anesth Analg*. 1998;87(3):661-665.

11. Maltby JR, Loken RG, Watson NC. The laryngeal mask airway: clinical appraisal in 250 patients. *Can J Anaesth*. 1990;37:509-513.

12. Apfelbaum JL, Hagberg CA. Practice guidelines for management of the difficult airway: an updated report by the American Society of Anesthesiologists Task Force on Management of the Difficult Airway. *Anesthesiology*. 2003;98:1269.

13. Ferson DZ, Rosenblatt WH, Johansen MJ, Osborn I, Ovassapian A. Use of the intubating LMA-Fastrach in 254 patients with difficult-to-manage airways. *Anesthesiology*. 2001;95(5):1175-1181.

14. Mizushima A, Wardall GJ, Simpson DL. The laryngeal mask airway in infants. *Anaesthesia*. 1992;47(10):849-851.

15. Rowbottom SJ, Simpson DL, Grubb D. The laryngeal mask airway in children. A fibreoptic assessment of positioning. *Anaesthesia*. 1991;46(6):489-491.

16. Morrison LJ, Deakin CD, Morley PT, et al. Part 8: advanced life support: 2010 International Consensus on Cardiopulmonary Resuscitation and Emergency Cardiovascular Care Science with Treatment Recommendations. *Circulation*. 2010;122(16 Suppl 2):S345-S421.

17. Ramachandran SK, Kumar AM. Supraglottic airway devices. *Respir Care*. 2014;59(6):920-931.

18. Brimacombe JR, Berry A. The incidence of aspiration associated with the laryngeal mask airway: a meta-analysis of published literature. *J Clin Anesth*. 1995;7(4):297-305.

19. Verghese C, Brimacombe JR. Survey of laryngeal mask airway usage in 11,910 patients: safety and efficacy for conventional and nonconventional usage. *Anesth Analg*. 1996;82(1):129-133.

20. Ramachandran SK, Mathis MR, Tremper KK, Shanks AM, Kheterpal S. Predictors and clinical outcomes from failed Laryngeal Mask Airway Unique: a study of 15,795 patients. *Anesthesiology*. 2012;116(6):1217-1226.

21. Bernardini A, Natalini G. Risk of pulmonary aspiration with laryngeal mask airway and tracheal tube: analysis on 65,712 procedures with positive pressure ventilation. *Anaesthesia*. 2009;64(12):1289-1294.

22. Rabey PG, Murphy PJ, Langton JA, Barker P, Rowbotham DJ. Effect of the laryngeal mask airway on lower oesophageal sphincter pressure in patients during general anaesthesia. *Br J Anaesth*. 1992;69(4):346-348.

23. Schmidbauer W, Genzwurker H, Ahlers O, Proquitte H, Kerner T. Cadaver study of oesophageal insufflation with supraglottic airway devices during positive pressure ventilation in an obstructed airway. *Br J Anaesth*. 2012;109(3):454-458.

24. Lloyd Jones FR, Hegab A. Case report. Recurrent laryngeal nerve palsy after laryngeal mask airway insertion. *Anaesthesia*. 1996;51(2):171-172.

25. Figueredo E, Vivar-Diago M, Munoz-Blanco F. Laryngo-pharyngeal complaints after use of the laryngeal mask airway. *Can J Anaesth*. 1999;46(3):220-225.

26. Inomata S, Nishikawa T, Suga A, Yamashita S. Transient bilateral vocal cord paralysis after insertion of a laryngeal mask airway. *Anesthesiology*. 1995;82(3):787-788.

27. Litman RS, Keon TP. Postintubation croup in children. *Anesthesiology*. 1991;75:1122-1123.

28. Koka BV, Jeon IS, Andre JM, MacKay I, Smith RM. Postintubation croup in children. *Anesth Analg*. 1977;56:501-505.

29. Holinger PH, Kutnick SL, Schild JA, Holinger LD. Subglottic stenosis in infants and children. *Ann Otol Rhinol Laryngol*. 1976;85:591-599.

30. Fearon B, Cotton R. Subglottic stenosis in infants and children: the clinical problem and experimental correction. *Can J Otolaryngol*. 1972;1:281-289.

31. Mossad E, Youssef G. Subglottic stenosis in children undergoing repair of congenital heart defects. *J Cardiothorac Vasc Anesth*. 2009;23:658-662.

32. Hawkins DB. Hyaline membrane disease of the neonate prolonged intubation in management: effects on the larynx. *Laryngoscope*. 1978;88:201-224.

33. Benjamin B. Prolonged intubation injuries of the larynx: endoscopic diagnosis, classification, and treatment. *Ann Otol Rhinol Laryngol*. 1993;160:1-15.

34. Liu H, Chen JC, Holinger LD, Gonzalez-Crussi F. Histopathologic fundamentals of acquired laryngeal stenosis. *Pediatr Pathol Lab Med*. 1995;15:655-677.

35. Fine GF, Borland LM. The future of the cuffed endotracheal tube. *Paediatr Anaesth*. 2004;14:38-42.

36. Weiss M, Dullenkopf A, Fischer JE, Keller C, Gerber AC. Prospective randomized controlled multi-centre trial of cuffed or uncuffed endotracheal tubes in small children. *Br J Anaesth*. 2009;103(6):867-873.

37. Weiss M, Dullenkopf A, Gysin C, Dillier CM, Gerber AC. Shortcomings of cuffed paediatric tracheal tubes. *Br J Anaesth*. 2004;92:78-88.

38. Litman RS, Weissend EE, Shibata D, Westesson PL. Developmental changes of laryngeal dimensions in unparalyzed, sedated children. *Anesthesiology*. 2003;98:41-45.

39. Dalal PG, Murray D, Messner AH, Feng A, McAllister J, Molter D. Pediatric laryngeal dimensions: an age-based analysis. *Anesth Analg*. 2009;108:1475-1479.

40. Ashtekar CS, Wardhaugh A. Do cuffed endotracheal tubes increase the risk of airway mucosal injury and post-extubation stridor in children? *Arch Dis Child*. 2005;90:1198-1199.

41. Cox RG. Should cuffed endotracheal tubes be used routinely in children? *Can J Anaesth*. 2005;52:669-674.

42. Weiss M, Gerber AC. Cuffed tracheal tubes in children—things have changed. *Paediatr Anaesth*. 2006;16:1005-1007.

43. Penlington GN. Letter: endotracheal tube sizes for children. *Anaesthesia*. 1974;29(4):494-495.

44. von Rettberg MI, Thil E, Genzwürker H, Gernoth C, Hinkelbein J. Endotracheal tubes in pediatric patients. Published formulas to estimate the optimal size. *Anaesthesist*. 2011;60:334-342.

45. Cole F. Pediatric formulas for the anesthesiologist. *Am J Dis Child*. 1957;94:672-673.

46. Eckenhoff JE. Some anatomic considerations of the infant larynx influencing endotracheal anesthesia. *Anesthesiology*. 1951;12:401-410.

47. Negus VE. *The Comparative Anatomy and Physiology of the Larynx*. New York, NY: Grune & Stratton; 1949.

48. Wilson TG. Some observations on the anatomy of the infantile larynx. *Acta Otolaryngol*. 1953;43:95-99.

49. Davenport HT, Rosales JK. Endotracheal intubation in infants and children. *Can Anaesth Soc J*. 1959;6:65-74.

50. Gillespie NA. Endotracheal anaesthesia in infants. *Br J Anaesth*. 1939;17:2-12.

51. Westhorpe RN. The position of the larynx in children and its relationship to the ease of intubation. *Anaesth Intensive Care*. 1987;15:384-388.

52. Shorten GD, Armstrong DC, Roy WI, Brown L. Assessment of the effect of head and neck position on upper airway anatomy in sedated paediatric patients using magnetic resonance imaging. *Paediatr Anaesth*. 1995;5:243-248.

53. Adnet F, Baillard C, Borron SW, et al. Randomized study comparing the "sniffing position" with simple head extension for laryngoscopic view in elective surgery patients. *Anesthesiology*. 2001;95:836-841.

54. Karsli C, Der T. Tracheal intubation in older children with severe retro/micrognathia using the GlideScope Cobalt Infant Video Laryngoscope. *Paediatr Anaesth*. 2010;20:577-578.

55. Hackell RS, Held LD, Stricker PA, Fiadjoe JE. Management of the difficult infant airway with the Storz Video Laryngoscope: a case series. *Anesth Analg*. 2009;109:763-766.

56. Vlatten A, Aucoin S, Gray A, Soder C. Difficult airway management with the STORZ video laryngoscope in a child with Robin sequence. *Paediatr Anaesth*. 2009;19:700-701.

57. Pean D, Desdoits A, Asehnoune K, Lejus C. Airtraq laryngoscope for intubation in Treacher Collins syndrome. *Paediatr Anaesth*. 2009;19:698-699.

58. Vlatten A, Soder C. Airtraq optical laryngoscope intubation in a 5-month-old infant with a difficult airway because of Robin sequence. *Paediatr Anaesth*. 2009;19:699-700.

59. Sbaraglia F, Lorusso R, Garra R, Sammartino M. Usefulness of Airtraq in a 3-month-old child with Apert syndrome. *Paediatr Anaesth*. 2011;21:984-985.

60. Hartmann SM, Farris RW, Di Gennaro JL, Roberts JS. Systematic review and meta-analysis of end-tidal carbon dioxide values associated with return of spontaneous circulation during cardiopulmonary resuscitation. *J Intensive Care Med*. 2015;30:426-435.

61. Hamrick JL, Hamrick JT, Lee JK, Lee BH, Koehler RC, Shaffner DH. Efficacy of chest compressions directed by end-tidal CO_2 feedback in a pediatric resuscitation model of basic life support. *J Am Heart Assoc*. 2014;3(2):e000450. doi:10.1161.

62. Sheak KR, Wiebe DJ, Leary M, et al. Quantitative relationship between end-tidal carbon dioxide and CPR quality during both in-hospital and out-of-hospital cardiac arrest. *Resuscitation*. 2015;89:149-154.

63. Brinsmead TL, Davies MW. Securing endotracheal tubes: does NeoBar availability improve tube position? *J Paediatr Child Health*. 2010;46:243-248.

64. Fearon B, Whalen JS. Tracheal dimensions in the living infant (preliminary report). *Ann Otol Rhinol Laryngol*. 1967;76:965-974.

65. Lau N, Playfor SD, Rashid A, Dhanarass M. New formulae for predicting tracheal tube length. *Peadiatr Anesth*. 2006;16:1238-1243.

66. Plummer AL, Gracey DR. Consensus conference on artificial airways in patients receiving mechanical ventilation. *Chest*. 1989;96:178-180.

67. Cooke J. Tracheostomy: care and management review. https://www.ccam.net.au/handbook/tracheostomy/. Accessed August 21, 2015.

68. Sherman JM, Davis S, Albamonte-Petrick S, et al. Care of the child with a chronic tracheostomy. *Am J Respir Crit Care Med*. 2000;161:297-308.

69. Restrepo RD, Brown JM, Hughes JM. AARC clinical practice guidelines. Endotracheal suctioning of mechanically ventilated patients with artificial airways 2010. *Respir Care*. 2010;55(6):758-764.

70. Gillies D, Spence K. Deep versus shallow suction of endotracheal tubes in ventilated neonates and young infants. *Cochrane Database Syst Rev*. 2011;7:CD003309.

71. Nasotracheal suctioning—2004 revision & update. American Association for Respiratory Care, clinical practice guidelines. *Respir Care*. 2004;49:1080-1084.

72. Kiraly NJ, Tingay DG, Mills JF, Morley CJ, Copnell, B. Negative tracheal pressure during neonatal endotracheal suctioning. *Pediatr Res*. 2008;64:29-33.

73. Argent AC. Endotracheal suctioning is basic or is it? *Pediatr Res*. 2009;66:364-367.

74. Dunne C, Spreckley C, Smith L. Suction. Great Ormond Street Hospital for Children. http://www.gosh.nhs.uk/health-professionals/clinical-guidelines/suction. Accessed August 21, 2015.

75. Taylor JE, Hawley G, Flenady V, Woodgate PG. Tracheal suctioning without disconnection in intubated ventilated neonates. *Cochrane Database Syst Rev*. 2011;12:CD003065.

76. Maggiore SM, Iacobone E, Zito G, Conti G, Antonelli M, Proietti, R. Closed verses open suctioning techniques. *Minerva Anestesiologica*. 2002;68:360-364.

77. Gillies D, Spence K. Deep verses shallow suction of endotracheal tubes in ventilated neonates and young infants. *Cochrane Database Syst Rev*. 2011;7:CD003309.

23

Oxygen Therapy

Teresa A. Volsko

OUTLINE

Introduction
Indications of Oxygen Therapy
  Clinical Signs and Symptoms of Hypoxemia and Hypoxia
Monitoring Oxygen Therapy
Hazards/Complications
Oxygen Delivery Devices
  Variable Performance Oxygen Delivery Devices
  Reservoir Devices
  Fixed Performance Oxygen Delivery Devices
  Enclosure Devices
References

OBJECTIVES

1. List the indications for oxygen therapy.
2. Describe the physiologic mechanisms and provide examples of conditions that contribute to hypoxemia.
3. Define normoxemic hypoxia.
4. Describe the signs and symptoms associated with hypoxemia.
5. Differentiate between central and peripheral cyanosis.
6. Explain the methods for evaluating the efficacy of oxygen therapy.
7. Compare and contrast the indications, contraindications, and hazards associated with variable performance oxygen delivery devices.
8. Describe how a nasal cannula is applied to an infant and child.
9. Describe the essential components of applying reservoir devices to infants and children.
10. Compare and contrast the indications, contraindications, and hazards associated with the various fixed performance oxygen delivery devices.
11. Describe the indications, contraindications, and hazards associated with the various enclosure devices.

KEY TERMS

air-entrainment mask
air-entrainment nebulizer
central cyanosis
enclosure devices
fixed performance devices
heated high-flow nasal
  cannula (HHFNC)
incubator
nasal cannula
nonrebreathing mask

normoxemic hypoxia
oxygen hoods
partial rebreathing
  mask
Qp/Qs ratio
reservoir device
retinopathy of
  prematurity (ROP)
simple mask
variable performance

Introduction

The administration of oxygen plays an essential role in the treatment and outcomes of infants and children with respiratory impairment. Oxygen therapy is administered across the continuum of care, from prehospital or emergency care during transport to definitive care though a variety of inpatient and outpatient settings, including acute care and intensive care units, physician offices, extended care facilities, and home. The devices used to administer oxygen therapy have evolved throughout the years. Technologic advances offer bedside clinicians a variety of devices to choose from and enable the caregiver to select a device that delivers the concentration and flow the patient needs while enhancing comfort and, ultimately, adherence to therapy.

Indications of Oxygen Therapy

The principal goal of oxygen therapy is to achieve adequate tissue oxygenation by preventing and/or treating documented or suspected hypoxemia.[1,2] Infants and children are particularly susceptible to hypoxemic events and, depending on the severity, they can lead to complications, including tissue hypoxia, metabolic abnormalities, acid–base disturbances, and even death.[3–5] Vital organs, such as the brain, heart, and kidneys, need high amounts of oxygen to adequately function. Exercise, injury (trauma, burns), and illness increase oxygen requirements and, because the human body does not have a store of oxygen in the body, require supplemental oxygen administration to treat hypoxemia.[6] In the absence of a respiratory or cardiac condition, exercise does not increase the oxygen requirements to the point where treatment is needed. However, children with chronic respiratory conditions, such as cystic fibrosis, may require oxygen for exercise-related activities. **Table 23-1** provides a list of physiologic mechanisms and examples of conditions that contribute to hypoxemia. For example, newborns have a higher concentration of fetal

hemoglobin, which has a greater affinity for oxygen. The presence of higher fetal hemoglobin concentrations shifts the oxygen dissociation curve to the left, allowing higher oxygen saturation for any given PaO_2. Therefore, a PaO_2 less than 60 mm Hg and an SpO_2 less than 90% would be indicative of hypoxemia in newborn infants. In children, hypoxemia is characterized by a PaO_2 of less than 80 mm Hg or an SpO2 of less than 94% to 95%.

There are conditions that require prompt administration of high concentrations of oxygen. The highest concentration of supplemental oxygen should be administered during cardiopulmonary arrest while resuscitation is provided.[7] After the return of spontaneous circulation, FiO_2 should be titrated to achieve and maintain an SpO_2 of 94%.[8]

Hypoxia is the most important indication for oxygen therapy. Hypoxia can result from different acute conditions, including but not limited to acute respiratory failure, severe anemia, low cardiac output, severe sepsis, trauma, surgical intervention, and anesthesia. Supplemental oxygen therapy is also required when **normoxemic hypoxia** is present or when tissue hypoxia is present despite normal arterial PaO_2 or SpO_2.[8] Cyanide poisoning is an example of normoxemic hypoxia.

Clinical Signs and Symptoms of Hypoxemia and Hypoxia

Several respiratory signs were found to be associated with hypoxemia. The literature reports that there is no single sign or symptom that can accurately predict hypoxemia in young children. Signs and symptoms include tachypnea, tachycardia, grunting, nasal flaring, chest retractions, and head bobbing.[9] Hypoxemia may also present as general signs of depression, manifested as poor feeding or the inability to feed, lethargy, and/or irritability. Infants may also present with poor muscle tone and, in extreme cases, flaccid with arms and legs in a frog-leg position (**Figure 23-1**).[9]

Clinicians often use the presence of **central cyanosis**, or bluish discoloration of the tongue or mucous membranes, as an indication for the need to administer supplemental oxygen. In children, central cyanosis does not occur until arterial hemoglobin concentrations drop to 4 to 6 g/dL. Children presenting with central cyanosis typically have a PaO_2 of approximately 50 to 60 mm Hg and an SpO_2 of 85% to 95%. Central cyanosis in a newborn infant is a late and often ominous sign.

Monitoring Oxygen Therapy

It is important to monitor the oxygenation status of children receiving oxygen therapy in the acute care setting. The clinical monitoring includes observation of the child's level of consciousness, vital signs, respiratory depth and pattern, and the color of the skin and mucosa. Pulse oximetry (SpO_2) is a convenient, noninvasive method for intermittent or continuous monitoring of oxygen therapy.[10] Pulse oximetry can be used to

TABLE 23-1
Physiologic Mechanisms Contributing to and Conditions That Often Result in Hypoxemia

Physiologic Mechanisms	Conditions
Decreased alveolar ventilation	Respiratory insufficiency Respiratory failure
Ventilation/perfusion mismatch	Asthma Lower respiratory tract infections
Right-to-left intracardiac or intrapulmonary shunt	Congenital heart defects
Reduced oxygen-carrying capacity	Anemia Carbon monoxide poisoning
Reduced inspired oxygen	Altitude

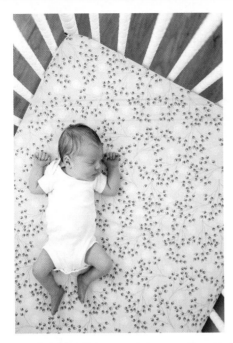

FIGURE 23-1 An infant with low muscle tone, positioned in the frog-leg position. Legs are flexed at the knees and arms at the elbows.
© Mint Images/Mint Images RF/Getty Images.

TABLE 23-2
Calculations Used to Assess Tissue Oxygenation

Assessment	Calculation
Arterial oxygen content (CaO_2)	$CaO_2 = (Hb. \times 1.34 \times SaO_2) + (PaO_2 \times 0.003)$
Venous oxygen content (CvO_2)	$CvO2 = (Hb. \times 1.34 \times SvO_2) + (PvO2 \times 0.003)$
Oxygen consumption (VO_2)	$CO \times (CaO_2 - CvO_2) \times 10$
Oxygen delivery (DO_2)	$(CaO_2 \times CO) \times 10$

CO = cardiac output; Hb = hemoglobin

monitor oxygen saturation levels as the concentration of oxygen is titrated to need. There are conditions where pulse oximetry is not reliable, including carbon monoxide poisoning and methemoglobinmia. Periodic measurements of arterial blood and analysis of PaO_2 and SaO_2 by hemoximetry can be used to accurately assess tissue oxygenation. **Table 23-2** provides calculations that can be used to assess, monitor, and trend the status of tissue oxygenation.

Hazards/Complications

Optimal strategies for the use of oxygen in preterm infants and young children remain controversial. It is often challenging to achieve a balance between attaining adequate tissue oxygenation and avoiding oxygen toxicity. There remains a paucity of clear evidence-based guidance for clinicians on safe oxygen saturation targets. What does seem apparent is that these targets vary over time in the life of a preterm infant.

Prolonged exposure to high concentrations of oxygen (i.e., FiO_2 >0.5) can cause cellular damage resulting from the formation of highly reactive oxygen free radicals (hydroxyl radicals and peroxynitrite) after prolonged exposure to oxygen therapy. Although oxidative damage can occur in any cell in the body, deleterious effects most often occur in the lungs, eyes, red blood cells, kidneys, and endocrine glands (thyroid and adrenal). Additionally, the rate of absorption atelectasis is accelerated when high concentrations of oxygen are delivered. The literature reports that higher saturation targets are associated with an increased number of babies requiring oxygen at 36 weeks' gestation[11] as well as increased exacerbations of chronic lung disease.[12]

Judicial use of supplemental oxygen should be considered for children with congenital large ventricular septal defects. The administration of oxygen in this population can cause pulmonary vasodilatation and a diversion of blood to the pulmonary circulation instead of systemic circulation. A high **Qp/Qs ratio**, or pulmonary blood flow/systemic blood flow ratio, results in and causes pulmonary overcirculation, which can lead to tissue ischemia, severe lactic metabolic acidosis, pulmonary edema, and even death if the hyperoxia is not reversed.

Caution should also be used when administering supplemental oxygen to children with chronic hypercapnia due to chronic obstructive lung disease or neuromuscular failure. Hyperoxia in these cases can lead to coma and death.

Oxygen therapy has a role in the development of **retinopathy of prematurity (ROP)**. The pathogenesis of ROP includes two phases. In the first phase, hyperoxia leads to vessel-growth cessation. The second phase, precipitated by the increasing metabolic demand of the developing retina with a compromised vascular supply, is characterized by relative hypoxia, which leads to pathologic neovascularization that extends into the vitreous.[13] The timing of the development of ROP is dependent on the infant's gestational age, which provides an estimation of the maturity of the retinal vasculature. Significant risk factors for ROP include the need for high levels of respiratory support, or high concentrations of oxygen, to stabilize the infant's clinical course.[14]

Oxygen Delivery Devices

The effectiveness of oxygen therapy depends on the ability to deliver the precise dose (FiO_2) with an interface that meets the flow and comfort needs of the child. Oxygen delivery devices or interfaces are broadly classified into four categories: low flow, high flow, reservoir, and enclosures. These devices are categorized by their ability to meet the inspiratory demands of the patient and to deliver a stable FiO_2. **Table 23-3** provides an overview of the performance characteristics of devices

TABLE 23-3
A Comparison of the Interfaces Used to Deliver Oxygen Therapy to Children

Device	Classification	FiO$_2$ Stability	FiO$_2$ Range	Illustration
Nasal cannula	Low flow	Variable	Low range <0.35	© lavizzara/Shutterstock.
Simple mask	Reservoir	Variable	Moderate range 0.35–0.60	© Fertnig/E+/Getty.
Partial rebreathing mask	Reservoir	Variable	Moderate range 0.50–0.60	© Jones & Bartlett Learning.
Nonrebreathing mask	Reservoir	Variable	High range >0.60	© lisafx/iStock/Getty Images Plus.

Air-entrainment mask	High flow	Fixed	Low–moderate range <0.35–0.60	
Heated high-flow nasal cannula	High flow	Fixed	Low–high range <0.35 to >0.60	
Oxygen hood	Enclosure	Fixed	Low–high range <0.35 to >0.60	
Incubator	Enclosure	Fixed	Low range <0.35	

© Fuse/Corbis/Getty Images.

Courtesy of Fisher & Paykel Healthcare.

© Steve Lovegrove/Shutterstock.

© Stoyan Yotov/Shutterstock.

or interfaces commonly used to deliver oxygen therapy to infants and children.

Variable Performance Oxygen Delivery Devices

Variable performance devices provide a portion of the total flow of gas a patient inhales per breath. These devices are also referred to as variable performance devices because the devices do not satisfy the patient's total flow needs; the patient entrains air as well as the flow of oxygen from the device. Therefore, depending on the child's tidal volume, inspiratory time, and the flow of oxygen from a low-flow device, the actual FiO_2 can vary from breath to breath. These devices typically deliver low to moderate concentrations of oxygen but can deliver higher concentrations as with the nonrebreathing mask. The nasal cannula, simple mask, partial rebreathing mask, and nonrebreathing mask are examples of variable performance oxygen delivery devices.

Nasal Cannula

A **nasal cannula** is commonly used to delivery low concentrations of oxygen to infants and children. It consists of small-bore oxygen tubing connected to two short prongs. The prongs are angled down to conform to the anatomic features of the nares.

Indications, Contraindications, and Hazards

A nasal cannula provides a method for continuous oxygen administration and allows direct caregivers the ability to provide care with ease. A nasal cannula allows an infant to receive supplemental oxygen while feeding and receiving routine nursing care, and parents are able to hold their infant and provide skin-to-skin care, also known as kangaroo care. Infants cared for with this delivery device also have increased mobility compared with those who receive oxygen therapy by a hood, which increases interactions with parents, caregivers, and environment and may be developmentally beneficial.[15] In children, the use of this oxygen delivery device allows the child to communicate, eat, and interact with their environment. As with infants, increased mobility is also facilitated.

The benefits derived from this oxygen delivery device are balanced by some drawbacks, including the instability of oxygen administration in transitions between oral and nasal breathing, drying of nasal mucosa, and lack of precise knowledge about the delivered oxygen concentration.[16]

Device Application

Nasal cannulas are available in a variety of sizes, one of which can be seen in (**Figure 23-2**). Prong length and the width or the space between the prongs varies with size to accommodate the anatomic features of a range

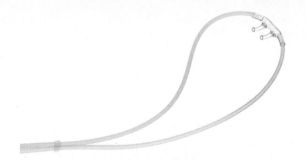

FIGURE 23-2 An example of a nasal cannula. This oxygen delivery device is available in a variety of sizes to accommodate the anatomical features of children as they grow and develop.

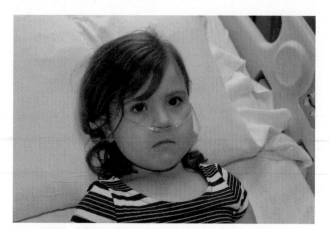

FIGURE 23-3 Proper application of a nasal cannula. The prongs fit in the nare, with the slant or curvature downward, and are not occlusive. The oxygen delivery tubing is looped over the ears and secured comfortably, not tightly, in place under the chin.

of patients, from a preterm infant to a developing child. The prongs should fit comfortably in the nares without being occlusive (**Figure 23-3**). The prong-to-nare ratio describes the amount of space the prong occupies in the nare. The literature reports that, for a standard nasal cannula, the prong-to-nare ratio should not exceed 50%.[17] Nasal cannulas are also available with only a single prong. This modification allows for oxygen to be delivery to patients with craniofacial conditions, such as choanal atresia or cleft lip, or to those requiring placement of a nasogastric tube.

The nasal cannula is a low-flow device and does not provide the total flow to meet the inspiratory needs of the patient. Therefore, the concentration of oxygen delivered through a nasal cannula is dependent upon the flow of oxygen through the device, the concentration of oxygen delivered to the patient (if blended gas is delivered), minute ventilation, and the amount of air the infant or child entrains through the nose and mouth.[18] The ratio of oxygen provided through the device and air entrained through the nose and mouth determine the concentration of oxygen delivered to the alveoli.[19] Neonatal and pediatric patients require much lower flow deliveries than those used for adults receiving oxygen by nasal cannula. Because of the anatomic features of the upper airway and the small tidal volumes in infants, oxygen delivery to the hypopharynx is more stable when flows of 1 L/minute or less are used to deliver oxygen by a traditional nasal cannula. As a result, predicting the concentration of oxygen delivered by a nasal cannula is not as easy in infants and small children. Therefore, the rule of 4s, which estimates a 4% change in delivered oxygen concentrations for each liter delivered by a nasal cannula, cannot be reliably applied. Finer et al.[20] described a regression equation to predict the inspired oxygen concentration delivered to neonates when using a low-flow flowmeter and nasal cannula. When a nasal cannula was connected to a flowmeter at 100% humidified oxygen by a simple bubble-through humidifier, and 5.5 mL/kg was used to estimate tidal volume, the regression formula described in **Table 23-4** was able to produce a wide range of predictable FiO$_2$s for neonates when compared to measured pharyngeal oxygen concentrations. Although the equation had acceptable correlation between the measured and predicted oxygen delivery for infants weighing more than 1500 grams, this equation had a greater predictive value when used with infants weighing less than 1500 grams.[20]

Often, specially designed low-flow flowmeters are used to deliver oxygen by nasal cannula. These flowmeters, depending on the design and manufacturer, have a maximum flow of 1 L/minute or 3 L/minute (**Figure 23-4**). A flowmeter connected to a blender is often used to deliver FiO$_2$s of less than 1.0 to preterm infants receiving oxygen therapy by nasal cannula.[21] When blenders are used, oxygen titration is typically accomplished by weaning the FiO$_2$ in addition to the flow. There are no standards for oxygen titration or weaning. Typically, when the FiO$_2$ reaches 0.23, a trial of room air is performed.[22]

Securing the device in place can be challenging for preterm infants. The cartilage of the ears may not be

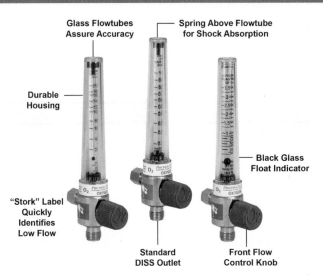

FIGURE 23-4 Low-flow flowmeters used to deliver oxygen to pediatric patients. An example of a flowmeter with a maximum flow of 3 L/min, graduated in 0.5-L increments.
Courtesy of Precision Medical.

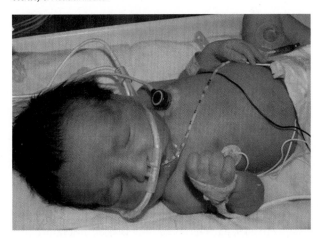

FIGURE 23-5 Application of a nasal cannula to an infant. The small-bore oxygen tubing is secured at the base of the neck, posteriorly.
Courtesy of Neotech Products.

well developed enough to hold the tubing in place, and securing the oxygen tubing around the small chin risks airway obstruction. Therefore, a common way to secure the small-bore oxygen tubing in place is at the base of the occiput (**Figure 23-5**). Because many infants are positioned supine, in the safe sleep position, it is important to ensure that the infant does not rest their head on the small-bore tubing. The tubing should rest at the base of the occiput to avoid the risk of skin breakdown due to the pressure of the head on the tubing. Figure 23-5 also illustrates the use of the Tender Grip skin fixation tab (Salter Labs, Arvin, CA). This skin fixation device has a round base, composed of microporous tape, attached to a securable flap. The flap opens to allow oxygen tubing from the cannula to rest against the fixation device and closes to secure it in place. There are a variety of fixation devices or cannula holders on the market. EZ-Hold (Neotech Products, Valencia, CA) uses a securable flap attached to a hydrocolloid base (**Figure 23-6**).

TABLE 23-4
Regression Equation Used to Predict the FiO$_2$ Delivered by Nasal Cannula to Infants

Predicted FiO$_2$ = (O$_2$ flow × 0.79) [(0.21 × VE) (VE × 100)]
Oxygen flow is expressed in mL/min
The flow of oxygen must be provided by a flowmeter connected to 100% oxygen rather than blended gas
Minute ventilation, or V$_E$, is calculated by multiplying the infant's respiratory rate by the predicted tidal volume, or V$_T$
Predicted V$_T$ is calculated by multiplying the infant's weight in kg by 5.5

Data from Finer NN, Bates R, Tomat P. Low flow oxygen delivery via nasal cannula to neonates. *Pediatr Pulmonol.* 1996;21(1):48-51.

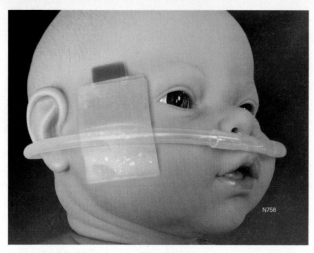

FIGURE 23-6 Application of a nasal cannula to an infant using a nasal cannula holder. The flap can be opened and closed to secure the small-bore tubing.
Courtesy of Neotech Products.

Nasal cannula holders are used to prevent inadvertent removal of the oxygen delivery device in active patients. These devices are also protective to the epidermal layers of the skin and minimize the skin irritation and epidermal stripping that can occur when tape is used to secure the cannula in place on the infant's fragile facial surface.

Reservoir Devices

A continuous flow of oxygen is accumulated within the interface of a **reservoir device**, allowing the patient to breathe in the flow of oxygen provided by the flowmeter in addition to the gas contained within the device. Simple masks, partial rebreathing masks, and nonrebreathing masks are examples of reservoir devices used to deliver oxygen to children. As the flow of oxygen through a reservoir device may not meet the total flow needs for pediatric patients, the oxygen concentration delivered to the patient is variable.

Simple Mask

A **simple mask** is a lightweight plastic mask designed to fit over the child's nose and mouth. The mask has exhalation ports located on either side of the mask that also allow the patient to entrain air to meet their total flow needs. The mask is held in place by a small, adjustable elastic band attached to the device's peripheral ends (**Figure 23-7**). A flexible metal strip, located at the proximal end of the mask, allows the caregiver to conform the mask to the contours of the nasal bridge to prevent the flow of oxygen from escaping and to minimize irritation to the child's eyes. Small-bore, smooth lumen tubing attaches the mask to the oxygen source. Similar to a nasal cannula, a variable concentration of oxygen is delivered. However, the simple mask does help increase the potential to deliver higher oxygen concentrations.

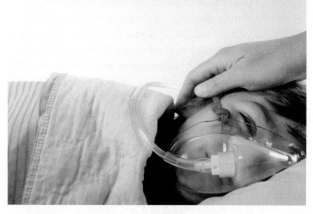

FIGURE 23-7 A simple mask in place on a child.
© Fertnig/E+/Getty.

Indications, Contraindications, and Hazards

A simple mask may be used to deliver moderate concentrations of oxygen, 35% to 60%, to children. This delivery device is commonly used for short-term therapy, such as during inter- or intrahospital transport, in the emergency department, postoperatively in the recovery or postanesthesia care unit, or during stabilization of the child during special procedures or emergency care. Because oxygen concentrations are variable and dependent upon minute ventilation and the flow of gas to the patient, this device is not recommended for children requiring precise oxygen concentration delivery or for those whose oxygen requirements may require titration over time.[23]

Children often have difficulty adhering to oxygen therapy delivered by this device. The simple mask muffles speech and interferes with the child's ability to communicate; limits their mobility; and makes eating, bottle feeding, or breastfeeding very difficult. Care should be taken when securing the mask to the child's face; the mask should fit snugly, but not tightly, against the face. A very tight fit increases the risk of skin irritation and breakdown, which can contribute to the formation of pressure ulcers.

The use of insufficient flow to the mask (i.e., flow rates less than those recommended for this device) may not provide a sufficient source of fresh gas and may limit the ability to flush the patient's exhaled CO_2 from the mask.

Device Application

After gently placing the mask against the patient's face, the adjustable elastic straps are secured around the patient's head, above the ears. Care should be taken to adjust the straps so that the mask is held in place, but is not tightly held against the skin, and that the straps do not fold or cause discomfort to the cartilage of the ears. A bubble humidifier may be used to provide additional humidity when this device is used postoperatively, during procedures, or for emergency care. However, during transport this device is connected directly to the oxygen source to prevent water from the humidifier from inadvertently entering the small-bore tubing.

The flow of oxygen to the mask varies and can range from 6 to 10 L/minute. It is important to maintain a sufficient flow of gas to the patient to minimize the propensity for CO_2 accumulation in the mask. Assessment of the patient's oxygen requirement is often accomplished noninvasively by trending SpO_2. Because the flow cannot be weaned, as with a nasal cannula, this device is discontinued and other delivery devices, such as an air-entrainment mask or a traditional or heated high-flow nasal cannula when FiO_2 titration is required, are used. Assessment of the patient's skin integrity around the periphery of the mask is also important. Any redness or indentations signify that the mask fit is not proper. When it is difficult to obtain proper fit without compromising skin integrity, even for very short-term therapy, a different delivery device should be considered.

Partial Rebreathing Mask

A **partial rebreathing mask** has a reservoir bag attached to the disposable plastic mask. Oxygen is delivered to this device through small-bore, smooth lumen tubing at the junction between the mask and the reservoir bag. Similar to a simple mask, a partial rebreathing mask has exhalation ports on either side of the mask to allow exhaled gas to escape and to provide a mechanism for the patient to entrain air should the oxygen source fail. The reservoir bag collects fresh gas from the oxygen source as well as a portion, typically the first third, of the patient's exhaled gas. Because the first third of the exhaled gas represents anatomic dead space, it is presumed that the child will not rebreathe exhaled CO_2.

Indications, Contraindications, and Hazards

A partial rebreathing mask is used when a child requires the delivery of moderate, 50% to 60%, concentrations of oxygen.[24] Similar to the simple mask, this delivery device is commonly used for short-term therapy. FiO_2 delivery is variable and dependent upon the child's minute ventilation. Hypo- and/or hyperventilation can change oxygen concentration delivery. The depth and rate of respirations should be observed, with strict attention to changes, because changes in minute ventilation will influence oxygen concentration delivery.

Children often have difficulty adhering to oxygen therapy delivered by this device as well. As with all reservoir devices, the mask will muffle speech and often interferes with the child's ability to communicate; limits their mobility; and makes eating, bottle feeding, or breastfeeding very difficult. Care should be taken when securing the mask to the child's face. To obtain moderate concentrations of oxygen, this mask must fit a bit more snuggly against the face. The flexible metal strip, which is located at the proximal end of the mask, allows the caregiver to conform the mask to the contours of the nasal bridge to prevent the flow of oxygen from escaping, maintain the delivery of moderate oxygen concentrations, and minimize irritation to the child's eyes from escaping gas flow. Because this mask fit is more snug than that needed with a simple mask, there is an increased risk of skin irritation and breakdown, both of which can contribute to pressure ulcer formation. For this reason, assessment of the patient's skin integrity around the periphery of the mask is very important. Any redness or indentations signify that the mask fit is not proper. As with the simple mask, a different delivery method should be chosen if skin integrity cannot be assured.

Device Application

Once the mask is held gently against the patient's face, the adjustable elastic straps are secured around the patient's head, just above the ears, to hold the mask snugly against the patient's face. While adjusting the elastic band, care should be taken to avoid folding or causing discomfort to the cartilage of the ears.

The flow of oxygen to the mask varies and can range from 6 to 15 L/minute. It is important to maintain a sufficient flow of gas to the reservoir bag. During inspiration, the bag should not deflate to more than one-half of its capacity. Assess the child for several minutes to ensure that flow is adequate to prevent the bag from completely deflating or deflating to more than one-half of the device's capacity during inspiration (**Figure 23-8**). It is also important to assess the patient's oxygen requirement. This is often accomplished noninvasively by trending SpO_2. Because the flow to this device cannot be weaned, it is often discontinued and the use of another delivery device, such as an air-entrainment mask or heated high-flow nasal cannula, is used when FiO_2 titration is required.

Nonrebreathing Mask

A **nonrebreathing mask** has a circular flap or valve at the juncture where the reservoir bag attaches to the disposable plastic mask. Oxygen is delivered to this device

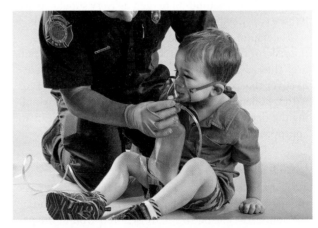

FIGURE 23-8 A partial rebreathing mask in place on a child.
© Jones & Bartlett Learning.

through small-bore, smooth lumen tubing below the flap or valve at the junction between the mask and the reservoir bag. The flap or valve between the reservoir bag and the mask prevents exhaled gas from entering the reservoir bag and diluting the concentration of oxygen available for delivery to the child. Similar to a partial rebreathing mask, the nonrebreathing mask has exhalation ports on either side of the mask that allow exhaled gas to escape and to provide a mechanism for the patient to entrain air should the oxygen source fail. However, depending on the manufacturer, circular flaps are used to cover the exhalation ports and to minimize the amount of air entrained by the patient. These flaps allow the nonrebreathing mask to be capable of delivering higher (>60%) concentrations of oxygen.[24]

Indications, Contraindications, and Hazards

A nonrebreathing mask is used when a child requires the delivery of higher concentrations, >60%, of oxygen.[24] Similar to the other reservoir masks discussed in this chapter, this delivery device is commonly used for short-term therapy. FiO_2 delivery is variable and dependent upon the child's minute ventilation. Hypo- and/or hyperventilation can change oxygen concentration delivery, although alterations in oxygen concentrations are much less than that of a partial rebreathing mask because of the flaps or valves. The depth and rate of respirations should be observed, with strict attention to changes, because changes in minute ventilation will influence oxygen concentration delivery. The mask may be connected to an oxygen blender to facilitate oxygen concentration titration. This type of mask may also be used to deliver helium and oxygen gas mixtures.[24]

As with the simple and partial rebreathing masks, the nonrebreathing mask limits the child's ability to communicate, move, and feed. Also, because a snug fit is required for the mask to properly deliver oxygen, care should be taken to ensure that the mask fits properly and is not too tight. Skin integrity must also be maintained, and alternative methods of oxygen delivery should be used if there is any evidence of skin irritation or breakdown.

The flap(s) covering the exhalation ports increase the risk for CO_2 accumulation in the event of a gas failure. The risk is minimized when only one flap is used to cover the exhalation port. For masks manufactured with two flaps, removing one of the flaps by gently pulling the flap away from the mask and discarding it in an appropriate receptacle can also minimize this risk.

Device Application

Similar to the application of a partial rebreathing mask, the mask is held gently against the patient's face and the adjustable elastic straps are secured around the patient's head, just above the ears, to hold the mask snugly against the patient's face. While adjusting the elastic band, take care to avoid folding or causing discomfort to the cartilage of the ears.

The flow of oxygen to the mask varies and can range from 6 to 15 L/minute and must be sufficient to keep the reservoir bag inflated to at least one-half of its capacity during inspiration. Because a child may be anxious when the mask is first applied, it is important to assess the child for several minutes to ensure that there is enough flow to prevent the bag from completely deflating or from deflating to more than one-half of the device's capacity during inspiration (**Figure 23-9**).

Assessing the child's oxygen requirement is often accomplished noninvasively by trending SpO_2. Because the flow to this device cannot be weaned, it is often attached to a blender to adjust the concentration of oxygen delivered to the child. Discontinuation of this device and initiation of a fixed performance device, such as an air-entrainment mask or heated high-flow nasal cannula, is also an option when FiO_2 titration is required.

Fixed Performance Oxygen Delivery Devices

Fixed performance devices deliver a precise concentration of oxygen at a flow rate that meets or exceeds the patient's inspiratory demands. Air-entrainment masks, air-entrainment nebulizers, and heated high-flow nasal cannulas are examples of fixed performance oxygen delivery devices.

Air-Entrainment Masks

An **air-entrainment mask** provides a range of low to moderate concentrations of oxygen through the use of jet port mixing of gas from the oxygen source and air entrained from the atmosphere. The total flow of gas delivered to the patient meets or exceeds the patient's

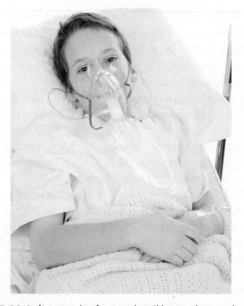

FIGURE 23-9 An example of a nonrebreathing mask properly positioned on a child.
© lisafx/iStock/Getty Images Plus.

inspiratory demands, allowing for precise FiO$_2$ delivery. An adaptor connects to the mask with a small segment of corrugated tubing. The adaptor has a jet port, which connects to the oxygen source by small-bore tubing. The flow of gas through the jet port and the size of the entrainment ports determine the amount of air entrained from the atmosphere. The ratio of oxygen delivered through the jet port and air entrained from the atmosphere determines the FiO$_2$ delivered through this device (**Figure 23-10**). The smaller the air-entrainment port, the less ambient air is entrained and a higher FiO$_2$ delivery occurs. The adaptor will specify the flow of oxygen required from the oxygen source. **Figure 23-11** illustrates two types of air-entrainment masks, one in which oxygen concentration can be changed by physically changing the adaptor, and the other by rotating the adaptor, which changes the size of the air-entrainment port.

Indications, Contraindications, and Hazards

Air-entrainment masks are indicated for children requiring precise delivery of low to moderate

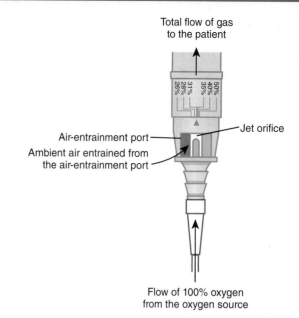

FIGURE 23-10 An illustration of the components of the adaptor used to provide precise oxygen concentrations for an air-entrainment mask.

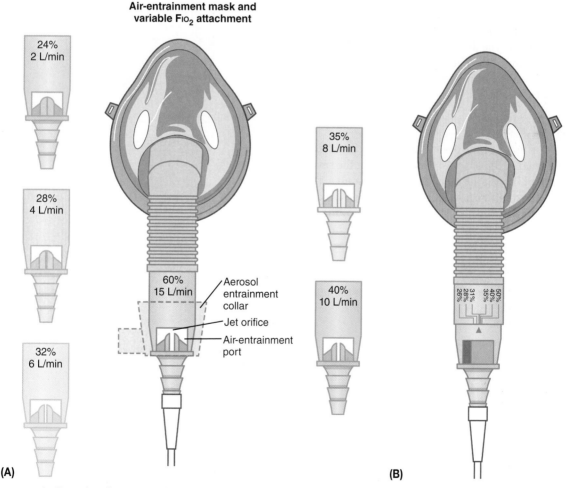

FIGURE 23-11 An illustration of two types of air-entrainment masks. (**A**) Oxygen concentration can be changed by physically changing the adaptor that attaches to the small segment of corrugated tubing. (**B**) Oxygen concentration is adjusted by rotating the adaptor, which changes the size of the air-entrainment ports.

concentrations of oxygen. Unlike the simple mask, the concentration of oxygen provided by an air-entrainment mask is known and can be varied, depending on the manufacturer, by either changing the FiO_2 selection on the adaptor or changing the adaptor. An air-entrainment mask allows for oxygen titration without the need to change to a different type of oxygen delivery device.

Similar to the variable performance reservoir masks, this device can be confining, can muffle speech and often interferes with the child's ability to communicate, and makes feeding difficult. The mask should be carefully secured snugly against the face. When it is difficult to obtain proper fit without compromising skin integrity, even for very short-term therapy, a different delivery device capable of providing fixed oxygen concentrations, such as a high-flow nasal cannula, should be considered.

Inadvertent occlusion of the air-entrainment ports can alter the oxygen concentration delivered to the child. Bed linens, such as blankets and sheets, can block the flow of ambient air through the air-entrainment ports. Depending on the patient's inspiratory flow demands, a higher FiO_2 will be delivered if the total flow delivered to the patient still meets or exceeds the patient's inspiratory demands. There are instances when the air-entrainment ports are completely occluded by bed linens or other supplies used in the care of the patient (sterile drapes, dressings, etc.). In these cases, FiO_2 delivery will be lower because the occluded air-entrainment ports prevent delivery of the expected total flow to the patient.

Device Application

Select the adaptor or the desired setting that matches the FiO_2 specified in the provider order. Connect the small-bore tubing from the adaptor to the oxygen source. It is important to set the flow of oxygen from the source to the amount specified on the adaptor. The flowmeter setting from the oxygen source will vary and, depending on the manufacturer, can be as low as 4 L/minute for an FiO_2 of 0.24 to as high as 12 to 15 L/minute for an FiO_2 of 0.50. Once gas is flowing through the device, gently hold the mask against the patient's face, place the adjustable elastic straps around the patient's head, just above the ears, to hold the mask snugly against the patient's face, and secure the mask in place by adjusting the elastic band on the periphery of the mask. While adjusting this elastic band, care should be taken to avoid folding or causing discomfort to the cartilage of the ears. The mask should fit snugly against the face.

Noninvasive monitoring of the child's oxygen requirement can be accomplished by assessing SpO_2. Oxygen can be titrated by changing the FiO_2 selection on the adaptor or by changing the adaptor, as shown in Figure 23-11.

Air-Entrainment Nebulizer

An **air-entrainment nebulizer** or large-volume nebulizer provides a precise oxygen concentration, using the principle of air entrainment described for air-entrainment masks, while delivering aerosol particulate to the child. The nebulizer directly connects to the oxygen flowmeter, and gas from the oxygen source flows through a jet nozzle surrounded by an air-entrainment port. The concentration of oxygen delivered to the patient depends on the flow of gas set on the flowmeter and by rotating the adaptor, which adjusts the size of the entrainment port (**Figure 23-12**). The air-entrainment nebulizer's reservoir is typically filled with sterile water.

Indications, Contraindications, and Hazards

Air-entrainment nebulizers are used with children requiring the delivery of high humidity or aerosol particulate. Postoperatively, an air-entrainment nebulizer

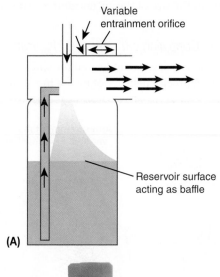

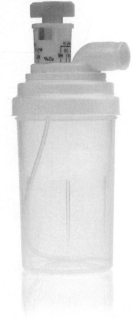

FIGURE 23-12 (**A**) An illustration of the principles of operation for an air-entrainment nebulizer. (**B**) A photo of an air-entrainment nebulizer.

(**A**) Modified from Cohen N, Fink J. Humidity and aerosols. In: Eubanks DH, Bone RC, eds. *Principles and Applications of Cardiorespiratory Care Equipment.* St. Louis, MO: Mosby; 1994.; (**B**) Image courtesy of Teleflex Incorporated. ©2018 Teleflex Incorporated. All rights reserved.

may be used to deliver cool aerosol particulate to an irritated or swollen upper airway after extubation or following a surgical procedure, such as a tonsillectomy. An air-entrainment nebulizer may also be used to deliver humidified supplemental oxygen to children whose upper airway is bypassed because of the presence of an artificial airway, such as a tracheostomy tube.

When a face mask is used to provide oxygen therapy, the mask can be confining and may cause the child to be anxious and irritable. Infants and young children may pull and tug at the mask, making it difficult for the mask to remain snuggly in place.

Because this device produces aerosol particulate, the potential exists for microbial contamination. Excessive condensation in the large-bore corrugated tubing that connects the nebulizer to the mask causes resistance to the flow of gas through the tubing and can alter the FiO_2 delivered to the patient in much the same way that obstructing the entrainment ports on an air-entrainment mask alters FiO_2 delivery. A water trap or water bag is helpful in capturing the condensate and in minimizing the potential for tubing occlusion. It is essential for the clinician to observe the water level in the nebulizer's reservoir and to ensure that the water does not fall below the minimum levels, as providing dry gas at high flows can dry airway secretions and cause mucosal irritation.

At FiO_2s of 0.50 or greater, the use of two air-entrainment nebulizers connected in parallel may be considered if the total flow from one nebulizer is not sufficient to meet the inspiratory demands of the patient. This is typically of concern with older children with larger tidal volumes and higher minute ventilation.

Device Application

A variety of interfaces can be connected to an air-entrainment nebulizer, including a face mask, face tent, and tracheostomy mask (**Table 23-5**). Generally, large-bore corrugated tubing connects the interface to the nebulizer. A water trap or drainage bag may be used to collect condensate, which minimizes the propensity for inadvertent lavage when the tubing is repositioned and prevents alterations in FiO_2 delivery. Care should be taken to secure the drainage bag or water trap to avoid tugging or tension on the interface, which can dislodge the device or cause pressure points on the face.

A heater can be used in conjunction with an air-entrainment nebulizer to provide warmed aerosol particulate for children with an artificial airway. When a heater is used in tandem with this device, the temperature of the delivered gas mixture must be monitored to minimize the chance for overheating the gas or providing humidified gas that is not sufficiently heated.

Heated High-Flow Nasal Cannula

A **heated high-flow nasal cannula (HHFNC)** provides a flow of heated, humidified gas through nasal prongs at flow rates that meet and/or exceed the patient's inspiratory demand. Currently, there is no single definition of what constitutes "high flow." The literature is conflicting for infants, with some studies reporting high flow as gas flow rates of greater than or equal to 2 L/minute[24,25] and others reporting flow rates of greater than 2 L/kg/minute.[26] Flow rates greater than 6 L/minute are generally considered high flow in children.[25] The gas is heated to at or near body temperature (34–37°C), allowing gas to be delivered at 100% relative humidity. This reduces the sensation of nasal dryness, which may enhance comfort and improve adherence to therapy.

Several studies report the positive effects of HHFNC use. The use of a HHFNC is reported to reduce work of breathing,[27,28] improve lung compliance,[29] enhance mucociliary clearance,[30] and increase functional residual capacity (FRC) by providing a continuous positive airway pressure (CPAP) effect.[31] The CPAP effect is unpredictable and difficult to quantify because it is determined by a combination of factors, including the nare-to-prong ratio, flow delivered to the patient, and whether the mouth is open or closed.

Compared to low-flow oxygen devices and reservoir masks, studies have demonstrated that the HHFNC was more effective in removing end-expiratory oxygen-depleted gas from anatomic dead space and subsequently provided better oxygen delivery.[32] In children, the extrathoracic dead space is proportionally two to three times greater than that of adults.[33] It is not until after age 6 years that this volume decreases to the volume seen in adults, or approximately 0.8 mL/kg.[33]

There are several commercially available HHFNC delivery systems. **Figure 23-13** provides examples of systems approved for use in children. Compared to a standard nasal cannula, the reservoir area preceding the prongs and connector tubing are larger in diameter to minimize resistance to the higher flows delivered through the device. The cannulas are available in a variety of sizes, and recommendations for nare-to-prong ratio mirror those for a standard nasal cannula.

Indications, Contraindications, and Hazards

An HHFNC can be used to treat hypoxemia and mild to moderate respiratory distress associated with a variety of conditions, including neonatal respiratory distress syndrome,[34] apnea of prematurity,[35] congenital heart defects,[36] obstructive sleep apnea,[37] bronchiolitis,[38] and asthma.[39] Therapy can be initiated in a variety of settings, including the general care unit, during interhospital transport, in the emergency department, and in intensive care settings. Commercially available systems are easy to use and require minimal technical skill to set up and apply.

Although there is a growing body of literature reporting the use of HHFNCs in the treatment of children with respiratory distress and hypoxemia, a dearth of high-quality evidence, in terms of randomized controlled trials, exists to support its use. The inability to directly measure and monitor distending pressures is a

TABLE 23-5
Interfaces Used to Deliver Oxygen Therapy by Air-Entrainment Nebulizer to Children

Interface	Illustration
Aerosol face mask	© Yongcharoen_kittiyaporn/Shutterstock.
Aerosol face tent	
Tracheostomy mask	Courtesy of Lacey Rugg.

clinical concern because of the risk of trauma secondary to the delivery of excessive pressures to the infant's or child's airway. There are systems that incorporate a pressure relief valve to stop flow when a predetermined pressure in the circuit is reached. However, the effect on oxygenation has not been well studied to determine the clinical consequences when flow is limited or stopped when the pressure relief is activated. Additionally, most commercially available systems require electricity to power the device. Although batteries are available to operate the devices during inter- and/or intrahospital transport, the batteries are heavy and may make the system cumbersome to navigate.

Device Application

The circuit and assembly required depend on the manufacturer or brand of device used. Regardless of the system used, the circuit and component parts are

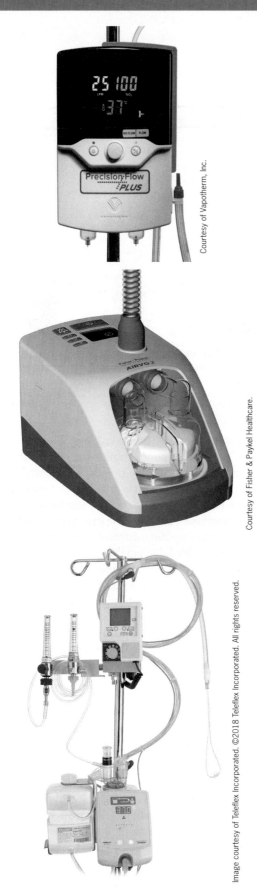

FIGURE 23-13 Examples of commercially available systems designed to deliver medical gas therapy through a heated high-flow nasal cannula.

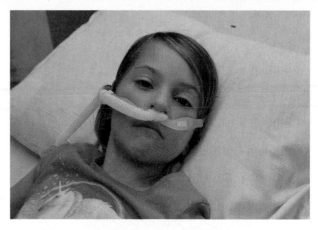

FIGURE 23-14 An HHFNC properly positioned on a child.

single-patient use and disposable. Cannulas are available in a variety of sizes, ranging from preterm to adult. As previously mentioned, the prong-to-nare ratio mirrors that for a standard nasal cannula and should not exceed 50%.[17] **Figure 23-14** shows a properly applied HHFNC.

Enclosure Devices

Enclosure devices deliver oxygen therapy in a device that envelops all or a part of the patient's body. Enclosure devices used to provide supplemental oxygen to neonates and infants include oxygen hoods and incubators.

Oxygen Hoods

Oxygen hoods are enclosure devices that encompass the infant's head and neck, typically to the shoulder area (**Figure 23-15**). An oxygen blender is used to provide the ordered or specified FiO_2 ranging from 0.21 to 1.0, which can be connected directly to the hood or to a circuit capable of providing heat and humidity. An oxygen analyzer is typically used to verify the oxygen concentration delivered to the infant.

Indications, Contraindications, and Hazards

Oxygen hoods are indicated for the delivery of low to high concentrations of oxygen to preterm and term infants. This delivery device is typically well tolerated and allows for care of the torso and upper and lower extremities without interruption of therapy. There is no increased risk of airway obstruction or gastric distention with this method of oxygen delivery.[40] The oxygen concentration contained within the device depends on the flow rate of oxygen to the hood and on the hood's size, shape, and volume.[41] For the smallest sizes, a minimum flow of 4 L/minute is required to clear the infant's exhaled CO_2 from the device and to provide a constant flow of fresh blended gas to fill the enclosure.[41] To avoid excessive noise from the delivery of gas at high flows to a small enclosure and cooling of the baby, flows greater than 10 L/minute should not be used.[40] There is a risk of

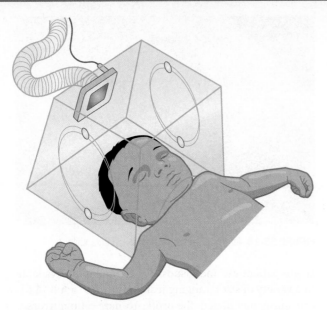

FIGURE 23-15 A schematic of an oxygen hood used to deliver oxygen therapy to an infant.

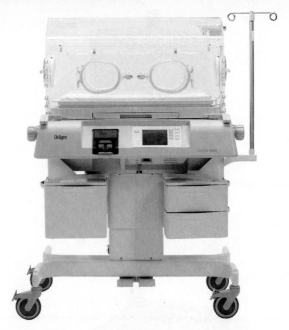

FIGURE 23-16 An incubator is used to provide low concentrations of oxygen in a temperature- and humidity-controlled environment.

CO_2 retention and hypoxemia if the tubing connecting the hood to the heated humidifier and oxygen source is disconnected.[42]

Feeding; oral care; airway care (i.e., nasopharyngeal suctioning); and assessment of the head, face, and neck are difficult to accomplish without disrupting the therapy. In these instances, the oxygen hood is partially lifted, or removed, reducing the FiO_2 delivered to the infant. Additionally, this oxygen delivery device does not allow the parents to provide kangaroo care and requires the use of an alternate delivery device, such as a nasal cannula, to provide this care.

Device Application

These plastic enclosures are commercially available as disposable or nondisposable products in a variety of sizes. The flow used to deliver blended oxygen to the patient ranges from 4 to 10 L/minute. This form of oxygen delivery also provides heated humidification. An oxygen analyzer should be used to verify the delivered oxygen concentrations. The temperature in the hood should be monitored and maintained within the infant's neutral thermal environment to minimize the propensity for exposing the infant to overheating and/or cold stress.[43]

Incubator

An **incubator** is a Plexiglas enclosure device that encompasses the infant's entire body and is capable of delivering a range of low concentrations of oxygen in a temperature- and humidity-controlled environment (**Figure 23-16**).[44]

Indications, Contraindications, and Hazards

Although an incubator is primarily used to provide a temperature- and humidity-controlled environment

for preterm infants, it offers a viable method for delivering low (<35%) concentrations of oxygen.[45] The temperature within the isolette is regulated by a servo-controlled mechanism attached to a small sensor affixed to the infant's skin. Care can be provided through portholes, allowing the caregiver's hands and arms to extend into the incubator to provide routine nursing care. Adjustable porthole covers are often used to reduce the size of the portholes to minimize variations in temperature and oxygen concentration. Specially designed shields can be attached to this enclosure to minimize transmission of noise levels from monitors and alarms common to the intensive care unit.[46]

Kangaroo care cannot be accomplished in an incubator and requires the use of an alternate delivery device, such as a nasal cannula, to provide this type of care. Variations in the concentration of oxygen, humidity level, and temperature can occur when the incubator door is opened, which increases the risk of cold stress and hypoxemia.[44]

Device Application

Supplemental oxygen therapy is provided by connecting small-bore oxygen tubing to a flowmeter. Some manufacturers incorporate the use of solenoid valves to regulate the flow of oxygen. Because the flow of oxygen needed to deliver a specific FiO_2 is manufacturer specific, clinicians should consult with and adhere to the manufacturer recommendations specific to the device in use. An oxygen analyzer can be used to verify and monitor the FiO_2 contained within the incubator.

Case Study 1

A previously healthy 7-month-old female presents to the emergency department with fever, congestion, and cough. She has had poor fluid intake for 48 hours. At daycare, a few children were absent due to a viral infection. Symptoms were getting worse, and over the past 8 hours she had no fluid intake. The past medical history showed nothing significant, and she had received an influenza vaccine. A physical exam assessed as follows: heart rate 130 beats per minute, respiratory rate 60 breaths per minute, blood pressure 90/50 mm Hg, temperature 38.5°C, and an oxygen saturation of 87% on room air. She had copious clear rhinorrhea and a loose cough. Lungs had mild wheezing. She had intercostal retractions and nasal flaring but no abdominal breathing. The remainder of her physical examination was normal. The diagnosis of likely respiratory syncytial virus (RSV) and hypoxia was made. She was placed on oxygen at 2 L/minute by nasal cannula, and her saturations increased to 95%. She was admitted to the hospital for oxygen therapy and supportive care. The laboratory evaluation confirmed RSV. Over the next 24 hours, her oxygen requirement and work of breathing increased. Heated high-flow nasal cannula therapy was initiated at 10 L/minute at an FiO_2 of 0.50 to maintain oxygen saturations >94%. Her condition stabilized, and within 48 hours the oxygen and flow were slow and oral rehydration commenced.

1. **What important clinical indication for oxygen therapy was present in this scenario?**

2. **Initially, was the nasal cannula the most appropriate choice of oxygen delivery device for this patient, or would you recommend a different one?**

3. **What physiologic mechanism was causing hypoxemia for this child?**

Case Study 2

A 13-year-old previously healthy boy was hit in the chest while playing baseball with friends and developed acute chest pain and dyspnea. Shortly after the injury, he had a brief syncopal episode. He was driven to the emergency department by his parents and taken immediately to the trauma room. Oxygen by nonrebreathing mask was administered per their trauma protocol and a full assessment was completed. A physical exam shows the boy in respiratory distress with mild petechiae isolated to his chest. Vital signs were as follows: heart rate 136 beats per minute, respiratory rate 40 breaths per minute, blood pressure 90/50 mm Hg, temperature 37.4°C, and oxygen saturation of 94% on nonrebreathing mask. The boy has been in good health and is physically active. He has a medical history of seasonal allergies and an acute episode of pharyngitis. There is no family history of cardiac diseases. Cardiac examination revealed normal heart sounds and no murmur. He has normal radial pulses with delayed capillary refill. Breath sounds are coarse bilaterally. The remainder of the physical examination findings were normal. The boy is later admitted to the hospital for suspected cardiac contusion.

1. **How would you evaluate the oxygenation status of this patient given the information presented in this case?**

2. **Could you recommend another oxygen delivery device given his presentation?**

3. **What are some hazards associated with the use of a nonrebreathing mask?**

References

1. Leach RM, Treacher DF. Oxygen transport-2. Tissue hypoxia. *BMJ.* 1998;317(7169):1370-1373.
2. American Association for Respiratory Care. Clinical practice guideline: oxygen therapy for adults in the acute care facility: 2002 revision and update. *Respir Care.* 2002;47(6):717-720.
3. Singh V, Gupta P, Khatana S, Bhagol A. Supplemental oxygen therapy: important considerations in oral and maxillofacial surgery. *Natl J Maxillofac Surg.* 2011;2(1):10-14.
4. Cherian S, Morris I, Evans J, Kotecha S. Oxygen therapy in preterm infants. *Paediatr Respir Rev.* 2014;15(2):135-141.
5. Usen S, Weber M. Clinical signs of hypoxaemia in children with acute lower respiratory infection: indicators of oxygen therapy. *Int J Tuberc Lung Dis.* 2001;5(6):505-510.
6. Bateman NT, Leach RM. ABC of oxygen. Acute oxygen therapy. *BMJ.* 1998;317(7161):798-801.
7. Atkins DL, de Caen AR, Berger S, et al. 2017 American Heart Association focused update on pediatric basic life support and cardiopulmonary resuscitation quality: an update to the American

Heart Association guidelines for cardiopulmonary resuscitation and emergency cardiovascular care. *Circulation*. 2018;137(1):e1-e36.

8. Jindal SK, Aggarwal AN. Oxygen therapy. In: Chawla R, Todi S, eds. *ICU Protocols: A Stepwise Approach*. New York: Springer Science & Business Media; 2012:107-112.

9. Zhang L, Mendoza-Sassi R, Santos JC, Lau J. Accuracy of symptoms and signs in predicting hypoxaemia among young children with acute respiratory infection: a meta-analysis. *Int J Tuberc Lung Dis*. 2011;15(3):317-325.

10. Hay WW Jr, Rodden DJ, Collins SM, Melara DL, Hale KA, Fashaw LM. Reliability of conventional and new pulse oximetry in neonatal patients. *J Perinatol*. 2002;22(5):360-366.

11. SUPPORT Study Group of the Eunice Kennedy Shriver NICHD Neonatal Research Network, Carlo WA, Finer NN, et al. Target ranges of oxygen saturation in extremely preterm infants. *N Engl J Med*. 2010;362(21):1959-1969.

12. Supplemental Therapeutic Oxygen for Prethreshold Retinopathy Of Prematurity (STOP-ROP), a randomized, controlled trial. I: primary outcomes. *Pediatrics*. 2000;105(2):295-310.

13. Lashkari K, Hirose T, Yazdany J, McMeel JW, Kazlauskas A, Rahimi N. Vascular endothelial growth factor and hepatocyte growth factor levels are differentially elevated in patients with advanced retinopathy of prematurity. *Am J Pathol*. 2000;156(4):1337-1344.

14. American Academy of Pediatrics Policy Statement. Screening examination of premature infants for retinopathy of prematurity. *Pediatrics*. 2013;131:189-195.

15. Pease P. Oxygen administration: is practice based on evidence? *Paediatr Nurs*. 2006;18(8):14-18.

16. Wettstein R, Shelledy D, Peters J. Delivered oxygen concentrations using low-flow and high-flow nasal cannulas. *Respir Care*. 2005;50(5):604-609.

17. Volsko TA, Fedor K, Amadei J, Chatburn RL. High flow through a nasal cannula and CPAP effect in a simulated infant model. *Respir Care*. 2011;56(12):1893-1900.

18. Benaron DA, Benitz WE. Maximizing the stability of oxygen delivered via nasal cannula. *Arch Pediatr Adolesc Med*. 1994;148:294-300.

19. Miller MJ, Martin RJ, Carlo WA, Fouke JM, Strohl KP, Fanaroff AA. Oral breathing in newborn infants. *J Pediatr*. 1985;107(3):465-469.

20. Finer NN, Bates R, Tomat P. Low flow oxygen delivery via nasal cannula to neonates. *Pediatr Pulmonol*. 1996;21(1):48-51.

21. Walsh M, Engle W, Laptook A, et al. Oxygen delivery through nasal cannulae to preterm infants: can practice be improved? *Pediatrics*. 2005;16(4):857-861.

22. Uygur P, Oktem S, Boran P, Tutar E, Tokuc G. Low- versus high-flow oxygen delivery systems in children with lower respiratory infection. *Pediatr Int*. 2016;58(1):49-52.

23. French W, Lewarski J. Administrating medical gases. In: *Equipment for Respiratory Care*. Burlington, MA: Jones & Bartlett Learning; 2016:31-54.

24. Lee JH, Rehder KJ, Williford L, Cheifetz IM, Turner DA. Use of high flow nasal cannula in critically ill infants, children, and adults: a critical review of the literature. *Intensive Care Med*. 2013;39(2):247-257.

25. Dysart K, Miller TL, Wolfson MR, Shaffer TH. Research in high flow therapy: mechanisms of action. *Respir Med*. 2009;103(10):1400-1405.

26. ten Brink F, Duke T, Evans J. High-flow nasal prong oxygen therapy or nasopharyngeal continuous positive airway pressure for children with moderate-to-severe respiratory distress? *Pediatr Crit Care Med*. 2013;14(7):e326-e331.

27. Pham TMT, O'Malley L, Mayfield S, Martin S, Schibler A. The effect of high flow nasal cannula therapy on the work of breathing in infants with bronchiolitis. *Pediatr Pulmonol*. 2015;50(7):713-720.

28. Saslow JG, Aghai ZH, Nakhla TA, et al. Work of breathing using high-flow nasal cannula in preterm infants. *J Perinatol*. 2006;26(8):476-480.

29. Milési C, Baleine J, Matecki S, et al. Is treatment with a high flow nasal cannula effective in acute viral bronchiolitis? A physiologic study. *Intensive Care Med*. 2013;39(6):1088-1094.

30. Metge P, Grimaldi C, Hassid S, et al. Comparison of a high-flow humidified nasal cannula to nasal continuous positive airway pressure in children with acute bronchiolitis: experience in a pediatric intensive care unit. *Eur J Pediatr*. 2014;173(7):953-958.

31. Kubicka ZJ, Limauro J, Darnall RA. Heated, humidified high-flow nasal cannula therapy: yet another way to deliver continuous positive airway pressure? *Pediatrics*. 2008;121(1):82-88.

32. Roca O, Riera J, Torres F, Masclans JR. High-flow oxygen therapy in acute respiratory failure. *Respir Care*. 2010;55(4):408-413.

33. Numa AH, Newth CJ. Anatomic dead space in infants and children. *J Appl Physiol*. 1996;80(5):1485-1489.

34. Kugelman A, Riskin A, Said W, Shoris I, Mor F, Bader D. A randomized pilot study comparing heated humidified high-flow nasal cannulae with NIPPV for RDS. *Pediatr Pulmonol*. 2015;50(6):576-583.

35. Sreenan C, Lemke RP, Hudson-Mason A, Osiovich H. High-flow nasal cannulae in the management of apnea of prematurity: a comparison with conventional nasal continuous positive airway pressure. *Pediatrics*. 2001;107(5):1081-1083.

36. Testa G, Iodice F, Ricci Z, et al. Comparative evaluation of high-flow nasal cannula and conventional oxygen therapy in paediatric cardiac surgical patients: a randomized controlled trial. *Interact Cardiovasc Thorac Surg*. 2014;19(3):456-461.

37. Tapia IE, Marcus CL. Newer treatment modalities for pediatric obstructive sleep apnea. *Paediatr Respir Rev*. 2013;14(3):199-203.

38. Bressan S, Balzani M, Krauss B, Pettenazzo A, Zanconato S, Baraldi E. High-flow nasal cannula oxygen for bronchiolitis in a pediatric ward: a pilot study. *Eur J Pediatr*. 2013;172(12):1649-1656.

39. Mayfield S, Jauncey-Cooke J, Bogossian F. A case series of paediatric high flow nasal cannula therapy. *Aust Crit Care*. 2013;26(4):189-192.

40. Frey B, Shann F. Oxygen administration in infants. *Arch Dis Child Fetal Neonatal Ed*. 2003;88(2):F84-F88.

41. Jain S, Johri A. Study of factors determining the oxygen concentration in the head box. *Indian Pediatr*. 1984;21(2):159-166.

42. Jatana SK, Dhingra S, Nair M, Gupta G. Controlled FiO$_2$ therapy to neonates by oxygenhood in the absence of oxygen analyzer. *Med J Armed Forces India*. 2007;63(2):149-153.

43. Pollock TR, Franklin C. Use of evidence-based practice in the neonatal intensive care unit. *Crit Care Nurs Clin North Am*. 2004;16(2):243-248.

44. St Clair N, Touch SM, Greenspan JS. Supplemental oxygen delivery to the nonventilated neonate. *Neonatal Netw*. 2001;20(6):39-46.

45. White J. Isolette. *Am J Nurs*. 2017;117(4):33.

46. Altuncu E, Akman I, Kulekci S, Akdas F, Bilgen H, Ozek E. Noise levels in neonatal intensive care unit and use of sound absorbing panel in the isolette. *Int J Pediatr Otorhinolaryngol*. 2009;73(7):951-953.

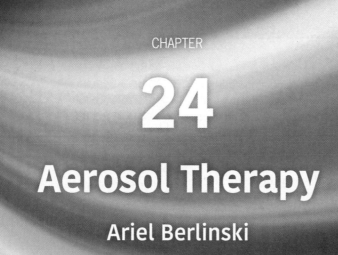

CHAPTER

24
Aerosol Therapy

Ariel Berlinski

© Anna Rubak/Shutterstock, Inc.

OUTLINE

OBJECTIVES

1. Describe mechanisms of lung deposition and the effects of aerosol and patient-related characteristics on lung deposition.

2. Compare and contrast the use of various aerosol devices with infants and children.
3. Differentiate between spacers and valved holding chambers.
4. Discuss the factors involved in selection of a device for aerosol delivery.
5. Explain the essential components included in patient and caregiver education for aerosol therapy.
6. Discuss the pertinent issues during aerosol delivery during noninvasive and invasive ventilation.

KEY TERMS

aerosol
breath-actuated nebulizers
breath-enhanced nebulizers
Brownian diffusion
continuous output
  jet nebulizers
dry powder inhalers (DPIs)
geometric standard
  deviation (GSD)
jet nebulizers
large-volume nebulizers
mass median aerodynamic
  diameter (MMAD)

nebulizers
pressurized metered dose
  inhalers (pMDIs)
residence time
residual volume (RV)
respirable fraction
smart nebulizers
soft mist inhalers
spacers
ultrasonic nebulizers
valved holding
  chamber (VHC)
vibrating mesh nebulizers

Introduction

Aerosol therapy is administered to infants and children to treat a variety of respiratory conditions. The inhaled route is usually preferred to treat respiratory conditions because it allows for the delivery of high concentrations of medication topically to the affected area(s). This allows inhaled medications to start working faster and requires lower drug doses to achieve the desired effect, decreasing the risk for side effects.[1]

Pediatric patients have unique anatomic, physiologic and behavioral characteristics that impact aerosol delivery efficiency. This chapter will focus on practical issues related to the administration of inhaled therapy to infants and children.

Aerosol Medicine: A Review of Basic Concepts

An **aerosol** is defined as a suspension of liquid or solid particles in a carrier gas. Aerosols could be generated by a variety of devices, which include nebulizers, pressurized metered dose inhalers (pMDIs), soft mist inhalers, and dry powder inhalers (DPIs).[2] Aerosols are generally characterized by a central tendency and a dispersion measurement as well as by the **respirable fraction** (proportion of particles <5 μm). The **mass median aerodynamic diameter (MMAD)** represents the particle diameter at which half of the mass of the particles in an aerosol are smaller than the MMAD and the other half of the particles are larger. The dispersion measurement is the **geometric standard deviation (GSD)**, or a measure of how spread the size of the particles are around the MMAD.[1] Although the respirable fraction is considered the fraction of the aerosol that this is highly likely to deposit in the lungs, it is not clear that this is true for pediatric patients. Some authors have suggested that the use of aerosols with smaller particle size will result in higher intrapulmonary deposition.[3] It is not clear, however, what the ideal size is for aerosols delivered through artificial airways. Most medical aerosols are composed of particles of different sizes, with MMADs of 3 to 6 μm, and are also heterodysperse (GSD <1.22).[1]

Factors Influencing Aerosol Deposition in Infants and Children

Factors affecting lung deposition can be divided into two categories: aerosol-related factors and patient-related factors, which are highlighted in **Table 24-1**.[4]

An understanding of the mechanisms of aerosol deposition will enable clinicians to select the most appropriate delivery device and to optimize inhalation technique. There are three main mechanisms of aerosol deposition: inertial impaction, gravitational sedimentation, and Brownian diffusion.[5]

TABLE 24-1
Factors Determining Aerosol Deposition

Aerosol Factors	Patient Factors
Particle size	Inspiratory flow rate
Velocity	Age
Hygroscopic properties	Breathing pattern (i.e., tidal volume, rate)
Drug viscosity and surface tension	Nasal vs. mouth breathing
Solution vs. suspension	Upper airway anatomy
	Disease severity
	Physical and cognitive abilities
	Adherence, contrivance

Data from Geller D, Berlinski A. Aerosol delivery of medication. In: Light MJ, Homnick DN, Schechter MS, Blaisdell CJ, Weinberger MM, eds. *Pediatric Pulmonology*. Elk Grove Village, IL: American Academy of Pediatrics; 2011.

There are a variety of factors that influence how long aerosol particles remain suspended and include particle size, density, and forward velocity. Inertial impaction is the main mechanism responsible for deposition of aerosols, with an MMAD between 3 μm and 5 μm. This occurs mainly in the upper and large airways as a result of sudden changes in the direction of the flow of the aerosol. Inertial impaction is also responsible for deposition of smaller particles at branch points in the airway when high inspiratory flows are used. Inhalation technique is important to aerosol deposition. The technique depends on the type of device generating the medicated aerosol. When a respiratory therapist is administering a medicated aerosol to a child by a jet nebulizer or pMDI, a slower inhalation will enhance intrapulmonary deposition of the medicated aerosol that is administered to the patient. This inhalation technique does not apply when a DPI is used, as a slow inhalation would not be sufficient to de-aggregate the dry powder medication from the device. Higher inspiratory flows are required to trigger medication release when a medicated aerosol is delivered by a DPI.[1] When reviewing an order for medicated aerosol therapy, it is important for the respiratory therapist to consider the child's ability to cooperate and perform the breathing technique necessary to enhance drug delivery.

Particles with an MMAD between 0.5 μm and 3 μm are mainly deposited by gravitational sedimentation, or they are deposited because gravity causes the aerosol particles to settle out of suspension. Gravitational forces will cause very large particles to settle out of suspension much earlier than smaller particles. Sedimentation rate affects the quantity of particles that are delivered to the lungs. Breathing pattern also plays an important role, as it affects the **residence time**, or how long aerosol particles remain in the lung, in particular the last six generations of the airways. A breath-holding maneuver increases the residence time. Therefore, a breath hold should be used when possible to increase intrapulmonary deposition, especially when medication is administered by pMDIs and DPIs.

Finally, particles smaller than 0.5 μm are deposited at the alveolar level by random motion, also known as **Brownian diffusion**. Very small aerosols, or those less than 0.1 μm, are likely to remain in suspension and are not deposited in the lungs. Rather, these aerosol particles are exhaled. Aerosols containing hygroscopic substances, such as sodium, experience growth as they travel through the airways.[6]

Age-Related Factors Affecting Aerosol Lung Dose

There are anatomic differences in infants and small children that affect aerosol delivery.[7,8] Compared to adults, the larynx of infants is situated much higher, and the epiglottis is closer to the palate. The pharynx and supraglottic tissues are less rigid in infants and more prone to inspiratory collapse. In children, the tongue is relatively larger and occupies a greater proportion of the oral airway compared to adults. Additionally, infants are preferred nose breathers until the age of 18 months; the nose is an excellent filter, and it decreases aerosol lung deposition by 50% when compared to aerosol particles inhaled through the mouth.[9]

The depth and rate with which children breathe also differ from adults and affect aerosol deposition. Infants and children breathe at much faster rates and have lower inspiratory flows, shorter inspiratory times, and lower tidal volumes than adults.[10] Infants and small children often cry during therapy, which causes a 4- to 10-fold reduction in intrapulmonary drug deposition.[11,12]

Device-Related Considerations

The type and fit of the interface used to deliver the medicated aerosol is another important factor to consider. Because infants and small children are unable to properly use a mouthpiece, a face mask is typically the interface of choice. A face mask that does not snuggly fit on the child's face results in a significant decrease in lung deposition.[13] Mask selection is crucial because masks made of a harder plastic material will not easily conform to the infant's or child's face. This may impair aerosol deposition by allowing aerosol particles to escape from the gaps or leaks between the face and mask. Masks made of harder plastic material also are uncomfortable to wear and may cause discomfort to the child during therapy.

The art of delivering aerosols to infants and young children is a learned skill that requires patience and family engagement. How a child breathes during aerosol therapy is also important. During administration of medicated aerosols by pMDI or nebulizer, slow inhalation maneuvers enhance pulmonary deposition of aerosols.[14] However, in small children, it may be difficult to teach them how to properly breathe in order to enhance aerosol deposition. This will inherently impact the efficiency with which aerosol particles are delivered to the airways and result in lower intrapulmonary deposition for particles with a larger MMAD.[15] Disease status also determines the amount and site of inhaled drug deposition because of the effects of the disease state on the airway.[16] For example, children with an acute exacerbation of asthma have constricted, inflamed airways that may reduce the efficiency of aerosol particle deposition.

Other Considerations

Our knowledge of aerosol drug delivery has been gathered through human, animal, and in vitro studies. There are concerns for radiation exposure and the need for repeated blood extractions, which have limited the number of human studies that are available. As a result, a vast amount of knowledge has been generated using in vitro models. Initially, these models were very simple. Technologic advances, such as the development of three-dimensional printing, enabled the construction of anatomically correct models derived from CT/MRI data.[8] These models have greater in vivo/in vitro correlation than their simple predecessors and allow scientists to test different delivery devices and interfaces under normal pulmonary characteristics and different disease states. This body of research provides practitioners with important information regarding aerosol delivery efficiency for specific devices, which determines the absolute amount of drug that reaches the desired place in the lung. Cost is also a factor that is often considered when selecting the medication and delivery device used. The costs of the drug delivered to the airway, as well as the cost of the aerosol delivery device and respiratory therapist's time to administer the medication, are the key factors used to define cost effectiveness.

Aerosol Devices

There are many different types of delivery devices available to nebulize medications for delivery to the respiratory track. Devices have different operational characteristics, and it is important for the respiratory therapist to understand how these devices work to best match the delivery device to the patient in need of medicated aerosol therapy.

Nebulizers

Nebulizers are devices that convert a solution/suspension in an inhalable mist. There are three main types of nebulizers: jet, ultrasonic, and vibrating mesh nebulizers.

Jet Nebulizers

Jet nebulizers use a gas source to convert a solution/suspension in a mist. The gas is forced through a very small orifice, resulting in a decrease in pressure at the sides of the high-velocity jet stream (Bernoulli effect). Solutions/suspensions present in the nebulizer cup are drawn up the capillaries and aerosolized. The mist impacts one or more baffles, resulting in further reduction of the particle size. Some of the drug impacts the walls of the nebulizer cup, and so tapping the nebulizer cup helps recirculate and re-aerosolize the liquid. **Table 24-2** outlines the advantages and disadvantages of the use of nebulizers with infants and children.[4]

There are different types of gas sources that can be used to power a nebulizer: room air, oxygen, and helium–oxygen gas mixtures also known as heliox. In settings outside of an acute care hospital, such as home care, long-term care, physician offices, and clinics, an air compressor is often used to power a nebulizer. Air compressors generate a wet gas while medical gases generate a dry gas. The pressure and flow delivered by an air compressor differs from that delivered by high-pressure gas systems (i.e., piped gas or high-pressure tanks).

Piped in gas, or central air and oxygen, are pressurized at 50 pounds per square inch (psi); a flowmeter reduces that working gas pressure and allows the clinician to adjust the flow of gas powering the nebulizer. Typically, gas flows of 6 to 10 L/minute are used to power a jet nebulizer, depending on brand/model specifications. It is important for the respiratory therapist to follow the specific manufacturer recommendations for use.[17] Conversely, in general, compressors generate gas at lower pressures (15–30 psi) and lower flows (3–9 L/min).[18,19] When the patient's inspiratory flow exceeds the driving flow of the nebulizer, the aerosol gets diluted with entrained air.[20]

Flow and pressure generated by the compressors decay over time, especially if the device is used to deliver inhaled medications several times per day.[19] As compressors age and begin to fail, the time it takes to nebulize medication increases. It is important for clinicians to ask patients and families about the duration of their nebulized therapy because an increase in nebulization time may represent a compressor failure. Higher gas flows result in faster nebulization times and smaller particle size.[21]

The use of heliox as a gas source to power the nebulizer results in smaller particle size and lower drug delivery than the use of oxygen at similar flows.[22] An increase in the heliox gas flow improves drug delivery.[23] Practitioners need to remember that if they use an oxygen-calibrated flowmeter to deliver heliox, the flow delivered to the patient will differ. When an oxygen-calibrated flowmeter is used to deliver oxygen–helium gas mixtures, conversion factors of 1.6 and 1.8 need to be applied for the 70:30 and 80:20 admixtures, respectively. Total flow calculations are found in **Table 24-3**.

Jet nebulizers are the most commonly used nebulizers. There are three main types of jet nebulizers: continuous output, breath-enhanced, and breath-actuated jet nebulizers.

Continuous output jet nebulizers have constant output of aerosol irrespective of the timing of the respiratory cycle.[24] **Figure 24-1** provides an example of a commercially available jet nebulizer used to deliver medicated aerosol therapy to a child. The design of nebulizers that continuously nebulize and deliver medication leads to significant waste of the aerosolized medication. The use of a mouthpiece and the addition of a 15-cm extension tube distal to the patient acts as a reservoir for aerosol particles and enhances drug delivery when a continuous nebulizer is used.[25] The length of therapy varies, but jet nebulizers are generally run until sputtering occurs, which is the point in which drug output drastically decreases.

Breath-enhanced nebulizers incorporate a one-way valve into their design that allows an increase of the airflow in the chamber during inspiration, leading to an increase in aerosol output.[24] Aerosol output still

TABLE 24-2
Advantages and Disadvantages of Nebulizers

Advantages	Disadvantages
Easy technique (tidal breathing)	Bulky, less-portable than pMDIs or DPIs
Can use at any age	Longer treatment times
Can use with any disease severity	Require cleaning and disinfection
Can use with artificial airways	Noisy (may disturb infants)
Can use with mechanical ventilation	Require power source
High doses possible (e.g., antibiotics)	High variability between brands

Data from Geller D, Berlinski A. Aerosol delivery of medication. In: Light MJ, Homnick DN, Schechter MS, Blaisdell CJ, Weinberger MM, eds. *Pediatric Pulmonology*. Elk Grove Village, IL: American Academy of Pediatrics; 2011.

TABLE 24-3
Calculating Total Flow to the Patient When Delivering Helium-Oxygen Gas Mixtures with an Oxygen-Calibrated Flowmeter

Gas Mixture	Conversion Factor	Formula
70:30 (70% helium: 30% oxygen)	1.6	1.6 × gas flow set on the oxygen-calibrated flowmeter
80:20 (80% helium: 20% oxygen)	1.8	1.8 × gas flow set on the oxygen-calibrated flowmeter

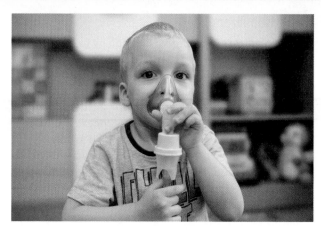

FIGURE 24-1 An example of a commercially available jet nebulizer used to deliver medicated aerosol therapy to a child.

© Piotr Adamowicz/Shutterstock.

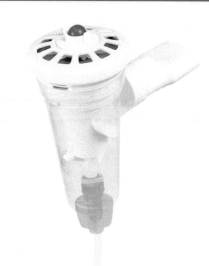

FIGURE 24-3 A breath-actuated nebulizer, the Monaghan AeroEclipse II.

Courtesy of Monaghan Medical Corporation.

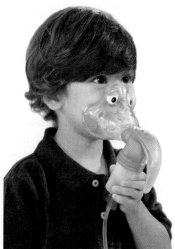

FIGURE 24-2 A breath-enhanced nebulizer, the PARI LC Sprint. The nebulizer may be used with a mouthpiece or a specially designed mask.

PARI LC® Sprint and Bubbles The Fish™ are trademarks of PARI GmbH and its affiliates. Used with permission.

occurs during expiration, and so some models have incorporated an expiratory valve into the mouthpiece while others offer a Y-shaped connector that allows the addition of an exhalation filter (**Figure 24-2**).

Finally, **breath-actuated nebulizers** use a one-way valve to deliver aerosol only during inspiration.[25] There are two different designs to this type of nebulizer. One design modifies a continuous output jet nebulizer by adding a one-way valve proximal to the patient and a reservoir bag distal to the patient that is filled with aerosol during exhalation.[26] The other design incorporates a spring-loaded valve that allows aerosol production only during inhalation.[26] Both of the designs result in zero waste to the environment. **Figure 24-3** provides an example of a breath-actuated nebulizer. It is important for providers who prescribe this type of device and for respiratory therapists who administer medication through this type of device to verify that the patient is able to generate an inspiratory flow of 15 L/minute, which is

needed to trigger the valve. Because the inspiratory flow of children is reduced during an exacerbation of their pulmonary condition, it is important for clinicians to evaluate a child's ability to trigger the valve both when their disease state is stable and during an exacerbation. The trade-offs associated with the use of breath-enhanced nebulizers are an increase in the nebulization time and the need to either adjust the dose or the nebulization time to avoid overdosing the patient.

Residual volume (RV) is the amount of drug left in the nebulizer cup after the nebulization process is complete.[21] The residual volume can vary from 0.5 to 2.2 mL. Prescribing a decrease in the loading volume, or the volume of drug that is instilled in the nebulizer cup, could result in significantly underdosing the patient because the residual volume remains constant.[27] In the absence of a lower-dose preparation, prescribing a shorter nebulization time while maintaining the loading dose could deliver a lower amount of medication to the infant or child. Another option includes reducing the amount of active solution/suspension but maintaining the same total volume by adding normal saline. This is especially important when using nebulizers with large residual volume, as increasing the fill volume also increases nebulization time.[21]

Ultrasonic Nebulizers

Ultrasonic nebulizers use a piezoelectric crystal that creates acoustic vibrations that cause the liquid or medication immediately above the transducer to disrupt air–liquid interface and form droplets.[24] The higher the vibration frequency, the smaller the particle size generated by the nebulizer. The nebulization process is generally noiseless and produces an aerosol particle size larger than those produced by jet nebulizers.

Also, the suspension/aerosol solution heats up over time and could lead to the denaturalization of proteins. These factors limit the type of medication that can be delivered by this device—for example, this technology is inefficient and should not be used to deliver budesonide.[28] The limitations of this device, as well as the development of less expensive vibrating mesh devices, make the ultrasonic nebulizer a less attractive option for drug delivery.

Vibrating Mesh Nebulizer

Vibrating mesh nebulizers are the newest addition to the nebulizer family. The liquid is forced through a membrane with laser-drilled holes. A piezoelectric crystal vibrates either a plate (active mesh), generating an upward/downward movement of the plate, or a horn (passive mesh), which generates an upward/downward movement of the liquid.[6,29] The diameter and shape of the holes, as well the characteristics of the medication (viscosity and surface tension), determine the aerosol particle size. These devices are quiet, efficient, and have a low residual volume. They are, however, relatively expensive. Although there are some devices that can be used with a variety of medications, also known as open source devices, many have been customized to match the characteristics of a specific medication. Devices customized to match the characteristics of a certain medication have been approved as a drug–device combination, such as Cayston® (Gilead, Foster City, CA). Cayston is an aerosolized antibiotic, commonly used in the treatment of patients with cystic fibrosis. **Figure 24-4** provides an illustration of the vibrating mesh device used to deliver Cayston®.

Adequate care of the mesh is essential for proper function. A poorly cleaned device will cause the orifices to clog, which decreases efficiency and increases nebulization time. Touching the mesh during cleaning will damage the unit. Patients should be asked about the length of therapy of their treatments during their clinic visits. Practitioners need to be aware of the high efficiency of these devices and adjust the dose of any drug that has dose-related side effects or a narrow therapeutic index.

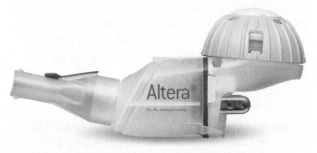

FIGURE 24-4 The proprietary vibrating membrane nebulizer used to deliver Cayston, or aerosolized aztreonam, an antibiotic used in the treatment of cystic fibrosis. Refer to the product's full prescribing information for details.
Altera® Nebulizer System is a trademark of PARI GmbH and its affiliates. Used with permission.

Smart Nebulizers

Smart nebulizers incorporate technology to allow control of drug delivery, and they also allow recording of adherence to therapy. This type of nebulizer is more precise because it interacts with the patient's breathing pattern. Smart nebulizers are ideal for the delivery of expensive drugs with low therapeutic index. The Akita Jet (Vectura Group PLC, Chippenham, UK) is an example of a nebulizer that uses either a breath-enhanced or a vibrating mesh nebulizer coupled to a system that releases aerosol at a controlled flow (12 L/min) during inspiration.[30] The system also allows a distal and a proximal airway delivery mode by releasing the aerosol at the beginning or the middle of the inspiratory cycle. Although more accurate and more efficient than other nebulizers, it is bulky and expensive. A portable version has been recently approved (Breelib, Vectura Group PLC, Chippenham, UK) and is commercialized in Europe to deliver inhaled iloprost, which is used in the treatment of pulmonary artery hypertension. The I-Neb AAD system is a portable, battery-operated passive vibrating mesh nebulizer that interacts with the patient and can be used for inhaling in either a tidal breathing mode or a targeted inhalation mode.[31] The targeted inhalation mode involves the use of a flow restrictor and tactile feedback to coach the patient to inhale slowly and deeply. This process changes the patient's inspiration–expiration ratio and results in significantly higher lung deposition compared to when the tidal breathing mode is used. The device continuously monitors inspiratory time during three consecutive breaths and then delivers the drug during the first half of the predicted duration of inhalation. The I-Neb AAD system is commercialized in the United States for the delivery of inhaled iloprost.

Large-Volume Nebulizers

Large-volume nebulizers are continuous output nebulizers typically used for continuous aerosol delivery of bronchodilators. Commonly, this type of nebulizer is used for the treatment of status asthmaticus. Research has suggested a favorable cost–benefit ratio when large-volume, rather than small-volume, nebulizers are used.[32] In the emergency department, the use of this type of nebulizer decreases the respiratory therapist's contact time with the patient, therefore increasing productivity.

In general, the reservoir can hold 200 to 240 mL of solution and could run for 8 hours.[33] The nebulizer is connected to the central oxygen supply through a Christmas tree or nipple adapter. The solution output varies and is dependent upon the make and model used. Drug output is determined by the amount of albuterol placed in the reservoir and the airflow used to aerosolize the solution. Some models allow the concomitant use of heliox. In vitro studies demonstrated that solution and drug output are not reliable after 5 hours of operation, suggesting that the solution needs to be changed if longer operation times are required.[33] Frequent determination of the volume remaining in the nebulizer is recommended during continuous nebulization.

Patient Interfaces

Drug delivery through mouthpieces or face masks has been shown to be clinically equivalent.[34,35] A mask is preferred for patients who, due to their age or cognitive impairment, are unable to properly use a mouthpiece. To use a mouthpiece correctly, the patient should be able to place it behind their teeth and seal their lips around it.

When a face mask is used, the seal around the face is important and plays a key role in optimizing drug delivery. Facemask seal is influenced or affected by the material used to build the mask: Rigid masks are less likely to achieve a good seal and are more likely to upset the child. The space between the face and mask, also known as dead space, does not seem to affect drug delivery during nebulization.[36] Face masks have holes that allow air entrainment when the inspiratory flow exceeds the nebulizer flow. The occlusion of these holes does not improve drug delivery and has the potential to result in CO_2 rebreathing.[36] When a mask does not fit properly, especially along the bridge of the nose, leak of aerosols results in facial and ocular deposition.[37–40] Mask design plays a role not only in ocular exposure but also in the delivery efficiency, especially whether the aerosol stream reaches the oronasal area as a straight stream from the nebulizer (front-loaded) or if a bottom-loaded mask is used. Moving a bottom-loaded mask away from the face results in a larger decrease in the amount of drug available for inhalation compared to a front-loaded one. Some authors reported the use of a hood to deliver aerosol therapy.[41] Although drug deposition is similar to traditional masks, this interface exposes the skin and eyes to the drug being nebulized. Newer interfaces have a hole to thread a pacifier and a funnel placed at the top to allow alignment with the nostrils (**Figure 24-5**).[42,43] The aerosol is inhaled through the nares, and the mask is kept in place by the suckling of the pacifier. Some children do not cooperate well with their prescribed aerosol therapy. As a result, rather than using a mouthpiece or face mask, some clinicians choose to use a blow-by technique.

The blow-by technique consists of directing the aerosol stream to the patient's face by either using a front-loaded mask placed away from the face or by capping the t-piece connector on one end and placing a 15-cm extension tube on the other. This technique is not recommended because it results in decreased intrapulmonary deposition and increased ocular and facial drug deposition.

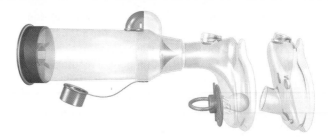

FIGURE 24-5 An interface used to deliver medicated aerosol to toddlers. This interface has a hole to thread a pacifier, which allows delivery of the mask to be held in place as the child sucks on the pacifier.
Courtesy of InspiRx.

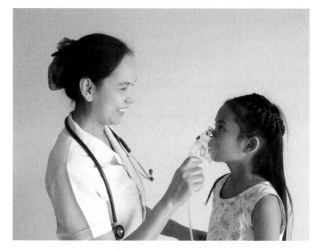

FIGURE 24-6 Proper technique for aerosol therapy. The child is sitting upright on the edge of the bed. The mask fits snuggly on the face, covering the nose and mouth but not the eyes. The respiratory therapist provides support and coaching to the patient as therapy is administered.
© ChooChin/Shutterstock.

Technique for Aerosol Delivery by Nebulizer

When a nebulizer is used to deliver medicated aerosol therapy, lower inspiratory flows (<12 L/min) are associated with increased lung delivery.[44] Because there are a variety of different types of nebulizers available for use, the clinician needs to be aware of how the different types of nebulizers operate and to ensure that the child can use the delivery device. For example, if a breath-actuated device is prescribed for a child, the therapist should verify that the child can develop enough flow to open the inspiratory valve. Similarly, a patient will not benefit from the increased drug if they are not able to open the inspiratory valve on a breath-enhanced nebulizer. Aerosol therapy should be administered with the child in a high Fowler position if in bed or in a sitting position when possible (**Figure 24-6**). The use of a sitting or high Fowler position leads to higher intrapulmonary deposition compared to aerosol delivery when a child is supine.

The clinician also needs to be aware of the acute side effects of the inhaled medication(s) that are administered. Cough and bronchoconstriction are common side effects associated with the administration of hyperosmolar solutions and antibiotics while tachycardia and tremor may occur with the administration of beta 2 agonists.

Cleaning, Disinfecting, and Assembling the Nebulizer

Cleaning and disinfecting nebulizers is crucial to avoid device malfunction and microbial contamination. The Cystic Fibrosis Foundation published rigorous infection control guidelines that specifically address the different disinfection techniques that have proven to be effective to kill *Pseudomonas aeruginosa* and are recommended for the respiratory care equipment.[45] The use of vinegar solutions is no longer recommended for nebulizer disinfection due to its poor killing power, especially with regard to *P. aeruginosa*. It is important to follow manufacturer recommendations for cleaning devices, especially those with nondisposable components.

Patient and family education is a very important part of patient care. For effective use of aerosol devices at home, patients and families need comprehensive training. Education should include the following: (1) how to assemble and operate the device, (2) which device is used or paired with a particular nebulizer, (3) the position to sit in and breathing technique used during aerosol administration, (4) recognizing side effects, (5) how to clean and disinfect the device, and (6) when to suspect malfunctioning. Teach-back is often used to validate the patient's and/or caregivers' retention of the education and training they receive. Teach-back provides the patient and/or caregiver with the ability to demonstrate their skills to the clinical team. Education on each of the previously mentioned points, as well as teach-back, can be incorporated into daily practice. Each time a respiratory therapist administers a medicated aerosol therapy, they provide a teachable moment for the patient and the caregivers. Prior to discharge, the patient and/or caregivers should be able to verbalize an understanding of how and when to use the medication and to recognize side effects. The patient and/or caregivers should also demonstrate proper assembly, use, and cleaning and disinfection of the prescribed device.

Metered Dose Inhalers

Metered dose inhalers deliver a precise dose of medication stores under pressure. These devices can be pressurized and contain propellants, or mechanical energy, to generate the aerosol and deliver the medication. Depending on the design, coordination between device actuation and the child's breathing pattern is required.

Pressurized metered dose inhalers (pMDIs) are inhalation devices that consist of a canister, containing a drug, propellants, and excipients stored under pressure, and a plastic actuator.[6,24] The metering valve is a key component of this device, and its precise matching to the actuator is responsible for the consistency of drug delivery with each actuation. The dose loaded in the metering chamber gets replenished after the release of the previous dose. The aerosol is released from the pMDI at a high speed, but if a distance is applied between the pMDI and the patient's mouth, the aerosol slows down and decreases in size due to evaporation. Chlorofluorocarbons (CFCs) were once widely used as propellants in pMDIs. Because of their detrimental effect on the ozone layer, CFCs have been replaced in pMDI propellants by hydrofluoroalkane (HFA).[46] Older inhalers (using CFCs) were colder than HFA inhalers and were responsible for the Freon effect, which interrupted the patient's inspiratory maneuver because the temperature of the aerosol was so low.[47] Commonly used medications administered to infants and children by pMDI include short-acting bronchodilators, anticholinergics, corticosteroids, and corticosteroid/long-acting bronchodilator combinations. The dose of these drugs, delivered by the pMDI, is in the µg range. The drugs are formulated as either solutions or suspensions. Therefore, before use, it is important to shake the canister to mix the medication and propellant. When the canister is not adequately shaken or there is a delay between shaking and actuation, the amount of drug delivered with the actuation will differ from the prescribed formulation of the suspension.[48,49] A delay between actuation and inhalation when using a pMDI with a valved holding chamber results in a decrease in delivered drug for both suspensions and solutions.[50,51] Shaking the canister has a more profound effect than the time intervals between canister actuations. Aerosol characteristics of albuterol delivered by pMDI remained unchanged when the interval between puffs, or canister actuations, changed from 60 seconds to either 30 or 15 seconds, provided the inhaler was shaken right before each actuation.[50] Corticosteroids formulated as solutions have a smaller MMAD (1.2 µm) than those formulated as suspensions, which results in low oropharyngeal and high intrapulmonary deposition.[51] A breath-hold maneuver after a full inhalation of medication administered by a pMDI increases intrapulmonary deposition of the aerosol.[51]

Many inhalers contain alcohol as their excipient and can transiently increase the breath alcohol exhalation test.[52] Studies done with inhalers containing CFC as a propellant demonstrated multiple actuations of the pMDI without re-shaking in between, and delays between actuation and inhalation impaired drug delivery.[53] It is crucial that the pMDI is operated in an upright position and is shaken right before actuation.

Although most of the new formulations have an incorporated dose counter, there are some that still do not. It is challenging for patients and caregivers to keep track of the doses administered and to recognize when the inhaler is empty. For inhalers containing 120 doses of a scheduled medication, used for 4 or 2 puffs per day, patients and families can be taught to discard the canister after 30 or 60 days, respectively. However, this cannot be done with medications that are taken on an as-needed basis, such as short-acting bronchodilators. In this case, the respiratory therapist should provide a chart to allow the patient to document their use of the pMDI. The practice of submerging the canister in water to know whether it was empty or not should not be used. This technique is not only inaccurate but also causes the metering valve to become blocked.[54] Whether a dose counter is used or not, the respiratory therapist has to advise the patient to discard the inhaler once the calculated or measured remaining doses reach zero.

HFA pMDIs have to be primed after opening and after certain circumstances. Care of the inhalers is required to avoid obstruction of the nozzle of the actuator. Unfortunately, each pMDI has different priming and care specifications. Respiratory therapists should be aware of manufacturer-specific instructions for priming and include priming in the education provided to patients and caregivers on pMDI use. Table 24-4 outlines the advantages and disadvantages of the use of pMDIs with infants and children.[4]

Soft Mist Inhalers

More recently, **soft mist inhalers** have been developed (Respimat, Boeringher Ingelheim, Ridgefield, CT). This device is propellant-free and uses the mechanical energy generated by a tensioned spring to generate the aerosol.[55] This aerosol delivery to the patient is slower and the mist lasts longer than the one generated by a pMDI HFA;

TABLE 24-4
Advantages and Disadvantages of Metered Dose Inhalers

Advantages	Disadvantages
Compact, portable	Difficult technique to learn/teach
Rapid delivery	Coordination for actuation and inhalation
Multidose convenience	High oropharyngeal dose (not with valved holding chamber)
Easy to clean	Dissatisfaction with hydrofluoroalkane propellant
Acceptable for any age (when used with a valved holding chamber)	Intolerance of tight face mask (young children)
Dose counters are now more common	Limited number of drugs available

Data from Geller D, Berlinski A. Aerosol delivery of medication. In: Light MJ, Homnick DN, Schechter MS, Blaisdell CJ, Weinberger MM, eds. *Pediatric Pulmonology*. Elk Grove Village, IL: American Academy of Pediatrics; 2011.

therefore, it is recommended to be used without a spacer or valved holding chamber.[56] Compared to a pMDI, the soft mist inhaler has lower upper airway deposition because the medication is delivered at a slower velocity.[57] The aerosol produced by this type of device lasts 1.5 seconds. When the dose release button is pressed, medication contained within the device's cartridge is released. After pressing the dose release button, the child should be instructed to seal their lips around the mouthpiece and to inhale slowly to total lung capacity. The mouthpiece has two lateral openings that need to remain patent during the inhalation maneuver. Inhalation technique is important because a shorter inhalation maneuver will result in decreased intrapulmonary deposition. A drawback of these devices is that they have to be discarded after 90 days of using the first dose. This device is commercially available in the United States to deliver different medications, including tiotropium bromide, ipratropium bromide/albuterol, tiotropium bromide/olodaterol, and olodaterol. Tiotropium bromide has been recently approved for maintenance asthma therapy for patients 12 years or older and is also indicated for adults with chronic obstructive pulmonary disease. The latter three formulations are indicated for chronic obstructive pulmonary disease and do not have a pediatric indication. The respiratory therapist should instruct the patient on how to assemble the device and when priming is required. Similar to nebulizers, when a mask is used to deliver medication with a soft mist inhaler, mask dead space does not affect aerosol drug delivery.

Valved Holding Chambers and Spacers

The two most common errors seen during inhalation therapy are lack of coordination between actuating the device and inhaling the medication and inhaling too fast. Improper technique results in poor disease control.[58] Manufacturers have addressed actuation-inhalation coordination in two different ways. Breath-actuated pMDI devices minimize coordination problems. This type of pMDI was very popular among adolescents and young adults. Unfortunately, breath-actuated pMDI devices are no longer made in the United States. Their use in the pediatric population had some limitations; the two most common problems were that patients needed to generate enough flow to trigger the valve and the stopping of the inhalation maneuver after getting startled by the noise produced by the device.

The use of an add-on device, specifically a **valved holding chamber (VHC)**, can minimize coordination problems between actuation and inhalation and facilitate medication delivery in children.[59] A VHC is a tubelike structure that incorporates low-resistance inspiratory and expiratory valves. The inspiratory valve helps to improve the coordination between actuation and inhalation while the expiratory valve allows the expiratory flow to be diverted out of the system without having to break the seal between the interface and the patient and without mixing with aerosol present in the chamber. The chamber also provides distance between the pMDI and the patient's mouth. **Spacers** are valveless tubes that provide distance between the pMDI and the patient's mouth. Currently, there is a pMDI with a corticosteroid solution that has a spacer incorporated into the design. Both VHCs and spacers allow deceleration of the aerosol and impaction of the large particles against their walls. This results in a decrease in oropharyngeal deposition, thus minimizing side effects, such as thrush when a corticosteroid is administered, or tremor with the administration of a beta 2 agonist.[60] Homemade spacers are used in developing countries with good success.[61]

VHCs are manufactured in a variety of different shapes and volumes. The most commonly used in the United States are of cylindrical shape and are small in volume, approximately 150 mL. Also, some VHCs require the pMDI canister to be removed from the plastic actuator, as the VHC has an actuator that the pMDI canister will seat against. The pMDIs with a dose counter placed around the stem valve require special adapters when used with a VHC. Other brands of VHCs require the canister and plastic actuator to be inserted in the distal portion of the VHC. The use of VHCs that do not require removal of the canister are preferred because an imperfect match of the stem and the actuator could affect drug output.[62]

The material used to build the spacer/VHC can significantly affect drug delivery. Most devices are made of plastic, and some of them can accumulate electrostatic charge in their internal walls.[63] This results in attraction of the aerosol particles to the walls, thus decreasing drug delivery. Different strategies have been used to overcome this problem. The electrostatic effect has been mitigated by coating the inner walls with an ionic detergent before its first use and periodically thereafter.[63] This can be easily achieved by washing the spacer/VHC with water and an ionic detergent and letting the VHC air dry. Some manufacturers have changed the material from plastic to metal, such as the Vortex (PARI Inc Midlothian, VA).[64] Although efficient, they have the disadvantage that the patient/caregiver cannot see the interior of the device and the aerosol going through it. More recently, many manufacturers have changed the plastic material to one that is nonelectrostatic.[65] Spacers and VHCs need to be cleaned weekly to minimize the risk of infection.[66]

Many VHCs incorporate a whistle that blows when the inspiratory flow exceeds 30 L/minute. Although the intention of the whistle is to coach the patient to take a slower inspiration, some children are amused that they can generate the whistle and continue to perform the technique incorrectly, thus defeating the intent to provide feedback.

Patient Interfaces for pMDIs

Similar to what occurs with nebulizers, pMDIs with spacers or VHCs could be used with either a mask

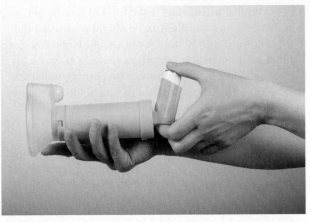

FIGURE 24-7 A VHC with a mask can be used to administer a pMDI to a small child.
© Laboko/Shutterstock.

or a mouthpiece. A mask is used when the infant or child cannot seal their lips around the mouthpiece (**Figure 24-7**). Unlike nebulizers and soft mist inhalers, the mask's dead space volume does matter and inversely affects drug delivery (i.e., larger mask, less drug delivery).[67] Some commercially available masks have a dead space that is larger than the tidal volume of a 6- to 12-month-old infant.[68] Moreover, some masks are rigid, making them unfit for pediatric use. More recently, a mask with a low dead space that allows a pacifier to be threaded through it and provides nasal delivery was introduced to the market.[69] This design takes advantage of the fact that infants and young children are obligate nose breathers; therefore, its effectiveness in older populations remains to be proven. The mask should fit snuggly against the infant's or child's face. Mask fit is also crucial because leaks produce a decrease in inhalation flow that impairs the patient's ability to open the inspiratory valve. Minor leaks have been associated with a decrease in drug delivery.[70] The use of the mask also could result in unwanted facial and ocular deposition.

Inhalation Technique for pMDIs

Many healthcare professionals have not mastered the technique for operating aerosol delivery devices.[71] Although the literature reports that respiratory therapists perform these techniques better than other professions, when administering medicated aerosols, there is always the opportunity to continue to improve.[72] Improper inhaler technique has been linked to poor clinical outcomes.[56]

Lack of patient cooperation makes aerosol delivery with pMDI and a VHC more challenging when administering medication to infants and children. Infants often cry when the mask is applied and may continue crying during medication administration. The literature reports a 10-fold decrease in lung deposition when radiolabeled albuterol was administered by pMDI to crying infants.[73] Administration of a pMDI with a VHC to sleeping toddlers resulted in their awakening and increased respiratory distress in most of the participants.[74] This resulted in a lower inhaled dose and a higher dose variability.[74] However, the use of a soft mist inhaler with a VHC with sleeping children did not awaken them or cause undue distress and resulted in acceptable lung deposition of the radiolabeled aerosol.[75]

Similar to the technique used for aerosol administration by nebulizer, the patient should be sitting upright, either in a chair, on the edge of the bed, or supported in a high Fowler position (Figure 24-6).

There are two different techniques that can be used when administering a pMDI to an infant or child. The first uses tidal breathing and the other uses a single slow inhalation. A breath-hold maneuver should be attempted when using a single slow inhalation technique. Spacers should be used only if the child can coordinate actuation with the start of inhalation and use a single breath inhalation technique. One study reported that 80% of 5-year-old children were able to perform the single inhalation maneuver.[76] The tidal breathing maneuver can be used with either a mask or a mouthpiece. This technique is often used to help children transition from a mask with tidal breathing technique to a mouthpiece with a single breath inhalation. Patients should be switched from face mask **(Figure 24-8)** to mouthpiece once they are able to seal their lips around the mouthpiece. This would improve aerosol delivery and minimize side effects.[35,67] The number of breaths that the patient needs to inhale during tidal breathing depends on their tidal volume and the chamber's volume. Fewer breaths than previously thought might be required to empty the VHC.[76,77] Patients are required as able to swish and spit after the administration of inhaled corticosteroids to minimize local side effects.

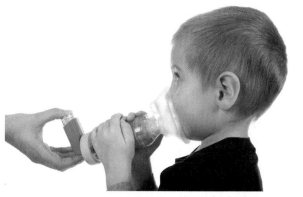

FIGURE 24-8 Administration of a pMDI to a child requires the child to be awake and sitting upright.
© LSOphoto/iStock/Getty Images.

Respiratory therapists need to provide comprehensive education to patients and caregivers that includes the following: (1) how to assemble the device, (2) how and when to prime, (3) proper inhalation technique, (4) how and when to clean and disinfect the device, and (5) how to track or determine the number of doses remaining in the device. Ideally, those skills should be reviewed prior to discharge from the hospital or emergency department and at every physician visit.

Dry Powder Inhalers

Dry powder inhalers (DPIs) allow drug delivery to the lungs without the need of a suspending medium,[2] which results in the delivery of larger drug amounts compared to pMDIs. Although the initial devices included a single-dose capsule, newer devices incorporate multidose functionality either in individually packed blister strips and disks or in a common reservoir.[6,78] Dose counters are incorporated into the design of the DPI. Some, such as the Diskus and Twisthaler, change with every dose, and others change every 10 doses. These devices are mainly used in pediatrics for the treatment of asthma to administer corticosteroids and corticosteroid/long-acting bronchodilator combinations and in cystic fibrosis to administer tobramycin. The drug is generally blended with an excipient carrier (lactose) or prepared as a macro-aggregate.[79] Newer technology (spray drying) has allowed the development of DPI formulations that do not require a carrier. The energy required to disaggregate the powder is directly related to the patient's inspiratory flow and the internal resistance of the device. For a given device, a higher inhalation flow results in smaller particle size. Devices with high resistance typically deliver more intrapulmonary dose.[78,79] All currently available devices are passive and require the patient to actuate the device by inhalation. It is important to note that a threshold inspiratory flow has to be met to actuate the device. Most devices show a positive relationship between inspiratory flow and lung deposition.[80] Newer drug formulations, such as tobramycin (TOBI Podhaler), do not benefit from inhaling at flow higher than the threshold.[81] Some pediatric patients might not be able to achieve the minimum required flow for a specific device.[82] Most DPI devices require a minimum peak inspiratory flow of 30 to 40 L/minute to actuate the device and to receive a dose of the prescribed medication. The child's lips must remain tightly sealed during inspiration, and they must be taught to achieve the peak inspiratory flow closer to the beginning of inhalation.

Patients must also load the dose of the DPI before inhalation.[78] This process involves piercing of the capsule or blister, twisting the base of the device (Flexhaler), or pressing a lever (Diskus). The Twisthaler loads the dose when the cap is untwisted, and the cap locks when all doses have been delivered. Several critical mistakes can occur during drug delivery with DPIs. Such errors as

TABLE 24-5
Advantages and Disadvantages of Dry Powder Inhalers

Advantages	Disadvantages
Compact, portable	Need strong inspiratory effort
Rapid delivery time	High oropharyngeal impaction
Breath actuated	Vulnerable to humidity
Dose counters in multidose devices	Limited to children >5 years
Easier to learn than pressurized metered dose inhalers	Multiple dry powder inhaler device types
No need for a valved holding chamber or spacer	Technique confusion with other devices

Data from Geller D, Berlinski A. Aerosol delivery of medication. In: Light MJ, Homnick DN, Schechter MS, Blaisdell CJ, Weinberger MM, eds. *Pediatric Pulmonology.* Elk Grove Village, IL: American Academy of Pediatrics; 2011.

tilting the device once loaded, not loading the device in an upright position, blowing inside the device before inhalation, and not generating enough inspiratory flow all reduce drug delivery to the patient. Increased humidity results in formation of large aggregates, so DPIs need to be kept in dry and cool places, and patients should be taught not to exhale into the device before sealing their lips around the mouthpiece and inhaling the medication.[83] Table 24-5 outlines the advantages and disadvantages of the use of DPIs with infants and children.[4]

The respiratory therapist needs to be familiar with each individual DPI that they plan to use with their patients. A step-by-step demonstration is necessary and the use of teach-back recommended when validating the caregivers' and/or patient's ability to properly administer the medication. The use of objective measurement of peak inspiratory flow is recommended to ensure that the patient can generate adequate inspiratory flow for any given device.[84]

How to Choose the Right Device for My Patient

Several factors should be considered when choosing an aerosol delivery device for an infant or child.[1,6] Factors include drug availability, cognitive ability of the patient, patient preference and cultural beliefs, provider preference and knowledge, the medications covered by the patient's insurance plan, cost, and reimbursement. The patient and/or caregiver should be able to demonstrate proficiency in the use and care of the device. When possible, a single type of device should be prescribed to avoid confusion.

Many drugs have been approved as a drug–device combination. The package insert of the medication

provides a list of all approved devices. Some examples include Bethkis (Tobramycin)/Pari LC Plus + Pari Vios compressor; Cayston/Altera; and Pulmozyme/six different nebulizer-compressor combinations and the eRapid. Every effort should be made to use the recommended device with the medication. If an alternative is needed, practitioners need to look for devices of similar performance and should monitor the clinical course of the patient because a change in device could potentially result in under- or overdosing.

Role of the Respiratory Therapist in the Outpatient Clinic

Respiratory therapists are uniquely skilled to educate patients and caregivers about the proper use and cleaning of devices and add-on devices, and they play an important role in the outpatient clinic. The respiratory therapist should observe the patient and/or caregiver perform a hands-on demonstration of device assembly and administration of medicated aerosol therapy. Repeated reinforcement of proper technique with the patient and caregivers at each visit helps the child and caregivers remain competent with their skills. Use of printed and/or electronic information provides patients and caregivers with a valuable resource in between clinic or office visits. Younger children might need to be desensitized to a mask. Practice and demonstration with a doll might increase their acceptance.

Aerosol Administration in Patients Receiving Respiratory Support

Pediatric patients receiving inhaled therapy under special circumstances include children receiving support with high-flow nasal cannula, noninvasive ventilation (NIV), tracheostomies, and invasive mechanical ventilation. Most current data are based on in vitro studies, thus removing physiologic response and biologic variability from the equation. Also, the actual amount of drug needed at the target site is usually unknown, making the interpretation of a two- or threefold difference in output between devices difficult. Classic descriptions of aerosol characteristics do not necessarily apply to aerosols delivered through tracheostomies and endotracheal tubes (ETT) because the upper airway is bypassed. Another important consideration is that the internal diameters (IDs) of ETTs, tracheostomies, and circuits are smaller than the adult ones.

Aerosol Administration with a High-Flow Nasal Cannula

High-flow nasal cannula systems are increasingly being used in patients in respiratory distress.[85] Many of these patients also have a concomitant need for aerosol therapy. The available literature on efficacy is limited. An in vitro study reported that with a vibrating mesh nebulizer placed on the dry part of the humidifier, deposition was 2% of the nominal dose when the cannula flow was 6 L/minute O_2 and 5.4% of the nominal dose when a 80:20 heliox mixture was used.[86] Another study, using similar device placement, reported a 0.5% deposition for vibrating mesh and jet nebulizers when the cannula flow was 8 L/minute.[87] Deposition increased to 3.3% for the vibrating mesh nebulizer when the flow was decreased to 4 L/minute. The same study included full-term macaques (neonatal model) and showed a 0.49% and 0.85% lung deposition for the vibrating mesh nebulizer operated at 4 L/minute and 2 L/minute, respectively.[87] Placing the vibrating mesh nebulizer before the cannula showed inspired doses of 0.6% and 0.6% to 12% for the neonatal and pediatric models, respectively.[88] All the aforementioned studies highlight the low lung deposition when an aerosol device is used in conjunction with a high-flow nasal cannula. This low lung deposition is consistent with previous studies evaluating transnasal aerosol delivery using anatomically correct models.[89] They highlight the importance of recognizing that the nose efficiently filters out aerosol particles. Additionally, aerosol particles exiting the cannulas had an MMAD lower than 1.43 μm.[87,88]

Limited clinical data are available, and the in vitro data suggest that, at the flows patients in respiratory distress are expected to receive, lung deposition is very low (0.5–1%). Although the use of high-flow nasal cannulas is increasing, it is not clear how they should be implemented. Future studies are necessary to help answer this question.

Aerosol Administration during Noninvasive Mechanical Ventilation

The use of NIV in the pediatric population has increased.[90] Patients might receive NIV as chronic ventilator support, before intubation, or after extubation. New ventilators can deliver NIV without needing to change the existing ventilator circuit. Patients should be disconnected from the interface to receive aerosol therapy if possible.[91] A schematic of aerosol delivery NIV can be seen in **Figure 24-9** and **Figure 24-10**.[17,91] Figure 24-9 shows possible placement of the aerosol device when a dual-limb circuit is used while Figure 24-10 shows possible placement of the aerosol device when a single-limb circuit is used.

The use of pressure support increased lung deposition from 11.5% to 15.3% without changing

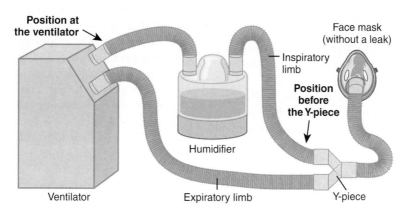

FIGURE 24-9 A schematic illustrating proper placement of an aerosol device when a dual-limb circuit is used to deliver NIV.

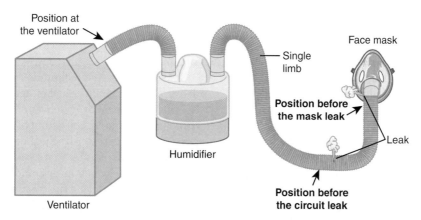

FIGURE 24-10 A schematic illustrating proper placement of an aerosol device when a single-limb circuit is used to deliver NIV.

deposition pattern.[90] These data have not been replicated. Conversely, in a study with adult patients, concomitant use of bilevel ventilation and aerosol therapy did not increase intrapulmonary deposition.[92]

Compared to a standard jet nebulizer, the literature reports that the use of vibrating mesh nebulizers increases intrapulmonary deposition. An in vitro study evaluated delivery efficiency using an anatomically correct pediatric model with a dual-limb circuit connected to the mask with an elbow without leak.[93] The authors reported that the vibrating mesh nebulizer achieved delivery efficiency of 18%, 17.6%, and 13.3% when placed before the mask, before the Y-piece, and at the ventilator, respectively.[93] The delivery efficiency of another vibrating mesh nebulizer inserted in the mask had a 10.7% delivery efficiency.[93] Delivery efficiency for the jet nebulizer was 3.8% and 3.5% when placed before the Y-piece and at the ventilator, respectively. Increasing the bilevel settings from 15/5 to 20/5 cm H_2O did not improve delivery efficiency.[93] Using a single-limb circuit, a pediatric in vitro study reported delivery efficiency of 4%, 5%, and 11% when a vibrating mesh nebulizer was placed on the dry side of the humidifier, right before the mask and the leak, and integrated into the mask after the leak, respectively.[94] Another study, also using a single-limb circuit, reported 16.6%, 4.7%, and 10% delivery efficiency when a vibrating mesh nebulizer was placed before the mask, at the ventilator, and incorporated into the mask, respectively.[95] Delivery efficiency for the jet nebulizer was 5.5% and 2.1% when placed before the mask (after the circuit leak) and at the ventilator, respectively.

In summary, during NIV with single- or double-limb circuits, the best placement for the nebulizer is before the mask. The use of a double-limb circuit improved aerosol delivery while increasing bilevel pressures did not improve delivery efficiency. The vibrating mesh was 3.5- to 5-fold more efficient than the jet nebulizer. Careful monitoring of the patient's response to therapy is necessary.

Aerosol Administration through Tracheostomy Tubes

Improvements in neonatal and pediatric critical services are responsible in part for the increase in the number of patients who undergo tracheostomy.[96] Infants and children with tracheostomies often require medicated aerosol and airway clearance therapy as a routine part of their ongoing care.[97] A survey regarding aerosol therapies in spontaneously breathing children with tracheostomies revealed that a majority, or 68%, used assisted technique with pMDI to administer aerosolized medications to the children, and 32% used it with a nebulizer.[97] The assisted technique requires the use of a resuscitation bag to provide a manually assisted breath during aerosol administration. **Figure 24-11** provides an

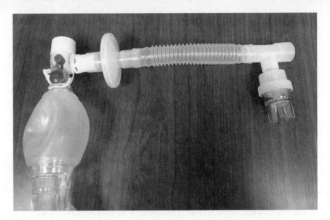

FIGURE 24-11 Example of a nebulizer setup used to provide medicated aerosol delivered by assisted technique through tracheostomies.

illustration of how a nebulizer connected to an extension tube and a bag-valve resuscitator are used to provide this technique.

Our current understanding of aerosol delivery through tracheostomies is mostly derived from in vitro studies.[97–105] A study including tracheostomized children compared different routes of administering gentamicin to the airway. Compared to aerosol delivery, instilling gentamicin directly into the airway resulted in a 24-fold higher concentration of gentamicin in the sputum and a 28-fold higher blood level of this drug.[98]

In vitro studies evaluated the effect of ID of the tracheostomy tube, breathing pattern, use of different aerosol generators, use of add-on devices, type of interface, type of formulation, and use of assisted technique on delivery through pediatric-size tracheostomies.[99–103] The size of the tracheostomy tube may affect aerosol drug delivery. A decrease in drug delivery by pMDI occurred when a tracheostomy tube was downsized, or reduced from 4.5 to 3.5 mm ID, but no change in drug delivery occurred when the ID of the tracheostomy tube changed from 5.5 to 4.5 mm.[99,100]

Nonelectrostatic VHCs are the best add-on devices to deliver pMDIs through tracheostomies.[99–101] The use of assisted technique with pMDIs and a VHC decreased drug delivery.[99,100,102] Soft mist inhalers with VHC delivered more drug than pMDIs with VHC.[101] In general, larger tidal volumes delivered more drug, but the effect decreased with tidal volumes equal to or larger than the VHC's volume.[100–102]

The use of assisted technique with aerosol therapy delivered by a nebulizer had either a neutral or a positive effect on distal drug delivery.[100,102,103] When a dual-compartment model consisting of proximal and distal parts was used, greater tracheal deposition was noted.[103] This study demonstrates that assisted techniques with aerosol therapy by nebulizer could be used to target the large airways during the treatment of bacterial tracheitis. A bacterial filter should be placed before the resuscitation bag to avoid retrograde escape of aerosol that could damage the bag. Bias flow decreased drug delivery in adult models and is expected to have the same consequences in pediatric ones.[105]

Practical aspects to enhance aerosol delivery through tracheostomies include cleaning the tracheostomy tube before the treatment, encouraging the child to take larger and slower breaths when possible, disconnecting the heated trach collar before aerosol administration, and avoiding the assisted techniques for pMDIs but considering the use of this technique for antibiotic treatment of intratracheal infections.[104]

Aerosol Administration during Invasive Mechanical Ventilation

Similar to patients receiving noninvasive ventilation, many intubated and mechanically ventilated pediatric patients receive inhaled medications. Administration of aerosol therapy inline with the ventilator circuit is preferred because it does not require the patient to be disconnected from the ventilator circuit, which decreases the risk for ventilator-associated pneumonia and also minimizes derecruitment.[106]

The position of the aerosol delivery device has been widely studied. In a study of intubated children receiving aerosol therapy, a pMDI with a spacer placed between the Y-piece and the ETT yielded equivalent results to a jet nebulizer placed on the inspiratory limb (10–20 cm before the Y-piece).[107] Animal models have been used to evaluate the use of ultrasonic and vibrating mesh nebulizers during invasive ventilation. Ceftazidime delivery in mechanically ventilated pigs showed no difference in aerosol deposition when an ultrasonic and a vibrating mesh nebulizer were used.[108] In another animal study, vibrating mesh and ultrasonic nebulizers placed at the ventilator inlet delivered significantly more drug than a pMDI via spacer or adapter placed before the Y-piece.[109] Our current understanding of aerosol delivery during mechanical ventilation is mostly derived from in vitro studies.[110–126]

Practitioners need to be aware that nebulization can affect ventilator function, and setting adjustments might be required.[110] The use of jet nebulizers adds flow and can increase tidal volume delivery. This can contribute to volutrauma in infants and small children. Therefore, it is important for the respiratory therapist to monitor tidal volume delivery during aerosol delivery with a jet nebulizer and to adjust the set tidal volume to deliver the prescribed amount during the treatment. It is equally important to readjust or to increase the tidal volume after completing the aerosol therapy to minimize the propensity for hypoventilation. Filters should be used at the ventilator to prevent aerosolized particles from entering into the ventilator's internal components. Some mechanical ventilators have a connection port to power the nebulizer. Nebulizers powered by ventilators can perform differently depending on the design of the respective ventilator.[111]

Several variables affect drug delivery and need to be considered when selecting a device: type of circuit, type of ventilator, type and amount of drug required, and bias flow.[110–126] Although many studies reveal several-fold differences in drug output among different aerosol generators, it is not clear if this is clinically relevant. Sometimes increasing either the loading dose or the volume might overcome the poor efficiency of the device.[112] Caution should be taken when increasing the loading dose or volume because, if done with a very efficient device, there is the potential for drug toxicity.

The use of heated-wired circuits limits the potential places where an aerosol generator could be placed. **Figure 24-12** provides a schematic of the different positions an aerosol delivery device can be positioned to deliver medicated aerosol therapy to an intubated infant or child.[17,91] During conventional mechanical ventilation, placing the nebulizer on the dry side of the humidifier enhances aerosol delivery if an adult-size ventilator circuit is used (Figure 24-12).[112–114] However, placement before the Y-piece optimizes drug delivery if a neonatal circuit is used (Figure 24-12).[115,116] Studies have

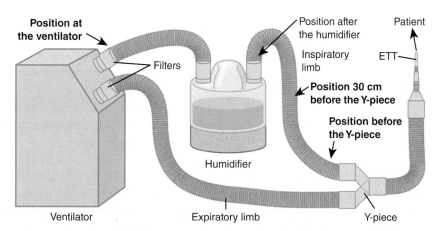

FIGURE 24-12 A schematic illustrating proper placement of an aerosol device when a dual-limb circuit is used to deliver mechanical ventilation to an intubated infant or child.

demonstrated no value in increasing the tidal volume during aerosol administration, as increasing tidal volume does not increase drug delivery during nebulization.[114] Additionally, the increase in tidal volume can contribute to alveolar overdistention and volutrauma.

The bias flow, often used when ventilating infants and small children, can reduce drug delivery to the airways.[113] Although studies using adult models reported a negative effect of humidity on drug delivery, a recent clinical study showed no difference in albuterol delivery when pMDI and nebulizers were used with dry and humid circuits.[117] Similar to what occurs with tracheostomy tubes, the size of the ETT affects drug delivery.[116–118] However, this does not hold true for submicronic aerosols.[118]

Vibrating mesh nebulizers are more efficient and more expensive than jet nebulizers.[112–114] The best timing (inspiration, expiration, or continuous) for aerosol delivery has not yet been defined, and results are conflicting.[119–120] During high-frequency oscillatory ventilation (HFOV), placing the nebulizer before the ETT enhanced drug delivery while placement in the dry side of the humidifier resulted in negligible drug delivery.[121]

Spacers, VHCs, and adapters are used to deliver pMDIs during mechanical ventilation. Adapters are very inefficient and their use is discouraged.[109,122] The pMDI should be actuated at the beginning of inhalation.[123] The add-on devices, specifically a spacer or VHS, can be placed between either the ETT and the Y-piece or the inspiratory limb and the Y-piece. Placing the spacer or VHC between the ETT and the Y-piece adds dead space to the system, is cumbersome, and can potentially contribute to ETT dislodgement during its manipulation. Some spacers can be collapsed when not in use, which reduces rainout in the spacer chamber. Similar to what occurs with nebulizers, the use of a pMDI with a smaller ETT size decreases drug delivery.[124] Specialty gas administration with mechanical ventilation and aerosol delivery has also been studied. The administration of oxygen–helium gas mixtures through a ventilator circuit increased drug delivery with pMDIs.[125] The use of pMDI aerosols with smaller MMAD also resulted in higher drug delivery.[126]

Aerosol Delivery Considerations with Neonatal Patients

Bronchodilators and inhaled corticosteroids are used in preterm newborns. Drug delivery is hindered in this population due to smaller airway and ETT size, lower tidal volumes, and smaller diameter of the ventilator circuit. Aerosols are delivered both to patients on respiratory support and to those who are not. Spontaneously breathing neonates might not be able to open the inspiratory valve of some VHCs; therefore, it is important for the respiratory therapist to verify that the valve is opening during therapy.[127] Studies have demonstrated aerosol deposition is less than 1% for ventilated and nonventilated neonates.[128,129] A nonvalved spacer with pMDI was more effective in reducing respiratory resistance compared to a jet nebulizer in spontaneously breathing nonventilated neonates.[130,131] In ventilated preterm newborns, an ultrasonic nebulizer was more effective in decreasing respiratory resistance than either a pMDI or a jet nebulizer.[132] The efficiency of a vibrating mesh nebulizer was demonstrated in animal models, which showed a 25-fold increase in drug delivery compared to a jet nebulizer (0.5% of loading dose).[133] A 10-fold reduction in aerosol deposition of beclomethasone HFA occurred when piglets either suffered lung injury or were ventilated at high settings compared to controls.[134] Drug delivery during high-flow nasal cannula, bubble continuous positive airway pressure (CPAP), and SiPAP (Carefusion, San Diego, CA) ranged from 0.7% to 1.3% and was best when the vibrating mesh nebulizer was placed on the dry side of the humidifier.[135] However, the opposite was found in a variable-flow CPAP system.[136]

Case Study 1

A 3-year-old male presents to his pediatrician with a complaint of coughing at night for 2 weeks. His parents have been using a decongestant/antihistamine syrup. Initially the cough improved, but it worsened over the last 3 days. He is noted to have morning sneezing and nasal congestion. He has had similar episodes in the past, but this episode is worse. His past history is notable for eczema and dry skin since infancy. He is otherwise healthy. His father and brother have a history of asthma; there are no smokers or pets in the home. At this time his vital signs are as follows: heart rate 98 beats per minute, respiratory rate 26 breaths per minute, blood pressure 84/65 mm Hg, temperature 38.1°C, and oxygen saturation 99% on room air. He is alert, cooperative, chest excursion is symmetrical, and no retractions are noted. His chest has an increased AP diameter and it is hyperresonant to percussion. Rhonchi and occasional wheezes are heard on auscultation. His skin is dry, with no evidence of eczema. The initial impression was an acute

Case Study 1 (*continued*)

exacerbation of asthma. He is treated with nebulized albuterol. His physician prescribed nebulized albuterol and nebulized corticosteroids, in addition to an antihistamine at night to reduce his morning allergy symptoms.

1. This patient will be receiving albuterol and an inhaled corticosteroid by jet nebulizer at home. During patient/family education on the medication and use of the delivery device, what information should the respiratory therapist provide the family about nebulization time and the residual volume?

2. What information should the family receive regarding cleaning the jet nebulizer?

3. Would an MDI be an appropriate alternative to a jet nebulizer for medication delivery in this patient? Provide the rationale for your response.

Case Study 2

A 2-year-old female with spinal muscular atrophy type 1 presented to the emergency department in moderate respiratory distress. Physical exam showed a bell-shaped configuration of thorax and ribs, and moderate intercostal and substernal retractions. The patient was receiving bilevel positive airway pressure (BiPAP) at home with the following settings: spontaneous mode, pressure 18/10 cm H_2O, room air, with 4-hour sprints twice a day. BiPAP was initiated on the following settings: spontaneous/timed mode rate of 22, pressure 20/10 cm H_2O, and FiO_2 0.40. Albuterol and hypertonic saline were administered by jet nebulizer and an aggressive secretion clearance regimen was ordered. Chest radiograph revealed diffuse left lung opacification consistent with left lower lobe pneumonia, clear visualization of the diaphragm, and left upper lobe atelectasis. The right lung was clear. The patient was transferred to the pediatric intensive care unit (PICU). Due to increased work of breathing, the patient settings were increased to BiPAP 24/12 x 28 60% FiO_2 around the clock for impending respiratory failure. Albuterol treatments were increased to Q2 hours followed by chest percussion, postural drainage, and cough assist.

The patient's respiratory status continues to deteriorate. She was intubated and mechanical ventilation initiated. A vibrating mesh nebulizer was used to deliver medicated aerosol therapy inline with the ventilator circuit.

1. What is different about the vibrating mesh nebulizer versus a jet nebulizer?

2. Why was the vibrating mesh nebulizer selected when the patient was intubated and switched from a noninvasive ventilator to an ICU ventilator?

3. Would a metered dose inhaler be an appropriate medication delivery choice for the patient during noninvasive ventilation?

References

1. Laube BL, Janssens HM, de Jongh FH, et al. What the pulmonary specialist should know about the new inhalation therapies. *Eur Respir J.* 2011;37(6):1308-1331.
2. Dolovich MB, Dhand R. Aerosol drug delivery: developments in device design and clinical use. *Lancet.* 2011;377(9770):1032-1045.
3. Amirav I, Newhouse MT, Minocchieri S, Castro-Rodriguez JA, Schüepp KG. Factors that affect the efficacy of inhaled corticosteroids for infants and young children. *J Allergy Clin Immunol.* 2010;125(6):1206-1211.
4. Geller D, Berlinski A. Aerosol delivery of medication. In: Light MJ, Homnick DN, Schechter MS, Blaisdell CJ, Weinberger MM, eds. *Pediatric Pulmonology.* Elk Grove Village, IL: American Academy of Pediatrics; 2011; 913-928.
5. Darquenne C. Aerosol deposition in health and disease. *J Aerosol Med Pulm Drug Deliv.* 2012;25(3):140-147.
6. Davidson N, Tong HJ, Kalberer M, et al. Measurement of the Raman spectra and hygroscopicity of four pharmaceutical aerosols as they travel from pressurised metered dose inhalers (pMDI) to a model lung. *Int J Pharm.* 2017;520(1-2):59-69.
7. Harless J, Ramaiah R, Bhananker SM. Pediatric airway management. *Int J Crit Ill Injury Sci.* 2014;4(1):65-70.
8. Xi J, Si X, Zhou Y, Kim J, Berlinski A. Growth of nasal and laryngeal airways in children: implications in breathing and inhaled aerosol dynamics. *Respir Care.* 2014;59(2):263-273.
9. Chua HL, Collis GG, Newbury AM, et al. The influence of age on aerosol deposition in children with cystic fibrosis. *Eur Respir J.* 1994;7(12):2185-2191.
10. Azouz W, Chetcuti P, Hosker HS, Saralaya D, Stephenson J, Chrystyn H. The inhalation characteristics of patients when they use different dry powder inhalers. *J Aerosol Med Pulm Drug Deliv.* 2015;28(1):35-42.

11. Murakami G, Igarashi T, Adachi Y, et al. Measurement of bronchial hyperreactivity in infants and preschool children using a new method. *Ann Allergy*. 1990;64(4):383-387.

12. Iles R, Lister P, Edmunds AT. Crying significantly reduces absorption of aerosolised drug in infants. *Arch Dis Child*. 1999;81(2):163-165.

13. Erzinger S, Schueepp KG, Brooks-Wildhaber J, Devadason SG, Wildhaber JH. Facemasks and aerosol delivery in vivo. *J Aerosol Med*. 2007;20(Suppl 1):S78-S83; discussion S83-S84.

14. Laube BL, Jashnani R, Dalby RN, Zeitlin PL. Targeting aerosol deposition in patients with cystic fibrosis: effects of alterations in particle size and inspiratory flow rate. *Chest*. 2000;118(4):1069-1076.

15. Mallol J, Rattray S, Walker G, Cook D, Robertson CF. Aerosol deposition in infants with cystic fibrosis. *Pediatr Pulmonol*. 1996;21(5):276-281.

16. Diot P, Palmer LB, Smaldone A, DeCelie-Germana J, Grimson R, Smaldone GC. RhDNase I aerosol deposition and related factors in cystic fibrosis. *Am J Respir Crit Care Med*. 1997;156(5):1662-1668.

17. Berlinski A. Pediatric aerosol therapy. *Respir Care*. 2017;62(6):662-677.

18. Smith EC, Denyer J, Kendrick AH. Comparison of twenty three nebulizer/compressor combinations for domiciliary use. *Eur Respir J*. 1995;8(7):1214-1221.

19. Awad S, Williams DK, Berlinski A. Longitudinal evaluation of compressor/nebulizer performance. *Respir Care*. 2014;59(7):1053-1061.

20. Collis GG, Cole CH, Le Souëf PN. Dilution of nebulised aerosols by air entrainment in children. *Lancet*. 1990;336(8711):341-343.

21. Hess D, Fisher D, Williams P, Pooler S, Kacmarek RM. Medication nebulizer performance. Effects of diluent volume, nebulizer flow, and nebulizer brand. *Chest*. 1996;110(2):498-505.

22. Hess DR, Acosta FL, Ritz RH, Kacmarek RM, Camargo CA Jr. The effect of heliox on nebulizer function using a beta-agonist bronchodilator. *Chest*. 1999;115(1):184-189.

23. O'Callaghan C, White J, Jackson J, Crosby D, Dougill B, Bland H. The effects of heliox on the output and particle-size distribution of salbutamol using jet and vibrating mesh nebulizers. *J Aerosol Med*. 2007;20(4):434-444.

24. O'Callaghan C, Barry PW. The science of nebulised drug delivery. *Thorax*. 1997;52(Suppl 2):S31-S44.

25. Pisut FM. Comparison of medication delivery by T-nebulizer with inspiratory and expiratory reservoirs. *Respir Care*. 1989;34(11):985-988.

26. Gardenhire DS, Burnett D, Strickland S, Myers TR. *A Guide to Aerosol Delivery Devices for Respiratory Therapists*. 4th ed. Irving, TX: American Association of Resipiratory Care; 2017.

27. Kradjan WA, Lakshminarayan S. Efficiency of air compressor-driven nebulizers. *Chest*. 1985;87(4):512-516.

28. Berlinski A, Waldrep J. Effect of aerosol delivery system and formulation on nebulized budesonide output. *J Aerosol Med*. 1997;10(4):307-318.

29. Waldrep JC, Dhand R. Advanced nebulizer designs employing vibrating mesh/aperture plate technologies for aerosol generation. *Curr Drug Deliv*. 2008;5(2):114-119.

30. Fischer A, Stegemann J, Scheuch G, Siekmeier R. Novel devices for individualized controlled inhalation can optimize aerosol therapy in efficacy, patient care and power of clinical trials. *Eur J Med Res*. 2009;14(Suppl 4):S71-S77.

31. Nikander K, Prince I, Coughlin S, Warren S, Taylor G. Mode of breathing-tidal or slow and deep-through the I-neb Adaptive Aerosol Delivery (AAD) system affects lung deposition of (99m)Tc-DTPA. *J Aerosol Med Pulm Drug Deliv*. 2010;23(Suppl 1):S37-S43.

32. Papo MC, Frank J, Thompson AE. A prospective, randomized study of continuous versus intermittent nebulized albuterol for severe status asthmaticus in children. *Crit Care Med*. 1993;21(10):1479-1486.

33. Berlinski A, Willis JR, Leisenring T. In-vitro comparison of 4 large-volume nebulizers in 8 hours of continuous nebulization. *Respir Care*. 2010;55(12):1671-1679.

34. Lowenthal D, Kattan M. Facemasks versus mouthpieces for aerosol treatment of asthmatic children. *Pediatr Pulmonol*. 1992;14(3):192-196.

35. Lipworth BJ, Jackson CM. Comparable efficacy of administration with face mask or mouthpiece of nebulized budesonide suspension for infants and young children with persistant asthma. *Am J Respir Crit Care Med*. 2001;163(5):1277-1278.

36. Berlinski A. Effect of mask dead space and occlusion of mask holes on delivery of nebulized albuterol. *Respir Care*. 2014;59(8):1228-1232.

37. Kumar P, Parashette KR, Noronha P. Perioral dermatitis in a child associated with an inhalation steroid. *Dermatology Online Journal*. 2010;16(4). http://escholarship.org/uc/item/0tq4z5z9.

38. Nakagawa TA, Guerra L, Storgion SA. Aerosolized atropine as an unusual cause of anisocoria in a child with asthma. *Pediatr Emerg Care*. 1993;9(3):153-154.

39. Sangwan S, Gurses BK, Smaldone GC. Facemasks and facial deposition of aerosols. *Pediatr Pulmonol*. 2004;37(5):447-452.

40. Harris KW, Smaldone GC. Facial and ocular deposition of nebulized budesonide: effects of face mask design. *Chest*. 2008;133(2):482-488.

41. Amirav I, Balanov I, Gorenberg M, Groshar D, Luder AS. Nebuliser hood compared to mask in wheezy infants: aerosol therapy without tears! *Arch Dis Child*. 2003;88(8):719-723.

42. Amirav I, Luder A, Chleechel A, Newhouse MT, Gorenberg M. Lung aerosol deposition in suckling infants. *Arch Dis Child*. 2012;97(6):497-501.

43. El Taoum KK, Xi J, Kim J, Berlinski A. In vitro evaluation of aerosols delivered via the nasal route. *Respir Care*. 2015;60(7):1015-1025.

44. Brand P, Friemel I, Meyer T, Schulz H, Heyder J, Häubetainger K. Total deposition of therapeutic particles during spontaneous and controlled inhalations. *J Pharm Sci*. 2000;89(6):724-731.

45. Saiman L, Siegel JD, LiPuma JJ, et al. Infection prevention and control guideline for cystic fibrosis: 2013 update. *Infect Control Hosp Epidemiol*. 2014;35(Suppl 1):S1-S67.

46. The Montreal Protocol on substances that deplete the ozone layer. Final Act (Nairobi:UNEP1987). Federal Register 1994; 59FR56276–56298.

47. Leach CL. The CFC to HFA transition and its impact on pulmonary drug development. *Respir Care*. 2005;50(9):1201-1208.

48. Hatley RH, Parker J, Pritchard JN, von Hollen D. Variability in delivered dose from pressurized metered-dose inhaler formulations due to a delay between shake and fire. *J Aerosol Med Pulm Drug Deliv*. 2017;30(1):71-79.

49. Berlinski A, von Hollen D, Pritchard JN, Hatley RH. Delay between actuation and shaking of a hydrofluoroalkane fluticasone pressurized metered-dose inhaler. *Respir Care*. 2018;63(3):289-293. doi: 10.4187/respcare.05782.

50. Berlinski A, Pennington D. Effect of interval between actuations of albuterol hydrofluoroalkane pressurized metered-dose inhalers on their aerosol characteristics. *Respir Care*. 2017;62(9):1123-1130.

51. Leach CL, Colice GL. A pilot study to assess lung deposition of HFA-beclomethasone and CFC-beclomethasone from a pressurized metered dose inhaler with and without add-on spacers and using varying breathhold times. *J Aerosol Med Pulm Drug Deliv*. 2010;23(6):355-361.

52. Bruce C, Chan HP, Mueller L, Thomas PS, Yates DH. Effect of hydrofluoroalkane-ethanol inhalers on estimated alcohol levels in asthmatic subjects. *Respirology*. 2009;14(1):112-116.

53. Wildhaber JH, Devadason SG, Eber E, et al. Effect of electrostatic charge, flow, delay and multiple actuations on the in vitro delivery of salbutamol from different small volume spacers for infants. *Thorax*. 1996;51(10):985-988.

54. Rubin BK, Durotoye L. How do patients determine that their metered-dose inhaler is empty? *Chest.* 2004;126(4):1134-1137.

55. Geller DE. New liquid aerosol generation devices: systems that force pressurized liquids through nozzles. *Respir Care.* 2002;47(12):1392-1404; discussion 1404-1405.

56. Hochrainer D, Hölz H, Kreher C, Scaffidi L, Spallek M, Wachtel H. Comparison of the aerosol velocity and spray duration of Respimat Soft Mist inhaler and pressurized metered dose inhalers. *J Aerosol Med.* 2005;18(3):273-282.

57. Newman SP, Brown J, Steed KP, Reader SJ, Kladders H. Lung deposition of fenoterol and flunisolide delivered using a novel device for inhaled medicines: comparison of Respimat with conventional metered-dose inhalers with and without spacer devices. *Chest.* 1998;113(4):957-963.

58. Al-Jahdali H, Ahmed A, Al-Harbi A, et al. Improper inhaler technique is associated with poor asthma control and frequent emergency department visits. *Allergy Asthma Clin Immunol.* 2013;9(1):8.

59. Nikander K, Nicholls C, Denyer J, Pritchard J. The evolution of spacers and valved holding chambers. *J Aerosol Med Pulm Drug Deliv.* 2014;27(Suppl 1):S4-S23.

60. Taylor SA, Asmus MJ, Liang J, Coowanitwong I, Vafadari R, Hochhaus G. Performance of a corticosteroid inhaler with a spacer fashioned from a plastic cold-drink bottle: effects of changing bottle volume. *J Asthma.* 2003;40(3):237-242.

61. Zar HJ, Liebenberg M, Weinberg EG, Binns HJ, Mann MD. The efficacy of alternative spacer devices for delivery of aerosol therapy to children with asthma. *Ann Trop Paediatr.* 1998;18(2):75-79.

62. Berlinski A, Waldrep JC. Metering performance of several metered-dose inhalers with different spacers/holding chambers. *J Aerosol Med.* 2001;14(4):427-432.

63. Piérart F, Wildhaber JH, Vrancken I, Devadason SG, Le Souëf PN. Washing plastic spacers in household detergent reduces electrostatic charge and greatly improves delivery. *Eur Respir J.* 1999;13(3):673-678.

64. Voeurng V, Andrieu V, Bun H, Reynier JP, Dubus JC. A new small volume holding chamber for asthmatic children: comparison with Babyhaler spacer. *Pediatr Allergy Immunol.* 2006;17(8):629-634.

65. Rau JL, Coppolo DP, Nagel MW, et al. The importance of nonelectrostatic materials in holding chambers for delivery of hydrofluoroalkane albuterol. *Respir Care.* 2006 May;51(5):503-510.

66. Cohen HA, Cohen Z, Pomeranz AS, Czitron B, and Kahan E. Bacterial contamination of spacer devices used by asthmatic children. *J Asthma.* 2005;42:169-172.

67. Chavez A, McCracken A, Berlinski A. Effect of face mask dead volume, respiratory rate, and tidal volume on inhaled albuterol delivery. *Pediatr Pulmonol.* 2010;45(3):224-229.

68. Shah SA, Berlinski AB, Rubin BK. Force-dependent static dead space of face masks used with holding chambers. *Respir Care.* 2006;51(2):140-144.

69. Amirav I, Luder AS, Halamish A, et al. Design of aerosol face masks for children using computerized 3D face analysis. *J Aerosol Med Pulm Drug Deliv.* 2014;27(4):272-278.

70. Esposito-Festen JE, Ates B, van Vliet FJ, Verbraak AF, de Jongste JC, Tiddens HA. Effect of a facemask leak on aerosol delivery from a pMDI-spacer system. *J Aerosol Med.* 2004;17(1):1-6.

71. Amirav I, Goren A, Pawlowski NA. What do pediatricians in training know about the correct use of inhalers and spacer devices? *J Allergy Clin Immunol.* 1994;94(4):669-675.

72. Alismail A, Song CA, Terry MH, Daher N, Almutairi WA, Lo T. Diverse inhaler devices: a big challenge for health-care professionals. *Respir Care.* 2016;61(5):593-599.

73. Tal A, Golan H, Grauer N, Aviram M, Albin D, Quastel MR. Deposition pattern of radiolabeled salbutamol inhaled from a metered-dose inhaler by means of a spacer with mask in young children with airway obstruction. *J Pediatr.* 1996;128(4):479-484.

74. Esposito-Festen J, Ijsselstijn H, Hop W, van Vliet F, de Jongste J, Tiddens H. Aerosol therapy by pressured metered-dose inhaler-spacer in sleeping young children: to do or not to do? *Chest.* 2006;130(2):487-492.

75. Amirav I, Newhouse MT, Luder A, Halamish A, Omar H, Gorenberg M. Feasibility of aerosol drug delivery to sleeping infants: a prospective observational study. *BMJ Open.* 2014;4(3):e004124.

76. Schultz A, Le Souëf TJ, Venter A, Zhang G, Devadason SG, Le Souëf PN. Aerosol inhalation from spacers and valved holding chambers requires few tidal breaths for children. *Pediatrics.* 2010;126(6):e1493-e1498.

77. Berlinski A, von Hollen D, Hatley RHM, Hardaker LEA, Nikander K. Drug delivery in asthmatic children following coordinated and uncoordinated inhalation maneuvers: a randomized crossover trial. *J Aerosol Med Pulm Drug Deliv.* 2017;30(3):182-189.

78. Berlinski A. Assessing new technologies in aerosol medicine: strengths and limitations. *Respir Care.* 2015;60(6):833-847; discussion 847-849.

79. Hoppentocht M, Hagedoorn P, Frijlink HW, de Boer AH. Technological and practical challenges of dry powder inhalers and formulations. *Adv Drug Deliv Rev.* 2014;75:18-31.

80. Nielsen KG, Skov M, Klug B, Ifversen M, Bisgaard H. Flow-dependent effect of formoterol dry-powder inhaled from the Aerolizer. *Eur Respir J.* 1997;10(9):2105-2109.

81. Haynes A, Geller D, Weers J, et al. Inhalation of tobramycin using simulated cystic fibrosis patient profiles. *Pediatr Pulmonol.* 2016;51(11):1159-1167.

82. De Boeck K, Alifier M, Warnier G. Is the correct use of a dry powder inhaler (Turbohaler) age dependent? *J Allergy Clin Immunol.* 1999;103(5 Pt 1):763-767.

83. Borgström L, Asking L, Lipniunas P. An in vivo and in vitro comparison of two powder inhalers following storage at hot/humid conditions. *J Aerosol Med.* 2005;18(3):304-310.

84. Adachi YS, Adachi Y, Itazawa T, Yamamoto J, Murakami G, Miyawaki T. Ability of preschool children to use dry powder inhalers as evaluated by In-Check Meter. *Pediatr Int.* 2006;48(1):62-65.

85. Milési C, Boubal M, Jacquot A, et al. High-flow nasal cannula: recommendations for daily practice in pediatrics. *Ann Intensive Care.* 2014;4:29.

86. Ari A, Harwood R, Sheard M, Dailey P, Fink JB. In vitro comparison of heliox and oxygen in aerosol delivery using pediatric high flow nasal cannula. *Pediatr Pulmonol.* 2011;46(8):795-801.

87. Réminiac F, Vecellio L, Loughlin RM, et al. Nasal high flow nebulization in infants and toddlers: an in vitro and in vivo scintigraphic study. *Pediatr Pulmonol.* 2017;52(3):337-344.

88. Perry SA, Kesser KC, Geller DE, Selhorst DM, Rendle JK, Hertzog JH. Influences of cannula size and flow rate on aerosol drug delivery through the Vapotherm humidified high-flow nasal cannula system. *Pediatr Crit Care Med.* 2013;14(5):e250-e256.

89. El Taoum K, Xi J, Kim J, Berlinski A. In-vitro evaluation of nebulized aerosols delivered via nasal route. *Respir Care.* 2015;60(7):1015-1025.

90. Lazner MR, Basu AP, Klonin H. Non-invasive ventilation for severe bronchiolitis: analysis and evidence. *Pediatr Pulmonol.* 2012;47(9):909-916.

91. Berlinski A. Inhaled drug delivery for children on long-term mechanical ventilation. In: Sterni LM, Carroll JL, eds. *Caring for the Ventilator Dependent Child: A Clinical Guide.* New York: Humana Press; 2016:217-239.

92. Galindo-Filho VC, Brandão DC, Ferreira Rde C, et al. Noninvasive ventilation coupled with nebulization during asthma crises: a randomized controlled trial. *Respir Care.* 2013;58(2):241-249.

93. Velasco J, Berlinski A. Albuterol delivery efficiency in a pediatric model of noninvasive ventilation with double-limb circuit. *Respir Care.* 2008;63(2):141-146.

94. White CC, Crotwell DN, Shen S, et al. Bronchodilator delivery during simulated pediatric noninvasive ventilation. *Respir Care.* 2013;58(9):1459-1466.

95. Velasco J, Berlinski A. Albuterol delivery efficiency during non-invasive ventilation in a model of a spontaneously breathing child [Abstract]. *Am J Respir Crit Care Med.* 2017:A2813.

96. Trachsel D, Hammer, J. Indications for tracheostomy in children. *Paediatr Respir Rev* 2006;7:162-168.

97. Baran D, Dachy A, Klastersky J. Concentration of gentamicin in bronchial secretions of children with cystic fibrosis of tracheostomy. (Comparison between the intramuscular route, the endotracheal instillation and aerosolization). *Int J Clin Pharmacol Biopharm.* 1975;12(3):336-341.

98. Willis LD, Berlinski A. Survey of aerosol delivery techniques to spontaneously breathing tracheostomized children. *Respir Care.* 2012;57(8):1234-1241.

99. Berlinski A, Chavez A. Albuterol delivery via metered dose inhaler in a spontaneously breathing pediatric tracheostomy model. *Pediatr Pulmonol.* 2013;48(10):1026-1034.

100. Cooper B, Berlinski A. Albuterol delivery via facial and tracheostomy route in a model of a spontaneously breathing child. *Respir Care.* 2015;60(12):1749-1758.

101. Berlinski A, Cooper B. Oronasal and tracheostomy delivery of soft mist and pressurized metered-dose inhalers with valved holding chamber. *Respir Care.* 2016;61(7):913-919.

102. Alhamad BR, Fink JB, Harwood RJ, Sheard MM, Ari A. Effect of aerosol devices and administration techniques on drug delivery in a simulated spontaneously breathing pediatric tracheostomy model. *Respir Care.* 2015;60(7):1026-1032.

103. Berlinski A. Nebulized albuterol delivery in a model of spontaneously breathing children with tracheostomy. *Respir Care.* 2013;58(12):2076-2086.

104. Berlinski A, Ari A, Davies P, et al. Workshop report: aerosol delivery to spontaneously breathing tracheostomized patients. *J Aerosol Med Pulm Drug Deliv.* 2017;30(4):207-222.

105. Piccuito CM, Hess DR. Albuterol delivery via tracheostomy tube. *Respir Care.* 2005;50(8):1071-1076.

106. Yokoe DS, Anderson DJ, Berenholtz SM, et al. A compendium of strategies to prevent healthcare-associated infections in acute care hospitals: 2014 updates. *Infect Control Hosp Epidemiol.* 2014;34(Suppl 2):S21-S31.

107. Garner SS, Wiest DB, Bradley JW, Habib DM. Two administration methods for inhaled salbutamol in intubated patients. *Arch Dis Child.* 2002;87(1):49-53.

108. Ferrari F, Liu ZH, Lu Q, et al. Comparison of lung tissue concentrations of nebulized ceftazidime in ventilated piglets: ultrasonic versus vibrating plate nebulizers. *Intensive Care Med.* 2008;34(9):1718-1723.

109. Berlinski A, Holt S, Thurman T, Heulitt M. Albuterol delivery during mechanical ventilation in an ex-vivo porcine model. *J Aerosol Med Pulm Drug Deliv.* 2013;26(2):1-57.

110. Hanhan U, Kissoon N, Payne M, Taylor C, Murphy S De Nicola LK. Effects of in-line nebulization on preset ventilator variables. *Respir Care.* 1993;38:474-478.

111. McPeck M, O'Riordan, TG, Smaldone GC. Choice of mechanical ventilator: influence on nebulizer performance. *Respir Care.* 1993;38(8):887-895.

112. Berlinski A, Willis JR. Albuterol delivery by 4 different nebulizers placed in 4 different positions in a pediatric ventilator in vitro model. *Respir Care.* 2013;58(7):1124-1133.

113. Ari A, Atalay OT, Harwood R, Sheard MM, Aljamhan EA, Fink JB. Influence of nebulizer type, position, and bias flow on aerosol drug delivery in simulated pediatric and adult lung models during mechanical ventilation. *Respir Care.* 2010;55(7):845-851.

114. Berlinski A, Willis JR. Effect of tidal volume and nebulizer type and position on albuterol delivery in a pediatric model of mechanical ventilation. *Respir Care.* 2015;60(10):1424-1430.

115. DiBlasi RM, Crotwell DN, Shen S, Zheng J, Fink JB, Yung D. Iloprost drug delivery during infant conventional and high-frequency oscillatory ventilation. *Pulm Circ.* 2016;6(1):63-69.

116. Berlinski A, Kumaran S. Particle size characterization of nebulized albuterol delivered by a vibrating mesh nebulizer through pediatric endotracheal tubes [Abstract]. *Am J Respir Crit Care Med.* 2016:A2191.

117. Moustafa IOF, Ali MRA, Al Hallag M, et al. Lung deposition and systemic bioavailability of different aerosol devices with and without humidification in mechanically ventilated patients. *Heart Lung.* 2017;46(6):464-467.

118. Ahrens RC, Ries RA, Popendorf W, Wiese JA. The delivery of therapeutic aerosols through endotracheal tubes. *Pediatr Pulmonol.* 1986;2(1):19-26.

119. Di Paolo ER, Pannatier A, Cotting J. In vitro evaluation of bronchodilator drug delivery by jet nebulization during pediatric mechanical ventilation. *Pediatr Crit Care Med.* Med 2005;6(4):462-469.

120. Wan GH, Lin HL, Fink JB, et al. In vitro evaluation of aerosol delivery by different nebulization modes in pediatric and adult mechanical ventilators. *Respir Care.* 2014;59(10):1494-500.

121. Fang TP, Lin HL, Chiu SH, et al. Using jet nebulizer and vibrating mesh nebulizer during high frequency oscillatory ventilation: an in vitro comparison. *J Aerosol Med Pulm Drug Deliv.* 2016;29(5):447-453.

122. Wildhaber JH, Hayden MJ, Dore ND, Devadason SG, LeSouëf PN. Salbutamol delivery from a hydrofluoroalkane pressurized metered-dose inhaler in pediatric ventilator circuits: an in vitro study. *Chest.* 1998;113(1):186-191.

123. Diot P, Morra L, Smaldone GC. Albuterol delivery in a model of mechanical ventilation. Comparison of metered-dose inhaler and nebulizer efficiency. *Am J Respir Crit Care Med.* 1995;152(4 Pt 1):1391-1394.

124. Garner SS, Wiest DB, Bradley JW. Albuterol delivery by metered-dose inhaler in mechanically ventilated pediatric lung model. *Crit Care Med.* 1996;24(5):870-874.

125. Habib DM, Garner SS, Brandeburg S. Effect of helium-oxygen on delivery of albuterol in a pediatric, volume-cycled, ventilated lung model. *Pharmacotherapy.* 1999;19(2):143-149.

126. Mitchell JP, Nagel MW, Wiersema KJ, Doyle CC, Migounov VA. The delivery of chlorofluorocarbon-propelled versus hydrofluoroalkane-propelled beclomethasone dipropionate aerosol to the mechanically ventilated patient: a laboratory study. *Respir Care.* 2003;48(11):1025-1032.

127. Fok TF, Lam K, Chan CK, et al. Aerosol delivery to non-ventilated infants by metered dose inhaler: should a valved spacer be used? *Pediatr Pulmonol.* 1997;24(3):204-212.

128. Fok TF, Monkman S, Dolovich M, et al. Efficiency of aerosol medication delivery from a metered dose inhaler versus jet nebulizer in infants with bronchopulmonary dysplasia. *Pediatr Pulmonol.* 1996;21(5):301-309.

129. Fok TF, Lam K, Ng PC, et al. Delivery of salbutamol to nonventilated preterm infants by metered-dose inhaler, jet nebulizer, and ultrasonic nebulizer. *Eur Respir J.* 1998;12(1):159-164.

130. Sivakumar D, Bosque E, Goldman SL. Bronchodilator delivered by metered dose inhaler and spacer improves respiratory system compliance more than nebulizer-delivered bronchodilator in ventilated premature infants. *Pediatr Pulmonol.* 1999;27(3):208-212.

131. Mazela J, Polin RA. Aerosol delivery to ventilated newborn infants: historical challenges and new directions. Eur J Pediatr. 2011 Apr;170(4):433-444. *Eur J Pediatr.* 2011;170(4):433-444.

132. Fok TF, Lam K, Ng PC, et al. Randomised crossover trial of salbutamol aerosol delivered by metered dose inhaler, jet nebuliser, and ultrasonic nebuliser in chronic lung disease. *Arch Dis Child Fetal Neonatal Ed*. 1998;79(2):F100-F104.

133. Dubus JC, Vecellio L, De Monte M, et al. Aerosol deposition in neonatal ventilation. *Pediatr Res*. 2005;58(1):10-14.

134. Dubus JC, Montharu J, Vecellio L, et al. Lung deposition of HFA beclomethasone dipropionate in an animal model of bronchopulmonary dysplasia. *Pediatr Res*. 2007;61(1):21-25.

135. Sunbul FS, Fink JB, Harwood R, Sheard MM, Zimmerman RD, Ari A. Comparison of HFNC, bubble CPAP and SiPAP on aerosol delivery in neonates: an in-vitro study. *Pediatr Pulmonol*. 2015;50(11):1099-1106.

136. Farney KD, Kuehne BT, Gibson LA, Nelin LD, Shepherd EG. In vitro evaluation of radio-labeled aerosol delivery via a variable-flow infant CPAP system. Respir Care. 2014;59(3):340-344.

25

Airway Clearance and Lung Expansion Therapy

Lisa L. Bylander

OUTLINE

OBJECTIVES

1. List the indications, contraindications, complications, and age-specific considerations for incentive spirometry, chest physiotherapy, oscillatory positive expiratory pressure therapy, autogenic drainage, high-frequency chest wall compression and oscillation, intrapulmonary percussive ventilation, and cough assistance therapy.
2. Describe the proper administration technique for incentive spirometry, chest physiotherapy, oscillatory positive expiratory pressure therapy, autogenic drainage, high-frequency chest wall compression and oscillation, intrapulmonary percussive ventilation, and cough assistance therapy.
3. Explain how chest physiotherapy, oscillatory positive expiratory pressure therapy, autogenic drainage, high-frequency chest wall compression and oscillation, intrapulmonary percussive ventilation, and cough assistance therapy achieve airway clearance.
4. Discuss the challenges to providing airway clearance and lung expansion therapy to infants and children.

KEY TERMS

airway clearance
  therapy (ACT)
autogenic drainage (AD)
chest physiotherapy (CPT)
cough assistance therapy
high-frequency chest wall
  compression (HFCWC)
high-frequency chest wall
  oscillation (HFCWO)
huff coughing
incentive spirometry

insufflation-exsufflation
intrapulmonary percussive
  ventilation (IPV)
mucociliary escalator
mucus hypersecretion
oscillatory positive
  expiratory pressure
  (OPEP) therapy
percussion
postural drainage
vibration

Introduction

Airway clearance therapy (ACT) is a general term that refers to several modalities having one goal: to clear retained pulmonary secretions from the airways. Retention of airway secretions is a common occurrence in many acute and chronic respiratory diseases of infants and children. This is most often due to dysfunction of the mucociliary escalator, hypersecretion of mucus, or an ineffective or absent cough. When the **mucociliary escalator** is functioning well, mucus and the debris trapped in the airways are propelled up the respiratory tract, where the secretions can be expectorated. When mucus is more viscous, as occurs with cystic fibrosis, dehydration, or infection, it becomes more difficult for the cilia to move mucus up the escalator. The thickness and depth of this mucus layer can slow, and even stop, the cilia from functioning properly. **Mucus hypersecretion** in a child is most often associated with asthma, cystic fibrosis, and bronchiectasis. This, in combination with a child's smaller airways, can lead to difficulty clearing secretions. An effective cough is the key to moving mucus in airways that are affected by an impaired mucociliary escalator or mucus hypersecretion. However, an ineffective or absent cough, as is found in neuromuscular diseases, high spinal cord injuries, and children with an artificial airway, can further impair the ability to clear pulmonary secretions.

The goals of ACT are listed in **Table 25-1**. It is important to note that the effectiveness of any lung expansion or ACT is dependent upon proper technique. This is particularly important in the pediatric population where the choice of ACT should be dependent upon the child's age, developmental/maturity level, ability to cooperate, and psychological adjustment to their condition.[1]

Incentive Spirometry

Lung expansion is essential to providing an effective cough. **Incentive spirometry**, also referred to as sustained maximal inspiration, uses a visual aid to encourage children to take a deep breath. With each breath, the spirometer provides feedback on the child's inspiratory volume. In 2011, the American Association for Respiratory Care published a clinical practice guideline recommending that incentive spirometry not be used alone in the treatment and prevention of postoperative complications. Instead, the guideline recommends combining it with proper pain control, early ambulation, coughing, and deep breathing.[2]

Indications and Contraindications

Incentive spirometry is indicated for the prevention and treatment of atelectasis and is most often provided to children who have undergone thoracic or abdominal surgery. It is also therapeutic in children who are predisposed to shallow breathing, whether as a result of their disease process, pain, immobility, or use of a thoracic or abdominal binder. Because cooperation and understanding are required for effective therapy, incentive spirometry is contraindicated in those who are unable to perform the maneuver. This includes very young children as well as those who are heavily sedated, have cognitive delays, or present with inspiratory volumes less than 33% of predicted values.

Administration

Box 25-1 provides instruction in administering incentive spirometry to a child. Children should be instructed to take their time with repeated maneuvers, as they may hyperventilate and become dizzy if done too quickly. Coughing is performed at any time necessary and is encouraged again at the end of the treatment to assure any loose secretions are expelled from the airway. It should be noted that a slow inspiration is best with this procedure. A fast inspiration will preferentially fill

---

TABLE 25-1
Goals of Airway Clearance Therapy

Clear greater volumes of excess secretions from the lungs
Improve cough
Improve mucociliary escalator function
Reduce air trapping and improve ventilation of the lungs

BOX 25-1 Administration of Incentive Spirometry

1. Explain the procedure to the child and family.
2. Assist the child into a sitting or semi-Fowler position.
3. Establish the volume goal.
4. Hold the incentive spirometer or place it on a flat surface in an upright position in front of the child.
5. Place the mouthpiece in the child's mouth and ask them to close their lips tightly around it.
6. Instruct the child to exhale normally and then to inhale slowly through the mouthpiece to a maximal inspiration, with a breath hold for 3 to 5 seconds.
7. Instruct the child to remove the mouthpiece and to then exhale normally.
8. After allowing the child to breathe normally for several breaths, repeat the maneuvers.

alveoli that are already open while a slow breath will more likely reinflate atelectatic alveoli. Some children may need nose clips to adequately perform the maneuvers. Incentive spirometry can be difficult for younger or developmentally delayed children. Patients with recent chest or abdominal surgery or trauma may experience pain. With these patients, it often proves beneficial to provide pain medication prior to therapy.

Chest Physiotherapy

Chest physiotherapy (CPT) uses percussion or vibration on the chest wall to mobilize secretions along with postural drainage to allow gravity to aid in draining those secretions to the large airways, where they can be coughed out and expectorated. There are various methods and devices that can be used to perform CPT. It is important to note that all forms of CPT should be followed by coughing to clear any secretions that have been mobilized. Tracheal suctioning or some form of assisted cough may be indicated when secretions are palpated or auscultated and the child is unable to effectively cough spontaneously or on command. Vibratory and percussive devices are available for all sizes of patients, ranging from the smallest premature infant to the teenager. It is important to adhere to manufacturer specifications regarding the appropriate use of all devices.

Indications and Contraindications

CPT may be indicated in any patient who has retained pulmonary secretions and is having difficulty clearing on their own. It should be used judiciously in extremely premature infants, as there may be increased risk for intraventricular hemorrhage. A review of the literature finds that CPT is not routinely recommended for the treatment of pneumonia in adults.[3] However, this is not well defined in children. It has also been noted that CPT may not be beneficial in the treatment of bronchiolitis.[4] Contraindications to CPT are listed in **Table 25-2**.

TABLE 25-2
Contraindications to Chest Physiotherapy

Elevated intracranial pressure (>20 mm Hg)
Nonstabilized head or neck injury
Active hemorrhage with hemodynamic instability
Recent spinal injury
Empyema
Distended abdomen
Uncontrolled hypertension
Large pleural effusion

Postural Drainage

Postural drainage is used to assist gravity in moving secretions from the lung. The child is placed in various positions to target drainage of specific lung segments. Some positions may be contraindicated in certain situations; for example, it may be contraindicated to use the Trendelenburg position in children who have increased intracranial pressure or gastroesophageal reflux disease.[5] **Figure 25-1** and **Figure 25-2** illustrate the positions used for postural drainage in infants and children.

Percussion and Vibration

With the purpose of loosening secretions from the bronchial walls, **percussion** or vibration is provided while the infant or child is in various degrees of postural drainage. The clinician may percuss on the chest using their cupped hand or a device made for percussion, focusing on the various segments of the lungs. Percussion should not be performed over the spine or sternum; below the rib cage; or over zippers, snaps, or buttons. Care should be taken when percussing around chest tubes, drains, catheters, and sutured areas.

In neonatal and pediatric care, **vibration** is most often performed using a vibratory device. This is especially true with premature neonates. Because their chest walls are very compliant, percussion on the chests may result in decreased lung volumes during therapy. Use of a vibratory device may also be an appropriate option for children who cannot tolerate percussion, as seen in **Figure 25-3**, **Figure 25-4**, and **Figure 25-5**. There are several devices marketed to use for percussion or vibration. Some of these devices are electrically or pneumatically powered.

Administration

To reduce the risk of vomiting and aspiration, food should be withheld and tube feedings stopped for 30 to 60 minutes prior to CPT or treatment delayed for 1 to 2 hours after eating. Drainage of the lung segments, along with percussion or vibration, can be performed in any order. Length of time spent in each segment or position is usually 30 seconds to 1 minute for neonates, infants, and young children and up to 5 minutes for the older child. The time required is dependent upon the patient's condition and tolerance and varies according to each institution's policies. Be aware that it may be difficult to keep toddlers and young children in one position for the allotted time, as they are not always cooperative.

Percussion can be frightening for infants and children as well as for their families. It is important to explain to the child and caregiver how the procedure is performed and the reason it is needed. Demonstrating the procedure by percussing on your own chest or using a doll or one of the child's stuffed animals can help

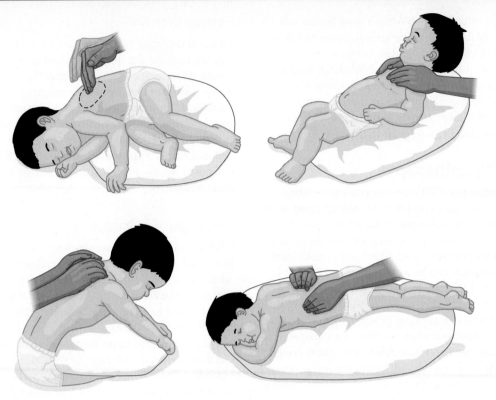

FIGURE 25-1 Positions for postural drainage of an infant.

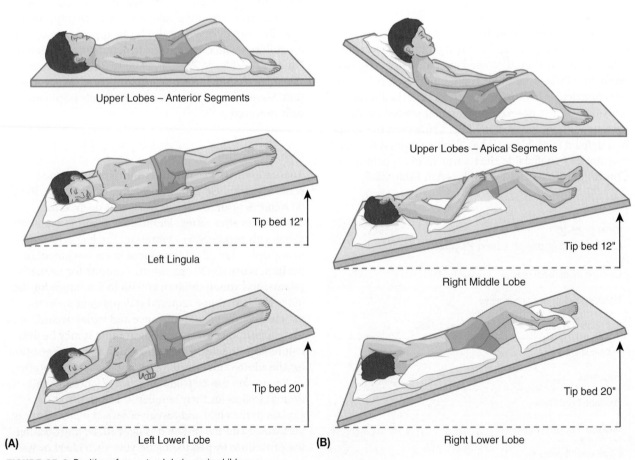

Upper Lobes – Anterior Segments

Upper Lobes – Apical Segments

Left Lingula

Tip bed 12"

Right Middle Lobe

Tip bed 12"

Left Lower Lobe

Tip bed 20"

Right Lower Lobe

Tip bed 20"

(A)

(B)

FIGURE 25-2 Positions for postural drainage in children.

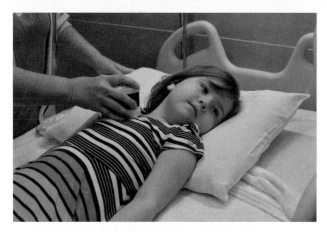

FIGURE 25-3 Child receiving percussion to anterior segment of the right upper lobe with a pneumatic percussor.

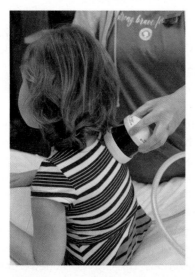

FIGURE 25-4 Child receiving percussion to posterior segment of the right upper lobe with a pneumatic percussor.

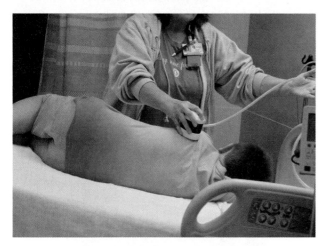

FIGURE 25-5 Child receiving percussion and postural drainage to the lateral basal segment of the left lower lobe using a pneumatic percussor.

alleviate fears. Distraction techniques may be helpful as well, such as listening to music, watching a movie, or singing a song during therapy.

TABLE 25-3
Complications Associated with Chest Physiotherapy

Position-related hypoxia
Excessive accumulation of secretions in the airway
Elevated intracranial pressure (>20 mm Hg)
Aspiration of secretions into other areas of the lung
Hypertension
Hypotension
Pulmonary hemorrhage
Pain or injury to the ribs, muscles, or spine
Nausea
Vomiting
Gastric reflux
Aspiration of secretions
Heart arrhythmias
Headache
Dizziness

Complications

CPT generally has few complications when techniques are appropriate for the child's condition. Most of the complications are dependent upon the child's health. **Table 25-3** lists complications associated with CPT.

Oscillatory Positive Expiratory Pressure Therapy

Positive expiratory pressure (PEP) therapy uses a device that provides back pressure during exhalation, hence the term positive expiratory pressure. This pressure helps distend the airways and gets air behind secretions that can then be moved to the large airways, where they are expectorated with a cough or huff maneuver. **Oscillatory positive expiratory pressure (OPEP) therapy**, also known as vibratory PEP, uses the resistance during exhalation while creating vibrations or oscillations at the airway opening. These vibrations shear mucus from the surface of the airways. After blowing through the device several times, **huff coughing** is performed to clear the mucus from the lungs. OPEP devices are commonly known by their brand names, including Flutter, Acapella, Aerobika, and Cornet.

Indications and Contraindications

OPEP therapy is indicated for use in children with disorders in which retained secretions are unable to be cleared effectively with coughing alone. Typical conditions include cystic fibrosis, bronchiectasis, and pneumonia. It may also be helpful in conditions in which there is air trapping secondary to mucus plugs, such as chronic lung disease and asthma.[6] Because OPEP therapy requires the child's cooperation and therapy effectiveness is dependent on technique, it is contraindicated in younger children and in children who are unable to follow directions due to developmental delay or diminished levels of consciousness. Other contraindications are listed in **Table 25-4**.

Administration

Box 25-2 provides directions on administering OPEP therapy to a child. There are many devices that offer various visual aids or audible sounds that may help a child perform the technique and hold their attention. Making the therapy into a game is helpful when working with the younger child. Although a mask may be necessary to use in some conditions, it is preferable to have children perform therapy with a mouthpiece, as shown in **Figure 25-6** and **Figure 25-7**.

Autogenic Drainage

Autogenic drainage (AD) is a form of ACT that uses a cycle of controlled breathing exercises at varying depths to loosen secretions in different areas of the lungs. The exercises consist of three phases, with the depth of inspiration increasing with each phase.[7] Expiration is slow and prolonged to mobilize secretions with less coughing and energy expenditure. Huff coughing is performed, which is gentler and less tiring.

BOX 25-2 Administration of Oscillatory Positive Expiratory Pressure (OPEP) Therapy

1. Explain the procedure to the child and family.
2. Assist the child into a sitting or semi-Fowler position.
3. Adjust the expiratory resistor dial to the appropriate setting.
4. If a mask is used, attach it to the device and hold it firmly over the child's face. If a mouthpiece is used, instruct the child to place the mouthpiece between the teeth, keeping their lips tightly around the mouthpiece.
5. Instruct the child to breathe in slowly and deeply, taking a slightly larger than normal breath through their nose, and to hold the breath for 2 to 3 seconds.
6. Instruct the child to blow out through their mouth into the device, exhaling actively but not forcefully. Explain that blowing out "should not be as hard as you can blow but just hard enough to make a fluttering sound, like a kitten purring." Remind the child to keep their cheeks stiff while blowing out. Encourage exhalation to be three times longer than inhalation.
7. Repeat these breaths for a total of 10 to 20 breaths, followed with huff coughing to clear any secretions. This counts as one set or cycle.
8. Repeat each set or cycle four to six (or the amount indicated per institutional policy) times with huff coughing after each cycle.

TABLE 25-4
Contraindications to Oscillatory Positive Expiratory Pressure Therapy

Untreated or unresolved pneumothorax
Active hemoptysis
Lung lobectomy or transplantation
Undrained empyema or lung abscess
Hemodynamic instability
Sinusitis
Middle ear infection
Acute increased work of breathing

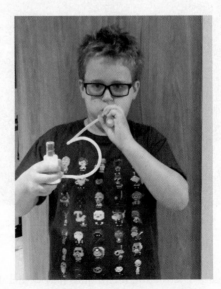

FIGURE 25-6 A child performing positive expiratory pressure (PEP) therapy.

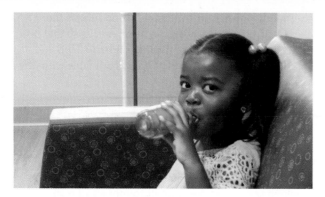

FIGURE 25-7 A child performing oscillatory positive expiratory pressure therapy using an Acapella device.

Once a child is properly trained, the technique can be used anytime and anywhere without assistance or equipment.

Indications and Contraindications

AD is indicated for the removal of thick or sticky retained secretions in children with cystic fibrosis or bronchiectasis. There are no absolute contraindications to AD; however, it is not indicated in children who are unable to follow complex instructions, who are not spontaneously breathing, or who do not have sufficient airflow to perform the maneuvers.

Administration

In comparison to other forms of ACT, AD is a slightly complex, time-consuming technique to learn and requires more training to effectively perform. Younger children may have difficulty understanding and performing it correctly; however, by the time they are 8 to 12 years of age, most children can effectively perform the therapy. It often takes more than one training session before therapy is fully mastered. There are many videos available online that may help in teaching children and their families. AD is performed in three phases:

- Phase 1 – Unsticking mucus in the small airways
- Phase 2 – Collecting mucus in the middle airways
- Phase 3 – Clearing mucus from the large airways

Box 25-3 provides directions on administering autogenic drainage. Dizziness secondary to hyperventilation may occur, especially when first learning to perform the therapy. Coughing spells, as well as wheezing, may present when exhaling forcefully.

High-Frequency Chest Wall Compression and Oscillation

High-frequency chest wall compression (HFCWC) uses an air-pulse generator that is attached by way of hoses to an inflatable garment (vest, jacket, or wrap) that wraps around the child's chest. The generator rapidly delivers

---

BOX 25-3 Administration of Autogenic Drainage

1. Explain the procedure to the child and family.

2. Assist the child in sitting upright or reclining with the head and neck slightly extended to keep the upper airway open.

3. Ask the child to blow their nose and to clear any upper airway secretions by huff coughing.

4. **Phase 1** ("unsticking" mucus from the airway walls): Instruct the child to **breathe in** slowly through the nose and to take a normal-size breath, actively using the diaphragm if possible. Encourage the child to **pause**, holding the breath for 3 seconds to allow air to evenly distribute in the lungs and get behind secretions. Instruct the child to **breathe out** through the mouth as long as possible with a sigh-like breath, maintaining a slow and prolonged exhalation. **Repeat** this maneuver for 2 to 3 minutes or until crackles are heard at the beginning of exhalation. When repeating the breaths, remind the child to inhale slowly without pulling secretions back into the lungs.

5. **Phase 2** (collecting mucus in the middle airways): Instruct the child to maintain the same position as

in Phase 1 but to **breathe in** with a slightly larger breath, **pause** again for about 3 seconds, and then **breathe out** a little faster this time but not to full exhalation. **Repeat** this for 2 to 3 minutes. Encourage the child to exhale faster during this phase but not so fast that cough or wheezing occurs.

6. **Phase 3** (clearing mucus from the large airways): Instruct the child to maintain the same position and to **breathe in** a slow, deep breath through the nose, **pause** to hold the breath for 3 seconds, and then **breathe out** forcefully through an open glottis and do two to three huff coughs to move the secretions to the mouth where they can be expectorated. **Repeat** this maneuver for 2 to 3 minutes until secretions are cleared.[5,6] This is the end of one cycle. After resting for a few minutes, repeat cycles for 20 to 30 minutes.

7. Each phase should last about 2 to 3 minutes. Remind the child to try not to cough during phases 1 and 2 but to wait until phase 3, or when mucus is felt in the large airways, and to use huff coughing.

small bursts of air into and out of the garment, inflating and then deflating the garment against the chest wall at selected frequencies and pressures. During inflation, as the chest wall is compressed, short bursts of expiratory flow are generated, which loosen mucus so that it can be moved to the large airways and expectorated.[8] There are no specific positions or breathing techniques required during therapy, which makes it ideal for children with neurologic impairment or those unable to perform such techniques because of weakness.[9] In similar fashion, **high-frequency chest wall oscillation (HFCWO)** is a form of ACT in which the child wears a garment or vest that delivers compression pulses to the chest wall. The alternating pulses quickly compress and release the chest wall, helping to loosen and thin mucus so that it is more easily removed from the lungs. **Figure 25-8** and **Figure 25-9** are examples of garments available with The Vest by Hill-Rom.

Table 25-5 provides information on four commercially available devices.

Indications and Contraindications

This therapy is indicated in the treatment of disorders in which secretions are difficult to move and result in airway obstruction. It is used most often to treat

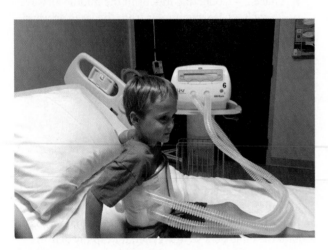

FIGURE 25-8 Child receiving high-frequency chest wall compression (HFCWC) wearing a wrap garment from The Vest by Hill-Rom.

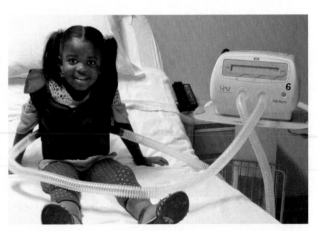

FIGURE 25-9 Child receiving high-frequency chest wall compression (HFCWC) wearing a vest garment from The Vest by Hill-Rom.

TABLE 25-5
High-Frequency Chest Wall Compression and Oscillation Devices

Device	The Vest	SmartVest	inCourage	AffloVest
Available chest circumference	16–75 inches	16–52 inches	16–60 inches	18–65 inches
Waveform	Sine	Sine	Triangle	N/A
System	• Inflatable vest • Two hoses • Air pulse generator	• Inflatable vest • One hose • Air pulse generator	• Inflatable vest • Two hoses • Pulsating therapy unit	• Vest containing eight oscillating motors • Battery
Hose system	Dual locking	Single hose	Dual locking	None
Weight (based off vest fitting a 52-inch chest)	2.4 lbs	2.2 lbs	1.8 lbs	10.3 lbs
Features	Garment available as a jacket (vest) or a wrap. Has Bluetooth technology that gives feedback about therapy through a health portal.	Has built-in wireless technology to track therapy. Provides color selection for both vests and generators.	Enables deep breaths during therapy. Provides selection of patterns for vests and custom decorative decals for the therapy unit.	Vest contains eight separate motors for vibration, percussion, or drainage. Powered by AC or battery. Patient can be entirely mobile when taking therapy.

TABLE 25-6
Contraindications to High-Frequency Chest Wall Compression or Oscillation

Absolute Contraindications
Active hemoptysis or pulmonary hemorrhage
Unstable head or neck injury
Relative Contraindications
Pulmonary embolism
Subcutaneous emphysema
Bronchopulmonary fistula
Esophageal surgery
Uncontrolled hypertension
Hemodynamic instability
Rib fractures
Empyema or large pleural effusion
Suspected tuberculosis
Burns, open wounds, or recent skin grafts on the thorax
Lung contusion
Recent spinal anesthesia or spinal surgery

children with cystic fibrosis and bronchiectasis. It is also effective in treating other disorders that present with excessive secretions, especially those with neurodisabilites. **Table 25-6** lists contraindications to HFCWC and HFCWO therapy. Therapy may be provided in the conditions listed as relative contraindications if the benefits of the therapy outweigh the dangers.

Administration

Box 25-4 provides directions on administering HFCWC and HFCWO therapy. For therapy to be effective, it is imperative that the garment is appropriately sized. **Figure 25-10** illustrates a child who has outgrown his vest garment. As the child grows, the garment must be replaced.

Many institutions have specific recommendations for settings used during therapy. At this time there is no consensus on settings. Most institutions use a range of frequencies in order to target the various-size airways. Therapy tends to be better tolerated when starting with lower frequencies and working up to the ordered settings.

Therapy is more easily accepted when the child is provided a demonstration of what it looks and sounds like. This can be done by placing the garment around a pillow or stuffed animal. Younger children often find it fun to hear themselves talk or sing during therapy. Playing board games, video games, or watching television can provide a distraction for the child.

Complications

Should any complication occur during HFCWC or HFCWO therapy, then therapy should be terminated and followed with reevaluation or the decision to discontinue it. **Table 25-7** lists complications that may result from providing this therapy.

BOX 25-4 Administration of High-Frequency Chest Wall Compression or Oscillation Therapy

1. Explain the procedure to the child and family.
2. Assist the child into a sitting or semi-Fowler position.
3. Place an appropriate-size garment (vest or wrap) on the child.
   - Position the vest to rest on the child's shoulders and extend to the waist, above the hips.
   - Position the wrap to lie just beneath the armpits and extend to the waist, above the hips.
   - A correctly fitted garment is one that, when deflated, does not restrict breathing and is loose enough to fit a closed fist beneath the back of the garment.
   - Foam or folded washcloths/towels may be placed around gastrostomy tubes, ports, and incisions for added comfort.
4. Assure that settings are correct, and with the garment in place, turn the generator on.
5. After 10 minutes of therapy (or per institutional policy), stop therapy and encourage the child to clear loosened secretions by performing three to five huff or active coughs. Suctioning may be necessary in some cases.
6. Restart therapy, using a higher speed or frequency, and again stop therapy after 10 minutes (or per institutional policy) and encourage the child to cough. Repeat this step one more time.

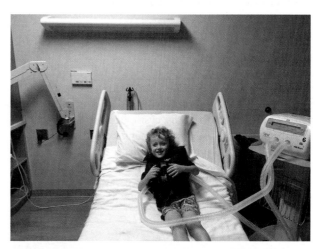

FIGURE 25-10 During a hospitalization, it was determined that this child's vest garment was too short for him.

TABLE 25-7
Complications Associated with High-Frequency Chest Wall Compression and Oscillation

Hypoxia
Vomiting with or without aspiration
Acute hypotension or hypertension during therapy
Bronchospasm
Cardiac arrhythmias
Chest, spinal, or abdominal pain
Bronchospasm
Arrhythmias

TABLE 25-8
Contraindications to Intrapulmonary Percussive Ventilation

Elevated intracranial pressure (>20 mm Hg)
Hemodynamic instability
Tracheoesophageal fistula
Recent esophageal fistula
Active hemoptysis
Recent pulmonary hemorrhage
Active or untreated tuberculosis
Pulmonary blebs
Bullous emphysema
Untreated pneumothorax

Intrapulmonary Percussive Ventilation

Intrapulmonary percussive ventilation (IPV) is an ACT that delivers small, rapid, high-flow bursts of air directly into the airway. These bursts of air oscillate, causing a wedge pressure to get behind secretions, loosening them so that they can then move to the large airways where they are expectorated or removed through suctioning. This provides airway clearance as well as hyperinflation. The IPV circuit includes a high-output nebulizer that provides a means to deliver inhaled medications, including bronchodilators and hypertonic saline, and hydrate secretions. Studies, however, debate the efficacy of medication deposition.[10–12] Therapy can be given by mouthpiece or mask, although this may be difficult and ineffective with younger children who cannot maintain a mouth seal or when unable to achieve a tight seal around the mask. It can also be delivered through an endotracheal or tracheostomy tube with or without mechanical ventilation.

Indications and Contraindications

IPV is indicated for use in infants and children who require mobilization of secretions and in whom other forms of ACT have been ineffective. Disorders that often benefit from therapy include neurodisabilities with pulmonary symptoms, cystic fibrosis, pneumonia, chronic lung disease, and mechanically ventilated infants and children with atelectasis or retained secretions. Although the only absolute contraindication to IPV is an untreated pneumothorax, other relative contraindications are listed in **Table 25-8**.

Administration

Regardless of age, IPV tends to be well tolerated when used with an artificial airway. Perhaps this better

tolerance is because these children do not need to focus on opening and closing their glottis. Therapy with a mouthpiece requires more instruction and is best tolerated by children who are at least 8 years of age. Mask treatments are usually reserved for those who are cognitively impaired or too young to correctly perform a mouthpiece treatment. Some children, however, prefer the mask over a mouthpiece, as seen in **Figure 25-11**. In this author's experience, mask treatments with IPV are not well tolerated because both infants and children tend to "fight" the treatment, which may prevent pressure from being delivered to the lower airways. Therapy can be somewhat uncomfortable in cognitively intact children; therefore, it is important to prepare them for what to expect.

A nebulized aerosol is always provided. This is typically normal saline, but hypertonic saline and bronchodilators may also be nebulized. A treatment usually lasts 10 to 15 minutes and often consists of stopping the treatment intermittently to allow coughing or suctioning. Treatment may consist of a gradual increase in pressure and frequency while others may maintain a high setting throughout the treatment. To reduce the risk of aspiration, tube feedings or meals should be held for one hour prior to therapy and the head of the bed should be at a minimum of 45 degrees.

Complications

Complications of IPV are often due to improper application. They include pneumothorax, hyperventilation, gastric insufflation, hemodynamic compromise, air trapping, and alveolar overdistention. The rapid positive pressure breaths may lead to a markedly reduced $PaCO_2$, which in turn may cause dizziness or may blunt

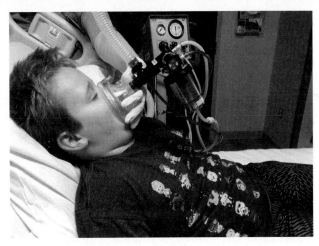

FIGURE 25-11 Child receiving intrapulmonary percussive ventilation (IPV).

the respiratory drive. The child should be observed for several minutes post therapy to assure that the respiratory drive is intact.

MetaNeb System

The MetaNeb System has three therapies in one: volume expansion, secretion clearance, and nebulized aerosol therapy. Using engineering similar to IPV, it provides continuous positive expiratory pressure (CPEP) to improve lung expansion and then immediately follows with continuous high-frequency oscillation (CHFO) to promote airway clearance. The system is powered using 50-pounds per square inch compressed gas and will provide supplemental oxygen if run off of compressed oxygen. Treatments usually consist of a 10-minute session with 4 alternating cycles of CPEP and CHFO. The nebulizer produces an aerosol throughout the treatment.

The MetaNeb System is indicated for use with children who have excessive secretion production, an inability to clear secretions, and inadequate lung expansion or clinically significant atelectasis. It can be used in spontaneously breathing patients as well as in those requiring mechanical ventilation.[13]

Cough Assistance Therapy

The goal of ACT is to mobilize secretions, which, to be effective, requires a strong cough. **Cough assistance therapy**, also referred to as mechanical **insufflation-exsufflation**, is beneficial for infants and children who have an ineffective or absent cough. This therapy consists of mechanical devices that simulate a cough. These devices provide positive pressure to inflate the lungs and at the end of inspiration quickly follow with a negative pressure. Therapies are given using a face mask or mouthpiece or the device is attached directly to an endotracheal or tracheostomy tube. The rapid switch from positive pressure to negative pressure

produces an expiratory flow that shears secretions from the airway walls and moves them to where they can be expectorated or suctioned. The fast, expiratory flow rate from the lungs simulates a natural cough.

Two commercial devices are currently available: the Hill-Rom VitalCough System and the Philips Respironics CoughAssist T70. They both function in about the same manner, having manual and automatic modes with positive and negative pressure controls. The VitalCough has the "PAP on Pause" feature that enables the clinician to dial in a CPAP of 1 to 15 cm H_2O that is active between machine breaths. This may be beneficial for patients who are positive end-expiratory pressure sensitive. The CoughAssist T70, which is known as the E70 outside the United States, includes the Cough-Trak feature that synchronizes with the patient's respiratory effort. This can be especially beneficial when using a mask interface. Both the E70 and the T70 may be used in an acute care or home care setting and have an external battery that is compatible with the company's Trilogy ventilator.

Indications and Contraindications

Children who will benefit most from cough assistance therapy are those with an ineffective cough or absent cough. This is often seen in neurodisabilities, such as muscular dystrophy, myasthenia gravis, and disorders with paralysis of the respiratory muscles as well as those with an artificial airway in place.[14] It is also indicated for the treatment of children in whom secretion removal is ineffective. This includes such conditions as bronchopulmonary dysplasia, cystic fibrosis, and bronchiectasis. Contraindications to cough assistance therapy are listed in **Table 25-9.**

Administration

In cough assistance therapy, a cough cycle is composed of an inspiratory phase, pause phase, and expiratory phase. Together, four to six cough cycles compose a sequence. Resting for 30 to 60 seconds between sequences allows time to expectorate secretions and to avoid hyperventilation. A total of four to six sequences with the resting periods are considered as one treatment. Treatments can be scheduled multiple times daily as well as on a PRN basis. **Box 25-5** provides information on administering therapy to an infant or child.

There are no established guidelines for setting the inspiratory and expiratory pressures; instead, they are set according to the child's condition, level of comfort, and therapeutic goals. It is recommended to begin the treatment with low positive and negative pressures, typically 10 to 15 cm H_2O for 1 to 2 seconds. As the child becomes more familiar with the therapy, the pressures can be gradually increased by 5 to 10 cm H_2O during each sequence. Pressures are adjusted to obtain good chest rise and secretion clearance. When an artificial airway

TABLE 25-9
Contraindications to Cough Assistance Therapy

Elevated intracranial pressure (>20 mm Hg)
Untreated or recent pneumothorax
Untreated or recent pneumomediastinum
Hemodynamic instability
Recent maxillofacial or skull surgery
Active hemoptysis
Bullous emphysema
Recent lobectomy
Known or suspected tympanic membrane rupture

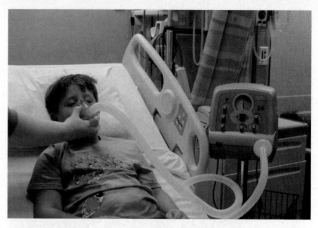

FIGURE 25-12 Child receiving cough assistance therapy with the Philips Respironics CA3200 CoughAssist device.

BOX 25-5 Administration of Cough Assistance Therapy

1. Explain the procedure to the child and family.
2. Assist the child into a sitting or semi-Fowler position.
3. Determine the interface needed—mask, mouthpiece, or connection to an artificial airway.
4. Adjust the settings: inspiratory and expiratory pressures, inhale and exhale times, and pause time.
5. Administer four to six breaths in a row. This is considered to be one cycle.
6. Remove the cough assistance device to allow time to pause and expectorate secretions. Encourage the child to cough. Provide suctioning if needed.
7. Allow a pause or rest period of at least 30 seconds to 1 minute for the child to recover.
8. Complete four to six more cycles (steps 5 through 7).
9. The treatment is complete when
   - 5 to 10 cycles have been completed;
   - secretions have been removed; or
   - the child is unable to tolerate further treatment.

with a cuff is in place, pressure may be better delivered if the cuff is inflated during the treatment. Higher pressures may be required when a mask is used. It is not uncommon to require pressures of 35 to 45 cm H_2O to be effective.

As with other forms of ACT, it is recommended that tube feedings and meals be held for 1 to 2 hours prior to therapy or to wait 1 hour following feedings before administering therapy. This will minimize the risk of vomiting and aspiration. Gastrostomy tubes may need to be vented before, during, or after a treatment.

Having negative pressure applied to the airway, along with a mask held tightly on a child's face, can be a frightening experience. Explaining therapy and demonstrating how the air feels can help alleviate some of the apprehension. It may help some children to know that the device will "push air into your chest" for a certain amount of time and then it will "pull it out of your chest" for a certain amount of time. Counting along with the in-and-out breaths helps some children better tolerate the treatment. The child in **Figure 25-12** is receiving cough assistance therapy with a mask.

Complications

Complications occurring with cough assistance therapy include barotrauma, tympanic membrane rupture, gastric insufflation with possible aspiration of gastric contents (especially with mask therapy), central airway collapse due to high exsufflation pressures, and loss of functional residual capacity following prolonged exsufflation times. Because this therapy delivers several repeated hyperinflation breaths, patients are at risk of hyperventilation or decreasing the respiratory drive.

Summary

ACT consists of various techniques, all with the purpose of removing secretions from the airways. The correct choice of therapy may be one that is cost effective and clinically relevant. Ultimately, however, the choice may come down to patient and/or family preference, which so often affects adherence and compliance at home. It is also important to note that the effectiveness of any lung expansion or airway clearance modality is dependent upon proper technique, especially in the pediatric population.

Case Study 1

A 22-month-old male with spinal muscular atrophy (SMA) type 1 presented to the pulmonary clinic in moderate to severe respiratory distress. His parent stated that he typically uses bilevel noninvasive ventilation (NIV) at night and during naps only. However, for the past 2 days he had "needed his BiPAP 24/7 and is unable to come off of it" due to respiratory distress. He was also receiving albuterol via small volume nebulizer and CPT every 4 hours. The child was admitted directly to the pediatric intensive care unit. Upon admission, a chest radiograph was ordered that revealed right upper lobe atelectasis and a right middle lobe opacification. The left lung was clear. It also showed a bell-shaped configuration of the thorax and ribs, which is typical for SMA 1. The inspiratory and expiratory pressures and breath rate for the NIV were increased. IPV was started with albuterol and hypertonic saline every 4 hours in addition to cough assist every 2 hours for airway secretion clearance. After 3 days, the child's X-ray showed mild improvement, but he still had atelectasis on the right. He continued to receive albuterol and cough assist treatments every 2 hours while alternating IPV and CPT every 4 hours. After 3 more days, the chest X-ray showed improvement in the atelectasis; he was able to be weaned from the increased NIV settings, and twice a day sprints were started. When he tolerated NIV settings close to his home regimen, albuterol and cough assist treatments were reduced to every 4 hours, and IPV and hypertonic saline were discontinued. On day 12 the patient was discharged home.

1. **Why is IPV indicated for this child?**
2. **Why were the NIV settings increased?**
3. **Why do most children with SMA need cough assistance therapy as part of their daily airway clearance regimen?**

Case Study 2

This patient is a 13-year-old, Caucasian, 8th-grade female with cystic fibrosis (CF). She was diagnosed with CF at 2 months of age, after newborn screening and genetic testing results confirmed the mutation. She has mild to moderate severity of disease, with a forced expiratory volume in 1 second (FEV_1) at 85% of predicted. She has been hospitalized 5 times in the last 10 years for pulmonary infections with *Pseudomonas aeruginosa*. She has not tested positive for methicillin-resistant *Staphylococcus aureus* or *Burkholderia cepacia*. She has missed approximately 6 school days this year due to CF. Her daily routine on school days includes waking up at 6 a.m., first taking her nebulized medications, which include a bronchodilator and a mucolytic agent. This is followed by her vest therapy, which takes approximately 45 minutes to adequately percuss every lung segment. This is usually interrupted by some coughing episodes, which may be prolonged, and she ends with a huff maneuver. The morning routine continues with eating breakfast and taking multiple medications that include a prophylactic antibiotic, nonsteroidal anti-inflammatory drug (NSAID), antihistamine agent, pancreatic enzymes, and vitamins. After school, her mother performs manual CPT with postural drainage. This therapy takes 45 minutes to 1 hour, during which time she may have several coughing episodes as well. She then relaxes and spends time with her family and friends. Before eating dinner she takes more medications, including NSAID, antibiotic, and pancreatic enzymes. Before bedtime she takes another nebulized bronchodilator treatment and follows that with the vest therapy for another 45 minutes while watching television.

1. **What is vest therapy?**
2. **Is there an alternative airway clearance device that could be used when the vest is not available?**
3. **What does postural drainage achieve for patients with cystic fibrosis?**

References

1. Michael S, Schechter MS. Airway clearance applications in infants and children. *Respir Care.* 2007;52:1382-1390.
2. Restrepo RD, Wettstein R, Wittnebel L, Tracy M. AARC Clinical Practice Guideline, Incentive Spirometry: 2011. *Respir Care.* 2011;56:1600-1604.
3. Yang M, Yan Y, Yin X, et al. Chest physiotherapy for pneumonia in adults. *Cochrane Database Syst Rev.* 2013;2:CD006338. doi:10.1002/14641858.CD006338.pub3.
4. Roqué I, Figuls M, Gine-Carriga M, et al. Chest physiotherapy for acute bronchiolitis in paediatric patients between 0 and 24 months old. *Cochrane Database Syst Rev.* 2012;2:CD004873. doi:10.1002/14651858.CD004873.pub4.
5. Button BM, Heine RG, Catto-Smith AG, et al. Postural drainage and gastro-esophageal reflux in infants with cystic fibrosis. *Arch Dis Child.* 1997;76:148-150.
6. Myers TR. Positive expiratory pressure and oscillatory positive expiratory pressure therapies. *Respir Care.* 2007;52:1308-1327.
7. Fink JB. Forced expiratory technique, directed cough, and autogenic drainage. *Respir Care.* 2007;52:1210-1223.
8. Chatburn RL. High-frequency assisted airway clearance. *Respir Care.* 2007;52:1224-1237.
9. Panitch HB. Respiratory implications of pediatric neuromuscular disease. *Respir Care.* 2017;62:826-848.
10. Reychler G, Keyeux A, Cremers C, et al. Comparison of lung deposition in two types of nebulization: intrapulmonary percussive ventilation vs jet nebulization. *Chest.* 2004;125:502-508.
11. Reychler G, Wallemacq P, Rodenstein DO, et al. Comparison of lung deposition of amikacin by intrapulmonary percussive ventilation and jet nebulization by urinary monitoring. *J Aerosol Med.* 2006;19:199-207.
12. Berlinski A, Willis RJ. Albuterol delivery via intrapulmonary percussive ventilator and jet nebulizer in a pediatric ventilator model. *Respir Care.* 2010;55:1699-1704.
13. Hill-Rom Services, Inc. *The MetaNeb System from Hill-Rom: User Manual.* Singapore: Hill-Rom; 2010.
14. Stehling F, Bouikidis A, Schara, U, Mellies U. Mechanical insufflations/exsufflation improves vital capacity in neuromuscular disorders. *Chronic Respir Dis.* 2015;12:31-35.

26

Mechanical Ventilation of the Neonate

Katherine L. Fedor

OUTLINE

OBJECTIVES

1. Describe the indications for noninvasive ventilation (NIV) and invasive ventilation.
2. List the contraindications for the use of NIV.
3. Describe the challenges to delivery of NIV.
4. Explain the importance of inspiratory positive airway pressure (IPAP), mandatory rate, expiratory positive airway pressure (EPAP), and inspiratory time in managing NIV.
5. Compare and contrast weaning strategies for continuous positive airway pressure (CPAP) and NIV.
6. Discuss the benefits of heated high-flow nasal cannula use.
7. Describe the strategies used to minimize complications associated with noninvasive and invasive mechanical ventilation.
8. List the factors that play a role in the development of ventilator-induced lung injury.
9. Differentiate among continuous mandatory ventilation (CMV), intermittent mandatory ventilation (IMV), and continuous spontaneous ventilation (CSV).
10. Describe the principles of operation for pressure support ventilation and neutrally adjusted ventilatory assist ventilation (NAVA).
11. Differentiate among pressure control, volume control, and volume targeted ventilation.
12. Explain the strategies used to minimize asynchrony.
13. Describe the operating principles for high-frequency oscillatory ventilation (HFOV) and high-frequency jet ventilation (HFJV).
14. Discuss the ventilator management strategies for HFOV and HFJV.
15. Describe the goals for mechanically ventilating infants with ductal dependent cardiac lesions.

KEY TERMS

atelectotrauma
biphasic positive pressure
bronchopulmonary
    dysplasia (BPD)
continuous mandatory
    ventilation (CMV)
continuous positive airway
    pressure (CPAP)
continuous spontaneous
    ventilation (CSV)
cycle time
demand flow
expiratory positive airway
    pressure (EPAP)
flow cycling
flow-triggered breath
heated high-flow nasal
    cannula (HHFNC)
high-frequency jet
    ventilation (HFJV)
high-frequency oscillatory
    ventilation (HFOV)
inspiratory positive airway
    pressure (IPAP)
intermittent mandatory
    ventilation (IMV)

machine-triggered
neutrally adjusted
    ventilatory assist
    ventilation (NAVA)
noninvasive ventilation (NIV)
patient-triggered
positive end-expiratory
    pressure (PEEP)
pressure control
    ventilation (PCV)
pressure support
    ventilation (PSV)
pressure-triggered breath
rise time
synchronized intermittent
    mandatory ventilation
    (SIMV)
trigger sensitivity
volume control
    ventilation (VCV)
volume targeted
    ventilation (VTV)
volutrauma

Introduction

Mechanical ventilation of the neonate can be extremely complicated. Differences in chest wall compliance, airway resistance, and pulmonary and circulatory pathophysiology affect the neonatal lung and present unique challenges in the overall approach to ventilatory support. It is important to understand the effects of positive pressure ventilation on pulmonary, systemic, and cerebral perfusion to maximize ventilation and minimize complications.

Medical advances and improved functionality of mechanical ventilators have contributed to improved neonatal outcomes over the past three decades, but much work remains. This chapter outlines the indications and goals for invasive and noninvasive mechanical ventilation of the neonate, including neonatal assessments, monitoring, and blood gas management. It will also review conventional modes of mechanical ventilation as well as nonconventional modes, such as high-frequency oscillatory ventilation and high-frequency jet ventilation. Complications specifically related to mechanical ventilation of the neonate are also included.

Noninvasive Ventilation

Noninvasive ventilation is used to treat acute and chronic conditions in neonates with impaired lung inflation and gas exchange. **Noninvasive ventilation (NIV)** refers to the delivery of intermittent or continuous assisted ventilation or to providing continuous positive pressure during spontaneous breathing to enhance lung expansion by restoring or improving functional residual capacity (FRC) and/or improving minute ventilation without the use of an artificial airway. Noninvasive ventilation is most commonly provided in the form of **continuous positive airway pressure (CPAP)**. CPAP does not provide assisted ventilation. This is a spontaneous mode of ventilation that enhances oxygenation and preserves lung inflation by improving the FRC. **Biphasic positive pressure** is also commonly used in neonates. Biphasic positive pressure, also known simply as NIV, improves ventilation and provides ventilatory support to the infant by delivering positive pressure during inspiration and **positive end-expiratory pressure (PEEP)** to improve minute ventilation.

CPAP

CPAP was first used in the early 1970s to treat respiratory distress syndrome (RDS) associated with prematurity. CPAP is administered by nasal prongs or nasal mask that provides an adequate distending pressure, which subsequently results in expansion and stabilization of collapsed alveoli secondary to surfactant deficiency.[1]

Infants with respiratory distress have heterogeneous lung disease. Lack of surfactant causes repeated collapse and reexpansion of the ventilating lung units, also known as **atelectotrauma**. Administering CPAP restores FRC by applying continuous positive pressure to the lung units during spontaneous breathing.[2] CPAP reduces the work of breathing by decreasing the amount of energy required to overcome alveolar opening pressure. Because CPAP does not provide ventilatory support, infants receiving CPAP must have an adequate neurologic drive to breathe.

Assisting Ventilation with the Use of NIV

NIV provides positive pressure, above the distending pressure, during inspiration to further reduce the work of breathing and to augment ventilation. NIV is indicated in neonates with respiratory insufficiency as evidenced by CO_2 retention. The interfaces required for NIV mirror those used for CPAP. Because NIV provides ventilatory support, the devices used to deliver NIV often differ from those used to deliver CPAP. NIV provides assisted ventilation, and so any uneven distribution of ventilation can potentially lead to regional overdistention of the lungs, or **volutrauma**, which must be avoided in all modalities of positive pressure ventilation.[3]

Indications and Goals

Table 26-1 outlines the common indications for the use of CPAP and NIV. The goals of therapy for preterm infants with surfactant deficiency are to increase FRC, decrease the work of breathing, improve pulmonary compliance, and improve the ventilation-to-perfusion ratio to enhance gas exchange.

TABLE 26-1
Indications for Neonatal CPAP and NIV

Indications	Modality
Delivery room management associated with alveolar recruitment	CPAP* or NIV**
Respiratory distress syndrome (prematurity)	CPAP* or NIV**
Apnea of prematurity	CPAP* or NIV**
Postextubation	CPAP* or NIV**
Hypotonia with respiratory depression and insufficiency	CPAP* or NIV**
Conditions associated with loss of lung volume, such as transient tachypnea of the neonate (TTN)	CPAP * or NIV **
Obstructive airway diseases	CPAP*

*Must have adequate respiratory drive to sustain adequate gas exchange
**Indicated when respiratory drive is insufficient to provide adequate gas exchange

Data from Mahmoud RA, Roehr CC, Schmalisch G. Current methods of non-invasive ventilatory support for neonates. *Paediatr Respir Rev.* 2011;12(3):196-205; and Fedor KL. Noninvasive respiratory support in infants and children. *Respir Care.* 2017;62(6):699-717.

Contraindications

Contraindications for the use of NIV in the neonatal patient include the following medical conditions or treatment failures associated with respiratory failure:[4]

- CPAP or NIV failure
  - $PaCO_2$ >65 mm Hg
  - pH <7.25
  - Frequent and severe apneas
- Congenital diaphragmatic hernia (CDH), unrepaired
  - Gastric insufflation
- Tracheoesophageal fistula (TE fistula)
- Cranial facial abnormalities
  - Prevents interface application
- Neuromuscular disorders associated with severe respiratory depression
- Untreated pneumothorax

Interfaces

Limitations associated with successful application and use of CPAP or NIV can be attributed to the patient interfaces, delivery devices, and available technology. Interfaces include nasal prongs, nasal masks, extended nasal prongs, or nasal pharyngeal tubes. The primary patient interfaces most often used in neonates are nasal prongs and nasal masks. Both nasal prongs and nasal masks are associated with system leaks, which may necessitate the use of a chin strap to maximize positive pressure delivery. The recent popularity of the RAM cannula poses an added delivery challenge. This is a nonocclusive nasal cannula interface, and when used to deliver CPAP, may limit the pressure delivered to the infant.[5] Additionally, its performance will not be significantly impacted by the use of a chin strap because the chin strap minimizes a leak only at the mouth. Because this device is noninclusive, it is difficult to control for the leaks around the nares. The presence of leaks with this or any interface will negatively affect the triggering capabilities, which are exaggerated by the neonate's inability to generate measurable inspiratory flow through the delivery system. **Table 26-2** provides a small sample of common neonatal interfaces used to deliver CPAP or NIV.

Delivery Devices

There are several stand-alone devices capable of delivering CPAP to neonatal patients. These neonatal devices are generally limited for use in patients weighing less than 5 kg. NIV may be delivered through a single stand-alone device or through the various intensive care unit (ICU) ventilators currently on the market.

Challenges

The biggest logistic clinical limitation related to the application of NIV in neonates is the ability to synchronize breath delivery to the patient. The combination of the device and interface used impacts the ability to synchronize the mechanical breath with an infant's inspiratory effort. Leaks in the system, often due to the type of interface used, reduce the ability of the device to detect inspiratory efforts. The device used to deliver NIV can contribute to triggering inefficiencies as well. If the device senses inspiratory effort at the patient wye (through the use of a flow sensor), synchronization is more likely to occur because the device can sense the small inspiratory efforts (or changes in pressure that occur during inspiration). The device is less likely to synchronize mechanical breaths with the patient's spontaneous efforts when the trigger mechanism is located within the device.

Flow delivery is a challenge during CPAP and NIV. Flow can be either continuous or demand. Continuous flow delivery provides an operator-set amount of flow during inspiration and expiration. Setting continuous flow can be challenging. If the flow is set too high, the patient will breathe against the resistance of the set flow provided by the ventilator or CPAP device, and work of breathing would increase.[6] When continuous flow is set too low, there is an insufficient flow of gas to the patient, which impairs CO_2 removal.

Demand flow is a feature that allows the patient to access additional flow of gas during inspiration. Triggering demand flow can also be problematic for the neonatal patient during CPAP and NIV delivery. Difficulty with triggering demand flow is a combination of several factors, including physiologic (infants have very small tidal volumes and weak respiratory muscle strength)

TABLE 26-2
A Small Sample of Common Neonatal Interfaces Used to Deliver CPAP or NIV

Manufacturer	Interface	Use	Illustration
Inca	Neonatal infant prongs	CPAP, NIV	
Hudson RCI	Neonatal infant prongs	CPAP, NIV	
Neotech	RAM cannulas	CPAP, NIV—Dual-limb circuits (mechanical ventilators)	
Fisher and Paykel	Neonatal infant prongs or mask	CPAP, NIV	

and equipment-related (variable leaks in the patient/ventilator circuit related to the fit of the interface) issues. Triggering capabilities improve as leaks are minimized. Adjuncts, such as chin straps and nasal prong–occluding devices, may help to reduce leaks and improve triggering performance. Some CPAP devices offer flow-variable, pressure-constant features to accommodate for variable system leaks, which will help to maintain a constant distending pressure and to meet patient flow demands. The ability or inability to trigger will influence how NIV is managed and must be evaluated on an individual basis.

There are patient safety factors to consider during the administration of NIV. Interfaces, including patient headgear, have the potential to cause skin ulcerations. Skin barriers help to protect the fragile skin of preterm and newborn infants. Use of a variety of interfaces, such as switching at regular intervals between prongs and masks, helps distribute the pressure of the interface to different points on the infant's face. It is important to evaluate the integrity of the skin when performing a patient ventilator assessment or check. Any redness or breakdown should be immediately evaluated by a clinician skilled in staging skin wounds. Because positive pressure is not applied to the lungs through an artificial airway, there is the risk of gastric insufflation, and because the airway is not protected during NIV, there is the risk of aspiration.

During NIV the delivered tidal volume will be influenced by the difference between the **inspiratory positive airway pressure (IPAP)** and the **expiratory positive airway pressure (EPAP)** settings, so clinical indicators should be used to evaluate the effectiveness of breath delivery. Clinical indicators of adequate tidal volume include assessment of chest rise, breath sounds, noninvasive assessment of oxygenation (pulse oximetry) and carbon dioxide (end-tidal or transcutaneous CO_2), and the level of consciousness. Ultimately, adequate evaluation of ventilation may require blood gas analysis.

Management of the Patient

It is important to keep the goals of therapy in mind when determining and implementing the respiratory plan of care. The goal of CPAP is to restore or improve FRC and to correct or prevent alveolar collapse. CPAP will effectively reduce the work of breathing as it unloads inspiratory muscles and provides an inflation pressure in excess of the opening pressure of the lungs.[7] Generally, CPAP levels of 5 to 8 cm H_2O will accomplish these goals. Because CPAP does not provide ventilatory assistance, it should only be used on patients with an adequate respiratory drive. CPAP pressures should be incrementally increased to achieve the targeted oxygen saturation goal (set by the provider, using criteria to

minimize retinopathy of prematurity) at a FiO_2 of less than 0.50 to 0.60.

The characteristics of CPAP devices often influence patient management. CPAP devices are pressure constant, flow variable, flow constant, or pressure variable. Pressure-constant delivery devices are preferred to sustain lung recruitment by preventing intermittent alveolar collapse. When adequate CPAP levels are achieved, the work of breathing should improve as evidenced by a decreased respiratory rate, fewer sternal or intercostal retractions, and improved oxygen saturations with the ability to wean the FiO_2.

When NIV is indicated, the clinician must determine the appropriate mode of ventilation to use. Traditional neonatal NIV devices are time cycled and pressure limited. These devices deliver a preset pressure at a preset rate with the ability to trigger additional breaths as needed, provided that patient triggering can be detected. This mode can lead to asynchrony when patient breathing efforts are undetectable, causing the delivery of a mandatory breath after the initiation of spontaneous effort (i.e., at mid-inspiration or during exhalation).

It takes time and patience to initiate NIV. It is very important to select the patient interface that minimizes the propensity for large leaks, which will maximize the infant's ability to trigger demand flow and a mechanical breath. It is equally important to ensure that the interface and headgear do not fit so snugly that skin breakdown can occur. The mandatory or operator-set respiratory rate will depend on patient need and is guided by noninvasive CO_2 monitoring and/or blood gases to determine the level of support needed to achieve and maintain adequate ventilation. The EPAP setting provides a resting distending pressure level that prevents alveolar collapse and should be increased if evidence of lung volume loss is present. The EPAP setting has a direct relationship with oxygenation and should be titrated based on oxygen saturation. When the FiO_2 has been minimized (≤ 0.40), EPAP settings should not exceed 7 to 8 cm H_2O.

IPAP is the positive airway pressure delivered to the lungs during inspiration. IPAP is applied above EPAP and directly controls volume delivery to the patient. There is a linear relationship between pressure and volume: the higher the IPAP setting, the larger the volume delivery. The IPAP setting should be titrated to achieve adequate chest expansion and CO_2 removal.

Inspiratory time determines the length of time inspiration occurs, or the time that inspiratory pressure is delivered to the lungs. Inspiratory time should be sufficient for breath delivery (typically 0.3–0.6 seconds). Excessively long inspiratory times will be uncomfortable for patients and may increase the work of breathing if patients are forced to exhale against inspiratory flow.

There are other parameters available on the ICU ventilators, specifically trigger sensitivity, rise time, and cycle time, that enable the respiratory therapist to improve breath synchrony. The **trigger sensitivity** should be set so that the patient can easily trigger a spontaneous or assisted breath. Variable leaks, which inherently occur during NIV, make it difficult to set the sensitivity. Sensitivity should be evaluated when the patient is repositioned or when adjusting or changing to a different interface. The aforementioned changes impact the amount of leak that occurs around the interface, which affects the ease with which the patient can trigger a mechanical breath or access additional or demand flow. A sensitivity level that is set too low will cause auto-triggering to occur, which places the patient at risk for hyperventilation. A trigger sensitivity that is not set high enough will prevent the device from sensing a patient's inspiratory efforts, contributing to patient ventilatory asynchrony and the risk for barotrauma. This will also reduce the patient's ability to trigger the demand flow.

The **rise time** reflects how aggressive inspiratory flow is delivered. Rise time should be set to meet the patient's inspiratory demands and to maximize comfort. The **cycle time** setting determines the transition period from inhalation to exhalation and may be flow or time based. In the presence of large system leaks, the cycle setting alters the threshold for transition to exhalation, which can enhance breath synchrony.

Safety Considerations

Alarms or patient safety features are incorporated into devices that deliver NIV. It is essential to set ventilator alarms appropriately. High tidal volume and high respiratory rate alarms should be set 20% to 30% above the respective ventilator setting. High-pressure alarms should be set at 5 to 10 cm H_2O above IPAP levels. The low-pressure alarm should be set above the EPAP setting but below the IPAP setting. Apnea times should be set at approximately 10 seconds for neonates but may be lower if patients have periodic apneas resulting in desaturation. Backup ventilation settings (if available) should mirror full ventilatory support.

Weaning and Liberation from CPAP and NIV

Weaning CPAP support should commence when there is resolution of the disease process requiring the use of CPAP. Initially, the FiO_2 should be weaned to ≤0.40. Once at a minimal level, the CPAP levels can be weaned. When CPAP is indicated to treat acute lung disease, FiO_2 and CPAP levels should be weaned as tolerated to maintain a predetermined oxygenation goal. Clinical (oxygenation, ventilation, vital signs, breath sounds, and work of breathing) and diagnostic (chest radiograph) indicators should be evaluated to determine the resolution of disease process and readiness for weaning. CPAP can be discontinued when the patient has been stable on a level of 5 cm H_2O with an FiO_2 of less than or equal to 40%.

Weaning a patient from noninvasive ventilatory support is a more complicated process. System leaks have a bigger impact on the weaning strategy and must be considered when developing the individualized plan of care. When patients can trigger a breath, the approach is similar to that used for weaning from invasive ventilation. However, when significant or large leaks are present and patients are unable to trigger spontaneous or assisted breaths, their spontaneous breaths are not supported. In this case, a traditional weaning strategy of incrementally reducing the mandatory respiratory rate is used. Weaning the mandatory rate shifts more work to the patient because it increases the number of breaths that are not supported by the set inspiratory pressure. The clinician must assess the patient frequently and monitor the infant's response as the mandatory rate is reduced. Weaning the mandatory rate can dramatically increase the work of breathing for patients with limited reserves, who may not tolerate this strategy.

When gradually reducing the mandatory rate is not tolerated, an alternate approach would be to set the mandatory rate at a physiologic level (normal respiratory rate for the infant or neonate according to adjusted gestational age) and gradually wean the IPAP setting until the IPAP and EPAP settings are nearly equal. This approach offers a more gradual shift of the respiratory muscle work.

Weaning is still very much an art. There is a need for more research before evidence-based recommendations can be made. Clinicians should always evaluate the efficiency of the current strategies and adjust as needed.

Heated High-Flow Nasal Cannula

Recent popularity and widespread use of the **heated high-flow nasal cannula (HHFNC)** have led to inclusion of this modality in the NIV discussion. The definition of high flow is not universally accepted, but flow rates of greater than 1 L/minute are generally considered high flow in the neonatal patient.[8] The assumed benefits of HHFNCs are realized from maximum mucociliary clearance, reduced inflammatory reactions, inhibition of bronchoconstrictor reflex, reduced airway resistance, and washout of the nasopharyngeal dead space.[9] The evidence for positive pressure delivery with HHFNCs is mixed and highly variable. The literature reports the limited utility of an HHFNC as efficacious and safe to use as nasal CPAP when applied immediately postextubation or early as initial noninvasive support for respiratory dysfunction.[10] However, in a systematic review evaluating the quality of available published evidence, there is a lack of convincing evidence suggesting that HHFNC is superior or inferior to usual care, especially when compared to nasal CPAP.[11] There is also uncertainty regarding whether HHFNC can be considered cost effective.[11] There are a few different delivery devices that can be used, all of which allow the FiO_2 to be easily adjusted between 0.21 and 1.0 in order to achieve patient-specific oxygenation goals.

Monitoring during NIV

Monitoring of patients on CPAP and NIV should include pulse oximetry with saturation targets that are patient specific and reflect the acuity of the disease process. Pulse oximetry is a good indicator of oxygenation status; however, it is of little value in evaluating the patient's ventilation status. Assessing the adequacy of ventilation must include a periodic evaluation of CO_2 measurement. Carbon dioxide measurements can be obtained noninvasively with transcutaneous monitoring or invasively by arterial, venous, or capillary blood gas analysis. Carbon dioxide targets will be disease specific, with a goal to normalize or achieve a compensated acid–base status. Evaluating the infant's work of breathing and the level of consciousness can also provide valuable clinical information on the overall effectiveness of NIV. It is helpful to have a clear picture of the patient's baseline clinical status when evaluating the effectiveness of treatment.

Chest radiographs can provide useful diagnostic information if clinical symptoms are present, will be a useful tool in evaluating the adequacy of lung inflation, and may also provide useful information regarding disease progression.

Invasive Mechanical Ventilation

The use of an artificial airway (i.e., endotracheal tube, tracheostomy tube) is required to provide continuous or intermittent invasive mechanical ventilatory support.

Indications and Goals

There are many physiologic and clinical indications for mechanical ventilation of the neonate. Primary indications include the presence of respiratory failure but can also be related to a number of clinical indications, which are outlined in **Box 26-1**.

The goals of mechanical ventilation will be patient specific and include the ability to maintain or maximize FRC by applying PEEP and to achieve and maintain adequate oxygenation and ventilation. The patient's diagnosis, disease state, and response to therapeutic intervention are considered when developing a ventilation management strategy. The strategy used should also minimize harm by aiming to reduce ventilator-induced lung injury (VILI) and ventilator-associated events (VAEs).

Neonatal conditions often change rapidly; therefore, frequent assessments are required. The mechanical ventilation plan of care should be reviewed frequently as well, allowing the patient's condition and response to ventilator parameter changes to influence decisions to modify the plan of care. Modification to the plan of care may include more frequent assessment of the patency of the artificial airway, change in the position of the artificial airway, change in patient positioning to enhance oxygenation, administration of surfactant due to changes in pulmonary compliance, or initiation of a different mode of ventilation because of the development of air leaks.

BOX 26-1 Indications for Mechanical Ventilation of the Neonate

Restrictive Disorders
- RDS associated with prematurity and surfactant deficiency
- Pulmonary hypoplasia
- Congenital pneumonia
- Pleural effusions (e.g., chylothorax, hydrops)
- Congenital diaphragmatic hernia
- Congenital pulmonary cysts (CPAM)
- Rib cage anomalies (achondroplasia)

Obstructive Disorders
- MAS (meconium aspiration syndrome)
- Pulmonary sequestration
- BPD (bronchopulmonary dysplasia)

Neurologic
- Hypotonia syndromes (central hypoventilation syndrome, mitochondrial disorders, congenital neuromuscular disorders)
- Apnea associated with intraventricular hemorrhages or intracranial hemorrhages
- Hypoxic ischemic encephalitis
- Neonatal seizure disorders

Airway Disorders
- Congenital tracheomalacia
- Choanal atresia
- Pierre Robin syndrome
- Congenital subglottic stenosis
- Nasopharyngeal tumors

Surgical
- Abdominal wall defects (omphalocele, gastroschisis)
- Neuro-tube defects (spina bifida, myelomeningocele, etc.)

Cardiovascular
- Congenital cardiomyopathy
- Congenital cardiac defects associated with intracardiac shunting requiring balanced circulation
- Apnea secondary to prostoglanin E (PGE) administration
- Sepsis resulting in cardiovascular compromise
- Primary pulmonary hypertension of the newborn

Strategies for Preventing Lung Injury

The unique characteristics of the preterm neonatal lung and the routine resuscitation of extremely low birthweight (ELBW) neonates have resulted in many randomized controlled studies designed to address strategies targeted at reducing VILI. Most of these strategies have explored the effects of different strategies of ventilation on long-term outcomes.

Ventilator strategies used to prevent lung injury in neonatal patients involve measures that reduce the need for positive pressure ventilation and supplemental oxygen delivery. This includes surfactant replacement, application of lung-protective ventilation strategies, and other pharmacologic and nonpharmacologic interventions.[12]

The strongest evidence for the prevention or reduction of lung injury is centered on surfactant administration with early and adequate lung recruitment, adequate oxygenation (SpO$_2$ of 90–95%), permissive hypercapnia (PaCO$_2$ of 45–55 mm Hg, pH >7.2), and gentle ventilation.[12] Studies have demonstrated that prophylactic surfactant replacement has been shown to reduce the rate of BPD by reducing the need for and duration of intubation and mechanical ventilation, especially in ELBW infants.[13] Approaches using surfactant administration, early extubation, and initiation of NIV show promising results in reducing the incidence of acute lung injury and development of BPD. Specifically, the incidence of BPD and air leak syndromes was lower with the INtubation SURfactant Extubation (INSURE) approach.[14] Expanded studies comparing synchronized intermittent mandatory ventilation and early extubation to nasal CPAP or NIV compared to the INSURE approach indicate that the INSURE approach lowered the incidence of BPD.[14]

In animal studies, the most important risk factors for VILI are the use of high tidal volumes, which result in overdistension of the alveoli (volutrauma), and inadequate PEEP, which causes atelectasis.[15] The use of inadequate PEEP results in atelectasis because gas flow is diverted to the open regions of the lung, which leads to regional overdistension and heterogeneous lung disease because of repetitive opening and collapse of unstable lung units (atelectictrauma).[15] The literature recommends limiting the delivered tidal volume (V$_T$) to 4 to 7 mL/kg, but limiting the V$_T$ can still result in overdistension if significant atelectasis persists and gas flow enters more compliant lung regions; therefore, optimal PEEP levels should be continually evaluated.[15]

Physiologic Challenges Influencing Mechanical Ventilation of the Preterm Infant

Respiratory distress syndrome (RDS) affects 60% to 80% of infants born at less than 28 weeks' gestation. In 1959, Avery and Mead established that the primary etiology of RDS was the lack of pulmonary surfactant.[16] The lack of pulmonary surfactant leads to a decreased FRC

TABLE 26-3
Classification of BPD

Classification	Days on Supplemental Oxygen	Oxygen Requirement at 36 Weeks Corrected Gestational Age
Mild	Required 28 days of supplemental oxygen	No oxygen requirement at 36 weeks' corrected gestational age or at discharge
Moderate	Required 28 days of supplemental oxygen	Oxygen requirement of ≤0.30 at 36 weeks' corrected gestational age or at discharge
Severe	Required 28 days of supplemental oxygen	Oxygen requirement of ≥0.30 at 36 weeks' corrected gestational age or at discharge

with widespread atelectasis and decreased pulmonary compliance, both of which contribute to ventilation/perfusion mismatch. These physiologic changes contribute to progressive hypoxia, hypercarbia, and acidosis. The interventions required to overcome the physiologic effects of RDS often lead to the development of **bronchopulmonary dysplasia (BPD)**, a chronic lung condition that is quantified as mild, moderate, or severe. **Table 26-3** outlines the classification criteria for BPD.[17]

In the preterm infant, a highly compliant state of the chest wall and the presence of low pulmonary compliance contribute significantly to the susceptibility of VILI and VAE. The high compliance of the chest wall is attributable to the cartilaginous structure of the rib cage. Poor pulmonary compliance is related to the lack of surfactant in the lung. Together these factors comprise the respiratory system compliance.[18] Additionally, immature alveolarization, dynamic elastic recoil, high airway resistance, and poor collateral ventilation are contributing factors that play a role in the development of VILI in the vulnerable neonatal lung.[18]

The prevention of premature birth is the best defense against RDS, but it is not always possible to avoid a preterm delivery. When preterm delivery is anticipated and cannot be avoided, antenatal steroids should be administered when the mother presents in labor between 24 and 34 weeks' gestation.[19] Treatment with betamethasone or dexamethasone should be administered 24 to 48 hours prior to delivery whenever possible, although treatment at less than 24 hours prior to delivery has also been shown to be beneficial.[19]

Management of the Patient

Permissive hypercapnia is a strategy that allows PaCO$_2$ levels to rise between 45 and 55 mm Hg while maintaining a pH of >7.20. It is widely believed that a higher CO$_2$ tolerance will lead to a decreased need for positive pressure ventilation and therefore lower the rates of BPD and VILI.[20] The concept of permissive hypercapnia can be applied to a variety of ventilator modes and breath delivery modalities. It must be noted that permissive hypercapnia may not be indicated for patients with primary pulmonary hypertension and that excessive hypercapnia can increase the incidence of neurodevelopmental impairment.[20] Adequate oxygenation is important for neurodevelopment and end-organ perfusion; however, excessive levels of oxygen have been associated with the development of retinopathy of prematurity (ROP)[21] and systemic inflammatory responses resulting in pulmonary complications.

Modes of Ventilation

A challenge to describing modes of ventilation is that no industry-standard naming convention exists. As a consequence, manufacturers give unique names to modes that may be identical and similar or nearly identical names to modes that function very differently. A mechanical ventilator assists breathing by controlling the breath sequence and the pressure or volume waveform.

Breath Sequence

Breath sequence describes the mechanism for breath delivery. There are two categories of breath: mandatory, or breaths that are delivered at a preset frequency by the ventilator, and spontaneous, or breaths that are not controlled by the ventilator. Spontaneous breaths are initiated (the patient's own breathing effort) and controlled (tidal volume and frequency) by the patient. Breath delivery can be terminated by time, pressure, volume, or flow. All modes of breath delivery have primary and secondary termination criteria.

Continuous Mandatory Ventilation (CMV)

Continuous mandatory ventilation (CMV), commonly referred to as assist control (AC), provides a fully supported or mandatory breath. The breath can be **patient-triggered** (the patient has an inspiratory effort that starts or initiates a mandatory breath) or **machine-triggered** (a breath initiates after a preset time elapses). All patient-triggered or machine-triggered breaths are delivered at preset parameters. This mode of ventilation may reduce the imposed work of breathing for the patient because each breath is maximally supported.

Synchronized Intermittent Mandatory Ventilation (SIMV)

Synchronized intermittent mandatory ventilation (SIMV) provides a preset number of mandatory breaths and allows the patient to take a spontaneous breath between the mandatory breaths. Spontaneous breaths can be unsupported or augmented with the addition of pressure support. Similar to CMV (or AC), the mandatory breaths can be machine- or patient-triggered. SIMV may allow patients to have better overall control of ventilation by allowing the patient to bear a portion of the work of breathing.

Variable leaks, inherent when uncuffed endotracheal tubes are used, may interfere with the ventilator's ability to sense patient triggering. When this happens, breath synchronization may not occur and **intermittent mandatory ventilation (IMV)** is delivered. IMV is SIMV without the synchronization. The common variations of SIMV or IMV are as follows: mandatory breaths are always delivered at an operator-set frequency, and mandatory breaths are only delivered when the patient's spontaneous respiratory rate falls below an operator-set threshold (i.e., the patient's respiratory rate is less than 30 breaths per minute). Most clinicians are very comfortable with this mode of ventilation and the ability to successfully wean ventilatory support by reducing the mandatory breath rate, set inspiratory pressure, or tidal volume.

Continuous Spontaneous Ventilation

The ability to spontaneously ventilate promotes diaphragmatic activity and lessens the propensity for diaphragm atrophy. **Continuous spontaneous ventilation (CSV)** modes used for neonatal patients include pressure support ventilation and neutrally adjusted ventilatory assist ventilation (NAVA). **Pressure support ventilation (PSV)** is a spontaneous mode of ventilation in which breaths are supported by an operator-set pressure target. The breath can be initiated by pressure or flow triggering. A **flow-triggered breath** occurs when the patient generates enough inspiratory effort (above a threshold or sensitivity setting) to start a flow of gas to the patient. Once a breath is triggered, gas flow and pressure are delivered to the patient until a preset pressure target is reached. Typically, the breath ends when flow decays to a predetermined setting, also known as **flow cycling**.

NAVA

Neutrally adjusted ventilatory assist ventilation (NAVA) is the name of a spontaneous mode of ventilation that is available on the Servo-I and Servo-U ventilators (Maquet, Rastatt, Germany). Similar to pressure support, the patient's own respiratory drive controls the rate of ventilation. This spontaneous mode of ventilation uses an orogastric catheter embedded with special sensors that detect electronic signals from the phrenic nerve to the diaphragm, sensing diaphragmatic contraction. These signals are used to synchronize the delivery of flow and preset pressure to the patient. The breath ends when the sensors embedded in the orogastric catheter sense diaphragmatic relaxation. These signals are transmitted to, and interface with, the ventilator to control flow delivery during the inspiratory phase of ventilation. When the diaphragm relaxes, flow ceases and the patient is permitted to exhale. Responsiveness of the ventilator is more effective because it is based on diaphragm contractility as opposed to flow requirements detected at the ventilator. Diaphragm activity is controlled by impulses sent to the phrenic nerve and is a true reflection of patient demand based on native neurologic responses. The NAVA level controls the amount of ventilator assist that is provided to the patient. The performance of the ventilator and delivery of flow while the patient is in NAVA is unaffected by leaks associated with endotracheal tubes. NAVA has been shown to improve patient synchrony, which may minimize patient work of breathing. **Figure 26-1** outlines the patient–ventilator interactions when using this proprietary spontaneous mode of ventilation.

NAVA can be used invasively or noninvasively. During invasive NAVA, there are safety backup ventilation features that ensure that the infant receives mechanical ventilatory support if the diaphragm catheter signal is lost or if the patient becomes apneic. If the diaphragm signal is lost, the patient receives pressure support ventilation. Should the patient become apneic or the ventilator unable to detect sufficient spontaneous effort to trigger a pressure-supported breath, a mechanism for backup ventilation is provided. Both pressure support and backup ventilation are determined by and have parameters set by the clinician. Pressure support and backup ventilation are available in invasive and noninvasive NAVA. Backup ventilation allows for full ventilatory support if all patient breathing efforts were

to cease. Terminology used for this proprietary mode of ventilation can be found in **Table 26-4**.

There are several steps required to prepare for the initiation of NAVA. The procedure for initiating this mode of ventilation is found in **Table 26-5**. Because a special orogastric catheter is needed to detect diaphragmatic signals, selecting the appropriate-size catheter is important. Catheter size is dependent on the patient's height and weight; a sizing chart can be found in **Table 26-6**. Once the clinician selects the correct catheter size, depth of insertion must be calculated to place the catheter in the location to detect a strong signal. **Table 26-7** provides guidelines for determining the catheter insertion depth. Once the catheter is inserted to the premeasured depth, ventilator graphics are used to adjust the catheter position. The graphics used to adjust the catheter position can be accessed through the NAVA menu, after which there is a selection softkey for Edi catheter positioning (**Figure 26-2**).

When initiating NAVA, the NAVA level can be determined by accessing the NAVA preview screen, which

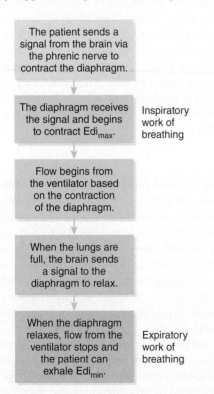

FIGURE 26-1 Patient–ventilator interaction during mechanical ventilation with NAVA.

TABLE 26-4
NAVA Terminology

NAVA level	The NAVA level is the overall level of support provided to the patient (higher levels indicate more ventilator assist).
Edi peak	This is an indication of the inspiratory work of breathing and indicates the contractility or energy expenditure of the diaphragm.
Edi min	This is an indication of the expiratory work of breathing and indicates the effectiveness of PEEP and the relaxation state of the diaphragm.
Trigger Edi	This is indicative of the amount of diaphragm exertion required to initiate a response from the ventilator.

TABLE 26-5
Procedure for the Initiation of NAVA

1. Place the NAVA module with cable into the designated slot on the side of the Servo I.

2. Select the appropriate Edi catheter (based on the size of the patient—6 Fr, 8 Fr, 12 Fr, and 16 Fr sizes are available—as outlined in Table 26-6).

3. Dip the end of the catheter into some sterile water or pour sterile water into the catheter tray prior to insertion (careful not to wet the cable connectors); do not use lubricant on the catheter. Wetting the catheter helps to activate the sensors within the catheter.

4. Insert the catheter to the premeasured depth (see NEX, Table 26-7) and plug into the NAVA cable.

5. Access the NAVA menu by depressing the NAVA softkey, then select Edi catheter positioning to determine catheter placement (Figure 26-5).

TABLE 26-6
NAVA Catheter Size

Edi Catheter Size	Inner Electrode Distance	Patient Weight	Patient Height
16 Fr: 125 cm	16 mm	–	>140 cm
12 Fr: 125 cm	12 mm	–	75–160 cm
8 Fr: 125 cm	16 mm	–	>140 cm
8 Fr: 100 cm	8 mm	–	45–85 cm
6 Fr: 50 cm	6 mm	1.0–2.0 kg	<55 cm
6 Fr: 49 cm	6 mm	0.5–1.5 kg	<55 cm

TABLE 26-7
Calculations Used to Estimate Nasal Catheter Insertion Distance

Size Fr/cm	Calculation
16 Fr	NEX (cm) × 0.9 + 18 = Y (at the nose)
12 Fr	NEX (cm) × 0.9 + 15 = Y (at the nose)
8 Fr: 125 cm	NEX (cm) × 0.9 + 18 = Y (at the nose)
8 Fr: 100 cm	NEX (cm) × 0.9 + 8 = Y (at the nose)
6 Fr: 50 cm	NEX (cm) × 0.9 + 3.5 = Y (at the nose)
6 Fr: 49 cm	NEX (cm) × 0.9 + 2.5 = Y (at the nose)

NEX (cm) = nose/earlobe/xyphoid
Y = insertion distance from tip to the nose

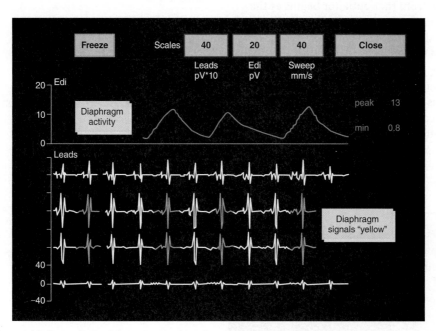

FIGURE 26-2 Graphics provide the necessary information used to adjust the NAVA catheter position.

allows the clinician to preview the level of support and compare it to the ventilator waveform in the current mode of ventilation. **Figure 26-3** shows the NAVA waveform superimposed on a pressure control breath. Note that the catheter detects diaphragm activity, allowing the ventilator to deliver a synchronized mandatory breath. Figure 26-3 also displays the NAVA level, which is adjusted in this illustration to match the pressure delivered during a mandatory pressure control breath. There are some basic NAVA signal observations that can be made during the initiation of this spontaneous mode of ventilation. These observations include the following:

- The Edi catheter signal should display from larger to smaller; if the signal goes from smaller to larger in size, the catheter may have looped around

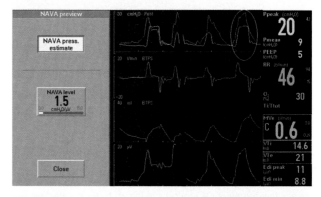

FIGURE 26-3 An illustration of how to use the NAVA preview screen to evaluate mandatory breath synchronization and to adjust the NAVA level to match the pressure delivered during a mandatory pressure control breath.

Courtesy of Getinge.

and the catheter should be pulled back and reinserted.

- If the blue signals are in the top two rows, the catheter is advanced too far and should be pulled back.
- If the blue signals are in the bottom two rows, the catheter should be advanced.

Alternatively, the clinician may choose to place the patient in NAVA ventilation and titrate the NAVA level to achieve a pre-NAVA peak inspiratory pressure (PIP), a predetermined V_T, or an Edi_{max} that is <20 mV and a delivered V_T that is within the prescribed target range. After the NAVA level is set, the PEEP can then be adjusted to produce an Edi_{min} of <2 mV.

There are other parameters the clinician must set, which include the trigger Edi, pressure support, and backup ventilation. The trigger Edi should be set so that flow from the ventilator begins as the diaphragm contracts; this is seen graphically as a lavender spike at the onset of the diaphragm waveform (**Figure 26-4**).

The settings for pressure support and backup ventilation will be patient specific and should be determined based on diagnosis and pulmonary condition. Other available settings can be seen in **Figure 26-5**. There is a dearth of information regarding ventilator management with this proprietary mode of ventilation. However, commonly used ventilator management guidelines are found in **Table 26-8**.

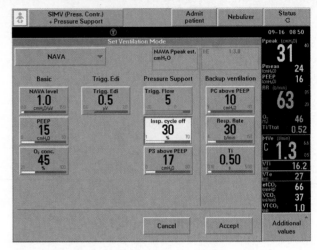

FIGURE 26-5 An illustration of how the pressure support and backup ventilation parameters are set.
Courtesy of Getinge.

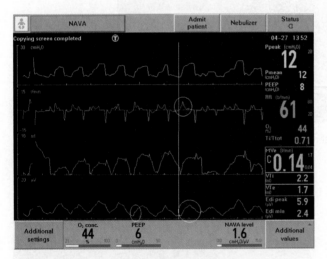

FIGURE 26-4 An example of using NAVA graphics to set the NAVA level. The lavender spike originates from the beginning of diaphragmatic contraction, indicating that the Edi trigger is appropriately set. A lavender spike that appears higher on the diaphragm signal means that trigger is set too high and the activity is not picked up until the diaphragm is partially contracted. A signal displayed on the down slope of the signal means that trigger is set too low and the ventilator is detecting diaphragmatic activity during the relaxation phase. When there is no detection of a diaphramatic signal with a flow-triggered response the ventilator will deliver a pressure-supported breath.
Courtesy of Getinge.

TABLE 26-8
Commonly Used Guidelines for Managing Ventilation with NAVA

Parameter	Increase	Decrease	Notes
Oxygenation (O_2)	Increase FiO_2 Increase PEEP	Decrease FiO_2 Decrease PEEP	Before changing PEEP levels, it is important to evaluate the Edi_{min}; increasing or decreasing PEEP levels can lead to overdistension or derecruitment
Ventilation (CO_2)	Increase NAVA level	Decrease NAVA level	It is important to evaluate the Edi_{max} before changing the NAVA level

Extubation may be considered when the PIP – PEEP is <10 cm H_2O.

Pressure Support Ventilation

Pressure support ventilation is a spontaneous mode of ventilation; therefore, use of this mode of ventilation is dependent on the patient having a sufficient respiratory drive. During inspiration, pressure reaches an operator-set value. All breaths are either pressure or flow triggered. Specifically, to initiate a **pressure-triggered breath**, the patient must make sufficient effort to generate an airway pressure drop below end-expiratory pressure larger than the operator-set sensitivity threshold. Flow-triggered breaths are initiated when the patient's inspiratory effort generates inspiratory flow above the trigger sensitivity setting. The breath ends or terminates when flow decays to a preset value, which is typically a percentage of the peak flow. There may be variable leaks in the system due to the use of uncuffed endotracheal tubes (ETTs) with newborn infants. Most ventilators allow the flow termination criteria to be adjusted, which minimizes the risk of a prolonged inspiration. As a safety mechanism, a secondary cycle mechanism—pressure or time—can be set, which also reduces the chances of a prolonged inspiration and the need for the patient to actively exhale to end the breath.

Because this is a spontaneous mode of ventilation, the patient determines the respiratory rate, inspiratory time, and flow. The V_T delivered to the patient depends on the amount of patient effort, the level of pressure support, and the resistance and compliance of the respiratory system. The pressure support level is typically titrated to a value that achieves a target tidal volume. Because the patient controls the respiratory rate, the clinician must monitor minute ventilation. Clinicians should also monitor mean airway pressure to prevent delivering exceedingly high mean airway pressures that can cause trauma to the lung.

Pressure support ventilation can be used as a method to wean the infant from ventilatory support and to reduce the work of breathing imposed by physiologic factors (increased chest wall compliance and reduced lung compliance) and increased airway resistance due to the use of very small ETTs.

Pressure versus Volume Control Ventilation

The breath is delivered in a distinctly different manner with pressure control ventilation than volume control ventilation. It is important for the respiratory therapist to understand the nuances of breath delivery when providing ventilatory assistance to critically ill infants.

Pressure Control Ventilation

Pressure control ventilation (PCV) has been used for decades and remains a common mode of ventilation used in preterm infants. PCV results in the delivery of a predetermined pressure during inspiration at a predetermined time and rate. PCV may be delivered with a CMV (or AC) or IMV breath sequence. Historically, this form of ventilation was delivered by infant ventilators (e.g., Sechrist, Sechrist Industries, Anaheim, CA) that were time cycled and pressure limited. Currently, pneumatically powered, time-cycled, pressure-limited ventilators (e.g., MVP-10, International Biomedical) are used for interfacility transport of infants and neonates. Because pressure remains constant during inspiration, there is the ability to have precise control of and deliver higher mean airway pressures, which have a direct effect on oxygenation.

Asynchrony may occur when the patient's demands are not met (inspiratory pressure is set too low, causing a very low tidal volume to be delivered) or if the inspiratory time is excessive (causing an increased work of breathing as the patient attempts to exhale against the delivery of flow and pressure). There are two common strategies to address asynchrony. Neuromuscular blocking agents and sedation can be used to achieve exact control of ventilation. The use of these agents would prevent any spontaneous breaths from occurring. However, the use of this strategy can contribute to diaphragmatic atrophy and impair mobilization of fluid, resulting in generalized tissue edema.[22] An alternate strategy is to deliver CMV (or AC) at a high mandatory frequency rate, between 60 and 120 per minute, to overcome spontaneous efforts.[23] This strategy meets or exceeds the ventilation requirements of the neonate, which in turn will limit or eliminate spontaneous effort.

When pressure-limited ventilation is used, flow decays during inspiration. This results in the delivery of more laminar flow, which may improve the distribution of gas and result in less dysynchrony and pressure overshoot. Because the set inspiratory pressure is controlled, or does not vary with every mechanical breath, tidal volume varies. V_T delivery is dependent on lung compliance; therefore, V_T delivery will vary as compliance changes. It is important for clinicians to monitor V_T delivery, as this monitored parameter will alert the clinical staff of changes to the patient's pulmonary status. When the patient's compliance decreases, V_T delivery decreases, increasing the risk of hypoventilation and/or atelectatrauma. As pulmonary disease resolves or after surfactant administration, compliance will increase and result in a higher V_T delivery with each mechanical breath. Large V_T delivery may result in lung injury and contribute to hyperventilation. The respiratory plan of care must include closely monitoring V_T delivery and a mechanism (individual orders or a protocol) to manipulate the pressure to maintain the desired V_T delivery.

Volume Control Ventilation

Volume control ventilation (VCV) delivers a consistent V_T and flow at a set mandatory breath rate. Pressure is not held constant and is dependent on lung compliance and airway resistance. Compared to pressure-limited ventilation, VCV often results in a higher peak airway pressure during mandatory breath delivery. Most ventilators do offer the ability to ramp the early phase of inspiration or to decelerate the flow pattern to mimic the flow characteristics seen in pressure-limited ventilation. The primary advantage for VCV is that volume delivery is guaranteed regardless of changes in lung compliance. The higher peak airway pressures that result from VCV may be undesirable if they exceed 25 cm H_2O.

Volume Targeted Ventilation

The nomenclature associated with volume targeted breath delivery is variable, and each manufacturer has a unique description of this breath type. **Volume targeted ventilation (VTV)** is also known as adaptive ventilation. All forms of VTV use algorithmic technology that monitors volume delivery and provides automatic pressure adjustment to maintain the preset targeted V_T. As a safety measure, the algorithm does not allow for pressure delivery changes that exceed 2 to 3 cm H_2O per breath. This breath delivery type relies on accurate V_T measurements to maximize the benefits of conditions associated with lung compliance changes. Based on manufacturer design, the reference point for delivered V_T may be measured at the inspiratory output of the ventilator, the expiratory transducer, or the patient airway. Airway leaks will impact functionality of breath delivery based on the reference point of delivered V_T. In the presence of significant airway leaks, the delivered V_T will be reduced when delivery is referenced at the inspiratory output of the ventilator. Because the leak is distal to where V_T delivery is referenced by the ventilation, the desired V_T will be reached at a lower pressure. Conversely, if the V_T measurement is referenced at the expiratory transducer, the ventilator will sense that the leak is reducing V_T delivery and respond by increasing the pressure delivered during inspiration in order to meet the desired V_T delivery. The amount of pressure increase is proportional to the effect the leak has on V_T delivery (i.e., the larger the leak, the higher the pressure increase over consecutive breaths). Patient airway measurements may offer the most consistent functionality, especially if leak compensation is available. If leak compensation is unavailable, then the ventilator's response to the leak will depend on whether the reference point is based on the inspiratory or expiratory volume at the airway sensor. Generally, volume targeted breath delivery is not advised in the presence of a significant airway leak unless using airway volume monitoring with leak compensation.

In an evaluation of infants born between 24 and 32 weeks' gestation requiring mechanical ventilatory support for respiratory distress syndrome, PSV + VTV provided tidal volume delivery that was closer to the desired or set value and was not associated with overventilation.[24]

Time Constants

Time constants reflect the efficiency of lung inflation and are the product of airway resistance and lung compliance. During mechanical ventilation of the neonate, mandatory respiratory rates can exceed 40 to 60 breaths per minute. This results in very a short total cycle time (TCT), typically of 1.5 seconds or less. Neonatal time constants are rarely calculated but range between 0.05 seconds in low lung compliance states versus 0.25 seconds in neonates with normal lung compliance.[25] Inspiration is an active process while expiration is passive; therefore, the clinician must ensure that sufficient time is allowed for expiration. The rule of thumb is at least 3 time constants are required to effectively exhale 95% of the breath. Allowing sufficient time for exhalation also helps prevent air trapping and

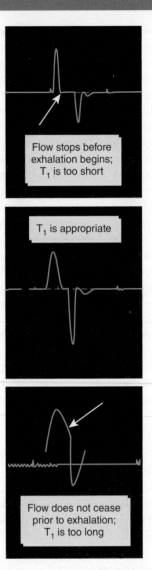

FIGURE 26-6 An illustration of how the flow-time waveform can be used to determine if inspiratory time (T_I) is set appropriately.

hyperinflation. For preterm infants, inspiratory time (T_I) generally ranges between 0.25 and 0.30 seconds when lung compliance is low and between 0.35 and 0.40 seconds in neonates with BPD or those with normal or near-normal lung compliance. Flow-time graphics often aid clinicians in setting appropriate inspiratory and expiratory times. The clinician can visualize how the breath is delivered to the patient. **Figure 26-6** illustrates how the flow time graphic can be used to determine if the inspiratory time is appropriately set for the patient. Flow will cease at the end of breath delivery when the inspiratory time is set appropriately. If flow ceases prior to exhalation, then the inspiratory time is too long. Conversely, if expiration starts before inspiratory flow ceases, then the inspiratory time is too short.

Trigger Sensitivity and Cycle Criteria

Trigger refers to the start of inspiration. During mechanical ventilation of a term or preterm infant, the patient's spontaneous inspiratory efforts can trigger a mechanical breath by either flow or pressure. (NAVA is the exception, where the trigger is a signal indicating diaphragm contraction.) The term or preterm infant's ability to trigger a breath depends on the strength of spontaneous inspiratory effort and the presence and magnitude of an existing ETT leak. It is important for the clinician to take the time necessary to assess the patient and to adjust the trigger sensitivity to a level that maximizes patient comfort and breath synchrony. A trigger sensitivity that is set too low (or too sensitive) will cause auto-triggering and deliver excessive minute ventilation. Auto-trigger can also occur when excess condensation (water) is present in the ventilator circuit. Water sloshing in the limbs of the patient circuit causes changes in pressure and flow and can trigger mechanical breaths.

A trigger sensitivity that is set too high (too insensitive) will prevent the ventilator from capturing or detecting patient breathing efforts. This may lead to an overall increased work of breathing and patient–ventilator asynchrony.

A closely related ventilator parameter is the cycle setting. The cycle setting is the criteria used to end or terminate inspiration. The terms for this ventilator parameter vary by ventilator manufacturer. Generally, this parameter adjusts the amount of flow decay, from peak flow, needed to end inspiration. Most ventilators have a default value of 25% to 30%, which means that inspiration can transition to exhalation when flow drops to 25% to 30% of the peak flow. Although there are default values, this parameter should be adjusted by the clinician. The amounts of leak present and total respiratory rate are important factors to consider when adjusting cycle criteria.

When the ETT leak is large, the value may need to be increased so that the inspiratory cycle time is not excessive. Ventilator graphics will aid the clinician in setting these values. The flow-time waveform is helpful when setting the flow trigger. The clinician should observe the flow trigger indicator at the onset of inspiratory flow, very similar to the observations made when adjusting inspiratory time (Figure 26-6). If patient effort is not detected at the onset of a spontaneous or assisted breath, then the trigger setting is not sensitive enough. Conversely, if the ventilator triggers inspiration before the preset time interval for a mandatory breath when no spontaneous effort is present, the trigger setting is too sensitive.

Nonconventional Modes of Ventilation

Nonconventional modes of ventilation are designed to provide the lowest possible tidal volume (often less than dead space) and ventilator frequencies much higher than conventional ventilators. Nonconventional modes of ventilation are often referred to as gentle ventilation and are designed to minimize the risk of volutrauma. Nonconventional modes of ventilation include **high-frequency jet ventilation (HFJV)** and **high-frequency oscillatory ventilation (HFOV)**. They are often used as a primary proactive strategy to limit exposure to excessive alveolar stretch to prevent lung injury when volutrauma exists (i.e., pulmonary air leaks) to allow the lung the opportunity to heal or as a ventilation method when conventional methods of ventilation fail.

High-Frequency Oscillatory Ventilation

HFOV is essentially a high-flow CPAP system with superimposed pressure oscillations. The pressure oscillations are created by an electronically driven diaphragm. HFOV incorporates a recruitment strategy by applying mean airway pressure to inflate the lung at or beyond the opening pressure and a lung protective strategy that uses rapid shallow delivery of active oscillation to provide minute ventilation, resulting in attenuated pressure delivery of gas to the lungs. CO_2 removal is enhanced by the active exhalation that occurs when the bellows retract, thus withdrawing gas during each backstroke of the piston. The active exhalation strategy is thought to reduce hyperinflation, although the evidence for its use is mixed.

The oscillation frequency can be set from 3 to 15 Hz. One Hz is 60 cycles or oscillations per second. Mean airway pressure can be adjusted between 5 and 55 cm H_2O. Mean airway pressure is adjusted with a control that varies the resistance of the exhalation manifold. Bias flow, which generates the high-flow CPAP effect, is adjustable from 0 to 60 L/minute. Oscillatory pressure amplitude is directly controlled by the "power" setting, which determines the power driving the oscillator piston. The actual pressure amplitude of the airflow oscillations is dependent on the patient's respiratory mechanics or airway resistance and lung compliance. The power can be adjusted to provide maximum pressure amplitude of 140 cm H_2O.

Lung protection is the primary goal during HFOV regardless of the indications for use; however, differences will be seen in the overall management of HFOV based on the primary strategy used. When initiating HFOV for a patient with severe RDS or radiologic evidence of lung volume loss, the clinician should set a mean airway pressure (mP_{AW}) equal to or slightly higher than the mP_{AW} provided by conventional ventilation. **Table 26-9** provides guidelines for the initiation of HFOV. Generally, the frequency (Hz rate) is set according to the age and weight of the patient. Amplitude is adjusted while observing chest wall movement and is increased until the pressure is sufficient to produce a chest wall wiggle. FiO_2 is titrated to obtain an SpO_2 within the prescribed range. Most often, FiO_2 is initially set at 1.0 and weaned afterward.

TABLE 26-9
Guidelines for the Initiation of HFOV

Settings	Lung Recruitment	Lung Protection (Air Leaks or Pulmonary Interstitial Emphysema)
Hz mP_{AW}	Patient specific: Preterm: 13–15 Hz Term: 8–10 Hz 2–4 above mP_{AW} of the conventional ventilator Increase mP_{AW} by 1 cm H_2O until desired SpO_2 is achieved, then wean FiO_2	Patient specific: Preterm: 13–15 Hz Term: 10–12 Hz Equal to mP_{AW} of the conventional ventilator Accept SpO_2 ≥88%
FiO_2	100%	100%
Amplitude	Enough to produce chest wiggle in the following manner: Infant to the umbilicus Adjust ΔP by 2–4 to change ventilation (↑ΔP to ↓CO_2)	Enough to produce chest wiggle in the following manner: Infant to the umbilicus Adjust ΔP to accept permissive hypercapnia in the absence of pulmonary hypertension
T_I	33% (never to exceed 50%)	33% (do not adjust)

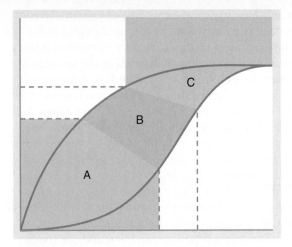

FIGURE 26-7 A pressure volume curve is used to illustrate lung recruitment. The red areas indicate (**A**) underinflation or (**C**) overinflation. (**B**) represents the desired inflation point at which ventilation is effective without risk of lung trauma.

TABLE 26-10
Examples of the Relationship among Oxygenation, Ventilation, and Changes in HFOV Parameters or Settings

Parameter	To Increase Oxygenation and Ventilation	To Decrease Oxygenation and Ventilation
O_2	Increase mP_{AW}	Decrease mP_{AW}
	Increase FiO_2	Decrease FiO_2
	Increase T_I (not very effective—do not use in lung protection strategy)	
	Initiate inhaled nitric oxide therapy in the presence of pulmonary hypertension	
CO_2	Decrease ΔP	Increase ΔP
	Increase Hz	Decrease Hz (results in higher gas delivery and is equivalent to increasing the V_T)

After the initial ventilator parameters are programed, the patient should be closely monitored for their response to ventilation. The SpO_2 may not initially be within the prescribed range. Should this occur, slowly increase the mP_{AW} until the SpO_2 begins to rise. A rise in SpO_2 indicates lung recruitment is occurring (**Figure 26-7**).

Once the lung is recruited and the SpO_2 is stabilized, the FiO_2 may be weaned as tolerated, keeping the SpO_2 within the prescribed range. While the primary control for oxygenation is related to the mP_{AW} and the FiO_2, ventilation is primarily controlled by amplitude.[26] During HFOV, the partial pressure of carbon dioxide ($PaCO_2$) can change rapidly. Monitoring the $PaCO_2$ is important. To minimize blood loss and reduce the frequency with which blood gases are obtained, noninvasive monitoring by a transcutaneous CO_2 monitor is helpful. Transcutaneous CO_2 monitoring allows for continuous evaluation of the efficacy of ventilation. Rapid and prolonged hypocarbia can reduce cerebral blood flow and result in cerebral ischemic events. Dramatic swings in cerebral perfusion contribute to intracranial hemorrhage. Ventilator adjustments based on oxygenation and ventilation are presented in **Table 26-10**.

It should be noted that HFOV often has a negative impact on the hemodynamic state of the patient secondary to high intrathoracic pressures. During incremental and/or decremental changes in continuous distending pressure during HFOV, changes in lung mechanics and right ventricular output can occur and affect hemodynamic stability.[27] The hemodynamic state of the patient should be monitored and supported to increase the likelihood of successfully ventilating the patient with HFOV.

Patients are frequently weaned to minimum HFOV settings and converted to conventional ventilation prior to extubation because clinicians find it easier to assess extubation readiness from a conventional means. It is, however, permissible to extubate directly from HFOV by weaning the mP$_{AW}$ to a minimal setting and the amplitude to "off," which is essentially providing only high-flow CPAP.

High-Frequency Jet Ventilation

HFJV is an alternative to HFOV. The Bunnell Life Pulse High-Frequency Ventilator is the device used to provide this nonconventional mode of ventilation. The ventilator is microprocessor controlled and capable of delivering and monitoring between 240 and 660 humidified breaths per minute. HFJV provides small pulses of fresh gas using high-velocity flow interruption during inspiration. Unlike HFOV, exhalation is passive. Small tidal breaths at rapid rates are injected through a side port of the ETT adapter using a proprietary adaptor, the Bunnell Inc. LifePort Adapter shown in **Figure 26-8**. HFJV is used in tandem with a conventional ventilator. During HFJV, the CV provides CPAP. If atelectasis is a concern, the conventional ventilator can provide low rate IMV breaths for the alveolar recruitment. PEEP is adjusted on the conventional ventilator to stabilize alveolar inflation, after which the mode can be switched from IMV back to CPAP.

HFJV provides delivery of a pressure-limited breath with a fixed inspiratory time. This differs from HFOV in that the inspiratory time is a percentage of total cycle. The principal of operation for HFJV closely mimics the strategy of PCV; therefore, ventilator adjustments are easily transferable to most clinicians. **Table 26-11** outlines the guidelines used to adjust ventilator parameters

when initiating HFJV. After the initiation of HFJV, adjustments to ventilator parameters on conventional ventilators and HFJV depend on the goals established for the management of the patient. Noninvasive assessment of oxygenation (SpO$_2$) and ventilation (transcutaneous CO$_2$) facilitate ventilator management. Chest radiography is useful in evaluating the presence of lung pathology and effectiveness of lung recruitment efforts. For example, delivery of larger tidal volume delivery by HFJV (use of higher PIPs to obtain a higher V$_T$) in conjunction with intermittent sigh breaths with the conventional ventilator may be a useful strategy for ventilating

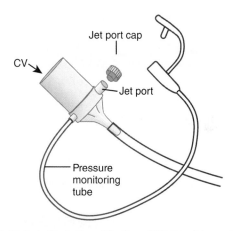

FIGURE 26-8 An illustration of the Bunnell LifePort Adapter. HFJV gas flow is injected through the jet port, and conventional ventilation is provided through the 22-mm ETT adapter. The pressure monitoring tube measures and transmits the PIP, PEEP, and Servo pressure to the HFJV.

Reproduced from Bunnell Incorporated, Life Pulse™ High Frequency Ventilator Operator's Manual, Figure 14, p. V-15, retrieved from www.bunl.com.

TABLE 26-11
General Guidelines for Ventilator Parameter Adjustment during the Initiation of HFJV

Parameter	HFJV Setting	Conventional Ventilator Setting	Comments
PIP	Equal to or 1–2 cm less than the PIP used before HFJV was initiated	Start with current PIP setting	Titrate HFJV PIP to desired PaCO$_2$
			Titrate PIP to recruit lung
PEEP	N/A	5–7 cm H$_2$O	Increase by 2 cm H$_2$O to preserve mP$_{AW}$
Frequency	420/min	0–5/min	Frequencies of 240–360/min can be used when lung disease requires long expiratory times (e.g., PIE, BPD, MAS) or patients have radiologic evidence of gas trapping (hyperinflation)
T$_I$	0.020 sec (minimum)	0.3–0.4 sec	HFJV inspiratory-expiratory ratio must allow for adequate expiratory time
FiO$_2$	Titrate to desired SpO$_2$ used to monitor oxygenation status	Titrate to desired SpO$_2$ used to monitor oxygenation status	Initial setting will be based on current conventional ventilator setting
	The identical FiO$_2$ should be set on the HFJV and conventional ventilator	The identical FiO$_2$ should be set on the HFJV and conventional ventilator	

Data from Bunnell Inspired Infant Care. www.bunl.com/uploads/4/8/7/9/48792141/hfjvguidelines.pdf.

a neonate with respiratory failure related to loss of lung volume. **Table 26-12** provides general guidelines for titrating HFJV and conventional ventilator settings.

Monitoring the servo working pressure alerts the clinician to changes in patient condition, such as an improvement in lung compliance, the need to suction, or when there are changes to the integrity of the patient–ventilator circuit. The servo pressure will increase when any of the following occur: lung compliance or airway resistance improves, there is an increase in the ETT leak, or a circuit leak is present. The servo pressure will decrease when lung compliance or airway resistance worsens, the ETT becomes obstructed, a tension pneumothorax has developed, or secretions are present that require suctioning.

The choice to provide HFOV or HFJV is usually determined by clinician or physician preference. However, there are some advantages of HFJV. One key advantage is that the mP_{AW} required to ventilate the patient is usually lower during HFJV, thus resulting in less hemodynamic compromise. **Figure 26-9** outlines the key pressure differences during HFOV and HFJV.

TABLE 26-12
General Guidelines for Adjusting Conventional and HFJV Parameters. Adjustments Are Based on Individual Patient Goals

Affected Parameter/Goal	To Increase Parameter/Goal	To Decrease Parameter/Goal
O_2	Increase FiO_2	Decrease FiO_2
	Increase PEEP	Decrease PEEP
CO_2	Decrease the rate on the HFJV	Increase the rate on the HFJV
	Decrease the PIP on the HFJV	Increase the PIP on the HFJV
Lung recruitment strategy	Increase the PIP on conventional ventilator	Decrease the PIP on the conventional ventilator (presence of air leaks or PIE)
	Increase the mandatory rate or frequency on conventional ventilator	Decrease the mandatory rate or frequency (presence of air leaks or PIE)
	Increase the T_I on conventional ventilator	
Lung protection strategy	Decrease the PIP on the conventional ventilator	N/A (lung protection is a primary goal of HFJV; therefore, we never decrease lung protective ventilation—follow increase lung recruitment strategy if there is a loss of lung volume)
	Decrease the mandatory rate or frequency on the conventional ventilator	

Data from Bunnell Inspired Infant Care. http://www.bunl.com/uploads/4/8/7/9/48792141/servopressure.pdf.

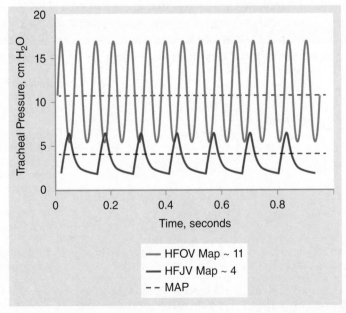

FIGURE 26-9 An illustration of the difference in tracheal and mean airway pressures that occur with HFVJ and HFOV.

Reproduced from Bunnell Incorporated, Advantages of Life Pulse HFJV Compared to Other HFV, p. 2, retrieved from www.bunl.com.

Ventilatory Management

Ventilatory management is complex and requires an evaluation of the infant's current pathophysiology and clinical presentation. The disease process, chest radiograph results, current respiratory status, and potential complications must all be considered when ventilator management decisions are made.

Adjusting Ventilator Parameters

It is also important for the clinician to understand how changes in ventilator parameters affect blood gas values. A summary of ventilator management for conventional and advanced modes of ventilation related to blood gas measurements is presented in **Table 26-13**. Blood gas targets for oxygenation and ventilation are shown in **Table 26-14**.

It should be noted that wide swings in $PaCO_2$ levels should be avoided. $PaCO_2$ levels that are too high are associated with increased cerebral blood flow while excessively low $PaCO_2$ levels are associated with limited cerebral blood flows. Wide swings in cerebral blood flows can contribute to intracranial hemorrhages or intraventricular hemorrhages. As ventilator parameter changes are made, it is also essential for the clinician to adjust ventilator alarms.

TABLE 26-13

General Guidelines for Adjusting Conventional and Nonconventional Ventilator Parameters to Achieve a Change in Blood Gas Values

Desired Effect	Conventional Ventilator	HFOV	HFJV
↑ PO_2	↑ FiO_2, ↑ PEEP, ↑ PIP	↑ FiO_2, ↑ MAP	↑ FiO_2, ↑ HFJV PIP, ↑ conventional PEEP, rate, or PIP
↓ PO_2	↓ FiO_2, ↓ PEEP, ↓ PIP	↓ FiO_2, ↓ MAP	↓ FiO_2, ↓ HFJV PIP, ↓ conventional PEEP, rate, or PIP
↑ PCO_2	↓ rate, ↓ PIP, ↓ set or target V_T	↓ amplitude	↓ HFJV PIP, ↓ conventional rate or PIP
↓ PCO_2	↑ rate, ↑ PIP, ↑ set or target V_T	↑ amplitude, ↓ hertz	↑ HFJV PIP, ↑ conventional rate or PIP
Comment	Target delivered V_T should be 4–6 mL/kg in all breath delivery types to avoid VILI.	MAP is used to recruit the lung while amplitude is used to eliminate CO_2.	The conventional vent is used to provide PEEP and a sigh is provided when a rate is employed.

PIP – PEEP = (ΔP) delivered V_T: There is a linear difference between the ΔP and the V_T, provided maximum inflation is not exceeded. Regardless of breath delivery type, the goal should be to maintain a delivered V_T of 4–6 mL/kg.

Oxygenation is a product of oxygen concentration and mean airway pressure (MAP). The MAP is related to any setting that is related to the amount or duration of positive pressure delivery (PIP, PEEP, and, to a lesser degree, rate and T_I).

CO_2 levels are influenced by minute ventilation (VE). Rate x V_T = VE

During HFOV, the T_I is a percentage of TCT; therefore, as hertz is ↓ T_I is ↑, resulting in increased gas delivery per piston stroke.

During HFJV, the T_I is fixed; therefore, changes in rate have no effect on delivered volume.

TABLE 26-14

Targeted Blood Gas Values for Different Lung Pathologies

Lung Pathology or Condition	pH	$PaCO_2$	PaO_2
Normal compliance	7.35–7.45	35–45 mm Hg	60–100 mm Hg
Decreased compliance (permissive hypercapnia)	Early 7.25–7.35	Early 45–55 mm Hg	50–70 mm Hg
	Late 7.30–7.35	Late 50–60 mm Hg	
Pulmonary hypertension	7.30–7.40	40–50 mm Hg	80–100 mm Hg

TABLE 26-15
Common Saturation Targets for Different Neonatal Disorders

Neonatal Disorder	Saturation Target
Preterm neonates	90–95%
Primary pulmonary hypertension of the newborn neonates	95–100%
Cyanotic heart defects	≥70–75%
Noncyanotic cardiac lesions	≥85%, depending on the severity of intracardiac shunting
CDH	≥85%, depending on functional lung volume and vascularization
Full-term infants with nonpulmonary or noncardiac disorders (abdominal wall disorders, neuro-tube disorders, etc.)	≥93–95%

Primarily, noninvasive monitoring incorporates the routine use of continuous pulse oximetry and often includes transcutaneous or end-tidal CO_2 monitoring. Pulse oximetry targets will be patient and disease specific. Oxygen saturations of common neonatal disorders are found in **Table 26-15**. Transcutaneous or end-tidal CO_2 values should closely mimic arterial CO_2 values. Oximetry responses are rapid and reflect the current oxygenation status of the patient while transcutaneous CO_2 responses are rapid once the monitor has stabilized.

Mechanical Ventilation of the Neonate with Cardiac Disease

Patients with ductal-dependent cardiac lesions require precise, balanced cardiopulmonary circulation. Goals for mechanical ventilation focus on promoting or limiting pulmonary blood flow by using strategies associated with oxygen delivery and pH management through CO_2 manipulation and inspired oxygen administration. High oxygen delivery will result in vasodilatation of the pulmonary vessels and should be provided in patients with right-sided cardiac defects that are associated with impaired pulmonary blood flow. A higher pH will also improve pulmonary circulation and is achieved with slightly lower CO_2 levels. It is important to limit pulmonary blood flow for infants with ductal-dependent left-sided lesions. Therefore, the strategy is to limit the concentration of oxygen delivered. Additionally, the pH should be maintained at a slightly higher level to achieve a mild respiratory acidosis. Balanced circulation is difficult to achieve and close monitoring of the patient's acid–base status is extremely important.

Weaning and Extubation

The ventilator-weaning plan will also be patient specific. Generally, the parameters that should be weaned are based on blood gas analysis or results obtained from noninvasive monitoring. The choice of which ventilator parameter to wean depends on which parameter or setting is most toxic to the lungs. Excessive pressures (PIP) and inspired oxygen level are considered the most damaging. The clinician must approach pressure weans with caution, as pressure changes can affect both oxygenation and ventilation. In most cases, only one parameter at a time should be weaned, with the exception of FiO_2. It is important to note that weaning strategy differs from the strategy used to adjust ventilator parameters during the initial stabilization following intubation.

Extubation criteria are also patient specific and include resolution of acute respiratory failure or active infection, the ability to sustain spontaneous respirations, and the ability to protect the airway. Most practitioners would consider extubation of the neonate if the FiO_2 were less than 40%, the mandatory respiratory rate was ≤15 breaths per minute, the PIP was ≤20 cm H_2O, and the PEEP was ≤5 cm H_2O. Postextubation interventions include nasal CPAP, noninvasive ventilation, or high-flow nasal cannula. The postextubation intervention will depend on the neonate's ability to maintain FRC, minute ventilation, or oxygenation status. CPAP is used when the neonate has a strong respiratory drive but has a lung condition associated with a loss of lung volume or tracheal malesia. Noninvasive ventilation is used when the patient has a weak respiratory drive or respiratory muscle fatigue. The high-flow nasal cannula is designed to flush out the anatomic dead space and to provide oxygen-enriched gas flow to the patient, improving oxygenation status. High-flow nasal cannulas must be heated and humidified and can be used at flows of 1 to 8 L/minute in the neonate.

Complications of Mechanical Ventilation

There are a number of complications or conditions related to mechanical ventilation, many of which can be minimized or prevented by carefully monitoring the patient. One of the most serious acute complications associated with the delivery of positive pressure ventilation is the development of pulmonary air leaks. Air leaks occur when excessive pressure is applied to the lungs, causing the alveolar wall to rupture and resulting in air accumulation in the pleural space. This causes the lung to collapse, impairs gas exchange, and can lead to hemodynamic compromise.

Chronic complications are also a concern for clinicians caring for neonates requiring mechanical ventilation. The most common chronic condition that results from mechanical ventilation is BPD, which affects approximately 50% of all neonates born at less than 25 weeks' gestation and results in altered lung function requiring long-term medical management. In the very low birthweight infant, it may not be possible to eliminate the risk of BPD, but it can be minimized by providing gentle ventilation by utilizing permissive hypercapnia in the absence of pulmonary hypertension. Gentle ventilation may include HFOV or HFJV to protect the lungs by limiting alveolar stretch.

Another complication associated with mechanical ventilation that is frequently encountered in the preterm population is retinopathy of prematurity. ROP involves partial or full detachment of the retina, affecting vision. This complication is associated with excessive fluctuation in oxygen levels of the neonate less than 37 weeks' gestation. **Table 26-16** presents other complications that are noted in preterm infants requiring mechanical ventilation.

TABLE 26-16
Complications Associated with Mechanical Ventilation of Preterm and Term Infants

Complication	Cause	Note
Necrotizing enterocolitis	Inflammatory process of the gastrointestinal tract that may result from prolonged hypoxia or perfusion to the organ	Treatment includes administration of broad-spectrum antibiotics and, in severe cases, surgical removal of the affected intestine.
Patent ductus arteriosis (PDA)	Continued flow through the PDA can result in excessive pulmonary blood flow resulting from left-to-right shunting from the aorta to the pulmonary artery and pulmonary edema	The PDA normally closes within the first hours or days of life; however, continued flow through the PDA prevents closure. Treatment includes administration of indomethacin or ibuprofen and fluid restriction or, in severe cases, surgical ligation of the vessel.
Feeding intolerance	Although early feeds are encouraged, they are often provided by orogastric tubes, thus bypassing the normal feeding mechanism. This can lead to feeding intolerance or the inability to swallow. If necrotizing enterocolitis is suspected, feeds are usually stopped and intolerance can develop or worsen when reintroduced.	Feeds can be supplemented with hyperalimentation, but when the normal feeding process cannot be re-established, surgical placement of a gastric tube or a juedenal tube can be performed to provide an alternate form of feeding.
Airway malacia (tracheal or bronchial)	The ETT can cause pressure on the wall of the trachea and lead to areas of weakness in the tracheal wall, which is composed of incomplete cartilaginous rings.	Use of appropriate-size ETTs can minimize the development of malacia.
Vocal cord dysfunction	Prolonged intubation affecting vocal cord function.	Long-term presence of an ETT may affect the ability of vocal cords to close completely once the ETT has been removed, thus affecting aspiration risk, voice quality, and ability to maintain FRC.
Ventilator-associated pneumonia	The presence of an artificial airway increases the risk of contaminants directly to the lungs.	The risk of infection can be reduced by limiting breaks in the ventilating circuit (closed suction systems, etc.).

Case Study 1

Jane was a preterm neonate born at 28 weeks' gestation, weighing 1.3 kg at birth. She was born by spontaneous vaginal delivery. Her mother received a course of antenatal steroids on admission to hospital to enhance surfactant maturation and to reduce the severity of respiratory distress syndrome (RDS). The neonate was rigorous at birth, spontaneously breathing, and required no resuscitation efforts except for some stimulation and prevention of heat loss. She was placed on nasal CPAP with a pressure of 5 cm H_2O and 35% FiO_2 to maintain an oxygen saturation between 89% and 93%. Her initial arterial blood gas (ABG) revealed the following: pH 7.32, PaO_2 62 mm Hg, CO_2 45 mm Hg, bicarbonate 23 mEq, and base excess mEq/L. However, 6 hours later, the neonate started to have increased work of breathing with tachypnea, chest retractions, and nasal flaring and an increasing oxygen requirement. The ABG showed a respiratory acidosis pH 7.24, PaO_2 57 mm Hg, CO_2 63 mm Hg, bicarbonate 21 mEq/L, and base excess 3. Therefore, the noninvasive ventilation was initiated at a PIP of 12 cm H_2O and a PEEP of 7 cm H_2O. With minimal improvement after an hour and worsening respiratory status, the patient was intubated. Mechanical ventilation was initiated on the following settings: SIMV PIP 24 cm H_2O, PEEP 6 cm H_2O, I-time 0.35 seconds, and a rate of 60 breaths per minute. She remained stable on this mode through the night. Weaning was initiated on day 2 of invasive ventilatory support. On day 4 the ventilator settings were weaned to SIMV PIP 18 cm H_2O, PEEP 4 cm H_2O, I-time 0.35 seconds, and a rate of 20 breaths per minute. The measured V_T was 4 to 6 mL/kg; spontaneous breathing rate was 50 to 60 breaths per minute and synchronized with the mechanical breath delivery. She was weaned to CPAP and extubated on day 6.

1. Why was a trial of biphasic positive pressure ventilation worthwhile for this patient? What was the rationale for initiating noninvasive ventilation?

2. What ventilator changes would you recommend if the ABG post intubation was pH 7.50, PaO_2 80 mm Hg, CO_2 32 mm Hg, and bicarbonate 19 mEq/b and base excess −3, L?

3. What change in ventilation strategy might you consider if the initial setting of SIMV PIP 24, PEEP 6, I-time 0.35, and a rate of 60 produced a blood gas classified as a respiratory acidosis?

Case Study 2

A term neonate (4 kg) was born with thick meconium following a prolonged and arduous labor. Apgar scores were 1 at 1 minute and 4 at 5 minutes of life. The neonate required full resuscitation measures at birth, was intubated and mechanically ventilated by t-piece resuscitator in the delivery suite, and transferred to the neonatal intensive care unit. He was ventilated in the SIMV mode on the following settings: PIP 26 cm H_2O, PEEP 5 cm H_2O, I-time 0.4 seconds, and a respiratory rate of 45 breaths per minute F_IO_2 0.80. The ABG revealed the following: pH 7.09, CO_2 74 mm Hg, PaO_2 35 mm Hg, bicarbonate 16 mEq/L, and base excess 8. The PIP was increased to 30 cm H_2O, and 5 minutes after the increase to the PIP, the following was observed: SpO_2 90% to 95% and the measured tidal volume 3 ml/kg. The measured MAP on the ventilator was 16 cm H_2O, and tidal volume was 12 mL (3 mL/kg). The mode of ventilation was switched to HFOV. The initial oscillator settings were MAP 18 cm H_2O, amplitude 38, frequency 10 Hz, and FiO_2 75%. This continued for 8 hours, during which time the clinical condition and blood gases started to improve. The chest X-ray showed good lung expansion. The amplitude was reduced as chest wiggle was pronounced and CO_2 started to decrease. Oxygenation also started to improve, so FiO_2 was reduced to 40% on day 2. Over the next 48 hours, the MAP was slowly reduced by increments of 1 to 2 cm H_2O until a MAP of 14 cm H_2O. The oxygen requirement was only 35%. On day 6 of life, the neonate was to be extubated to nasal CPAP at 4 cm H_2O and an F_IO_2 of 0.28.

1. What was the rationale for transitioning from conventional ventilation to HFOV?

2. How do you approach setting the mean airway pressure when transitioning from conventional ventilation to HFOV?

3. What ventilator parameters are used to increase or decrease CO_2 on the HFOV?

4. What is an important aspect of setting the amplitude when transitioning to HFOV?

References

1. Wiswell TE, Srinivasa P. Continuous positive airway pressure. In: Goldsmith JP, Karotkin EH, eds. *Assisted Ventilation of the Neonate.* 4th ed. Philadelphia: Elsevier; 2003:127-129.

2. Diblasi RM. Nasal continuous positive airway pressure (CPAP) for the respiratory care of the newborn infant. *Respir Care.* 2009; 54(9):1209-1235.

3. Mahmoud RA, Roehr CC, Schmalisch G. Current methods of non-invasive ventilatory support for neonates. *Paediatr Respir Rev.* 2011;12(3):196-205.

4. Fedor KL. Noninvasive respiratory support in infants and children. *Respir Care.* 2017;62(6):699-717.

5. Gerdes JS, Sivieri EM, Abbasi S. Factors influencing delivered mean airway pressure during nasal CPAP with the RAM cannula. *Pediatr Pulmonol.* 2016;51(1):60-69.

6. Bailes SA, Firestone KS, Dunn DK, McNinch NL, Brown MF, Volsko TA. Evaluating the effect of flow and interface type on pressures delivered with bubble CPAP in a simulated model. *Respir Care.* 2016;61(3):333-339.

7. Loh LE, Chan YH, Chan I. Noninvasive ventilation in children: a review. *J Pediatr (Rio J).* 2007;83(2 Suppl):S91-S99.

8. Cummings JJ, Polin RA, The Committee on Fetus and Newborn. Noninvasive respiratory support. *Pediatrics.* 2016;137(1):e20153758.

9. Chao KY, Chen YL, Tsai LY, Chien YH, Mu SC. The role of heated humidified high-flow nasal cannula as noninvasive respiratory support in neonates. *Pediatr Neonatol.* 2017;58(40):295-302.

10. Yoder BA, Stoddard RA, Li M, King J, Dirnberger DR, Abbasi S. Heated, humidified high-flow nasal cannula versus nasal CPAP for respiratory support in neonates. *Pediatrics.* 2013;131(5): e1482-e1490.

11. Fleeman N, Mahon J, Bates V, et al. The clinical effectiveness and cost-effectiveness of heated humidified high-flow nasal cannula compared with usual care for preterm infants: systematic review and economic evaluation. *Health Technol Assess.* 2016;20(30):1-68.

12. Berger TM, Fontana M, Stocker M. The journey towards lung protective respiratory support in preterm neonates. *Neonatology.* 2013;104(4):265-274.

13. Stevens TP, Harrington EW, Blennow M, Soll RF. Early surfactant administration with brief ventilation vs. selective surfactant and continued mechanical ventilation for preterm infants with or at risk for respiratory distress syndrome. *Cochrane Database Syst Rev.*2007;4:CD003063.

14. Rigo V, Lefebvre C, Broux I. Surfactant instillation in spontaneously breathing preterm infants: a systematic review and meta-analysis. *Eur J Pediatr.* 2016;175(12):1933-1942.

15. Kaam A. Lung-protective ventilation in neonatology. *Neonatology.* 2011;99(4):338-341.

16. Avery ME, Mead J. Surface properties in relation to atelectasis and hyaline membrane disease. *AMA J Dis Child.* 1959;97 (5, Part 1):517-523.

17. Kugelman AM. A comprehensive approach to the prevention of bronchopulmonary dysplasia. *Pediatr Pulmonol.* 2011;46:1153-1165.

18. Gleason CA. *Avery's Diseases of the Newborn.* 9th ed. Philadelphia: Elsevier; 2012.

19. American College of Obstetricians and Gynecologists' Committee on Obstetric Practice; Society for Maternal–Fetal Medicine. Committee Opinion No. 677. Antenatal corticosteroid therapy for fetal maturation. *Obstet Gynecol.* 2016;128(4):e187-e194.

20. Van Marter LJ. Progress in discovery and evaluation of treatments to prevent bronchopulmonary dysplasia. *Biol Neonate.* 2006;89(4):303-312.

21. Ludwig CA, Chen TA, Hernandez-Boussard T, Moshfeghi AA, Moshfeghi DM. The epidemiology of retinopathy of prematurity in the United States. *Ophthalmic Surg Lasers Imaging Retina.* 2017;48(7):553-562.

22. Zimmerman KO, Smith PB, Benjamin DK, et al. Sedation, analgesia, and paralysis during mechanical ventilation of premature infants. *J Pediatr.* 2017;180:99-104.

23. Shetty SG, Greenough A. Neonatal ventilation strategies and long-term respiratory outcomes. *Early Human Dev.* 2014;90(11):735-739.

24. Unal S, Ergenekon E, Aktas S, et al. Effects of volume guaranteed ventilation combined with two different modes in preterm infants. *Respir Care.* 2017;62(12):1525-1532.

25. Kamlin C, Davis PG. Long versus short inspiratory times in neonates receiving mechanical ventilation. *Cochrane Database Syst Rev.* 2004;18(4):CD004503.

26. Zannin E, Dellaca' RL, Dognini G, et al. Effect of frequency on pressure cost of ventilation and gas exchange in newborns receiving high frequency oscillatory ventilation. *Pediatr Res.* 2017;82(6): 994-999.

27. Zannin E, Doni D, Ventura ML, et al. Relationship between mean airways pressure, lung mechanics, and right ventricular output during high-frequency oscillatory ventilation in infants. *J Pediatr.* 2017;180:110-115.

Mechanical Ventilation of the Pediatric Patient

Katherine L. Fedor

Teresa A. Volsko

© Anna Rubak/ShutterStock, Inc.

OUTLINE

OBJECTIVES

1. Discuss the indications for CPAP and noninvasive ventilation (NIV).
2. List the interfaces used to administer NIV.
3. Differentiate between spontaneous, spontaneous/timed, and timed modes of NIV.
4. Discuss how weaning strategies differ when a patient can and cannot trigger a breath during NIV.
5. List the alarms and parameter ranges used for NIV.
6. Explain the problems and complications associated with NIV use.
7. Discuss the strategy used to initially set ventilator parameters for invasive ventilation in children.
8. Explain the problems that can occur with flow rates that are set too low or high during volume control ventilation.
9. Describe how pressure volume curves can be used to set and adjust PEEP and inspiratory pressure.
10. Explain the importance of appropriately setting trigger and cycle sensitivity.
11. Discuss the ventilator management strategies used to minimize lung injury.
12. Describe how ventilator strategies differ when high-frequency oscillatory ventilation and high-frequency jet ventilation are used.
13. Differentiate between biphasic ventilation and airway pressure release ventilation.
14. List the modes of ventilation frequently used for weaning.

KEY TERMS

adaptive support
  ventilation (ASV)
airway pressure release
  ventilation (APRV)
atelectotrauma
auto-mode
auto-trigger
beaking
biphasic ventilation
continuous positive airway
  pressure (CPAP)
cycle sensitivity
cycle time
delta P
delta pressure (ΔP)
Edi_{max}
Edi_{min}
expiratory positive airway
  pressure (EPAP)
heated high-flow nasal
  cannula (HHFNC)

inspiratory positive airway
  pressure (IPAP)
inspiratory time
invasive mechanical
  ventilation
mandatory minute
  ventilation (MMV)
neurally adjusted
  ventilatory assist
  ventilation (NAVA)
noninvasive biphasic positive
  pressure ventilation
noninvasive ventilation (NIV)
ramp time
rise time
smart care
spontaneous mode
spontaneous/timed mode
timed mode
trigger
volutrauma

Introduction

Mechanical ventilation of the pediatric patient closely mimics the indications and strategies used to ventilate adults. The strategies employed are based on the severity and origin of respiratory failure as well as on the best available evidence in the literature. Technologic advances and implementation of evidence-based care have contributed to improved outcomes in terms of reduced morbidity and mortality for children requiring ventilatory support.

This chapter presents indications and strategies for noninvasive and invasive mechanical ventilation; it outlines the application and use of invasive and noninvasive patient monitoring devices, patient assessment, and ventilatory management. Advanced modes of mechanical ventilation strategies, including high-frequency oscillatory ventilation, high-frequency jet ventilation, and neurally adjusted ventilatory assist (NAVA) in the pediatric patient population, will be addressed. Complications specifically related to mechanical ventilation of the pediatric patient are also reviewed in this chapter.

Noninvasive Ventilation

Noninvasive ventilation (NIV) offers an alternative to intubation and mechanical ventilation in the treatment of acute or chronic respiratory disorders commonly encountered in infants and children. There are many distinct challenges associated with the application, management, and safety of NIV in the pediatric population. Recent evidence highlights the complications associated with invasive ventilation. Noninvasive ventilation refers to the delivery of intermittent or continuous assisted ventilation or providing continuous positive pressure during spontaneous breathing to enhance lung expansion by restoring or improving functional residual capacity (FRC) and/or improving minute ventilation without the use of an artificial airway. Noninvasive ventilation is most commonly provided in the forms of **continuous positive airway pressure (CPAP)** or **noninvasive biphasic positive pressure ventilation**. Noninvasive biphasic positive pressure ventilation is often referred to as NIV. Unlike NIV, CPAP does not provide assisted ventilation. CPAP is a spontaneous mode of ventilation that enhances oxygenation and preserves lung inflation by improving the FRC. Because CPAP does not provide tidal breathing support, patients receiving CPAP must have an adequate neurologic drive and the necessary respiratory reserve to breathe spontaneously.

Biphasic positive pressure or NIV improves minute ventilation by providing ventilatory support without the use of an artificial airway, and it improves FRC through the application of positive end-expiratory pressure (PEEP). Positive pressure applied above the distending pressure or PEEP further reduces the work of breathing and augments ventilation when respiratory insufficiency or failure is present as evidenced by CO_2 retention. Although the

interfaces required for biphasic ventilation mirror those used for CPAP, the delivery devices often differ.

Indications for CPAP and NIV

The primary advantage of NIV is avoidance of an artificial airway, which in turn reduces the propensity for oral and mucosal injury associated with intubation, tracheal injury secondary to endotracheal tube cuff trauma, reduced risk of nosocomial infections, decreased need for sedation, increased tolerance for enteral feeds, the potential for care outside of the ICU, and an improved ability to ambulate.[1] Common indications for the use of CPAP and NIV in pediatric patients are outlined in **Table 27-1**.

TABLE 27-1
Indications for the Use of CPAP and NIV in Children

Indications	Modality
Respiratory insufficiency associated with acute lung injury/disease/condition	
• Pneumonia	CPAP, NIV
• Asthma	CPAP, NIV
• Bronchiolitis	CPAP, NIV
• Pediatric acute respiratory distress syndrome (PARDS; mild to moderate)	CPAP or NIV
• Atelectasis	CPAP or NIV
Pulmonary edema associated with cardiomyopathy	CPAP, NIV
Heart failure associated with congenital heart disease	CPAP, NIV
Respiratory insufficiency associated with chronic lung disease/conditions	
• Cystic fibrosis	
• Neuromuscular diseases	CPAP or NIV
• Neurologic disorders associated with respiratory depression	
• Chest wall deformities (e.g., scoliosis)	
Anatomical airway obstruction/collapse	
• Obstructive sleep apnea (OSA)	CPAP or NIV
• Tracheal malacia	CPAP or NIV
• Bronchial malacia	
• Upper airway obstruction (e.g., enlarged tonsils)	CPAP
• Postextubation or prevention of intubation	CPAP, NIV

- CPAP: Must have adequate respiratory drive to sustain adequate gas exchange
- NIV: Indicated when respiratory drive is insufficient to provide adequate gas exchange

Data from Cheifetz IM. Invasive and noninvasive pediatric mechanical ventilation. *Respir Care.* 2003;48(4):442-453.
Basnet S, Mander G, Andoh J, Klaska H, Verhulst S, Koirala J. Safety, efficacy, and tolerability of early initiation of noninvasive positive pressure ventilation in pediatric patients admitted with status asthmaticus: a pilot study. *Pediatr Crit Care Med.* 2012;13(4):393-398.
Ganu SS, Gautam A, Wilkins B, Egan J. Increase in use of non-invasive ventilation for infants with severe bronchiolitis is associated with decline in intubation rates over a decade. *Intensive Care Med.* 2012;38(7):1177-1183.

NIV is primarily used for the treatment of impending respiratory failure associated with acute or chronic respiratory insufficiency secondary to pulmonary disease, neuromuscular disease, airway obstruction, or infectious processes; for postextubation management; or to avoid intubation. NIV may be administered intermittently or continuously, based on patient need and the reversibility of the primary indication for ventilatory assistance.

Published studies reporting the efficacy of NIV in children suggest that proper timing and patient selection have a direct impact on outcomes of children with respiratory failure. In a pilot study evaluating the use of NIV in patients admitted with status asthmaticus, Basnet et al.[2] found children treated with NIV and standard treatment (short acting β-agonists and systemic steroids) had lower clinical asthma scores compared to those receiving standard treatment alone. Clinical asthma scores evaluated objective and subjective data that included respiratory rate, accessory muscle use, air exchange, wheeze, and inhalation/exhalation ratios. Although the clinical asthma scores at baseline were identical, the NIV group had clinical asthma scores that were 15% to 35% lower at each subsequent interval of the study compared to standard care alone.[2] Ganu et al.[3] evaluated the impact NIV had on intubation rates and length of stay in infants with severe bronchiolitis. Children treated with NIV had fewer ventilated days (2.38 days ± 2.43) compared to those who were intubated and mechanically ventilated (5.19 ± 6.34). Overall, an increase in the use of NIV, 2.8% per year, and a decrease in invasive ventilation, 1.4% per year, was realized over the period.[3]

Recently, the Pediatric Acute Lung Injury Consensus Conference Group published recommendations related to the use of NIV in children with acute respiratory distress syndrome. These recommendations included various components of noninvasive support with a consensus ranging from 80% agreement (weak) to 100% agreement (strong).[4] NIV was not recommended for children with severe disease. Although the evidence was weak, immunodeficient patients were identified to be at a greater risk of complications from invasive ventilation and may benefit from early intervention with NIV.[4]

Patient Interfaces

The patient interface is important to the successful implementation of NIV. Manufacturers are increasing their selection of patient interfaces for the pediatric population. There are a variety of interfaces to choose from, including nasal prongs, nasal pillows, nasal masks, oronasal masks, full-face masks, and face shields. Nasal tubes positioned in the pharyngeal airway are also used to provide NIV. All noninvasive interfaces are associated with system leaks, which may influence the performance of the delivery device related to triggering and cycling capabilities. The RAM cannula (Neotech

Inc., Valencia, CA) is a popular interface choice for NIV. This interface is not FDA approved for use as a CPAP or NIV delivery device, and it presents an added delivery challenge for the clinician. The RAM cannula is a high-resistance, nonocclusive interface. Laboratory investigations report that when leaks are ≤30%, the RAM cannula interface resulted in clinically acceptable transmission of pressures. However, when leaks exceed 50%, a clinically negligible amount of pressure was transmitted to the artificial lungs.[5] In the outpatient setting, the use of the RAM cannula in children with chest wall weakness, central control abnormalities, or obstructive and restrictive lung disease contributing to chronic respiratory failure resulted in a significant decrease in arterial $PaCO_2$, a reduced incidence of interface intolerance, and a greater tracheostomy avoidance compared to the use of oronasal or nasal masks to administer NIV.[6]

Factors to consider when selecting the patient interface will include patient headgear and patient safety risks related to the potential for development of skin ulcerations, gastric insufflation, and aspiration. When the risk of aspiration is present, it is best to select a nasal interface, such as a nasal mask or pillows, if possible, to minimize exposure to the accumulation of secretions and/or gastric contents and to reduce the potential for suffocation. The risk of gastric insufflation can be reduced by placement of a vented nasogastric tube while the risk of skin ulcerations can be to reduced by alternating patient interface devices and the use of protective skin barriers. Commonly used pediatric interfaces are presented in **Table 27-2**.

Challenges and Contraindications for the Use of NIV in Pediatric Patients

The most challenging logistical and clinical limitations of NIV in children are reducing interface intolerance and asynchronized breath delivery secondary to triggering and cycling inefficiencies. When a mask is used, proper fit is important. Masks with a substantial volume of gas contained within the interface will reduce trigger sensitivity and make it difficult for the child to initiate a supported breath. Impaired respiratory muscle strength will also reduce the ability to trigger a breath, even when the amount of gas contained within the interface is minimized and leak compensation is employed. Under these conditions, it may be necessary to use a spontaneous timed mode of NIV to achieve and maintain adequate minute ventilation.

All patient interfaces can be associated with air leaks; similar to the RAM cannula, nasal masks are also nonocclusive and often result in excessive air leaks through the mouth. Chin straps can be used to keep the mouth closed and to improve the child's ability to trigger a supported breath. Similarly, nasal prong–occluding devices may help to reduce leaks when nasal prongs are used, especially with smaller patients. Large leaks (>30%)

TABLE 27-2
Common Patient Interfaces Used for NIV

Vendor	Interface	Use	Patient Range	Image
Neotech	RAM cannulas	CPAP, NIV—dual-limb circuits (mechanical ventilators)	Infant / Child (small, medium, large)	 Courtesy of Neotech Products.
Respironics	Simplicity nasal mask	CPAP, NIV (single- and dual-limb devices)	Infant, toddler	 Used with permission of Philips Respironics, Murrysville, PA.
	Performa full-face shield		Toddler, school age, adolescent	 Used with permission of Philips Respironics, Murrysville, PA.
	Performa oral nasal mask		Infant, toddler, school age, adolescent	 Used with permission of Philips Respironics, Murrysville, PA.

Vendor	Interface	Use	Patient Range	Image
ResMed	Pixi	Nasal mask	Toddler, school age	
Sleepnet	MiniMe 2 nasal mask	CPAP, NIV (single- and dual-limb devices)	Infant, toddler	
Circadiance	Sleepweaver cloth nasal mask	CPAP	Toddler, school age, adolescent	

contribute to trigger ineffectiveness by reducing a child's ability to generate an adequate measurable inspiratory flow. Leaks can compromise minute ventilation due to flow and volume that are lost through the leak during inspiration. Leaks can make it difficult to reach the set inspiratory pressure, which in turn reduces tidal volume delivery to the patient. Leaks impair the ability to terminate the breath by compromising the flow cycling threshold, which alters the transition from inspiration to expiration. The aforementioned issues negatively affect patient–ventilator synchrony and contribute to NIV intolerance.

Many noninvasive delivery devices do offer the ability to compensate for interface leaks, which can improve triggering and cycling capabilities and reduce the propensity for NIV intolerance. Some ventilators allow the user to adjust the threshold for transition to exhalation.

However, in the presence of significant leaks, adjustments to the transition threshold may sacrifice effective pressure delivery during NIV. Most commercially available NIV delivery devices are approved for use in patients greater than 20 kg. Therefore, mechanical ventilators are often used to deliver NIV, especially in children weighing 5 to 20 kg. If NIV is required for use outside the pediatric ICU, in long-term care facilities, or in the home, portable ventilators approved for patients ≥5 kg are usually employed.

Management of the Patient Using CPAP and NIV

The goal of CPAP is to restore adequate FRC to correct, reverse, or minimize alveolar collapse. CPAP will effectively reduce the work of breathing as it unloads the work of the inspiratory muscles and allows effective inflation in excess of the opening pressure of the lungs.[7] The level of CPAP required to accomplish this goal in pediatric patients can range from 5 to 15 cm H_2O but varies with the severity of disease. Disorders associated with low lung compliance may require CPAP levels in excess of 10 cm H_2O. CPAP should be used only on patients with an adequate respiratory drive, and when pressures higher than 10 cm H_2O are needed, small (1–2 cm H_2O) adjustments should be incrementally increased to achieve a targeted oxygen saturation goal at an FiO_2 of less than or equal to 0.50 to 0.60. When adequate CPAP levels are achieved, the work of breathing should improve as evidenced by a decreased respiratory rate, fewer sternal or intercostal retractions, and improved oxygen saturations.

When CPAP is used to treat acute lung disease, FiO_2 and CPAP levels should be adjusted as tolerated to maintain oxygenation levels within the specified or provider-ordered ranges. Weaning from CPAP support should commence when the disease process causing the oxygenation problem has or is resolving. Clinical (i.e., work of breathing, hemodynamic stability) and diagnostic (chest radiography, noninvasive oxygen saturation) indicators should be evaluated to determine resolution of disease process and readiness to wean. If CPAP is applied intermittently for nocturnal use for the treatment of obstructive sleep apnea (OSA), the CPAP level is maintained while the FiO_2 is titrated to maintain the provider ordered saturation range. Weaning of CPAP may involve intermittent trials of a high-flow nasal cannula (HFNC) or standard nasal cannula at increasing intervals. CPAP may be discontinued when the patient has been stable on a level of 5 to 6 cm H_2O with an FiO_2 of less than or equal to 40%. Patients are commonly transitioned to HFNC first, as an intermediate step following CPAP, before transitioning to a standard nasal cannula.

NIV adds inspiratory pressure (IP) to the distending pressure, enhancing ventilation and thus CO_2 removal. NIV is required when respiratory insufficiency or respiratory failure is present as evidenced by elevated levels of CO_2. NIV can be administered in spontaneous, spontaneous/timed, or timed mode. The clinician must determine the appropriate mode to use to ensure the effectiveness of NIV and to maximize patient comfort. The **spontaneous mode** is a patient-triggered mode that provides an inspiratory pressure assist without a backup rate. When choosing this mode, the patient must have a good respiratory drive and be able to effectively trigger breaths. The **timed mode** offers a set pressure delivery at a preset mandatory rate and allows additional patient-triggered breaths as needed. This mode can lead to asynchrony when patient breathing efforts conflict with the preset rate. The **spontaneous/timed mode** is a patient-triggered mode that provides inspiratory pressure assist with a backup time-based rate. This mode may offer a combination of patient safety and patient comfort, provided that triggering is effective. Each of these modes can be provided by most noninvasive and invasive delivery devices.

Initial NIV settings should be individualized. This often requires the clinician to have patience and to spend time at the bedside to evaluate tolerance and adjust ventilator settings to optimize ventilation and patient–ventilator synchrony. It will be important to select the interface that facilitates patient tolerance and maximizes triggering capabilities. If a set respiratory rate is used, the rate will be age specific and reflect the level of support needed to provide adequate minute ventilation. The **expiratory positive airway pressure (EPAP)** setting should provide a resting pressure level that minimizes alveolar collapse and should be increased if evidence of lung volume loss is present. The EPAP setting has a direct relationship with oxygenation and should be titrated based on oxygen saturation. EPAP settings should not exceed 7 to 8 cm H_2O for infants or 10 to 12 cm H_2O for older children. **Inspiratory positive airway pressure (IPAP)** is applied to the resting expiratory pressure and translates to volume delivery to the patient. The difference between the IPAP and EPAP settings, or the **delta P**, is the key determinant of volume delivery because there is a linear relationship between pressure and volume. The IPAP setting should be titrated to achieve adequate chest expansion and CO_2 removal. **Inspiratory time**, or the amount of time devoted to inspiration, should be age appropriate and sufficient for breath delivery. Excessively long inspiratory times (>0.8 seconds in infants and 1 second in children) will be uncomfortable and may increase the work of breathing, especially if the patient exhales against inspiratory flow while a breath continues to be delivered. Excessively long inspiratory times may also impair passive exhalation and result in air trapping.

There are other secondary settings available to tailor the way a breath is delivered and may include trigger sensitivity, rise time, breath transition cycle, and pressure ramp time. However, the availability of these settings is manufacturer specific and dependent on the device used. Trigger sensitivity should be set so that the patient can easily initiate a spontaneous or assisted breath without auto-triggering. This can be difficult to achieve secondary to nonuniform leaks around the NIV interface, which have a significant impact on the triggering mechanism. **Rise time** reflects the amount of time required to reach the maximum flow during pressure support ventilation (PSV) or pressure control ventilation (PCV) and should be set to maximize patient comfort. Patients with restrictive lung disease often tolerate a slower rise to pressure. This slower rise to pressure also improves the distribution of ventilation. Patients with increased airway resistance often prefer a more aggressive rise, which shortens inspiratory time and allows for a longer exhalation period. The **cycle time** setting determines the threshold for transition from inhalation to exhalation. Cycle time is important to consider during PSV to improve breath synchrony. It may be either flow or time based. Increasing the cycle time setting should lower the threshold for transition in the presence of large system leaks. The **ramp time**, if available, will allow for a gradual increase in pressure delivery. Adjustments in ramp time are made to assist with patient tolerance and comfort.

Titrating or managing NIV support is a much more complicated process than management strategies used for CPAP. System leaks have a much bigger impact in the initiation of, management of, and liberation from NIV. The approach to weaning is similar to that used for invasive ventilation, if the patient is able to trigger a breath. However, when patients are unable to trigger spontaneous or assisted breaths, a traditional weaning strategy of incrementally reducing the mandatory respiratory rate often does not work. This strategy often fails because it shifts much more of the work of breathing to the patient because spontaneous breaths are not supported and mandatory breaths are not synchronized. This increased work of breathing, especially for patients with limited reserves, contributes to intolerance and weaning failure. To avoid the aforementioned issue, an alternate approach would be to set the mandatory rate to a physiologic level, based on patient age and severity of disease process, and to wean the IPAP setting until the IPAP and EPAP settings are nearly equal. This liberation approach may offer a more gradual shift of the respiratory muscle work from the machine to the patient. There is little evidence in the literature with regard to an optimal weaning strategy. This is a gap that needs more research before evidence-based recommendations can be made. **Table 27-3** provides general management strategies for NIV.

The general success or failure of NIV is difficult to predict. Failure of NIV is often attributed to the lack of interfaces available to minimize leaks, enhance comfort, and minimize intolerance. Bernet and colleagues[8] suggest that the FiO_2 level after 1 hour of NIV may be a predictive factor for success. In the first hour following initiation of NIV, nonresponders had a higher median FiO_2 requirement (0.8) compared to responders (0.48).[8] Patient compliance also plays a role in the success of NIV. Compliance in pediatric patients receiving CPAP has been studied and often is a predictor of NIV success or failure. Poor compliance often contributes to increasing respiratory compromise, leading to respiratory insufficiency and the need for invasive ventilatory support. Hawkins et al.[9] found poor overall compliance, only 49%, in a cohort of patients requiring NIV nocturnally.

All forms of ventilation require patient safety features to be employed. This translates to appropriately adjusting the alarm settings. If available, high tidal volume and high respiratory rate alarms should be set 20% to 30% above baseline. High-pressure alarms should be set at 5 to 10 cm H_2O above IPAP. Low-pressure alarms

TABLE 27-3
General NIV Management Guidelines

Goal	Parameter Adjustment	Comment
Improve oxygenation	↑ FiO_2, ↑ EPAP, ↑ IPAP	Increase if FiO_2 ≤0.50 or EPAP ≥10 cm H_2O.
		Increase EPAP if ≤10 cm H_2O or FiO_2 ≥0.50.
		IPAP will increase mean airway pressure (mP_{AW}) and improve oxygenation.
Wean oxygenation	↓ FiO_2, ↓ EPAP, ↑ IPAP	FiO_2 should be weaned if ≥0.50.
		EPAP should be weaned if ≥10 cm H_2O.
		IPAP should be weaned if ≥25 cm H_2O or excessive chest rise or tidal volume (V_T) is noted.
Improve ventilation	↑ rate, ↑ IPAP	Increase rate if IPAP is ≥20–25 cm H_2O or if V_T is ≥6–8 mL/kg.
		Increase IPAP if V_T is <4–5 mL/kg or set rate is high for age group.
Wean ventilation	↓ rate, ↓ IPAP	Decrease rate if IPAP is ≤15–18 cm H_2O or if V_T is <4–5 mL/kg.
		Decrease IPAP if V_T is ≥6–8 mL/kg or set rate is minimum for age group.
Changing oxygenation and ventilation	Change FiO_2 and rate	FiO_2 will affect oxygenation and rate will affect ventilation.
	Change ΔP	ΔP will increase or decrease ventilation and oxygenation.*

ΔP = delta P
* ΔP affects V_T and mP_{AW}; therefore, pressure changes will affect oxygenation and ventilation.

should be set above the EPAP setting but below the IPAP setting. Apnea time intervals should not exceed 15 seconds for most pediatric patients or 20 seconds for adolescents. Backup ventilation settings, if available, should mirror full ventilatory support settings. Other safety measures clinicians may consider are the use of remote alarm monitoring, including video monitoring, and central nurse call monitoring for heart rate, saturation, and disconnect, especially if the patient is cared for outside of the pediatric ICU.

The Use of Sedation During NIV

The use of sedation to improve tolerance in patients receiving noninvasive ventilation should be given careful consideration. Patients may not tolerate application of the interface or the delivery of inspiratory flow, often perceived as excessive, which prompts providers to contemplate the use of pharmacologic intervention. When all efforts to maximize comfort (e.g., ventilator parameter adjustments, trial of different interfaces) fail, it is essential to select an agent that will enhance comfort and not impair ventilation. Midazolam (Versed) is often used because it produces minimal respiratory depression.

Patient Monitoring During CPAP and NIV

In addition to cardiorespiratory monitoring, surveillance of patients requiring CPAP and NIV should include pulse oximetry monitoring with individualized saturation or patient-specific targets reflective of disease acuity. Pulse provides a good indication of oxygenation status; however, it is of little value for assessing the patient's ventilation status. The adequacy of ventilation must include some periodic form of carbon dioxide measurement. CO_2 measurements can be obtained noninvasively with transcutaneous monitoring or invasively by arterial, venous, or capillary blood gas analysis. CO_2 targets will be disease specific and should account for a compensated acid–base status. End-tidal CO_2 monitoring is rarely used; measurements are often inaccurate due to a dilution effect caused by high inspiratory flows within the patient interface. Assessment of work of breathing and level of consciousness can also provide valuable clinical information on the overall effectiveness of NIV. A change from the baseline clinical and neurologic status provides clinicians with important information needed to determine therapeutic effectiveness.

Chest radiographs are useful in evaluating the adequacy of lung inflation. Chest radiographs may also be used to monitor disease progression. However, they will not reflect the adequacy of oxygenation or ventilation.

Adjuncts or Alternative Approaches to Noninvasive Ventilation

Technologic advances offer clinicians tools to enhance the effectiveness of NIV. These advances offer novel ways to trigger inspiration and improve patient–ventilator interaction, particularly with infants and young children who have rapid respiratory rates and small tidal volumes. To complicate matters, breath delivery in NIV is generally pressure limited and does not accommodate variability in respiratory demand.[10]

A manufacturer proprietary mode, neurally adjusted ventilatory assist (NAVA; Getinge, Wayne, NJ; Maquet Critical Care) uses a specially designed catheter to detect and use diaphragmatic electrical activity as a trigger mechanism. **Figure 27-1** displays a line drawing of the catheter used to connect and send the electrical signals to the Servo-I or Servo-U ventilator (Getinge, Wayne, NJ; Maquet Critical Care) to trigger flow at the start of inspiration. The signals (Edi) exist at two levels. The **Edi**$_{max}$ represents diaphragmatic contraction, or the start of inspiratory effort. The **Edi**$_{min}$ represents diaphragmatic relaxation, or the expiratory effort required to maintain FRC. When the Edi catheter is properly placed, signals provide feedback that controls the flow of gas from the ventilator. The literature reports the utility of this trigger mechanism in infants and children with sporadic breathing patterns and large interface leaks.[11] **Figure 27-2** shows the ability to trigger in the presence of a large patient interface leak. In a cross-over study, Baudin and colleagues[11] compared pressure control NIV and NIV-NAVA in a cohort of children admitted to the pediatric ICU with respiratory failure secondary to bronchiolitis. Asynchrony, in terms of auto-triggering, double triggering, or nontriggered breaths, was scored using an objective asynchrony index and found to be lower during NIV-NAVA ($3 \pm 3\%$) compared to pressure control NIV ($38 \pm 21\%$).[11] Trigger delay was also shorter during NIV-NAVA (43.9 ± 7.2 ms) compared to pressure control NIV (116.0 ± 38.9 ms).[11] There were also statistically significant fewer ineffective efforts when NIV-NAVA was used (0.54 ± 1.5) than when pressure control NIV was used (21.8 ± 16.5 events/min).[11]

Successful use of NIV-NAVA is limited by the functionality of the NAVA catheter and the neurologic respiratory drive of the patient. However, NAVA does provide a backup safety feature to delivery ventilation

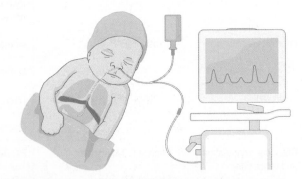

FIGURE 27-1 Illustration of an infant with a NAVA Edi Catheter in place and the signal response to diaphragmatic activity.
Courtesy of Getinge.

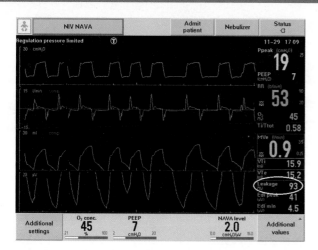

FIGURE 27-2 Graphical representation of NIV-NAVA with large patient interface leak.
Courtesy of Getinge.

when an Edi signal cannot be detected. The ventilator, in this instance, will provide backup noninvasive pressure control ventilation.

The use of a **heated high-flow nasal cannula (HHFNC)** to support the work of breathing in children with respiratory distress has gained popularity in recent years. Data, however, are limited and conflicting with regard to the efficacy with which a CPAP effect is produced. It is important to distinguish the intended goals of therapy when implementing HHFNC therapy. One theory is that the flow rates used during HHFNC administration will be sufficient enough to produce a CPAP effect. In a small cohort of children (n = 10) with obstructive sleep apnea and CPAP interface and/or device intolerance, Hawkins et al.[12] found that the use of an HHFCN at flows of 10 to 50 L/minute were effective in reducing the median number of obstructive apnea hypopnea events per hour (11.1 to 2.1 events/hour), improving oxyhemoglobin saturation (mean SpO_2 of 91.3% to 94.9%), and reducing heart rate (88 bpm to 74 bpm). It is also hypothesized that the high flow rates delivered by the HHFNC are sufficient enough to meet all, the patient's inspiratory flow demands, will flush CO_2 out of the anatomic dead space, and will replace it with a fresh gas source provided by the high-flow system.[13] Therefore, the nasopharyngeal anatomic dead space is used as a reservoir of fresh gas, which in effect reduces rebreathing and decreases the contribution of the anatomic dead space to breathing inefficiency.[13] Rebreathing of exhaled CO_2 is reduced and the conducting airways become a reservoir for fresh gas, which is particularly important in small children, considering that the extrathoracic anatomic dead space of a newborn is as high as 3 mL/kg and does not approximate that of an adult (0.8 mL/kg) until after 6 years of age.[14] There are other assumed benefits of HHFNC use, including maximizing mucociliary clearance, reducing inflammatory reactions, inhibiting the bronchoconstrictor reflex, and reducing airway resistance.[15,16] High flow may be delivered

at whatever FiO_2 is necessary to achieve the designated patient-specific oxygenation goals, at flows of 2 to 20 L/minute in pediatric patients at a recommended temperature of 34°C to 35°C.[16]

Complications and Safety During NIV

Complications associated with NIV are most often seen in the most fragile patients and include but are not limited to gastric distension, aspiration, pneumothorax, and pressure ulcerations. Of these, pressure ulcerations or skin breakdown are the most preventable. Pressure ulcers develop from pressure applied to the skin when the NIV interface is placed. Excessive pressure from a tight-fitting interface results in periods of ischemia, which in turn causes damage to the epidermis and, depending on the severity, may also cause damage to the underlying deeper tissue.[17] The extent of damage is characterized by stage and can be found in **Table 27-4**.

The use of skin barriers, such as hydrocolloid and/or foam products, assessing interface fit to assure a small leak is present, frequent skin integrity assessments, and the use of a different device type to offload the pressure on the bridge of the nose or around the nares, are helpful in minimizing the formation of pressure ulcers.[18] In addition to routine inspection, cleansing of the face and interface are effective in minimizing rubbing friction.[18] Maintaining normal skin hydration is also an important factor for protecting skin tissue integrity.[19] In a sample of 50 children, Visscher et al.[19] investigated factors contributing to pressure ulcer formation. Skin breakdown was most commonly noted and was more severe with the use of oronasal masks.[19] The bridge of the nose represented the area most vulnerable to pressure injury.[19] Caregivers should be trained to recognize the stages of skin breakdown and be knowledgeable in the measures aimed at minimizing pressure injury risk.

The risk for gastric distension can be reduced by ensuring that all patients receiving NIV have vented gastric tubes in place to circumvent excess air from the stomach. It is also important to employ aspiration precautions, which include strict feeding schedules, elevating the head of the bed, careful suctioning procedures to reduce gagging and emesis, and close patient monitoring.[20]

Pneumothoraces can be reduced by minimizing pressure delivery and careful clinical observation and monitoring of chest rise, compliance changes resulting in trends in volume delivery, and appropriate alarm settings.

Invasive Mechanical Ventilation

Invasive mechanical ventilation requires the use of an artificial airway (e.g., endotracheal tube, tracheostomy tube) to provide continuous or intermittent mechanical ventilatory support.

TABLE 27-4
Characterization of Pressure Ulcers by Stage

Stage	Description	Illustration
Stage I	Nonblanchable erythema that may be painful, soft, and warmer or cooler than adjacent tissue	
Stage II	Partial dermal loss that often can be seen as a shallow open ulcer or an intact blister	
Stage II	Dermal loss to the extent where subdermal elements can be seen	
Stage IV	Full-thickness tissue loss with exposed bone, tendon, or muscle	
Unstagable	Full thickness wounds covered by slough and/or eschar	

Indications and Goals

The indications for invasive mechanical ventilatory support in children mirror those reported for adults. Respiratory failure is the disease process most often requiring the use of invasive ventilatory support. In children, respiratory failure can be categorized into either restrictive pathology (characterized by decreased FRC and decreased lung compliance [C_L]) or obstructive pathology (characterized by increased FRC and normal to decreased C_L secondary to hyperinflation).[4] The obstructive pathology can involve the upper and/or lower airways. Other indications for invasive ventilation include neurologic disorders, neuromuscular disorders, cardiovascular collapse, and postsurgical procedures involving stabilization of the patient's cardiorespiratory system. **Table 27-5** provides a detailed list of clinical indications for invasive ventilatory support in children.

When mechanical ventilation is required, the goals are individualized and dependent upon patient condition and the underlying disease causing the need for respiratory support. Strategies should be determined by diagnosis, disease state, and patient response. In all cases, goals for mechanical ventilation will include the ability to maintain or maximize FRC by applying continuous distending pressure and should include provisions to ensure adequate oxygenation and ventilation based on the current patient condition. The strategies used should minimize ventilator-induced lung injury (VILI) and ventilator-associated events (VAEs). Frequent evaluation of the patient is required as the patient's condition(s) may change rapidly. The patient plan of care should specify time-sensitive goals related to invasive ventilatory support. Interventions may result in modifications to the established goals and strategies or may involve evaluation and modification of mechanical ventilation adjuncts. Often, goals and milestone projections for goal attainment are modified because of patency or position problems encountered with the artificial airway, new onset of air leaks, changes in lung compliance and/or airways resistance, or the addition of alterations in the function of other organs. Plans of care should be updated to reflect alterations in the goal or projected timeline to goal attainment. **Figure 27-3** provides an illustration of a plan of care documented in the electronic medical record.

Ventilator Modes

The spectrum of patients and variation of lung disease are vastly different in children as compared to term and preterm infants. As infants grow and develop, chest wall compliance is less affected by body position and becomes less compliant (although it is still more compliant than the chest wall of an adult).[21] Airway resistance, in both the upper[22] and lower airways,[23] is also much higher in children. These physiologic characteristics contribute to the pulmonary time constants (T_C) of the individual patient (T_C = airways resistance (R_{AW}) $\times$ lung compliance (C_L)) and influence ventilator settings related to inspiratory time or flow. A summary of the detailed descriptions of breath sequence is presented in **Table 27-6**, and modes of ventilation are provided in **Table 27-7**.

TABLE 27-5
Indications for Mechanical Ventilation of the Pediatric Patient

Restrictive Disorders	**Neurologic Disorders**
• ARDS (pediatric respiratory distress syndrome) • Scoliosis • Pneumonia • Pleural effusions (e.g., chylothorax, hemothorax) • Chronic or acute aspiration • Chest wall tumors or masses • Rib cage anomalies (achondroplasia)	• Central hypoventilation syndrome, mitochondrial disorders, congenital neuromuscular disorders • Brain tumors resulting in increased intracranial pressure or apnea • Encephalitis or encephalopathy syndromes • Traumatic brain injuries • Neurologic infections (meningitis) • Drug overdose
Obstructive Disorders (Upper Airway)	**Neuromuscular Disorders**
• Croup • Epiglottitis • Laryngomalacia • Trachealmalacia • Subglottic stenosis • Neck masses	• Myasthenia gravis • Guillain-Barre syndrome • Spinal cord injury • Mitochondrial disorders • Diaphragm paralysis (e.g., phrenic nerve damage)
	Surgical
	• Hypoventilation (postsurgical recovery)
Obstructive Disorders (Lower Airway)	**Cardiovascular Disorders**
• Asthma • Bronchiolitis • Cystic fibrosis • Bronchopulmonary dysplasia (BPD)	• Cardiomyopathy (e.g., myocardial dysfunction) • Congenital cardiac defects (postoperative recovery) • Shock • Sepsis resulting in cardiovascular compromise

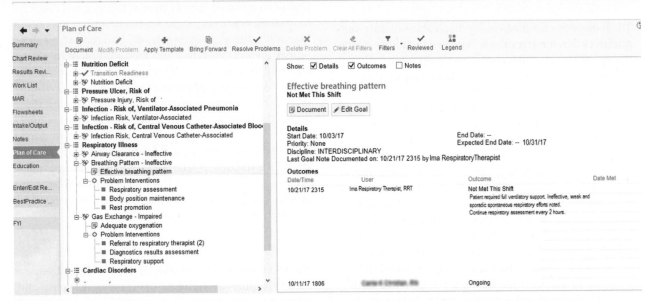

FIGURE 27-3 An illustration of documentation used to communicate progress toward goal attainment. Note the goal of achieving adequate spontaneous respiratory support is projected in 10 days. The respiratory therapist provided a summary of the barriers to goal attainment. In this case, the supporting evidence can be found in the patient's flow sheet documentation. The flowsheet provides the spontaneous respiratory rate and V_T details at the time of the assessment.

TABLE 27-6
Breath Sequence Comparison

Breath Sequence	Advantages	Disadvantages
Continuous mandatory ventilation, also known as assist control (AC)	Shifts the work of breathing to the ventilator	Patient's spontaneous triggering may result in inadvertent or unintentional hyperventilation
Synchronized intermittent mandatory ventilation (SIMV)	Divides the work of breathing between the patient and the ventilator Easier to wean Spontaneous breaths can be supported to facilitate spontaneous breathing effort	May shift too much work of breathing to the patient if not monitored closely May result in dysnchrony when spontaneous breaths compete with mandatory breaths
Continuous spontaneous ventilation	Patient controls breath and allows for greater patient comfort	Patients may tire or have apneic episodes, resulting in hypoventilation

TABLE 27-7
A Summary of the Advantages and Disadvantages Associated with Modes of Ventilation

Mode	Advantages	Disadvantages
Volume control ventilation (VCV)	Every mandatory breath delivered by the ventilator at a preset volume	Constant flow pattern characteristics result in a more turbulent flow and higher peak pressures
Pressure control ventilation (PCV)	Decelerating flow pattern results in a more laminar flow and desired tidal volumes can be achieved at lower peak pressures	Volume delivery is based on lung compliance and can change, resulting in variable tidal volume delivery
Volume targeted ventilation	Combines the advantages of VCV and PCV by targeting a tidal volume and delivering it in a decelerating flow pattern	Breath delivery is based on feedback to the ventilator and will be affected by endotracheal tube (ETT) leaks (caution should be taken if the leak exceeds 30%)

TABLE 27-8
Recommendations for Initial Mandatory Breath Rate Settings by Age

	Infant	Toddler	Small Child	Child	Adolescent
Age range	30 days to 1 year	>1–3 years	>3–5 years	>5–10 years	>10 years
Mandatory breath rate (breaths/min)	25–40	20–35	20–30	18–25	12–20

Setting Mandatory Breath Rate

Pediatric patients can be classified as infant, toddler, small child (preschool), child (school age), and adolescent. The initial mandatory rate set on a mechanical ventilator depends on the normal respiratory rates for each of the aforementioned age-based classifications and the disease process contributing to the need for ventilatory support. Some commonly used initial respiratory rate settings by age group are presented in **Table 27-8**.

The set mandatory rate will be dependent upon severity and progression of disease. Children with high airway resistance and air trapping require respiratory rates at the lower range of normal and a longer expiratory time. Because respiratory rate is a component of minute ventilation ($V_E = RR \times V_T$), there is an inverse relationship with CO_2 removal. Increasing the mandatory rate should reduce arterial CO_2 provided that the delivered V_T is unchanged. During weaning, the mandatory rate may be weaned to a minimum rate (i.e., 4–6 breaths/min depending on the patient's age) or to CPAP with or without pressure support in all age groups.

Setting Tidal Volume (V_T) or Inspiratory Pressure (IP)

Lung protective strategies recommend limiting the delivered V_T to 6 to 8 mL/kg. Tidal volume can either be directly set (as with VCV) or will be a result of inspiratory pressure delivery applied to baseline PEEP (during PCV). When PCV is used, V_T delivery will vary and is based on the compliance and resistance of the respiratory system. As lung compliance worsens, V_T delivery will decrease. Conversely, as the disease process and lung compliance improve, the V_T delivered with each mandatory pressure controlled breath will increase. Careful V_T monitoring is necessary when PCV is used to avoid hypoventilation or potential lung injury from the delivery of excessive volumes. There is an inverse relationship between V_T and CO_2 removal: Increasing the V_T should reduce arterial CO_2 provided that the respiratory rate is unchanged.

Limiting V_T to avoid alveolar overdistention is a component of lung protective strategy. It is important to note that regional overdistension can still occur if significant atelectasis persists and gas flow patterns are diverted to the more compliant areas of the lung.[24]

Adjusting Inspiratory Time, Flow, and I:E Ratios

Inspiratory time (T_I) is an operator-set parameter during PCV and will be dependent on the mandatory breath rate setting and age of the patient. To allow sufficient time to exhale, the T_I should allow for an I:E ratio of at least 1:2. When VCV is used, the clinician will either adjust the flow rate to achieve the target T_I or set the T_I to produce a constant flowrate. The aforementioned adjustments depend on the specific brand of ventilator used.

The general starting point for setting the inspiratory flowrate is 10 L/minute per 100 mL of V_T. There is an inverse relationship between flowrate and T_I: Higher set inspiratory flowrates result in a shorter T_I. Because time constants are longer in children compared to preterm or term newborn infants, the T_I set for pediatric patients is longer than that set for term or preterm newborns. The total cycle time influences inspiratory and expiratory times. It is important for the clinician to set the T_I at a target that is age appropriate and to allow for sufficient time to achieve complete exhalation before the next breath occurs.

Ventilator graphics can be a valuable tool in evaluating the appropriateness of T_I and/or flowrates during mechanical ventilation. **Figure 27-4** represents the flow

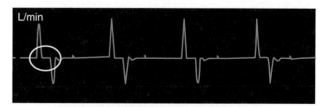

Inspiration ends before exhalation begins, resulting in a breath hold if the T_I is too long

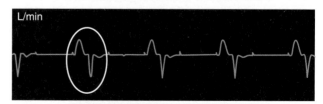

Inspiration will end when expiration begins when the T_I is set appropriately

FIGURE 27-4 Examples of flow-time waveforms during PCV when T_I is not set appropriately for the patient's age and disease condition.

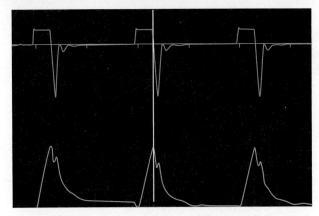

FIGURE 27-5 Evaluation of the flow-time and volume-time waveforms during VCV to determine the appropriateness for the flow setting. The white line represents end inspiration and the transition to passive exhalation. Flow stops as exhalation begins. There is no evidence of a breath hold or premature breath termination. This indicates that the flowrate set is providing a T_I that is appropriate for the patient.

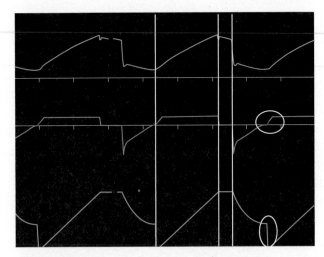

FIGURE 27-6 Evaluation of the flow-time and volume-time waveforms during VCV. This graphic illustrates the effect set flow has on T_I when set too low.

waveforms during PCV that occur when T_I settings are and are not appropriately set.

During VCV, the clinician must observe the flow-time scalar and compare the end of inspiratory flow to the start of exhalation. T_I is set appropriately when flow stops as exhalation begins and there is no evidence of a breath hold or premature breath termination (**Figure 27-5**).

When inspiratory flowrates are set too slow, prolonged T_I results and a plateau will occur on the volume waveform, indicating a breath hold (**Figure 27-6**). If the inspiratory time is too short or flowrates are too aggressive, the clinician will observe premature breath termination before the volume is delivered. Flowrates that are set too high will contribute to turbulent flow delivery to the airways, which may compromise the distribution of ventilation. Graphically, this can be seen by the delivery

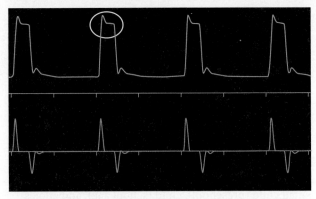

FIGURE 27-7 A graphical example of pressure overshoot, resulting from the delivery of high inspiratory flows, which also results in a very short T_I.

of higher peak inspiratory pressures and the presence of pressure overshoot (**Figure 27-7**).

The Use of PEEP

PEEP is used to recruit and maintain FRC. As FRC is restored and approaches the opening pressure of the lung, less positive pressure will be required to deliver volume during a breath. This is an important concept in the application of lung protective ventilation strategies.[24] Inadequate PEEP results in atelectasis, allowing gas flow to follow the path of least resistance into open regions of the lung, leading to regional overdistension in the presence of heterogeneous lung disease.[25] When PEEP levels are less than the opening pressure of the lungs, the pressure applied to the lungs does not result in volume delivery until the opening pressure is reached (**Figure 27-8A**). When the lungs are overdistended, pressure applied at the end of the breath does not result in additional volume delivery because the alveoli are maximally stretched. The pressure volume curve is helpful in identifying overdistension. The portion of the curve where pressure continues to rise but volume plateaus is referred to as **beaking** (**Figure 27-8B**).

Pressure–volume curves can be difficult to obtain when the patient is not paralyzed. As a result, clinicians often set PEEP to the level that produces the smallest change in pressure, or **delta pressure (ΔP)**. ΔP is calculated as PIP – PEEP at a specific V_T and provides the set level of PEEP of best compliance. When PEEP is set too high, intrathoracic pressure rises to a point where hemodynamic compromise can occur. Therefore, it is important to monitor systemic blood pressure and to evaluate the effect that titrating PEEP levels has on hemodynamic stability. Changes in blood pressure (i.e., hypotension) during PEEP titration are a sign that PEEP is set too high and should be reduced.

Setting and Adjusting Inspired Oxygen Concentration (FiO₂)

Adequate oxygenation is important for neurodevelopment and end-organ perfusion; however, excessive

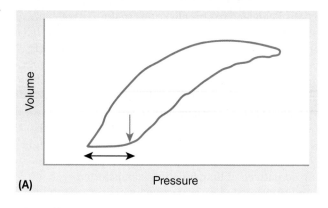

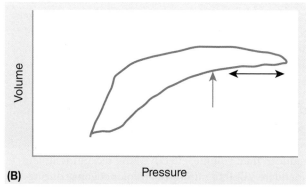

FIGURE 27-8 Pressure volume curves illustrating the opportunity to appropriately set PEEP and inspiratory pressure. (**A**) PEEP in this case is set too low. PEEP should be increased to "Opening Pressure" or the PEEP should be increased to the pressure level at the point when volume begins to increase (depicted by the red arrow). (**B**) Beaking (depicted by the black arrow) is a sign of overdistention and can contribute to volutrauma. The inspiratory pressure, in this case, should be decreased to the pressure at which volume ceases to produce additional volume (red arrow).

levels of oxygen have been associated with systemic inflammatory responses resulting in pulmonary complications.[26] The goals related to oxygen delivery should be diagnosis based and provide adequate tissue oxygenation at the lowest possible FiO_2. **Table 27-9** provides

an example of target saturation ranges based upon diagnosis or condition-specific considerations.

Setting and Adjusting Trigger and Cycle Sensitivity

Trigger refers to the initiation of an inspiratory breath. Mechanical breaths can be initiated or triggered by the patient's spontaneous effort or by the ventilator when no patient effort exists or is detected. Breaths that are ventilator or machine triggered occur after a preset time elapses and depends on the set mandatory rate, inspiratory time, or flow. For example, during pressure control ventilation, a breath will be delivered every 3 seconds when the mandatory rate is set to 20 breaths per minute and the inspiratory time is set at 1 second.

The use of flow triggering is common in infants and children while pressure triggering may be seen in older children and adolescents. It is easier for infants and younger children to flow trigger because this trigger mechanism is referenced to the bias flow the ventilator delivers. Commonly, a flow sensor placed at the patient wye or connection is used to sense inspiratory effort. This allows the ventilator to sense small changes in flow and to use that mechanism to sense inspiratory effort to synchronize breath delivery with patient need or effort.

It is important to adjust the inspiratory trigger setting to a level that is sensitive enough to detect inspiratory effort. The inspiratory trigger setting is patient specific and based on the strength of spontaneous inspiratory effort as well as on the presence and magnitude of an ETT leak. If the trigger is set too low, the ventilator will **auto-trigger**. Auto-triggering can also occur when excess condensation is present in the ventilator circuit. Depending on the trigger sensitivity setting, excessive condensation can slosh in the circuit and cause frequent and rapid changes in bias flow, which in turn are interpreted by the ventilator as patient effort. When the trigger is not set sensitive enough to detect patient

TABLE 27-9
Oxygen Saturation Targets for Children Based on Diagnosis or Specific Conditions

Diagnosis or Condition	Saturation Target	Considerations
Passive pulmonary blood flow (Glenn, Fontan)	70–75% (Glenn)	Liberal use of oxygen will lower pulmonary pressures and enhance pulmonary blood flow.
	85–90% (Fontan)	
Conditions associated with pulmonary hypertension	95%	Liberal use of oxygen will lower pulmonary pressures and enhance pulmonary blood flow.
Acute lung disease (PARDS)	≥88%[4]	Targeting normal oxygen saturations will result in the use of higher inspiratory pressures and risk VILI.
Normal lung function	93–99%	When mechanical ventilation is required for patients with normal lung function, the saturation target should be within the normal range and the FiO_2 requirement should be ≤0.40.

breathing effort, the ventilator will not respond to the patient's inspiratory efforts and will contribute to an increased work of breathing. Auto-triggering and trigger sensitivity that are set below a level that prevents the ventilator from detecting inspiratory effort contribute to patient–ventilator dysynchrony.

Cycle sensitivity refers to the setting that terminates the inspiration, transitioning the breath to exhalation. The term used for this setting is not standard and varies by ventilator manufacturer. Cycle sensitivity is used to control the duration of the breath during pressure support breaths. Most ventilator manufacturers use a general default value that requires a drop in peak flow of 25% to 30% of the maximum flow. The cycle sensitivity setting allows the clinician to adjust the default setting, based on the respiratory pattern of the patient, to improve patient–ventilator synchrony. For example, if a large or significant ETT leak is present, inspiratory time may be prolonged during a pressure supported breath. In this case, the ventilator senses the leak and interprets it as volume loss. In response to the ventilator's interpretation, additional flow is delivered over a longer period of time to compensate for the perceived volume loss, which increases total inspiratory time. To minimize the risk for prolonged inspiratory times when large or significant ETT leaks are present, the clinician can increase the cycle sensitivity, which in turn will synchronize the transition from inspiration to expiration with the patient's breathing pattern.

Ventilator graphics are very helpful and can assist the clinician in setting trigger and cycle sensitivity. The flow-time waveform allows the clinician to visualize the onset of inspiratory flow by observing the flow-trigger indicator at the onset of inspiratory flow. When a patient is making inspiratory effort and a deflection in flow is noted on the flow-time waveform but a mechanical breath is not triggered, the setting is not sensitive enough. Conversely, when there is no detectible deflection in flow but the ventilator is delivering breaths above the set mandatory rate, the trigger sensitivity setting is set too sensitively.

The clinician should also observe the transition from inspiration to expiration. When inspiration is prolonged and the patient is making active efforts to exhale, the cycle sensitivity is not set sensitive enough.

Strategies for Preventing Lung Injury

Factors related to VILI are barotrauma, volutrauma, hyperoxia, and the underlying disease process.[27] Strategies used to prevent lung injury are targeted at reducing alveolar overinflation by minimizing the duration and intensity of positive pressure delivered to the lungs and include ventilator management strategies that incorporate permissive hypercapnia; early extubation; nonconventional ventilation, such as high-frequency ventilation; and alternative therapies, such as extracorporeal membrane oxygenation.

VILI can lead to complications that negatively impact patient outcomes and contribute to increased ICU and hospital lengths of stay. The process of repeated collapse and re-expansion of the ventilating lung units, or **atelectotrauma**, is often heterogeneous and results in uneven distribution of ventilation.[28] Heterogeneous atelectasis can potentially lead to regional overdistention of the lungs and result in **volutrauma**, which, when combined with underinflated areas of the lung, contribute to ventilation/perfusion mismatch.[28] This mixed pattern of lung inflation is most often seen in conditions related to restrictive lung disease with low lung compliance, but obstructive lung diseases can have a restrictive component that will complicate ventilator management.[28] Lung recruitment maneuvers and PEEP management can maximize lung inflation and improve ventilation/perfusion match and gas exchange.[29]

Permissive hypercapnia is a strategy that allows $PaCO_2$ levels to rise above normal values while maintaining a pH of 7.20 to 7.25 or greater. The literature reports that a higher CO_2 tolerance in combination with reduced tidal volume, effective lung recruitment, and adequate PEEP to minimize alveolar collapse during expiration will lead to a reduction in positive pressure ventilation and therefore lower the rates of VILI and VAEs.[30] It is important to note that permissive hypercapnia may not be indicated for patients with pulmonary hypertension, hemodynamic instability, or elevated intracranial pressures.

Advanced Modes of Ventilation and Concepts: High-Frequency Jet Ventilation and High-Frequency Oscillatory Ventilation (HFJV, HFOV)

The indications and concepts of gentle ventilation using high-frequency oscillatory ventilation (HFOV) or high-requency jet ventilation (HFJV) for pediatric patients are similar to those for neonatal patients. The use of HFJV and HFOV in pediatric patients is controversial and often used when children are failing conventional ventilation.[31] Indicators that conventional ventilation has failed include plateau pressures of greater than 28 cm H_2O or oxygenation index (OI) of greater than 12 to 15 (OI = $mP_{AW} \times FiO_2/PaO_2$).[31]

The hertz setting in HFOV is typically lower in pediatric patients. Because inspiratory time is based on a percentage of cycle time, and tidal volumes are larger in children compared to neonates, the piston has a longer time for forward movement to deliver the volume required to ventilate a child, therefore necessitating a lower hertz rate.[32] Pediatric patients weighing more than 35 kg require the use of the Sensormedics 3100B (Cardinal Health, Dublin, OH). The concept of lung recruitment and lung protection during HFOV provides ventilation in the safe lung zone (**Figure 27-9**).

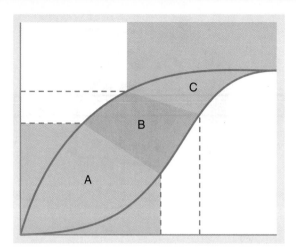

FIGURE 27-9 An illustration of the safe zone, or the area of ventilation HFOV targets. The red areas indicate (A) underinflation or (C) overinflation. (B) The desired inflation point or safe zone at which ventilation is effective without risk of lung trauma

There are several factors to consider when transitioning a child from conventional ventilation to HFOV. **Table 27-10** provides guidelines for initial HFOV settings, mirroring those used for neonates and infants, and outlines the factors to consider. Gas exchange can change rapidly during HFOV, and clinicians need to be able to recognize and react to those changes to avoid complications. Ventilator adjustment strategies are similar to those used for neonates and are presented in **Table 27-11**. Pediatric patients are frequently weaned to minimum HFOV settings and are much more likely to be converted to conventional ventilation prior to extubation.

HFJV is an alternative to HFOV in pediatric patients and is commonly provided by the Bronchotron or VDR 4, both manufactured by Percusionaire (Sandpoint, ID) (**Figure 27-10**). These HFJVs provide time-cycled and pressure-limited high-frequency pulsations over a baseline pressure. Tidal volumes delivered during

TABLE 27-10
Guidelines for Initial HFOV Settings in Children

Settings	Lung Recruitment	Lung Protection (Minimizing the Chance for Air Leaks or Hyperinflation)
Hz	Patient specific:	Patient specific:
	Infant: 8–10 Hz	Infant: 10–12 Hz
	Child: 6–10 Hz	Child: 6–10 Hz
	Adolescent: 3–5 Hz	Adolescent: 3–5 Hz
mP_{AW}	2–4 above mP_{AW} of the conventional ventilator	Equal to mP_{AW} of the conventional ventilator
	Increase mP_{AW} by 1 cm H_2O until desired SpO_2 is achieved, then wean FiO_2	Accept $SpO_2 \geq 88\%$
FiO_2	100%	100%
Amplitude	Enough to produce chest wiggle in the following manner:	Enough to produce chest wiggle in the following manner:
	Infant: The abdomen	Infant: The abdomen
	Child: The hip	Child: The hip
	Adolescent: The thigh	Adolescent: The thigh
	Adjust ΔP by 2–4 to change ventilation (áΔP to âCO_2)	Adjust ΔP to accept permissive hypercapnia in the absence of pulmonary hypertension
T_I	33% (never to exceed 50%)	33% (do not adjust)
Monitoring transcutaneous CO_2 and oxygen saturation by pulse oximetry	Highly recommended	Highly recommended
	Rapid changes in $PaCO_2$ levels may occur, affecting cerebral perfusion	Rapid changes in $PaCO_2$ levels may occur, affecting cerebral perfusion
	As mP_{AW} approaches opening pressure of the lung, oxygenation will improve	As mP_{AW} approaches opening pressure of the lung, oxygenation will improve

TABLE 27-11
Ventilator Adjustment Strategies Used to Manage Children Requiring HFOV

Parameter	To Increase	To Decrease
O_2	↑ mP_{AW}	↓ mP_{AW}
	↑ FiO_2	↓ FiO_2
	↑ T_I (not very effective—do not use in lung protection strategy)	
	Initiate inhaled nitric oxide therapy in the presence of pulmonary hypertension	
CO_2	↓ amplitude	↑ amplitude
	↑ Hz	↓ Hz (this results in higher gas delivery and is equivalent to increasing the V_T)

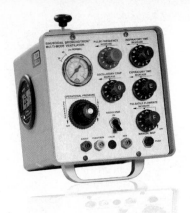

(A)

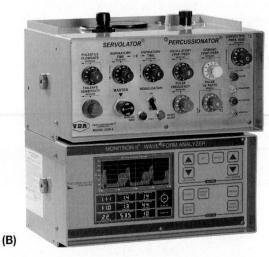

(B)

FIGURE 27-10 The **(A)** Bronchotron and **(B)** VDR 4 high-frequency ventilators.
Courtesy of Percussionaire Corp.

HFJV are higher and mandatory rates are lower than ventilation with HFOV. Exhalation differs as well. Exhalation is passive during HFJV and active during HFOV. The VDR 4 differs from the Bronchotron in that the pulsatile flowrate and demand CPAP settings are separate controls, which allows the clinician to have greater control of breath delivery. The literature reports that airway patency may be better maintained with the use of HFJV because gas is not actively withdrawn during exhalation, therefore reducing the potential for airway collapse.[33] Additionally, HFJV is the preferred mode in the presence of bronchopleural fistulas.[33]

Oxygenation with HFJV is controlled by mean airway pressure (mP_{AW}), which is a product of the demand CPAP/PEEP, the oscillatory CPAP/PEEP, and the frequency. Ventilation is controlled by the frequency and pressure settings. The management strategy related to titrating ventilation and oxygenation mimics that of pressure control ventilation.

HFOV and HFJV are more common in centers that care for critically ill pediatric patients than centers that care only for critically ill neonates. The choice related to which device to use should be based on diagnosis and the overall goals of ventilation.

Biphasic Ventilation and APRV

Biphasic ventilation is a pressure control breath delivery type and applies two distinct PEEP levels (high and low), which allows for spontaneous ventilation throughout the ventilation cycle and the availability to add pressure support to augment a spontaneous breath. **Airway pressure release ventilation (APRV)** differs from biphasic ventilation in that the high PEEP setting is applied for a longer duration of time than the time applied

at the low PEEP setting. APRV provides an inverse I:E and is most commonly used in conditions associated with hypoxic respiratory failure and low lung compliance. When the lung compliance is low, exhalation occurs rapidly and air trapping is not a concern. Biphasic APRV should be considered when conventional ventilation efforts are failing as evidenced by increasing respiratory acidosis and hypoxemia. The clinician can quantify the severity or progression of hypoxemia by following the child's calculated OI.

The maximum I:E ratio used during APRV is 4:1, which significantly increases mP_{AW}. There is a risk for hemodynamic comprise secondary to the high transpulmonary pressures produced by the high mP_{AW}. Therefore, careful consideration should be given to patients with cardiac compromise prior to employing this strategy. Minute ventilation and CO_2 removal are a result of the number of transitions (rate) between high and low PEEP and the volume of gas that is produced (V_T) during those transactions. Oxygenation is a product of the mP_{AW} pressure and FiO_2. Graphic representation of APRV is provided in **Figure 27-11**.

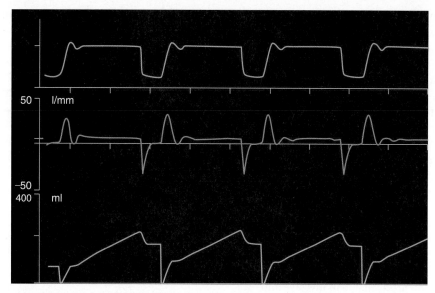

FIGURE 27-11 A graphic illustration of mechanical ventilation with APRV. Note the inverse I:E ratio.

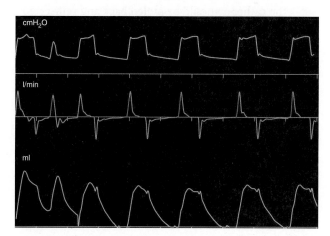

FIGURE 27-12 A graphic illustration of biphasic ventilation. Note that the I:E ratio is not inverse.

Biphasic ventilation delivers high and low pressures with I:E ratios that are not inverse and is graphically represented in **Figure 27-12**. This strategy might be useful in a patient with a leaky ETT or mild to moderate hypoxemia.

Neurally Adjusted Ventilatory Assist (NAVA)

Neurally adjusted ventilatory assist ventilation (NAVA) is the proprietary name of a spontaneous mode of ventilation available on the Servo-I and Servo-U ventilators (Maquet, Rastatt Germany). This mode of ventilation was reviewed in Chapter 26. This use of NAVA in children is similar to its use with neonates and newborn infants. However, there are some nuances for its particular use in children. Similar to pressure support, the patient's own respiratory drive controls the rate of ventilation. This spontaneous mode of ventilation uses an orogastric catheter embedded with special sensors that detect electronic signals from the phrenic

nerve to the diaphragm, sensing diaphragmatic contraction. These signals are used to synchronize the delivery of flow and to preset pressure to the patient. The breath ends when the sensors embedded in the orogastric catheter sense diaphragmatic relaxation. These signals are transmitted to and interface with the ventilator to control flow delivery during the inspiratory phase of ventilation. When the diaphragm relaxes, flow ceases and the patient is permitted to exhale. Responsiveness of the ventilator is more effective because it is based on diaphragm contractility as opposed to flow requirements detected at the ventilator. Diaphragm activity is controlled by impulses sent to the phrenic nerve and is a true reflection of patient demand based on native neurologic responses. The NAVA level controls the amount of ventilator assist that is provided to the patient. The performance of the ventilator and delivery of flow while the patient is in NAVA is unaffected by leaks associated with endotracheal tubes. However, this is not as important in the pediatric population as it is with neonates and newborn infants. This is because endotracheal tubes with cuffs are typically used with pediatric patients and uncuffed tubes with neonates and newborn infants. Because NAVA uses signals from the diaphragm to determine inspiratory effort, this proprietary mode of ventilation has been shown to improve patient synchrony, which may minimize patient work of breathing. **Table 27-12** provides a review of NAVA terminology.

The use of NAVA with children is identical to its use with neonates and newborn infants in that this mode of ventilation can be used invasively or noninvasively. During invasive NAVA, there are safety backup ventilation features that ensure the child receives mechanical ventilatory support if the diaphragm catheter signal is lost or the child becomes apneic. If the diaphragm signal is lost, the child will receive pressure support ventilation. Backup ventilation is provided if the child becomes apneic or if the ventilator is unable to detect spontaneous effort that is sufficient enough to trigger pressure supported breaths. The length of time and frequency with which the child receives backup ventilation may be important to the care of children with neurodegenerative disorders receiving this form of ventilatory support. Monitoring backup ventilation trends may provide an indication that the child's muscle weakness is worsening. When NAVA is used in conjunction with a ventilator liberation strategy, monitoring backup ventilation trends may provide the clinical team with information useful for evaluating how the patient tolerated the ventilator management plan of care. Both pressure support and backup ventilation are determined by and parameters are set by the clinician. Pressure support and backup ventilation are available in invasive and noninvasive NAVA. Backup ventilation allows for full ventilatory support if all patient breathing efforts were to cease.

Preparing the child for this mode of ventilation is important. The procedure for initiating this mode of ventilation is found in Table 27-13. Since a special orogastric catheter is needed to detect diaphragmatic signals, selecting the appropriate-size catheter is important. Catheter size is dependent on the patient's height. A sizing chart can be found in Table 27-14. Once the clinician selects the correct catheter size, depth of insertion must be calculated to place the catheter in the location to detect a strong signal. Table 27-15 provides guidelines for determining the catheter insertion depth. Once the catheter is inserted to the premeasured depth, ventilator graphics are used to adjust the catheter position. The graphics used to adjust the catheter position can be accessed through the NAVA menu, after which there is a selection softkey for the Edi catheter positioning, as shown in Figure 27-13. Basic NAVA preview signal observations shown in Figure 27-13 should include verification of the following:

- The Edi catheter signal should display from larger to smaller; if the signal goes from smaller to larger in size, the catheter may have looped around and the catheter should be pulled back and reinserted.
- If the blue signals are in the top two rows, the catheter is advanced too far and should be pulled back.
- If the blue signals are in the bottom two rows, the catheter should be advanced.

TABLE 27-12
NAVA Terminology

Term	Meaning
NAVA level	The NAVA level is the overall level of support provided to the patient (higher levels indicate more ventilator assist).
Edi peak	This is an indication of the inspiratory work of breathing and indicates the contractility or energy expenditure of the diaphragm.
Edi min	This is an indication of the expiratory work of breathing and indicates the effectiveness of PEEP and the relaxation state of the diaphragm.
Trigger Edi	This is indicative of the amount of diaphragm exertion required to initiate a response from the ventilator.

TABLE 27-13
Procedure for the Initiation of NAVA

1. Place the NAVA module with cable into the designated slot on the side of the Servo I or U ventilator.
2. Select the appropriate Edi catheter (based on size of the patient).
3. Dip the end of the catheter into some sterile water or pour sterile water into the catheter tray prior to insertion (careful not to wet the cable connectors)—do not use lubricant on the catheter. Wetting the catheter helps to activate the sensors within the catheter.
4. Insert the catheter to the premeasured depth (see NEX—Table 27-15) and plug into the NAVA cable.
5. Access the NAVA menu by depressing the NAVA softkey, then select Edi catheter positioning to verify catheter placement (Figure 27-13).

TABLE 27-14
Pediatric and Adolescent NAVA Catheter Sizes

EDI Catheter Size	Inner Electrode Distance (IED)	Patient Weight	Patient Height
16 Fr: 125 cm	16 mm	–	>140 cm
12 Fr: 125 cm	12 mm	–	75–160 cm
8 Fr: 125 cm	16 mm	–	>140 cm
8 FR: 100 cm	8 mm	–	45–85 cm

TABLE 27-15
Estimated Nasal Catheter Insertion Depth

Size Fr/cm	Calculation
16 Fr	NEX (cm) × 0.9 + 18 = Y (at the nose)
12 Fr	NEX (cm) × 0.9 + 15 = Y (at the nose)
8 Fr: 125 cm	NEX (cm) × 0.9 + 18 = Y (at the nose)
8 Fr: 100 cm	NEX (cm) × 0.9 + 8 = Y (at the nose)

NEX (cm) = nose/earlobe/xyphoid
Y = insertion distance from tip to the nose

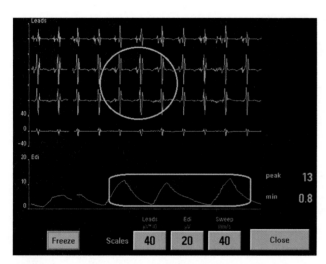

FIGURE 27-13 Graphical illustration of the signals obtained and trended during NAVA catheter positioning.
Courtesy of Getinge.

NAVA level and PEEP determinations mirror those used in the neonatal patient. Alternatively, the clinician may choose to place the patient in NAVA ventilation and titrate the NAVA level to achieve a pre-NAVA peak inspiratory pressure (PIP), a predetermined V_T, or an Edi_{max} that is <20 mV and a delivered V_T that is within the prescribed target range. After the NAVA level is set, the PEEP can then be adjusted to produce an Edi_{min} of <2 mV.

There are other parameters, the clinician must set, which include the trigger Edi, pressure support, and backup ventilation. The trigger Edi should be set so that flow from the ventilator begins as the diaphragm contracts; this is seen graphically as a lavender spike at the onset of the diaphragm waveform (**Figure 27-14**).

Settings for pressure support and backup ventilation during NAVA will be patient specific and should be determined based on age, weight, diagnosis, and pulmonary condition of the patient. Pressure support (PS) and pressure control (PC) settings should be sufficient enough to provide full ventilator support; the peak pressure observed during NAVA ventilation will serve as a guide to the PS and PC settings. When setting the trigger for NAVA and PS, it is important to note that the ventilator will provide the spontaneous breath based

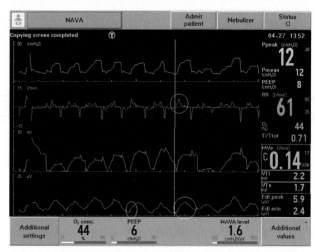

FIGURE 27-14 An example of using NAVA graphics to set the NAVA level. The lavender originates from the beginning of diaphragmatic contraction, indicating that the Edi trigger is appropriately set. If the lavender spike appears higher on the diaphragm signal, the trigger is set too high and the activity is not picked up until the diaphragm is partially contracted; conversely, if the signal is displayed on the down slope of the signal, the trigger is set too low and the ventilator is picking up activity during the relaxation phase. Note the lack of diaphragm signal with a flow-triggered response will cause the ventilator to deliver a pressure-supported breath.
Courtesy of Getinge.

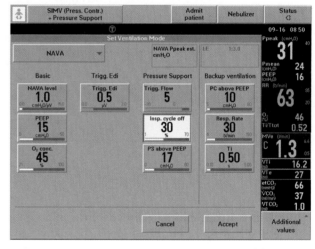

FIGURE 27-15 An illustration of the ventilator screen displaying pressure support and backup ventilation settings.
Courtesy of Getinge.

on the trigger signal that is sensed first. This becomes more important in the presence of an ETT leak and may require adjustment of the flow trigger (increase the flow threshold) and the inspiratory cycle (increase the percentage) settings to maximize NAVA triggering. An illustration of the ventilator screen displaying backup settings is seen in **Figure 27-15**.

There is a dearth of information regarding ventilator management with this proprietary mode of ventilation. Although ventilator management in the NAVA mode needs more study, commonly used guidelines are presented in **Table 27-16**.

TABLE 27-16
Commonly Used Guidelines for Managing Patients Using NAVA

Parameter	Increase	Decrease	Notes
Oxygenation (O_2)	Increase FiO_2	Decease FiO_2	Before changing PEEP levels, it is important to evaluate the Edi_{min}, as increasing or decreasing PEEP levels can lead to overdistension or derecruitment.
	Increase PEEP	Decrease PEEP	
Ventilation (CO_2)	Increase NAVA level	Decrease NAVA level	It will be important to evaluate the Edi_{max} before changing the NAVA level.

*Extubation may be considered when the PIP – PEEP is <10 cm H_2O.

TABLE 27-17
Basic Conventional and Nonconventional Ventilator Management Strategies

Desired Effect	Conventional Ventilator	HFOV	HFJV
↑ PO_2	↑ FiO_2, ↑ PEEP, ↑ PIP	↑ FiO_2, ↑ MAP	↑ FiO_2, ↑ HFJV PIP, ↑ demand PEEP, ↑ oscillatory PEEP, ↑ I:E ratio settings
↓ PaO_2	↓ FiO_2, ↓ PEEP, ↑ PIP	↓ FiO_2, ↓ MAP	↓ FiO_2, ↓ HFJV PIP, ↓ demand PEEP, ↓ oscillatory PEEP, ↓ I:E ratio settings
↑ $PaCO_2$	↓ rate, ↓ PIP, ↓ set or target V_T	↓ amplitude	↓ HFJV PIP, ↓ HFJV frequency
↓ $PaCO_2$	↑ rate, ↑ PIP, ↑ set or target V_T	↑ amplitude, ↓ hertz	↑ HFJV PIP, ↑ HFJV frequency
Comment	Target delivered V_T should be 4–6 mL/kg in all breath delivery types to avoid VILI.	MAP is used to recruit the lung while amplitude is used to eliminate CO_2.	The VDR 4â virtually applies oscillations over biphasic pressures controlled by I:E ratio settings.

PIP – PEEP = (ΔP) delivered V_T: There is a linear difference between the ΔP and the V_T, provided maximum inflation is not exceeded. Regardless of breath delivery type, the goal should be to maintain a delivered V_T of 6–8 mL/kg.
Oxygenation is a product of oxygen concentration and mean airway pressure (MAP). The MAP is related to any setting that is related to the amount or duration of positive pressure delivery (PIP, PEEP, and, to a lesser degree, rate and T_I).
CO_2 levels are influenced by minute ventilation (VE): Rate × V_T = VE.
During HFOV, the T_I is a percentage of TCT; therefore, as hertz is ↓ T_I is ↑, resulting in increased gas delivery per piston stroke.
During HFJV, pressure and rate adjustments mimic PC adjustments and T_I is variable.

Prone Positioning

Prone positioning changes the distribution of alveolar ventilation by redistributing blood flow and altering the regional lung compliance.[34] This redistribution of blood flow and increased regions of improved lung compliance result in improved ventilation/perfusion match and better gas exchange. Other effects of prone positioning include less left lower lung compression by the heart and enhanced secretion removal.[34] Studies have shown significant improvements in PaO_2/FiO_2 ratios following prone positioning at interval time points. The improvement in PaO_2/FiO_2 ratios and a reduction in mortality were associated with the use of prone positioning.[35]

Maintaining the airway patency and position of the ETT or tracheostomy tube and intravenous lines while positioning the patient prone is technically difficult. It takes a multidisciplinary team with a highly coordinated approach to safely change the patient from a supine to a prone position. The Pediatric Acute Lung Injury Consensus Conference Group does not routinely recommend the use of prone positioning, although they do recommend that it is considered in cases of severe pediatric ARDS.[4]

Management of the Patient Requiring Invasive Ventilation

Ventilatory management is complex and principles cannot be universally applied to all patients. Management requires evaluation of current pathophysiology and clinical presentation. Several factors should be considered when making decisions regarding ventilator management. The disease process, chest radiograph results, current respiratory status, and potential complications must all be considered. A summary of ventilatory management for conventional and nonconventional modes of ventilation related to the desired effect on ventilation and oxygenation are presented in **Table 27-17**.

Wide swings in CO_2 levels should be avoided. CO_2 levels that are too high are associated with acidosis, pulmonary vasoconstriction, and increased cerebral blood flow and may be harmful to patients with elevated intracranial pressures and patients with pulmonary hypertension. Excessively low CO_2 levels are associated with limited cerebral blood flows. Targeted values for arterial blood gas tensions are found in **Table 27-18**.

TABLE 27-18
Targeted Values for Arterial Blood Gas Tensions

Pediatric Lung Condition	pH	$PaCO_2$	PaO_2
Normal compliance	7.35–7.45	35–45 mm Hg	70–100 mm Hg
Decreased compliance (permissive hypercapnia)	7.15–7.25[3]	60–70 mm Hg (to maintain pH)	50–70 mm Hg
Pulmonary hypertension	7.35–7.40	40–50 mm Hg	80–100 mm Hg in the absence of cyanotic heart disease

Weaning and Extubation

Ventilator weaning should be individualized and outlined in the patient plan of care. Ventilator parameters that should be weaned are based on results from blood gas analysis or noninvasive monitoring. Weaning should be targeted first on the ventilator parameters or settings that are most toxic to the lungs. Excessive pressures and inspired oxygen level are considered the most damaging and should be adjusted first when weaning is considered.

Extubation criteria vary by center and include criteria related to resolution of acute respiratory failure or active infection, the ability to sustain spontaneous respirations, and the ability to protect the airway. Most practitioners would consider extubation of the pediatric patient if the FiO_2 were <0.40, the mandatory respiratory rate is minimal for age, the PIP is ≤20 to 25cm H_2O, and the PEEP is ≤5 cm H_2O. Postextubation interventions include the use of nasal CPAP, noninvasive ventilation, or high-flow nasal cannula. The postextubation intervention will depend on the patient's ability to maintain FRC, minute ventilation, or oxygenation status. CPAP is used when the patient has a strong respiratory drive but the lung condition is associated with a loss of lung volume or airway malacia. Noninvasive ventilation is often used when the patient has a weak respiratory drive or respiratory muscle fatigue. The high-flow nasal cannula is designed to flush out the anatomic dead space and to provide an oxygen-enriched gas flow to the patient, improving the oxygenation status. High-flow nasal cannulas must be heated and humidified and can be used at flows of up to 20 L/minute in pediatric patients and up to 40 L/minute in adolescent patients.

Ventilator weaning time can approach 40% of the total duration of mechanical ventilation, and advanced weaning tools are fueling the desire to improve efforts focusing on liberation from mechanical ventilation.[36] Weaning techniques range from protocols to the many closed loop ventilator modes commercially available. Automatic weaning modes available in the United States include **mandatory minute ventilation (MMV)**, **auto-mode**, **adaptive support ventilation (ASV)**, and **smart care**. MMV involves setting a target minute ventilation that is the reference point for support. The ventilator predicts the minute ventilation over 8 to 10 breaths and provides support based on that prediction. Auto-mode monitors the spontaneous breathing efforts and automatically switches to a spontaneous mode of pressure support or volume support, provided the patient does not violate the trigger timeout. ASV uses a percentage of minute ventilation to determine the level of ventilator support provided. The percentage of minute ventilation support provided is determined by the user. Smart care adjusts pressure support levels based on V_T, respiratory rate, end-tidal carbon dioxide, and patient condition. Not all closed loop features are available for pediatric patients and the evidence is mixed.

Complications of Mechanical Ventilation

There are a number of complications or conditions related to mechanical ventilation, many of which can be minimized or prevented by careful monitoring of the patient. One of the most serious acute complications associated with the delivery of positive pressure ventilation is the development of pulmonary air leaks. Air leaks occur when excessive pressure is applied to the lungs, causing the alveolar wall to rupture and resulting in an accumulation of air in the pleural space. This causes the lung to collapse and impairs gas exchange and can lead to hemodynamic compromise.

Summary

Mechanical ventilation is complex and cannot be universally applied to all patients equally. The variations and complexity of the pediatric patient require that all patients be evaluated individually with careful consideration given to diagnosis, severity of illness, complications, and patient response. There is a much broader range of age and weight in the pediatric population and treatment is complicated by the presence or absence of congenital abnormalities affecting cardiopulmonary blood flow or physiologic development. The clinician must have a strong understanding of the unique challenges associated with pediatric disorders and the unique mechanical ventilation strategies that should be applied.

Case Study 1

A 5-month-old male infant was admitted to the pediatric intensive care unit for severe bronchiolitis. The patient was initially managed on high-flow nasal cannula but, due to worsening respiratory distress, progressed to the use of noninvasive positive pressure ventilation at an inspiratory pressure of 22 cm H_2O, expiratory pressure of 4 cm H_2O, and an FiO_2 of 0.48. V_T is approximately 3.8 mL/kg. Arterial blood gas analysis 2 hours after the initiation of noninvasive ventilatory support reveals the following: pH 7.12, $PaCO_2$ 78 mm Hg, PaO_2 50 mm Hg, HCO_3 24 mEq/L, and base excess -4. SpO_2 was 88%.
  Classify the ABG:

a. Uncompensated respiratory acidosis

b. Uncompensated metabolic acidosis

c. Compensated respiratory acidosis

d. Compensated metabolic acidosis

Physical examination revealed grunting and significant suprasternal and intercostal retractions. Respiratory rate was 72 breaths per minute and heart rate was 130 beats per minute.
  What would the respiratory therapist recommend?

a. Intubate and initiate mechanical ventilation

b. Change the FiO_2 to 6.0

c. Increase the inspiratory pressure to 24 cm H_2O

d. Decrease the expiratory pressure to 2 cmH_2O

Case Study 2

An 11-year-old male with leukemia presented with septic shock, acute respiratory distress syndrome (ARDS), and multiorgan dysfunction. He became progressively hypoxemic, with an OI of 28 on pressure control (PC) ventilation despite the following settings: Fio_2 1.0, SIMV mode with PIP 38 cm H_2O, and PEEP 14 cm H_2o. He had a MAP of 24 cm H_2O. SpO_2 ranged from 84% to 86% and $P_{ET}CO_2$ ranged from 50 to 54 mm Hg. The patient remained hypotensive, and was unresponsive to fluid administration and vasopressors.

  Which of the following should the respiratory therapist recommend?

a. Change to HFOV

b. Switch to APRV

c. Increase the PEEP to 18 cm H_2O

d. Initiate heliox gas therapy

  Conventional ventilation in the APRV mode was initiated with the following settings: Phigh 36 cm H_2O, PLow 0 cm H_2O, Thigh 4 seconds, TLow 0.5 seconds, with an FiO_2 of 60%. The patient was able to breath spontaneously on the APRV mode.
  What is the maximum I:E ratio used during APRV?

a. 1:4

b. 1:5

c. 1:6

d. 1:7

1. **What is the maximum ratio of time high (thigh) and time low (tlow)?**

References

1. Cheifetz IM. Invasive and noninvasive pediatric mechanical ventilation. *Respir Care.* 2003;48(4):442-453.
2. Basnet S, Mander G, Andoh J, Klaska H, Verhulst S, Koirala J. Safety, efficacy, and tolerability of early initiation of noninvasive positive pressure ventilation in pediatric patients admitted with status asthmaticus: a pilot study. *Pediatr Crit Care Med.* 2012;13(4):393-398.
3. Ganu SS, Gautam A, Wilkins B, Egan J. Increase in use of non-invasive ventilation for infants with severe bronchiolitis is associated with decline in intubation rates over a decade. *Intensive Care Med.* 2012; 38(7):1177-1183.
4. Khemani RG, Smith LS, Zimmerman JJ, Erickson S; Pediatric Acute Lung Injury Consensus Conference Group. Pediatric acute respiratory distress syndrome: definition, incidence, and epidemiology. *Pediatr Crit Care Med.* 2015;16(5 Suppl 1):S23-S40.
5. Iyer NP, Chatburn RL. Evaluation of a nasal cannula in noninvasive ventilation using a lung simulator. *Respir Care.* 2015;60(4):508-512.
6. De Jesus Rojas W, Samuels CL, Gonzales TR, et al. Use of nasal non-invasive ventilation with a RAM cannula in the outpatient home setting. *Open Respir Med J.* 2017;21(11):41-46.
7. Loh LE, Chan YH, Chan I. Noninvasive ventilation in children: a review. *J Pediatr.* 2007;83(2 Suppl):S91-S99.
8. Bernet V, Hug MI, Frey B. Predictive factors for the success of noninvasive mask ventilation in infants and children with acute respiratory failure. *Pediatr Crit Care Med.* 2005;6(6):660-664.
9. Hawkins SM, Jensen EL, Simon SL, Friedman NR. Correlates of pediatric CPAP adherence. *J Clin Sleep Med.* 2016;12(6):879-884.
10. Stein H, Beck J, Dunn M. Noninvasive ventilation with neutrally adjusted ventilator assist in newborns, *Semin Fetal Neonatal Med.* 2016;21(3):154-161.
11. Baudin F, Pouyau R, Cour-Andlauer F, Berthiller J, Robert D, Javouhey E. Neurally adjusted ventilator assist (NAVA) reduces asynchrony during non-invasive ventilation for severe bronchiolitis. *Pediatr Pulmonol.* 2015;50(12):1320-1327.

12. Hawkins S, Huston S, Campbell K, Halbower A. High-flow, heated, humidified air via nasal cannula treats CPAP-intolerant children with obstructive sleep apnea. *J Clin Sleep Med*. 2017;13(8): 981-989.

13. Dysart K, Miller TL, Wolfson MR, Shaffer TH. Research in high flow therapy: mechanisms of action. *Respir Med*. 2009;103(10):1400-1405.

14. Numa AH, Newth CJ. Anatomic dead space in infants and children. *J Appl Physiol*.1996;80(5):1485-1489.

15. Rea H, McAuley S, Jayaram L, et al. The clinical utility of long-term humidification therapy in chronic airway disease. *Respir Med*. 2010;104(4):525-533.

16. Ward JJ. High-flow oxygen administration by nasal cannula for adult and perinatal patients. *Respir Care*. 2013;58(1):98-122.

17. Cornelissen LH, Bronneberg D, Bader DL, Baaijens FP, Oomens CW. The transport profile of cytokines in epidermal equivalents subjected to mechanical loading. *Ann Biomed Eng*. 2009;37(5):1007-1018.

18. Acorda DE. Nursing and respiratory collaboration prevents BiPAP-related pressure ulcers. *J Pediatr Nurs*. 2015;30(4):620-623.

19. Visscher MO, White CC, Jones JM, Cahill T, Jones DC, Pan BS. Face masks for noninvasive ventilation: fit, excess skin hydration, and pressure ulcers. *Respir Care*. 2015;60(11):1536-1547.

20. Bambi S, Mati E, De Felippis C, Lucchini A. Noninvasive ventilation: open issues for nursing research. *Acta Biomed*. 2017;88(1-S):32-39.

21. Ingimarsson J, Thorsteinsson A, Larsson A, Werner O. Lung and chest wall mechanics in anesthetized children. Influence of body position. *Am J Respir Crit Care Med*. 2000;162(2 Pt 1):412-417.

22. Laine-Alava MT, Murtolahti S, Crouse UK, Warren DW. Upper airway resistance during growth: a longitudinal study of children from 8 to 17 years of age. *Angle Orthod*. 2016;86(4):610-616.

23. Lambert RK, Castile RG, Tepper RS. Model of forced expiratory flows and airway geometry in infants. *J Appl Physiol*. 2004; 96(2):688-692.

24. Broche L, Perchiazzi G, Porra L, et al. Dynamic mechanical interactions between neighboring airspaces determine cyclic opening and closure in injured lung. *Crit Care Med*. 2017;45(4):687-694.

25. van Kaam A. Lung-protective ventilation in neonatology. *Neonatology*, 2011;99(4):338-341.

26. Priestley MA, Helfaer MA. Approaches in the management of acute respiratory failure in children. *Curr Opin Pediatr*. 2004;16(3):293-298.

27. Jauncey-Cooke JI, Bogossian F, East CE. Lung protective ventilation strategies in paediatrics—a review. *Aust Crit Care*. 2010;23(2):81-88.

28. Wiswell TE, Srinivasan P. Continuous positive airway pressure. In: Goldsmith JP, Karotkin EH, eds. *Assisted Ventilation of the Neonate*. 4th ed. Philadelphia: Elsevier;2003:128.

29. Jauncey-Cooke J, East CE, Bogossian F. Paediatric lung recruitment: a review of the clinical evidence. *Paediatr Respir Rev*. 2015;16(2):127-132.

30. Rotta AT, Steinhorn DM. Is permissive hypercapnia a beneficial strategy for pediatric acute lung injury? *Respir Care Clin N Am*. 2006;12(3):371-387.

31. Arnold JH, Anas NG, Luckett P, et al. High-frequency oscillatory ventilation in pediatric respiratory failure: a multicenter experience. *Crit Care Med*. 2000;28(12):3913-3919.

32. Custer JW, Ahmed A, Kaczka DW, et al. In vitro performance comparison of the Sensormedics 3100A and B high-frequency oscillatory ventilators. *Pediatr Crit Care Med*. 2011;12(4):e176-e180.

33. Baumann MH, Sahn SA. Medical management and therapy of bronchopleural fistulas in the mechanically ventilated patient. *Chest*. 1990;97(3):721-728.

34. Johnson NJ, Luks AM, Glenny RW. Gas exchange in the prone posture. *Respir Care*. 2017;62(8):1097-1110.

35. Scholten EL, Beitler JR, Prisk GK, Malhotra A. Treatment of ARDS with prone positioning. *Chest*. 2017;151(1):215-224.

36. Branson RD. Modes to facilitate ventilator weaning. *Respir Care*. 2012;57(10):1635-1648.

28

Surfactant Replacement Therapy

Amanda L. Roby

OUTLINE

OBJECTIVES

1. Define surfactant replacement therapy.
2. Describe the role of surfactant in the lungs and surfactant replacement agents.
3. Describe the indications for surfactant administration.
4. Explain the methods of administering surfactant.
5. Discuss the various surfactant preparations.
6. Explain the clinical considerations with surfactant replacement therapy.
7. List the common hazards and complications of surfactant replacement therapy.
8. Discuss the limitations of surfactant replacement therapy.

KEY TERMS

antenatal steroids
fetal lung maturity testing
preterm
respiratory distress
  syndrome (RDS)
respiratory failure
surfactant
term

Introduction

The infants in the neonatal intensive care unit (NICU) often require unique and specialized complex care. Long-term outcomes related to **respiratory distress syndrome (RDS)** are critically dependent on early assessment and intervention from the entire healthcare team. Surfactant replacement therapy (SRT) is the standard of care for most premature and term infants experiencing various types of respiratory distress.[1]

Surfactant replacement was established as an effective and safe therapy for immaturity-related surfactant deficiency by the early 1990s.[1] **Surfactant** is a compound found between the alveolar surfaces and gases in the lungs. During exhalation, surfactant-deficient alveoli do not inflate properly, which may cause the lung to collapse completely or may require great pressure to inflate the lung efficiently. Premature infants are often surfactant deficient and have an increased risk of RDS, a condition associated with morbidity and mortality.[2] Systemic reviews of randomized controlled trials confirmed that surfactant administration in preterm infants with established RDS reduces mortality, decreases the incidence of pulmonary air leaks (pneumothoraces and pulmonary interstitial emphysema), and lowers the risk of chronic lung disease or death at 28 days of age.[3–8] RDS due to surfactant deficiency is the most common cause of **respiratory failure** in preterm infants.[1]

Description

Surfactant replacement therapy is one of the few treatments that has evolved in clinical neonatology and one in which tremendous research progress continues to be made. In addition to RDS, surfactant deficiency has been observed in many other clinical cases in preterm and term infants, opening the doors to further surfactant replacement therapy opportunities.

Physiology in Normal Term Infants

The transition from a fetus to a newborn is the most complex process that occurs in human experience. Lung capabilities require the coordinated clearance of fetal lung fluid, surfactant secretion, and the onset of consistent breathing. A new infant, whether born at **term** or **preterm**, must quickly adapt to this complex transition. At birth, many infants will need assistance in the delivery room. The essential component of this transition at birth is the maintenance of an adequate respiratory effort.

The development of the fetal lung to support gas exchange is essential in preparation for birth (**Figure 28-1**). During the last third of gestation, or the third trimester of pregnancy, the fetal lung separates into about 4 million distal saccules known as respiratory bronchioles and alveolar ducts. At approximately 32 weeks' gestation, separation occurs to form alveoli.[9] Earlier in fetal development, around 22 weeks' gestational age, surfactant lipid and the lipophilic proteins SP-B and SP-C begin to be synthesized and aggregated into lamellar bodies in the maturing type II cells.[10] The lamellar bodies are essential active components in the storage and secretion of surfactant. As the lung matures, more and more of the lamellar bodies are released into fetal lung fluid and subsequently mix with amniotic fluid or are swallowed.[10] By 38 weeks' gestation, type II cells in the fetal lung contain much more surfactant than the adult lung. The major function of type II cells is secretion of pulmonary surfactant, which decreases the surface tension within the alveoli (**Table 28-1**). As 40 weeks' gestation approaches, fetal lung fluid secretion will diminish and fetal lung fluid volume may decrease. Simultaneously, surfactant is secreted into the fetal lung fluid during labor, which will increase the surfactant concentration in the fetal lung fluid.[11] Subsequently, the initiation of ventilation following birth causes alveolar stretch and deformations of type II cells, another secretion

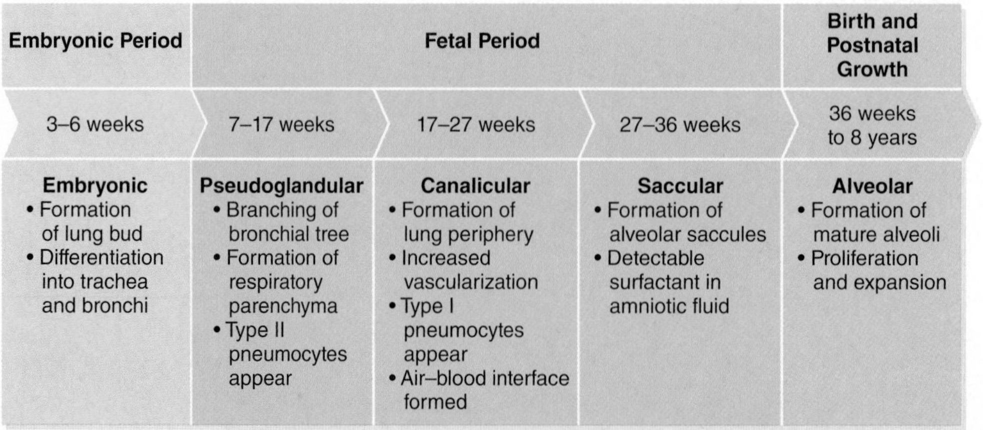

Embryonic Period	Fetal Period			Birth and Postnatal Growth
3–6 weeks	7–17 weeks	17–27 weeks	27–36 weeks	36 weeks to 8 years
Embryonic • Formation of lung bud • Differentiation into trachea and bronchi	**Pseudoglandular** • Branching of bronchial tree • Formation of respiratory parenchyma • Type II pneumocytes appear	**Canalicular** • Formation of lung periphery • Increased vascularization • Type I pneumocytes appear • Air–blood interface formed	**Saccular** • Formation of alveolar saccules • Detectable surfactant in amniotic fluid	**Alveolar** • Formation of mature alveoli • Proliferation and expansion

FIGURE 28-1 Key components of fetal lung development from conception to transition to extrauterine life.

TABLE 28-1
Description and Function of Type I and Type II Pneumocytes

Type I Pneumocytes	Type II Pneumocytes
• Involved in the process of gas exchange between the alveoli and the capillaries • Are squamous (flattened) in shape and extremely thin (~0.15 μm), minimizing diffusion distance for respiratory gases • Connected by occluding junctions, which prevent the leakage of tissue fluid into the alveolar air space • Are amitotic and unable to replicate; however, type II cells can differentiate into type I cells if required	• Responsible for the secretion of pulmonary surfactant, which reduces surface tension in the alveoli • Are cuboidal in shape and possess many granules (for storing surfactant components) • Comprise only a fraction of the alveolar surface (~5%) but are relatively numerous (~60% of total cells)

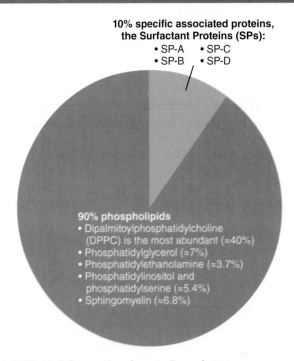

FIGURE 28-2 Composition of mammalian surfactant.

signal.[10] The type II cells act as alveoli caretakers and are essential for term infants to transition to gas exchange and air breathing. The secretory events concurrent with birth do not appreciably deplete surfactant stores in type II cells because surfactant synthesis and packaging into lamellar bodies continues, and the surfactant that has been secreted also is recycled back into type II cells to be secreted again as needed.[12]

Premature infants and other very sick newborns face some of the same medical issues. Premature infants often have breathing problems because their lungs are not fully developed. Generally, the earlier an infant is born, the higher the risk of complications. The preterm lung has several disadvantages for transition at birth. The structurally immature lung has less potential lung volume relative to body weight and metabolic needs, and secretion of fetal lung fluid may not cease prior to or after birth, which will delay clearance of fetal lung fluid. Further, the amount of surfactant stored in type II cells is low, and less surfactant can be secreted in response to birth. Many preterm lungs can adapt with help from new medical modalities.

Components of Pulmonary Surfactant

The composition, metabolism, and function of surfactant have been studied in depth. Surfactant is a complex phospholipid produced and secreted by the type II alveolar cells in the lung. It is synthesized and recycled through complex metabolic pathways. Surface-active properties decrease the surface tension at the air–water interfaces in the alveoli, preventing collapse during the entire respiratory cycle.[13–15] Surfactant also plays a role in host defense and improves mucociliary clearance with removal of particles from the lungs.[14,16]

Surfactant is composed of six phospholipids and four proteins. The components of surfactant are 80% to 86% phospholipids, 8% neutral lipids, and 6% to 12% proteins (**Figure 28-2**).[17–19] Saturated phosphatidylcholine (or lecithin) accounts for 70% of the phospholipid portion of surfactant, with dipalmitoylphosphatidylcholine (DPPC) accounting for 60% of the phosphatidylcholine.[17] This desaturated phospholipid, DPPC, is critical for lowering the surface tension and can reduce it to almost zero.[17] Although DPPC is the primary component for surface activity, alone it adsorbs poorly to the air–liquid interfaces within the alveoli. During exhalation, there is a reduction in surface tension and the monolayer becomes enriched with DPPC. The presence of the surfactant proteins and other unsaturated phospholipids aid in the adsorption and surface-active properties of surfactant.[17] The amount of DPPC in the lungs is dependent on lung development, with an increase seen at 22 weeks' gestation.[17] Sphingomyelin is a phospholipid seen in inverse proportions relative to phosphatidylcholine, with levels of sphingomyelin decreasing with lung maturity. In utero, the ratio of lecithin to sphingomyelin (L:S ratio) is used to determine lung maturity. An L:S ratio of greater than 2.0 to 2.5 is indicative of fetal lung maturity in most assays.[20]

Phosphatidylglycerol (PG) and phosphatidylinositol (PI) are acidic phospholipids that aid in DPPC adsorption, with the amounts of each of these substances affected by lung development and lung injury. They account for about 10% of total lipids.[14] During initial surfactant development in the fetus, PI is the primary acidic phospholipid, with increases of PG seen in the more mature lung after 34 to 35 weeks' gestation.[17,21] The presence of PG in the amniotic fluid is an important determinate of lung maturity.

There are four unique surfactant proteins (SP-A, SP-B, SP-C, and SP-D) that have been identified in extracted lung fluid (Table 28-2). SP-A and SP-D are hydrophilic, related to the collagenous lectins, and, although not critical to surface activity, are involved with down-regulating the inflammatory response of the lung.[15–17] SP-A, discovered in 1972, accounts for most of the surfactant proteins and functions as a host defense molecule in the alveoli, interacting with the immune cells of the lungs.[17] It binds endotoxins as well as a wide range of gram-positive and gram-negative organisms and promotes phagocytosis by alveolar macrophages.[17] In the presence of SP-B and SP-C, it plays a major role in promoting the adsorption of surfactant phospholipids at the air–liquid interface. SP-A plays a key role in the regulation of secretions and recycling of surfactant by alveolar type II cells and increases the resistance to surface inhibition.[22] SP-D is similar to SP-A in structure and function, binding bacteria and fungi.[17] Although it does not play a role in surface activity, SP-D plays an important role in phospholipid homeostasis and in lung defense against bacteria, fungi, and viruses.[16,19] SP-B and SP-C are hydrophobic proteins that improve the surface activity of surfactant phospholipids and are thought to be a critical component of natural surfactants. Both of these proteins are important for the rapid spreading and adsorption of phospholipids onto the alveolar surface. SP-B and SP-A are essential for tubular myelin formation and, along with SP-C, promote the adsorption of DPPC.[13,15,17] SP-B is critical for the stability of surfactant and, because of this stabilizing ability, an SP-B deficiency is fatal in infants.

The process of surfactant metabolism and recycling is complex. There are two types of alveolar cells. Type I cells are the gas-exchanging units, and type II cells are responsible for surfactant synthesis and release. About 90% to 95% of surfactant is recycled and reprocessed into the type II alveolar cells for continuous secretion.[15,17] This is a dynamic process, and with the surface-area changes during the respiratory cycle, there is continual turnover of surfactant at the alveolar level.

Fetal Lung Maturity Testing

The pulmonary system is among the last of the fetal organ systems to mature, both functionally and structurally. Advances in **fetal lung maturity testing** assist the medical world in determining the course of complicated as well as uncomplicated pregnancies. The fetus's gender and race/ethnicity appear to play a role in this process; respiratory problems near term are more common among white male fetuses than among female fetuses, blacks, and South Asians.[23,24]

Because the immature pulmonary system may not oxygenate the neonate adequately, preterm birth can lead to significant neonatal morbidity or mortality. Therefore, fetal lung maturity is sometimes assessed before iatrogenic preterm delivery and can be a factor in determining the timing of delivery in these cases. **Table 28-3** outlines the laboratory tests available for this purpose. All involve testing amniotic fluid and provide an indirect assessment of the likelihood of lung maturity; direct studies of fetal lung function are not possible.

A test for fetal lung maturity is performed before 39 weeks' gestation when this information can be used to assess the maternal-fetal risks of continuing the pregnancy versus the maternal-fetal risks of preterm birth. This is an infrequent occurrence. In most clinical settings, the test is omitted either because delaying delivery due to lung immaturity may place the mother or fetus at significant risk, or because the fetus would benefit from delaying delivery, even if lung maturity is documented, and delaying delivery does not place the mother at significant risk.[25] However, these assessments

TABLE 28-2
Function of the Four Unique Surfactant Proteins

SP-A: Hydrophilic	SP-B: Hydrophobic	SP-C: Hydrophobic	SP-D: Hydrophilic
• Formation of tubular lattice • Regulatory function • Defense function	• Reformation of layer after compression	• Spreading function	• Regulatory function • Defense function

TABLE 28-3
Tests Used to Evaluate Fetal Lung Maturity

Test	Normal Value	Significance
L:S ratio	≥2.0	FLM
Amniostat-FLM	Positive	FLM/phosphotidyl glycerol
Foams stability index	≥47	FLM
Microviscosity	≥55 mg/g	FLM
Lamellar body count	≥32,000 mL	FLM
OD at 650 nm	≥0.150	FLM
Bilirubin scan	A 450 less 0.025	FLM

FLM = fetal lung maturity

are not always black and white, and information about lung maturity may be helpful in the balance.[26] Also, the information may be helpful in estimating the level of newborn care that will be required. Tests for fetal lung maturity are generally not performed before 32 weeks' gestation, given the high prevalence of fetal pulmonary immaturity and the lower predictive value of a mature test result at this gestational age.[26]

There is another factor to consider when addressing the relevance of fetal lung maturity testing. The number of newborn deaths due to RDS has continued to decline because of improvements in the medical care of preterm infants. Most laboratories have noted a decline in the number of fetal lung maturity tests that they perform each year. This trend reflects the decreased use of the tests by obstetricians, many of whom indicate that the tests are no longer needed for patient care.[27]

Antenatal Steroids and Surfactant Production

Two main strategies are available for the prevention of neonatal RDS in cases of preterm delivery: antenatal administration of hormones that accelerate fetal lung maturation and prophylactic treatment with surfactant soon after birth. The efficacy of each of these therapeutic regimens has been well documented in large randomized clinical trials. Corticosteroids and surfactant operate by different mechanisms. **Antenatal steroids** are medications administered to the mother when preterm delivery is expected. They have been shown to reduce morbidity and mortality related to surfactant-deficient diseases.[28] They have also been shown to have definite beneficial effects, even in conditions of preterm premature rupture of membranes.[29] Dexamethasone and betamethasone are the corticosteroids used for the purpose, although the former is recommended over the latter based on its efficacy, safety, wide availability, and low cost in spite of some counter-logic.[30] Betamethasone is preferred over dexamethasone because it is thought to have better prophylaxis of brain softening of the premature fetus[30] (**Table 28-4**). Antenatal steroids are used with the intention to help the lungs of a premature fetus develop before birth occurs.[1] They are given when the fetus is expected to be delivered within 24 to 48 hours. Treatment can consist of 2 doses of 12 mg of betamethasone given intramuscularly 24 hours apart or 4 doses of 6 mg of dexamethasone given intramuscularly 12 hours apart. Optimal benefit begins 24 hours after initiation of therapy and lasts 7 days.[1] The time between administration of steroids and delivery may alter the effectiveness of the steroids.[31]

Antenatal steroids accelerate development of type I and type II pneumocytes, leading to structural and biochemical changes that improve both lung mechanics (maximal lung volume, compliance) and gas exchange.[30,31] The steroids stimulate production

TABLE 28-4
Dose and Frequency of Antenatal Steroid Administration

Antenatal Steroids	
Betamethasone (Celestone)	Dexamethasone (Decadron)
2 doses of 12 mg given 24 hours apart	4 doses of 6 mg given 12 hours apart
Given to mothers between 24–34 weeks' gestation who are expected to go into labor within the next 7 days; if labor does not occur within 7 days, do not repeat.	

of surfactant phospholipids by alveolar type II cells, enhance the expression of surfactant-associated proteins, reduce microvascular permeability, and accelerate the overall structural maturation of the lungs.[31] The increment in pool size of surfactant resulting from antenatal treatment with corticosteroids has been shown to be trivial relative to the dose of exogenous surfactant required for successful prophylaxis at birth.[31]

Indications

Currently, the only approved clinical indication for surfactant replacement therapy is neonatal RDS, although additional indications are likely to be approved in the near future. RDS is characterized by the presence of acute respiratory distress with disturbed gas exchange in a preterm infant. A typical chest radiograph shows a ground-glass appearance, air bronchograms, and reduced lung volume. The lungs of preterm babies with RDS are both anatomically and biochemically immature because they neither synthesize nor secrete surfactant well.[31] Surfactant normally lines the alveolar surfaces in the lung, thereby reducing surface tension and preventing atelectasis.[31] Surfactant replacement therapy, either as a rescue treatment or a prophylactic natural surfactant therapy, reduces mortality and several aspects of morbidity in infants with RDS.[30,31] Morbidities include deficits in oxygenation, the incidence of pulmonary air leaks (pneumothorax and pulmonary interstitial emphysema), and prolonged duration of ventilatory support.[30] Infants treated with surfactants have shorter hospital stays and lower costs of intensive care treatment compared with randomized control infants receiving no surfactants. The increase in survival is achieved with no increase in adverse neurodevelopmental outcome. Surfactant replacement increases the likelihood of surviving without bronchopulmonary dysplasia (BPD), largely by improving survival rather than the incidence of BPD.

The following steps should be used to validate the indication for surfactant replacement therapy:[32]

- Assess lung immaturity prior to prophylactic administration of surfactant by gestational age and birth weight and/or by laboratory evaluation of tracheal or gastric aspirate.

- Establish the diagnosis of neonatal RDS by chest radiographic criteria and the requirement for mechanical ventilation in the presence of short gestation and/or low birth weight.

The following should be used in assessing the outcomes of surfactant administration:[32]

- Reduction in FiO_2 requirement
- Reduction in work of breathing
- Improvement in aeration, as indicated by chest radiograph
- Improvement in pulmonary mechanics (compliance, airways resistance) and lung volume (functional residual capacity)
- Reduction in ventilator support (peak inspiratory pressure, positive end-expiratory pressure [PEEP], airway pressure)
- Improvement in ratio of arterial to alveolar PaO_2 and oxygen index

Preparations

Endogenous pulmonary surfactant is a phospholipoprotein containing DPPC that is produced by type II pneumocytes or alveolar cells. The compound's main function is to reduce surface tension within the alveoli of the lung, thus improving pulmonary compliance through reducing the work required to expand these alveolar units.[33] In turn, this process drastically increases the stability of the alveolar lining layer and ultimately prevents its collapse.

Conversely, according to West and Luks,[33] "surfactant is formed relatively late in fetal life, and babies born without adequate amounts develop respiratory distress" characterized by reduced lung compliance, subsequent atelectasis of alveolar units, and resulting noncardiogenic pulmonary edema. Therefore, it is imperative to

understand the two primary preparations available for exogenous surfactant replacement therapy and the general effectiveness of each method with regard to reversing the clinical manifestations of RDS.

Natural preparations of exogenous pulmonary surfactant used in surfactant replacement therapy are directly derived from animal sources. Human surfactant consists of surfactant associated proteins, specifically SP-A, SP-B, SP-C, and SP-D, which function to enhance the effectiveness of human surfactant.[34] SP-B has been shown to reduce surface tension within the alveolar lining layer to a greater degree in comparison to SP-C.[32] As a result, SP-B maintains the highest degree of significance in the prevention and treatment of RDS in premature infants. Essentially, the protein functions to enhance the rate of adsorption of phospholipids at the air–water interface and to retain anti-inflammatory properties.[35] Suitably, a major portion of animal-derived and naturally prepared surfactants consists of this specific surfactant protein, owing to the suggestion that natural surfactants maintain a greater efficacy over first-generation, synthetically produced surfactant that is protein-free.[34] **Figure 28-3** provides a timeline of the availability of the different surfactant preparations.

The actual sources of naturally extracted surfactant are adapted or purified from either bovine (cow) or porcine (pig) lungs. Among those that are commercially available are poractant alfa (Curosurf) derived from minced porcine lung tissue, calfactant (Infasurf) derived from lung lavage of newborn calves by centrifugation or organic solvent extraction, and beractant (Survanta) derived from minced bovine lung tissue.[36] Of the three aforementioned preparations, Infasurf retains all the hydrophobic characteristics and composition that are present within human surfactant and is therefore more closely associated with human biologic surfactant produced by type II pneumocytes within the alveoli.

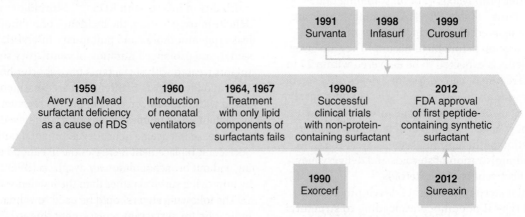

FIGURE 28-3 Significant milestones in surfactant preparations and use in the care for neonates with RDS.

However, Curosurf is made up of a larger portion of SP-B at 0.45 mg/mL within the 1.25 to 2.5 mL/kg dosage. Infasurf contains 0.26 mg/mL of SP-B within the 2 mL/kg dosage and Survanta retains less than 1 mg/mL of SP-B within its 4 mL/kg dose.[32] The literature reports that Curosurf reduces the need for repeat dosing, is associated with fewer complications of administration, leads to better short-term oxygenation, and may reduce the risk of mortality compared to Survanta.[34] Thus, both Curosurf and Infasurf are considered the most effective natural preparations of animal-derived surfactant.

As previously stated, these naturally extracted surfactants preserve a vital benefit over first-generation, protein-free synthetic surfactants in the retained composition of SP-B. Recent evidence suggests that natural surfactants offer several advantages when compared to synthetic surfactant preparations, which include more rapid supplemental oxygen weaning, lower mean airway pressures, reduced duration of mechanical ventilation, and decreased rate of mortality.[36] Natural surfactants have also displayed a more substantial absorption by premature infants, significant lowering of alveolar surface tension, and reduced risks of both pneumothorax and BPD in comparison to laboratory-derived synthetic surfactants.[32]

However, natural surfactants also maintain a variable degree of concern. For instance, the actual amount of SP-B available within the dosages of natural surfactants tends to vary considerably between formulations, specifically referred to as batch-to-batch variations.[32] Additionally, animal-derived surfactants contain foreign proteins that are potential immunogens, which can result in an immune response within premature infants that ultimately rejects the administered natural surfactant or possibly prion disease processes.[36] Lastly, there are obvious religious and cultural considerations regarding the use of bovine or porcine natural preparations of surfactant, as some demographic groups of patients may completely refuse the administration of these formulations.

Apart from naturally prepared and extracted formulations of surfactant, there is a variety of synthetic surfactant that is produced within the laboratory. First-generation synthetic surfactants are considered protein-free, lacking the vital SP-B that is a major component of animal-derived natural surfactants. For example, colfosceril (Exosurf) contains the phospholipid of DPPC yet lacks any protein component and has subsequently been discontinued.[35] However, newer synthetic surfactants have been developed that are largely made of SP-B–mimicking proteins. Lucinactant (Surfaxin) is a synthetic surfactant that consists of a 21-amino acid peptide known as KL4 that has recently been approved for the treatment of RDS in premature infants.[35]

A new synthetic surfactant described as CHF 5633 is the first laboratory-derived surfactant that contains both SP-B and C analogs as well as DPPC.[37] Through an animal study, a number of preterm lambs were administered either CHF 5633 or Curosurf. The pulmonary structure of the preterm lambs treated with CHF 5633 was considerably more compliant and maintained larger alveolar spaces with thinner alveolar walls in comparison to the group that was treated with Curosurf, indicating that this new synthetic surfactant expressed significant benefit over animal-derived surfactant.[37] However, the superiority of this synthetically produced surfactant still requires confirmation through an extensive clinical trial outside of the animal model, although the results reported are undoubtedly promising.

Newer synthetic surfactants, such as Surfaxin, offer a particular benefit in comparison to animal-derived surfactants. Synthetic preparations may have better quality control than natural surfactants because the synthetic preparations lack batch-to-batch formulation variability.[32]

Recent evidence suggests that when compared with animal-derived surfactant, Surfaxin is as efficacious as a laboratory-derived synthetic surfactant in the treatment of RDS in preterm infants.[35,36] Further research is required to explore the overall efficiency of these synthetically produced surfactants, especially those including CHF 5633, in this premature disease process in comparison to animal-derived surfactants. However, this most current research suggests that both naturally derived and newer synthetically derived surfactants maintain equivalent effectiveness in treating RDS in premature infants, and it is the responsibility of the clinician to ultimately compare the differences between these two preparations of exogenous surfactant. **Table 28-5** provides a comparison of the different surfactant preparations that are currently available.

Administration

Administration of surfactant therapy depends on the strategy the medical team will use. That strategy will determine the setting and timing of surfactant administered to the newborn.

Rescue Use versus Prophylactic Use

Two strategies for surfactant replacement therapy are available: rescue and prophylactic. However, whether surfactant should be given as soon as the infant is born or withheld until the infant has demonstrated respiratory distress remains controversial. Prophylactic treatment is defined as surfactant given down an endotracheal tube at initial resuscitation. Rescue treatment is when the surfactant is given to an intubated infant several hours after birth, when RDS has been diagnosed.

TABLE 28-5
A Comparison of Currently Available Surfactant Preparations

Trade Name	Survanta	Curosuf	Infasurf	Surfaxin
Generic	Beractant	Poractant alfa	Calfactant	Lucinactant
Source	Bovine	Porcine	Bovine	Synthetic
Indication	Prevention and treatment of RDS	Treatment of RDS	Prevention and treatment of RDS	Prevention of RDS
Phospholipid	25 mg/mL	76 mg/mL	35 mg/mL	30 mg/mL
Dosage	100 mg/4 mL/kg	200 mg/2.5 mL/kg	105 mg/3 mL/kg	175 mg/5.8 mL/kg
Interval	Not <q6 hr	1.25 mL/kg q12 hr	3 mL/kg q12 hr	Not <q6 hr
Dosing	4 aliquots	2 aliquots	2–4 aliquots	4 aliquots

Timing

A prophylactic or preventive surfactant therapy strategy is often initiated in infants at high risk of developing RDS. The primary purpose for surfactant administration is to prevent worsening RDS rather than treatment of established RDS. Prophylactic surfactant administration is dosed in the delivery room before initial resuscitation efforts begin, before the diagnosis of RDS has been identified, or after initial resuscitation but within a short the time frame after birth.

Rescue surfactant is given only to preterm infants with identified RDS. Rescue surfactant is most often administered within the first 12 hours after birth, when specified threshold criteria of severity of RDS are met. Although there are no statistically significant benefits to prophylactic use of surfactant when compared with prophylactic continuous positive airway pressure (CPAP), several studies have investigated whether administration of surfactant early in the course of respiratory insufficiency improves clinical outcomes. Early rescue is defined as surfactant treatment within 1 to 2 hours of birth, and late rescue is defined as surfactant treatment 2 or more hours after birth.[6] **Figure 28-4** outlines the timing of surfactant administration for prophylactic and rescue use.

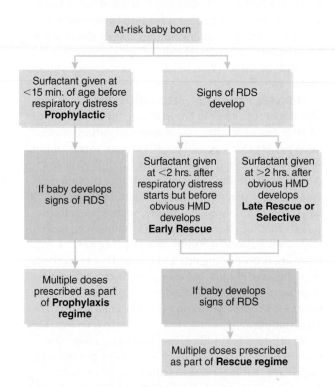

FIGURE 28-4 Timing of surfactant administration.

Preparation and Dosage

Surfactant administration has been studied using bolus, lavage, and aerosol delivery. Most of the surfactant studies calculate the dose or total volume of surfactant to be given by patient body weight and use an intratracheal bolus in divided doses to administer the therapy.[38] Administering the bolus of surfactant using an endotracheal tube or catheter is effective and has fewer reported adverse effects.[39] A Bodai valve can be inserted between the endotracheal tube and the ventilator circuit, which allows mechanical ventilation to be uninterrupted during surfactant administration. A catheter is inserted through the value, into the endotracheal tube. The bolus of surfactant is administered through the catheter, and the catheter is withdrawn after the surfactant bolus has completed.

Studies using aerosolized surfactant are still controversial in nature. Lavage therapy uses larger volumes of dilute surfactant in a washing-out procedure, where surfactant is removed by suctioning at the end of the procedure.[40]

Frequency of Administration

Repeat doses of surfactant are contingent upon the continued diagnosis of neonatal RDS. The frequency with which surfactant replacement is performed should depend upon the clinical status of the patient and the indication for performing the procedure. Additional doses of surfactant, given at 6- to 24-hour intervals, may be indicated in infants who experience increasing ventilator requirements or whose conditions fail to improve after the initial dose.

Patient Positioning

When surfactant is administered slowly (slow infusion and/or slow rate of ventilation) with the patient in an upright position, the distribution is dependent on the orientation of the airways with respect to gravity.[41-43] This could lead to overinflation of the parts of the lung receiving surfactant and result in lung injury.[44] Improved homogeneity is achieved when the patient is positioned supine rather than upright during surfactant administration. Animal models also show greater epithelial cell injury at slower propagating speeds.[45] In a randomized controlled trial, there was no difference in clinical outcomes when two fractional doses of surfactant were given in two different body positions, compared with four fractional doses given in four positions.[46] The practical ways to improve distribution are to position the infant to minimize the effects of gravity and to give surfactant in a reasonable volume with sufficient ventilator support to quickly clear the airways of fluid.

Monitoring

Manufacturer recommendations for administering surfactant differ. Therefore, it is important to follow the procedures outlined by the manufacturer for the specific preparations of surfactant used.[32] The equipment used to deliver surfactant and monitor the infant during surfactant administration are listed in **Table 28-6**.

Surfactant replacement therapy should be performed by healthcare providers who are proficient at administering surfactant and capable of handling adverse events. Staff should have an understanding of the proper use of the therapy and a mastery of the equipment and technical aspects of surfactant replacement therapy. It is also important for clinicians to have a comprehensive knowledge and understanding of ventilator management and pulmonary anatomy and pathophysiology. During administration, clinicians should continually assess the infant in order to respond to adverse reactions and/or complications during the procedure in a timely manner.

The following should be monitored as part of surfactant replacement therapy:[32]

- Proper placement and position of delivery device and ETT
- FiO_2 and ventilator settings

TABLE 28-6
Equipment Used during Surfactant Replacement Therapy

Administration Equipment

- Syringe containing the ordered dose of surfactant, warmed to room temperature or manufacturer's recommendation
- Appropriately sized feeding tube or catheter, endotracheal tube (ETT) connector with delivery port, or closed catheter system
- Mechanical ventilator with tidal volume monitoring capability

Resuscitation Equipment

- Laryngoscope and appropriately sized ETT
- Manual resuscitator that is capable of providing positive end-expiratory pressure/continuous positive end-expiratory pressure (PEEP/CPAP) and airway manometer
- Blended oxygen source capable of delivering FiO_2 of 0.21–1.0
- Suction equipment (i.e., catheters, sterile gloves, collecting bottle and tubing, and vacuum generator)
- Radiant warmer ready for use as applicable

Monitoring Equipment

- Tidal volume monitor, if available (if not within ventilator)
- Pulse oximeter
- Cardiorespiratory monitor

- Reflux of surfactant into the ETT
- Position of patient
- Chest wall movement
- Oxygen saturation by pulse oximetry
- Vital signs
- Pulmonary mechanics and tidal volumes
- Breath sounds

After administration, the following may be obtained:

- Invasive and/or noninvasive measurements of arterial blood gases
- Chest radiograph

Clinical Considerations for Therapeutic Administration

The most important physiologic function of surfactant is the effect it has on lung mechanics. By lowering the surface tension within the alveolus at the air–liquid interface, there is stabilization of lung volumes at low transpulmonary pressures. Surfactant will prevent collapse of the airways on expiration and allow for lower opening pressures to inflate the lung. Overall, there is less overdistension of alveoli, decreasing the risks of alveolar rupture as surfactant decreases the negative pressure needed to open the airways and reducing the work of breathing.[47] Surfactant promotes gas exchange between the alveoli and capillaries and plays a role in host defense mechanisms through the action of SP-A and SP-D. It is essential to monitor the infant's exhaled tidal volumes following surfactant replacement therapy.

As pulmonary compliance improves, the infant's tidal volumes will increase. To minimize overdistention, peak inspiratory pressures must be lowered. Adverse effects of surfactant therapy include transient decreases in blood pressure, cerebral blood flow velocity, and oxyhemoglobin concentration and activity as well as an increase in intraventricular hemorrhage.[18]

The INSURE (INtubation, SURfactant, and Extubation) technique is a very effective and useful method that reduces the need for mechanical ventilation, decreases side effects, shortens the hospitalization time, and eliminates extra hospital expenses. When the INSURE technique is used, the infant is intubated to administer the surfactant, then extubated to either CPAP or noninvasive ventilation.

Less invasive surfactant administration (LISA) is a method of surfactant administration that involves brief tracheal catheterization and has been extensively studied. The surfactant is administered through a flexible feeding tube and a semirigid vascular catheter while the infant receives nasal continuous positive airway pressure (nCPAP). The LISA method has been found to reduce the need for subsequent intubation and ventilation and to improve short-term respiratory outcomes. Despite the relatively small number of clinical trials involving LISA, this technique has found its way into clinical practice in some clinical facilities.

Minimally invasive surfactant therapy (MIST) is an alternative route for surfactant therapy. The current evidence regarding noninvasive surfactant delivery techniques in premature infants is limited to pilot data and feasibility studies. This is further complicated by varying delivery methods and availability of smaller devices for use in very preterm infants. With the growing interest in noninvasive respiratory support techniques, until conclusive data on superiority of approach is documented, the gold standard of respiratory support is endotracheal intubation, administration of surfactant, and optimal mechanical ventilation.

Hazards/Complications

Complications can occur during or following surfactant administration. Procedural complications resulting from the administration of surfactant include the following:[32]

- Plugging of the ETT by surfactant
- Hemoglobin desaturation and increased need for supplemental O_2
- Bradycardia due to hypoxia
- Tachycardia due to agitation, with reflux of surfactant into the ETT
- Pharyngeal deposition of surfactant
- Administration of surfactant to only one lung (i.e., right mainstem intubation)
- Administration of a suboptimal dose

Table 28-7 provides a comprehensive list of procedural and physiologic complications of surfactant replacement therapy. Complications can be prevented by slowly administering the surfactant, by closely monitoring oxygenation and lung mechanics (i.e., S_pO_2, mean airway pressures, and exhaled tidal volume), and by adjusting ventilator parameters (i.e., FiO_2 and PIP) following surfactant administration.

Limitations

Although surfactant replacement therapy has improved outcomes for preterm infants with RDS, there are some limitations. These include basic elements of bedside

TABLE 28-7
Complications of Surfactant Therapy

Procedural Complications	Physiologic Complications
ETT plugging (during surfactant administration)	Apnea
Transient hypoxemia	Right-to-left shunting resulting in pulmonary hemorrhage
Hypoxemia-related bradycardia	Increased shunting through a patent ductus arteriosus
Agitation due to reflux of surfactant in the endotracheal tube	Marginal increase in risk for retinopathy of prematurity
Agitation-induced tachycardia	Volutrauma risk (inattention to compliance changes and the need to reduce set inspiratory pressure)
Pharyngeal deposition during surfactant administration	Alterations in intracranial blood flow
Unilateral deposition of surfactant due to an endobronchial intubation	
Administering a suboptimal dose	

Data from Agarwal, A. Respiratory Distress in New born. SlideShare. 2015. https://www.slideshare.net/dragarwalankit/respiratory-distress-in-new-born

care, such as the inability to suction the endotracheal tube after administration, positioning problems, and inadvertent administration of surfactant to the stomach or to only one lung.[32]

Suctioning should be avoided immediately after therapy, and this could be a limitation in use for a patient who has a lot of secretions. Prophylactic administration may delay time to patient stabilization, and inability to closely monitor changes in pulmonary compliance and respond by reducing mechanical ventilatory support can lead to lung injury. Additionally, surfactant administered in the delivery room rarely has radiologic confirmation that the ETT is properly positioned. Esophageal and endobronchial intubations reduce the effectiveness of therapy by delivering the surfactant to the stomach or to only one lung.

Because bradycardia is often associated with bolus administration, infants with a slower heart rate should be monitored closely while receiving treatment to minimize the propensity for life-threatening bradycardia.[35]

The optimal method of surfactant administration has yet to be proven clearly after a few clinical trials.

Summary

The infants in the NICU require unique and specialized care. Surfactant treatment in preterm infants and term newborns with acute respiratory distress syndrome–like severe respiratory failure has become part of an individualized treatment strategy in many NICUs around the world. These infants constitute diverse groups of gestational ages, lung maturity, underlying disease processes, and postnatal interventions. An understanding of the complex processing of surfactant is key to the management of RDS and surfactant-deficient defects in the neonatal population. The development of newer research and newer surfactant products hold much promise for improved outcomes in neonatology.

Case Study 1

A term (41 weeks) female weighing 3100 g was born to a 30-year-old healthy gravida 2 para 1 mother by cesarean. Apgar scores were 9 and 9 at 1 and 5 minutes. The infant was initially well until day 3 of life, when she presented with tachypnea and increased work of breathing, including retractions and nasal flaring. The infant was transferred to the NICU. A complete sepsis workup was done and antibiotics were given as protocol. The infant was placed on a nasal cannula for oxygen saturations which ranged from 89-91%. A capillary blood gas was performed and revealed the following: pH 7.30, $PaCO_2$ 56 mm Hg, PaO_2 45 mm Hg, HCO_3 27 mEq/L, and BE 1. A chest radiograph showed mild hyperinflated lungs and mild perihilar interstitial markings. An echocardiogram was also ordered at this time, which showed an anatomically normal heart with no structural malformation. During the next 24 hours, the infant's respiratory status worsened, with progressive increases in work of breathing with increasing oxygen requirement. Continuous positive airway pressure was initiated by nasal mask at 6 cm H_2O and an FiO_2 of 0.50. A follow-up chest radiograph was performed, which showed increasing haziness of both lung fields with air bronchograms. Capillary blood gases obtained 12 hours after nasal CPAP therapy

revealed the following: pH 7.19, $PaCO_2$ 80 mm Hg, PO_2 40 mm Hg, HCO_3 29.5 mEQ/L, BE 1.8, and oxygen saturation 88%. Physical assessment revealed the following: temperature 37.1°C, heart rate 175 beats per minute, respiratory rate 90 breaths per minute, and blood pressure 70/40 mm Hg. The infant was intubated and mechanically ventilated with an inspiratory pressure of 20 cm H_2O, PEEP 6 cm H_2O, set rate of 60 breaths per minute, and FiO_2 of 0.80. Systemic examination was unremarkable except for respiratory distress. There was no clinical evidence of pulmonary hypertension. A complete sepsis workup was repeated. The white blood cell count was unremarkable. Chest radiograph following intubation revealed diffuse ground-glass appearance with air bronchograms. The endotracheal tube was 2 cm above the carina.

1. **What therapeutic recommendation would you make based on the infant's clinical presentation and chest radiograph?**

2. **Given this presentation, what diagnosis should be considered for this infant?**

3. **What information obtained by chest radiograph would indicate that this infant may benefit from surfactant replacement therapy?**

Case Study 2

You are called to the delivery room at 2:00 a.m. for a laboring gravida 1 para 0 mother at 28 weeks' gestation. The mother had good antenatal care and had a normal integrated prenatal screening (IPS), normal 20-week ultrasound, and protective serology, including rubella immune, human immonodeficiency virus (HIV) negative, venereal disease research laboratory (VDRL) negative, hepatitis negative. Group B *Streptococcus* (GBS) status is unknown as the woman had not yet had swabs done. Social history was negative for tobacco, alcohol, or recreational drug use during the pregnancy. She has gestational diabetes mellitus, which was reasonably controlled by diet and exercise alone. You arrive to the delivery room moments before the baby is born and prepare equipment for a potential resuscitation, which includes oxygen, bag and mask, suction, towels to dry, and intubation equipment. At birth, the newborn cries spontaneously. She is placed on the warmer to be dried and stimulated; her heart rate is 120 beats per minute and her respiratory rate is 60 breaths per minute. The infant grunts intermittently. At 4 minutes of age, the newborn has both subcostal and intercostal retractions, nasal flaring, and continuous grunting. Her respiratory rate is now 82 breaths per minute and her heart rate is 190 beats per minute. Oxygen saturation by pulse oximetry is 84% with blow-by oxygen. You begin providing CPAP at 6 cm H_2O by mask with a t-piece resuscitator. A systolic murmur gr 2/6 is auscultated loudest at the left upper sternal boarder (LUSB). The infant is transferred to the NICU where she continues to receive nasal CPAP at 6 cm H_2O and an FiO_2 of 0.45. The chest X-ray shows diffuse ground-glass appearance with air bronchograms. An arterial umbilical catheter (UAC) is inserted. Arterial blood gas reveals the following: pH 7.23, CO_2 60, PaO_2 40, HCO_3 27, BE +1, and lactate 4.8. Blood work shows white blood cell count 20.3, neutrophils 12.3, no left shift, hemoglobin 16.5, platelets 260.

1. **What is the first line of therapy for this premature infant considering her presentation?**

2. **What are the chemical components that make up surfactant?**

3. **How does surfactant work in the lung?**

References

1. Engle W. Surfactant-replacement therapy for respiratory distress in the preterm and term neonate. *Pediatrics.* 2008;121(2):419-432. doi:10.1542/peds.2007-3283.

2. Walsh B, Daigle B, DiBlasi R, Restrepo R. AARC clinical practice guideline. Surfactant replacement therapy: 2013. *Respir Care.* 2013;58(2):367-375. doi:10.4187/respcare.02189.

3. Stevens T, Harrington EW, Blennow M, Soll RF. Cochrane review: early surfactant administration with brief ventilation vs. selective surfactant and continued mechanical ventilation for preterm infants with or at risk for respiratory distress syndrome. *Cochrane Database Syst Rev.* 2007;17(4):CD003063.

4. Pfister R, Soll R, Wiswell T. Protein containing synthetic surfactant versus animal derived surfactant extract for the prevention and treatment of respiratory distress syndrome. *Evid Based Child Health.* 2010;5(1):17-51. doi:10.1002/ebch.517.

5. Stevens T, Blennow M, Myers E, Soll R. Cochrane review: early surfactant administration with brief ventilation vs. selective surfactant and continued mechanical ventilation for preterm infants with or at risk for respiratory distress syndrome. *Evidence-Based Child Health.* 2010;5(1):82-115. doi:10.1002/ebch.519.

6. Soll R. Early versus delayed selective surfactant treatment for neonatal respiratory distress syndrome. *Neonatology.* 2013;104(2):124-126. doi:10.1159/000353673.

7. Soll R. Prophylactic versus selective use of surfactant in preventing morbidity and mortality in preterm infants. *Neonatology.* 2012;102(3):169-171. doi:10.1159/000338551.

8. Rojas-Reyes MX, Morley CJ, Soll R. Prophylactic versus selective use of surfactant in preventing morbidity and mortality in preterm infants. *Cochrane Database Syst Rev.* 2012;14(3):CD000510.

9. Burri P. Structural aspects of postnatal lung development–alveolar formation and growth. *Neonatology.* 2006;89(4):313-322. doi:10.1159/000092868.

10. Clements J. Lung surfactant: a personal perspective. *Ann Rev Physiol.* 1997;59(1):1-21. doi:10.1146/annurev.physiol.59.1.1.

11. Faridy E, Thliveris J. Rate of secretion of lung surfactant before and after birth. *Respir Physiol.* 1987;68(3):269-277. doi:10.1016/s0034-5687(87)80012-9.

12. Jobe A. Pharmacology review: why surfactant works for respiratory distress syndrome. *NeoReviews.* 2006;7(2):e95-e106. doi:10.1542/neo.7-2-e95.

13. Lewis J, Jobe A. Surfactant and the adult respiratory distress syndrome. *Am Rev Respir Dis.* 1993;147(1):218-233. doi:10.1164/ajrccm/147.1.218.

14. Poynter S, LeVine A. Surfactant biology and clinical application. *Crit Care Clin.* 2003;19(3):459-472. doi:10.1016/s0749-0704(03)00011-3.

15. Morton N. Exogenous surfactant treatment for the adult respiratory distress syndrome? A historical perspective. *Thorax.* 1990;45(11):825-830. doi:10.1136/thx.45.11.825.

16. Crouch E, Wright J. Surfactant proteins A and D and pulmonary host defense. *Ann Rev Physiol.* 2001;63(1):521-554. doi:10.1146/annurev.physiol.63.1.521.

17. Jobe A, Ikegami M. Biology of surfactant. *Clin Perinatol.* 2001;28(3):655-669. doi:10.1016/s0095-5108(05)70111-1.

18. Suresh G, Soll R. Current surfactant use in premature infants. *Clin Perinatol.* 2001;28(3):671-694. doi:10.1016/s0095-5108(05)70112-3.

19. Ainsworth S, Milligan D. Surfactant therapy for respiratory distress syndrome in premature neonates. *Am J Respir Med.* 2002;1(6):417-433. doi:10.1007/bf03257169.

20. James D, Tindall V, Richardson T. Is the lecithin/sphingomyelin ratio outdated? *Obstetr Gynecol Surv.* 1984;39(8):485-486. doi:10.1097/00006254-198408000-00004.

21. Merritt T, Hallman M, Spragg R, Heldt G, Gilliard N. Exogenous surfactant treatments for neonatal respiratory distress syndrome and their potential role in the adult respiratory distress syndrome. *Drugs.* 1989;38(4):591-611. doi:10.2165/00003495-198938040-00006.

22. Coalson J, King R, Yang F, et al. SP-A deficiency in primate model of bronchopulmonary dysplasia with infection. In situ mRNA and immunostains. *Am J Respir Crit Care Med.* 1995;151(3):854-866. doi:10.1164/ajrccm.151.3.7881683.

23. Balchin I, Whittaker J, Lamont R, Steer P. Timing of planned cesarean delivery by racial group. *Obstetr Gynecol.* 2008;111(3):659-666. doi:10.1097/aog.0b013e318163cd55.

24. Anadkat J, Kuzniewicz M, Chaudhari B, Cole F, Hamvas A. Increased risk for respiratory distress among white, male, late preterm and term infants. *J Perinatol.* 2012;32(10):780-785. doi:10.1038/jp.2011.191.

25. ACOG Practice Bulletin No. 97: Fetal lung maturity. *Obstetr Gynecol.* 2008;112(3):717-726. doi:10.1097/aog.0b013e318188d1c2.

26. Towers C, Freeman R, Nageotte M, Garite T, Lewis D, Quilligan E. The case for amniocentesis for fetal lung maturity in late-preterm and early-term gestations. *Am J Obstetr Gynecol.* 2014;210(2):95-96. doi:10.1016/j.ajog.2013.10.004.

27. Grenache D, Wilson A, Gross G, Gronowski A. Clinical and laboratory trends in fetal lung maturity testing. *Clinica Chimica Acta.* 2010;411(21-22):1746-1749. doi:10.1016/j.cca.2010.07.025.

28. Mwansa-Kambafwile J, Cousens S, Hansen T, Lawn J. Antenatal steroids in preterm labour for the prevention of neonatal deaths due to complications of preterm birth. *Int J Epidemiol.* 2010;39 (Suppl 1):i122-i133. doi:10.1093/ije/dyq029.

29. Vidaeff Aramin S. Antenatal corticosteroids after preterm premature rupture of membranes. *Clin Obstetr Gynecol.* 2011;54(2):337-343. doi:10.1097/grf.0b013e318217d85b.

30. Lee B. Adverse neonatal outcomes associated with antenatal dexamethasone versus antenatal betamethasone. *Pediatrics.* 2006;117(5):1503-1510. doi:10.1542/peds.2005-1749.

31. McEvoy C, Schilling D, Spitale P, Peters D, O'Malley J, Durand M. Decreased respiratory compliance in infants less than or equal to 32 weeks' gestation, delivered more than 7 days after antenatal steroid therapy. *Pediatrics.* 2008;121(5):e1032-e1038. doi:10.1542/peds.2007-2608.

32. Walsh B, Daigle B, DiBlasi R, Restrepo R. AARC clinical practical guideline. Surfactant replacement therapy: 2013. *Respir Care.* 2013;58(2):367-375. doi:10.4187/respcare.02189.

33. West J, Luks A, West J. *West's Pulmonary Pathophysiology.* 9th ed. Philadelphia: Wolters Kluwer; 2017.

34. Fox G, Sothinathan U. The choice of surfactant for treatment of respiratory distress syndrome in preterm infants: a review of evidence. *Infant.* 2005;1(1):8-12.

35. Polin R, Carlo W. Surfactant replacement therapy for preterm and term neonates with respiratory distress. *Pediatrics.* 2013;133(1):156-163. doi:10.1542/peds.2013-3443.

36. Zhang H, Fan Q, Wang Y, Neal C, Zuo Y. Comparative study of clinical pulmonary surfactants using atomic force microscopy. *Biochim Biophys Acta.* 2011;1808(7):1832-1842. doi:10.1016/j.bbamem.2011.03.006.

37. Seehase M, Collins J, Kuypers E, et al. New surfactant with SP-B and C analogs gives survival benefit after inactivation in preterm lambs. *PLoS ONE.* 2012;7(10):e47631. doi:10.1371/journal.pone.0047631.

38. Holm BA, Matalon S. Role of pulmonary surfactant in the development and treatment of adult respiratory distress syndrome. *Anesth Analg.* 1989;69(6):805-818.

39. Valls-i-Soler A, Fernandez-Ruanova B, y Goya J, Etxebarria L, Rodriguez-Soriano J, Carretero [Caceres] V. A randomized comparison of surfactant dosing via a dual-lumen endotracheal tube in respiratory distress syndrome. *Pediatrics.* 1998;101(4):e4. doi:10.1542/peds.101.4.e4.

40. Wiswell T. Expanded uses of surfactant therapy. *Clin Perinatol.* 2001;28(3):695-711. doi:10.1016/s0095-5108(05)70113-5.

41. Fernández Ruanova M, Alvarez F, Gastiasoro E, et al. Comparison of rapid bolus instillation with simplified slow administration of surfactant in lung lavaged rats. *Pediatric Pulmonol.* 1998;26(2):129-134. doi:10.1002/(sici)1099-0496(199808)26:23.3.co;2-1.

42. Segerer H, van Gelder W, Angenent F, et al. Pulmonary distribution and efficacy of exogenous surfactant in lung-lavaged rabbits are influenced by the instillation technique. *Pediatr Res.* 1993;34(4):490-494. doi:10.1203/00006450-199310000-00021.

43. Hentschel R, Brune T, Franke N, Harms E, Jorch G. Sequential changes in compliance and resistance after bolus administration or slow infusion of surfactant in preterm infants. *Intensive Care Med.* 2002;28(5):622-628. doi:10.1007/s00134-002-1277-7.

44. Ikegami M, Jobe A, Tabor B, Rider E, Lewis J. Lung albumin recovery in surfactant-treated preterm ventilated lambs. *Am Rev Respir Dis.* 1992;145(5):1005-1008. doi:10.1164/ajrccm/145.5.1005.

45. Ghadiali S, Gaver D. Biomechanics of liquid–epithelium interactions in pulmonary airways. *Respir Physiol Neurobiol.* 2008;163(1-3):232-243. doi:10.1016/j.resp.2008.04.008.

46. Zola E, Gunkel J, Chan R, et al. Comparison of three dosing procedures for administration of bovine surfactant to neonates with respiratory distress syndrome. *J Pediatr.* 1993;122(3):453-459. doi:10.1016/s0022-3476(05)83440-7.

47. Wildeboer-Venerma F. Influence of nitrogen, oxygen, air and alveolar gas upon surface tension of lung surfactant. *Respir Physiol.* 1984;58(1):1–14.

29

Specialty Gas Administration

Craig Wheeler

Robin Connolly

OUTLINE

OBJECTIVES

1. List the specialty medical gases administered in neonatal and pediatric intensive care units.
2. Describe the rationale for heliox use with asthma, bronchiolitis, and upper airway obstruction.
3. Identify the role of endogenous nitric oxide.
4. List the indications, application, and limitations of inhaled nitric oxide.
5. Describe how inhaled carbon dioxide or nitrogen can be used to augment pulmonary vascular resistance in neonates with hypoplastic left heart syndrome.
6. Discuss the effect of anesthetic gases on the nervous system.
7. Explain how isoflurane might be helpful in managing intubated patients with status asthmaticus.

KEY TERMS

heliox
inhaled nitric oxide (iNO)
inspired carbon dioxide
isoflurane
methemoglobin (MetHb)
nitric oxide (NO)

nitrogen dioxide (NO_2)
pulmonary hypertension (PH)
Reynold's equation
Reynold's number (Re)
subambient gas mixtures

Introduction

Oxygen has been the cornerstone of respiratory care since its first use to the present day. Although the majority of patients do not typically require administration of specialty medical gases, subsets of neonatal and pediatric patients have etiologies and pathophysiologic conditions whose treatment may be optimized by specialty gas therapy, such as helium–oxygen mixtures, inhaled nitric oxide, subambient oxygen concentrations, inspired carbon dioxide, and anesthetic gas mixtures. An understanding of the physiologic basis of action is important to the selection and concentration of specialty gas. Some gas mixtures are selected for their gas density and viscosity and for the effect the gas has on the movement of gases during ventilation. The density of a gas can be calculated by the following equation:

$$p = M/V$$
where p = density, M = mass, and V = volume

Other gases are selected for their effect on pulmonary smooth muscle and the ability to alter pulmonary and systemic blood flow by manipulating pulmonary vascular resistance.

Helium–Oxygen Mixtures

Pediatric and neonatal patients have an assortment of physiologic conditions that may require adjunctive inhaled gases to treat a variety of conditions. Inhaled helium oxygen mixtures have been used to deliver gas to the lungs when pulmonary physiology is altered. It is important for clinicians to consider the therapeutic potential, possible adverse effects, and technical aspects of delivering this gas mixture.

Gas Physics

Helium–oxygen mixtures are often referred to as **heliox**. Helium is a colorless, odorless, tasteless, inert gas. It has a molecular weight of 4 grams, and it occupies 22.4 liters of volume under normal conditions.

Helium has a lower gas density than air and oxygen (**Table 29-1**). According to gas physics, the lower the density of a gas, the greater the benefit to gas flow during ventilation under turbulent conditions.[1] Helium also has a low viscosity. Viscosity describes the magnitude to which a fluid in motion resists flow. The higher a fluid's viscosity, the stronger its resistance to flow. A concentration of 80% helium and 20% oxygen, often represented as heliox 80/20, has a viscosity of 203.6 poise (µP).

Mechanism of Action

During heliox therapy, a conversion of turbulent gas flow to laminar flow occurs because of the administration of a gas with a low density. **Reynold's equation** for turbulent flow explains this phenomenon. Reynold's equation is the product of the velocity of gas flow, the diameter of the tube the gas is flowing through, and the gas density, divided by the viscosity of the gas. Solving this mathematical equation will yield a **Reynold's number (Re)**, whose value will determine whether flow is laminar or turbulent. An Re >4000 describes turbulent flow through a tube while an Re <2000 represents laminar flow through a tube.[1,2] Heliox has a lower Re, which facilitates laminar gas flow and reduces the pressure required to ventilate or move air in and out of the lungs. Heliox administration reduces the overall load or work of breathing.

Effect on the Respiratory System

The tracheobronchial tree comprises the trachea, carina, left and right mainstem bronchi, lobar bronchus, segmental bronchus, bronchi, and the alveolar ducts and sacs. Each generation down the tracheobronchial tree provides a different challenge to airflow by means of airway caliber, angles, the density and viscosity of the inspired gas, and flow rate.[3] The conducting airways for the trachea to the 10th generation of bronchi have a larger radius. During inspiration, the velocity of gas flow is higher in the conducting airways between the trachea and the 10th generation of bronchi and tends to travel in the center of the airway. Therefore, gas flow is more turbulent. As gas flows to the small airways and to the alveolar ducts and sacs, the radius of the airways is smaller; the velocity lessens and is more streamlined, or closer to the sides of the conducting airways, and characterized as laminar. Heliox reduces the work of breathing associated with conditions that exacerbate turbulent flow conditions in the lungs.

Safety

Helium is inert gas, meaning that it is not chemically reactive or toxic, even after prolonged exposure.[1] Helium is never administered alone—it must be combined with oxygen for a mixture that is compatible with life. The two most commonly available helium–oxygen mixtures are found in **Table 29-2**. No major adverse events have been reported in any of the larger randomized controlled trials when commercially available gas mixtures are used as a therapeutic adjunct.[4] Caution should be exercised when using 100% helium, 0% oxygen, and

TABLE 29-1
Comparison of the Gas Densities of Helium with Oxygen and Air

Gas	Density (g/L)	Viscosity (µP)
Helium	0.179	188.7
Oxygen	1.42	192.6
Air	1.29	170.8

TABLE 29-2
The Most Commonly Administered Commercially Available Heliox Concentrations

Commercially Available Concentration	Oxygen Concentration	Helium Concentration
70:30	30%	70%
80:20	20%	80%

100% oxygen, and/or air mixtures in a blending system. Failure of the air or oxygen gas source will result in the administration of 100% helium, which can result in profound hypoxemia and/or death.

Indications

Helium–oxygen gas mixtures are used in the treatment of a variety of conditions that impair normal gas flow through the airways. This specialty gas mixture facilitates laminar gas flow and reduces the pressure required to ventilate as well as the overall load or work of breathing.

Asthma

The role heliox plays in supplementing the treatment of asthma, particularly in the severe acute phase known as status asthmaticus, has been widely discussed. Severe acute asthma is the most common childhood respiratory condition responsible for pediatric intensive care unit (PICU) admissions yearly.[5] Airways inflammation and bronchospasm cause airflow in the narrowed airways of children with an asthma exacerbation to become more turbulent. Patients presenting in status asthmaticus are refractory to standard bronchodilator and corticosteroid therapies. Heliox is used to alleviate work of breathing while more definitive therapy is administered because it has a low density and allows gas flow to be delivered to the distal airways easier than with air or pure oxygen. Graham's law explains this gas mixture's mechanism of action: The flow rate of any gas is inversely proportional to the square root of its density. Based upon Graham's law, medicated aerosol administered during the delivery of heliox therapy can theoretically result in faster aerosolized medication and more effective delivery through narrowed airways.[6] Furthermore, heliox in conjunction with conventional mechanical ventilation can lower peak inspiratory pressure and improve ventilation for intubated asthmatics.[7]

Upper Airway Obstruction

The anatomy of the neonatal and pediatric airway results in a greater susceptibility to respiratory distress than the adult airway, especially when upper airway obstruction occurs. Infants and young children have a narrower, funnel-shaped airway compared to the cylinder-shaped airway of an adult. Compared to an adult, the upper airway in an infant or child has a higher airway resistance and more turbulent flow. According to Poiseuille's law, flow through a tube is directly related to the pressure difference between its two ends and its radius to the fourth power while inversely related to its length and viscosity of the fluid. Although heliox has a higher viscosity than air, it has a lower viscosity than oxygen and a lower density than both. Theoretically, gas will flow with greater ease through the more narrow airways of any child affected by postextubation stridor, croup, or any other form of upper airway obstruction. By decreasing airway turbulence, inhaled heliox as low as 60/40 has shown promise to alleviate increased work of breathing within minutes in the neonatal/pediatric population.[8] However, other trials have shown that it is not more effective than standard therapy with corticosteroids, humidified oxygen, and racemic epinephrine.[9,10] Currently, there is some evidence that is suggestive of short-term clinical benefits in children with moderate to severe croup who have also been given corticosteroids.[11]

Bronchiolitis

Bronchiolitis is the most common lower respiratory tract infection that affects infants. Approximately 90% of infants are affected within the first 2 years of life, mainly due to respiratory syncytial virus (RSV) and less commonly to parainfluenza, adenovirus, and human metapneumovirus.[12] The classic markers of this infection are airway edema, acute inflammation, bronchospasm, increased mucus production, sloughing, and necrosis of the epithelial lining of the small airways. This constellation of symptoms leads to the inevitable narrowing of the airways, which will create a higher resistance and turbulent flow in the infant's airway.[13] Providing 80/20 or 70/30 heliox as an inhaled gas therapy to an infant affected with bronchiolitis may lessen turbulent flow and in effect decrease the infant's work of breathing. This may reduce the propensity for progressive respiratory failure due to muscle fatigue. The literature reports that inhalation of a 70/30 concentration of heliox through a nonrebreather mask can improve the respiratory status of infants with RSV bronchiolitis within the first hour of treatment and shorten PICU lengths of stay.[14] Studies have also shown that heliox therapy for RSV bronchiolitis more effectively reduces respiratory distress when compared with standard care, including supplemental oxygen, intravenous hydration therapy, and nebulized epinephrine.[13]

Delivery Devices

Helium–oxygen gas mixtures may be delivered to infants and children who do not require mechanical ventilatory support as well as to those receiving ventilatory assistance. Several common types of respiratory care equipment can be used to deliver this specialty gas mixture. Some are more effectively used than others.

Nonrebreathing Mask

For spontaneously breathing patients, nonrebreathers are reliable delivery devices that can reduce room air entrainment and prevent an increase in gas density. Nonrebreathing masks are capable of delivering sufficient gas flow to meet a child's inspiratory flow demands. However, this device has its limitations. Most young children do not tolerate a snug-fitting mask on their face, and the fit of the mask is vital to prevent air entrainment and to deliver accurate concentrations of this specialty gas mixture to the patient. Additions to a nonrebreathing mask can be made to facilitate continuous bronchodilator therapy in conjunction with heliox administration. **Figure 29-1** illustrates the setup required to monitor oxygen delivery during heliox administration in conjunction with continuous medicated bronchodilator nebulization. Pulse oximetry is a useful method for monitoring oxygen status during heliox therapy. If a patient has a supplemental oxygen requirement, small-bore tubing can be connected to an oxygen source to change the oxygen concentration. Figure 29-1 shows how the FiO_2 can be monitored by placing an oxygen analyzer inline. Because gas supplied to the patient

is from a helium–oxygen tank, it is presumed that the oxygen analyzer will provide a measured FiO_2 that is a reflection of the oxygen concentration in the tank and the additional oxygen administered through small-bore tubing into the system; thus, the balance of gas delivered to the patient is assumed to be helium. The heliox concentration can be calculated by subtracting the FiO_2 from 100.

Example: FiO_2 analyzed at 40%
Helium concentration = 100 − 40 = 60
Heliox concentration = 60:40

High-Flow Nasal Cannula

High-flow nasal cannula (HFNC) is another method of heliox delivery. The primary advantage of using HFNC to deliver heliox is based on this device's ability to meet or exceed the patient's inspiratory flow demand. With this method, the nasopharynx becomes a reservoir for gas, which conceptually limits room air entrainment and allows for more precise delivery.

HFNC systems can be modified to deliver heliox using an H cylinder of gas, a flowmeter, and O_2 tubing to bleed heliox into the circuit. When using systems that require heated high-flow gas through a standard flowmeter, a conversion factor must be used to determine the flow of gas that is actually delivered to the patient. This is because standard oxygen flowmeters are not calibrated for the delivery of gas that has a lighter density than oxygen. **Table 29-3** provides an example of how to calculate gas flow with the two commercially available heliox concentrations using conversion factors.

There are commercially manufactured HFNC systems that are calibrated for heliox delivery and that provide a blender to adjust FiO_2. It should be noted that whatever the FiO_2 is set to, helium makes up the balance of the mixture (e.g., FiO_2 of 0.4 would result in the delivery of a 60/40 heliox mixture).

Ventilator

Most mechanical ventilators are not calibrated for the administration of heliox. When using helium–oxygen

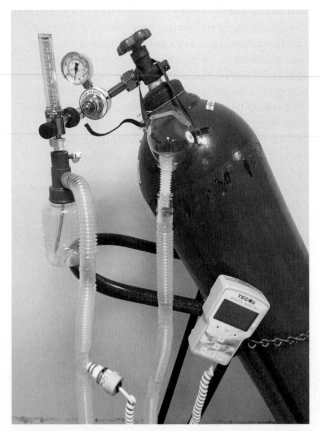

FIGURE 29-1 An illustration of the setup required to monitor oxygen delivery during heliox administration during continuous medicated aerosol administration.

TABLE 29-3
Conversion Factors for the Most Commonly Administered Commercially Available Heliox Concentrations

	Heliox Concentration	
	80/20	70/30
Conversion factor	1.8	1.6
Flow calculation formula	1.8 × set flow	1.6 × set flow
Example: set flow = 10 L/min	= 1.8 × 10 = 18 L/min	= 1.6 × 10 = 16 L/min

gas mixtures with ventilators that are not calibrated for this type of gas administration, there will be discrepancies between the set tidal volume and the exhaled tidal volumes and minute ventilation. Helium–oxygen gas mixtures are lighter than oxygen or air, which allows gas to flow faster and more erratically, which alters flow and volume calculations.[15] Ventilators calibrated to deliver heliox have a special adaptor, allowing the gas to be delivered as a driving gas. **Figure 29-2** shows the adaptor used to connect a high-pressure hose to a heliox tank and the 50 pounds per square inch (psi) air inlet on a ventilator. The clinician can then adjust the concentration of heliox delivered to the patient by adjusting the ventilator's oxygen concentration control. Setting the ventilator's oxygen control on 21% allows the clinician to deliver a heliox concentration equal to the concentration contained in the heliox tank. Increasing the oxygen control will increase the concentration of oxygen and reduce the concentration of helium delivered to the patient.

Gas Mixtures

Heliox is commercially available in H and E cylinders. The most common mixtures are 80/20 and 70/30. High-pressure cylinders with a gas mixture of 60/40 are also available.

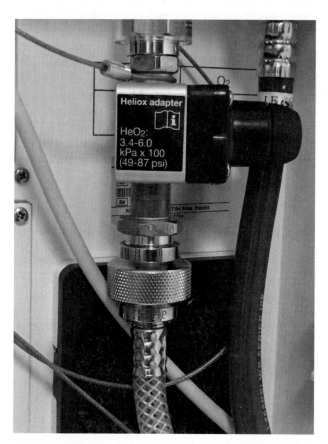

FIGURE 29-2 A special adaptor is used to connect a high-pressure hose to a heliox tank and the 50 psi air inlet on a ventilator.

Monitoring

A cardiorespiratory monitor should be used to continuously evaluate the heart rate, respiratory rate, blood pressure, and oxygen saturation of patients receiving heliox therapy. End-tidal ($ETCO_2$) or volumetric (VCO_2) carbon dioxide monitoring and respiratory mechanics are helpful in determining intrinsic positive end-expiratory pressure (PEEP) and how well intubated patients receiving this specialty gas mixture are ventilated.

Because high-pressure tanks are used to deliver heliox therapy, it is important to assess tank contents frequently. This will minimize an interruption in therapy because the tank is empty. A spare tank should be stored in close proximity to allow for easy transition from the empty to the full tank.

Limitations

There are no large randomized controlled trials to further elucidate indications or to identify the therapy limitations. Heliox does not affect the underlying pathophysiology responsible for airway obstruction. However, it may provide symptomatic relief in severe airway obstruction, and it is useful as an adjunct to more definitive treatment.[16]

Hazards/Complications

The potential hazards of heliox delivery are generally related to the devices used to deliver therapy. Inappropriately set flow rates may compromise nebulizer functions and affect drug delivery and particle size when heliox is used as the gas to power nebulizers.[17,18] The use of heliox with mechanical ventilators not calibrated for heliox delivery should be avoided, as errors in delivered and measured volumes will occur, potentially impacting patient safety.[19,20]

Nitric Oxide

The clinical use of inhaled nitric oxide has increased over the past several decades. This specialty gas has a profound effect on pulmonary vascular tone with minimal systemic adverse effects.

Gas Physics

Nitric oxide (NO) is a colorless, odorless gas consisting of one nitrogen and one oxygen atom. NO is a free radical and highly reactive gas that is unstable in the presence of air and undergoes oxidation to form **nitrogen dioxide (NO_2)**, a toxic environmental pollutant.[21]

Mechanism of Action

The identification of NO as an endothelial-derived vasodilator led to the investigation of **inhaled nitric oxide (iNO)** as a pulmonary vasodilator.[22,23] A substantial amount of evidence exists suggesting that the regulation of vascular muscle tone occurs at the cellular level. NO is synthesized as a byproduct following the conversion of L-arginine to L-citruline by nitric oxide synthase. NO rapidly diffuses across cell membranes, where it comes in contact with smooth muscle and activates guanylate cyclase, resulting in increased cyclic guanosine 3', 5'-monophosphate (cGMP).[24] Increased cGMP levels are accompanied by decreased intracellular calcium and the concomitant relaxation of vascular smooth muscle. Exogenous iNO enters the alveoli, diffuses across the alveolar–capillary membrane to the pulmonary smooth muscle cells, and results in vasodilation. iNO has a high affinity for hemoglobin, where it is bound and deactivated. It also has a very short half-life of 3 to 5 seconds, making it a selective pulmonary vasodilator, which may limit the vasodilatory effects to ventilated lung regions and therefore limit the effects on systemic circulation.[25-27]

Effect on the Cardiopulmonary System

The physiologic effects of iNO on **pulmonary hypertension (PH)** are multifactorial. The patient's response to therapy depends on the underlying cause of the PH. In neonates with PH, iNO can reverse hypoxic vasoconstriction by improving the balance of ventilation and perfusion (V/Q). The pulmonary vasodilatory effects decrease pulmonary vascular resistance (PVR), which in turn increases pulmonary blood flow to ventilated lung areas. Reducing PVR and improving V/Q matching decreases the amount of intracardiac shunting through the ductus arteriosus and/or the foramen ovale.[28,29] Physiologic responses to iNO typically occur within minutes of therapy initiation and are reflected in an increase in PaO_2 and/or SpO_2 and improved hemodynamic stability.

Safety

Multiple randomized and quasi-randomized controlled trials have evaluated the efficacy and safety of iNO therapy in term or near-term newborns with hypoxic respiratory failure. Current evidence suggests that it is safe and reasonable to administer iNO with PH and hypoxic respiratory failure. The literature does not support the use of iNO with hypoxic respiratory failure secondary to congenital diaphragmatic hernia.[30] The available evidence also does not support the routine or rescue use of iNO in premature infants <34 weeks' gestational age (WGA), and some reports suggest deleterious neurologic consequences.[31] Despite potential adverse outcomes and recommendations against using iNO therapy in infants <34 WGA, off-label use has increased and accounts for nearly half of all iNO use in the United States.[32-34]

Indications

Currently, the treatment of term neonates with acute hypoxic respiratory failure associated with pulmonary hypertension is the only indication for iNO approved by the Food and Drug Administration (FDA). Any other use of this specialty gas is considered off-label. Off-label use of iNO will not be addressed in this chapter.

Persistent Pulmonary Hypertension of the Newborn

Persistent pulmonary hypertension of the newborn is characterized by the failure of the pulmonary circulation to transition normally following birth, which results in PH. Intracardiac right-to-left shunting of blood across the foramen ovale and ductus arteriosus results in hypoxemia. Disorders that delay the normal relaxation of the pulmonary bed may be primary (e.g., idiopathic) or secondary conditions, such as congenital diaphragmatic hernia, meconium aspiration syndrome, and respiratory distress syndrome.[35] Methods of optimizing lung expansion include increasing mean airway pressure, initiating high-frequency ventilation, and administering surfactant, which should be employed prior to initiating iNO. iNO has been approved only by the FDA for therapy in term and near-term neonates (>34 WGA) with hypoxic respiratory failure associated with persistent pulmonary hypertension of the newborn and/or echocardiographic diagnosis of PH.[36,37] Although multiple large studies have demonstrated that iNO improves oxygenation and reduces the need for extracorporeal membrane oxygenation (ECMO), none has shown a decrease in mortality.[36-38] It should be noted that approximately 40% of neonates with persistent pulmonary hypertension of the newborn do not respond or sustain a response to iNO. If oxygenation and hemodynamic parameters do not improve despite these interventions, ECMO should be considered.[39]

Acute Respiratory Distress Syndrome (ARDS)

Numerous trials have investigated strategies for improving oxygenation and outcomes in pediatric ARDS. Despite the extensive adoption of lung-protective ventilation strategies, the mortality in pediatric patients with ARDS ranges from 22% to 35%.[40-42] The therapeutic aim for iNO administration to pediatric patients with ARDS is to reduce PH and intrapulmonary shunting by diverting pulmonary blood flow to better-ventilated areas of the lung. In a study of adult patients with ARDS, iNO has been shown to improve oxygenation for 1 to 3 days; however, these results were not sustained and did not have a beneficial impact on outcomes (e.g., duration of ventilation or mortality).[43] Similar to findings in adults, transient improvements in oxygenation were found when iNO was administered to pediatric patients with ARDS, but these studies did not evaluate the impact of iNO on morbidity or mortality.[44,45] Bronicki et al.[46] found that iNO decreased the duration of mechanical ventilation in pediatric patients with ARDS, which resulted in an improved survival rate without the use of ECMO. These results must be interpreted with caution: The sample size in this study was relatively small, and the study was terminated early for low enrollment.[46] A recent meta-analysis found no beneficial effects of iNO on mortality in either adult or pediatric patients with ARDS, regardless of the degree of hypoxemia. The routine use of iNO for acute hypoxic respiratory failure due to ARDS is not recommended.[47,48] Considering that most patients with ARDS demonstrate a short-lived response to iNO, administering this therapy to patients with ARDS should be considered only as a bridge to alternative ventilator strategies and/or ECMO.[49]

Congenital Heart Disease

Although iNO is only FDA approved for treatment of persistent pulmonary hypertension of the newborn, the literature reports therapeutic benefits of using iNO during the perioperative management of infants and children with PH and hypoxia associated with congenital heart disease. Preoperatively, iNO is used in the cardiac catheterization lab to reduce pulmonary vascular resistance, and response to therapy is used to delineate the operative plan and timing of corrective surgery.[50–52]

Clinically, PH is often described as the ratio of systolic pulmonary artery pressure relative to systolic systemic artery blood pressure (e.g., more than half of the systemic blood pressure).[55] A pulmonary hypertensive crisis occurs when the mean pulmonary artery pressure acutely exceeds the mean systolic arterial pressure.

In adults, PH has been defined as a mean pulmonary artery pressure (PAP) of ≥ 25 mm Hg, a pulmonary artery wedge pressure of ≤ 15 mm Hg, and an indexed pulmonary vascular resistance of >3 woods units.[53,54] Pulmonary hypertension in the pediatric perioperative patient is related to anatomic substrates that are not seen in adults, rendering these criteria less applicable.[55] Congenital heart disease is responsible for about 50% of PH cases in children, and the postoperative incidence of severe PH has been reported at 2% to 5%.[56–58]

The use of cardiopulmonary bypass during surgical repair of congenital heart defects has been associated with pulmonary vascular damage and the impairment of endothelial function, resulting in the transient loss of NO production and the presence of PH.[59] The goal for using iNO in infants and children with congenital heart defects is to improve right ventricular function and cardiac output by decreasing pulmonary artery pressure and pulmonary vascular resistance.[60,61]

Postoperative risk of PH can be assessed based on the type of cardiac lesion and then can be loosely categorized into four causative mechanisms: (1) increased pulmonary vascular resistance, (2) increased pulmonary blood flow, (3) combined increased pulmonary blood flow and pulmonary vascular resistance, and (4) increased pulmonary venous pressure.[62] PH is associated with high mortality and poor clinical outcomes. There are challenges in conducting large randomized controlled studies to evaluate the efficacy of using iNO before and after surgical correction of a congenital heart defect. The patient population is small, and there are ethical considerations with study design. As a result, most of the evidence base for iNO use in cardiac surgery stems from small observational, single-center randomized trials. A few studies have identified hemodynamic improvement with iNO administration following the bidirectional Glenn and Fontan operations, but clinical benefits have been variable.[63–65] A Cochrane review concluded that routine iNO administration in the postoperative period did not show any significant benefit to treat PH in children with congenital heart disease.[66] It was difficult to derive valid conclusions because of the methodological quality, sample size, bias, and heterogeneity of the four studies included in the meta-analysis.[66] Despite the lack of FDA approval and evidence in the literature, use of iNO to mitigate the effects of pulmonary vascular reactivity and postoperative PH in patients with congenital heart disease continues.

iNO is contraindicated in infants who are dependent on a right-to-left ductal shunt, such as an unrepaired hypoplastic left heart syndrome or interrupted aortic arch, as lowering pulmonary vascular resistance in these cases may result in pulmonary overcirculation and decreased systemic perfusion. iNO should be used cautiously in patients with left-sided obstructive lesions, such as obstructed total anomalous pulmonary venous return or left ventricular failure, because the increase in pulmonary blood flow may cause pulmonary edema without improving cardiac output.[67,68]

Application

Currently, the iNOmax DS$_{IR}$(Ikaria/Mallinckrodt Pharmaceuticals, Ellicott City, MD) is the only FDA-approved iNO delivery device. The iNOmax DS$_{IR}$ houses two aluminum canisters that contain pharmaceutical-grade NO (800 parts per million [ppm]) mixed with N_2 balance gas. This delivery device is capable of delivering iNO doses ranging from 0.1 to 80 ppm with conventional, anesthesia, and high-frequency ventilators. The iNOmax DS$_{IR}$ provides a constant dose of iNO to the inspiratory limb of the circuit through the use of a flow controller and injection module. Clinicians must be aware of the effects associated with using the iNOmax DS$_{IR}$ with various devices (e.g., conventional ventilation, anesthesia machines, and high-frequency ventilation), as each has subtle nuances to consider.

Delivery Devices

iNO may be delivered to infants and children receiving conventional invasive or noninvasive mechanical ventilatory support as well as high-frequency jet and high-frequency oscillatory ventilation. The nuances of proper equipment setup, patient monitoring, and safety considerations will be reviewed.

Conventional Ventilator

To assure accuracy of the iNO dose during delivery to mechanically ventilated patients, the manufacturer recommends positioning the injector module where there are minimal fluctuations in gas flow. Positioning the injector module between the inspiratory outlet and the dry side of the humidifier allows adequate mixing time along the inspiratory limb of the ventilator circuit and delivers a more stable dose to the patient.[69]

Oxygen dilution is inherent when delivering iNO to mechanically ventilated patients. Independent of the injection module position, the delivery system adds a proportional amount of NO gas based upon set dose and ventilator flow rate. As the iNO dose is increased, more gas is added to the inspiratory limb, resulting in a dilution of the O_2 concentration. **Table 29-4** illustrates the effect that increasing an iNO dose has on FiO_2.[70]

There are synchrony and safety considerations when delivering iNO during mechanical ventilation. The delivery device's monitoring system continuously samples gas at a rate of 230 mL/minute, which may affect trigger sensitivity and/or cause discrepancies in inhaled versus exhaled volumes (tidal volume and minute volume) and PEEP. These disparities may be clinically insignificant in larger patients; however, it may be necessary to adjust ventilator settings to adequately ventilate neonates.

Should the iNOmax DS_{IR} inadvertently fail, a backup delivery system and manual ventilation blender are available for short-term use until the delivery device can be replaced.

During manual ventilation with iNO delivery through a self-inflating bag, clinicians should be cognizant of the potential for NO_2 to build up within the manual resuscitation bag's reservoir and tubing.

High-Frequency Ventilators

Both high-frequency jet ventilation (HFJV) and high-frequency oscillatory ventilation (HFOV) are commonly used in combination with iNO therapy. Typically, with HFJV, the jet ventilator is functioning in tandem with the conventional ventilator. The HFJV supports a majority of the patient's minute volume while the conventional ventilator provides an exhalation valve, intermittent mandatory ventilation (IMV) breaths, and PEEP. As the conventional ventilation has a minimal role in ventilation, place the iNO injector module before the HFJV humidifier to allow for adequate time to mix with the gas delivered by the HFJV and to minimize exposure to pulsatile flow. **Figure 29-3** illustrates the position of the iNO injector module when used with the Bunnell Life Pulse HFJV (Bunnell Incorporated, Salt Lake City, UT). As the IMV rate on the conventional ventilator increases, air entrainment from the conventional ventilation circuit increases. HFJV strategy generally focuses on optimizing PEEP and minimizing the IMV rate to ≤5 breaths per minute. An IMV rate of ≤5 breaths per minute may still result in fluctuations in iNO concentration; however, the literature reports this difference as ≤10% of the set concentration.[71]

The iNO injector module should also be placed on the dry side of the circuit, before the humidifier, during HFOV. Because exhalation is active during HFOV, flow through the iNO injector module may move in a bidirectional manner. Placing a one-way valve between the injector module and the dry side of the humidifier will prevent retrograde flow and limit the potential for excessive iNO dose delivery to the patient. It is optimal to place the sampling line at the proximal port on the HFOV circuit as this allows for adequate mixing and provides more accurate monitoring.[72]

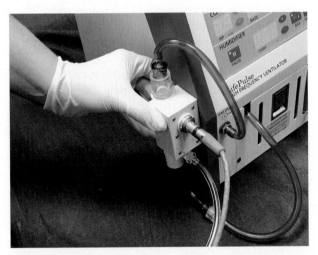

FIGURE 29-3 Position of the iNO injector module when used with the Bunnell Life Pulse HFJV.

Courtesy of Bunnell Inc.

TABLE 29-4
Dilution Effect That Increasing iNO Doses Has on Delivered Oxygen Concentrations

iNO Dose (ppm)	Percentage Oxygen Is Diluted from Its Intended Concentration
20	10
40	5
80	10

Noninvasive Applications

The majority of published data focusing on the use of iNO during invasive ventilatory support assume there is a negligible difference between the set and delivered iNO dose.[73,74] iNO delivery during noninvasive ventilation (NIV) with a traditional or high-flow nasal cannula results in the entrainment of air through the mouth or nares, which can decrease the NO dose delivered to the patient by approximately one-half.[75,76] Diblasi et al.[77] evaluated various NIV devices and occlusive nasal prongs to minimize leak during simulated iNO delivery and found a more accurate iNO delivery with nasal continuous positive airway pressure and NIV compared to delivery by HFNC. The HFNC has nonocclusive prongs, and the reduction in iNO dose delivery was outside of the recommended range by >20%.[77] Given the variability in NIV flow characteristics and leaks with patient interfaces, clinicians cannot assume that the set iNO dose is always equivalent to the dose delivered to the patient.

Anesthesia Machine

iNO is frequently used in the cardiac catheterization lab and in the operating room during repair of congenital cardiac lesions. An anesthesia ventilator is typically used to deliver iNO in these situations. Anesthesia ventilators employ a partial rebreathing circuit and a CO_2 scrubber to conserve the amount of anesthetic gas used. This results in partial rebreathing of fresh and exhaled gases that pass through the CO_2 scrubber. When delivering iNO inline with an anesthesia ventilator circuit, place the injector module on the inspiratory outlet of the ventilator and then add 6 to 12 inches of corrugated tubing after the module. This will allow for adequate mixing prior to the sample line. It is imperative to deliver a fresh gas flow rate that is higher than the patient's minute volume to avoid excessive recirculation of gases. Insufficient fresh gas flows will result in higher levels of NO and NO_2 as well as reduced O_2 concentrations.[78]

Dose Titration

Initial iNO doses between 2 and 80 ppm have been studied; however, most randomized clinical trials support 20 ppm as a routine starting dose.[30,39,79] iNO doses above 40 ppm have failed to demonstrate improved oxygenation in patients who did not respond to therapy at 20 ppm.[80] Sustained treatment at 40 to 80 ppm has been associated with adverse effects.[80] Typically, clinicians evaluate the effect of iNO 30 minutes after initiation of therapy. A positive response to therapy will result in an improvement in oxygenation and/or hemodynamic parameters. If the patient demonstrates a considerable clinical improvement, a stepwise reduction in iNO dose transpires. The iNO dose titration continues until the lowest dose maintaining the positive response to therapy is reached. If the patient fails to respond to therapy, titrate the iNO dose to a very low level and discontinue therapy.[79]

Monitoring

The INOmax system samples gas from downstream on the distal portion of the inspiratory limb, which allows gas concentrations of NO, NO_2, and O_2 to be continuously monitored using electrochemical cells for each respective gas.

Nitric Oxide

High concentrations of NO are associated with potential toxic effects, including methemoglobinemia, NO_2 formation, and decreased platelet aggregation.[81,82] The iNOmax DS_{IR} is equipped with a safety mechanism that terminates drug delivery when the monitoring system measures an NO concentration of $\geq$100 ppm.

FiO2

To account for the O_2 dilution that occurs during iNO administration, it is important to monitor and document the FiO_2 delivered by the iNOmax DS_{IR}. The FiO_2 monitored by the ventilator may not be accurate because the FiO_2 is measured before NO is introduced into the circuit. As the iNO dose increases, discrepancies between set and delivered FiO_2 become more significant, making it nearly impossible to deliver an FiO_2 of 1.0.[74]

Nitrogen Dioxide

The combination of O_2 and NO forms a toxic byproduct, NO_2, which has been associated with airway damage and inflammation.[83] NO_2 production increases exponentially when high FiO_2 and iNO concentrations are used simultaneously. Bouchet et al.[84] demonstrated that the use of an FiO_2 of 0.9 during iNO delivery was capable of producing 5 ppm of NO_2 in less than 2 seconds. The quantity of NO_2 formed can also be influenced by the delivery system (e.g., self-inflating resuscitator) and the amount of time left for iNO to oxidize within the circuit (e.g., partial rebreathing anesthesia circuit).

Methemoglobinemia

Methemoglobin (MetHb) is formed when iNO binds with hemoglobin (Hb), which reduces the availability of Hb to transport O_2. Factors associated with an increased risk for the development of methemoglobinemia include concurrently using high concentrations of both iNO and FiO_2 and iNO doses >20 ppm. Clinical trials report that MetHb levels peak approximately 8 hours after initiation of therapy. Monitoring MethHb levels by co-oximetry 4 to 8 hours after the initiation of iNO therapy, and every 24 hours thereafter, can aid in the early detection of methemoglobinemia.[37,39,79] Cyanosis and hypoxia can occur with MetHb concentrations greater than 10%. However, levels exceeding the clinically accepted threshold of 5% are unlikely to occur with the administration of iNO doses $\leq$20 ppm. MetHb levels ≤5% may be of little clinical significance and are often lower on follow-up measurements regardless of intervention (e.g., discontinuation or dose reduction) when doses are lower or therapy is discontinued.[85]

Weaning

Weaning of the iNO dose occurs after the patient demonstrates a positive response to therapy (improved SpO_2 and/or PaO_2) and is hemodynamically stable. Weaning minimizes the cost of care and reduces the potential for adverse effects. Typically, iNO is weaned by a series of stepwise dose reductions, such as a decrease in the iNO dose from 20 to 10 to 5 to 2.5 to 1 ppm, after which it is discontinued. Weaning protocols vary considerably in the duration of treatment, dose reductions, and time intervals between iNO dose changes. The literature reports that a 4-hour time period between weaning steps is a safe titration method.[37,86] It may be necessary to transiently increase the FiO_2 when iNO reaches 1 ppm or is discontinued.[86,87] Sildenafil has been shown to ameliorate rebound PH during weaning and discontinuation of iNO therapy for neonates with congenital heart defects who previously failed iNO weaning trials.[87,88]

Limitations

The primary disadvantages of iNO are the high cost of the gas and the complex delivery system required to deliver the therapy.[89–91] iNO has a very short half-life, which requires continuous administration, making it difficult to administer as a long-term therapy. When used in conjunction with mechanical ventilation, it is very important to optimize alveolar recruitment during iNO administration, as poorly ventilated alveoli impede NO from passing through the alveolar–capillary membrane, limiting the dilation effect on the pulmonary vasculature. Synergistic improvements in oxygenation have been observed when iNO was combined with recruitment measures, optimal PEEP, and high-frequency ventilation.[92–96]

Hazards/Complications

Rebound PH after discontinuation of therapy can occur, especially when therapy is administered for a longer duration of time. This results from a down-regulation of endogenous NO production. Transient increases in pulmonary artery pressure and decreases in PaO_2 have been observed shortly following discontinuation of iNO therapy, which lasts approximately 30 minutes before a new steady state is achieved. During this transitional period from 1 ppm to discontinuation, alternative therapeutic interventions, including sildenafil administration and increased FiO_2, are effective in preventing rebound PH.[87,97]

Subambient Oxygen and Inhaled Carbon Dioxide

Hypercarbic gas mixtures have been used for their pulmonary vasoconstrictive effects. This section describes the specialty gas mixtures that may be used to balance the pulmonary and systemic circulation in infants with certain congenital cardiac lesions.

Gas Physics

Nitrogen (N_2) is an inert, colorless, odorless gas that accounts for 78.09% of the Earth's atmosphere by volume. Carbon dioxide (CO_2) is colorless, odorless, and, under normal atmospheric conditions, has a concentration of 0.03%.

Mechanism of Action

The pulmonary vasculature is sensitive to acidosis and hypoxia, which increase pulmonary vascular resistance and limit pulmonary blood flow. Inspired nitrogen and carbon dioxide are gases that promote potent pulmonary vasoconstriction and are used to limit pulmonary blood flow in the perioperative management of infants with single ventricle physiology. Although not widely used, these inhaled specialty gases are helpful in balancing pulmonary and systemic blood flows, preserving the function of a single right-ventricle function, maximizing oxygen delivery to the tissues, and minimizing the need for intubation prior to surgical correction of the cardiac defect.[98]

Nitrogen

Inspired N_2 is used to dilute the concentration of oxygen in inspired air or to deliver subambient gas mixtures. **Subambient gas mixtures** deliver FiO_2 in the range of 0.14 to 0.20 to increase pulmonary vascular resistance by inducing hypoxic vasoconstriction.[99,100]

Carbon Dioxide

Inspired carbon dioxide, delivered in the range of 2% to 5%, induces hypercarbia and increases pulmonary vascular resistance, which limits pulmonary blood flow in neonates with hypoplastic left heart syndrome.[99,100]

Nitrogen versus Carbon Dioxide

Small interventional studies using a randomized crossover design compared the effectiveness of 17% inspired O_2 versus ~3% inspired CO_2 in neonates diagnosed with single ventricle physiology. Both methods reduced the ratio of pulmonary to systemic blood flow (Q_p:Q_s); however, systemic oxygen delivery increased during hypercarbia induced through inspired CO_2.[101] Inspired CO_2 was also found to improve cerebral oxygenation and mean arterial blood pressure, whereas a subambient gas mixture, FiO_2 of 0.17, did not have similar hemodynamic benefits.[102]

Effect on the Cardiopulmonary System

In the structurally normal cardiovascular system, the pulmonary and systemic circuits are connected in series and managed by two pumps, the right and left ventricles. Neonates with hypoplastic left heart syndrome typify a variant of the univentricular heart that is characterized by a hypoplastic left ventricle, stenosis or atresia of the mitral and aortic valves, and severe aortic arch hypoplasia. These patients require corrective surgery (Stage 1 pallation) within the first week of life, which includes reconstruction of the aortic arch, atrial septectomy, and creation of a stable source of pulmonary blood flow. Pulmonary blood flow is typically supplied through a restrictive systemic to pulmonary artery shunt (Blalock-Taussig or Central shunt) or a right ventricle to pulmonary artery shunt (Sano).

Because the hypoplastic left ventricle is essentially nonfunctional, the right ventricle manages cardiac output. The distribution of blood flow in infants with hypoplastic left heart syndrome is parallel and divided between the systemic and pulmonary circuits. One of the primary perioperative challenges in this patient population is maintaining a balance between Q_p and Q_s. Mathematical and simulation models of the univentricular heart have demonstrated that optimum systemic oxygen delivery (DO_2) occurs when the Q_p and Q_s are nearly equal. In contrast, a $Q_p{:}Q_s$ of <1 may lead to insufficient Q_p and potentially systemic hypoxemia[103,104] The $Q_p{:}Q_s$ is dependent upon the relative vascular resistances of both the pulmonary and the systemic circulations. Decreases in pulmonary vascular resistance may result in too much pulmonary blood flow, or overcirculation, at the expense of systemic perfusion. Decreased systemic perfusion can result in decreased coronary artery perfusion, multisystem organ failure, metabolic acidosis, and eventually cardiopulmonary collapse.[105]

Medical management focuses on maintaining an adequate balance of $Q_p{:}Q_s$ and maximizing DO_2 to the tissues. Mechanical ventilation is generally avoided preoperatively but may be required to support patients with apnea related to prostaglandin infusion, during interfacility transport to a quaternary care center, when respiratory failure is suspected. Mechanical ventilation strategies typically employ low FiO_2 (0.21–0.25), hypoventilation, and mild respiratory acidosis (e.g., CO_2 40–50) to achieve pulmonary vasoconstriction and improve systemic perfusion Q_s.[106,107]

Indications

When conventional strategies fail to limit high $Q_p{:}Q_s$, subambient oxygen concentrations or inspired CO_2 may be used as temporizing adjuncts for patients with hypoplastic left heart syndrome who are at risk for hemodynamic decompensation prior to surgery. Their use in the postoperative period following surgical correction and placement of a restrictive shunt as an optimal means of controlling pulmonary blood flow varies.[108,109]

Delivery Devices

Currently, there are no commercially available delivery devices for the administration of N_2 or CO_2.

Application

The administration of N_2 or CO_2 therapy can be delivered through a heated high-flow nasal cannula or a mechanical ventilator. Safety and monitoring are two important aspects to consider when N_2 or CO_2 gas mixtures are delivered to infants and children.

N_2 Administration and Conventional Ventilator

Administration of subambient oxygen concentrations to patients receiving mechanical ventilation requires the connection of an N_2 tank to the 50 psi air gas inlet of the ventilator. The ventilator's internal oxygen analyzer must be turned off, or in some cases disconnected, to avoid continuous alarms during hypoxic gas administration. It is imperative to connect an O_2 analyzer capable of measuring $FiO_2 \leq 0.15$ in order to provide accurate target FDO_2 delivery (e.g., 0.15–0.19) and monitoring. FiO_2 is incrementally adjusted on the ventilator while monitoring the O_2 analyzer for the desired set FDO_2 level. FDO_2 is then titrated to target oxygen saturations between 75% and 85%.

N_2 Administration through a High-Flow Nasal Cannula

Subambient oxygen therapy can also be administered by a high-flow nasal cannula by titrating N_2 into the HFNC circuit using small-bore tubing and a flowmeter. The blender, connected to the high-flow cannula, should be set at an FiO_2 of 0.21. During N_2 titration, an O_2 analyzer capable of analyzing subambient concentrations of oxygen is used to target and monitor the FDO_2. The nonocclusive prongs of the cannula allow for some air entrainment, making it difficult to set a precise FDO_2 level.

Carbon Dioxide

When administered to mechanically ventilated patients, CO_2 is bled into the humidifier or inspiratory limb of the conventional ventilator. An end-tidal CO_2 monitor may be used to monitor the delivered concentration of CO_2. When used, the end-tidal CO_2 monitor is placed after the humidifier to measure and monitor the concentration of CO_2 delivered to the patient. Because the CO_2 is bled into the ventilator circuit, ventilator parameter changes that affect minute ventilation may require titration of CO_2 flow to maintain prescribed inspired CO_2 levels. The targeted therapeutic range is generally 1% to 4% or 8 to 30 mm Hg, and adjustments are made in increments using the flow meter connected to the CO_2 tank.[110]

Monitoring

Patients receiving supplemental N_2 or CO_2 require cardiorespiratory monitoring and noninvasive monitoring of ventilation and oxygenation by capnography and pulse oximetry, respectively. Arterial blood gas sampling can be used to assess pH, PaO_2, mixed venous O_2, CO_2, and lactate. During subambient oxygen delivery, it is imperative to set the alarms on the O_2 analyzer for a tight range to avoid potentially disastrous swings in Q_p:Q_s resulting from a delivery error. If no beneficial changes in hemodynamics are noted (e.g., improved cardiac output), hypoxic gas administration should be discontinued. Patients receiving supplemental CO_2 must be monitored closely by capnography to ensure that the appropriate fraction of inspired CO_2 ($FiCO_2$) is delivered. High- and low-inspired CO_2 alarms on the ventilator (if applicable) should be set within 1 or 2 mm Hg of ordered inspired CO_2 levels.

Limitations

Both subambient oxygen delivery and inspired CO_2 are temporizing measures used on a short-term basis to limit overcirculation in the perioperative period. The efficacy of these therapies is supported by mid- to lower-grade evidence, and some controversy exists about the long-term effects and impact on cerebral blood flow.[111–113] Using inspired CO_2 to induce vasoconstriction requires the patient to be intubated, sedated, and paralyzed to avoid stimulation of the patient's respiratory drive. A compensatory metabolic alkalosis will develop over time in response to exogenous CO_2.

Hazards/Complications

The primary hazard using the aforementioned methods to increase pulmonary vascular resistance is the potential for error in gas delivery and subsequent effect on patient safety.

Anesthetic Gas Mixtures

Typically, inhalation is the primary route of anesthesia in the operating room. However, there are occasions when sedative and anesthetic medications are to provide anesthesia and amnesia to mechanically ventilated children in the ICU.

Gas Physics

Anesthetic gases are known as volatile liquids because they are easily vaporized at room temperature. Many exist that are most commonly used intraoperatively for sedation and include halothane, enflurane, **isoflurane**, desflurane, and sevoflurane. Although anesthetic gases are generally administered, they can also be used for their bronchodilator properties. Anesthetic gas mixtures may be used to treat patients with status asthmaticus who fail to improve or continue to clinically deteriorate with conventional methods of treatment. Typically, when used for this indication, isoflurane is the safest anesthetic of choice.[114]

Mechanism of Action

The benefits that anesthetic gases have within respiratory care stems from stimulation of the beta-adrenergic receptors of the sympathetic nervous system.[115] The stimulation of beta-1 receptors causes heart rate and contractility to increase. Beta-2 receptor stimulation causes bronchial and vascular smooth muscle relaxation. Anesthetic gases are not selective, and so both beta 1 and 2 responses occur.

Isoflurane is a clear, colorless liquid containing no additives or chemical stabilizers. This anesthetic gas has a mildly pungent, musty, ethereal odor and has a lower limit of flammability when used in an oxygen-rich environment. Isoflurane is used in the treatment of status asthmaticus for its bronchial dilation properties.

Effects on the Respiratory System

General anesthesia can increase the propensity for upper airway obstruction by relaxing pharyngeal muscles and can suppress respiratory function by decreasing airway protective cough and gag reflexes, decreasing minute ventilation, and stunting the peripheral chemoreceptors in the brain's response to hypercarbia.[116] Monitoring respiratory function is an essential part of safe administration. When used for bronchodilation, patients require intubation and mechanical ventilation. As the pharyngeal muscles are relaxed, the tongue can become displaced posteriorly and obstruct the airway.

Safety

Although anesthetic gases have been used in the treatment of status asthmaticus, there are no randomized controlled studies available to determine efficacy, outcomes, safety, or optimal timing of initiation compared to conventional treatment.

Indications

Inhaled isoflurane during mechanical ventilation is a modality used in the treatment of pediatric patients with status asthmaticus. The literature reports that when used for ventilatory failure refractory to conventional asthma therapy, improvements in pH and $PaCO_2$ were seen within the initial few hours of beginning treatment, providing time for traditional treatment to take effect.[117] Ventilation with lower peak inspiratory pressures and minimal renal toxicity were also realized.[118] Case reports of rapid recovery after the discontinuation of the anesthetic gas and successful extubation have been reported.[118]

Delivery Devices

Isoflurane is administered through a machine approved to administer anesthetic gas. The Occupational Health and Safety Administration's guidelines for workplace exposures state that specialty machines delivering anesthesia have two gas sources: a pipeline supply and a compressed gas cylinder supply. Gas sources used are typically oxygen, air, and/or nitrous oxide.[119] A central piping system from bulk storage is a hospital's main supply of anesthetic gases that connect to anesthesia machines at 50 to 55 psi through Diameter Indexed Safety System fittings. Compressed gas cylinders can be used but are generally reserved for emergency use, such as a central pipeline system failure. Compressed gas cylinders are attached to the back of the anesthesia machine by a hanger yoke assembly with the Pin Index Safety System. The Pin Index Safety System prevents accidental attachment of a cylinder to a yoke designed for another gas.

The anesthesia machine has ventilating capabilities. Fresh gases enter the machine's ventilator through an internal pipeline and travel to the vaporizer, where a concentration-calibrated specific agent is mixed with the fresh gas. Gas then exits a common gas outlet and into the patient's breathing circuit. Exhaled gases travel to the reservoir bag, then to the adjustable pressure-limiting valve, and exit into the scavenging system where waste gases are removed.

Titration

Anesthesia machines have vaporizers that are specifically labeled, color-coded, and calibrated for a specific anesthetic agent. Included on a standard vaporizer is a filling level sight glass to allow the operator to monitor the amount of liquid agent remaining during delivery, a control dial with numerical markers measured in volume percentage for agent titration, and a filling container to pour the liquid agent into. End-tidal concentrations of isoflurane are typically titrated slowly, in doses ranging from 0.5% to 1.5%, until clinical or laboratory improvement is noted or hypotension ensues.[117,120] In one large retrospective study, isoflurane was found to improve pH and $PaCO_2$ clearance within 4 hours in a series of patients with severe bronchospasm.[121]

Monitoring

A sample line placed into the inspiratory limb during agent delivery allows the clinician to monitor FiO_2, minimum alveolar concentration, $FiCO_2$, agent volume percentage, and $ETCO_2$. The minimum alveolar concentration is the alveolar concentration of an inhaled anesthetic in which 50% of patients will no longer respond to painful or surgical stimuli.

Limitations

Administration of isoflurane in the intensive care unit poses human resources issues. The most commonly debated topic is which clinicians should assume responsibility for filling the vaporizer, titration, and anesthetic delivery. The scope of practice defined by licensure may limit a respiratory therapist's ability to manage the delivery of this anesthetic gas under the direction of a physician. The lack of evidence-based clinical practice guidelines and infrequent use of this therapy in the ICU warrants developing a comprehensive infrastructure in which roles and responsibilities are defined and guidelines established for the safe administration of isoflurane under the supervision of an anesthesiologist.

Hazards/Complications

Anesthetic gas delivery can result in operator and/or patient decompensation. Volatile liquid spills are harmful to the operator, especially when the spill occurs in a poorly ventilated workplace environment. Spills can be contained by immediately covering the liquid with towels and absorbents and evacuating the area until properly trained personnel can effectively clean the spill.[119] During the containment and cleaning of a spill, staff handling volatile anesthetic gases and bystanders in the confined/affected area must wear personal protective equipment.

Clinicians must be knowledgeable of the signs and symptoms of adverse reactions during isoflurane gas delivery. Hypotension is the most commonly reported side effect, which is typically managed with vasoactive medications and fluid boluses.[118,121] Malignant hyperthermia, caused by an excess release of calcium to the body's skeletal muscles, can also occur.[122] Patients experiencing malignant hyperthermia are in a hypermetabolic state resulting from increased oxygen consumption and anaerobic metabolism and may also experience tachycardia and respiratory acidosis.[123] Malignant hyperthermia may be identified early in its onset by a sudden rise in $ETCO_2$. Continuous temperature monitoring is an important component of the care of patients receiving isoflurane in the ICU setting. When malignant hyperthermia is suspected, it is essential to disconnect the patient from the breathing circuit and to provide manual ventilation with 100% oxygen. Cardiorespiratory monitoring is also essential, as hypotension and cardiac arrhythmias can also occur.[114]

Case Study

A 3-year-old boy presented to the emergency department (ED) with sudden onset of cough and difficulty breathing that woke him from sleep. He has a history of mild intermittent asthma, and he had never been hospitalized. Vital signs in the ED were as follows: temperature 38.9°C, heart rate 110 beats per minute, blood pressure 90/60 mm Hg, respiratory rate 30 breaths per minute, and oxygen saturation by pulse oximetry 98% on room air. Exam is remarkable for stridor at rest, tracheal tug, and moderate intercostal retractions. The boy appeared fatigued and he refused to speak. Upon auscultation, breath sounds were clear with decreased aeration throughout. A mild scattered erythematous rash was noted on his chest and arms. A chest X-ray and respiratory viral panel were ordered. Racemic epinephrine 0.5 mL of nebulized 2.25% solution, diluted in 3 mL of normal saline was administered by small volume nebulizer. A dose of dexamethasone was also administered at that time. The patient was noted to have decreased stridor and decreased work of breathing following the racemic epinephrine treatment. Within 30 minutes the child had more notable stridor and noticeable increase in his work of breathing. The physician ordered heliox gas treatment at 80/20 mixture composition by heated high-flow nasal cannula. Within a few minutes, the child's work of breathing lessened, as did his stridor. The patient was admitted to the intensive care unit on the gas mixture and aerosolized racemic epinephrine every 2 hours.

1. **Why was heliox indicated in this case?**

2. **Describe the reasoning for using an 80/20 mixture instead of a 70/30 in this case.**

3. **Name another oxygen delivery device that you could have used in this case to deliver the heliox mixture.**

References

1. Hess DR, Fink JB, Venkataraman ST, Kim IK, Myers TR, Tano BD. The history and physics of heliox. *Respir Care.* 2006;51(6):608-612.
2. Reuben AD, Harris AR. Heliox for asthma in the emergency department: a review of the literature. *Emerg Med J.* 2004;21(2):131-135.
3. Barnett TB. Effects of helium and oxygen mixtures on pulmonary mechanics during airway constriction. *J Appl Physiol.* 1967;22(4):707-713.
4. Rodrigo G, Pollack C, Rodrigo C, Rowe BH. Heliox for nonintubated acute asthma patients. *Cochrane Database Syst Rev.* 2006;4:CD002884.
5. Nievas IF, Anand KJ. Severe acute asthma exacerbation in children: a stepwise approach for escalating therapy in a pediatric intensive care unit. *J Pediatr Pharmacol Ther.* 2013;18(2):88-104.
6. Frazier MD, Cheifetz IM. The role of heliox in paediatric respiratory disease. *Paediatr Respir Rev.* 2010;11(1):46-53; quiz 53.
7. Abd-Allah SA, Rogers MS, Terry M, Gross M, Perkin RM. Helium-oxygen therapy for pediatric acute severe asthma requiring mechanical ventilation. *Pediatr Criti Care Med.* 2003;4(3):353-357.
8. Grosz AH, Jacobs IN, Cho C, Schears GJ. Use of helium-oxygen mixtures to relieve upper airway obstruction in a pediatric population. *Laryngoscope.* 2001;9:1512-1514.
9. Terregino CA, Nairn SJ, Chansky ME, Kass JE. The effect of heliox on croup: a pilot study. *Acad Emerg Med.* 1998;5(11):1130-1133.
10. Weber JE, Chudnofsky CR, Younger JG, et al. A randomized comparison of helium-oxygen mixture (heliox) and racemic epinephrine for the treatment of moderate to severe croup. *Pediatrics.* 2001;107(6):E96.
11. Moraa I, Sturman N, McGuire T, van Driel ML. Heliox for croup in children. *Cochrane Database Syst Rev.* 2013;12:CD006822.
12. American Academy of Pediatrics Subcommittee on Diagnosis and Management of Bronchiolitis. Diagnosis and management of bronchiolitis. *Pediatrics.* 2006;118(4):1774-1793.
13. Liet JM, Ducruet T, Gupta V, Cambonie G. Heliox inhalation therapy for bronchiolitis in infants. *Cochrane Database Syst Rev.* 2015;9:CD006915.
14. Martinon-Torres F, Rodriguez-Nunez A, Martinon-Sanchez JM. Heliox therapy in infants with acute bronchiolitis. *Pediatrics.* 2002;109(1):68-73.
15. Brown MK, Willms DC. A laboratory evaluation of 2 mechanical ventilators in the presence of helium-oxygen mixtures. *Respir Care.* 2005;50(3):354-360.
16. Kallet RH. Adjunct therapies during mechanical ventilation: airway clearance techniques, therapeutic aerosols, and gases. *Respir Care.* 2013;58(6):1053-1073.
17. Anderson M, Svartengren M, Bylin G, Philipson K, Camner P. Deposition in asthmatics of particles inhaled in air or in helium-oxygen. *Am Rev Respir Dis.* 1993;147(3):524-528.
18. Kim IK, Phrampus E, Venkataraman S, et al. Helium/oxygen-driven albuterol nebulization in the treatment of children with moderate to severe asthma exacerbations: a randomized, controlled trial. *Pediatrics.* 2005;116(5):1127-1133.
19. Hurford WE, Cheifetz IM. Respiratory controversies in the critical care setting. Should heliox be used for mechanically ventilated patients? *Respir Care.* 2007;52(5):582-591; discussion 591-594.
20. Myers TR. Use of heliox in children. *Respir Care.* 2006;51(6):619-631.
21. Weinberger B, Laskin DL, Heck DE, Laskin JD. The toxicology of inhaled nitric oxide. *Toxicol Sci.* 2001;59(1):5-16.
22. Ignarro LJ, Buga GM, Wood KS, Byrns RE, Chaudhuri G. Endothelium-derived relaxing factor produced and released from artery and vein is nitric oxide. *Proc Natl Acad Sci U S A.* 1987;84(24):9265-9269.
23. Palmer RM, Ferrige AG, Moncada S. Nitric oxide release accounts for the biological activity of endothelium-derived relaxing factor. *Nature.* 1987;327(6122):524-526.
24. Arul N, Konduri GG. Inhaled nitric oxide for preterm neonates. *Clin Perinatol.* 2009;36(1):43-61.
25. Frostell CG, Blomqvist H, Hedenstierna G, Lundberg J, Zapol WM. Inhaled nitric oxide selectively reverses human hypoxic pulmonary vasoconstriction without causing systemic vasodilation. *Anesthesiology.* 1993;78(3):427-435.
26. Fratacci MD, Frostell CG, Chen TY, Wain JC Jr., Robinson DR, Zapol WM. Inhaled nitric oxide. A selective pulmonary vasodilator

of heparin-protamine vasoconstriction in sheep. *Anesthesiology.* 1991;75(6):990-999.

27. Hsu CW, Lee DL, Lin SL, Sun SF, Chang HW. The initial response to inhaled nitric oxide treatment for intensive care unit patients with acute respiratory distress syndrome. *Respiration.* 2008;75(3):288-295.

28. Bin-Nun A, Schreiber MD. Role of iNO in the modulation of pulmonary vascular resistance. *J Perinatol.* 2008;23(Suppl 3):S84-S92.

29. Griffiths MJ, Evans TW. Inhaled nitric oxide therapy in adults. *N Engl J Med.* 2005;353(25):2683-2695.

30. Finer NN, Barrington KJ. Nitric oxide for respiratory failure in infants born at or near term. *Cochrane Database Syst Rev.* 2006;4:CD000399.

31. Barrington KJ, Finer NN. Inhaled nitric oxide for respiratory failure in preterm infants. *Cochrane Database Syst Rev.* 2006;1:CD000509.

32. Kumar P, Committee on Fetus and Newborn, American Academy of Pediatrics. Use of inhaled nitric oxide in preterm infants. *Pediatrics.* 2014;133(1):164-170.

33. Cole FS, Alleyne C, Barks JD, et al. NIH Consensus Development Conference statement: inhaled nitric-oxide therapy for premature infants. *Pediatrics.* 2011;127(2):363-369.

34. Ellsworth MA, Harris MN, Carey WA, Spitzer AR, Clark RH. Off-label use of inhaled nitric oxide after release of NIH consensus statement. *Pediatrics.* 2015;135(4):643-648.

35. Lakshminrusimha S, Steinhorn RH. Pulmonary vascular biology during neonatal transition. *Clin Perinatol.* 1999;26(3):601-619.

36. Neonatal Inhaled Nitric Oxide Study G. Inhaled nitric oxide in full-term and nearly full-term infants with hypoxic respiratory failure. *N Engl J Med.* 1997;336(9):597-604.

37. Clark RH, Kueser TJ, Walker MW, et al. Low-dose nitric oxide therapy for persistent pulmonary hypertension of the newborn. Clinical Inhaled Nitric Oxide Research Group. *N Engl J Med.* 2000;342(7):469-474.

38. Roberts JD Jr., Fineman JR, Morin FC 3rd, et al. Inhaled nitric oxide and persistent pulmonary hypertension of the newborn. The Inhaled Nitric Oxide Study Group. *N Engl J Med.* 1997;336(9):605-610.

39. Nair J, Lakshminrusimha S. Update on PPHN: mechanisms and treatment. *Semin Perinatol.* 2014;38(2):78-91.

40. Flori HR, Glidden DV, Rutherford GW, Matthay MA. Pediatric acute lung injury: prospective evaluation of risk factors associated with mortality. *Am J Respir Crit Care Med.* 2005;171(9):995-1001.

41. Erickson S, Schibler A, Numa A, et al. Acute lung injury in pediatric intensive care in Australia and New Zealand: a prospective, multicenter, observational study. *Pediatr Crit Care Med.* 2007; 8(4):317-323.

42. Khemani RG, Smith LS, Zimmerman JJ, Erickson S, Pediatric Acute Lung Injury Consensus Conference. Pediatric acute respiratory distress syndrome: definition, incidence, and epidemiology: proceedings from the pediatric acute lung injury consensus conference. *Pediatr Crit Care Med.* 2015;16(5 Suppl 1):S23-S40.

43. Afshari A, Brok J, Moller AM, Wetterslev J. Inhaled nitric oxide for acute respiratory distress syndrome and acute lung injury in adults and children: a systematic review with meta-analysis and trial sequential analysis. *Anesth Analg.* 2011;112(6):1411-1421.

44. Day RW, Allen EM, Witte MK. A randomized, controlled study of the 1-hour and 24-hour effects of inhaled nitric oxide therapy in children with acute hypoxemic respiratory failure. *Chest.* 1997;112(5):1324-1331.

45. Dobyns EL, Cornfield DN, Anas NG, et al. Multicenter randomized controlled trial of the effects of inhaled nitric oxide therapy on gas exchange in children with acute hypoxemic respiratory failure. *J Pediatr.* 1999;134(4):406-412.

46. Bronicki RA, Fortenberry J, Schreiber M, Checchia PA, Anas NG. Multicenter randomized controlled trial of inhaled nitric oxide for pediatric acute respiratory distress syndrome. *J Pediatr.* 2015;166(2):365-369.

47. Adhikari NK, Dellinger RP, Lundin S, et al. Inhaled nitric oxide does not reduce mortality in patients with acute respiratory distress syndrome regardless of severity: systematic review and meta-analysis. *Crit Care Med.* 2014;42(2):404-412.

48. Afshari A, Brok J, Moller AM, Wetterslev J. Inhaled nitric oxide for acute respiratory distress syndrome (ARDS) and acute lung injury in children and adults. *Cochrane Database Syst Rev.* 2010;7:CD002787.

49. Mok YH, Lee JH, Rehder KJ, Turner DA. Adjunctive treatments in pediatric acute respiratory distress syndrome. *Expert Rev Respir Med.* 2014;8(6):703-716.

50. Barst RJ, Agnoletti G, Fraisse A, Baldassarre J, Wessel DL, Group NODS. Vasodilator testing with nitric oxide and/or oxygen in pediatric pulmonary hypertension. *Pediatr Cardiol.* 2010;31(5):598-606.

51. Ricciardi MJ, Knight BP, Martinez FJ, Rubenfire M. Inhaled nitric oxide in primary pulmonary hypertension: a safe and effective agent for predicting response to nifedipine. *J Am Coll Cardiol.* 1998;32(4):1068-1073.

52. Barr FE, Macrae D. Inhaled nitric oxide and related therapies. *Pediatr Crit Care Med.* 2010;11(2 Suppl):S30-S36.

53. Wheller J, George BL, Mulder DG, Jarmakani JM. Diagnosis and management of postoperative pulmonary hypertensive crisis. *Circulation.* 1979;60(7):1640-1644.

54. Hoeper MM, Bogaard HJ, Condliffe R, et al. Definitions and diagnosis of pulmonary hypertension. *Turk Kardiyol Dern Ars.* 2014;42(Suppl 1):55-66.

55. Hawkins A, Tulloh R. Treatment of pediatric pulmonary hypertension. *Vasc Health Risk Manag.* 2009;5(2):509-524.

56. Gorenflo M, Gu H, Xu Z. Peri-operative pulmonary hypertension in paediatric patients: current strategies in children with congenital heart disease. *Cardiology.* 2010;116(1):10-17.

57. Bando K, Turrentine MW, Sharp TG, et al. Pulmonary hypertension after operations for congenital heart disease: analysis of risk factors and management. *J Thorac Cardiovasc Surg.* 1996;112(6):1600-1607; discussion 1607-1609.

58. Lindberg L, Olsson AK, Jogi P, Jonmarker C. How common is severe pulmonary hypertension after pediatric cardiac surgery? *J Thorac Cardiovasc Surg.* 2002;123(6):1155-1163.

59. Wessel DL. Managing low cardiac output syndrome after congenital heart surgery. *Crit Care Med.* 2001;29(10 Suppl):S220-S230.

60. Miller OI, Tang SF, Keech A, Pigott NB, Beller E, Celermajer DS. Inhaled nitric oxide and prevention of pulmonary hypertension after congenital heart surgery: a randomised double-blind study. *Lancet.* 2000;356(9240):1464-1469.

61. Journois D, Baufreton C, Mauriat P, Pouard P, Vouhe P, Safran D. Effects of inhaled nitric oxide administration on early postoperative mortality in patients operated for correction of atrioventricular canal defects. *Chest.* 2005;128(5):3537-3544.

62. Taylor MB, Laussen PC. Fundamentals of management of acute postoperative pulmonary hypertension. *Pediatr Crit Care Med.* 2010;11(2 Suppl):S27-S29.

63. Goldman AP, Delius RE, Deanfield JE, et al. Pharmacological control of pulmonary blood flow with inhaled nitric oxide after the fenestrated Fontan operation. *Circulation.* 1996;94(9 Suppl): II44-II48.

64. Yoshimura N, Yamaguchi M, Oka S, et al. Inhaled nitric oxide therapy after Fontan-type operations. *Surg Today.* 2005;35(1):31-35.

65. Khambadkone S, Li J, de Leval MR, Cullen S, Deanfield JE, Redington AN. Basal pulmonary vascular resistance and nitric oxide responsiveness late after Fontan-type operation. *Circulation.* 2003;107(25):3204-3208.

66. Bizzarro M, Gross I, Barbosa FT. Inhaled nitric oxide for the postoperative management of pulmonary hypertension in infants and children with congenital heart disease. *Cochrane Database Syst Rev.* 2014;7:CD005055.

67. Loh E, Stamler JS, Hare JM, Loscalzo J, Colucci WS. Cardiovascular effects of inhaled nitric oxide in patients with left ventricular dysfunction. *Circulation.* 1994;90(6):2780-2785.

68. Semigran MJ, Cockrill BA, Kacmarek R, et al. Hemodynamic effects of inhaled nitric oxide in heart failure. *J Am Coll Cardiol.* 1994;24(4):982-988.

69. Hiesmayr MJ, Neugebauer T, Lassnigg A, Steltzer H, Haider W, Gilly H. Performance of proportional and continuous nitric oxide

delivery systems during pressure- and volume-controlled ventilation. *Br J Anaesth.* 1998;81(4):544-552.

70. Ikaria. Operation Manual for INOmax DSIR. New Jersey; 2012.

71. Platt DR, Swanton D, Blackney D. Inhaled nitric oxide (iNO) delivery with high-frequency jet ventilation (HFJV). *J Perinatol.* 2003;23(5):387-391.

72. Fujino Y, Kacmarek RM, Hess DR. Nitric oxide delivery during high-frequency oscillatory ventilation. *Respir Care.* 2000;45(9):1097-1104.

73. Kirmse M, Hess D, Fujino Y, Kacmarek RM, Hurford WE. Delivery of inhaled nitric oxide using the Ohmeda INOvent Delivery System. *Chest.* 1998;113(6):1650-1657.

74. Young JD, Roberts M, Gale LB. Laboratory evaluation of the I-NOvent nitric oxide delivery device. *Br J Anaesth.* 1997;79(3):398-401.

75. Kinsella JP, Cutter GR, Steinhorn RH, et al. Noninvasive inhaled nitric oxide does not prevent bronchopulmonary dysplasia in premature newborns. *J Pediatr.* 2014;165(6):1104-1108.

76. Kinsella JP, Parker TA, Ivy DD, Abman SH. Noninvasive delivery of inhaled nitric oxide therapy for late pulmonary hypertension in newborn infants with congenital diaphragmatic hernia. *J Pediatr.* 2003;142(4):397-401.

77. DiBlasi RM, Dupras D, Kearney C, Costa E Jr., Griebel JL. Nitric oxide delivery by neonatal noninvasive respiratory support devices. *Respir Care.* 2015;60(2):219-230.

78. Ceccarelli P, Bigatello LM, Hess D, Kwo J, Melendez L, Hurford WE. Inhaled nitric oxide delivery by anesthesia machines. *Anesth Analg.* 2000;90(2):482-488.

79. DiBlasi RM, Myers TR, Hess DR. Evidence-based clinical practice guideline: inhaled nitric oxide for neonates with acute hypoxic respiratory failure. *Respir Care.* 2010;55(12):1717-1745.

80. Kinsella JP, Abman SH. Inhaled nitric oxide therapy in children. *Paediatr Respir Rev.* 2005;6(3):190-198.

81. George TN, Johnson KJ, Bates JN, Segar JL. The effect of inhaled nitric oxide therapy on bleeding time and platelet aggregation in neonates. *J Pediatr.* 1998;132(4):731-734.

82. Radomski MW, Palmer RM, Moncada S. Endogenous nitric oxide inhibits human platelet adhesion to vascular endothelium. *Lancet.* 1987;2(8567):1057-1058.

83. Saugstad OD. Inhaled nitric oxide for preterm infants—still an experimental therapy. *Lancet.* 1999;354(9184):1047-1048.

84. Bouchet M, Renaudin MH, Raveau C, Mercier JC, Dehan M, Zupan V. Safety requirement for use of inhaled nitric oxide in neonates. *Lancet.* 1993;341(8850):968-969.

85. Hamon I, Gauthier-Moulinier H, Grelet-Dessioux E, Storme L, Fresson J, Hascoet JM. Methaemoglobinaemia risk factors with inhaled nitric oxide therapy in newborn infants. *Acta Paediatr.* 2010;99(10):1467-1473.

86. Kinsella JP, Walsh WF, Bose CL, et al. Inhaled nitric oxide in premature neonates with severe hypoxaemic respiratory failure: a randomised controlled trial. *Lancet.* 1999;354(9184):1061-1065.

87. Namachivayam P, Theilen U, Butt WW, Cooper SM, Penny DJ, Shekerdemian LS. Sildenafil prevents rebound pulmonary hypertension after withdrawal of nitric oxide in children. *Am J Respir Crit Care Med.* 2006;174(9):1042-1047.

88. Lee JE, Hillier SC, Knoderer CA. Use of sildenafil to facilitate weaning from inhaled nitric oxide in children with pulmonary hypertension following surgery for congenital heart disease. *J Intensive Care Med.* 2008;23(5):329-334.

89. Brunner N, de Jesus Perez VA, Richter A, et al. Perioperative pharmacological management of pulmonary hypertensive crisis during congenital heart surgery. *Pulm Circ.* 2014;4(1):10-24.

90. Angus DC, Clermont G, Watson RS, Linde-Zwirble WT, Clark RH, Roberts MS. Cost-effectiveness of inhaled nitric oxide in the treatment of neonatal respiratory failure in the United States. *Pediatrics.* 2003;112(6 Pt 1):1351-1360.

91. Todd Tzanetos DR, Housley JJ, Barr FE, May WL, Landers CD. Implementation of an inhaled nitric oxide protocol decreases direct cost associated with its use. *Respir Care.* 2015;60(5):644-650.

92. Dobyns EL, Anas NG, Fortenberry JD, et al. Interactive effects of high-frequency oscillatory ventilation and inhaled nitric oxide in acute hypoxemic respiratory failure in pediatrics. *Crit Care Med.* 2002;30(11):2425-2429.

93. Coates EW, Klinepeter ME, O'Shea TM. Neonatal pulmonary hypertension treated with inhaled nitric oxide and high-frequency ventilation. *J Perinatol.* 2008;28(10):675-679.

94. Hoehn T, Krause MF. Synergistic effects of high-frequency ventilation and inhaled nitric oxide in the treatment of hypoxemic respiratory failure in infancy. *Pediatr Pulmonol.* 1998;26(3):228-230.

95. Okamoto K, Kukita I, Hamaguchi M, Motoyama T, Muranaka H, Harada T. Combined effects of inhaled nitric oxide and positive end-expiratory pressure during mechanical ventilation in acute respiratory distress syndrome. *Artif Organs.* 2000;24(5):390-395.

96. Park KJ, Lee YJ, Oh YJ, Lee KS, Sheen SS, Hwang SC. Combined effects of inhaled nitric oxide and a recruitment maneuver in patients with acute respiratory distress syndrome. *Yonsei Med J.* 2003;44(2):219-226.

97. Davidson D, Barefield ES, Kattwinkel J, et al. Safety of withdrawing inhaled nitric oxide therapy in persistent pulmonary hypertension of the newborn. *Pediatrics.* 1999;104(2 Pt 1):231-236.

98. Graham EM, Bradley SM, Atz AM. Preoperative management of hypoplastic left heart syndrome. *Expert Opin Pharmacother.* 2005;6(5):687-693.

99. Day RW, Barton AJ, Pysher TJ, Shaddy RE. Pulmonary vascular resistance of children treated with nitrogen during early infancy. *Ann Thorac Surg.* 1998;65(5):1400-1404.

100. Shime N, Hashimoto S, Hiramatsu N, Oka T, Kageyama K, Tanaka Y. Hypoxic gas therapy using nitrogen in the preoperative management of neonates with hypoplastic left heart syndrome. *Pediatr Crit Care Med.* 2000;1(1):38-41.

101. Tabbutt S, Ramamoorthy C, Montenegro LM, et al. Impact of inspired gas mixtures on preoperative infants with hypoplastic left heart syndrome during controlled ventilation. *Circulation.* 2001;104(12 Suppl 1):I159-I164.

102. Ramamoorthy C, Tabbutt S, Kurth CD, et al. Effects of inspired hypoxic and hypercapnic gas mixtures on cerebral oxygen saturation in neonates with univentricular heart defects. *Anesthesiology.* 2002;96(2):283-288.

103. Migliavacca F, Pennati G, Dubini G, et al. Modeling of the Norwood circulation: effects of shunt size, vascular resistances, and heart rate. *Am J Physiol Heart Circ Physiol.* 2001;280(5):H2076-H2086.

104. Barnea O, Austin EH, Richman B, Santamore WP. Balancing the circulation: theoretic optimization of pulmonary/systemic flow ratio in hypoplastic left heart syndrome. *J Am Coll Cardiol.* 1994;24(5):1376-1381.

105. Rossano JW, Chang AC. Perioperative management of patients with poorly functioning ventricles in the setting of the functionally univentricular heart. *Cardiol Young.* 2006;16(Suppl 1):47-54.

106. Nelson DP, Schwartz SM, Chang AC. Neonatal physiology of the functionally univentricular heart. *Cardiol Young.* 2004;14 (Suppl 1): 52-60.

107. Chang AC, Zucker HA, Hickey PR, Wessel DL. Pulmonary vascular resistance in infants after cardiac surgery: role of carbon dioxide and hydrogen ion. *Crit Care Med.* 1995;23(3):568-574.

108. Yildiz M. Hypoxia is/is not the optimal means of reducing pulmonary blood flow in the preoperative single ventricle heart. *J App Physiol.* 2008;104(6):1840; author reply 1843.

109. Liske MR, Aschner JL. Counterpoint: hypoxia is not the optimal means of reducing pulmonary blood flow in the preoperative single ventricle heart. *J App Physiol.* 2008;104(6):1836-1838; discussion 1838-1839.

110. Myers TR. Therapeutic gases for neonatal and pediatric respiratory care. *Respir Care.* 2003;48(4):399-422; discussion 423-395.

111. Reddy VM, Liddicoat JR, Fineman JR, McElhinney DB, Klein JR, Hanley FL. Fetal model of single ventricle physiology: hemodynamic effects of oxygen, nitric oxide, carbon dioxide, and hypoxia in the

early postnatal period. *J Thorac Cardiovasc Surg*. 1996;112(2): 437-449.

112. Bradley SM, Simsic JM, Atz AM. Hemodynamic effects of inspired carbon dioxide after the Norwood procedure. *Ann Thorac Surg*. 2001;72(6):2088-2093; discussion 2093-2094.

113. Li J, Zhang G, Holtby H, et al. Carbon dioxide—a complex gas in a complex circulation: its effects on systemic hemodynamics and oxygen transport, cerebral, and splanchnic circulation in neonates after the Norwood procedure. *J Thorac Cardiovasc Surg*. 2008;136(5):1207-1214.

114. Basak B. Isoflurane as a general anesthetic: will it displace all other volatile anesthetics? *J Am Assoc Nurse Anesth*. 1984:614-618.

115. Guarino RD, Perez DM, Piascik MT. Recent advances in the molecular pharmacology of the alpha 1-adrenergic receptors. *Cell Signal*. 1996;8(5):323-333.

116. Davison R, Cottle D. The effects of anesthesia on respiratory function. *ATOTW*. 2010;205:1-8.

117. Shankar V, Churchwell KB, Deshpande JK. Isoflurane therapy for severe refractory status asthmaticus in children. *Intensive Care Med*. 2006;32(6):927-933.

118. Johnston RG, Noseworthy TW, Friesen EG, Yule HA, Shustack A. Isoflurane therapy for status asthmaticus in children and adults. *Chest*. 1990;97(3):698-701.

119. Administration OSH. Anesthetic Gases: Guidelines for Workplace Exposures. https://www.osha.gov/dts/osta/anestheticgases/index .html. Accessed July 1, 2018.

120. Carrie S, Anderson TA. Volatile anesthetics for status asthmaticus in pediatric patients: a comprehensive review and case series. *Paediatr Anaesth*. 2015;25(5):460-467.

121. Turner DA, Heitz D, Cooper MK, Smith PB, Arnold JH, Bateman ST. Isoflurane for life-threatening bronchospasm: a 15-year single-center experience. *Respir Care*. 2012;57(11):1857-1864.

122. Kim TW, Nemergut ME. Preparation of modern anesthesia workstations for malignant hyperthermia-susceptible patients: a review of past and present practice. *Anesthesiology*. 2011;114(1):205-212.

123. Nelson P, Litman RS. Malignant hyperthermia in children: an analysis of the North American malignant hyperthermia registry. *Anesth Analg*. 2014;118(2):369-374.

Extracorporeal Membrane Oxygenation

Peter Betit

John Priest

OUTLINE

OBJECTIVES

1. Describe the fundamental role of ECMO.
2. List the therapeutic modalities that contributed to the decline in ECMO use and improved neonatal mortality.
3. Describe the clinical indications for ECMO.
4. List the therapeutic goals for ECMO as respiratory support.
5. State the criteria used for selecting ECMO as a therapeutic option for neonates requiring respiratory support.
6. List the therapeutic goals for ECMO as cardiac support.
7. Explain the component of the ECMO circuit.
8. List the factors used to determine the type of ECMO support.
9. Describe the differences between venous-arterial and venous-venous ECMO support.
10. Differentiate between roller and centrifugal pumps.
11. Describe the relationship between sweep gas flow rate and $PaCO_2$.
12. Explain the goals of pulmonary support during ECMO.
13. Provide the treatable causes of hypotension and hypertension during ECMO.
14. List the complications associated with ECMO.

KEY TERMS

centrifugal pumps
extracorporeal cardiopulmonary resuscitation (ECPR)
extracorporeal membrane oxygenation (ECMO)
impeller
membrane oxygenator

oxygenation index (OI)
Pediatric Risk of Mortality Score (PRISM)
recirculation
roller pumps
transthoracic cannulation
venous-arterial (VA)
venous-venous (VV)

Introduction

Extracorporeal membrane oxygenation (ECMO) is a form of mechanical circulatory support that incorporates an artificial lung or membrane oxygenator and is used to support neonates, infants, and children with severe cardiac, respiratory, or cardiorespiratory failure.[1] The technique requires vascular access, to which a customized circuit is connected, and blood is circulated by means of a pump while artificial gas exchange occurs in the membrane oxygenator. ECMO systems are essentially adaptations of devices used for cardiopulmonary bypass, but they have evolved into more streamlined systems designed to provide prolonged support in a critical care setting.[2] The aim of this chapter is to describe the technical aspects, clinical application, physiologic effects, patient monitoring, and complications associated with ECMO.

Background

In 1977, Bartlett and colleagues[3] first described the lifesaving potential of ECMO and its ability to support newborns with respiratory failure. In the mid-1980s and over the subsequent decade, the role of ECMO in the management of newborns with hypoxemic respiratory failure was confirmed as several studies demonstrated safety, efficacy, and improved survival.[4-6] During this time, ECMO centers were being developed around the United States and Europe, and ECMO became an important adjunct in newborn intensive care.

In 1989, the Extracorporeal Life Support Organization (ELSO) was formed with the mission to coordinate clinical research in extracorporeal techniques, to develop guidelines, and to maintain a database of ECMO cases. This organization continues to expand with the addition of international affiliates, and the ELSO registry has maintained data and compiled statistics for over 69,000 cases.[7]

By the mid-1990s, less invasive techniques, including surfactant replacement therapy, high-frequency ventilation, and inhaled nitric oxide, also contributed to a decrease in neonatal mortality, and the need for ECMO declined.[8] Despite this decreased use, extracorporeal technology continued to evolve and other indications for ECMO were being considered, including support for such conditions as congenital heart disease and respiratory failure in children (Table 30-1). In the present decade, the application of ECMO continues to broaden as catheters and vascular access techniques have improved, and ECMO systems continue to be refined and their safety enhanced.[9]

Clinical Application

The fundamental role of ECMO is to provide well-perfused blood and to preserve organ function until the patient recovers from the underlying condition and is

TABLE 30-1
Indications for ECMO in Infants and Children

Type of Support	Goals of Therapy	Clinical Conditions
Respiratory	Support organ function, normalize gas exchange, and allow time for recovery	Meconium aspiration syndrome; Congenital diaphragmatic hernia; Sepsis, refractory septic shock; Persistent pulmonary hypertension; Respiratory failure refractory to other therapies; Pneumonia; Pulmonary air leaks; Acute respiratory distress syndrome; As a bridge to lung transplantation in chronic respiratory failure
Cardiac	Augment cardiac function in conditions resulting in low cardiac output or to provide complete support when there is no native cardiac output	During resuscitation (extracorporeal cardiopulmonary resuscitation); Cardiac failure; Severe and complex congenital heart disease

able to transition to more conventional critical care management or until alternative medical or surgical options can be pursued. ECMO should not be considered a therapeutic or curative option; it benefits patients most when the condition is reversible, but it has emerged as an important rescue measure when quite often the alternative outcome is mortality, and it has also become a viable option as a bridge to organ transplantation.[10] Because ECMO is being offered to a more heterogeneous population, historic indications and contraindications are not as strictly adhered to, provided that the risks of ECMO are carefully considered.

Selection Criteria

As ECMO is quite invasive and has associated risks, clinicians have strived to identify clear indications and to develop objective criteria, including the **oxygenation index (OI)**.[11] The OI is a calculation that helps gauge disease severity. Mean airway pressure (mPaw) and FiO_2 information obtained from the mechanical ventilator are used to calculate the OI, which is determined as follows: $OI = mPaw \times (FiO_2 / PaO_2) \times 100$. An OI in excess of 40 while using conventional mechanical ventilation has been associated with mortality risk greater than 80%.[12] When high-frequency oscillatory ventilation

(HFOV) is the mode of support, an OI greater than 60 is the threshold where the risk of mortality increases as higher mean airway pressures are used.

The decision to initiate ECMO is considered when the patient does not respond to maximum medical management, there is no associated morbidity, and the underlying condition is reversible. As an example, a newborn with severe respiratory failure associated with meconium aspiration that continues to be hypoxemic despite HFOV and inhaled nitric oxide, who has an OI >60 for several hours, would be a good candidate for ECMO. Broad indications for ECMO include respiratory failure in the newborn, acute respiratory failure in infants and children, cardiac disease, and chronic respiratory failure.

Newborn Respiratory Failure

A number of conditions affecting newborns may be unresponsive to standard treatment—conventional mechanical ventilation, high-frequency ventilation, inhaled nitric oxide—and can progress to severe respiratory failure. These conditions include persistent pulmonary hypertension of the newborn (PPHN), meconium aspiration syndrome (MAS), sepsis, pneumonia, respiratory distress syndrome, pulmonary air leak, and congenital diaphragmatic hernia (CDH). In these conditions, the application of ECMO supports organ function, normalizes gas exchange, and allows time for recovery (Table 30-1). As an example, with PPHN there is failure of the transitional circulation leading to right-to-left shunting, hypoxemia, and eventual right heart failure, but support with ECMO allows time for the pulmonary hypertension to reverse. When ECMO is used to support pulmonary conditions, such as MAS or air leaks, the lungs are given time to heal as lung-protective ventilator strategies are employed. Over the past decade, the average number of newborn respiratory failure cases reported in the ELSO registry is around 500, with a survival rate of 82%.[7]

Newborns with CDH have varying degrees of respiratory insufficiency, which is primarily influenced by the magnitude of lung hypoplasia and pulmonary hypertension.[13] In the most severe cases, ECMO may be used with the goal of promoting lung rest, lessening pulmonary hypertension, and improving right heart function.[14] The number of CDH cases reported to the ELSO registry averages about 250 each year, and survival rates averaging around 50% have not significantly changed since ECMO was first used in this population.[7]

Pediatric Respiratory Failure

There has been a steady increase since 2001 in the number of pediatric respiratory failure cases reported in the ELSO registry, with an average of about 250 per year and an increasing annual survival rate approaching 70%.[7] This increase is due in part to improvements in ECMO technology, which affords longer durations with fewer complications, and a willingness of clinicians to explore the boundaries of advanced medical-surgical options.[15] The principal diagnoses that have been reported are infectious pneumonia and acute respiratory distress syndrome. In 2009, the influenza A (H1N1) pandemic compelled hospitals to develop emergency preparedness measures that ranged from basic supportive care to advanced measures, including ECMO.[16] During this time, there was a renewed interest in developing ECMO programs and, since then, there has been an annual increase in the number of centers reporting data to the ELSO registry, now topping 250 worldwide.[7]

Following the success of ECMO in newborns, pediatric intensivists attempted to identify a population that would benefit from ECMO, but clinical trials and research efforts were difficult to conduct. In 1996, a multicenter trial was undertaken and the **Pediatric Risk of Mortality Score (PRISM)** was used to stratify which patients would receive ECMO.[17] PRISM is a prognostic scoring system used to determine the risk for mortality. This tool, derived from 14 physiologic variables, assesses mortality risk for pediatric patients during their first 24 hours of care in the intensive care unit (ICU). There were 38 patients in the ECMO group of this multicenter study, which suggested that ECMO was more beneficial.[17] The evidence for using ECMO in pediatric respiratory failure has largely been described in case series and retrospective reviews, including cases of refractory septic shock[18] and, although somewhat controversial, patients with immunocompromised conditions.[19]

ECMO has generally been considered a rescue modality for acute and reversible respiratory failure, but it has become an acceptable mode to support children with chronic respiratory failure as a bridge to lung transplantation.[20] The goals of this approach are to minimize sedation and promote mobility, including ambulation and physical therapy, which may improve the rate of recovery following lung transplantation.[21]

In general, the use of ECMO in the management of respiratory failure in children should be reserved for patients with a reversible condition or if suitability for lung transplantation has been determined, and if lung-protective ventilator strategies fail to provide clinically acceptable gas exchange.[22]

Cardiac Support

The use of ECMO to support infants and children with cardiac failure continues to evolve, with over 1000 cases reported to the ELSO registry annually.[7] The goals of ECMO are to augment cardiac function in conditions resulting in low cardiac output or to provide complete support when there is no native cardiac output (Table 30-1). Infants with severe and complex congenital heart disease may be supported with ECMO in the preoperative period as surgical strategies are being contemplated and as an extension of cardiopulmonary bypass in the postoperative period.[23]

The rapid initiation of ECMO during resuscitation is known as **extracorporeal cardiopulmonary resuscitation (ECPR)**; it is considered early in the resuscitative process, when it is clear that standard measures may be unsuccessful.[24] ECPR requires readily deployable systems and coordinated clinical teams to establish quick surgical access and mechanical circulatory support as advanced cardiac life support is simultaneously provided. Favorable outcomes are dependent on the quality of CPR, and survival rates approaching 40% have been reported by ELSO.[25]

Types of ECMO Support

The method of ECMO support is chosen based on a number of factors, including the patient's size, underlying condition, and severity and type of illness. ECMO is typically described by the route of drainage, which is always the venous system, and the route of reinfusion, which can either be the venous system or the arterial system; accordingly, the two main modes of ECMO support are venous-arterial and venous-venous[26] (**Table 30-2**).

Venuous-Arterial

Venous-arterial (VA) is the original approach to ECMO support and is the most commonly used.[27] The classic configuration for VA support in newborns and infants is cannulation of the right internal jugular vein, from where deoxygenated blood is drained, and the right common carotid artery, where oxygenated blood is returned. Because the patient's blood exits the body on the venous side and reinfuses on the arterial or systemic side, this type of ECMO provides both cardiac and respiratory support. One drawback to this approach is carotid ligation, which is tolerated in newborns, but the potential neurologic sequelae in older patients are

less understood. VA ECMO can also be accomplished through the femoral vein and artery or direct cannulation of the aorta and right atrium, referred to as central or **transthoracic cannulation**. Because reinfused blood is returned to the systemic circulation, VA ECMO can augment and even substitute for cardiac function.

A disadvantage of VA ECMO is the potential for poorly oxygenated blood being ejected from the left ventricle and delivered to the coronary arteries as the blood flow from the reinfusion cannula is in the distal aortic arch. This mainly occurs because blood that remains in the native pulmonary circulation may not be well oxygenated as it returns to the left side of the heart due to poor gas exchange in the lungs.

Venous-Venous

The **venous-venous (VV)** form of support involves the drainage and reinfusion of blood by way of the venous system or right side of the heart. This mode provides pulmonary support only and requires the patient to have sufficient cardiac function. VV support is established through various cannulation techniques, including the use of a venous-venous double-lumen cannula, referred to as VVDL, which is inserted in the right internal jugular vein. VVDL cannulae are oriented such that blood returning to the right atrium is directed toward the tricuspid valve, thus introducing well-oxygenated blood into the pulmonary circulation (**Figure 30-1**). One drawback of this approach is **recirculation**, or the tendency of reinfused oxygenated blood to mix with venous blood, reducing the overall amount of oxygen delivered.[28] This is typically managed by ensuring a gradient between SvO_2 and SpO_2, by assessing cannula and patient position, and by adjusting ECMO pump flow rates. The use of one catheter to accomplish both drainage and reinfusion is attractive, as carotid ligation is not required. Although VVDL is the preferred form of support for infants with pulmonary disease, conversion to VA is sometimes required if lung

TABLE 30-2
Comparison of the Two Modes of ECMO

Type	Cannulation Sites	Type of Support	Hazards/Disadvantages
Venous-arterial	Right internal jugular vein (deoxygenated blood is drained) and right common carotid artery (oxygenated blood is returned) Femoral vein and artery Direct cannulation of the aorta and right atrium	Respiratory cardiac	Potential neurologic sequelae with carotid ligation Potential for lower systemic PaO_2 Reduced pulmonary blood flow
Venous-venous	Double-lumen cannula inserted into the right internal jugular vein Bi-caval dual-lumen cannula inserted into the right internal jugular vein Cannulation of one or both femoral veins for drainage purposes and a catheter placed in the right internal jugular vein for reinfusion	Respiratory	Patients must have sufficient cardiac function Tendency of reinfused oxygenated blood to mix with venous blood Conversion to venous-arterial is sometimes required

development of ECMO systems, roller pumps were primarily used as they were commonly used in cardiopulmonary bypass devices, were widely available, and centrifugal technology was not well developed. In the most recent decades, centrifugal pump design has improved and has become prevalent in many institutions.

Roller Pumps

Blood is displaced with a roller pump by means of two spinning rollers that glide over a segment of tubing positioned in the pump head, commonly referred to as the raceway. The rollers are positioned opposite each other, with one roller always in contact with the raceway so that the tubing is always compressed or occluded. The rotating pump head and the spinning rollers propel blood forward and establish the blood flow rate or output of the ECMO system.

The output of a roller pump is influenced by three variables: the number of rotations of the pump head; the raceway diameter; and the degree of compression, or occlusion, of the rollers on the tubing. Roller pumps are typically calibrated to the diameter of the raceway, which is most commonly 3/8 inch, and the displayed output is reflected in liters per minute. This displayed output is used to gauge the degree of support that the patient is receiving and is fixed unless the rotations are manipulated. One drawback of roller pumps is the potential for the tubing to split or rupture, which may be minimized by using tubing with a higher durometer, or durability factor, and periodically shifting the raceway so that the rollers are not in constant contact with the same section of tubing.

Roller pumps provide a constant output that does not vary with changes in patients' hemodynamics or changes in circuit resistance, as the rotations are fixed. Thus, unless properly monitored, excessive pressure can develop on the pump outlet, leading to circuit rupture. Additionally, the inlet of the pump must be closely monitored to ensure that the blood being drained from the patient is sufficient; otherwise, excessive negative pressure could develop. To ensure adequate venous drainage, compliant reservoirs with integral pressure monitoring are incorporated, which signal the pump to automatically slow down in the presence of reduced drainage, thus prompting the clinician to investigate the cause of the decreased venous return. Likewise, pressures measured on the outlet side of the pump inform the clinician of circuit resistance.

Centrifugal Pumps

In contrast to roller pumps, centrifugal pumps are nonocclusive and respond to changes in circuit resistance and patient hemodynamics. Centrifugal pumps operate by entraining blood into the pump head by a vortex action produced by spinning **impeller** blades or rotating

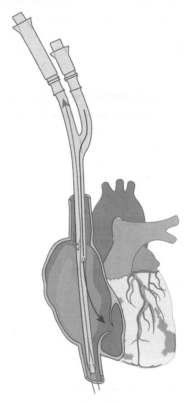

FIGURE 30-1 Schematic of a venous-venous dual-lumen cannula placed in the right internal jugular vein and positioned in the right atrium.

Reproduced from Rais-Bahrami K, VanMeurs KP. Venoarterial versus venousvenous ECMO for neonatal respiratory failure. *Seminars in Perinatology.* 2014;38(2):71–77, with permission of Elsevier.

function is significantly impaired, pulmonary hypertension is resulting in decreased right ventricular function, or cardiac output is insufficient.

Similar to a VVDL catheter is a bi-caval dual-lumen cannula, which is also inserted into the right internal jugular vein and also provides the routes for drainage and reinfusion but contains two drainage ports located at the level of the inferior and superior vena cava.[29] The availability of this catheter has expanded the use of VV ECMO to older patients and has been an important advancement as long-term ECMO support has become more feasible, with femoral vessels, historically used to provide VV support, being spared and allowing for improved patient mobility, including ambulation.[20]

Femoral VV ECMO entails the cannulation of one or both femoral veins for drainage purposes and a catheter placed in the right internal jugular vein for reinfusion. This may be suitable for shorter-duration ECMO and can typically be accomplished with a percutaneous technique.[30]

ECMO Circuits and Systems

The displacement of blood through an ECMO circuit is achieved by two types of mechanical pumps: **roller pumps,** which are occlusive, and **centrifugal pumps,** which are nonocclusive.[31] During the early cones. These impellers or cones are magnetically paired with an electric motor, and the rotation of the motor causes a pressure differential that urges the forward flow of blood—the higher the revolutions per minute, the higher the output or flow rate. The energy created by the pump creates active drainage, pulling blood into the pump head, unlike roller pumps, in which drainage is passive and by gravity. The impellers or cones also do not create any occlusion, so flow will vary in the presence of resistance and is preload and afterload dependent. As an example, in the presence of a reduced preload or decreased venous drainage, flow will decrease. Flow will also decrease with increased afterload due to increased systemic vascular resistance.

One of the perceived benefits of centrifugal pumps is the ability to create shorter and more compact ECMO circuits as compared to roller pumps, as a fair amount of the drainage limb can be eliminated.[32] Further advances in ECMO technology have yielded more compact and portable devices that incorporate enhanced safety features, improved blood compatibility, and a unique integrated centrifugal pump head and artificial membrane oxygenator.[33]

Extracorporeal Physiology

The ECMO circuit consists of tubing that joins the drainage and reinfusion cannulas and a membrane oxygenator. The pump circulates venous blood drained from the patient through the membrane where artificial gas exchange occurs, whereupon oxygenated blood exits and is returned to the patient (**Figure 30-2**).

Membrane Oxygenators

The principal **membrane oxygenator** used for many decades contained a silicone sheet arranged in a spool that separated blood and gas compartments. Gas exchange across the silicone sheet was dependent on the driving pressures of oxygen and carbon dioxide, and it was influenced by the composition of the supply gas, referred to as sweep gas; the degree of desaturation of the blood; and the rate at which it flowed through the membrane. These membranes were available with different surface areas to accommodate the full range of patients but were somewhat difficult to de-air and had fairly high resistance in the blood path.

Although the silicone membrane was the mainstay of the ECMO circuit, microporous or hollow-fiber membranes were being used during cardiopulmonary bypass, with ease of preparation and low resistance being the main attributes.[34] Because of these benefits, the microporous membrane was incorporated into ECMO circuits, but one drawback was that the fibers would degrade and leak plasma over time, necessitating replacement. The small woven fibers used in microporous membranes have improved with the addition of a polymethylpentene coating that preserves the fibers' integrity and minimizes oversaturation and leaking of fluid.[35] Gas exchange in these membranes occurs by diffusion, with gas running through the fibers and blood running adjacently and outside of the fibers.

Blood Pathway and Gas Exchange

Blood traverses the ECMO circuit in a continuous and closed loop, with venous blood entering the circuit by gravity if a roller pump is being used or actively by the negative draw of a centrifugal pump. Blood then passes through the membrane oxygenator where oxygen and carbon dioxide are exchanged, which occurs by the driving pressures and gradients between gas and blood compartments. The membrane oxygenator is supplied with a fresh gas source, called sweep gas. The sweep gas flow rate and oxygen concentration are titrated to achieve clinically acceptable blood gases—for example, increasing the sweep gas flow rate will cause more CO_2 to be removed. Depending on the patient size in relation to oxygenator surface area, carbon dioxide may need to be added to the sweep gas to lessen the driving pressure for CO_2; thus, the composition is a mixture of oxygen and carbon dioxide commonly known as carbogen.

The rate and concentration of the sweep gas primarily affect the patient's $PaCO_2$, whereas oxygenation is more influenced by the blood flow rate and the contribution of the patient's native cardiopulmonary function. Oxygen delivery is the product of the oxygen-carrying capacity and cardiac output and is supplemented by the ECMO support in which the hemoglobin concentration and the ECMO blood flow can be manipulated to augment oxygen delivery and to ultimately restore tissue perfusion and preserve end-organ function, the principal benefits of ECMO.

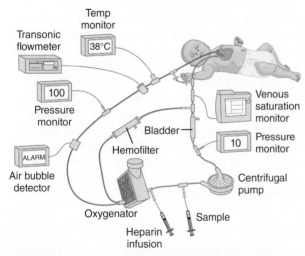

FIGURE 30-2 Schematic of a venous-arterial ECMO circuit with a centrifugal pump.

Reproduced from Rais-Bahrami K, VanMeurs KP. Venoarterial versus venousvenous ECMO for neonatal respiratory failure. *Seminars in Perinatology.* 2014;38(2):71–77, with permission of Elsevier.

Clinical Management

Once ECMO support is established and the patient is stabilized, all physiologic functions are closely evaluated through ongoing hemodynamic monitoring, laboratory and radiologic tests, and physical examination to ensure that the ECMO circuit is functioning properly, that the goals of support are being attained, and that complications are avoided.

Anticoagulation

The interaction of blood with the nonendothelial surface of an ECMO circuit results in thrombosis and requires anticoagulation to be established, typically accomplished with the use of unfractionated heparin, an antithrombotic mediator that inhibits the activation of clotting factors in the intrinsic pathway of the clotting cascade.[36] As blood is introduced into the ECMO circuit, a layer of protein adheres to the foreign material of the ECMO circuit and the generation of a thrombus occurs, activating both intrinsic and extrinsic coagulation pathways of the clotting cascade.

Managing anticoagulation is an important aspect of monitoring the ECMO circuit, as areas of stagnation may be prone to clotting. Anticoagulation has been monitored through a variety of tests, including activated clotting time (ACT), prothrombin time, activated partial thromboplastin time, and the anti-factor Xa assay.[37] ACT is one of the most common tests used to adjust unfractionated heparin dosages, typically to maintain an ACT range of 160 to 180 seconds. A more complete assessment of unfractionated heparin dosing may be determined by evaluating the anti-factor Xa with the cofactor antithrombin III (ATIII).[38] Unfractionated heparin exerts its anticoagulant effect by binding to antithrombin, a natural anticoagulant that plays an important role in hemostasis by inhibiting thrombin and factor Xa and greatly accelerating the neutralization of the coagulation proteins. With this mechanism of action, a deficiency of antithrombin will greatly reduce the effect of unfractionated heparin on coagulation.[39]

Patient Monitoring

Ongoing evaluation of the patient requiring ECMO support is focused on the preservation of organ function, recovery from the illness, and the mitigation of complications and uses standard and systematic critical care assessments and management.

Because of the potential for bleeding, hematologic parameters are closely monitored to determine which blood components need replacement. Hematologic and coagulation studies are used in tandem to assist with bleeding and thrombosis.[40]

Pulmonary support during ECMO is generally aimed at providing lung-protective ventilation, particularly if the reason for support is a primary respiratory condition, an approach that is often referred to as lung rest.[41] This approach allows the bulk of the gas exchange to occur through the membrane oxygenator and allows the reduction of ventilator settings to minimal levels, which vary depending on the underlying condition and the trajectory of the illness. One approach is to maintain a constant distending pressure by applying positive end-expiratory pressure (PEEP) of 10 to 12 cm H_2O, a method that theoretically prevents complete lung collapse. Another strategy is to provide phasic ventilation with a low mean airway pressure. No specific approach has been shown to be superior.

When the reason for ECMO usage is primarily for cardiac support, lung function is essentially normal, in which case the ventilator strategy is focused on maintaining lung function near normal or at the patient's baseline. Increased PEEP levels may be indicated if the reason for ECMO was heart failure and subsequent pulmonary edema and is usually needed short term once the heart is supported and the pulmonary edema clears.

Cardiovascular monitoring is accomplished by routine continuous hemodynamic monitoring, including heart rate, blood pressure, and sometimes central venous and pulmonary artery pressures in certain cardiac conditions. The main objective is to maintain a stable blood pressure, which is influenced by the native cardiac output, vasoactive medications, electrolyte derangements, preload and afterload, and the ECMO pump rate when using VA support.

Treatable causes of hypertension include patient discomfort, increase in afterload, neurologic changes, and increases in ECMO flow rate. Hypotension can be caused by a decrease in afterload; acute changes, such as cardiac tamponade or tension pneumothorax; or changes in volume status, such as increased urine output or bleeding. Hypotension can also be caused by an inadvertent wean of ECMO flow, a loosening of roller pump occlusion on the ECMO tubing, or excessive hemofiltration.

Neurologic evaluation of the ECMO patient is often limited, as sedation and in some cases muscle relaxation may preclude a complete neurologic evaluation, but some standard bedside diagnostic techniques are available, including electroencephalograms, head ultrasounds for newborns and small infants, and near-infrared spectroscopy.[42] Additionally, portable computerized tomography scans are available and can provide critical information.[43]

Maintaining appropriate levels of analgesia and sedation are important in maintaining patient comfort and in minimizing patient movement to prevent a malpositioning of cannulae and interruption ECMO flow. Historically, patients supported with ECMO have been heavily sedated and even muscle relaxed, but this has shifted to the use of minimal levels of sedation without muscle relaxation. This change has been predominantly in patients being supported for chronic conditions as a bridge to recovery or transplantation in order to support rehabilitative activities, including ambulation.[10]

Standard doses of medications may not be sufficient during ECMO as pharmacokinetics may vary due to volume distribution of the ECMO circuit. Even with more biocompatible circuits and coated membranes, drug sequestration occurs.[44]

Renal function can be impaired during ECMO and is associated with a decrease in renal perfusion and inflammatory damage.[45] Often, patients become fluid overloaded, which is attributed to fluid resuscitation prior to ECMO and the need for blood product replacement during ECMO.[46] Hemofiltration or continuous renal replacement therapy may be incorporated into the ECMO circuit and when used judiciously can assist with maintaining appropriate fluid balance.[47]

Weaning and Separation from ECMO

As the patient's condition begins to improve, assessing their readiness to be separated from ECMO becomes the priority. This assessment can be approached in two ways: by weaning or by periodic separation trials. Weaning encompasses the gradual reduction of ECMO flow rates as mechanical ventilator support is increased, a process that may occur over several days. Periodic trials occur later in the ECMO course and as signs of disease reversal are apparent. In this method, ECMO flow rates are reduced and ventilator support is increased in a much shorter time frame, typically over a couple of hours, following which the ECMO circuit is isolated from the patient. These methods are well suited to assessing patients requiring ECMO for a primary respiratory condition where improvement can be gauged by evaluating chest radiographs and dynamic lung compliance.

Patients requiring ECMO for a primary cardiac problem have similar weaning techniques; however, the return of heart function is used to determine weaning readiness. Gradual weaning may allow the heart to recondition and transition to the patient's native circulation. Echocardiograms are often used to assess the functionality of the heart during ECMO, while weaning, and during the trial of separation. If the heart has good function with acceptable hemodynamics, the patient meets the criteria for separation.

Despite the technique used, the decision to discontinue ECMO is made based on these trials and the trajectory of the patient's illness. If trial separation is unsuccessful, which may be indicated by poor cardiac function or the need for nonprotective ventilator support, then more time on ECMO may be indicated; alternative strategies also may need to be considered, such as organ transplantation. Rarely do patients require a second ECMO course, which is associated with poor outcomes.[48]

Complications

Complications associated with ECMO can be categorized as either patient complications or mechanical complications. Bleeding continues to be the most prevalent complication reported in the ELSO registry, with cannula and surgical site bleeding rates of 15% and 29%, respectively, in cardiac ECMO cases.[49] The risk of bleeding is high because anticoagulation is required to maintain ECMO circuit patency.

Neurologic complications may occur during ECMO, particularly in the neonatal population as the risk of intracranial hemorrhage is higher. The incidence of intracranial hemorrhage in infants less than 30 months of age is 7% to 10%.[49] Additional neurologic complications include clinical seizures and ischemic stroke.

Infection is another complication to be considered during extracorporeal support, seen most in patients who require ECMO for >14 days.[50] Infection risk is minimized with proper aseptic technique while accessing the patient and the circuit as well as antibiotic therapy.

Mechanical complications associated with ECMO include the failure of components, such as the membrane oxygenator, or adjunct equipment. One of the principal duties of an ECMO specialist is to closely monitor the function of the ECMO circuit, be able to identify problems, and employ well-rehearsed troubleshooting procedures. This includes periodic inspections of the entire ECMO system and monitoring thrombus formation.

Fleming and colleagues[51] reviewed complications in over 28,000 ECMO cases and found mechanical component failure had occurred in about 15% of cases, with oxygenator failure occurring in 6.5%, air in the circuit in 4.3%, pigtail cracks in 2.3%, and pump failures in 1.8%.

Outcomes

As of early 2016, the overall rate of survival to discharge, determined from over 42,000 patients in the ELSO registry, was 58%.[7] Infants supported with ECMO had a survival rate of 74% if the primary diagnosis was respiratory in nature and 41% with cardiac conditions.[7] In the pediatric category, in patients between the ages of 30 days and 18 years, survival rates were 58% and 51% for respiratory and cardiac diagnoses, respectively.[7]

Factors influencing mortality include primary diagnosis, the need for cardiopulmonary resuscitation, bleeding complications, and the weight of the patient.[49,52] Direct comparisons of outcomes between conventional therapy and ECMO demonstrate improved survival for neonates but are lacking for pediatrics.[21,53] Despite the application of ECMO for an increasingly acute and complex patient population across all age groups from 1993 to 2007, survival has remained unchanged, at approximately 68% for neonates and 57% for pediatrics.[21]

Case Study 1

A 9-year-old girl weighing 32 kg with a diagnosis of aplastic anemia was an inpatient on the oncology floor of a large pediatric hospital. She received a hematopoietic stem cell transplant. At that time, she developed an acute myocarditis that resulted in cardiorespiratory failure and secondary chemotherapy using cyclosporine and cyclophosphamide. Vital signs are as follows: respiratory rate of 36 breaths per minute, heart beat of 130 beats per minute, and blood pressure 90/55 mm Hg. She was subsequently transferred to the pediatric intensive care unit. Laboratory tests showed an increased N-terminal pro-B-type natriuretic peptide level of 10,000 pg/mL (normal, <125 pg/mL) and hyperlactemia (4.2 mmol/L). Dobutamine was administered intravenously. A chest radiograph showed bilateral diffuse pulmonary infiltrates and pleural effusions. The hemodynamic state of the patient rapidly deteriorated with progressive hypotension (85/50 mm Hg), tachycardia (155 beats/min), and hyperlactemia (8.1 mmol/L) despite increasing doses of dobutamine. Arterial blood gas analysis revealed the following: pH 7.46, $PaCO_2$ 32 mm Hg, PaO_2 80 mm Hg, HCO_3 27.2, and base excess –1. The patient was intubated and mechanically ventilated. Echocardiography showed severe left ventricular hypokinesis with an ejection fraction of 30%. To support her worsening cardiorespiratory failure, she was placed on VA ECMO.

1. **Explain the difference between VV ECMO and VA ECMO.**

2. **Why is VA ECMO indicated for the patient?**

3. **Describe one disadvantage of VA and VV ECMO.**

Case Study 2

A Caucasian male weighing 4950 g, born of vaginal delivery at 40 weeks gestation, presented with severe respiratory insufficiency due to meconium aspiration syndrome (MAS). He was immediately transferred to the neonatal intensive care unit for supportive care. There he was treated for a left-sided pneumothorax with a water-sealed chest tube. He was intubated and received mechanical ventilation on the following settings: peak inspiratory pressure 25 cm H_2O, PEEP 8 cm H_2O, mandatory rate 60 breaths per minute, inspiratory time 0.4 seconds, and FiO_2 of 1.0. The mean airway pressure as measured at 20 mm Hg. Arterial gas analysis showed the following: pH 7.29, PaO_2 39.4 mm Hg, $PaCO_2$ 52.7 mm Hg, HCO_3 24.5 mEq/L, BE -1.5, and oxygen saturation 84%. The echocardiogram showed severe pulmonary hypertension. Inhaled nitric oxide was started at 20 ppm. Cranial ultrasound scanning and blood coagulation tests yielded normal results. Dopamine and dobutamine were administered due to low blood pressure and impaired peripheral perfusion. After 12 hours of treatment, a number of ventilator changes were made to improve respiratory status, and inhaled intric oxide was increased to 30 ppm, but there was no improvement of the patient's respiratory status. Because no improvement in oxygenation or ventilation occurred, ECMO was considered. Venous-arterial ECMO by roller pump was initiated. The initial ECMO flow was 120 cc/kg and reduced according to the child's tolerance. The objective was to maintain PaO_2 between 70 and 90 mm Hg and $PaCO_2$ between 40 and 50 mm Hg. Mechanical ventilator settings were minimal to rest the lungs. The patient received ECMO for 6 days, was successfully weaned from ECMO support, and discharged home a month later.

1. **List two clinical conditions of the newborn that may be unresponsive to standard treatment.**

2. **Calculate the oxygenation index (OI) for this patient.**

3. **Describe the two types of ECMO circuits and systems.**

References

1. Makdisi G, Wang I. Extra corporeal membrane oxygenation (ECMO) review of a lifesaving technology. *J Thorac Dis.* 2015;7: E166-E176.

2. Palanzo D, Qui F, Baer L, Clark JB, Myers JL, Undar A. Evolution of the extracorporeal life support circuitry. *Artif Organs.* 2010;34:869-873.

3. Bartlett RH, Gazzaniga AB, Huztable RF, Schippers HC, O'Connor MJ, Jefferies MR. Extracorporeal circulation (ECMO) in neonatal respiratory failure. *J Thorac Cardiovasc Surg.* 1977;74:826-833.

4. Bartlett RH, Roloff DW, Cornell RG, Andrews AF, Dillon PW, Zwischenberger JB. Extracorporeal circulation in neonatal respiratory failure: a prospective randomized study. *Pediatrics.* 1985;76: 479-487.

5. O'Rourke PP, Crone RK, Vacanti JP, et al. Extracorporeal membrane oxygenation and conventional medical therapy in neonates with persistent pulmonary hypertension of the newborn: a prospective randomized study. *Pediatrics.* 1989;84:957-963.

6. UK Collaborative ECMO Trial Group. The report of the UK collaborative randomized trial of neonatal extracorporeal membrane oxygenation. *Lancet.* 1996;348:75.

7. Extracorporeal Life Support Organization. International Registry. http://www.elso.org. Accessed June 2016.

8. Fliman PJ, deRegnier RA, Kinsella JP, et al. Neonatal extracorporeal life support: impact on new therapies on survival. *J Pediatr.* 2006;148:595-599.

9. Gadepalli SK, Hirschl RB. Extracorporeal life support: updates and controversies. *Semin Pediatr Surg.* 2015;24:8-11.

10. Mohite PN, Sabashnikov A, Reed A, et al. Extracorporeal life support in "awake" patients as a bridge to lung transplant. *Thorac Cardiovasc Surg.* 2015;63(8):699-705.

11. Ortega M. Oxygenation index can predict outcome in neonates who are candidates for extracorporeal membrane oxygenation. *Pediatr Res.* 1987;22:462A.

12. Bayrakci B, Josephson C, Fackler J. Oxygenation index for extracorporeal membrane oxygenation: is there predictive significance? *J Artif Organs.* 2007;10:6-9.

13. Seetharamaiah R, Younger JG, Bartlett RH, Hirschl RB. Factors associated with survival in infants with congenital diaphragmatic hernia requiring extracorporeal membrane oxygenation: a report from the Congenital Diaphragmatic Hernia Study Group. *J Pediatr Surg.* 2009;44:1315-1321.

14. Waag K-L, Loff S, Zahn K, et al. Congenital diaphragmatic hernia: a modern day approach. *Semin Pediatr Surg.* 2008;17:244-254.

15. Zabrocki LA, Brogan TV, Staler KD, Poss WB, Rollins MD, Bratton SL. Extracorporeal membrane oxygenation for pediatric respiratory failure; survival and predictors of mortality. *Crit Care Med.* 2011;39:364-367.

16. Turner DA, Rehder KJ, Peterson-Carmichael SL, et al. Extracorporeal membrane oxygenation for severe refractory respiratory failure secondary to 2009 H1N1 influenza A. *Respir Care.* 2011;56:941-946.

17. Green TP, Timmons OD, Fackler JC, Moler FW, Thompson AE, Sweeney MF. The impact of extracorporeal membrane oxygenation on survival in pediatric patients with acute respiratory failure. *Crit Care Med.* 1996;24:323-329.

18. MacLaren G, Butt W, Best D. Extracorporeal membrane oxygenation for refractory septic shock in children: one institution's experience. *Pediatr Crit Care Med.* 2007;8:447-451.

19. Gupta M, Shanley TP, Moler FW. Extracorporeal life support for severe respiratory failure in children with immune compromised conditions. *Pediatr Crit Care Med.* 2008;9:380-385.

20. Lehr CJ, Zaas DW, Cheifetz IM, Turner DA. Ambulatory extracorporeal membrane oxygenation as a bridge to lung transplantation. *Chest.* 2015;147:1213-1218.

21. Rehder KJ, Turner D, Cheifetz IM. Extracorporeal membrane oxygenation for neonatal and pediatric respiratory failure: an evidence-based review of the past decade (2002-2012). *Pediatr Crit Care Med.* 2013;14:851-861.

22. Dalton HJ, Macrae DJ; for the Pediatric Acute Lung Injury Consensus Conference Group. Extracorporeal support with pediatric acute respiratory distress syndrome: proceedings from the Pediatric Acute Lung Injury Consensus Conference. *Pediatr Crit Care Med.* 205;16:S111-S117.

23. Thourani VH. Venoarterial extracorporeal membrane oxygenation (VA-ECMO) in pediatric cardiac support. *Ann Thorac Surg.* 2006;82:138-145.

24. Kane DA, Thiagarajan RR, Wypij D, et al. Rapid-response extracorporeal membrane oxygenation to support cardiopulmonary resuscitation in children with cardiac disease. *Circulation.* 2010;122(Suppl 1):S241-S248.

25. Thiagarajan RR, Laussen PC, Rycus PT, Bartlett RH, Bratton SL. Extracorporeal membrane oxygenation to aid cardiopulmonary resuscitation in infants and children. *Circulation.* 2007;116:1693-1700.

26. Sidebotham D, Allen SJ, McGeorge A, Ibbott N, Willcox T. Venovenous extracorporeal membrane oxygenation in adults: practical aspects of circuits, cannulae, and procedures. *J Cardiothorac Vasc Anesth.* 2012;26(5):893-909.

27. Kotani Y, Honjo O, Davey L, Chetan D, Guerguerian AM, Gruenwald C. Evolution of technology, establishment of program, and clinical outcomes in pediatric extracorporeal membrane oxygenation: the "sickkids" experience. *Artif Organs.* 2013;37(1):21-28.

28. Broman M, Frenckner B, Bjällmark A, Broomé M. Recirculation during veno-venous extracorporeal membrane oxygenation—a simulation study. *Artif Organs.* 2015;1:23-30.

29. Abrams D, Brodie D, Javidar J, et al. Insertion of bicaval dual-lumen cannula via the left internal jugular vein for extracorporeal membrane oxygenation. *ASAIO J.* 2012;58(6):636-637.

30. Spurlock DJ, Toomasian JM, Romano MA, Cooley E, Bartlett RH, Haft JW. A simple technique to prevent limb ischemia during veno-arterial ECMO using the femoral artery: the posterior tibial approach. *Perfusion.* 2012;27(2):141-145.

31. Barrett CS, Jaggers JJ, Cook EF, et al. Pediatric ECMO outcomes: comparison of centrifugal versus roller blood pumps using propensity score matching. *ASAIO J.* 2013;59(2):145-151.

32. Luciani GB, Hoxha S, Torre S, et al. Improved outcome of cardiac extracorporeal membrane oxygenation in infants and children using magnetic levitation centrifugal pumps. *Artif Organs.* 2016;40(1):27-33.

33. Alwardt CM, Wilson DS, Alore ML, Lanza LA, DeValeria PA, Pajaro OE. Performance and safety of an integrated portable extracorporeal life support system for adults. *JECT.* 2015;47:38-43.

34. Thiara APS, Noel TN, Kristiansen F, Karlsen HM, Fiane AE, Svennevig JL. Evaluation of oxygenators and centrifugal pumps for long-term pediatric extracorporeal membrane oxygenation. *Perfusion.* 2007;22:323-326.

35. Rambaud J, Guilbert J, Guellec I, Renolleau S. A pilot study comparing two polymethylpentene extracorporeal membrane oxygenators. *Perfusion.* 2012;28(1):14-20.

36. Annich GM. Extracorporeal life support: the precarious balance of hemostasis. *J Thromb Haemost.* 2015;13(Suppl 1):S336-S342.

37. Stocker CF, Horton SB. Anticoagulation strategies and difficulties in neonatal and paediatric extracorporeal membrane oxygenation (ECMO). *Perfusion.* 2016;31(2):95-102.

38. O'Meara LC, Alten JA, Goldberg KG, et al. Anti-xa directed protocol for anticoagulation management in children supported with extracorporeal membrane oxygenation. *ASAIO J.* 2015;61(3):339-344.

39. Saini A, Spinella PC. Management of anticoagulation and hemostasis for pediatric extracorporeal membrane oxygenation. *Clin Lab Med.* 2014;34(3):655-673.

40. Protti A, L'Acqua C, Panigada M. The delicate balance between pro-(risk of thrombosis) and anti-(risk of bleeding) coagulation during extracorporeal membrane oxygenation. *Ann Transl Med.* 2016;4(7):139.

41. Marhong JD, Telesnicki T, Munshi L, Del Sorbo L, Detsky M, Fan E. Mechanical ventilation during extracorporeal membrane oxygenation. An international survey. *Ann Am Thorac Soc.* 2014;11(6):956-961.

42. Tyree K, Tyree M, DiGeronimo R. Correlation of brain tissue oxygen tension with cerebral near-infrared spectroscopy and mixed venous oxygen saturation during extracorporeal membrane oxygenation. *Perfusion.* 2009;24(5):325-331.

43. LaRovere KL, Brett MS, Tasker RC, Strauss KJ, Burns JP; The Pediatric Critical Nervous System Program (cCNSp). Head computed tomography scanning during pediatric neurocritical care: diagnostic yield and the utility of portable studies. *Neurocrit Care.* 2012;16(2):251-257.

44. Hartham A, Buckley K, Heger M, Fortuna R, Mays K. Medication adsorption into contemporary extracorporeal membrane oxygenator circuits. *J Pediatr Pharmacol Ther.* 2014;19(4):288-295.

45. Villa G, Katz N, Ronco C. Extracorporeal membrane oxygenation and the kidney. *Cardiorenal Med.* 2015;6(1):50-60.

46. Kilburn DJ, Shekar K, Fraser JF. The complex relationship of extracorporeal membrane oxygenation and acute kidney injury: causation or association? *Biomed Res Int.* 2016; 2016:1094296.

47. Antonucci E, Lamanna I, Fagnoul D, Vincent JL, De Backer D, Silvio Taccone F. The impact of renal failure and renal replacement therapy on outcome during extracorporeal membrane oxygenation therapy. *Artif Organs.* 2016;40(8):746-754.

48. Shuhaiber J, Thiagarajan RR, Laussen PC, Fynn-Thompson F, del Nido P, Pigula F. Survival of children requiring repeat extracorporeal membrane oxygenation after congenital heart surgery. *Ann Thorac Surg.* 2011;91(6):1949-1955.

49. Paden ML, Rycus PT, Thiagarajan RR. Update and outcomes in extracorporeal life support. *Semin Perinatol.* 2014;38(2):65-70.

50. Bizzarro MJ, Conrad SA, Kaufman DA, Rycus P. Infections acquired during extracorporeal membrane oxygenation in neonates, children, and adults. *Pediatr Citi Care Med.* 2011;12(3):277-281.

51. Fleming GM, Gurney JG, Donohue JE, Remenapp RT, Annich GM. Mechanical component failures in 28,171 neonatal and pediatric extracorporeal membrane oxygenation courses from 1987 to 2006. *Pediatr Crit Care Med.* 2009;10(4):439-444.

52. Bairdain S, Betit P, Craig N, et al. Diverse morbidity and mortality among infants treated with venoarterial\extracorporeal membrane oxygenation. *Cureus.* 2015;7(4):e263.

53. Mosca MS, Narotsky DL, Liao M, et al. Survival following venovenous extracorporeal membrane oxygenation and mortality in a diverse patient population. *J Extra Corpor Technol.* 2015;47(4): 217-222.

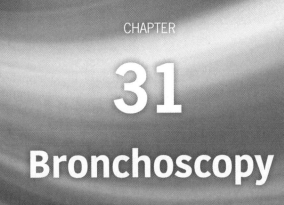

CHAPTER

31

Bronchoscopy

Pamela K. Leisenring
Kimberly D. Robbins

OUTLINE

OBJECTIVES

1. Distinguish between rigid bronchoscopy and flexible airway endoscopy.
2. Discuss the benefits of flexible airway endoscopy compared to rigid bronchoscopy in children.
3. List common indications for performing flexible airway endoscopy in children.
4. List the equipment and supplies used during flexible airway endoscopy.
5. Discuss clinical factors to consider when evaluating a child for flexible airway endoscopy.
6. Discuss recommendations for personnel safety during flexible airway endoscopy.
7. Describe the routes for entering the pediatric airway with a flexible endoscope.
8. List common medications used during flexible airway endoscopy procedures.
9. Discuss the various diagnostic and therapeutic techniques for airway endoscopy.
10. Recognize possible complications of flexible airway endoscopy.
11. Define high-level disinfection and explain its importance regarding rigid bronchoscopes and flexible airway endoscopes.

KEY TERMS

airborne infection isolation room
airway biopsy
airway brushing
bronchoalveolar lavage (BAL)
bronchoscopy
conscious sedation
endoscope
flexible airway endoscope
flexible airway endoscopy (FAE)
hemoptysis
high-level disinfection (HLD)
lung biopsy
personal protective equipment (PPE)
rigid bronchoscopy
Spaulding Classification Scheme
therapeutic lavage

527

Introduction

Bronchoscopy is a procedure that allows direct visualization and assessment of upper and central airway anatomy for diagnostic, therapeutic, or research purposes.[1] The procedure was once limited to the use of rigid bronchoscopes that accommodated only adult patients, but technology has evolved significantly. Now permanent flexible bronchoscopes of varying sizes are available so that even very small children may undergo the procedure. The instrument contains an eyepiece through which the bronchoscopist may directly visualize the airways. Most systems today connect to a camera source that displays the image of the airways on a computer screen for even better assessment.

Endoscope is the general term for an instrument with a slim, flexible tube attached to a camera source used to look somewhere inside the body.[2] There are various types of endoscopes, with the one used to evaluate the lungs referred to as a **flexible airway endoscope**. The procedure of evaluating the lungs with this instrument is called **flexible airway endoscopy (FAE)**, often interchangeably referred to as bronchoscopy. Both permanent and disposable bronchoscope systems with data management programs are readily available.

Indications for Bronchoscopy

Rigid bronchoscopy and FAE are complementary procedures, with each having advantages and disadvantages.[3]

Rigid Bronchoscopy

As illustrated in **Figure 31-1**, **rigid bronchoscopy** is performed by inserting the scope into the mouth, along the base of the tongue. It is then passed through the vocal cords and into the trachea. Pediatric-size rigid bronchoscopes provide a large working channel and the ability to optimally manage the child's airway and ventilation requirements during the bronchoscopy procedure. Rigid bronchoscopy also allows evaluation of suspected lesions in the intra-arytenoid portion of the glottis and better visualization of the subglottis than FAE.[1] However, as a surgical procedure requiring general anesthesia, rigid bronchoscopy is not preferred when FAE can safely meet the objectives of the procedure.[1,4] Rigid bronchoscopy is indicated mainly for retrieval of a foreign body and for control of massive hemoptysis.[1]

Flexible Airway Endoscopy

The flexible endoscope can be inserted either through the nose or mouth, as illustrated in **Figure 31-2**, where it is then passed through the vocal cords and into the trachea. FAE can be performed under **conscious sedation**, making it preferred over rigid bronchoscopy whenever feasible. Flexible endoscopes range from 2.8-mm outer diameter (OD) to 6.3-mm OD with internal working channels ranging from 1.2 mm to 3.2 mm. An endoscope with a 4.4-mm OD may be the largest size practical in pediatrics. This larger scope has the benefit of a 2.0-mm internal working channel, but the OD may be too large even for some adolescents. All sizes allow visual inspection of the anatomy and dynamics of the upper and central airways while the internal working channels provide the ability to obtain samples of secretions or tissue from the lower airways.[1,4]

According to the American Academy of Pediatrics, the most common indications for FAE are stridor or noisy breathing, chronic wheezing, persistent atelectasis, and recurrent radiographic densities.[1] **Table 31-1** lists a number of anatomic or infection-related issues that may be evaluated with bronchoscopy as well as diagnostic and therapeutic indications.[1,5]

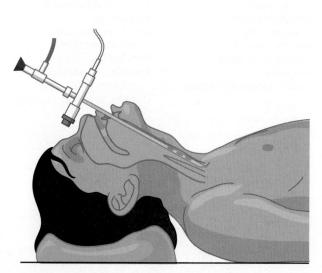

FIGURE 31-1 Rigid bronchoscopy.

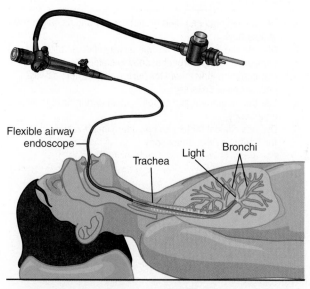

FIGURE 31-2 Flexible airway endoscopy.

TABLE 31-1
Indications for Performing Pediatric Flexible Airway Endoscopy

Stridor or noisy breathing
Chronic wheezing
Recurrent or persistent atelectasis
Recurrent radiographic densities
Congenital anomalies
Recurrent pneumonia
Mucus plugging
Respiratory failure
Failure to extubate
Suspected foreign body
Hemoptysis
Pulmonary hemorrhage
Inhalation injury
Interstitial lung disease
Unexplained cough
Tracheostomy evaluation
Post-lung transplantation
Suspected airway compression

TABLE 31-2
Equipment and Supplies Used during Flexible Airway Endoscopy

Appropriate-size flexible airway endoscope with transportation container
"Clean" and "Dirty" biohazard endoscope bags
Manufacturer-approved external lubricant for endoscope insertion tube
Airway medications for upper and lower airway anatomy
Nonbacteriostatic normal saline for specimen lavage
Suction
Specimen traps
Disposable cytology brushes
Biopsy forceps
Bite block
Ventilator, if indicated
Bronchoscopy system with data and imaging capabilities
Bedside heart monitor with pulse oximetry
Emergency response equipment and supplies
Bedside cleaning supplies
High-level disinfection supplies and equipment
Personal protection equipment for personnel

Preparing for Flexible Airway Endoscopy

The equipment and supplies needed to perform flexible airway endoscopy may vary slightly depending upon the objective of each procedure. **Table 31-2** lists the common items needed during FAE.

Lack of informed consent is the only contraindication for performing FAE.[5] Regardless of the child's clinical presentation, a thorough medical history helps determine if the benefit of FAE outweighs the potential risks. **Table 31-3** lists the factors that must be considered when evaluating a child for FAE.

The room in which FAE is performed is typically a bronchoscopy suite or intensive care unit. It should be of adequate size and location for personnel and patient safety during the procedure, including the multitude of activities that occur should emergency treatment be necessary.

As with all patient care procedures, safety precautions for personnel must be observed. **Personal protective equipment (PPE)** must be worn by all staff involved at the bedside during the FAE. This includes face masks and eye protection, nitrile gloves, and gowns. As a general safety precaution for personnel, the use of an **airborne infection isolation room** is the optimal choice at any time, but it is especially recommended when tuberculosis is suspected. In such cases, a PPE face mask with maximal particulate filtration should be worn by all personnel.

Performing Flexible Airway Endoscopy

Despite it being an invasive procedure, FAE is safe when performed by competent medical personnel. Several

TABLE 31-3
Evaluation of the Child Prior to Flexible Airway Endoscopy

Current symptoms
Clinical status
Current medications
Allergies
History of airway disorders
Pulmonary function test results
Arterial blood gas analysis
Chest radiography/CT scan/MRI results
Clotting factor results
Previous bronchoscopy findings

techniques are used to examine airway anatomy and to obtain samples from the airways, yielding information that aids in the diagnosis of airway disease.

Personnel

A bronchoscopist who is trained and certified to meet the institution's credentialing requirements will perform the procedure. Pediatric specialists who commonly perform bronchoscopy include pulmonologists, intensivists, trauma surgeons, and ear, nose, and throat (ENT) specialists. The American Thoracic Society (ATS) Technical Standards for FAE in Children describe a number of core competencies recommended for the pediatric bronchoscopist.[5] These competencies prepare the physician for all aspects of the procedure, including patient safety and management considerations, recognition of both normal and abnormal airway anatomy and functions, and cleaning and disinfection of equipment. The remaining personnel involved in performing the FAE are typically nonsurgical healthcare professionals.

Each bronchoscopy requires an anesthesia or sedation provider. In some cases, the bronchoscopist may be credentialed for conscious sedation while some institutions require a second provider to handle sedation or anesthesia needs. Collaboration between these two providers is essential to plan the procedure, decide the best choice of sedation for the child's clinical condition and goals of the procedure, and manage subsequent patient care needs.

The FAE team also includes a respiratory therapist and a nurse. Performing within their scopes of practice and institutional policies, these team members help ensure patient safety and optimal performance of the procedure.[5] The respiratory therapist manages airway medications, lavage, and specimens while also performing computer tasks and video imaging during the procedure. The nurse's role is to assist in monitoring the child and to administer sedation.

FAE team members are skilled in managing the airway and ventilation, providing emergency response, cleaning and disinfecting equipment, and maintaining accurate records of these processes. Meticulous monitoring of the bronchoscopy process and timely updates are paramount to patient safety and quality of care.[6] Periodic competency evaluations (e.g., annually) should be required to demonstrate maintained skills.

Examining the Airway

The upper airway, nasopharynx, oropharynx, hypopharynx, and larynx are evaluated and cultured during FAE.[1] While viewing the larynx, vocal cord function is assessed during phonation by the child.[4] FAE supports evaluation of the anterior glottis, but a rigid scope is required to view the intra-arytenoid area of the glottis. FAE also allows for examination of the trachea, main and lobar bronchi, and segmental and subsegmental bronchi. Although passing the endoscope through an endotracheal or tracheostomy tube bypasses the upper airway anatomy, it still allows for assessment of artificial airway placement and the central airway structures as well as allowing bronchoalveolar lavage (BAL) or other therapeutic treatments.

Insertion of the endoscope into the child's airways may be accomplished through the nose or mouth (with a bite block in place), an endoscopy mask, a laryngeal mask airway, a tracheostomy tube, or an endotracheal tube.[5] Artificial airways must be of adequate size to accommodate the OD of the flexible endoscope while allowing sufficient working space around its insertion tube. Patient circumstances will vary, so the bronchoscopist will determine the optimal size scope that permits proper ventilation of the child.

In addition to conscious sedation drugs, medications often used for patient safety and comfort are listed in **Table 31-4**.[5]

TABLE 31-4

Medications Delivered to the Airway during Flexible Airway Endoscopy

Beta-2 agonists: Administered prior to endoscopy
Injectable lidocaine, 1% or 2%: Applied to the vocal cords and/or carina to reduce incidence of cough and bronchospasm
Nasal decongestant: Administered to nares when indicated
2% lidocaine jelly: Administered to nares when indicated
Epinephrine: Administered for potential airway bleeding
Nonbacteriostatic normal saline: Administered when obtaining bronchoalveolar lavage specimens

---

Flexible Airway Endoscopy Techniques

A number of methods may be used to obtain samples of airway secretions or tissue for clinical laboratory diagnostic studies or therapeutic interventions.[5] The suspected underlying pathology helps determine which of the following techniques to employ in each procedure.

- **Bronchoalveolar lavage (BAL)** is used to obtain samples of airway secretions to diagnose infection.[1] After wedging the tip of the scope into distal airways, premeasured aliquots of nonbacteriostatic saline are instilled through the channel of the scope. Subsequent suctioning of the saline collects the sample for lab analysis.
- **Airway brushing** is performed by inserting a specimen brush through the working channel and gently scrubbing the airway mucosa. The brushing sample can be used to identify pulmonary dyskinesia or to enhance a lung biopsy performed to identify pulmonary dyskinesia. Airway lesions may be brushed to examine for cytology and may also be processed for cultures.[1]
- An **airway biopsy** is obtained by inserting a biopsy forceps through the working channel of the bronchoscope and obtaining a sample of airway tissue.
- A **lung biopsy** is performed by inserting biopsy forceps through the working channel and into the airway wall to obtain a sample of transbronchial lung tissue. In children it is used primarily post-lung transplantation and is the gold standard in diagnosing acute cellular rejection.[1] Biopsies are obtained under fluoroscopy for histologic examination. They may also be cultured if infection is suspected.[1]
- **Therapeutic lavage** involves systematically instilling large volumes of solutions throughout the lungs or into a particular area of interest followed by thorough suctioning. This technique helps remove mucous plugs and airway clots and may help relieve atelectasis.[5]
- Other therapeutic procedures include instillation of medications, endoscopic intubation, airway stent placement, balloon dilation of the airway, endobronchial ultrasound, and laser therapy with electrosurgery.[1]

Postprocedure Care

Children are closely monitored during the postsedation recovery phase of FAE. This includes monitoring their heart rate and rhythm, respiratory rate, oxygen saturation, and blood pressure. They are also observed for possible postprocedure complications. Upon satisfactory recovery, the child's caregivers are instructed to observe for delayed complications at home, such as **hemoptysis**, fever, or infections, and advised of the appropriate steps to take if such occur.

Complications Associated with Flexible Airway Endoscopy

As with any invasive procedure, the decision to perform FAE should be based on the benefits outweighing the risks. However, when performed by well-trained personnel who observe a detailed protocol, FAE is a relatively safe procedure with infrequent complications.[1] Complications related to instrumentation or inadequate topical anesthesia can occur on occasion. Possible complications during and after FAE are listed in **Table 31-5**.[1,5]

Infection Control

The level of disinfection required for contaminated medical devices is based on the **Spaulding Classification Scheme**. This system, developed by Dr. Earle H. Spaulding, classifies medical devices as noncritical, semicritical, or critical. The classification is based on the amount of risk the patient has of being contaminated by the device. Bronchoscopes are classified as semicritical equipment. This requires a minimum of **high-level disinfection (HLD)** after every use.[6]

The two common methods of HLD for bronchoscopes include automated reprocessing, in which peracetic acid is used to disinfect the equipment, and manual reprocessing, where the disinfectant is 2% glutaraldehyde. Whichever method is used, ensuring strict adherence to manufacturer's instructions for high-level disinfection is imperative. The Centers for Disease Control and Prevention provides detailed recommendations for the cleaning and HLD processes in healthcare facilities. These may be helpful in establishing protocols.

Thorough records regarding each HLD event should be maintained for such purposes as outbreak investigations and site visits by regulatory bodies.[5] In some institutions, the HLD process is provided by a central sterile processing department while in others it is the responsibility of the respiratory therapist, nurse, or other personnel.

TABLE 31-5
Complications of Flexible Airway Endoscopy

During Procedure	Postprocedure
Excessive coughing	Hemoptysis
Laryngospasm	Fever
Oxygen desaturation	Infection
Bronchospasm	
Epistaxis	
Pneumothorax	
Hemorrhage	
Nausea	

Summary

Over time, advances in the design of appropriately sized bronchoscopes, along with airway management options, have improved the feasibility and safety of pediatric bronchoscopy. Other contributing factors include improved anesthesia drugs, established national and international recommendations by expert panels, and advancement in professional skills for respiratory therapists and nurses. Although these developments promote the benefits of pediatric bronchoscopy, the number of controlled studies in this population remains limited and warrants further investigation and collaborations for the future.[5]

Case Study

A 2.5-year-old male weighing 9 kg was referred to the pulmonary clinic with a history of recurrent episodes of fever, cough, and respiratory distress. Viral labs and a variety of blood tests were done, but all were negative. Chest radiograph was performed, which showed left lower lobe consolidation. A CT scan of the chest showed 4-mm intraluminal soft tissue in the left main bronchus, causing atelectasis of the medial basal segment and air trapping in the rest of the lower lobe. A foreign body was suspected by the pulmonologist; an ENT surgeon was consulted to perform an urgent bronchoscopy. The preoperative evaluation revealed a heart rate of 136 beats per minute, blood pressure of 100/60 mm Hg, a respiratory rate of 36 breaths per minute, and oxygen saturation of 94% on room air. On auscultation, course breath sounds were present bilaterally. Air entry was decreased in the left lower base. Retractions and nasal

(continues)

Case Study (*continued*)

flaring with increased work of breathing were present. The child's hemoglobin was 13 g/dL; all other parameters were within normal limits. His condition was explained to the parents at length, as were all the risks of having a bronchoscopy procedure. The parents signed a high-risk consent document. On arrival in the surgery suite, the child was prepped for the procedure and all standard monitors were attached. A 5-mm rigid bronchoscope was introduced into the trachea after he was fully anesthetized. Anesthesia was maintained on oxygen, air, and sevoflurane at 2%, which was given through the side port of the rigid bronchoscope. A foreign body was visualized in the left main bronchus. After repeated attempts, the ENT surgeon was able to use the forceps to remove the foreign body. The child tolerated the procedure well and recovered in the postanesthesia care unit. He was admitted as an inpatient overnight for observation and discharged the following day.

1. **Why was a rigid bronchoscope used in this case?**

2. **In what clinical situations would a flexible airway endoscopy be preferred over a rigid bronchoscopy?**

3. **What types of techniques can be used to obtain specimens and labs using a bronchoscope?**

References

1. Goldfaub S, Panitch HB. Bronchoscopy. In: Light MJ, Blaisdell CJ, Homnick DN, eds. *Pediatric Pulmonology*. Itasca, IL: American Academy of Pediatrics; 2011:163-186.

2. Walters DM, Wood DE. Operative endoscopy of the airway. *J Thorac Dis*. 2016;8:S130-S139.

3. Holinger LD, Green CG, Gartian MG. Technique. In: Holinger LD, Lusk RP, Green CG, eds. *Pediatric Laryngology and Bronchoesophagology*. Philadelphia: Lippincott Williams & Wilkins; 1997:97-116.

4. Stradling P. *Diagnostic Bronchoscopy: A Teaching Manual*. 5th ed. Edinburgh, NY: Churchill Livingstone; 1986.

5. Faro A, Wood RE, Schechter MS, et al. Official American Thoracic Society technical standards: flexible airway endoscopy in children. *Am J Respir Crit Care Med*. 2015;191:1066-1080.

6. Centers for Disease Control and Prevention. (2016). Disinfection and Sterilization. https://www.cdc.gove/infectioncontrol/guidelines/disinfection/index.html. Accessed January 23, 2018.

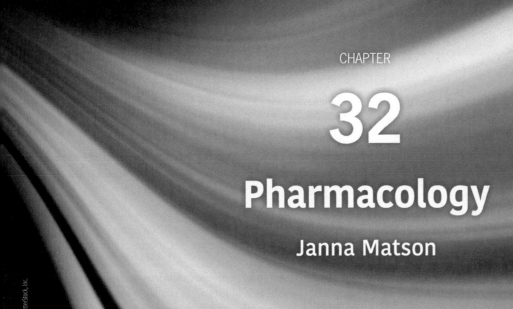

CHAPTER

32

Pharmacology

Janna Matson

OUTLINE

KEY TERMS

alpha-adrenergic receptors
anticholinergic
  bronchodilators
antimicrobials
beta-adrenergic
  receptor agonists
corticosteroids
leukotriene modifiers
long-acting beta-agonists
  (LABAs)

methylxanthines
mucolytics
neuromuscular blocking
  agents (NMBAs)
short-acting beta-agonists
  (SABAs)
skeletal muscle relaxants

OBJECTIVES

1. Describe the mechanism of action and side effects for the bronchodilators indicated for bronchospasm prophylaxis.
2. Compare the side effects of administering systemic corticosteroids and inhaled corticosteroids to children.
3. Discuss the indications, mechanism of action, and side effects of dornase-alfa.
4. Explain how leukotriene modifiers are used for the prophylaxis and treatment of asthma in children.
5. Discuss the antibiotics that are given to children through nebulizer therapy.
6. Explain the use of skeletal muscle relaxants in children.

Introduction

Key concepts in pharmacology are knowing what a drug does and understanding the consequences of administration of a drug. In neonatal and pediatric patients especially, dosing is difficult because there are few trials establishing safety and efficacy in a population so young and variable. The substantial changes in growth and development of infants and children impact the effectiveness of a drug and make this population more vulnerable to adverse drug reactions. Drug therapy can be paramount in improving outcomes, but careful consideration is required regarding dosing and side effect profiles when providing patient care. Patient monitoring and selection of appropriate agents for treatment based on the individual patient is paramount in a successful intervention.[1]

Bronchodilators

Bronchodilators are used in infant and pediatric care to both prevent and treat bronchospasm. They are divided into the following classifications:

- beta-adrenergic receptor agonists
- anticholinergics
- methylxanthines

Indications

Beta-adrenergic receptor agonists, such as albuterol, are indicated for both the treatment and the prophylaxis of acute bronchospasm.[2] Methylxanthines, such as theophylline and aminophylline, are indicated for asthma, neonatal apnea, and status asthmaticus.[3,4] Racemic epinephrine is indicated for the use of laryngotracheobronchitis, also known as croup.[5]

Beta-Adrenergic Receptor Agonists

The two types of beta-adrenergic bronchodilators are **short-acting beta-agonists (SABAs)** and **long-acting beta-agonists (LABAs)**. SABAs are for acute exacerbations and to prevent exercise-induced bronchospasm. LABAs are for maintenance therapy to control symptoms. Beta-agonists activate adrenergic receptors of the smooth muscle in the lungs and vasculature supplying the skeletal muscle system, which relaxes the bronchial and tracheal smooth muscles to relieve bronchospasms.[2] Beta-adrenergic receptors are expressed mostly in the alveolar region but also on many proinflammatory and immune cells. On the cellular level, beta-adrenergic receptors are activated by beta-agonists, which stimulate adenylcyclase and increase intracellular cyclic-3′,5′-adenosine monophosphate (cAMP). Increased cAMP leads to the activation of protein kinase A, which inhibits the phosphorylation of

BOX 32-1 Beta-Agonists

- SABAs are used as needed in all patients with asthma.
- Most albuterol inhalers have 200 puffs/inhaler.
- LABAs are used for maintenance therapy in conjunction with inhaled corticosteroids.

myosin and lowers intracellular ionic calcium concentrations, resulting in relaxation of the smooth muscles of the airway.[6]

Both SABAs and LABAs are administered via oral inhalation. Although albuterol is available as a tablet and syrup, it is mostly used with a nebulizer or as an inhaler. Short-acting beta-2-selective drugs are preferred via the inhaled route and should be used only as needed in all patients. Long-acting beta-2-agonists should be used as adjunctive therapy in asthma patients who are currently receiving an inhaled corticosteriod but whose symptoms are not adequately controlled (**Box 32-1**).[3,6] Dosages are listed in **Table 32-1**.

The most common side effects associated with SABAs are bronchospasm, excitability, palpitations, sinus tachycardia, headache, infection, nausea, pharyngitis, rhinitis, throat irritation, and tremor.[2] The most common side effect associated with LABAs is headache.[8]

Alpha-Adrenergic Receptors

Racemic epinephrine stimulates **alpha-adrenergic receptors**, leading to the constriction of precapillary arterioles and reduction in airway edema.[9] It is administered via oral inhalation and is available as a nebulizer solution. Dosages are listed in **Table 32-2**.

Palpitations and, in one case report, ventricular tachycardia and myocardial infarction in a previously healthy patient who received three doses of nebulized epinephrine in 1 hour are side effects of racemic epinephrine administration.[11]

Anticholinergic Bronchodilators

Anticholinergic bronchodilators block muscarinic cholinergic receptors, which hinders the action of acetylcholine. This decreases the formation of cyclic guanosine monophosphate, which results in decreased contractility of the smooth muscle.[12,13] These bronchodilators are administered via oral inhalation. Ipratropium bromide is available in a metered dose inhaler and nebulizer solution. Dosages are listed in **Table 32-3**.

Dry mouth, upper respiratory tract infections, cough, and bitter taste are side effects of anticholinergic bronchodilator use.[13]

TABLE 32-1
Dosing of Inhaled Beta-2-Agonist Bronchodilators[3,7]

Inhaled Beta-2-Agonists	Route of Administration	Dosage	Maximum Dosage
Albuterol (inhalation solution)	Small-volume nebulizer	Initial: 0.15 mg/kg per dose every 20–30 minutes for three doses, then 0.15–0.3 mg/kg every 30 minutes to 4 hours as needed	Initial: 5 mg/dose, then 10 mg/dose thereafter
Albuterol (inhalation solution)	Large-volume nebulizer for continuous use	0.5 mg/kg per hour or by weight: 5–10 kg = 7.5 mg/hour 10–20 kg = 11.25 mg/hour >20 kg = 15 mg/hour	20 mg/hour
Albuterol (90 mcg/actuation)	Metered dose inhaler with spacer	One-fourth to one-third actuation/kg or 4–8 actuations every 20–30 minutes for three doses, then every 1–4 hours as needed	8 actuations per dose
Levalbuterol (45 mcg/actuation)	Metered dose inhaler with spacer	90 mcg (2 actuations) every 4–6 hours; 45 mcg (1 inhalation) every 4 hours may be sufficient	2 actuations per dose
Levalbuterol (0.31-mg, 0.63-mg, and 1.25-mg vials)	Small-volume nebulizer	1 unit-dose vial every 6–8 hours as needed	1.25 mg three times daily

Data from National Asthma Education and Prevention Program Expert Panel 3. *Guidelines for the Diagnosis and Management of Asthma: Expert Panel Report 3.* Bethesda, MD: National Institutes of Health and National Heart, Lung, and Blood Institute; 2007; 07-4051; and Global Initiative for Asthma (GINA). *Global Strategy for Asthma Management and Prevention.* Updated 2017.

TABLE 32-2
Dosing of Inhaled Alpha-Adrenergic Bronchodilators[10,11]

Alpha-Adrenergic Bronchodilators	Route of Administration	Dosage	Comments
Racemic epinephrine (inhalation solution)	Small-volume nebulizer	2.25% solution: 0.05 mL/kg up to a maximum of 0.5 mL per dose	Given over 15 minutes May be repeated every 15–20 minutes, as needed

Data from Ledwith C, Shear L, Mauro R. Safety and efficacy of nebulized racemic epinephrine in conjunction with oral dexamethasone and mist in the outpatient treatment of croup. *Ann Emergo Med.* 1995;25:331-337; and Bjornson C, Russell K, Vandermeer B, et al. Nebulized epinephrine for croup in children. *Cochrane Database Cyst Rev.* 2013;CD006619.

TABLE 32-3
Dosing of Inhaled Anticholinergic Bronchodilators[3]

Anticholinergic Bronchodilators	Route of Administration	Dosage	Comments
Ipratropium bromide (17 mcg/actuation)	Metered dose inhaler with spacer	Severe exacerbation (0–12 years): 4–8 actuations every 20 minutes as needed for up to 3 hours	Severe exacerbation: ipratropium is added to short-acting beta-2 agonist Use holding chamber and face mask for children ≤4 years old
Ipratropium bromide (inhalation solution)	Small-volume nebulizer	Severe exacerbation (0–12 years): 0.25- to 0.5-mg inhalations via nebulizer every 20 minutes for 3 doses, then as needed	

Data from National Asthma Education and Prevention Program Expert Panel 3. *Guidelines for the Diagnosis and Management of Asthma: Expert Panel Report 3.* Bethesda, MD: National Institutes of Health and National Heart, Lung, and Blood Institute; 2007:07-4051.

TABLE 32-4
Dosing of Methylxanthines[15]

Methylxanthines	Route of Administration	Dosage	Comments
Theophylline	IV	Loading dose: Neonates: 5–8 mg/kg IV infused over 30 minutes Maintenance dose: Postnatal age up to 24 days: 1 mg/kg every 12 hours Postnatal age after 24 days: 1.5 mg/kg every 12 hours Total daily dose (mg) = [(0.2 × age in weeks) + 5] × (body weight in kg) every 8 hours	Therapeutic range: 5–15 mcg/mL Dosing is based on ideal body weight
Aminophylline	IV	Loading dose: Neonates: 4–6.4 mg/kg IV infused over 30 minutes Maintenance dose: Postnatal age up to 24 days: 0.8 mg/kg every 12 hours Postnatal age after 24 days: 1.2 mg/kg every 12 hours	Aminophylline contains 80% theophylline

IV = intravenous

Data from Theophylline in 5% dextrose IV injection, theophylline in 5% dextrose IV injection [package insert]. Deerfield, IL: Baxter Healthcare; 2003.

BOX 32-2 Methylxanthines

- Theophylline has several drug–drug interactions.
- Methylxanthines follow zero order kinetics, so a small dose increase can result in a large concentration increase.

Methylxanthines

Methylxanthines inhibit phosphodiesterase and histone deacetylase-2 activation, causing an increase in cAMP and resulting in the deactivation of inflammatory genes, which leads to bronchodilation. Theophylline may be useful as an add-on therapy, but its use is limited due to decreased effectiveness, adverse effects, and drug interactions.[14] The methylxanthine bronchodilators are available to use in an intravenous formulation or as a syrup, tablets, and capsules. Dosages are listed in **Table 32-4**.

Side effects include gastrointestinal upset, headache, tachycardia, insomnia, tremor, and nervousness. Signs of toxicity include persistent vomiting, ventricular tachycardia, and seizures.[16] Theophylline levels should be monitored to determine optimum blood levels and to avoid toxicities (**Box 32-2**).

Corticosteroids

Corticosteroids are anti-inflammatory drugs that are frequently used in the treatment of respiratory disease in neonatal and pediatric patients. They are the most effective anti-inflammatory medications for asthma. Systemic corticosteroids are given orally and by injection. Inhaled corticosteroids are available as pressurized metered dose inhalers, dry powder inhalers, and in liquid form for nebulization.

Indications

Corticosteroids are indicated for the maintenance treatment of asthma. They are the first-line treatment for long-term control of persistent asthma of any age. Inhaled corticosteroids are not indicated for the treatment of acute bronchospasm. They are also not indicated for the immediate treatment of status asthmaticus due to the delayed onset of relief, which can range from hours to days. However, short courses of systemic corticosteroids, or steroid "bursts," are used in asthma exacerbations.[7,17]

Mechanism of Action

Corticosteroids inhibit the inflammatory response by depressing the cell types and mediators involved in inflammation. Specifically, corticosteroids slow the migration of polymorphonuclear leukocytes and fibroblasts and inhibit the release of mediators associated with the inflammatory response, leading to attenuated mucous secretion and suppression of inflammatory processes. Consequently, corticosteroids reduce bronchial hyperresponsiveness, block late phase reaction to allergens, and improve lung function.[18]

Systemic Corticosteroids

Short courses of systemic corticosteroids may be used to establish control when beginning therapy or during a period where there is gradual deterioration in the patient's clinical status. In patients with long-term severe, persistent asthma, low doses of systemic corticosteroids may be used daily or every other day.[3] Dosages are listed in **Table 32-5**.

TABLE 32-5
Dosing of Systemic Corticosteroids[19–21]

Systemic Corticosteroid	Route of Administration	Dosage	Maximum Dosage
Prednisone/prednisolone	PO	1–2 mg/kg for the first dose, and then 0.5–1 mg/kg twice daily for subsequent doses starting the following day for 3–10 days	60 mg/day
Methylprednisolone	IV	1–2 mg/kg	125 mg/day
Dexamethasone	PO IV IM	0.6 mg/kg	16 mg/day

PO = by mouth; IV = intravenous; IM = intramuscular

Data from PredniSONE tablets, USP (prednisone) [package insert]. Salisbury, MD: Cadista Pharmaceuticals Inc.; 2016; Solu-medrol® IV, IM injection (methylprednisolone sodium succinate IV, IM injection) [package insert]. New York, NY: Pharmacia & Upjohn Co.; 2011; and Keeney G, Gray M, Morrison A, et al. Dexamethasone for acute asthma exacerbations in children: A meta-analysis. *Pediatrics.* 2014;133:493–499.

When corticosteroids are used for less than 1 month, side effects include weight gain, fluid retention, emotional instability, insomnia, and indigestion. Higher doses of short-term corticosteroids can cause increases in blood pressure and blood glucose. When corticosteroids are used for greater than 1 month, side effects may include Cushing syndrome, hypokalemia, sodium and water retention, hyperglycemia, weight gain, immunosuppression, glaucoma, growth retardation, acne, and gastrointestinal bleeding.[19]

Inhaled Corticosteroids

Inhaled corticosteroids are the mainstay for maintenance therapy in asthma. Many of the inhaled corticosteroids have no established usage in patients aged 4 years and younger who are unable to provide sufficient inspiratory flow for adequate lung deposition. A trial period of 4 to 6 weeks may be warranted to determine maximum benefit. Once control is achieved, the frequency of dosing may be reduced.[3] Dosages are listed in Table 32-6.

Side effects of inhaled corticosteroids are fewer when compared with systemic corticosteroids, as inhaled corticosteroids have limited systemic absorption. Side effects include difficulty speaking, hoarse voice, oral candidiasis, and cough (**Box 32-3**).[3]

Mucolytics

Mucoactive agents, or **mucolytics**, are drugs that change the biophysical properties of secretions. They are capable of modifying mucus production, secretion, nature and composition, and interactions with mucociliary epithelium.[27] Dornase alfa reduces the viscosity of infected sputum. It is indicated for the management of mucus in patients with cystic fibrosis who have a forced vital capacity that is ≥40% of the predicted value. It has been shown to reduce the risk of respiratory tract

BOX 32-3 Corticosteroids

- To prevent oral candidiasis after use of a steroid inhaler, rinse the mouth and throat with warm water and wipe the inside of an infant's or child's mouth with a wet cloth.

- If a mask is used, wash the skin around the mouth after use of a steroid inhaler with a face-mask spacer.

- Use a spacer or holding chamber if inhalation is with a pressurized metered dose inhaler.

infections requiring parenteral antibiotics in these patients.[28] This drug is Food and Drug Administration approved for patients older than age 5 years; however, some small studies suggest that its use may be extended to patients as young as 3 months old at the same dose as patients 5 years and older, resulting in similar safety and efficacy profiles.[29]

Dornase alfa is a recombinant human enzyme, deoxyribonuclease I (rhDNase), that hydrolyzes the DNA in sputum found in cystic fibrosis patients and reduces sputum viscosity and surface adhesiveness. The DNA released from broken-down neutrophils increases mucus viscosity, which obstructs the airway. Dornase alfa promotes airway clearance and thins mucus by degrading this extracellular DNA.[30]

Dornase alfa is available for nebulization as a preservative-free solution that should be kept refrigerated prior to use. Dosages are listed in **Table 32-7**, with a frequency of once per day. However, some patients may benefit from twice daily dosing.

Side Effects

The most common side effect is cough. Chest pain, fever, rash, dyspnea, and infection may also occur.[28]

TABLE 32-6
Dosing of Inhaled Corticosteroids[22–26]

Inhaled Corticosteroid	Low Daily Dosage	Low Daily Dosage	Medium Daily Dosage	Medium Daily Dosage	High Daily Dosage	High Daily Dosage
Age in years	0–4	5–11	0–4	5–11	0–4	5–11
Beclomethasone HFA 40 or 80 mcg/actuation	NA	40 mcg/actuation, 1–2 actuations twice daily	NA	40 mcg/actuation, 2–4 actuations twice daily 80 mcg/actuation, 1–2 actuations twice daily	NA	80 mcg/actuation, 3–4 actuations twice daily
Budesonide DPI 90 or 180 mcg/inhalation	NA	90 mcg/inhalation, 1–2 inhalations twice daiy	NA	180 mcg/inhalation, 1–2 inhalations twice daily	NA	180 mg/inhalation, 3–4 inhalations twice daily
Budesonide nebulization suspension 0.25 mg/2 mL, 0.5 mg/2 mL, or 1 mg/2 mL	0.25–0.5 mg once daily or as 2 divided doses	0.5 mg once daily or as 2 divided doses	0.75–1 mg once daily or as 2 or 3 divided doses	1 mg once daily or as 2 divided doses	1.25–2 mg once daily or as 2 divided doses	2 mg once daily or as 2 divided doses
Fluticasone DPI 50, 100, or 250 mcg/inhalation	NA	50 mcg/inhalation, 1–2 inhalations twice daily	NA	50 mcg/inhalation, 3–4 inhalations twice daily 100 mcg/inhalation, 1 inhalation in AM and 2 inhalations in PM to 2 inhalations twice daily	NA	100 mcg/inhalation, 2 inhalations in AM and 3 inhalations in PM 250 mcg/inhalation, 1 inhalation twice daily
Mometasone aerosol DPI (breath activated) 110 or 220 mcg/inhalation	NA	110 mcg/inhalation, 1 inhalation once daily	NA	110 mcg/inhalation, 2–3 inhalations once daily	NA	110 mcg/inhalation, 4 inhalations once daily or 2 inhalations twice daily 220 mcg/inhalation, 2 inhalations once daily or 1 inhalation twice daily

NA = not applicable
HFA = hydrofluoroalkane
DPI = dry powder inhaler

Data from QVAR® (beclomethasone dipropionate HFA) [package insert]. Horsham, PA: Teva Specialty Pharmaceuticals LLC; 2008; Pulmicort Flexhaler™ (budesonide inhalation powder) [package insert]. Wilmington, DE: AstraZeneca LP; 2008; Pulmicort Respules™ (budesonide inhalation suspension) [package insert]. Wilmington, DE: AstraZeneca LP; 2008; Flovent Diskus (fluticasone propionate inhalation powder) for oral inhalation. [package insert]. Research Triangle Park, NC: GlaxoSmithKline; 2017; and Asmanex® Twisthaler (mometasone furoate inhalation powder) [package insert]. Whitehouse Station, NJ: Merck & Co, Inc.; 2011.

TABLE 32-7
Dosing of Mucolytics[28]

Mucolytics	Route of Administration	Dosage	Comments
Dornase alfa (Pulmozyme)	Nebulizer	2.5 mg once daily	Do not mix with any other drug in nebulizer

Data from Pulmozyme® (dornase alpha) [package insert]. San Francisco: Genentech; 2014.

TABLE 32-8
Dosing of Leukotriene Receptor Antagonists[32,33]

Leukotriene Receptor Antagonist	Route of Administration	Dosage	Comments
Montelukast	Tablet	Ages 1–5 years: 4 mg once daily Ages 6–14 years: 5 mg once daily Ages 15 years and older: 10 mg once daily	Administer in the evening
Zafirlukast	Tablet	Ages 5–11 years: 10 mg twice daily 12 years and older: 20 mg twice daily	Take 1 hour before or 2 hours after meals Store in the original container

Data from Accolate® (zafirlukast) [package insert]. Wilmington, DE: AstraZeneca; 2013; and Accolate® oral tablets (zafirlukast oral tablets) [package insert]. Wilmington, DE: AstraZeneca Pharmaceuticals LP; 2011.

Leukotriene Modifiers

Leukotriene modifiers are used for the prophylaxis and chronic treatment of asthma in adults and children. Zafirlukast is indicated for the prevention and chronic treatment of asthma in pediatric patients 5 years of age and older. Montelukast is indicated for the prevention of exercise-induced bronchoconstriction in patients 15 years of age and older, in pediatric patients with asthma 12 months of age and older, and in pediatric patients 2 years of age and older for symptom relief of allergic rhinitis.

Leukotriene receptor antagonists inhibit the formation of leukotrienes, which are proinflammatory mediators produced from arachidonic acid. This inhibition helps decrease bronchoconstriction, vasoconstriction, and inflammation.[31]

Leukotriene modifiers are administered in tablet form, and the dosage frequency is dependent upon the medication (**Table 32-8**).

Headache is the most common side effect. Other side effects reported include dizziness, abdominal pain, and muscle weakness.[32,33]

Antimicrobials

The upper respiratory tract harbors a broad spectrum of potential pathogens, including *Streptococcus pneumoniae*, *Haemophilus influenzae*, *Moraxella catarrhalis*, and *Staphylococcus aureus*, which all have the potential to cause infection.[34] **Antimicrobials**, also known as antibiotics, fight infection either by destroying the bacteria or preventing it from growing and multiplying. The disease state being treated is indicative of the bacteria that is being targeted by the antimicrobial therapy. Cystic fibrosis patients are susceptible to infections caused by a broader range of bacteria that include *Pseudomonas aeruginosa*. Studies suggest that nebulized antibiotics are better than no treatment for early infection with *P. aeruginosa*, but there is still insufficient evidence supporting which strategy is more effective for the eradication of *P. aeruginosa* in cystic fibrosis.[35]

Inhaled Antibiotics

Tobramycin is an aminoglycoside with antipseudomonal activity and is the first-line treatment for patients with this infection.[36] Tobramycin is bactericidal and works by binding to the 30 S ribosomal subunit of susceptible bacteria and interfering with messenger RNA, resulting in a defective bacterial cell membrane.[37] Tobramycin is indicated for patients 6 years and older for patients colonized with *P. aeruginosa* to reduce infection and hospitalization. The side effects associated with tobramycin include ototoxicity, tinnitus, voice alteration, dizziness, and bronchospasms.[38]

Aztreonam lysine is a monobactam that has properties like beta-lactams. Aztreonam is bactericidal and inhibits bacterial cell wall synthesis by binding to penicillin-binding proteins located within the bacterial cell wall. The inhaled formulation of aztreonam is indicated to improve respiratory symptoms in cystic fibrosis patients with *P. aeruginosa*. This drug is recommended for patients older than 7 years for the inhalation formulation, but it can be also used intravenously in patients 9 months and older for the treatment of pulmonary exacerbations in cystic fibrosis. The side effects associated with aztreonam are allergic reactions, bronchospasms, decrease in forced expiratory volume at 1 second (FEV_1), fever, wheezing, cough, and chest discomfort.[37] Dosages are listed in **Table 32-9**.

Oral Antibiotics

Azithromycin is a macrolide antibiotic that binds to the 50 S ribosomal subunit of bacterial ribosomes and

TABLE 32-9
Dosing Information for Inhaled Antimicrobials[39,40,42–44]

Antimicrobial	Route of Administration	Dosage	Comments
Tobramycin inhalation solution	Nebulizer or podhaler	TOBI, Bethkis, Kitabis Pak: 300 mg via nebulizer every 12 hours for 28 days, followed by a 28-day off cycle TOBI Podhaler: 112 mg via podhaler every 12 hours for 28 days, followed by a 28-day off cycle	Doses should be at least 6 hours apart Do not use if FEV_1 is <40% predicted, FEV_1 is >80% predicted, or colonized with *B. cepacia*
Aztreonam lysine inhalation solution	Nebulizer	Cayston: 75 mg 3 times daily for 28 days, followed by a 28-day off cycle	Doses should be administered at least 4 hours apart Use Altera nebulizer system Delivers dose in less than 3 minutes

FEV_1 = forced expiratory volume in 1 second

Data from Cayston® (aztreonam) inhalation solution [package insert]. Foster City, CA: Gilead Science, Inc; 2014; Mogayzel J, Peter J, Naureckas E, et al. Cystic fibrosis pulmonary guidelines. Chronic medications for maintenance of lung health. *Am J Respir Crit Care Med.* 2013; 87:680–689; TOBI® Podhaler (tobramycin) [package insert]. East Hanover, NJ: Novartis Pharmaceuticals Corporation; 2014; TOBI® (tobramycin inhalation solution) nebulizer solution [package insert]. East Hanover, NJ: Novartis Pharmaceuticals Corporation; 2015; and Kitabis™ Pak (tobramycin inhalation solution) for oral inhalation use [package insert]. Midlothian, VA: PARI Respiratory Equipment, Inc; 2014.

BOX 32-4 Antimicrobials

- Tobramycin is not indicated for patients colonized with *Burkholderia cepacia*.
- Azithromycin is not indicated for patients with nontuberculous mycobacteria lung infections.

BOX 32-5 Muscle Relaxants

- Succinylcholine is the only depolarizing agent.
- Patients must be sedated and analgesia must be provided prior to administration of NMBAs.

inhibits protein synthesis in bacterial cells. Azithromycin is indicated for cystic fibrosis patients 6 years and older who are chronically colonized with *P. aeruginosa* to improve pulmonary function. It is primarily used to decrease inflammation and reduce exacerbations. Side effects associated with azithromycin include diarrhea, abdominal cramping, tinnitus, and nausea (**Box 32-4**).[40,41]

Skeletal Muscle Relaxants

Neuromuscular blocking agents (NMBAs) are indicated for the induction of neuromuscular blockade and provide skeletal muscle relaxation during surgery or mechanical ventilation. These agents do not provide analgesia or sedation and should be administered only after the patient is sedated and after analgesia is provided (**Box 32-5**).[45]

NMBAs can be divided into two categories: depolarizing and non-depolarizing. Succinylcholine is the only depolarizing agent available; all other agents are non-depolarizing. Succinylcholine works by binding to and activating acetylcholine receptors, producing a Phase I block, desensitizing the ion channels to further action potentials.[46] The non-depolarizing agents directly compete with acetylcholine and bind to the acetylcholine receptors on the motor-end plate, preventing neurotransmitters from binding to the receptor.[45]

Flushing, bradycardia, hypotension, tachyarrhythmia, and rash are side effects seen with administration of **skeletal muscle relaxants**.[47–50] Dosages are listed in **Table 32-10**.

TABLE 32-10
Dosing of Skeletal Muscle Relaxants[47-50]

Skeletal Muscle Relaxant	Dosage		Comments	Action	
	Initial	**Maintenance**		**Onset**	**Duration**
Succinylcholine	Neonates and infants up to 6 months: 2 mg/kg IV 6 months and older: 1 mg/kg IV	Not used for maintenance due to risk of malignant hyperthermia	Use in children should be limited to emergency intubation Short-acting	45–60 seconds	4–10 minutes
Atracurium	Age 1 month to 2 years: 0.3–0.4 mg/kg IV Ages 2 years and older: 0.4–0.5 mg/kg IV bolus	Age 1 month and older: 0.08–0.1 mg/kg IV bolus 20–45 minutes after initial dose, then every 15–25 minutes as needed 5–9 mcg/kg/min (range 2–15 mcg/kg/min) continuous IV infusion after initial dose, upon early evidence of spontaneous recovery	Independent of renal and hepatic function for metabolism Intermediate-acting	1–4 minutes	20–35 minutes
Cisatracurium	Age 1–23 months: Initial, 0.15 mg/kg IV over 5–10 seconds	Initial continuous IV infusion of 3 mcg/kg/min to rapidly counteract spontaneous recovery from initial bolus dose; thereafter, 1–2 mcg/kg/min continuous IV infusion	Independent of renal and hepatic function for metabolism Intermediate-acting	2–3 minutes	Up to 70 minutes
Pancuronium	Test dose of 0.02 mg/kg IV to measure responsiveness	Initial: 0.04–0.1 mg/kg IV (endotracheal intubation, 0.06–0.1 mg/kg IV); later incremental doses starting at 0.01 mg/kg may be used	May accumulate in renal or hepatic dysfunction Long-acting	4–6 minutes	120–180 minutes
Vecuronium	Ages 10–16 years: 0.08–0.1 mg/kg IV bolus	Ages 10–16 years: 0.01–0.015 mg/kg IV 25–40 minutes after initial dose, repeat every 12–15 minutes as needed	Doses should be individualized, patients ages 1–10 years may require a higher initial dose and more frequent supplemental doses May accumulate in renal or hepatic dysfunction	2–3 minutes	45–60 minutes

IV = intravenous

Data from Atracurium besylate injection, USP (atracurium besylate) for intravenous injection [package insert]. Bedford, OH: Bedford Laboratories; 2010; Pancuronium bromide injection (pancuronium bromide) [package insert]. Irvine, CA: Gensia Sicor Pharmaceuticals; 2003; CISATRCURIUM intravenous injection solution (cisatracurium besylate intravenous injection solution) [package insert]. Lake Zurich, IL: Fesenius Kabi USA (per DailyMed); 2015; and Vecuronium bromide intravenous injection lyophilized powder for solution (vecuronium bromide intravenous injection lyophilized powder for solution) [package insert]. Lake Zurich, IL: Fresenius Kabi USA (per DailyMed); 2016.

Case Study 1

A 10-year-old boy presented to a new pulmonary physician for evaluation. His mother stated that his primary condition was asthma. He had developed respiratory symptoms at 2 months of age, had been seen by many specialists, and had been on multiple medications since that time. The pregnancy was uneventful. When he was 2 months old, he developed a recurrent cough. He was started on albuterol and then, at 6 years of age, switched to levalbuterol hydrochloride. At various times he has also been treated with cromolyn sodium, fluticasone proprionate and salmeterol, and montelukast as well as with a short course of prednisolone for exacerbations. His last course of oral steroids was 9 months ago. The hallmark of his illness was that a cold would always trigger his asthma. He had approximately one emergency department visit per year, but he had never been hospitalized. His asthma symptoms would typically worsen with the weather changes in the spring and fall; the cold winter months were often particularly difficult. In addition to his asthma, his medical history was remarkable for several events of otitis media, seasonal mold allergies, occasional headaches, and croup. One or more of the events occurred about three times a year, lasting approximately 3 days for each episode. His current medications include 1 inhalation of combination fluticasone proprionate and salmeterol in the 250/50 strength twice daily and 2 to 4 inhalations of levalbuterol as needed. This visit was scheduled in the hopes of decreasing this child's episodes of illness, assessing the current medication regimen, and discussing new treatment opportunities.

1. **What is the difference between albuterol and levalbuterol?**

2. **What is the mechanism of action of montelukast, and should it be a part of this child's daily medication regimen?**

3. **What role does fluticasone proprionate and salmeterol serve in controlling this child's asthma symptoms?**

Case Study 2

A 9-year-old female with cystic fibrosis presented to the pulmonary clinic with persistent exertional dyspnea and cough with scant sputum production. Physical examination revealed normal vital signs, but she had an oxygen saturation of 91% while breathing room air. Her weight had fallen from 68.2 kg to 65.5 kg over the last 3 months. Cardiovascular exam was completely normal. Lungs demonstrated coarse breath sounds bilaterally and were moderately decreased. The abdomen was normal, extremities demonstrated mild clubbing, and there was no peripheral edema. FEV_1 had decreased from 70% to 50%. The chest radiograph resembled baseline findings with no obvious infiltrate or pneumothorax. Her standard inhaled treatment regimen was albuterol, 7% hypertonic saline, dornase alfa, and Flovent followed by vest therapy twice daily. She was prescribed a month-long course of azithromycin, aztreonam, and inhaled tobramycin for suspected pulmonary exacerbation with an acute superinfection. One month later she returned to the clinic for a follow-up visit. Physical exam revealed moderate improvement in dyspnea as well as her FEV_1, which now was back to baseline, and her oxygen saturation improved to 95% on room air.

1. **Why do you think multiple antibiotics were prescribed for this child?**

2. **What is the mechanism of action of dornase alfa?**

3. **What is the advantage of an inhaled corticosteroid versus oral systemic administration?**

References

1. Allegaert K, van den Anker JN. Clinical pharmacology in neonates: small size, huge variability. *Neonatology*. 2014;105:344-349.

2. Ventolin HFA (albuterol sulfate) inhalation aerosol for oral inhalation [package insert]. Research Triangle Park, NC: GlaxoSmithKline; 2014.

3. National Asthma Education and Prevention Program Expert Panel 3. *Guidelines for the Diagnosis and Management of Asthma: Expert Panel Report 3.* Bethesda, MD: National Institutes of Health and National Heart, Lung, and Blood Institute; 2007:07-4051.

4. Aminophylline (aminophylline dihydrate) [package insert]. Lake Forest, IL: Hopsira; 2009.

5. Epinephrine oral inhalation aerosol [package insert]. West Roxbury, MA: Armstrong Pharmaceuticals; 2004.

6. Cazzola M, Page C, Calzetta L, Matera M. Pharmacology and therapeutics of bronchodilators. *Pharmacol Rev*. 2012;64:450-504.

7. Global Initiative for Asthma (GINA). *Global Strategy for Asthma Management and Prevention.* Updated 2017.

8. Serevent Diskus (salmeterol xinafoate inhalation powder) for oral inhalation [package insert]. Research Triangle Park, NC: GlaxoSmithKline; 2016.

9. Rosekrans J. Viral croup: current diagnosis and treatment. *Mayo Clin Proc*. 1998;73:1102-1106.

10. Ledwith C, Shear L, Mauro R. Safety and efficacy of nebulized racemic epinephrine in conjunction with oral dexamethasone and mist in the outpatient treatment of croup. *Ann Emerg Med*. 1995;25:331-337.

11. Bjornson C, Russell K, Vandermeer B, et al. Nebulized epinephrine for croup in children. *Cochrane Database Cyst Rev*. 2013;CD006619.

12. Atrovent HFA (ipratropium bromide) inhalation aerosol [package insert]. Ridgefield, CT: Boehringer Ingelheim; 2012.

13. Atrovent (ipratropium bromide) solution [package insert]. Zanesville, OH: Cardinal Health; 2012.

14. Barnes P. Theophylline. *Am J Respir Crit Care Med*. 2013;188:901-903.

15. Theophylline in 5% dextrose IV injection, theophylline in 5% dextrose IV injection [package insert]. Deerfield, IL: Baxter Healthcare; 2003.

16. Elixophyllin (theophylline, anhydrous) liquid [package insert]. Detroit, MI: Caraco Pharmaceutical Laboratories; 2010.

17. Szefler SJ. Glucocorticoid therapy for asthma: clinical pharmacology. *J Allergy Clin Immunol*. 1991;88:147-165.

18. Stahn C, Löwenberg M, Hommes D, Buttgereit F. Molecular mechanisms of glucocorticoid action and selective glucocorticoid receptor agonists. *Mol Cell Endocrinol*. 2007;275:71-78.

19. PredniSONE tablets, USP (prednisone) [package insert]. Salisbury, MD: Cadista Pharmaceuticals; 2016.

20. Solu-medrol IV, IM injection (methylprednisolone sodium succinate IV, IM injection) [package insert]. New York: Pharmacia & Upjohn; 2011.

21. Keeney G, Gray M, Morrison A, et al. Dexamethasone for acute asthma exacerbations in children: a meta-analysis. *Pediatrics*. 2014;133:493-499.

22. QVAR (beclomethasone dipropionate HFA) [package insert]. Horsham, PA: Teva Specialty Pharmaceuticals; 2008.

23. Pulmicort Flexhaler (budesonide inhalation powder) [package insert]. Wilmington, DE: AstraZeneca; 2008.

24. Pulmicort Respules (budesonide inhalation suspension) [package insert]. Wilmington, DE: AstraZeneca; 2008.

25. Flovent Diskus (fluticasone propionate inhalation powder) for oral inhalation [package insert]. Research Triangle Park, NC: GlaxoSmithKline; 2017.

26. Asmanex Twisthaler (mometasone furoate inhalation powder) [package insert]. Whitehouse Station, NJ: Merck & Co; 2011.

27. Henke M, Ratjen F. Mucolytics in cystic fibrosis. *Paedtr Respir Rev*. 2007;8:24-29.

28. Pulmozyme (dornase alpha) [package insert]. San Francisco: Genentech; 2014.

29. Wagener J, Rock M, McCubbin M, et al. Aerosol delivery and safety of recombinant human deoxyribonuclease in young children with cystic fibrosis: a bronchoscopic study. *J Pediatr*. 1998;133:486-491.

30. Task Group on Mucoactive Drugs. Recommendations for guidelines on clinical trials of mucoactive drugs in chronic bronchitis and chronic obstructive pulmonary disease. *Chest*. 1994;106:1532-1537.

31. Dahlén S. Treatment of asthma with antileukotrienes: first line or last resort therapy? *Eur J Pharmacol*. 2006;533:40-56.

32. Accolate (zafirlukast) [package insert]. Wilmington, DE: AstraZeneca; 2013.

33. Accolate oral tablets (zafirlukast oral tablets) [package insert]. Wilmington, DE: AstraZeneca; 2011.

34. Bosch AATM, Biesbroek G, Trzcinski K, et al. Viral and bacterial interactions in the upper respiratory tract. *PLoS Pathog*. 2013;9(1): e1003057. https://doi.org/10.1371/journal.ppat.1003057.

35. Langton HS, Smyth A. Antibiotic strategies for eradicating *Pseudomonas aeruginosa* in people with cystic fibrosis. *Cochrane Database Syst Rev*. 2014;CD004197.

36. Flume P, O'Sullivan B, Robinson K, et al. Cystic fibrosis pulmonary guidelines. Chronic medications for maintenance of lung health. *Am J Respir Crit Care Med*. 2007;176:957-969.

37. Tobramycin (tobramycin sulfate vials for injection) [package insert]. Schaumberg, IL: American Pharmaceutical Partners; 2008.

38. Bethkis (tobramycin) [package insert]. Woodstock, IL: Chiesi USA; 2017.

39. Cayston (aztreonam) inhalation solution [package insert]. Foster City, CA: Gilead Science; 2014.

40. Mogayzel J, Peter J, Naureckas E, et al. Cystic fibrosis pulmonary guidelines. Chronic medications for maintenance of lung health. *Am J Respir Crit Care Med*. 2013;187:680-689.

41. Saiman L, Marshall B, Mayer-Hamblett N, et al. Azithromycin in patients with cystic fibrosis chronically infected with *Pseudomonas aeruginosa*: a randomized controlled trial. *JAMA*. 2003;290:1749-1756.

42. TOBI Podhaler (tobramycin) [package insert]. East Hanover, NJ: Novartis Pharmaceuticals; 2014.

43. TOBI (tobramycin inhalation solution) nebulizer solution [package insert]. East Hanover, NJ: Novartis Pharmaceuticals; 2015.

44. Kitabis Pak (tobramycin inhalation solution) for oral inhalation use [package insert]. Midlothian, VA: PARI Respiratory Equipment; 2014.

45. Farooq K, Hunter J. Neuromuscular blocking agents and reversal agents. *Anaesth Intensive Care Med*. 2014;15:295-299.

46. Anectine (succinylcholine chloride injection) [package insert]. Research Triangle Park, NC: GlaxoWellcome; 1999.

47. Atracurium besylate injection, USP (atracurium besylate) for intravenous injection [package insert]. Bedford, OH: Bedford Laboratories; 2010.

48. Pancuronium bromide injection (pancuronium bromide) [package insert]. Irvine, CA: Gensia Sicor Pharmaceuticals; 2003.

49. CISATRCURIUM intravenous injection solution (cisatracurium besylate intravenous injection solution) [package insert]. Lake Zurich, IL: Fesenius Kabi USA (per DailyMed); 2015.

50. Vecuronium bromide intravenous injection lyophilized powder for solution (vecuronium bromide intravenous injection lyophilized powder for solution) [package insert]. Lake Zurich, IL: Fresenius Kabi USA (per DailyMed); 2016.

Michael T. Bigham

Kendra Paxton

OUTLINE

OBJECTIVES

1. List the essential components of well-developed transport systems.
2. Describe the circumstances that affect crew configuration.
3. Explain the skills necessary for crew members to achieve and maintain to provide quality specialty care on transport.
4. Differentiate between crew resource management and a safety management system.
5. Explain the considerations used when choosing the mode of transport.
6. List the equipment and supplies important to the care of mechanically ventilated children during air/ground transport.
7. Discuss the effect altitude has on the care of critically ill infants and children.
8. Explain the importance of family presence on transport.

KEY TERMS

crew resource
  management (CRM)
fixed wing
post accident incident
  plan (PAIP)

rotor wing
safety management
  system (SMS)

Introduction

Complex ill and injured children and infants present with distinctly different anatomic, physiologic, and behavioral needs than their adult counterparts. Regionalization of neonatal and pediatric specialty services has necessitated the development of specialized interfacility transport services to transfer critically ill infants and children to hospitals equipped to care for their distinct needs. In the United States, hospital-based transport teams emerged in the 1960s for transport of neonatal patients and have grown to include specialty pediatric transport. In this chapter, we summarize some key elements of neonatal and pediatric critical care transport.

Transport Team

Critical care transport teams are designed to meet local needs for interhospital transfer. Transport teams generally complement the emergency medical services (EMS) and local nonpediatric hospitals, providing continued care of the injured/ill child in need of transport to a higher level of care. In certain circumstances, such as traumatic injury, it is clinically preferable to stabilize the infant and/or child and to provide prompt transfer from the scene. The majority of sick or injured pediatric patients benefit from a more methodical approach to transport that is focused less on speed of return to the tertiary hospital and more on rapidity of response to the bedside, clinical stabilization, and ongoing resuscitation prior to and during transport. The neonatal/pediatric patient population can be diverse and can range from premature newborns to late adolescents and even young adults receiving long-term care for a childhood disease. Although the transport environment may have some constraints, the same level of care provided to critically ill or injured children at a tertiary/quaternary care facility should be provided during transport. An evolving belief is that access to a skilled neonatal/pediatric transport team is optimal for the critically injured/ill pediatric patient being treated at institutions with fewer resources, and development of specialized teams should be tailored to meet the needs of the region served.[1] In a single-center study, Orr et al.[1] reported that infants and children transported by a pediatric specialty team had fewer unplanned events during transport when compared to an adult nonspecialty transport team (61% versus 1.5%) and had a lower in-hospital mortality, even after adjustment for illness severity (23% versus 9%). It was speculated that the pediatric specialty team's priority around stabilization and advanced early intervention at the referring facility perhaps minimized the risks of deterioration and/or unplanned events during transport, subsequently impacting the hospital mortality. A study evaluating adherence to sepsis resuscitation prior to admission to a regional children's hospital affirms this association of better preadmission resuscitation and better survival.[2] This notion of improved outcomes for specialty pediatric transport teams, commonly debated among the nonspecialty critical care transport services, was also studied in a 2016 report by Meyer et al.[3] Although the cohort of patients transported by the specialty pediatric transport cohort were younger and more acutely ill, the researchers found no difference in adjusted severity of illness or mortality 48 hours after admission to the pediatric intensive care unit (PICU). The evidence remains unclear on whether the use of a dedicated team proficient in pediatric and neonatal critical care is an important aspect of improved patient outcomes. Less debate exists around the fact that specialty pediatric/neonatal teams and nonspecialized teams must function within a developed transport system having the following essential components: (1) online medical control by qualified physicians, (2) ground and air ambulance capabilities, (3) a coordinated communications system, (4) written clinical and operational guidelines, (5) a comprehensive program for quality and performance improvement, (6) a database to track activity and permit patient follow-up, (7) medical and nursing leadership, (8) administrative resources, and (9) institutional endorsement and financial support.[4]

Crew Configuration

Critical care transport team composition varies widely by region, patient population, availability of resources, financial support, and other considerations, such as weight limitations during air medical transport. Several models of neonatal/pediatric specialty teams exist and more often are hospital-based teams supported by the receiving hospital; these include the use of either dedicated team members or the use of on-duty, unit-based staff. Each model for team composition has advantages and disadvantages, including costs, mobilization times, and personnel used. Crew configuration varies and is typically based on the institution's internal and regional resources and patient volume. Studies examining team types and team personnel describe crews to include the following caregivers: physicians, physicians in training, advanced nurse practitioners, critical care pediatric and/or neonatal nurses, respiratory therapists, paramedics, or basic emergency medical technicians (EMTs).[5,6] There is little evidence to support improved outcomes with the use of a physician, and the financial implications may preclude teams from using the physician resource. In a recent study, van Lieshout et al.[7] showed no difference in critical events during transport when non-physician-led critical care transports were compared to physician-led critical care transports (16.3% versus 15.2%). Many pediatric/neonatal teams with a high volume of transports primarily function without the use of an onboard physician and reserve the use for the very select and extremely critical patient transports. Local and state regulations may influence team composition, but it is essential that the crew maintain expertise in the management of pediatric respiratory conditions, as this is primarily the most common problem encountered. All transport teams should have staff with expertise in establishing and maintaining a neonatal/pediatric airway, advanced assessment skills, vascular access skills, resuscitation, and knowledge of dosing and administration of high-risk medications. The team members must also have in-depth knowledge of physiology, appropriate safety training, and exceptional communication skills. Regardless of the crew configuration, the literature supports the importance of training in reducing adverse events; specifically, adverse events during transport occurred in only 2%, or 1 in 49, of pediatric transports by a specialized team compared to 20%, or 18 of 92, of children transported by a nonspecialized team.[8]

Team Requirements

Team requirements include the type of clinical experience the respective team member must have before he/she is hired into a transport position as well as the clinical and safety training requirements. Team requirements depend on the population served (adult versus pediatric specialty), type of transport provided (scene versus intra-facility), accrediting body requirements, and mode of transport the crew will use (air, ground).

Clinical Experience

The selection of team members is best determined by the team's mission profile and patient clinical needs. Current Commission on Accreditation of Medical Transport Systems (CAMTS) accreditation standards recommend that team members have a minimum of 3 years' relevant critical care experience.[9] Although it is not clear if 3 years of critical care experience is superior to 2 years or inferior to 5 years, it is reasonable to believe that the practice of critical care medicine in the off-campus/highly stressed setting of critical care transport would benefit from a solid foundation of critical care expertise. Additionally, transport teams that respond to scene runs will benefit from prehospital experience. All personnel should meet certain physical requirements and will generally be evaluated in the pre-employment period on the ability to perform certain physical tasks, such as lifting heavy equipment and mobility in and out of the transport vehicles.

Transport team members, depending on demographics of the population the team serves, should have successful completion of certification courses, such as Pediatric Advanced Life Support (PALS), Advanced Cardiac Life Support (ACLS), and Neonatal Resuscitation Program (NRP). Completion of a trauma course with advanced skills lab, such as Transport Nurse Advanced Trauma Course (TNATC), Pediatric Fundamentals of Critical Care Support (PFCCS), or an audit of Advanced Trauma Life Support (ATLS), are worthy considerations for augmentation of transport-specific clinical care. Additional certifications may be necessary, such as EMT certification for the registered nurse and/or respiratory

therapist, and should be guided by mission profile, state licensure for ambulances, and accreditation standards.

The CAMTS requires crew members to attain specialty credentials to validate their more advanced skills. The commission will accept the specialty credential for clinicians working in transport, Certified Neonatal Pediatric Transport (CNPT), or Certified Flight Registered Nurse (CFRN). Credentials validating special critical care skills, such as Certified Critical Care Registered Nurse (CCRN) or Neonatal Pediatric Specialist (NPS), are also among the credentials CAMTS will accept.

Aside from the descriptions in the team composition section and the certifications listed earlier, some intangibles are consistently found in the outstanding critical care transport clinician. Commonly observed personality traits include independence, leadership, flexibility, adaptability, initiative, intelligence, the ability to problem solve, and utility of sound clinical judgment. Team members must also have excellent communication and interpersonal skills and must have the ability to diffuse tense and stressful situations. These are important because a majority of the clinical work the crew provides is on the scene or at a referral hospital, where resources are limited. Collectively, all selected personnel should be sufficiently trained and knowledgeable to assume the role of the team leader, and each member of the team must understand the principles of one another's roles in order to assist and complement one another during the transport.

Training Requirements

Guidelines for training are succinctly described by the American Academy of Pediatrics (AAP) Guidelines for Air and Ground Transport of Neonatal and Pediatric Patients and include cognitive, procedural, communication, and other skills.[10] Transport personnel are typically selected from experienced providers and have already acquired the extensive variety of necessary certifications. Generally, new transport personnel need to gain additional training to enhance their knowledge base to include advanced assessment, such as laboratory analysis, radiologic interpretation, and diagnostics, often not expected in their current job role. Although this text will not thoroughly address concepts of adult learning theory or other strategies to impart knowledge and skills for staff, common mechanisms for developing cognitive and procedural skills include didactic training in the classroom environment, self-learning modules, and individualized one-on-one instruction. The prevailing skill that must be reinforced in the new transport personnel is the ability to recognize and differentiate between "sick" and "not sick" pediatric/neonatal illnesses. The ability to recognize and predict the most common causes of patient deterioration and then appropriately intervene is only obtained through initial training, significant experience, and ongoing education. Procedural skills that are potentially lifesaving interventions, such as vascular access, advanced airway management, and needle decompression, are important in the transport environment.[10,11]

Competency-Based Training

Most critical care transport programs conceptualize training and competency in two categories: initial and ongoing competency. Initial competency represents the body of knowledge, procedural skill, and teamwork that is new and transport specific. Ongoing competency represents the body of knowledge, skill, and teamwork that requires retraining or simply practicing to ensure expertise when that knowledge, skill, and teamwork need to be applied. The field of critical care transport has been early to adopt strategies for initial and ongoing competency. As a result, there is a terrific amount of experience in the transport field regarding venues to optimize knowledge and skill acquisition, including simulation, cadaver labs, animal labs, or in the operating room under direct supervision.[12–16]

Initial competencies are often guided by an orientation pathway for the new neonatal/pediatric transport team member. Initial competencies vary widely among programs, so much so that in a recent analysis of pediatric/neonatal transport listserv posts, the topic of education of staff was a "top five" category.[17] Samples of orientation pathways are available, although it is important to understand that initial competency training should prepare the transport team personnel to function in the local environment, so orientation should be to specific equipment (isolette, IV pumps), vehicles (rotor and fixed wing, ground mobile intensive care unit [MICU]), and physical locations (frequently visited referral hospitals, emergency, inpatient, and neonatal resuscitation areas). Another vital initial competency often focuses on teamwork and communication. Transport members must be taught the ability to clearly communicate the plan of care with the treatment team members in what is often a highly emotional environment. Communication skills can be taught through a **crew resource management (CRM)** course in addition to practicing with closed-loop communication in simulation and certification courses.[18] CRM has a focus on

leadership, interpersonal communication, and decision making and was developed in 1979 from the NASA training workshops. Maintaining ongoing competency is somewhat more difficult, as it is resource intensive, and where orientation is often a full-time proposition, maintaining competencies must fit in around the work of transport. Content for ongoing competencies can also be difficult to identify and prioritize, although, generally, ongoing competency training prioritizes low-frequency but high-risk situations (e.g., cricothyroidectomy, transcutaneous pacing), high-frequency events (intubation, ventilator setup/management), and communication or even recent cases (run review to inform simulation content). Accreditation standards also exist for additional guidance on maintaining competency.[9]

Safety

Most hospitals have heard the call from the Institute for Healthcare Improvement to make hospitals safer for patients and have built cultures targeting safety and high-reliability behaviors.[19] Although the airline industry and the nuclear power industries are the most commonly shared examples of high reliability, the critical care transport field is not. Most ambulance and helicopter EMS incidents and accidents can be attributed to human factors and systems designs that can lead to poor decision making. Air ambulance accidents occur at an unfortunate rate of 8.3 to 12.75 accidents per year and result in a 30% fatality rate.[20] Data regarding ground ambulance accidents is less accurate, as there is no official reporting mechanism, but are estimated to be more prevalent and with a wide variety of injuries to the crew/patients. Safety is defined by the International Civil Aviation Organization as "the state in which the possibility of harm to persons or of property damage is reduced to, and maintained at or below, an acceptable level through a continuing process of hazard identification and safety risk management."[21] A commonly used transport tool is a **safety management system (SMS)**. An SMS is vital to create a culture of safety that supports risk assessment, accountability, professionalism, and organizational dynamics. SMSs integrate safety risk

TABLE 33-1
The Four Functional Components of a Safety Management System

Component	Goals
Safety policy	Establishes senior management's commitment to continually improve safety. Defines the methods, processes, and organizational structure needed to meet safety goals.
Safety risk management	Determines the need for, and adequacy of, new or revised risk controls based on the assessment of acceptable risk.
Safety assurance	Evaluates the continued effectiveness of implemented risk control strategies. Supports the identification of new hazards.
Safety promotion	Includes training, communication, and other actions to create a positive safety culture within all levels of the workforce. Promotion of safety is everyone's responsibility.

management and safety assurance concepts into repeatable, proactive systems. SMS is all about safety decision making throughout the organization and is composed of four functional components, which are listed in **Table 33-1**.

Safety Management Training Academy is provided through the Association of Air Medical Services; it offers a certification as a Certified Medical Transportation Safety Professional (MTSP-C) and provides a comprehensive foundation in the science and application of the discipline of safety systems for leaders in the medical transport industry. Programs with a robust SMS often identify a safety officer to promote best safety practices, systematically track and trend data in an effort to reduce emerging problems, and identify and mitigate threats to transport safety.

Environmental factors and fatigue can influence the safety of the transport environment. Air medical vendors operate under federal weather minimums that influence the decision to complete a mission; however, the same standards do not exist for ground ambulances. Ice, snow, and heavy rain can negatively impact the road safety of the crew, and a risk assessment tool can help provide objective guidance for the crew to determine the safety of the ground mission. Sleep deprivation, lengthy shifts, and night shifts can influence crew alertness and can affect the overall safety of the transport environment. Attention should be taken to minimize day-to-night shift rotations and to ensure adequate rest time between shifts for the pilots, drivers, and medical crew.

Despite mature safety management systems, safety events may still occur. Safety training should include vehicle breakdown, scene safety, and survival training. Drills should be conducted to test the safety system for all modes of transport. A developed **post accident incident plan (PAIP)** can guide staff, management, dispatch, and local law enforcement in the process in the event of an accident or incident. Finally, it is intended that safety management integrate with the quality management systems to contribute to the organization's safety performance as a result of using defined processes to identify and mitigate safety hazards and risks.

Transport Modes

Critically ill children are transported by ground critical care ambulances, rotor wing or helicopters, or fixed wing planes. The nature of the injury or illness, distance traveled, and environmental conditions are considered when determining the mode of transport.

Ground

Ground ambulance is the most commonly used mode for interfacility and prehospital transport (**Figure 33-1**). The advantages include low costs, high availability, and ability to respond in most weather conditions. Ground ambulances offer multiple levels of service, such as critical care, advanced life support, and basic life support,

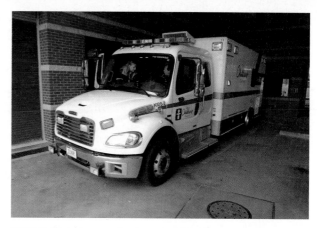

FIGURE 33-1 An example of a neonatal/pediatric specialty ground ambulance. The ambulances are equipped to be mobile ICUs.

and are typically readily available. The interior of the ambulance is more spacious and provides easier access to the patient to perform clinical interventions. With the larger cabins, ambulances can accommodate up to four crew members and often a parent or family member. Ambulances have the ability to be configured for special pediatric/neonatal circumstances, such as transporting twins or siblings. Unlike helicopters, there are no weight limitations and more equipment can be carried in the ambulance. Ground ambulances provide door-to-door service, and there is no need for a helipad or runway. Disadvantages can include traffic conditions, long travel times, and weather conditions. The ground speed of the ambulance is limited, and detours, inclement weather, and poor road conditions can delay or stop a ground transport. A functional service range for ground is between 0 and 150 miles, although any distance over 100 miles may become costly, time consuming, and inefficient. Another limitation to ground ambulances is the high potential for a rough ride to cause painful bouncing and the possibility of motion sickness. Despite the limitations, they currently remain the dominant vehicle in patient transport and are often the most preferred modality for critical care pediatric/neonatal patients.

Rotor Wing

According to the Association of Air Medical Services, there are approximately 400,000 **rotor wing** or helicopter transports annually in the United States.[22] The advantages include the speed of the helicopter, the ability to cover long distances, access into remote locations, and even the ability to bypass ground traffic in busy urban locales. A helicopter, as shown in **Figure 33-2**, can decrease travel times by one-third to one-fourth of that required for equal distance traveled by a ground ambulance and offers a typical range is up to 150 miles from the base of operations. The helicopter has the ability to provide door-to-door service, but it requires either a helipad or a clear 100-feet × 100-feet landing area free

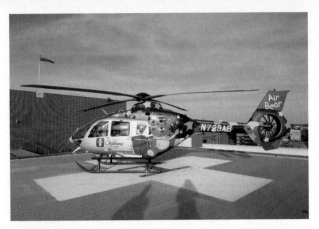

FIGURE 33-2 An example of a branded neonatal/pediatric air ambulance. Although equipped for specialized transports, the exterior appears friendly and nonintrusive.

TABLE 33-2
Appropriate Reasons to Use an Air Medical Helicopter in the Out-of-Hospital Setting[24]

Patient has a significant potential to require high-level life support available from an air medical helicopter, which is not available by ground transport.
Patient has a significant potential to require a time-critical intervention, and an air medical helicopter will deliver the patient to an appropriate facility faster than ground transport.
Patient is located in a geographically isolated area, which would make ground transport impossible or greatly delayed.
Local EMS resources are exceeded.

Data from American College of Emergency Physicians. Air Medical Transport Section. https://www.acep.org/how-we-serve/sections/air-medical-transport/. Accessed September 1, 2018.

of obstructions. Weather can impact helicopter operations more profoundly than other transport modalities, with specific limitations of visibility, precipitation, icing, and wind. The cabin of the helicopter is considerably smaller and more limiting than a ground ambulance and can make in-flight clinical interventions very difficult. Weight and balance is extremely important in helicopters and can limit the amount of equipment onboard and the size/configuration of the medical crew. Helmets and headsets are necessary for the crew to provide both hearing protection and to facilitate communication over the loud aircraft; methods to provide hearing protection to the patient are essential, as there is a large amount of noise. Altitude and flight physiology are factors associated with the use of a helicopter, and the crew must be educated on these factors. The costs associated with the use of a helicopter are significantly higher than ground transport. The cost effectiveness and overuse have been called into question for both adult and pediatric patients and should be monitored closely by the program administrators.

Fixed Wing

There are approximately 150,000 **fixed wing** (airplane) transports annually in the United States.[22] The use of fixed wing transport is typically reserved for long distances often greater than 150 miles, building on ability to cover greater distances and travel at high speeds. Additional advantages include a pressurized cabin, lessening the risk of high altitudes. The cabin space is relatively large and can accommodate specialized equipment and several crew members. Fixed wing aircraft can often fly in weather conditions that are suboptimal for helicopters. The most notable disadvantage of fixed wing transport is the need to land at and depart from an airport, requiring a secondary patient transfer, usually using a ground ambulance, to and from the location of the patient. Additionally, fixed wing transport often requires more extensive time to mobilize and initiate the transport.

The Role of Medical Control

Although many transport teams may function without a physician or mid-level provider on board, medical control of the team during transport is critical. The medical control physician helps to guide decisions for mode of transport (in collaboration with the referring facility) and provides medical leadership and oversight for clinical care.

Triage and Mode of Transportation

Critical care transport of the neonatal or pediatric patient is generally initiated in one of two circumstances: scene transport or interfacility transport. Scene transport calls are generally initiated by the EMS crews at the scene of the accident or injury. Triage of scene transports is generally managed by local EMS protocols or recommendations of national EMS agencies.[23] Table 33-2 outlines the most succinct policy statement on the use of air medical helicopters, although not specific to infants or children, which was put forth by the American College of Emergency Physicians.[24]

More commonly, neonatal and pediatric transports are interfacility in nature. The intake or triage of referrals from community hospitals or ambulatory care facilities is often fielded through a centralized communication center. The centralized communication center is usually staffed with a communication specialist, often with nursing or EMS training, who serves as the valuable communication link among the referring facility, the receiving facility, the medical team, the pilots, and the medical control physician.[25] The referral call generally results in direct communication between the receiving medical control physician and the referring clinician, allowing the medical control physician to understand the nature of the clinical care that may be necessary for the patient, understand the resources that may be necessary to provide the clinical care upon return to the receiving facility, and provide additional clinical management recommendations. Furthermore, the nature of the referral can help facilitate decisions around the use of air transport or ground transport. The primary decision around preferred mode of transportation is managed by the referring clinician, specifically that the transfer must be made with qualified personnel and the appropriate medical equipment.

Medical Control Communication

After the initial triage communication between the referring facility and the medical control physician or accepting physician, the role of the medical control physician transitions to the oversight of the clinical management of the care for the transferred patient. In many instances, appropriately trained residents in emergency medicine or pediatrics, fellowship trainees, or even attending physicians provide direct, hands-on medical control as a member of the transport team. Commonly, however, the medical control physician is simply the remote clinical oversight for the critical care transport team who is at the bedside of the patient. In those instances, immediate availability of the medical control physician is expected to provide clinical guidance and to make treatment recommendations in accordance with critical care transport clinical protocols that govern the team's care. In order to optimize this role of the remote medical control physician, some teams have adopted video telemedicine to augment either the initial triage conversation or the ongoing medical control communication.[26,27] The medical director may sometimes serve as medical control physician, although the medical director's responsibilities extend further and include development of clinical protocols, quality improvement activities, oversight of training and competencies, and clinical case reviews.

Equipment

Transport teams should be equipped with medications and supplies to be self-sufficient. Dedicated supplies for the care for injured or ill pediatric/neonatal patients should be organized and ready for quick access. State regulations in most instances identify the minimum needs for licensure as a mobile intensive care unit; however, critical care teams typically exceed those needs based on their mission profile. Comprehensive lists of recommended transport equipment are available for review in multiple publications.[10,28] Supplies and medications should be ample enough to last the entire transport time, and it is not recommended that the teams rely on borrowing from the sending facilities. **Table 33-3** provides an example of the equipment stored in a respiratory care flight bag. It is important to note that many teams have an additional pouch or bag specific to airway management, which includes laryngoscope blades, handles, endotracheal tubes, airway adjuncts, and medications for rapid sequence intubation. There are also

bags specific to nursing and general medical-surgical supplies. Medication bags are particularly relevant for neonatal/pediatric patients, as pediatric or neonatal specialty medications are often not available in typical concentrations or formulations at the referring facility. Equipment and medication bags should be checked on a routine basis to ensure that equipment is available and properly maintained.

The equipment needs to be portable, rugged, lightweight, and easy to clean, and it needs to meet hospital, state, and federal requirements. Additional

---

TABLE 33-3

Example of the Contents of a Ventilator-Specific Respiratory Care Flight Bag (the bag is assembled with a series of pouches to keep contents organized and easily accessible)

Pouch 1: Adaptor Bag

Christmas tree adaptor
Red cap
15-mm adaptor
22-mm adaptor
Pediatric omni flex
Adult omni flex
Infant heat moisture exchanger (HME)
Pediatric HME
Adult HME
O_2 tubing
Preemie RAM cannula
Newborn RAM cannula
Infant RAM cannula
Peds RAM cannula

Pouch 2: Pediatric Specialty Laryngoscope Blades

Six #1 to #4 macintosh (MAC) blades

Pouch 3: NIV Masks

Small BiPAP mask
Medium BiPAP mask
Large BiPAP mask

Pouch 4: High-Pressure Adaptors and Hoses

Quick connect adaptors for oxygen and air (i.e. Fairfield, Chemtron)
Air flowmeter
Air pigtail

Pouch 5: Oxygen and ETCO$_2$ Adaptors and Ventilator Circuits

O_2 high-pressure hose
Neonatal transport ventilator circuit
Adult mainstream ETCO$_2$ adaptor
Infant/pediatric mainstream ETCO$_2$ adaptor
Pediatric transport ventilator circuit
Adult transport ventilator circuit

Inside Top Pocket

Ventilator quick reference cards

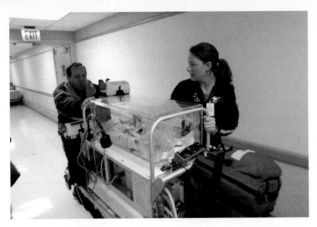

FIGURE 33-3 An example of a transport isolette used for ground critical care transport.

consideration is required for equipment onboard aircraft, as it needs to adhere to the Federal Aviation Administration requirements and needs to have been tested in the transport environment. Various types of isolettes with stretchers are available and must provide regulated temperature, oxygen, and humidity as well as allow for easy access during transport. **Figure 33-3** provides an example of a transport isolette. The safety of equipment storage in transport is mandatory. There are approved methods for securing equipment in the transport vehicles. Different devices for securing patients exist and are based on the patient's age and weight. Proper storage and dispensing of medications is essential for safe and effective care, and some medications, such as surfactant and prostaglandins, require special procedures for storage. Some highly specialized neonatal and pediatric critical care transport teams carry nitric oxide, heliox, blood products, and even extracorporeal membrane oxygenation equipment. In these circumstances, devices to facilitate proper gas mixture and measurements are required, additional power and space requirements exist, and proper refrigeration of blood products is necessary.

Oxygen and air cylinders must be labeled and checked, and there must be enough onboard to meet at least twice the anticipated needs for supply. Just like the equipment, medications need to be checked and restocked routinely before and after every transport. High-pressure cylinders should be stored in a safe, dedicated place between transports and in accordance with manufacturer's recommendations for the temperature and humidity of the storage room. Transport teams should come prepared and always assume that the sending facility does not carry the specialized medications or fluids. The medications lists should include intravenous fluids, inotropic agents, resuscitative medications, rapid sequence intubation induction and paralytic medications, antibiotics, prostaglandins, surfactant preparations, asthma and croup medications, and anticonvulsants. For hospital-based transport teams, institutional policies govern the

documentation requirements for controlled substances and the process for replenishing supplies after use.

Clinical Care in Pediatric and Neonatal Critical Care Transport

Clinical management of the acutely ill or injured child is both similar and dissimilar from inpatient neonatal intensive care unit (NICU), PICU, and emergency department care. The overlap with hospital-based, often tertiary, care lies in the physiology of the patients. Generally, the extremes of weather and/or altitude are unique to transport care. However, the physiology and principles of clinical management of the transported neonate or child mirror the care provided in hospital-based settings. Neurologic, cardiac, and pulmonary management concepts are different when considering physical settings for the care (unfamiliar space and resources at a referring hospital or even in a remote wilderness setting), the equipment options are generally fewer, and the depth of backup clinical expertise is often nonexistent. Here we will highlight a few specific clinical management priorities in the transport setting.

Airway Care

Airway management is lifesaving and has been studied in multiple settings. Tracheal intubation (TI) is generally the primary means for definitive airway management. In the pediatric prehospital setting, first TI attempt success rate was 66%, with 11% of attempts having associated major complications.[29,30] A 2016 study in pediatric emergency departments demonstrated 83% first-pass TI success, with a 15% adverse event rate.[31] More recently, Bigham et al.[32] describe first-attempt intubation success in transport, including in specific patient populations. First attempt TI success rate was 59.3% in neonates, 81.7% in pediatric patients, and 87% adults.

Alternative airway management devices are growing in popularity, with the most popular being supraglottic airways. Supraglottic airways are appealing for both ease of use and effectiveness. In the neonatal/pediatric population, large-scale studies using supraglottic airways do not exist, although numerous small studies confirm that in complex airways, failed intubations, and rescue from failed intubations, there is a valuable role for supraglottic airways.

Mechanical Ventilation

Airway management is valuable only when coupled with mechanical ventilation. Two broad mechanical ventilation categories exist: noninvasive and invasive ventilation. It is, however, important to clarify that mechanical ventilation is an essential tool for the critical care transport team—so much so that Delphi-achieved consensus quality metrics identified the use of mechanical ventilation in an intubated transport patient as a key quality metric.[33] In the transport setting, such issues as power and gas supplies and isolette-embedded ventilators are among some of the key transport-unique considerations.

Altitude

Issues related to the impact of altitude in the critical care management of an infant and/or child are important features of any transport clinical discussion. At altitude, the partial pressure of oxygen and barometric pressure are lower. The two biggest implications of this topic are related to gas expansion within a contained space and hypoxia. Boyle's law reminds us that *pressure × volume = constant*. Thus, gas volume expands under conditions where pressure is lower. This can impact tracheal tube cuff volume (increased volume at altitude with lower pressure), with resulting increasing cuff pressure that increases linearly with increasing altitude. The clinical impact on a cuff that is inflated to minimally occlusive pressure at ground level is that when flying, either by helicopter or fixed wing transport, it may expand, causing increased mucosal pressure on the intubated child. Based on the same physics, a pneumothorax, pneumopericardium, or even gaseous distended stomach/bowel will expand with decreased atmospheric pressure at higher altitude. Based on the alveolar gas equation where P_{atmos} is atmospheric pressure, P_{H2O} is water pressure, and RQ is the respiratory quotient ($PaO_2 = (FiO_2 \times (P_{atmos} - P_{H2O})) - (PaCO_2 / RQ)$), the lower atmospheric pressure at higher altitude can impact oxygenation, clinically requiring an increase in FiO_2 to achieve the same PaO_2.

Family on Transport

Clinical, operational, and safety elements of a critical care transport team are paramount. However, issues of patient/family-centered care cannot be discounted. The impact of family presence during resuscitation and in the hospital-based care setting has consistently demonstrated the value of family presence on transport. Application of that concept to the critical care transport setting has been more difficult. For the transported neonate immediately following birth, the mother is often still receiving medical care herself, making it unsafe for her to transport. In fact, many programs standardly disallow a mother to ride with the critically ill newborn until she has been both cleared by her physician and is 24 hours postpartum. Air transport adds another layer of family presence complexity due to the close proximity of the family member to the crew, the consistently high stress of the situation, and family anxiety with unfamiliarity of helicopter or fixed wing travel. Joyce[34] reported family presence in an Ohio pediatric/neonatal transport as ranging from 23% to 66%. It is imperative that programs develop their own process for family presence on transport and that the policies and standard work to accomplish that in a way that is safest for the crew, the patient, and the family member.

Neonatal/pediatric transport has many features and challenges similar to adult transport, along with many additional unique clinical and operational entities. These differences reinforce the mantra that holds true on the inpatient care of infants and children as well: Children are not just little adults.

Case Study

A female infant weighing 650 g was born vaginally at 24 6/7 weeks of gestation in a small rural hospital. Her mother was admitted a few hours prior to delivery for ruptured membranes and sudden onset of premature labor. The Apgar scores were 5 at 1 minute and 8 at 5 minutes. Arrangements were made for transport to a Level 3 NICU. Once the rotor wing transport was confirmed, the team consisting of a registered nurse, paramedic, and respiratory therapist prepared for transport by gathering and loading their equipment in the aircraft and performing pre-flight safety checks. The team discussed a plan of care during the transport with the medical control physician and referring physician by conference call. During the 75-mile flight to the referring hospital, the team reviewed an emergency response plan by discussing their response to such scenarios as endotracheal tube malposition, hypoxemia, and hemodynamic instability during flight. Team members reviewed their roles and agreed to the plan prior to arriving at the referral facility. After assuming care, based on the clinical assessment, chest radiograph and arterial blood gas results and consultation with the medical control physician, the infant was intubated, surfactant replacement therapy was administered, and mechanical ventilatory support was initiated. The neonate was also given 250 mL/kg of fluid by IV to stabilize the blood pressure. During the return flight to the tertiary care center, the infant was hemodynamically stable, ventilator parameters were adjusted as needed based on vital signs, SpO_2 and $pETCO_2$ values, and the protocol outlined for this patient's plan of care. On arrival of the team to the NICU, handoff of care was provided, which included a report of clinical care and assessing the patient before care was transferred to the NICU team.

1. **Describe the varying models of crew configuration.**

2. **What type of skills/requirements are important for a member of the transport team?**

3. **Compare and contrast ground mobile ICU and fixed and rotor wing transport modes. Could this transport have been done using a different mode of transport?**

References

1. Orr RA, Felmet KA, Han Y, et al. Pediatric specialized transport teams are associated with improved outcomes. *Pediatrics*. 2009;124(1):40-48.

2. Han YY, Carcillo JA, Dragotta MA, et al. Early reversal of pediatric-neonatal septic shock by community physicians is associated with improved outcome. *Pediatrics*. 2003;112(4):793-799.

3. Meyer MT, Mikhailov TA, Kuhn EM, Collins MM, Scanlon MC. Pediatric specialty transport teams are not associated with decreased 48-hour pediatric intensive care unit mortality: a propensity analysis of the VPS, LLC database. *Air Med J*. 2016;35(2):73-79.

4. American Academy of Pediatrics. Section on Transport Medicine. *Guidelines for Air and Ground Transport of Neonatal and Pediatric Patients*. 3rd ed. Elk Grove Village, IL: American Academy of Pediatrics; 2007.

5. Tanem J, Triscari D, Chan M, Meyer MT. Workforce survey of pediatric interfacility transport systems in the United States. *Pediatr Emerg Care*. 2016;32(6):364-370.

6. Karlsen KA, Trautman M, Price-Douglas W, Smith S. National survey of neonatal transport teams in the United States. *Pediatrics*. 2011;128(4):685-691.

7. van Lieshout EJ, Binnekade J, Reussien E, et al. Nurses versus physician-led interhospital critical care transport: a randomized non-inferiority trial. *Intensive Care Med*. 2016;42(7):1146-1154.

8. Edge WE, Kanter RK, Weigle CG, Walsh RF. Reduction of morbidity in interhospital transport by specialized pediatric staff. *Crit Care Med*. 1994;22(7):1186-1191.

9. Commission on Accreditation of Medical Transport Systems. http://www.camts.org/10th_Edition_Standards_For_Website.pdf. Accessed October 21, 2016.

10. American Academy of Pediatrics. Section on Transport Medicine. *Guidelines for Air and Ground Transport of Neonatal and Pediatric Patients*. 4th ed. Elk Grove Village, IL: American Academy of Pediatrics; 2016.

11. Kuszajewski ML, O'Donnell JM, Phrampus PE, Robey WC 3rd, Tuite PK. Airway management: a structured curriculum for critical care transport providers. *Air Med J*. 2016;35(3):138-142.

12. Alfes CM, Steiner SL, Manacci CF. Critical care transport training: new strides in simulating the austere environment. *Air Med J*. 2015;34(4):186-187.

13. Abrahamsen HB, Sollid SJ, Öhlund LS, Røislien J, Bondevik GT. Simulation-based training and assessment of non-technical skills in the Norwegian Helicopter Emergency Medical Services: a cross-sectional survey. *Emerg Med J*. 2015;32(8):647-653.

14. LeFlore JL, Anderson M. Effectiveness of 2 methods to teach and evaluate new content to neonatal transport personnel using high-fidelity simulation. *J Perinat Neonatal Nurs*. 2008;22(4):319-328.

15. Bigelow AM, Gothard MD, Schwartz HP, Bigham MT. Intubation in pediatric/neonatal critical care transport: national performance. *Prehos Emerg Care*. 2015;19(3):351-357.

16. Air Medical Physician Association. Position Papers. https://www.ampa.org/?page_id=11372. Accessed September 1, 2018.

17. Krainz T. AAP Transport LISTSERV™: A Mechanism to Inform Research and Educational Agendas. AAP Transport Listserve. Accessed October 20, 2016.

18. Helmreich RL, Merritt AC, Wilhelm JA. The evolution of crew resource management training in commercial aviation. *Int J Aviat Psychol*. 1999;9(1):19-32.

19. National Institutes of Health. *Crossing the Quality Chasm: A New Health System for the 21st Century*. Washington, DC: National Institutes of Health; 2001.

20. Huber, M. AIN Special Reports. https://www.ainonline.com/aviation-news/special-reports. Accessed September 1, 2018.

21. International Civil Aviation Organization. *Safety Management Manual*. Quebec, Canada: International Civil Aviation Organization; 2009.

22. Association of Air Medical Services. http://aams.org/member-services/fact-sheet-faqs/. Accessed October 22, 2016.

23. American College of Emergency Physicians. Policy Statements. https://www.acep.org/patient-care/policy-statements/#sm.00014oj3jul8we6oy8m1ji6ybs67u. Accessed September 1, 2018.

24. American College of Emergency Physicians. Air Medical Transport Section. https://www.acep.org/how-we-serve/sections/air-medical-transport/#sm.00014oj3jul8we6oy8m1ji6ybs67u. Accessed September 1, 2018.

25. International Association of Medical Transport Communication Specialists. http://www.iamtcs.org/resources.html. Accessed November 3, 2016.

26. Tsai SH, Kraus J, Wu HR, et al. The effectiveness of video-telemedicine for screening of patients requesting emergency air medical transport (EAMT). *J Trauma*. 2007;62(2):504-511.

27. Patel S, Hertzog JH, Penfil S, Slamon N. A prospective pilot study of the use of telemedicine during pediatric transport: a high-quality, low-cost alternative to conventional telemedicine systems. *Pediatr Emerg Care*. 2015;31(9):611-615.

28. American College of Surgeons. Equipment for Ambulances. https://www.facs.org/~/media/files/quality%20programs/trauma/publications/ambulance.ashx. Accessed September 1, 2018.

29. Prekker ME, Delgado F, Shin J, et al. Pediatric intubation by paramedics in a large emergency medical services system: process, challenges, and outcomes. *Ann Emerg Med*. 2016;67(1):20-29.

30. Gausche M, Lewis RJ. Out-of-hospital endotracheal intubation of children. *JAMA*. 2000;283(21):2790-2792.

31. Bigelow AM, Gothard MD, Schwartz HP, Bigham MT. Intubation in pediatric/neonatal critical care transport: national performance. *Prehosp Emerg Care*. 2015;19(3):351-357.

32. Dwyer RC, Walls RM, Brown CA 3rd; NEAR III Investigators. Techniques and trends, success rates, and adverse events in emergency department pediatric intubations: a report from the National Emergency Airway Registry. *Ann Emerg Med*. 2016;67(5):610-615.

33. Ground and Air Medical Quality in Transport. The Vision. http://gamutqi.org. Accessed October 22, 2016.

34. Joyce CN, Libertin R, Bigham MT. Family-centered care in pediatric critical care transport. *Air Med J*. 2015;34(1):32-36.

34

The Respiratory Technology–Dependent Infant and Child

L. Denise Willis

OUTLINE

OBJECTIVES

1. List the benefits of caring for a respiratory technology–dependent child at home.
2. Recognize the risks of caring for a respiratory technology–dependent child at home.
3. Define the role of a multidisciplinary discharge planning team.
4. List the criteria that must be met before a respiratory technology–dependent child may be discharged home.
5. Discuss the preparation and education required of the respiratory technology–dependent child's caregivers.
6. Describe what is included in a home evaluation and what preparations should be made in the home prior to a respiratory technology–dependent child's discharge from the hospital.
7. List the medical equipment that may be used in the home of a respiratory technology–dependent child.
8. Describe the activities that will occur on the day of discharge.
9. Identify barriers to discharge from the hospital.
10. Discuss outpatient care of the respiratory technology–dependent child.
11. Explain the process of transitioning a respiratory technology–dependent child from pediatric to adult care.

KEY TERMS

discharge planning
home evaluation
home medical equipment company
home nursing agency
home ventilator

primary caregiver
rooming-in
secondary caregiver
technology-dependent child
trach go bag
transition to adult care

Introduction

In 1987, the Office of Technology Assessment defined the **technology-dependent child** as one who requires both a life-sustaining medical device and ongoing nursing care.[1] This includes children dependent upon respiratory technology in the home setting, such as those who have a tracheostomy and/or require mechanical ventilation to maintain pulmonary stability. Other types of respiratory technology used in the home include aerosol and airway clearance devices and non-invasive ventilator support. This chapter will focus on the child who is both tracheostomy dependent and ventilator dependent.

To be safely managed at home, respiratory technology–dependent children must have committed, trained caregivers to provide direct care and supervision 24 hours a day, 7 days a week. Using a multidisciplinary team approach, extensive preparation, time, and effort is invested in training caregivers and planning the discharge home for these medically fragile children. Once transitioned home, they require ongoing care from outpatient specialists, home nursing services, and home equipment providers. One of the major challenges in the management of respiratory technology–dependent children is that they are not a homogenous group of individuals. They are medically complex and have a wide variety of diagnoses, such as neuromuscular disease, neurologic conditions, chronic lung disease of prematurity, or conditions affecting control of breathing. Many typically also have one or more comorbidities further complicating their care.

The American Association for Respiratory Care (AARC) defines the goals of home mechanical ventilation as to sustain and prolong life, enhance quality of life, reduce morbidity, improve or maintain physical and psychological function, and provide cost-effective care.[2] Specifically for pediatrics, there is an additional goal to enhance growth and development.[2]

There are two groups of children who discharge home with a tracheostomy and ventilator. One group eventually weans from the ventilator and may be able to have the tracheostomy removed, such as may be the case with chronic lung disease of prematurity. Due to the nature of their diagnosis, as is often seen with progressive neuromuscular disease or spinal cord injury, the other group receives the tracheostomy and requires the ventilator for their lifetime. Regardless of the need for respiratory technology, the primary goal is for a discharge home and to integrate the child as part of the family unit.

The Maternal and Child Health Bureau estimates that 15% of all youth aged 0 to 17 years in the United States have special healthcare needs.[3] As a result of improved medical care and advancements in technology, there is a growing population of respiratory technology–dependent children. They are living longer and often surviving into adulthood. This has

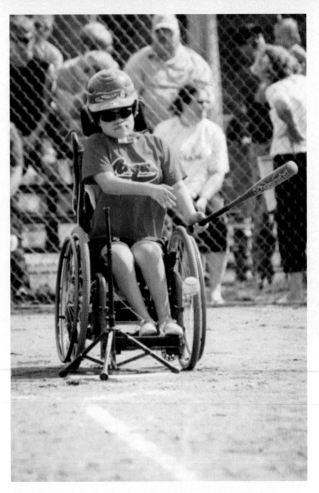

FIGURE 34-1 Respiratory technology–dependent child enjoying a family outing.

created the need for adult providers with experience in caring for young adults with special health needs. It is not uncommon for some respiratory technology–dependent young adults to attend college and enter the workforce.

Having a tracheostomy and requiring a ventilator does not mean the child is resigned to the home environment. Depending on the circumstances, these children attend public school, participate in community activities, and take family vacations when possible. However, there are special considerations and preparations required for these children to go outside the home. **Figure 34-1** pictures a respiratory technology–dependent child enjoying activities outside the home.

Preparing for Discharge

In regard to preparing for discharge home, the single difference between the child with only a tracheostomy and the child who also requires mechanical ventilation is simply the ventilator equipment itself. All the same requirements for caregiver training, monitoring, and home preparation remain regardless of whether a ventilator is needed. The only additional requirement for the ventilator-dependent child is caregiver instruction in operating and troubleshooting equipment specific to the ventilator. Although the ventilator is considered life-support equipment, tracheostomy education is perhaps the most vital element that must be mastered to safely care for these children in the home setting.

There is an extensive amount of training that caregivers must undergo before the child requiring a tracheostomy and long-term mechanical ventilation can safely discharge home. However, prior to any training or home preparations being initiated, it will need to be determined who will be the direct care providers and if the home is adequate for the child and can support the equipment. Family meetings with the medical team are helpful to discuss the requirements. Some institutions develop a contract agreement for caregivers to sign that outlines the expectations for training and all requirements that must be met before discharge home can occur. In an ideal situation, caregivers will have already been informed of all requirements before the decision is made to place a tracheostomy and provide long-term mechanical ventilation in the home.

Planning for the discharge home of the tracheostomy- and/or ventilator-dependent child is a process that takes time. Nurses and respiratory therapists attend specialized schools for several years to learn how to care for patients. Caregivers are often expected to become experts and competent with the skills in just a matter of weeks. It is vitally important to tailor the education to the individual caregiver and to ensure that they fully comprehend the information provided and can demonstrate the knowledge and skills necessary to care for their child at home.

Transition from Hospital to Home

The ultimate goal for the respiratory technology–dependent child is to transition home, when and if that option is available. There are multiple benefits to caring for the child at home. However, there are also risks that must be recognized.

Benefits of Providing Care at Home

The child's home is preferred over the hospital for several reasons, including a reduced risk of infection, decreased cost, and improved quality of life. The home also provides a better atmosphere for addressing psychosocial and developmental needs. Although the aim of the hospital setting is to maintain medical stability during acute illness, it was never intended to be a permanent residence. The hospital can be a noisy environment, with little distinction between night and day, limited social interaction, restricted mobility, and sterile surroundings.[4] On the contrary, home is more personable, with established routines and schedules as well as familial interaction and nurturing that is often limited in the hospital due to demands of staff providing medical care. Once deemed medically stable, the healthcare team should begin developing a plan for discharge home.

Children who have a tracheostomy and/or require mechanical ventilation are at high risk for recurrent respiratory infections and related complications, emergency department visits, and hospital readmissions. The probability of infection is theoretically less at home due to decreased exposure to nosocomial illnesses. Other children in the community admitted to the hospital with infectious disease pose a threat to the respiratory technology–dependent child. Minimizing potential sick contacts when possible is an important step in ensuring optimal health.

Compared to hospitalization, providing long-term mechanical ventilation at home is less costly. Although the initial expense for the equipment, supplies, nursing services, and ongoing maintenance may be elevated, the overall cost is lower compared to remaining in the hospital.[4,5] When readmissions can be avoided and/or decreased, costs can be further reduced. Many institutions manage medically stable ventilator-dependent children in the intensive care unit (ICU) as the wards are generally not equipped to handle ventilator equipment. As expected, ICU stays cost more than the regular hospital wards. However, there are some institutions that have designated units, similar to a step-down unit, that are specially designed for long-term ventilated children. Such a unit can provide a more structured environment for the discharge planning process to be initiated and accomplished. These chronic ventilator-dependent units may also be used when hospital readmission is necessary but an ICU admission is not warranted.

Ventilator-dependent children often thrive in their home environment and will meet developmental milestones sooner than if hospitalized, as prolonged hospitalization can delay growth and development. Studies have shown that improvements occur in physical, emotional, psychological, and social aspects when these children are cared for at home.[6] Many ventilator-dependent children attend school and enjoy recreation and leisure activities, such as watching television, listening to music, playing games, and attending sporting events.[7] Family and community integration, as well as peer interaction, are important for developing social skills and help to instill a sense of normalcy. Children with chronic health problems often yearn to be regarded as "normal" and to be treated as such.[6]

Risks of Providing Care at Home

Although discharge home is the ultimate goal, it is not without inherent hazards. These children are extremely vulnerable and have an increased risk of death due to the presence of the tracheostomy tube. The ventilator further increases risk, especially if the child is unable to maintain any spontaneous breathing efforts. Despite advances in technology and care, preventable deaths of the tracheostomy- and ventilator-dependent child have not considerably improved in the past 20 years.[8] Caregivers who did not receive adequate training or who cannot demonstrate the required skills necessary to care for the tracheostomy- and ventilator-dependent child present considerable danger to the child's safety. Insufficient staffing of home nursing can also jeopardize care. This is especially true in those circumstances where caregivers heavily depend on the home nurse to provide the majority of the child's care.

Home nursing services are never guaranteed for many reasons, and therefore the caregiver must have an alternate plan in the event the home nurse is unable to be present. For example, the home nurse could become acutely ill or may be suddenly unable to report to work due to a personal emergency. The caregivers will then have to either provide the care themselves or have other trained individuals attend to the child. The child with a tracheostomy should never be left with an untrained caregiver, as this has a high potential for a very unfortunate and disastrous outcome. Sadly, this has happened when caregivers became desperate due to lack of help at home. Additionally, some caregivers may become overly confident or complacent and forget the reality of how fragile their respiratory technology–dependent child remains despite being relatively stable.

Nurses seeking employment often do not consider private duty home nursing and prefer the hospital or clinic setting. This has resulted in a shortage of home nurses and those who are proficient in caring for the respiratory technology–dependent child. A survey of caregivers of ventilator-dependent children identified that home care was often disrupted due to a lack of nursing staff as well as nurses being deficient in knowledge and skills.[8] A study assessing the skills of home care nurses revealed that the majority were not proficient in respiratory assessment, tracheostomy care and tube change, suctioning, managing tracheostomy emergencies, and troubleshooting the ventilator.[8] To address this issue, some programs have created education curricula geared toward home nurses, as currently most of the training received may be through video or online instruction.[8] Ongoing education, including updates in clinical practice for caring for the tracheostomy- and ventilator-dependent child, is an important consideration for all nursing agencies.

The availability of night nursing in particular can directly impact the health and well-being of caregivers. A study examining the relationship between home nursing coverage and daytime function of caregivers found that those who had regular night nursing coverage slept more than those who did not.[9] Additionally, caregivers who had less night nursing hours exhibited more signs of depression and sleepiness.

No standards of care exist for determining how many hours of nursing should be provided at home and it varies greatly from state to state, depending upon the payer. Some state-funded insurance programs approve nursing services in the home for children who have a tracheostomy alone and do not require a ventilator while others will only authorize nursing hours for those requiring both a tracheostomy and a ventilator. In some instances, it is further restricted to only when the child requires the ventilator—for example, nursing hours are approved only for the hours when the child uses the ventilator at night.

Other risks for home care include caregiver stress and fatigue, financial loss, and lack of community and financial resources. Attending to the ventilator-dependent child is demanding and can consume the caregiver as it is a 24-hour-a day, 7-day-a week continuous occupation. The care burden can impact families by creating marital discord, draining financial resources, and enhancing sibling rivalry. Because trained caregivers must always be available in the event that the home nurse cannot be present, this may affect the caregiver's ability to continue employment outside the home, therefore directly impacting the ability to support the family unit. Caregivers of these children are at high risk for burnout and fatigue. Caregivers often suffer from disrupted sleep and lack of social interaction. Their livelihood becomes centered on the child's technology and can lead to social isolation and depression when there is no time for personal interests or other outlets for coping.[10] Caregivers still need to devote time to themselves or they will be unable to efficiently care for their child. Networking with other caregivers of ventilator-dependent children can be a means of social support and a venue for sharing frustrations as well as obtaining helpful information and resources about which some caregivers may not be fully informed. However, it can also be a source of misinformation, so caution must be taken when making networking recommendations.

Home is supposed to be a place of security, privacy, and comfort where individuals are surrounded by familiar faces, sights, sounds, and daily rituals.[6] As accommodations are made for the medical equipment and there is a near-constant presence of nurses and medical equipment company personnel in the home, privacy is invaded and the traditional meaning of home is altered.[6] The lines between hospital and home can become blurred with the constant medical needs and presence of technology. The home equipment can also be noisy, causing disruption to other family members.

In cases where there are inadequate resources to provide care at home, the medical team, including the social worker, should become involved to address the issue. If for any reason the caregivers are unable or unwilling to provide their child's care, and home nursing services cannot be reasonably staffed, then an alternative site of care must be considered, such as a skilled nursing facility with experience in caring for ventilator-dependent children.

Multidisciplinary Discharge Planning Team

To achieve a successful transition home, discharge planning requires a truly dedicated team of individuals devoted to caring for the ventilator-dependent child. There are many disciplines involved, including physicians, nurses, respiratory therapists, discharge planners, nutritionists, child life specialists, and social workers. Some facilities even have psychology services available. The home care agencies, as well as the child and caregivers, should also be considered part of the multidisciplinary team. Each team member has a specific role in planning for the discharge home. **Table 34-1** lists possible members of a multidisciplinary discharge planning team.

The role of the **discharge planning** team is not only to ensure that education and training are provided for home but also to define caregiver expectations that must be met so that the child can safely be cared for at home. Communication between team members is vital to make certain that all participants are aware of the plan of care and goals for discharge. Medical rounds and discharge planning meetings provide a useful means for multidisciplinary team member interaction and for updating the plan of care. Prior to any meetings with caregivers, it is prudent for the medical team to convene in advance and to confirm that all members are knowledgeable about the child and informed of the discharge plan. Poorly planned meetings portray disorganization, cause caregiver confusion, and may lead to distrust of the medical team. Therefore, a preconference discussion with the medical team prior to meeting with caregivers is highly encouraged.

The physician manages the child's care by prescribing ventilator settings, respiratory treatments, and other related medications. Depending on the underlying diagnosis, there will most likely be more than one physician and/or specialty involved that will focus on the related aspect of care. A pulmonologist will typically manage the ventilator and respiratory issues. An otolaryngologist may manage tracheostomy care while a cardiologist may be needed to address heart disorders. The ventilator-dependent child will still require a primary care physician (PCP) once discharged to address general care issues as well as to coordinate care and referrals to specialists when indicated.

The role of the hospital nurse and respiratory therapist is multifaceted in caring for the ventilator-dependent child. Generally they not only provide direct care at the bedside but also may be involved in training and education for the family. While the respiratory therapist assists with ventilator evaluation and management and administers aerosol and airway clearance therapies, this presents a unique opportunity to help prepare caregivers for administering the care at home. Those who provide education for home should remain cognizant of the variations and/or modifications in how some modalities may be done in the home setting compared to the hospital, such as clean versus sterile technique for suctioning. More on this subject is discussed later within this chapter.

The discharge planner is responsible for arranging all the home medical equipment, supplies, and services, including home nursing and any therapies, such as physical, occupational, and speech therapy, that may be prescribed after discharge. Some institutions are fortunate to have a nurse discharge planner and a respiratory therapy discharge planner who both work closely with the home care providers. In these instances, the respiratory discharge planner will ensure that all the home respiratory equipment and supplies are obtained while the nurse discharge planner will make arrangements for home nursing services, therapies, enteral formula, and related equipment and supplies as well as nonrespiratory equipment, such as wheelchairs and beds.

Other important members of the multidisciplinary team caring for the ventilator-dependent child include the nutritionist, child life specialist, social worker, speech therapist, occupational therapist, physical therapist, and sometimes psychology where available. Each of these disciplines brings an area of expertise to provide value-added service for these medically fragile children. There is consistency and continuity of care when these team members are assigned specifically to respiratory technology–dependent children.

An often overlooked group of individuals also dedicated to caring for tracheostomy- and ventilator-dependent children are the home care agencies, which similarly includes respiratory therapists, nurses, and various other therapists, such as physical, occupational, and speech. Although these entities may not be directly involved until the child is discharged, it is important for the inpatient team to

TABLE 34-1
Multidisciplinary Discharge Planning Team

Hospital Team	Home Care Team
• Physician • Nurse practitioner • Nurses • Respiratory therapist • RN case manager/discharge planner • Respiratory care case manager/discharge planner • Social worker • Nutritionist • Child life specialist • Physical therapist • Speech therapist • Occupational therapist • Pharmacist • Chaplain • Insurance case manager	• Medical equipment company • Home nursing agency • Outpatient therapies in the community

collaborate and partner with them, as they are often the eyes and ears once the child is at home. Open communication between home agencies and the inpatient team is vital during the discharge planning process in order to avoid potentially preventable problems once the child is home. When the child is home, the agencies will also need access to the medical team who will follow the child in the outpatient clinic setting.

In the era of family-centered care, arguably the most important members of the team are the child and their caregivers. The role of good communication with caregivers cannot be overstressed. Consideration should also be given to allow caregivers to participate in discharge planning meetings. If caregivers are unable to physically attend, technology has made possible other means of interaction, such as phone or video conferencing. This encourages active participation from caregivers in the care of their child.

Criteria for Discharge Home

In order for the tracheostomy- and ventilator-dependent child to be safely cared for at home, several criteria must first be met, including medical stability, identified caregivers, training and education, and availability of home services. Inadequacy in one or more of these areas can prolong hospitalization, delaying discharge. Although caregivers are always eager to take their child home, it is the responsibility of the medical team to ensure that it can be done safely and without harm. The best interests of the child should always be the primary consideration regardless of any other circumstances.

Medical Stability

To be considered medically stable for discharge home with a ventilator, the child must demonstrate cardiopulmonary stability as well as the absence of any physiologically unstable medical conditions that would require a greater degree of care and resources beyond what is accessible in the home.[2] This includes a fraction of inspired oxygen (FiO_2) requirement of less than 0.40, partial pressure of oxygen in arterial blood (PaO_2) greater than 60 mm Hg, positive end-expiratory pressure (PEEP) setting less than 10 cm H_2O, and a stable tracheostomy.[2,11] Oxygen systems for the home are generally not designed to deliver high liter flows. Additionally, an elevated FiO_2 need above 0.40 may imply low pulmonary reserve, meaning that a mild illness may lead to acute deterioration and hospital readmission instead of being able to be cared for at home.[11]

To be considered stable for discharge, there should be no need to make changes in the ventilator settings and FiO_2 in the 1 to 2 weeks prior to discharge.[12] High PEEP settings may also indicate a lack of stability. Complete airway collapse or lung decruitment can occur with ventilator disconnect in the presence of high PEEP requirements. Some children with airway issues, such as tracheal or subglottic stenosis, may be heavily dependent upon PEEP to maintain a patent airway.

Growth and nutrition are another consideration for medical stability, as nutritional status can directly impact pulmonary health. In most cases, the child should weigh at least 5 kg before attempting to trial the **home ventilator**, as most home ventilators have Food and Drug Administration approval for a minimum weight requirement of 5 kg. Previously, older models that are no longer available had a lower limit of 10 kg. Therefore, the newer technology allows medically stable children to attempt transition to the home ventilator sooner.

Skilled Caregivers

The standard of care for most institutions is that a minimum of two trained caregivers must be able to demonstrate the required skills and be available to devote their full attention to caring for the tracheostomy- and ventilator-dependent child. It can be more demanding than a full-time career, as the reality is there is no "time off" on weekends or holidays. Caring for a young child without special healthcare needs is already challenging in itself. Factor in the medical issues, tracheostomy and ventilator care, and all the medical equipment and it can become quite overwhelming. Although there must be at least two trained caregivers, both caregivers are not required to be present with the child at all times, but they must be readily available.

A minimum of two caregivers must be identified before discharge home can be considered. Caregivers may or may not be the biological parents. It is not uncommon that, for various reasons, the parents may be unable to provide care and grandparents, other family members, or friends may become involved. For example, one parent may be employed full-time while the other stays home with the child and takes on the role of **primary caregiver**. In this situation a grandparent, aunt or uncle, or personal friend may decide to train as the **secondary caregiver** to assist when needed. These children require constant supervision and monitoring, and the primary caregiver will need to run errands at some point or help care for other children in the home as well, so a secondary caregiver who can share responsibilities is necessary. In families with abundant social support, several family members or friends may decide to undergo training. Although private-duty home nursing services can be obtained, they are never a guarantee and should not be relied upon as the primary or sole source of care.

The designated caregivers must then receive extensive training and education in tracheostomy, ventilator equipment and troubleshooting, and other related aspects of care. A list of required skills should be provided to caregivers. Training is typically done by a member of the medical team. Caregivers are encouraged to practice skills under supervision as often as possible to become proficient and confident enough to eventually provide them without the assistance of the medical team. Before being allowed to discharge home, each caregiver who will be responsible for providing direct care to the child must demonstrate the skills and be validated by the medical team. Following successful demonstration and validation of all required skills, caregivers are then expected to assume care of the child for 24 to 72 hours, often referred to as **rooming-in**, depending upon institutional requirements. This rooming-in period occurs while the child remains in the hospital setting under supervision of the medical team. This is the final test to determine if the caregivers are competent to care for the child at home.

Available Home Medical Equipment and Nursing Staff

Throughout the course of education and training, the discharge planning team will assist caregivers with identifying home care providers, including the **home medical equipment company**, often referred to as the durable medical equipment (DME) company; **home nursing agency**; and any therapy services that may be indicated. All these services must be established and in place before discharge can be considered. The home must have passed inspection and any issues addressed and resolved before equipment can be delivered. All required home medical equipment, including respiratory devices and supplies, should be obtained before the child is ready for discharge. The follow-up plan with the PCP, otolaryngologist, pulmonologist, and other required specialists must also be in place.

Caregiver Education and Preparation

The discharge planning process begins once the decision is made to place a tracheostomy tube or provide mechanical ventilation at home. Discharge plans should be initiated as soon as possible to allow time for training and arrangement of all home services. When the child is a candidate for going home, a tentative discharge date should be set to allow caregivers adequate time for training and for preparing the home. At this point, a meeting between the medical team and caregivers should be held to define expectations for training and to outline all the required skills that must be completed before discharge can occur. The expectation of being available to train should be clearly defined. Caregivers should be fully informed of all the skills they will be

required to master and all the services that must be in place before discharge can occur.

Caregivers should be given information regarding how to prepare the home as well as the plan for outpatient follow-up. It should also be understood that although the tentative discharge date is a goal, it is subject to change depending on how the child tolerates the home ventilator and how caregiver training and home preparation progress. The discharge planning process can take weeks to months depending on individual circumstances. To prevent unnecessary delays in discharge, the medical team should routinely consult with caregivers, ensuring that training is ongoing and home preparations are continuing.

Caregivers should be encouraged to be present at the hospital as much as possible to learn the care required at home and to practice newly learned skills. It cannot be overstated or stressed enough that the more time caregivers are present to learn the care and practice skills while in the hospital, the more competent and comfortable they will become to provide the care at home. They should communicate with their child's nurses and respiratory therapists as to when they will be available to perform bedside care. By doing so, the child's daily schedule can be planned with time allowed for the caregivers to provide care. Learning about the ventilator is only one aspect of care. **Table 34-2** provides a complete listing of all respiratory-related training and education that must be completed before discharge home. Depending on the diagnosis and condition, caregivers may also be required to learn how to administer enteral feeds, use a feeding pump, and dispense medications through a gastrostomy tube. Additionally, there may be wheelchair, hospital bed, patient lift, and other related equipment in the home that caregivers must learn to operate.

Education Skill Proficiencies

From a respiratory standpoint, caregivers must be able to demonstrate proficiency in both routine and emergency tracheostomy tube change, routine tracheostomy care, and troubleshooting and maintaining the ventilator and related home equipment. It is essential that caregivers are able to recognize signs and symptoms of respiratory distress as well as to take appropriate action when increased work of breathing or changes in the child's condition have been identified. Although all the skills are important to master, the tracheostomy education and training could arguably be considered one of the most vital components. **Table 34-3** includes a complete listing of required elements for tracheostomy education and training. Ensuring caregiver competence through education and skills validation is an essential part in transitioning the respiratory technology–dependent child from hospital to home.

TABLE 34-2
Respiratory-Related Training and Education

Signs and symptoms of respiratory distress • Recognition • Response	Home ventilator • Settings and monitored parameters • Responding to alarms • Troubleshooting • Circuits and disposable supplies • External battery and charger • Emergency plan for electrical power outage

Humidification
• Heated humidifier
  • Proper placement relative to child
  • Adequately secured
• Heat and moisture exchanger (artificial nose)
• Speaking valve
• Air compressor with tracheostomy collar
	Suction device
	• Suction canister and tubing
	• Suction catheters
	• Suction pressure
	• Portability
	• Suction using sterile technique
	• Suction using clean technique
	• Suction using a mucus trap

Oxygen • Stationary and portable devices • Prescription for liter flow setting • Location for placing oxygen • Increasing and decreasing liter flow • Using only as needed	Pulse oximeter • Applying probe • Probe site rotation • Responding to alarms • Causes of false readings • Acceptable range
Resuscitation bag • Manual ventilation • Lung expansion therapy • Cleaning and disinfection	Airway clearance therapy • Chest physiotherapy • High-frequency chest wall compression or oscillation • Intrapulmonary percussive ventilation • Mechanical insufflation-exsufflation
Medication administration	

TABLE 34-3
Elements of Tracheostomy Education

Routine tracheostomy care
Routine and emergency tracheostomy tube change
Securing the tube
Frequency of tube change
Cleaning the tube
Cuffed and uncuffed tubes
Cuff volume and inflation method (sterile water, air)
Humidification
Use of self-inflating manual resuscitation bag and mask
Suctioning technique: shallow and deep
Tracheostomy bag and supplies
Tracheostomy-modified CPR
Emergency care
Accidental decannulation
Mucus plug
Inability to replace tube

Tracheostomy Tube Care

Practicing tracheostomy care and tube change on a manikin is helpful in preparing for validation. However, caregivers must be able to demonstrate the skills on the child as well. Caregivers should become comfortable and confident in managing the tracheostomy at home. They must also be prepared to handle emergency situations, such as accidental decannulation and mucus plugs. Practicing emergency scenarios is important in preparing for how to deal with possible tracheostomy crises. Classes in tracheostomy-modified cardiopulmonary resuscitation (CPR) and proof of competency are also required.

Frequency of routine tracheostomy care and tube change must be established prior to discharge. To reduce the risk of accidental decannulation, two trained caregivers should always assist with tracheostomy interventions, including changing the tracheostomy tube and stoma care. Caregivers should be instructed to communicate with each other to determine who will be responsible for removing the old tube and who will insert the new tube. Instructions for cleaning and disinfecting tubes should also be provided as well as information on the expected lifetime of the tube and when it should be changed. Additionally, instruction is needed if the child is requiring a cuffed tube. Caregivers should understand the purpose of the cuff and what is used to fill it, as the cuff may be filled with air or sterile water, depending upon the brand of tube.

Every tracheostomy-dependent child must have a bag, or any type of portable satchel or backpack, that contains all the necessary supplies to perform a tracheostomy tube change. Often referred to as a **trach go bag**, this should be transported with the child at all times. Required contents of the bag are listed in **Table 34-4**. Accidental decannulation can occur at anytime and anywhere. Infants and young children who are active will not hesitate to pull out their tracheostomy tube if given the opportunity. In the event that the tracheostomy tube cannot be replaced, a smaller size tube should be attempted. If the smaller tube cannot be placed and the child is in distress, emergency services

TABLE 34-4
Contents of a Tracheostomy Bag

Current-size tracheostomy tube
One size smaller tracheostomy tube
Obturator
Tracheostomy ties
Water-soluble lubricant
Heat moisture exchanger
Stethoscope
Scissors
Normal saline vials
Suction catheters
Mucus trap for emergency suction
Self-inflating manual resuscitation bag and mask

should be contacted and, if indicated, caregivers must begin administering tracheostomy-modified CPR.

Manual Resuscitation Bag

Caregivers must be trained in the use of a manual resuscitation bag and must be able to demonstrate correct technique with both the bag connected to the tracheostomy tube and connected to a mask in the event the tracheostomy tube cannot be replaced. Manual resuscitation bags are either flow-inflating or self-inflating. Flow-inflating bags are generally used only in the hospital setting as they require a higher flow of oxygen or air to inflate the bag than is generally available at home. Additionally, they are not always equipped with a pressure manometer to monitor peak inspiratory pressure during bagging. In contrast, a self-inflating resuscitation bag is preferred for home. This bag does not require additional flow to operate and has a pop-off valve so that only a limited amount of pressure can be exerted. Self-inflating bags have the option to add oxygen flow. The physical feel of providing ventilation with a self-inflating bag is different from the flow-inflating bag; therefore, caregivers should learn to use the self-inflating bag and then practice using the bag while in the hospital. Ideally, once a discharge date has been set, the flow-inflating bag should be removed from the child's hospital room and only the self-inflating bag is used.

Suctioning the Tracheostomy Tube

Suctioning the tracheostomy tube is another skill required of caregivers. Instruction should include choosing the appropriate catheter size and the correct suction pressure setting. To preserve the integrity of the airway, shallow suctioning is now preferred for routine clearing of secretions. This involves premeasuring the suction catheter depth to avoid repeated passing of the catheter past the tip of the tracheostomy tube. However, deep suctioning may be necessary when there are thick secretions or when attempting to remove a mucus plug. Routine instillation of saline is no longer recommended.

Sterile technique for suctioning is used in the hospital, but it is not always feasible in the home. Funds may be limited for the amount of suction catheters provided at home and therefore it becomes necessary to disinfect and reuse catheters. There is literature supporting the use of this practice, and it has been deemed safe.[13,14] Additionally, sterile gloves may not be readily available in the home suction catheter kits or when the catheter is being reused after disinfection. In this instance, it is acceptable to use nonsterile gloves or simply clean, washed hands.

Humidification

Because the tracheostomy tube bypasses the upper airway, humidification should always be used. The goal of humidification is to attempt to match the normal physiologic state in the airway. This can be accomplished in several ways, including heated humidification, a heat and moisture exchanger (HME), or a speaking valve. The method that is selected will depend on the child's condition and needs.

In patients with a tracheostomy only, the HME is often placed while the child is awake, and heated humidification is used only during sleep.[15] The HME is adequate for humidification needs during the day but may not be sufficient for continuous use, hence the use of heated humidification at night.[16] For patients requiring mechanical ventilation, the HME allows for mobility within the home as well as when traveling outside the home. HMEs are available in both pediatric and adult styles and the appropriate size must be ensured. An adult-size HME used with an infant may create increased dead space in the ventilator circuit.

In the hospital setting, sterile water is used in the heated humidifier, but it may not be readily available at home as it is often not covered by insurance or Medicaid. A common and acceptable practice is to use boiled tap water in the humidifier. If distilled water is preferred, it should still be boiled to avoid potential contamination.[17] Caregivers should be provided with instruction on appropriate temperature settings and cautioned to not allow the humidifier chamber to become dry, as this can enhance the risk of mucus plugging. Circuit condensation is considered contaminated and should never be drained back into the water chamber.[18] Instead, condensation should be emptied onto a towel or into a water trap. If the humidifier water chamber is reusable, disinfection instructions should be provided.

Speaking Valves

A main concern of caregivers regarding placement of a tracheostomy tube is loss of their child's voice and the inability to hear their child. A speaking valve is often used to assist with phonation. The valve works by redirecting exhaled air through the vocal cords to produce sound. There are various types of speaking valves. One valve is designed to be used with a tracheostomy alone and should not be used with mechanical ventilation. There are other styles that are designed to be used inline with the ventilator circuit. Speaking valves should never be used with an inflated tracheostomy cuff or while the child is sleeping. Before using a speaking valve at home, the child should be evaluated to determine if they are able to tolerate it. A speech therapist often assists with this process. There are some children with a tracheostomy who, due to an air leak around the tube, are able to produce vocal sounds without the use of a speaking valve.

Mechanical Ventilator

Caregivers must be instructed on use of the mechanical ventilator. The education varies with each hospital, but it is usually provided by hospital staff as well as staff from the home medical equipment company. This includes understanding ventilator function and what the ventilator settings represent, checking ventilator settings, providing oxygen, and monitoring the child with such devices as a pulse oximeter or apnea monitor.

It is imperative that caregivers correctly respond to ventilator alarms and any signs of respiratory distress. Instruction regarding appropriate alarm settings should be provided, as setting alarm parameters too high or too low can be dangerous. Ideally, alarm settings in the hospital should be identical to what will be set at home. Possible causes of the alarm should be discussed and common scenarios simulated or witnessed. Typically, a leak within the system is a common cause for a low-pressure alarm to be activated. This could be due to loose connections, small holes or cracks within the circuit, or a leak around the tracheostomy tube. If the low-pressure alarm is constantly sounding due to a leak, the low pressure alarm setting should not be decreased. Instead, it should be determined if the child needs a larger tube or a cuffed tracheostomy tube. The same is true for activation of the high-pressure alarm. Kinks, secretions, or excess condensation in the ventilator tubing can all cause the alarm to sound; setting the alarm to a higher pressure will not solve the underlying problem. Alarm settings in the hospital should never be manipulated to avoid nuisance alarms. The underlying cause of the alarm should be addressed rather than adjusting the setting outside the normal range. This can be confusing to caregivers and may cause them to believe that doing so is acceptable. It also reduces their ability to learn the proper response to alarms. Alarm fatigue is a common occurrence in the hospital setting and can carry over to the home if the medical team sets a bad example.

Sometimes alarms will self-correct, such as a high-pressure alarm during coughing or crying. However, most will not cease until corrected. Caregivers should be taught to quickly respond to all alarms each time they sound, beginning with visualizing their child and the airway. From there they should ensure that all connections are secure, examining the ventilator circuit from their child and back to the ventilator.

Caregivers should be made aware that in some scenarios low-pressure and disconnect alarms may not be activated, even though their child is disconnected from the ventilator. One study of simulated tracheal decannulations reported that home ventilators may not detect a low pressure when using pediatric tracheostomy tubes. As a result, the low-pressure alarm may not activate following decannulation.[19] This may also occur if the ventilator circuit becomes disconnected from the tracheostomy tube and is lodged against bedding with enough of an obstruction to cause the machine to continue to sense positive pressure. This further justifies

setting appropriate alarm parameters as well as continuously monitoring the child with a pulse oximeter or apnea monitor.

Spending time at the bedside is invaluable in exposing caregivers to scenarios that require troubleshooting and quick response. For example, it is at the bedside that the caregiver learns quickly that an increase in the peak inspiratory pressure usually indicates the need for suction. It is also at the bedside that they may witness an emergent tracheostomy tube change due to a mucus plug, which is valuable experience in preparation for an emergency at home.

Ideally, the child should use the actual ventilator that will be used at home prior to discharge. Often there are some differences between the hospital and home ventilator. The same is true for other equipment, such as the pulse oximeter, suction, and oxygen devices. The initial day at home should not be the first time the home equipment is used. Caregivers should be given an opportunity to have hands-on experience prior to the day of discharge to avoid potentially preventable problems at home.

Monitoring Devices

Besides the trained caregiver, the pulse oximeter is one of the most important monitoring tools used at home. The pulse oximeter must be used continuously during sleep, including daytime naps, and anytime the child is not being directly monitored. Caregivers must be educated as to proper probe placement, changing probe sites, monitoring skin integrity, alarm settings, response to alarms, and technical limitations. The pulse oximeter probe should be moved to a different site periodically to avoid skin breakdown. This is especially important in infants and those with delicate skin, as burns from the pulse oximeter sensor have occurred.[20,21] Many of the disposable probes come packaged with a cover for the light to protect skin.

Caregivers should demonstrate the appropriate action to take in the presence of valid decreased oxygen saturation values. They should be provided with an acceptable range for oxygen saturation as well as how to respond when the saturation drops below that threshold. Caregivers should be made aware that there are signs and symptoms of respiratory distress and increased work of breathing that may occur long before the pulse oximeter value decreases. Therefore, it is important to closely monitor for these signs without solely relying on the pulse oximeter reading.

Supplemental Oxygen

Instructions for the use of supplemental oxygen, including when to increase and decrease the prescribed liter flow, are included in caregiver training. Additionally, caregivers will need to identify where to connect the supplemental oxygen. Options for oxygen placement include a tracheostomy ring, which is an extension connected directly to the tracheostomy tube; an accessory oxygen port placed within the inspiratory limb of the circuit; or a designated port on the ventilator. Depending on the ventilator, adding flow through the ventilator circuit instead of using the designated oxygen port on the ventilator may cause erroneous readings for certain monitored parameters on the ventilator, including exhaled volumes.

Aerosol and Airway Clearance Devices

Some children may also require aerosol and airway clearance devices at home to maintain pulmonary stability. If inhaled medications are prescribed for home, caregivers will not only need to learn how to administer them but also the indications and considerations for sequence of therapy. Types of inhaled medications that may be used at home include bronchodilators, corticosteroids, antibiotics, and mucolytics. These medications are commonly available in the form of a metered dose inhaler or nebulizer solution. Delivery devices, such as a holding chamber, aerosol compressor, and nebulizer, may be required depending on the medication prescribed. Caregivers must be instructed on proper device technique as well as equipment cleaning and disinfection. A survey of aerosol administration practices for children with a tracheostomy found that delivery device technique is highly variable depending on the institution.[22] More research is needed in this area to standardize the use of aerosol delivery devices for this population of technology-dependent children.

Airway clearance devices may also be prescribed for home. Manual chest physiotherapy, high-frequency chest wall compression or oscillation, and mechanical insufflation-exsufflation for cough assistance are some of the more common modalities used at home. Other devices and methods available include positive expiratory pressure (PEP) and vibratory PEP devices and active cycle breathing. These are generally not age appropriate for young children or those with developmental delay due to the level of skill and cooperation required to effectively perform the therapy. Moreover, older children who may be age appropriate may still be unable to use these devices due to neuromuscular weakness. Regardless of the airway clearance device prescribed for home, caregivers must demonstrate correct technique prior to discharge.

Rooming-In

Once caregivers have been validated on all skills, they should be prepared for a room-in or family care stay. This involves the caregivers staying in the room with their child and assuming all medical care with supervision from the medical team to determine if they are ready and competent to provide safe care at home. During this time, caregivers will be expected to administer all feedings and all medications, including both inhaled and through the gastrostomy tube; provide

airway clearance therapy; perform ventilator checks; and respond to all ventilator and monitor alarms. In institutions in which a minimum of two caregivers are required, they may take turns sleeping and monitoring the child to simulate how it would be at home, as there should always be at least one trained caregiver awake and monitoring the child at all times.

Practices vary among institutions for the final room-in as the time may last anywhere from 24 to 72 hours. It should be noted that the room-in is not a time for learning skills: This is a test of the caregivers to ascertain if they are ready for discharge. Some programs offer an initial 24-hour room-in that is completed prior to the final stay to allow practice and to help caregivers gain an understanding of the expectations at home.

Transportation Home

How the ventilator-dependent child is transported from the hospital at discharge varies widely among different institutions. Some require the initial discharge home for the child who is both tracheostomy- and ventilator-dependent to be accomplished with non-emergency ambulance transport. Others plan for caregivers to use their personal vehicle for the transport home. When a personal vehicle is used for transportation, at least one trained caregiver must not drive but instead sit near and monitor the child. That caregiver should be readily available to address any tracheostomy- or ventilator-related issue that may arise. An untrained individual can serve as the driver.

Regardless of the mode of transportation, if a car seat or wheelchair will be used, it must be determined if the child can tolerate being seated in it for the duration of the ride home. A practice test of remaining in the seat or chair is performed prior to the day of discharge. For those unable to tolerate the full length of time, it should be trialed frequently so that they can gradually increase the amount of time it would take for the drive home. Consideration should also be given to children using a stroller for travel outside the home. A double stroller can help facilitate carrying all the equipment. It should be noted that a front-to-back stroller is preferred over the side-by-side style as the latter may be unbalanced with the weight of equipment, causing it to overturn.

Ventilator-dependent children often require extended hospitalizations. Once the child has transitioned to the portable home ventilator and is medically stable, short excursions outside of the hospital room with either a trained caregiver or medical staff should be considered. This will allow the child to become acclimated so that the time of discharge is not the first time outside of the hospital room. Some institutions have caregivers practice taking the child to the car or to the hospital cafeteria to practice for discharge. This not only helps the child have a short respite from the hospital room but also helps the caregivers become more comfortable with managing the child outside of the room but still within the confinements of the hospital.

Preparing the Home

Once the caregivers have been established, a **home evaluation** must be performed to determine if it can adequately support all prescribed equipment. This should be done long before discharge so that any identified issues can be addressed and resolved without delaying discharge. Typically, both the medical equipment supplier and the nursing provider will inspect the home prior to discharge. Any identified deficiencies must be corrected before the child can go home. In many cases, the medical equipment supplier may not provide equipment or begin any form of caregiver training and the nursing agency may not provide nurses if a home has not passed inspection. The home nursing agency examines many of the same aspects as the medical equipment company. However, they also want to ensure that the home offers a clean, safe environment for the nurse and that there is a comfortable chair for the nurse to sit in and a table or designated area where charting can be performed.

Evaluation by the medical equipment company consists of assessing the electrical outlets, observing for overall cleanliness and safety, and determining if utilities are working. Grounded outlets help to protect against electric shock and are necessary to operate the ventilator and other respiratory equipment. Older, two-pronged outlets cannot accommodate power cords with three prongs. It is never advisable to use an outlet adapter in a two-pronged outlet for a three-pronged cord, as this may cause potential risk for shock and/or electrocution. If the home does not have grounded outlets, an electrician is required to install a ground wire and upgrade the outlets to three-pronged.

Overall cleanliness of the home is assessed, as excess clutter can pose a fire hazard and attract pests. The home must have a working smoke detector as well as a fire extinguisher. Larger homes may require more than one smoke detector, depending upon the square footage. A plan of escape in the event of fire needs to be discussed and arranged with the caregivers if there is not one already in place. **Table 34-5** includes a checklist of required home components.

If the child requires a wheelchair, a ramp may be needed for entry into the home. The Americans with Disabilities Act provides specifications for building wheelchair ramps. These guidelines help determine the proper slope and length of the ramp. Ramps may be constructed of concrete, pressure-treated wood, or steel and must be able to support the weight of the wheelchair, the child, and the caregiver. Hallways in the home must be wide enough to allow the wheelchair to pass through. If the home has more than one level and the child's room is not on the ground floor, special accommodations should be made with either an elevator or

TABLE 34-5
Home Evaluation Checklist

All utilities working • Electricity • Water • Gas • Telephone
Smoke detector
Fire extinguisher
Fire escape plan
Bed for child
Adequate space for child's bed, equipment, and supplies
Designated area to clean, disinfect, and dry equipment
Overall cleanliness
Wheelchair accessibility (if indicated) • Wheelchair ramp • Hallways and doorways wide enough

stair lift. Consideration must also be given to children residing in an apartment with multiple stories.

For nursing staff to provide careful monitoring during the night, technology-dependent children require their own room and bed that is not shared with parents or siblings. There are various reasons this may or may not be a bedroom. Bedrooms in the home may not be spacious enough to contain all the equipment. Medical equipment generates heat, and when multiple pieces are grouped together it may become quite warm in a small room. Caregivers may prefer to have the child situated closer to their bedroom or, for privacy matters when nursing personnel are in the home, caregivers may prefer to have it situated farther away. The family may opt to convert a dining room or other living space into the child's room.

Ventilator equipment is commonly placed on a bedside table or microwave cart that is sturdy enough to support the weight of the equipment. Consideration also must be given to placement of the heated humidifier. It is critical that the humidifier be maintained at a level below the child's airway and either mounted on a pole or secured using a plate with screws. This is to ensure that circuit condensation does not inadvertently enter the tracheostomy tube and even more importantly prevents water from spilling into the child's airway should the humidifier be accidentally turned over. **Figure 34-2** provides examples of a secured humidifier.

A room or an area within the child's room should be designated to store the equipment and supplies. Storing supplies can be accomplished with cabinets, drawers, or a wheeled cart to provide quick, easy access when needed. **Figure 34-3** is an example of how supplies may

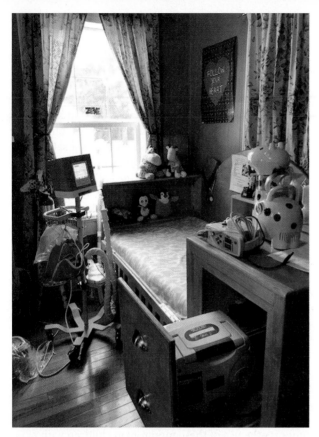

FIGURE 34-2 Home ventilator with the humidifier secured to the pole.

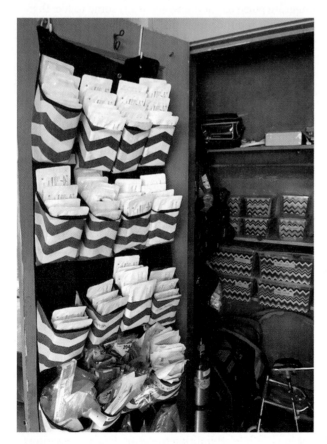

FIGURE 34-3 Supplies organized within a closet.

be organized within a closet. Often located near a sink, an area should be allocated for cleaning, disinfecting, and drying equipment.

Home Medical Equipment

All home respiratory equipment and disposable supplies are provided by a home medical equipment company. Caregivers should be provided with a list of potential home medical equipment providers to choose from. The choice of provider should first be determined by caregiver preference and availability of services. Services vary by company and not all may be able to provide the prescribed items—for example, some suppliers provide respiratory equipment only while others may have respiratory equipment as well as mobility equipment and enteral supplies. Insurance may also dictate which company can be selected, as some may be considered out of network and result in higher co-pays than an in-network provider.

Caregivers will need to be aware of how to obtain replacement supplies, including tracheostomy tubes, ventilator tubing, suction catheters, oxygen refills, enteral feeds, and related provisions. Once they have selected their choice of provider for these items, caregivers should be given the contact information for that company. This may end up being more than one company depending on the needs of the child and the availability of resources.

Mechanical ventilators used in the home differ from hospital models in several ways. They are portable and do not require a 50 pounds per square inch (psi) gas source for operation as do hospital models. Home ventilators have an internal battery as well as an external battery source for travel outside the home. An external battery source is also necessary for backup use in the event of an electrical power failure. Battery life must be long enough to use during follow-up clinic appointments, school attendance, and other activities outside the home.

Having a second ventilator in the home is not as common as it once was, mostly due to reimbursement issues. Some pay sources provide compensation for a backup device to remain in the home, but many do not. In cases that do not, it is at the discretion of the medical equipment company as to whether they deem it necessary to have a backup source of ventilation. The AARC Clinical Practice Guideline regarding long-term invasive mechanical ventilation in the home recommends a second ventilator for those patients who are unable to maintain spontaneous ventilation for 4 or more consecutive hours, those residing in an area where a replacement device cannot be provided within 2 hours, and those requiring ventilation during mobility.[2] A self-inflating manual resuscitation bag can be considered a second source of ventilation.

The company providing the respiratory equipment will also furnish disposable supplies. Ventilator circuits, suction catheters, tracheostomy tubes, ties to secure the tube, HMEs, a manual self-inflating resuscitation bag, oxygen tubing, and pulse oximeter probes are disposable supplies that are needed for the home. The frequency of ventilator circuit changes in the home varies depending on an individual institution's policy. This may range anywhere from weekly to monthly or when visibly soiled. Many inpatient practices have shifted to changing ventilator tubing less frequently to decrease the rate of ventilator-associated pneumonia. More often than weekly is not recommended unless the circuit has malfunctioned or has been soiled.[2]

The heated humidification system for the home consists of a heater and water chamber and is usually quite similar to the hospital model. As mentioned previously, excess circuit condensation should not be drained back into the humidifier chamber. A cooler temperature setting in the home may increase circuit condensation. Ways to decrease rainout in the tubing include avoiding drafts from a fan or air vent or insulating the circuit with a wrap specially designed for ventilator tubing.

For children with a tracheostomy who do not require a ventilator, a heated tracheostomy collar is typically used for nighttime humidification. When used without a ventilator, the heated humidification system for the home differs from that in the hospital and requires an air compressor. The medical equipment company should ensure that a passover humidifier is provided and not a heated aerosol. Bland aerosol administration for long-term humidification is not recommended as it can cause overhydration and poses an infection risk.[23]

A suction device is needed to assist with removing tracheal secretions. Although there are some children who may have sufficient cough effort to expel secretions, it is still necessary to have a suction device in the home. It is not uncommon to have both a portable suction machine that uses an internal battery system and a stationary suction machine that remains in the home. Suction canisters and tubing are also provided. In the event of an emergency where the suction device has malfunctioned or is not available, a mucus trap can be used to provide manual suction.

Tracheostomy emergencies can occur suddenly and often without warning. Therefore, oxygen should remain available in the home, whether it is required or just on standby. Home systems are designed to provide oxygen measured in liter flow rather than through blenders with an adjustable FiO_2. Oxygen equipment used in the home includes a concentrator, liquid system, or tanks/cylinders. If the child requires oxygen on a routine basis, then a portable system must be available. The choice of liquid, concentrator, and/or cylinders typically depends on the individual child's needs and availability of equipment provided by the home equipment company. Many portable systems incorporate conserving devices that provide oxygen flow only when triggered. Infants and small children are usually unable to adequately trigger these devices and should instead use continuous flow regulators.

A pulse oximeter is required for monitoring oxygen saturations at home. Although this device and other monitors are extremely useful tools to have available at home, they can never replace the vigilant, trained caregiver. Most home pulse oximeters have an internal battery so that it can be used during travel outside the home. Probe-type oximeters may be disposable or permanent depending on the equipment supplier but should be appropriately sized for the child.

End-tidal carbon dioxide ($ETCO_2$) devices are commonly used in the hospital to monitor exhaled CO_2 and to observe trends. They are not routinely used at home for the general population of ventilator-dependent children as data are lacking to justify the use of it, and most insurers will not reimburse for them. There is, however, evidence to support the routine use of an $ETCO_2$ monitor at home for children with congenital central hypoventilation syndrome.[24]

The routine use of apnea or cardiorespiratory monitors at home for the ventilator-dependent child is not standard practice by all institutions and may not be reimbursed for this purpose by all state-funded payers. However, a 2003 policy statement from the American Academy of Pediatrics, which was reaffirmed in 2007, supports the use of these monitors in children with a tracheostomy and those requiring mechanical ventilation.[25] Many of the newer cardiorespiratory monitors integrate pulse oximetry, which leads some to feel that their use is redundant as there is generally a pulse oximeter already in use and newer ventilator technology incorporates additional alarm features for apnea. Furthermore, obstruction due to a plugged tracheostomy tube or decannulation may not be recognized on the cardiorespiratory monitor because it uses impedance technology to sense apnea.

Depending on the child's need for aerosol and/or airway clearance modalities at home, there are a variety of possible options. Nebulizer supplies, an aerosol compressor, metered dose inhaler chambers, "boppers" or percussors for manual chest physiotherapy, high-frequency chest wall compression vest, or mechanical insufflation-exsufflation are examples of the types of devices and supplies that may be needed at home for the respiratory management plan. These treatments and modalities should always be trialed with the child prior to using at home, as occasionally there are differences in device models. Other techniques and devices may be available for home but are generally not as common as those previously described.

Day of Discharge

Although caregivers have been eagerly awaiting the day to finally go home, they are often very anxious and nervous. While attempting to ensure final preparations are complete, including securing all home equipment and supplies and having the home prepared, the day of discharge may become a hectic, emotional event. Discharge day is not a time to learn new skills or obtain new information. All training and education should have been provided and completed prior to this day. Ideally, caregivers should be well rested so that they are able to focus all their attention and efforts on caring for their child as they are about to assume total care outside of the hospital setting.

One way to reduce the chaos of discharge day is to have a meeting with the caregivers and the discharge planning team 1 to 2 weeks prior to discharge to make all final preparations and to inform caregivers what to expect on this day. This discharge meeting should include the multidisciplinary team as well as home nursing and home medical equipment personnel. Taking a checklist approach will help make certain that all equipment has been obtained, follow-up appointments made, and home nursing secured. The discharge meeting is also the time to discuss what equipment must be at the hospital ready to use during the transport home. This includes the home ventilator, portable oxygen, pulse oximeter, portable suction machine, and tracheostomy supply bag. Likewise, there should be discussion of required equipment and supplies for anytime the child will travel outside the home. The discharge meeting also provides an opportunity for caregivers to ask last-minute questions and for the medical team to review the plan of care. Additionally, this conference is a good forum to introduce the outpatient team who will assume the care after discharge home.

The method of transportation home will need to be determined and plans made well in advance of the day of discharge. In some practices, the home equipment company personnel and home nurses will either meet the child at the home or follow them from the hospital to home. If caregivers are transporting the child home in their personal vehicle, having the home care team follow them home may be helpful in the event there are issues encountered en route. They may also assist with transferring the child and all the equipment from the vehicle to inside the home.

Barriers to Discharge

There are many factors that can prolong or delay discharge. It is quite rare that the discharge process is executed perfectly as planned and that issues are not encountered along the way. Although the eventual goal is to go home, caregivers should be aware that barriers are common and occur despite all best efforts. Even when caregiver training is progressing, the child may become acutely ill or home nursing services are not established and the discharge date must be postponed.

Medical instability, lack of availability of home nursing services, poor collaboration and communication between services, caregiver social circumstances, lack of reimbursement, and loss of funding are some of the many barriers that may arise throughout the discharge process. Technology-dependent children who are not medically stable for discharge must remain hospitalized until they are well enough to transition home. This may unfortunately give caregivers a false sense of extra time to train for the skills needed for home. Even if the expected discharge date is delayed, caregivers can still participate in the child's care and focus on what can be learned at the present time.

Home nursing services may be difficult to establish but must be in place before the ventilator-dependent child can go home. Unfortunately, lack of communication or miscommunication between the hospital providers and home agencies can be a source of delay. Both sides must work together in the best interests of the child to facilitate transition to home.

Social issues tend to be one of the main barriers to discharge home. If the home is not adequate to support the child and the equipment, then attempts must be made to correct the problems or another home option must be attained. This can also impact the financial aspect as caregivers may not have the resources or funds to move to another home or repair the existing one. A social worker can typically assist caregivers with finding information and resources to address these issues.

Healthcare coverage often dictates the services and equipment that can be obtained at home. There are situations in which the child could benefit from having certain pieces of equipment in the home, but the payer will not reimburse for it and caregivers do not have the financial ability to secure it. Until it can be determined that alternatives are available, the child should remain hospitalized although they may be deemed medically stable for discharge.

In some unfortunate situations, the caregivers love and care deeply for their child, yet they simply cannot comprehend the necessary information, or they are unable to perform the skills proficiently to provide safe care in the home. Or, in some circumstances, they may be physically or emotionally unable to care for the child. When home is not an option, another plan will need to be determined, as the hospital is not the ideal place for a child to stay. There are long-term care facilities that may be considered or, in some situations, other family members may take custody of the child.

Outpatient Care

Children with tracheostomies need regular follow-up with a PCP, otolaryngologist, and pulmonologist after discharge.[26] If the child did not have a PCP established before the hospitalization, one must be identified before going home. The pulmonologist will manage the ventilator in the outpatient clinic. Other specialists may also be required depending upon the diagnosis and other comorbidities. The frequency of follow-up appointments with all physicians and specialty clinics should be established and discussed with the caregivers prior to discharge home. Routine visits with the pulmonologist should be scheduled at regular intervals ranging from 1 to 6 months depending on the diagnosis, severity of illness, reason for need of the ventilator, and ability to wean.[11]

Caregivers need instructions regarding whom to contact concerning problems or questions that arise once they are home. For issues or concerns not related to respiratory matters, caregivers may be instructed to contact the PCP or the specialist associated with the issue. If the outpatient team is not yet familiar with the child, caregivers may be instructed to contact the hospital. For home equipment malfunction, the medical equipment provider should be contacted.

When attending outpatient clinic appointments, caregivers should be prepared to be away from the home for an extended period of time. They should ensure that they have everything with them they may potentially need, such as extra supplies and feeds. It cannot be assumed that the clinic will have a suction device or oxygen available if needed. It is helpful to provide caregivers with a checklist of items they may need to have with them for outings.

Due to the nature of their diagnosis, not all children will be candidates for ventilator weaning and may require mechanical ventilation for the duration of their lives. Currently there is not a standardized approach to use to begin weaning, when and if that is an option. Practices vary considerably for this and may range from decreasing settings to trialing off the ventilator for short periods of time while awake. The pulmonologist will determine the best method for the child and formulate a plan. Time off the ventilator may initially be as short as 10 to 15 minutes or to allow time for certain activities of daily living, such as bathing. Some institutions refer to the time off the ventilator as a sprint. Sprints should be done under close supervision and never without an order from the physician. If the child is not tolerating the sprint, or has increased work of breathing, the ventilator should be immediately restarted. The physician should be made aware of any difficulties or intolerance with the prescribed time off the ventilator.

Once the child is able to remain off the ventilator while awake during the day, the next step is to decrease nighttime support. Often a sleep study, or polysomnography testing, is used to determine if mechanical ventilation during sleep can be reduced or removed altogether. It is important to note that although the child may be able to spend increased amounts of time without ventilator support, it may need to be reinstituted during an acute illness.

When the ventilator can be discontinued, consideration is given to removing the tracheostomy tube. One of the first steps toward tracheal decannulation is to downsize the tracheostomy tube. This is followed by capping the tube. Capping the tracheostomy tube is generally only attempted when decannulation is an option. Not all children with a tracheostomy are candidates for capping. Capping the tracheostomy tube forces both inhalation and exhalation to be done through the upper airway. Capping should never be done with a cuffed tube or during sleep unless otherwise directed. In some cases, it is months to years before tracheostomy capping is a consideration.

Transition from Pediatric to Adult Care

Advances in medical care and technology have improved survival of the respiratory technology–dependent child. Many children who would have normally not survived are now living longer and becoming young adults. It is estimated that annually nearly 500,000 youth with special healthcare needs turn 18 years of age.[3] The Maternal and Child Health Bureau defines children with special healthcare needs as those who "have or are at increased risk for a chronic physical, developmental, behavior, or emotional condition who also require health and related services beyond that required by children generally."[27] This definition includes the ventilator-dependent child. As this ever-increasing population becomes young adults, the need for adult healthcare providers with expertise in caring for the ventilator-dependent individual continues to grow.

Transition from pediatric to adult care is a process and not a single transfer event. Early discussion, planning, and preparation help to prevent potential problems that may occur when it is time for the actual transfer to take place. Although the concept may at first seem frightening, **transition to adult care** should be approached positively. It is the role of the pediatric team to empower these young adults with the knowledge and tools they need to be successful in the future. Not encouraging them to learn their care if they have the ability to do so is setting them up for failure. In cases where the young adult may be unable to learn care or to have the capacity to make decisions, guardianship will need to be established.

The Society for Adolescent Medicine first defined healthcare transition in 1993 as "the purposeful, planned movement of adolescents and young adults with chronic physical and medical conditions from child-centered to adult-oriented health-care systems."[28] A 2002 consensus statement from the American Academy of Pediatrics (AAP) defined transition as "a dynamic, lifelong process that seeks to meet their individual needs as they move from childhood to adulthood. The goal is to maximize lifelong functioning and potential."[29]

The first question usually asked in regard to transition is why it is necessary. Why must the child who has been cared for by the same pediatric healthcare team who knows them best not maintain their care there? Pediatricians are not trained to care for adults. Screening for disease prevention and issues related to reproduction are two examples of areas that are best addressed by an adult provider. The goal of transition to adult care is to ensure that young people receive developmentally and medically appropriate health care.[29] For the child in which the odds were against them to reach adulthood, having a future as a young adult is an exciting possibility.

There are several barriers that may hinder transition. Preconceived notions and misconceptions are generally the main factors. When leaving an environment in which they have received care for the majority of their lives, patients, caregivers, and the pediatric healthcare team may be reluctant to transition due to lack of trust or confidence in the adult system. The pediatric healthcare team often lacks the knowledge and training for beginning the transition process, and adult providers may not be prepared to assume the care of these medically complex young adults. There is also poor reimbursement for transition services, as evidenced by the fact that less than half of youth with special healthcare needs receive the transition support services for which they are entitled.[30] A survey of pediatric pulmonary programs found that 78% did not use a standardized transition process for respiratory technology–dependent children.[31] Poorly coordinated healthcare transitions may lead to gaps in care and potential loss to follow-up. In addition to the pediatric team needing a standardized approach to transition, the adult providers must also prepare. It is often challenging to identify adult providers willing to accept the ventilator-dependent young adult into their practice. This population is best served when the pediatric and adult providers partner together and collaborate to ensure that these individuals receive the care they need.

To provide education, guidance, and tools for transitioning youth with special healthcare needs, the Got Transition Center in cooperation with the Maternal and Child Health Bureau and the National Alliance to Advance Adolescent Health developed the Six Core Elements of Transition.[32] The elements include creating a transition policy, tracking and monitoring, assessing readiness to transition, planning, transfer of care, and transfer completion. The Got Transition Center has resources and tools available for both pediatric and adult providers as well as youth and families. Additionally, information regarding different models of care is also included.

The first step in developing a transition program is to create a transition policy. This involves defining the process for how transition will occur, setting the upper age limit for which patients will be followed, and identifying who will be responsible for initiating the process. The medical team must be familiar with the policy and understand their role as it relates to transition. The

AAP recommends sharing the institutional policy with patients and caregivers between the ages of 12 and 14 years.[33] This may seem young to begin the process, but it is never too early to start planning for the future. Early discussions allow youth and their family time to accept the idea so that it is not a surprise when the time comes for the actual transfer. The majority of unsuccessful transitions have occurred due to poor planning and failure to inform the patient and family in a timely manner.

Planning is the key ingredient for a successful transition. It is also important to ensure that the entire team is in agreement with the process that is used. If all team members are not sharing the same message with patients and caregivers, it becomes confusing and causes problems. For example, if the pediatric pulmonary division's plan for transition is that all ventilator-dependent young adults transition between the ages of 19 and 20 years, yet another physician disagrees and tells the patient that they do not have to transition until they turn 21 years of age, the family is now confused and distrustful of the team despite them following the transition policy.

Tracking and monitoring involves identifying those youth who are ready to begin the process as well as documenting progression. Sample tracking logs are available from the Got Transition Center to assist with this procedure. Because the pulmonary department may be one of several specialties involved in a young adult's care, tracking can be helpful in monitoring outcomes and assisting with coordination of care with other services. All discussions regarding transition to adult care should be documented in the medical record.

It is recommended to begin assessing readiness to transition at 14 years of age. This allows time to determine what the child knows about their healthcare needs and to establish goals for self-care if they will be managing their own care in the future. Even if not physically able to provide their own care, if the child has the cognitive ability to understand their condition and treatment, then it may be feasible to begin shifting some of the responsibility. One example of beginning this is to have the child name all their medications and then move to explaining the purpose of each medication. Once the knowledge of medications has been grasped, attention is then moved to learning about the ventilator and other respiratory devices. Readiness assessments should be done annually to compare from year to year, gauge understanding, and determine where reinforcement is needed. These assessments should be documented in the plan of care. Unfortunately, not all respiratory technology–dependent children are candidates for self-care. In many cases the goal is simply to maintain stability and to ensure that the caregiver is knowledgeable about the medical needs and care.

Transition planning is ongoing up until the time of the actual transfer of care. The ventilator-dependent young adult and/or their caregivers should be informed of the available options for adult pulmonologists. Once they have identified an adult provider, the pediatric team should begin communicating with the adult team regarding the impending transfer.

Regardless of the child's ability to understand or participate in their own care, once 18 years of age is reached, they are legally considered an adult. It must be determined prior to turning 18 years of age if legal guardianship is needed. This should be addressed before the 18th birthday. If not dealt with in a timely manner, the responsible guardian will not have legal access to records and information and may be unable to make informed decisions about medical care.

The time frame for transfer should be discussed throughout the course of planning. Many institutions use 21 years of age as the upper age limit. However, it is not good practice to wait until reaching the upper age limit to transfer. Ideally, the transfer to adult care should occur before the maximum age is reached to avoid gaps in care related to insurance coverage or other issues. Delaying transition after attaining the upper age limit is a recipe for disaster. For example, a ventilator-dependent young adult who has turned 21 years of age may become acutely ill prior to a planned appointment with an adult pulmonologist. Being unable to return to the pediatric hospital, this individual's only option is to go to the emergency department of an adult hospital that has no medical records or history about them. Establishing care with the adult provider before reaching the upper age limit of the pediatric institution can help prevent such a fiasco from occurring.

Transfer of care is the actual physical move to adult care. This is usually noted as being the first adult pulmonary clinic appointment. It is important to plan for this transfer to occur during a stable clinical state, as the middle of an acute exacerbation is not an ideal time to attempt to establish new relationships with physicians, nurses, and therapists. Once the first appointment has been scheduled with the adult pulmonologist, the pediatric team should ensure that there are enough prescriptions and supplies to last until that appointment time and that appointment details, including date, time, and location, have been relayed. Some of the biggest fears about transition are related to being uncertain of where to go and where to park. It is helpful to ensure that the adult team has received all medical records needed to care for the young adult. A plan for interim care should also be determined at the time of the last appointment or encounter with the pediatric team. Although this may vary by institution, most pediatric pulmonary practices will assume responsibility for the ventilator-dependent young adult until care has been established with the adult pulmonologist. For example, if the young adult becomes ill or needs medication refills before being seen in the adult clinic, the pediatric team is the contact.

Transfer completion involves communicating with either the adult provider or the ventilator-dependent young adult to confirm attendance of the first appointment so that there is no loss to follow-up or interruptions in care. This is also included as part of the tracking and monitoring process. Once transfer of care has been completed, the young adult is considered officially transitioned to the adult pulmonary provider. Collaboration between the pediatric and adult groups is as equally as important as planning to ensure a seamless transition.

Summary

Planning for the initial hospital discharge of the tracheostomy- and ventilator-dependent child is a process that takes time and careful preparation for a successful transition to home. There are many aspects that must be taken into consideration, including adequate number of caregivers available to care for the child, caregiver training and education, home preparation, and obtaining home equipment and nursing services. When any of these areas are not satisfactory, discharge can be delayed. Caregivers need adequate time for training and skills validation. They also need realistic expectations prior to the training process so that they will be fully informed of everything they will be required to learn. Unfortunately, not all ventilator-dependent children are candidates to discharge home. It may take weeks or months before they are deemed medically stable for discharge. At times caregivers may be unable to demonstrate proficiency of the skills or lack the resources to care for the child at home. Caring for these children can be quite stressful and overwhelming at times.

Some ventilator-dependent children may eventually be able to wean from the ventilator and have the tracheostomy removed. Others may require the tracheostomy and ventilator for their lifetime. For those who become young adults, planning for eventual transition to adult care should begin in the early teen years. The mission of the healthcare team should be to prepare and equip both the children and their caregivers to be successful at home so that they can attempt to assume a sense of normalcy. Although there has been improved care and technology, as evidenced in the increased lifespan of technology-dependent children, more research and published standards of care are needed to standardize the approach to managing their long-term care.

Acknowledgments

The author would like to thank Tammy Hall, RRT, for sharing expertise from the home care perspective.

Case Study 1

A 2-year-old girl with Pompe disease, a rare and often terminal disorder that affects the heart and skeletal muscles, is admitted to the hospital due to progression of the disease. Her past medical history is significant for hypotonia, developmental delay, feeding difficulties, and significant dilated cardiomyopathy with cardiac hypertrophy, which led to the diagnosis of Pompe disease at 8 months of age. She lives in a one-bedroom apartment with her mother and 4-year-old brother. She attends day care while her mother works. In the past 12 months, she developed a progressive sleep disorder and respiratory insufficiency, requiring noninvasive ventilation (NIV). During this hospitalization her cardiorespiratory status could not be stabilized, and she required a tracheostomy and continuous invasive mechanical ventilation. This intervention reduced her chronic cardiac failure, but the respiratory muscle function remained severely compromised. After a month she became a candidate for investigative interventions, which were started and well tolerated. Her respiratory status improved, and she began sprints from the ventilator for 10 minutes, three times a day. While preparing for discharge, the child's mother told the social worker that she had lost her job due to missing multiple workdays while staying at the hospital with her daughter. She also shared that she was fearful she would not have financial resources to pay her apartment rent and that she had very little family support to help her. The multidisciplinary medical team met weekly with the mother to strategize on successfully transitioning her daughter home with a tracheostomy and continuous mechanical ventilation. Several weeks later this child was discharged home where she is expected to continue to need this level of care indefinitely due to her disease process.

1. **What are the benefits of being home for this patient?**

2. **Who should be included in the multidisciplinary discharge planning team?**

3. **What barriers to discharge did this family face?**

Case Study 2

A 15-year-old male with Duchenne's muscular dystrophy is admitted to the hospital due to increased oxygen requirement following a viral infection. He had been stable and managed at home with NIV by mask at night and a cough assist device for most of his adolescent years. Over the next 24 hours, his PCO_2 levels increased and he required continuous mechanical ventilation. On hospital day 14, the decision was made for him to receive a tracheostomy and percutaneous endoscopic gastrostomy tube. Considering his diagnosis, the patient and family expressed a desire to return home as soon as possible. A hospital interdisciplinary team worked to identify his needs and to achieve financial approval from his health insurance. Resources were outlined to cover home equipment, patient care, education/training, and other miscellaneous costs. A targeted discharge date was proposed, and a training schedule for the home care nurses and the family was developed. Weekly interdisciplinary meetings were held to update and review discharge plans. Home visits were completed to examine elements of the home environment. Before discharge, the patient was transitioned to home equipment, including the ventilator and various devices to mimic the home environment. The family then provided 48 hours of continuous care, which was observed by nursing and respiratory staff. Any concerns were addressed in real time. One week later the patient was transported home via ambulance.

1. **Now that this patient has a tracheostomy tube, what equipment should be provided in the home?**

2. **What are some risks of providing care at home?**

3. **What training must the family/caregivers successfully complete before discharge can occur?**

References

1. United States Congress, Office of Technology Assessment. *Technology-Dependent Children: Hospital v. Home Care- A Technical Memorandum.* Publication # OTA-TM-H-38. Washington, DC: US Government Printing Office; May 1987.

2. American Association for Respiratory Care, Respiratory Home Care Focus Group. AARC clinical practice guideline: long-term invasive mechanical ventilation in the home – 2007 revision and update. *Resp Care.* 2007;52(8):1056-1062.

3. Lotstein DS, McPherson M, Strickland B, Newacheck PW. Transition planning for youth with special health care needs: results from the national survey of children with special health care needs. *Pediatrics.* 2005;115(6):1562-1568.

4. King AC. Long-term home mechanical ventilation in the United States. *Resp Care.* 2012;57(6):921-932.

5. Taylor JH. Children who require long-term ventilation: staff education and training. *Intensive Crit Care Nurs.* 2004;20:93-102.

6. Wang KW, Barnard A. Technology-dependent children and their families: a review. *J Adv Nurse.* 2004;45(1):36-46.

7. Dumas H. Rehabilitation considerations for children dependent on long-term mechanical ventilation. *ISRN Rehabilitation.* 2012;756103.

8. Boroughs D, Dougherty JA. Decreasing accidental mortality of ventilator-dependent children at home. *Home Health Nurse.* 2012;30(2):103-111.

9. Meltzer LJ, Boroughs DS, Downes JJ. The relationship between home nursing coverage, sleep and daytime functioning in parents of ventilator-assisted children. *J Pediatr Nurs.* 2010;25(4):250-257.

10. Cockett A. Technology dependence and children: a review of the evidence. *Nurs Child Young People.* 2012;24(1):32-35.

11. Panitch HB. Home ventilation. In: Light MJ, Blaisdell CJ, Homnick DN, Schechter MS, Weinberger MM, eds. *Pediatric Pulmonology.* Elk Grove Village, IL: American Academy of Pediatrics; 2011:1091-1110.

12. Barnhart SL, Carpenter A. Transition from hospital to home. In: Sterni LM, Carroll JL, eds. *Caring for the Ventilator Dependent Child.* New York: Springer Science+Business Media; 2016:89-120.

13. Shabino CL, Erlandson AL, Kopta LA. Home cleaning-disinfection procedure for tracheal suction catheters. *Pediatr Infect Dis J.* 1986;5(1):54-58.

14. Scoble MK, Copnell B, Taylor A, Kinney S, Shann F. Effect of reusing suction catheters on the occurrence of pneumonia. *Heart Lung.* 2001;30(3):225-233.

15. Willis D, Barnhart SL. Troubleshooting common ventilator and related equipment issues in the home. In: Sterni LM, Carroll JL, eds. *Caring for the Ventilator Dependent Child.* New York: Springer Science+Business Media; 2016:185-216.

16. Restrepo RD, Walsh BK. AARC clinical practice guideline: humidification during invasive and noninvasive mechanical ventilation. *Respir Care.* 2012;57:782-788.

17. Saiman L, Siegel J. Infection control in cystic fibrosis. *Clin Microbiol Rev.* 2004;17:57-71.

18. Branson RD. Humidification for patients with artificial airways. *Respir Care.* 1999;44:630-641.

19. Kun S, Nakamura CT, Ripka JF, Ward SLD, Keens TG. Home ventilator low-pressure alarms fail to detect accidental decannulation with pediatric tracheostomy tubes. *Chest.* 2001;119(2):562-564.

20. Bunker DL, Kumar R, Martin A, Pegg SP. Thermal injuries caused by medical instruments: a case report of burns caused by a pulse oximeter. *J Burn Care Res.* 2014;35(2):e132-e134.

21. Ceran C, Taner OF, Tekin F, Tezcan S, Tekin O, Civelek B. Management of pulse oximeter probe-induced finger injuries in children: report of two consecutive cases and review of the literature. *J Pediatr Surg.* 2012;47:e27-e29.

22. Willis LD, Berlinski A. Survey of aerosol delivery techniques to spontaneously breathing tracheostomized children. *Respir Care.* 2012;57(8):1234-1241.

23. Kallstrom TJ. AARC clinical practice guideline. Bland aerosol administration – 2003 revision & update. *Respir Care.* 2003;48:529-533.

24. Weese-Mayer DE, Berry-Kravis EM, Ceccherini I, et al. An official ATS clinical policy statement: congenital central hypoventilation syndrome: genetic basis, diagnosis and management. *Am J Respir Crit Care Med.* 2010;181:626-644.

25. American Academy of Pediatrics, Committee on Fetus and Newborn Apnea. Sudden infant death syndrome, and home monitoring. *Pediatrics.* 2003;111:914-917.

26. Benson RC, Newaskar M. Tracheostomies. In: Light MJ, Blaisdell CJ, Homnick DN, Schechter MS, Weinberger MM, eds. *Pediatric Pulmonology.* Elk Grove Village, IL: American Academy of Pediatrics; 2011:1077-1090.

27. Mcpherson M, Arango P, Fox H, et al. A new definition of children with special health care needs. *Pediatrics.* 1998;102:137-140.

28. Blum RW. Transition to adult health care: setting the stage. *J Adolesc Health.* 1995;17:3-5.

29. American Academy of Pediatrics, American Academy of Family Physicians, American College of Physicians-American Society of Internal Medicine. A consensus statement on health care transitions for young adults with special health care needs. *Pediatrics.* 2002;110:1304-1306.

30. McManus MA, Pollack LR, Cooley WC, et al. Current status of transition preparation among youth with special needs in the United States. *Pediatrics.* 2013;131:1090-1097.

31. Agarwal A, Willis D, Tang X, et al. Transition of respiratory technology dependent patients from pediatric to adult pulmonology care. *Pediatr Pulmonol.* 2015;50(12):1294-1300.

32. The National Alliance to Advance Adolescent Health. www.gottransition.org. Accessed February 5, 2016.

33. Cooley WC, Sagerman PJ. Supporting the health care transition from adolescence to adulthood in the medical home. *Pediatrics.* 2011;128:182-200.

35

Pediatric Palliative and Hospice Care

Eve deMontmollin

OUTLINE

OBJECTIVES

1. Differentiate between palliative care and hospice care.
2. List the goals of pediatric palliative care.
3. Recognize patient disorders that may benefit from palliative care.
4. Discuss the importance of providing psychosocial and spiritual guidance during palliative care.
5. Explain how pain may be managed during palliative care.
6. Explain how the Concurrent Care for Children Requirement of the Affordable Care Act has affected the care of terminally ill children.

KEY TERMS

celebration of life
concurrent curative care
hospice care
palliative care

Patient Protection and
   Affordable Care
   Act (PPACA)
quality of life

Introduction

A life-limiting illness is one that limits normal life expectancy. Examples include cancer, heart disease, cystic fibrosis, and muscular dystrophy. When children develop such a chronic or life-threatening illness, dramatic life changes occur. Not only do they experience physical suffering but also their lives, along with the lives of their family, are often filled with fear, anxiety, confusion, and sadness. This creates unique challenges, especially when that condition persists for months and sometimes years. Pediatric **palliative care** involves developing a plan of care that is as individual as the child and family it serves and includes all measures taken to lessen suffering and to improve **quality of life** at every stage of the illness.

Pediatric Palliative Care

The essential difference between adult and pediatric palliative care is the age of the patient. In adult medicine, typically the patient (adult) provides consent. In pediatric medicine, consent is provided by the child's primary caregiver(s), typically one or both parents.

Definition

Pediatric palliative care is specialized care for infants and children who have a life-limiting or terminal illness. It includes comprehensive medical, psychosocial, and spiritual care aimed at relieving symptoms and suffering, slowing the progression of the disease, and achieving the best possible quality of life for the child while also providing emotional support to the family.[1] Palliative care ideally begins when the illness is diagnosed. It can be provided at any stage of the illness—at diagnosis, during active treatment, when all treatment has been completed, or near the end of life—and alongside concurrent disease-modifying curative treatment plans. It does not replace the active treatment team but instead works with this team. Palliative care is provided in hospitals, community-based health centers, long-term care facilities, and in a child's home.[2,3] Services provided by a palliative care team are listed in **Table 35-1**.

Goals

Palliative care focuses on supporting children and their families, on both an inpatient and outpatient basis, while enhancing their quality of life. **Table 35-2** lists the goals of pediatric palliative care.

Indications

Palliative care is appropriate for children (birth to 21 years of age) with a wide range of conditions, even when cure remains a distinct possibility.[4] It is not only indicated by a specific diagnosis but also when physical and psychosocial stressors occur as a result of the life-limiting illness. Children and their families can suffer physically and emotionally with pain caused by anxiety from a diagnosis or fear of an uncertain future at all stages of chronic and life-limiting conditions. **Table 35-3** and **Table 35-4** provide indications that may call for a palliative care consult.[5,6]

Communication

Communication is the key to building a trusting relationship when providing palliative care to children and their families. A systematic, individualized, and compassionate approach is essential when invited into their medically complex world. Effective communication requires the palliative care team to be emotionally available and to honestly discuss physical and emotional suffering, treatment strategies, and the possibility of death.

TABLE 35-2
Goals of Pediatric Palliative Care

Manage symptoms caused by illness and treatment
Minimize suffering
Improve quality of life for the child and family
Provide support for the child and family during transition and loss
Assist the child and family in making difficult decisions
Customize care for specific needs
Collaborate with providers, community resources, and schools
Prevent and alleviate unnecessary hardships and suffering

TABLE 35-1
Possible Services from a Palliative Care Program

Pain and symptom management
Emotional, psychological, and spiritual support
Coordination of care
Identification of available community resources
Assistance with complex decision making
Assistance with communication between the child/family and medical staff
Memory-making
Sibling support
Anticipatory grief support
Advanced care planning
Bereavement follow-up

TABLE 35-3
Pediatric Disorders That May Indicate the Need for Palliative Care

Cancer
Congenital heart disease
Congenital malformations
Chronic respiratory failure
Cystic fibrosis
Cerebral palsy
Muscular dystrophy
Chromosomal abnormalities (e.g., trisomy 13, trisomy 18)
Hypoxic or traumatic brain injury
Sickle cell anemia
Severe brain malformation

TABLE 35-4
Child/Family Stressors That May Indicate a Need for Palliative Care

Multiple unplanned hospitalizations
Difficulty managing pain or symptoms
Prolonged hospitalizations or intensive care admissions without medical improvement
Requests for futile care
Family with limited social support (e.g., homeless, chronic mental illness)
Psychological or spiritual distress
Declining ability to complete activities of daily living
Difficulty controlling physical or emotional symptoms
Uncertainty regarding prognosis
Uncertainty regarding goals of care (e.g., resuscitation, nutrition, chemotherapy)
Request for information regarding hospice appropriateness

TABLE 35-5
Adjunctive Therapies for Symptom Management during Palliative Care

Therapeutic play using child life specialists
Aromatherapy
Guided imagery
Massage
Music therapy

As the child and family are guided through the hospital experience, they are educated about what to expect during treatment and given assistance in identifying goals of care and making decisions as the illness changes.

Psychosocial and Spiritual Concerns

A chaplain, social worker, and child life specialist who are trained in family systems and childhood development are included in an interdisciplinary palliative care team. These team members bring assessment and intervention tools unique to the needs of the child with a life-limiting illness. When addressing psychosocial and spiritual needs, special attention is given to developmentally appropriate interventions. A child's developmental age and chronological age may not be the same due to an illness. If an illness begins at infancy, the child may not reach developmental milestones as would be expected with normal development. How a child understands their illness and death depends upon their level of development. Careful assessment of what a child can currently do is required to estimate developmental age. Moreover, the impact that the illness has on the entire family will alter the parents' hopes and dreams for their child. Stress on the family may cause and/or exacerbate conflict among family members. The family's spiritual beliefs and cultural values and beliefs influence the plan of care and how they view death. These beliefs and values must be carefully assessed.

Symptom Management

Management of symptoms and pain in the pediatric population is a top concern for both the child and the family. When asked what worries parents the most about their child's illness, parents typically list pain management as their biggest concern. Being cognizant of the family's fears related to pediatric pain management ensures that a child receives appropriate and effective pain relief. Education and support regarding the treatment of a child's pain is provided by the palliative care physician. The palliative care team provides a thorough assessment of pain and can assist with recommendations for the most appropriate route for medication administration and compounded medicine preparations. Educating the child and family about the body's physiologic response to the end of life is essential in relieving them of the anxiety related to symptom management.[7] **Table 35-5** includes adjunctive therapies that may be used along with pharmacologic pain interventions.

Pediatric Hospice Care

The goals of care are similar in palliative care and hospice care medicine. However, palliative care is open-ended, and although support is ongoing during palliative care, it may be sought alongside goals of a cure. In a typical hospice setting, in contrast, a cure is no longer an option. To be eligible for **hospice care**, a physician must attest that the child's life expectancy is approximately 6 months or less.

Concurrent Care for Children

Concurrent curative care occurs when a child receives curative care to treat a disease or normalize an underlying health condition while also receiving hospice care for pain and symptom management and psychosocial end-of-life needs. For many years, children whose illnesses became life threatening were unable to receive concurrent curative care. They were unable to receive hospice services while getting curative treatment or they had to discontinue curative treatments in order to be eligible for hospice services. On March 23, 2010, when President Obama signed the **Patient Protection and Affordable Care Act (PPACA)** into law, it enacted a new provision known as the Concurrent Care for Children Requirement (CCCR). This small provision has significantly affected concurrent curative care for terminally ill children. The law now mandates that children with a life-limiting illness can receive hospice care concurrently with full medical management and hopes for a cure. Today, all state Medicaid programs pay for both curative and hospice services for qualifying children younger than 21 years of age. Children who are eligible for and receive hospice care must also have available all other services related to treatment.[8]

When Goals of Care Change

When treatment of an illness involves risk versus benefit, a child's quality of life becomes a significant issue. The family may question current medical management. At this point, a family-centered approach that includes discussion with the multidisciplinary team is imperative. The focus now shifts from treatment of an illness to symptom and pain management, with an emphasis on comfort and the child's retention of dignity. This redirection of care emphasizes continual recognition of the family's perception of care delivered. Withdrawal of medical devices and technology may take place simultaneously with an increase in delivery of psychosocial and emotional care.

A Case Study: Assisting with End-of-Life Care

The following case study is representative of a child who received both palliative and hospice care services.

Medical History and Present Illness

Taylor was an 8-year-old female with a genetic disorder nearing the projected life expectancy of this disease. She was referred to palliative care at 2 years of age. The consult goal at that time was to assist the family in identifying goals of care and to provide overall support to Taylor and her family. Since her diagnosis, Taylor had received care from several specialists that required multiple outpatient clinic visits. This also included biweekly enzyme infusions at the infusion center, which were an all-day endeavor. At the age of 4 years, Taylor developed chronic respiratory failure and required placement of a tracheostomy tube and 24-hour mechanical ventilation. Gastrostomy tube feedings were needed to maintain her nutrition. At this time, Taylor lived at home with her family, who felt that their daughter's quality of life was good. She received in-home therapies, went on family trips, and smiled often when interacting with others.

Escalation of Care

Approximately 3 months prior to her 9th birthday, Taylor required frequent admissions to the critical care unit. Each time she presented with various acute illnesses related to the progression of her disease. With each illness, her family noted that Taylor was less responsive to them. She no longer smiled at the people and things that used to bring her joy. As both Taylor and her family's needs changed during this time, the palliative care team increased their visits. One month prior to her 9th birthday, while admitted to the critical care unit, the family requested to take Taylor home.

Wishes Honored

A multidisciplinary team meeting with the family was arranged. Attending the meeting were Taylor's family and a palliative care physician, pulmonologist, nurse, respiratory therapist, social worker, child life specialist, chaplain, and hospice coordinator. The palliative care team directed the meeting while the family's questions and concerns were answered by the appropriate specialist. The family did not wish to discontinue use of the ventilator at that time. The palliative care team, in conjunction with the pulmonary and hospice teams, honored the family's wishes and developed a plan to transition Taylor to her home. A detailed plan of care included ventilator management by the pulmonologist while all other symptoms were managed by the palliative care and hospice teams. Focus was placed on making each day of Taylor's life meaningful. Once she was home, the palliative care team worked closely with the hospice team. The child life specialist with hospice used play therapy with Taylor's siblings to help them understand death and made memory and legacy items. The hospice chaplain assisted the family with their spiritual needs and pre-death funeral arrangements.

Celebration of Life

Upon discharge from the hospital, Taylor's family was hopeful that she would be more responsive once she returned to her home environment. However, this did not occur, and Taylor had fewer and fewer moments of wakefulness. Through building rapport with the hospice team, the family decided that Taylor's death at home would not be in the best interests of Taylor and her siblings. The parents' wish was to plan removal of the ventilator with Taylor in the hospital on her 9th birthday, surrounded by staff the family had built relationships with during Taylor's life. With new goals established and in conjunction with the hospice team, the palliative care team made arrangements for Taylor's admission to the hospital.

On the morning of her 9th birthday, a **celebration of life** party was held. Many of the physicians, nurses, respiratory therapists, and other medical support staff were present. Pictures and banners lined Taylor's room. Taylor woke up momentarily during the celebration. Once the guests had left, the family closed the door of Taylor's room, leaving only Taylor and her parents inside the room. After 30 minutes of quiet time with Taylor, her parents requested removal of the ventilator. The palliative care team stood quietly by as the physician prepared to administer comfort medication, should it be needed. Taylor's parents requested that a respiratory therapist who had provided care to Taylor throughout the years be present. This therapist, at the direction of the physician, turned off the ventilator, removed the ventilator circuit, and gently laid Taylor in the arms of her parents. Within 2 minutes, Taylor took her last breath. With tears in the eyes of everyone present, Taylor's parents were allowed the controlled, dignified death they had hoped for their daughter.

Palliative and Hospice Care Projections

Children are living longer as advancements in medical technology and research in pediatric medicine evolve. Technology is enabling families to care for their children outside of an acute care setting. Through the expanded use of telemedicine, medical access is more widely available than ever before. Families have the option to continue to "do everything possible" or to choose to limit what is done and, with available outpatient resources, children are able to receive more advanced care in their homes. If the family wishes, children no longer need to die in hospitals. Instead they can remain at home surrounded by family, friends, and all things familiar.

Case Study

A mother of two had an extremely difficult birth with her third child, a son, which resulted in a diagnosis of hypoxic ischemic encephalopathy. He received feedings through a gastrostomy tube, required frequent suctioning and secretion clearance therapy, and had frequent seizures. The medical team, which included palliative care, explained to the family that the infant's life would be difficult and likely shorter than other newborns going home. He had an increased likelihood of having recurrent pneumonia and frequent hospitalizations. His parents talked about coordinating care and how they wanted to give him the best possible life without adding to his suffering. Over the next couple of months, he was hospitalized twice after discharge from the neonatal intensive care unit. During each admission, the infant's condition seemed to be worsening. The family expressed concern that he was suffering and experiencing a decreasing number of "good days." The possibility of placing the infant in hospice care was discussed, but at this time the infant was too sick to leave the hospital. An empathetic communication about prognosis and goals of care allowed the parents to embrace the concept of a good death. At the family's request, their son was baptized. Photos, handprints, and footprints were also taken. Time was allotted for other family members to arrive. Many family members were able to hold him in his final moments, and he died peacefully in his mother's arms.

1. **What are the goals of palliative care?**
2. **What is the key to building trust between the medical team and the family?**
3. **What is the difference between palliative care and hospice care?**

References

1. Klick JC, Hauer J. Pediatric palliative care. *Curr Probl Pediatr Adolesc Health Care*. 2010;40:120-151.
2. Mack JW, Wolfe J. Early integration of pediatric palliative care: for some children, palliative care starts at diagnosis. *Curr Opin Pediatr*. 2006;18:10-14.
3. Ullrich CK, Wolfe J. Caring for children living with life-threatening illness: a growing relationship between pediatric hospital medicine and pediatric palliative care. *Pediatr Clin North Am*. 2014;61:xxi-xxiii.
4. Himelstein BP, Hilden JM, Boldt AM, Weissman D. Pediatric palliative care. *N Engl J Med*. 2004;350:1752-1762.
5. Kaye EC, Rubenstein J, Levine D, et al. Pediatric palliative care in the community. *CA Cancer J Clin*. 2015;16:315-333.
6. Carter B, Levetown M. *Palliative Care for Infants, Children, an Adolescents: A Practical Handbook*. Baltimore: Johns Hopkins University Press; 2004.
7. Kenyon B. Current research in children's conceptions of death: a critical review. *Omega J Death Dying*. 2001;43:63-91.
8. Keim-Malpass J, Hart TG, Miller JR. Coverage of palliative and hospice care for pediatric patients with a life-limiting illness: a policy brief. *J Pediatr Health Care*. 2014;27:511-516.

Glossary

A

acinus A region of lung supplied by a first-order respiratory bronchiole and includes the respiratory bronchioles, alveolar ducts, and alveolar sacs distal to a single terminal bronchiole.

acrocyanosis A bluish color of the hands and feet caused by decreased extremity circulation for the first few minutes of life in newborns.

adaptive support ventilation (ASV) An automatic weaning mode that uses a percentage of minute ventilation to determine the level of ventilator support provided.

adenotonsillar hypertrophy A condition in which the adenoids and tonsils are enlarged. It is a common cause of obstructive sleep apnea in children.

Adenotonsillectomy (AT) An operation to remove both the adenoids and the tonsils; the primary treatment for adenotonsillar hypertrophy in children.

adherence programs Programs that have been developed to improve adherence with positive airway pressure (PAP) in the inpatient and outpatient settings. These programs attempt to build a positive, supportive relationship with patients and families by implementing behavioral interventions and desensitization protocols that will facilitate PAP introduction and maintain long-term adherence.

advanced maternal age (AMA) Women older than 35 years at a stage of reproduction that is associated with greater odds of complications, such as preterm labor and delivery, preeclampsia, poor fetal growth, fetal distress, postpartum hemorrhage, and intrauterine fetal demise.

aerosol A suspension of liquid or solid particles in a carrier gas.

afterload The resistance the heart must overcome to eject blood from the ventricle. It is elevated in some congenital heart defects, such as aortic stenosis.

air leak syndrome The accumulation of air or gas, particularly in the space found between the chest wall and the lung of an infant. The common conditions are pneumothorax, pneumomediastinum, and pneumopericardium.

airborne infection isolation room A patient-care room used to isolate persons with a suspected or confirmed airborne infectious disease, such as tuberculosis.

air-entrainment mask A fixed performance oxygen delivery device that provides a range of low to moderate concentrations of oxygen through the use of jet port mixing of gas from the oxygen source and air entrained from the atmosphere.

air-entrainment nebulizer A large-volume nebulizer that provides a precise oxygen concentration, using the principle of air entrainment, while delivering an aerosol. The nebulizer directly connects to the oxygen flowmeter, and oxygen flows through a jet nozzle surrounded by an air-entrainment port. The concentration of oxygen delivered to the patient depends on the flow of gas set on the flowmeter and the size of the entrainment port.

airway biopsy A biopsy obtained by inserting a biopsy forceps through the working channel of a bronchoscope and obtaining a sample of airway tissue.

airway brushing A methodology performed by inserting a specimen brush through the working channel of a bronchoscope and gently scrubbing the airway mucosa. The brushing sample can be used to identify pulmonary dyskinesia or to enhance a lung biopsy performed to identify pulmonary dyskinesia.

airway clearance therapy (ACT) Airway clearance techniques that may include percussion, vibration, deep breathing, and huff coughing; used to clear retained pulmonary secretions from the airways.

airway pressure release ventilation (APRV) An alternative mode of mechanical ventilation in which the high positive end-expiratory pressure setting is applied for a longer duration of time than the lower positive end expiratory pressure with the majority of the respiratory cycle spent at the high pressure. It provides an inverse I:E ratio and is most commonly used in conditions associated with hypoxic respiratory failure and low lung compliance.

airway secretion overload A clinical picture created by the introduction, production, and retention of secretions in the airway. Airway secretions naturally occur in the airway and are responsible for maintaining normal airway function

alert verbal painful unresponsiveness (AVPU) algorithm A method of rapidly assessing level of consciousness during a neurologic assessment. It is a simplification of the Glasgow Coma Scale used to assess the level of consciousness and/or deterioration in the mental status of infants and children.

allergic bronchopulmonary aspergillosis (APBA) A hypersensitive immune response to airway colonization of fungi and molds, such as *Aspergillus.*

alpha-adrenergic receptors Autonomic receptors that when activated, generally produce excitatory responses of the smooth muscle in which they are located.

amniocentesis The most common invasive diagnostic test performed during pregnancy in which the amniotic fluid is sampled using a hollow needle inserted into the uterus. It is performed between 16 and 18 weeks' gestation to screen for chromosome abnormalities in the developing fetus.

amniotic fluid A watery fluid, usually clear or light yellow in color, in which the fetus is completely surrounded.

anastomosis A new surgical connection between two body structures.

animal-assisted therapy A therapeutic intervention that incorporates animals, such as horses, dogs, cats, pigs, and birds, into the treatment plan. It is used to enhance and complement the benefits of traditional therapy.

antenatal steroids Medications administered to the mother when preterm delivery is expected. They have been shown to reduce morbidity and mortality related to surfactant-deficient diseases.

antepartum period The period before childbirth, with reference to the mother.

anteroposterior (AP) A radiographic projection position in which the radiographic beam enters the chest from front to back.

anticholinergic bronchodilators Bronchodilators that block muscarinic cholinergic receptors, which hinders the action of acetylcholine. This decreases the formation of cyclic guanosine monophosphate, which results in decreased contractility of the smooth muscle.

antimicrobials Drugs used to treat a broad spectrum of potential pathogens that are harbored in the upper respiratory tract.

aortic stenosis A congenital heart defect with narrowing of the aortic valve; it is a defect that primarily involves an obstruction to the left ventricular outflow. This occurs because the aortic valve, positioned between the left ventricle and the aorta, does not properly open and close.

Apgar score An assessment tool for the evaluation of the newborn in the delivery room. This scoring system evaluates the presence and characteristics of five parameters: heart rate, respiratory rate, skin color, reflex irritability, and muscle tone.

apnea A pause in breathing of longer than 20 seconds, often associated with bradycardia, cyanosis, or both; resulting in pathological changes in heart rate and oxygen saturation.

apnea of prematurity A developmental disorder common to infants born before 35 weeks' gestation; it is the result of an immature respiratory control. It is characterized by apneic events that last more than 20 seconds or shorter apneic periods associated with oxygen desaturation and/or bradycardia.

arterial blood gas analysis A blood test for the evaluation of oxygenation, gas exchange, and acid–base balance; often used in diagnostic evaluation and to assess the patient's response to therapeutic interventions.

arterial catheters A thin catheter inserted into an artery to continuously measure blood pressure or to obtain arterial blood. It is useful when frequent sampling of arterial blood is required.

asthma A chronic inflammatory disorder of the airways in which many cells and cellular elements play a role: in particular, mast cells, eosinophils, neutrophils (especially in sudden onset, fatal exacerbations, occupational asthma, and patients who

smoke), T lymphocytes, macrophages, and epithelial cells. In susceptible individuals, this inflammation causes recurrent episodes of coughing (particularly at night or early in the morning), wheezing, breathlessness, and chest tightness. These episodes are usually associated with widespread but variable airflow obstruction that is often reversible either spontaneously or with treatment.

asthma action plan A set of written instructions based on zones defined by the child's peak flow and symptoms that direct the actions a child and family need to take in response to changes in the child's peak flow or asthma symptoms.

atelectotrauma An injury to the lung due to repeated collapse and reexpansion of the under-recruited alveoli, associated most often with mechanical ventilation.

atretic plate The anatomical thin tissue plate that separates the nasal cavity from the pharynx.

atrial septal defect (ASD) A congenital heart defect with a hole in the wall (septum) between right and left atria (upper chambers of the heart). At birth, a small atrial septal defect may not cause any symptoms, but a larger atrial septal defect could lead to heart failure.

atrioventricular canal (AVC) defect A congenital heart defect with incomplete development of the septa involving both atria and both ventricles, resulting in a large hole that allows oxygenated and deoxygenated blood to mix.

autogenic drainage (AD) A form of airway clearance therapy that uses a cycle of controlled breathing exercises at varying depths to loosen secretions in different areas of the lungs. The exercises consist of three phases, with the depth of inspiration increasing with each phase.

auto-mode An automatic weaning mode that monitors the spontaneous breathing efforts and automatically switches to a spontaneous mode of pressure support or volume support, when the patient makes a respiratory effort and then reverts to a mandatory breath if no effort is recognized.

auto-trigger The delivery of a breath during mechanical ventilation above the breathing rate set on the ventilator and without a spontaneous inspiratory effort; also known as self-cycling.

Avian influenza The H5N1 influenza virus; a virus infection is transmitted to humans primarily through direct contact with diseased or deceased birds infected with the virus. Contact with excrement from infected birds or contaminated surfaces or water are also considered mechanisms of infection.

B

bacterial colonization A condition in which bacteria are identified in the airway, even though the patient is stable and free of acute respiratory illness.

beaking The portion of the pressure–volume curve where pressure continues to rise but volume plateaus.

bedside pulmonary function testing Standard pulmonary functions tests, which are performed in the laboratory, are also performed at the patient's bedside. This is an important option in evaluating critically ill patients in the intensive care unit, patients in isolation, and those who are unable to go to the laboratory.

beta-adrenergic receptor agonists Bronchodilators that are used to both prevent and treat bronchospasm. Activation of adrenergic receptors of the smooth muscle in the lungs and vasculature supplying the skeletal muscle system relaxes the bronchial and tracheal smooth muscles and relieves bronchospasm.

bicycle ergometer A device with saddle, pedals, and some form of handlebars arranged as on a bicycle to use in children as they are more familiar with bicycles than treadmills. It is easier to monitor oxygen saturation, blood pressure, and electrocardiogram with fewer artifacts from motion.

biphasic positive pressure A noninvasive ventilation technique that delivers positive pressure during inspiration to improve ventilation and provide ventilatory support.

biphasic ventilation A mode of ventilation that applies two distinct positive end-expiratory pressure levels (high and low), which allows for spontaneous ventilation throughout the ventilation cycle and the availability to add pressure support to augment a spontaneous breath.

blastocyte An undifferentiated embryonic cell.

body plethysmography Also known as a body box; the most common measurements obtained are airway resistance and static lung volumes.

bonding The formation of a close relationship between a parent and an infant or child.

breath-actuated nebulizers A jet nebulizer that uses a one-way valve to deliver aerosol only during inspiration. There are two different designs to this type of nebulizer. One design modifies a continuous output jet nebulizer by adding a one-way valve proximal to the patient and a reservoir bag distal to the patient that is filled with aerosol during exhalation. The other design incorporates a spring-loaded valve that allows aerosol production only during inhalation. Both designs result in zero waste to the environment.

breath-enhanced nebulizers A jet nebulizer that incorporates a one-way valve into the design that allows an increase of the airflow in the chamber during inspiration, leading to an increase in aerosol output. Aerosol output still occurs during expiration, and so some models have incorporated an expiratory valve in the mouthpiece, while others offer a Y-shaped connector that allows for the addition of an exhalation filter.

bronchiolitis An acute inflammatory disease of the lower respiratory tract, resulting in obstruction of the small airways, or bronchioles. It is a common seasonal viral infection, with incidence peaking in the winter, that causes wheezing and congestion in infants up to 2 years of age.

bronchoalveolar lavage (BAL) A procedure to obtain samples of airway secretions to diagnose infection.

bronchogenic cyst An abnormal growth of lung tissue characterized as a malformation of the bronchial tree.

bronchoprovocation A test that assesses bronchial hyperresponsiveness or airway hyperresponsiveness.

bronchoprovocation challenge test A diagnostic test used to differentiate asthma from other diseases; it is performed in a clinic setting using either methacholine or mannitol.

bronchopulmonary dysplasia (BPD) A chronic lung disease that most often affects premature babies who received oxygen and/or positive pressure ventilation.

bronchoscopy A procedure that allows direct visualization and assessment of upper and central airway anatomy for diagnostic, therapeutic, or research purposes.

Broselow tape A commercially available, color-coded, length-based tape that can be used to quickly select the proper size of equipment and dosage of emergency medications in the pediatric patient.

Brownian diffusion A mechanism that affects aerosol deposition; random motion of particles immersed in a fluid, in which particles smaller than 0.5 μm are deposited at the alveolar level.

C

capillary blood gas A blood sample obtained from a capillary is a useful alternative for assessing acid–base balance and ventilation in infants and children. A capillary blood gas sample correlates well with the pH, $PaCO_2$, HCO_3, and base excess (BE) obtained from an arterial sample and provides a less invasive sampling method.

capillary refill A valuable initial physiologic parameter, in which the finger or toe should be lifted slightly above the level of the heart to assure assessment of arteriolar capillary refill and not venous stasis. Light pressure is applied to blanch the nail bed. The pressure is released and the amount of time until color returns is measured. In neonates, the skin over the sternum is compressed. Capillary refill is normal if color returns in fewer than 2 seconds. Volume depletion or hypotension can cause a delay in capillary refill of more than 3 seconds.

capillary refill time A method to assess cardiac output and peripheral circulation. It is the time it takes for the skin color to return to normal after the capillaries have been compressed. In a neonate, it is checked by compressing the skin over the sternum. In others it is done by pressing on the toe or finger. Normal capillary refill time is fewer than 2 seconds.

capnography The continuous noninvasive measurement, analysis, and recording of the partial pressure of CO_2 at the end of a tidal breath. It is the graphical representation of ventilation. Most capnographs have the ability to display a breath-to-breath waveform in addition to a trend graph of end-tidal CO_2 values over time.

capnometry The noninvasive measurement (digital) of the partial pressure of CO_2 at the end of a tidal breath, without a graph or continuous waveform.

cardiomegaly A medical condition in which the heart is enlarged; and it is often an indication of a congenital for enlarged, indicating acyanotic heart defect.

celebration of life A memorial service to pay tribute to a life lived.

central cyanosis Bluish discoloration of the tongue or mucous membranes due to poor blood oxygenation.

central sleep apnea A heterogeneous group of sleep disorders in which respiratory effort is repetitively diminished or absent.

central venous catheter A catheter inserted via a large vein into the superior vena cava or right atrium to provide a direct route for fluid, medication, and nutritional support to the central circulation.

central venous line (CVL) A central venous catheter.

centrifugal pumps Nonocclusive mechanical pumps used for the displacement of blood through an extracorporeal membrane oxygenation (ECMO) circuit; it responds to changes in circuit resistance and patient hemodynamics.

cepacia syndrome A combination of necrotizing pneumonia, respiratory failure, and bacteremia as a result of infection with *Burkholderia cepacia*.

cerebral palsy (CP) A group of nonprogressive neurodisability disorders that appear in infancy or early childhood and permanently affect body movement and muscle coordination.

cystic fibrosis transmembrane conductance regulator (CFTR) A membrane protein and A chloride channel expressed in the apical membrane of epithelial cells lining the lung, pancreas, gut, sweat duct, reproductive tract, kidney, liver, and submucosal glands. It regulates several ion conductance pathways, including epithelial sodium, chloride, and potassium channels, as well as bicarbonate transport.

chest compressions An act of applying pressure on the chest to help blood flow through the heart during cardiopulmonary resuscitation.

chest physiotherapy (CPT) An airway clearance therapy that uses percussion or vibration on the chest wall to mobilize secretions along with postural drainage to allow gravity to aid in draining those secretions to the large airways, where they can be coughed out and expectorated.

chief complaint (CC) The health problem or concern, described in the child's or parent's own words, that caused the individual to seek medical attention.

child life specialists Pediatric healthcare professionals who help children and families cope with the stress and uncertainty of acute and chronic illness, injury, trauma, disability, loss, and bereavement during hospitalization.

choanal atresia A congenital disorder in which there is a narrowing of the back of the nasal cavity (choanae), resulting in a lack of continuity between the nasal cavity and the pharynx; it is the most common form of congenital nasal obstruction and infants often present with difficulty breathing.

chronic lung disease (CLD) A term used interchangeably with bronchopulmonary dysplasia, it is a lung disease of the premature infant who has received oxygen therapy and positive pressure ventilation.

chylothorax Also known as chylopleura, it is the presence of chyle in the pleural space secondary to leakage from the thoracic duct. It can be caused by trauma to the neck or thorax or by an obstruction of the thoracic duct.

coarctation of the aorta A congenital heart defect with narrowing of the aorta, ranging in severity from mild to severe, that causes increased work of the heart to pump blood to the lower portion of the body.

compliance The change in volume divided by the change in pressure; it is used to describe the elastic properties of the respiratory system.

computerized tomography scan An imaging procedure that generates and records many radiographic images as the detector moves around the patient's body. A computer reconstructs the individual images into cross-sectional images or "slices" of internal organs and tissues.

concurrent curative care Curative and hospice care; it is when a child receives curative care to treat a disease or normalize an underlying health condition while also receiving hospice care for pain and symptom management and psychosocial end-of-life needs.

congenital central hypoventilation syndrome (CCHS) Also known as Ondine's curse; a rare genetic disorder characterized by severe alveolar hypoventilation and autonomic nervous system dysfunction. It is due to a mutation in the PHOX2B gene that is essential in the migration of neural crest cells and development of the autonomic nervous system.

congenital diaphragmatic hernia (CDH) A complex congenital disorder with high mortality due to a hole in the diaphragm that allows abdominal organs to move into the chest, which hinders lung development; infants suffer a combination of various degrees of insufficient lung growth and pulmonary hypertension.

congenital pulmonary airway malformation A rare, disorganized overgrowth of fetal lung tissue, formally known as congenital cystic adenomatoid malformation.

congenital pulmonary anomalies A collection of uncommon lung deformities that affect the airway, parenchyma, and vasculature of infants who require intervention at birth or later in life.

conscious sedation Administrating a combination of medicines (anesthesia) without loss of consciousness but to help the patient relax and to block pain during a medical procedure.

continuous mandatory ventilation (CMV) Commonly referred to as assist control; a mode of mechanical ventilation that provides a fully supported or mandatory breath. The breath can be patient-triggered or machine-triggered.

continuous output jet nebulizers Jet nebulizers that have constant output of aerosol irrespective of the timing of the respiratory cycle. The design of nebulizers that continuously nebulize and deliver medication leads to significant waste of the aerosolized medication. The use of a mouthpiece and the addition of a 15-cm extension tube distal to the patient acts as a reservoir for aerosol particles and enhances drug delivery when a continuous nebulizer is used.

continuous positive airway pressure (CPAP) A spontaneous mode of ventilation that enhances oxygenation and preserves lung inflation by improving the functional residual capacity to treat acute and chronic conditions in neonates with impaired lung inflation and gas exchange.

continuous spontaneous ventilation (CSV) A mode of ventilation in which every breath is spontaneous, it includes pressure support ventilation and neutrally adjusted ventilatory assist ventilation.

contraction stress test (CST) A test to evaluate the fetus's ability to tolerate changes in blood flow and oxygenation during contractions; fetal heart rate response to uterine contractions is measured.

corticosteroids Anti-inflammatory drugs that are frequently used in the treatment of respiratory disease in neonatal and pediatric patients.

cough assistance therapy Also referred to as mechanical insufflation-exsufflation; an airway clearance therapy that consists of mechanical devices that simulate a cough. These devices provide positive pressure to inflate the lungs and at the end of inspiration quickly follow with a negative pressure, which produces an expiratory flow that shears secretions from the airway walls and moves them to where they can be expectorated or suctioned. The fast, expiratory flow rate from the lungs simulates a natural cough.

cough peak flow (CPF) A measurement of the velocity of air as a patient coughs into a flow measuring device, such as a peak flow meter. This measurement represents the effectiveness of a patient's cough for clearing secretions.

crew resource management (CRM) A course developed in 1979 from the NASA training workshops that taught communication skills in addition to practicing with closed-loop communication in simulation and certification courses. It has a focus on leadership, interpersonal communication, and decision making.

cricothyrotomy An incision made through the skin and cricothyroid membrane to secure a patent airway during certain life-threatening situations.

Cushing's triad A sign of increased intracranial pressure. It is a triad of hypertension, bradycardia, and widening pulse pressure.

cut-down procedure A procedure in which a central venous catheter is placed percutaneously or through surgical cannulation to access the internal and external jugular, common facial, brachial, femoral, and saphenous veins.

cyanotic The bluish appearance of the skin that occurs because blood is not oxygenated. Patients with cyanotic cardiac defects will have lower than normal oxygen saturations.

cyberbullying Covert psychological bullying conveyed through electronic means; it can result in physical and psychological harm with emotional distress, symptoms of depression, and adverse coping mechanisms, such as withdrawal and substance abuse.

cycle sensitivity The setting that terminates the inspiration, transitioning the breath to exhalation. The term used for this setting is not standard and varies by ventilator manufacturer. It is used to control the duration of the breath during pressure support breaths.

cycle time A parameter available on ventilators that determines the transition period from inhalation to exhalation and may be flow- or time-based.

cystic fibrosis (CF) A life-limiting autosomal recessive disorder.

cytokines Regulatory proteins, such as lymphokines and interleukins, that are produced by immune system cells and act as intercellular mediators in the modulation of immune response.

D

decannulation Removal of the tracheostomy tube.

deformational plagiocephaly A physical condition whereby the soft bones of the head become misshapen or flat as a result of frequently laying in the same position for prolonged periods of time.

delta P The difference between the inspiratory positive airway pressure and the expiratory positive airway pressure settings; a key determinant of volume delivery in non-invasive ventilation because there is a linear relationship between pressure and volume.

delta pressure (ΔP) The calculation of PIP – PEEP at a specific tidal volume; it provides the set level of PEEP of best compliance (PIP denotes peak inspiratory pressure).

demand flow A ventilator feature that allows the patient to access additional flow of gas during inspiration.

developmental milestones Behaviors and tasks that most children can do by a certain age. Like growth, developmental milestones are built upon the experience and mastery of the behaviors before them.

diaphragm pacing A treatment option for patients with congenital central hypoventilation syndrome. It provides daytime ventilatory support for those who are 24-hour ventilator dependent, allowing for mobility and independence from the ventilator during the day. It can be the sole source of ventilation, permitting tracheal decannulation for those patients who are ventilator dependent only during sleep.

diffusing capacity (DLco) A pulmonary function test that indirectly measures gas transport at the alveolar level.

digital clubbing A deformity of the finger- or toenails; it is often associated with chronic respiratory or cardiac diseases in which there has been long-term hypoxia.

dipalmitoylphosphatidylcholine (DPPC) The most abundant phospholipid in pulmonary surfactant, often referred to as lecithin, that may be used as a marker for fetal lung maturity.

discharge planning A multidisciplinary process that involves a child's transition from a healthcare setting to home.

distal intestinal obstruction syndrome (DIOS) An intestinal obstruction in the distal or terminal ileum; it is associated with the passage of large amounts of food that are not completely digested into the small bowel. Symptoms include right lower quadrant pain, anorexia, nausea, vomiting, and occasionally fever.

distraction osteogenesis A treatment option to correct mandibular hypoplasia by making a longer bone out of a very short bone.

dry powder inhalers (DPIs) Devices that allow delivery of a drug to the lungs without the need of a suspending medium, which results in the delivery of larger drug amounts compared to pressurized metered dose inhalers.

ductus arteriosus An anatomic shunt that serves to enhance the efficacy and distribution of blood flow to the developing fetus; this short, broad vessel connects the trunk of the pulmonary artery to the aorta. It is a normal part of a baby's circulatory system before birth that usually closes shortly after birth.

ductus venosus   An anatomic shunt connecting the intra-abdominal umbilical vein to the inferior vena cava at its inlet to the heart; this vein channels 70% to 80% of umbilical blood through the liver before entering the inferior vena cava.

Dunn formula   The measurement of shoulder to umbilicus length. A method used to determine the umbilical arterial catheter insertion length.

E

Ebstein's anomaly   A rare congenital heart defect in which the tricuspid valve does not properly close. As a result, blood flow does not move in the right direction, causing the heart to work less efficiently.

eclampsia   A complication of pregnancy in which a mother with hypertension from preeclampsia develops seizures, after other seizure disorders or causative factors have been ruled out.

ectoderm   The outermost of the three germ layers of an embryo formed by the 3rd week of life; it forms the nervous system, skin or epidermis, glandular tissue, and many of the sensory organs.

Edi_{max}   A signal that represents diaphragmatic contraction; the start of inspiratory effort.

Edi_{min}   A signal that represents diaphragmatic relaxation, or the expiratory effort required to maintain functional residual capacity.

embryoblast   A compact mass of approximately 46 cells inside the primordial embryo that form the embryonic tissues.

encephalopathy   A term that means brain disease, damage, or malfunction.

enclosure devices   Devices that deliver oxygen therapy by enveloping all or a part of the patient's body and are supplemental oxygen to neonates and infants; included are oxygen hoods and incubators.

endoderm   The innermost of the three germ layers of an embryo formed by the 3rd week of life; it produces the cecum, intestine, stomach, thymus, liver, pancreas, thyroid, prostate, and lungs.

endoscope   The general term for an instrument with a slim, flexible tube attached to a camera source used to look somewhere inside the body.

endotracheal tube   A tube that is inserted into the trachea to provide positive pressure ventilation, effective suctioning of pulmonary secretions, or protection from pulmonary aspiration. It is made of polyvinylchloride (PVC) and designed with a slight curve, making it easier to pass around the tongue without the need for a stylet.

epiglottitis   A serious airway emergency that can be life threatening. It results from a bacterial infection that causes acute inflammation of the supraglottic region of the oropharynx and is seen in children between 2 and 5 years of age.

epinephrine   The primary vasopressor for use in resuscitation. It is used with neonates in the delivery room to increase the rate and force of cardiac contractions and is recommended for a heart rate of fewer than 60 beats per minute after 30 seconds of adequate positive pressure ventilation with 100% oxygen and chest compressions.

Epworth Sleepiness Scale (ESS)   A scale intended to measure routine sleep practice. It is a questionnaire that asks caregivers to rate how often their child will doze off or fall asleep in different situations, such as watching television, doing homework, and riding in a car.

esophageal atresia   A congenital defect that affects the alimentary tract in which the upper esophagus ends and does not connect with the lower esophagus and stomach.

esophageal manometry   A diagnostic test used to identify problems with movement and pressure in the esophagus.

eucapnic voluntary hyperpnea (EVH)   A bronchoprovocation test performed in a pulmonary function laboratory to identify exercise-induced bronchospasm.

excessive daytime sleepiness (EDS)   Persistent sleepiness and often a general lack of energy that is present even during the day after apparently adequate or even prolonged nighttime sleep.

exercise-induced bronchospasm (EIB)   A condition in which the airways in the lungs narrow in response to physical exercise.

expiratory positive airway pressure (EPAP)   Positive airway pressure applied during the expiratory phase of mechanically assisted ventilation.

expiratory reserve volume (ERV)   The maximal amount of air that can be exhaled from the lungs.

extracorporeal cardiopulmonary resuscitation (ECPR)   Rapid initiation of extracorporeal membrane oxygenation (ECMO) during cardiopulmonary resuscitation.

extracorporeal membrane oxygenation (ECMO)   A form of mechanical circulatory support that incorporates an artificial lung or membrane oxygenator and is used to support neonates, infants, and children with severe cardiac, respiratory, or cardiorespiratory failure.

exudate   The fluid that accumulates within a pleural effusion that characteristically has a high protein count and some white and red blood cells; usually associated with increased capillary permeability due to infection, inflammation, or malignancy.

exudative phase   The acute phase in acute respiratory distress syndrome characterized by disrupted fluid balance following injury to the alveolar–capillary barrier.

F

failure to thrive   A term used in pediatric medicine to indicate inadequate weight gain or inappropriate weight loss.

family-centered care   An innovative approach to the planning, delivery, and evaluation of health care that is grounded in a mutually beneficial partnership among children, their families, and the clinical practitioners and professionals caring for the child who recognize the importance of the family in the patient's life.

family-centered rounds A process in which a hospitalized child's medical teams often meet in the child's room (to discuss current plan of care) where they speak with the family and child, incorporating their opinions, questions, suggestions, and beliefs into the plan—that is, including family in clinical rounds.

fetal biophysical profile (BPP) A noninvasive test that uses observations obtained during an ultrasound and the results of a nonstress test (NST) to evaluate the well-being of a fetus and to determine if a fetus is at risk of fetal death.

fetal lung maturity testing Tests performed on fetal amniotic fluid to provide an indirect assessment of the likelihood of lung maturity and that assists in determining the course of complicated as well as uncomplicated pregnancies.

FEV1 Forced expiratory volume in 1 second (FEV_1); measurement that in children is reflective of the degree of small-airway obstruction. It is measured prior to a bronchodilator treatment and again 15 minutes after bronchodilator administration, to determine reversibility of airway obstruction.

FEV_1/FVC ratio A calculated ratio used in the diagnosis of obstructive and restrictive lung disease.

fibroproliferative phase A phase in acute respiratory distress syndrome characterized by continued inflammatory response, fibrosis, and scarring of the alveolar–capillary unit.

fixed performance devices Devices that deliver a precise concentration of oxygen at a flow rate that meets or exceeds the patient's inspiratory demands.

fixed wing An airplane used to transport critically ill children, typically reserved for long distances often greater than 150 miles.

flail chest A fracture of two or more contiguous ribs in two or more places. The segment of fractured ribs creates a paradoxical breathing pattern, moving inward with inspiration and outward with expiration.

flexible airway endoscope An instrument with a slim, flexible tube attached to a camera source used to evaluate the lungs.

flexible airway endoscopy (FAE) The procedure of evaluating the lungs with a flexible airway endoscope, interchangeably referred to as bronchoscopy.

flow cycling A variable used to determine when a mechanical ventilator cycles to exhalation in which inspiration ends when air flow decreases.

flow-triggered breath A breath that occurs when the patient generates enough inspiratory effort (above a threshold or sensitivity setting) to initiate a flow of gas to the patient.

flow-volume loop A graph that plots measured flow on the Y axis and volume on the X axis for pulmonary function.

fluoroscopy An imaging technique that uses X-rays to examine tissues and deep structures of the body.

focal bronchiectasis A condition that occurs when a large airway becomes obstructed. The resulting inability to clear secretions leads to a cycle of infection, inflammation, and airway wall damage.

foramen ovale A small hole located in the septum between the two upper chambers of the heart that allows oxygenated blood to go from the left atrium to the left ventricle to the aorta to supply blood to the brain.

forced expiratory flow rate over the midportion of exhalation (FEF$_{25-75\%}$) Measurement that represents the flow rate measured over the midportion of a maximal exhalation. It is accurate only if the patient consistently blows to residual volume and produces multiple repeatable from efforts that have evidence of upper airway tension or glottis closure are not accurate.

forced expiratory volume in 1 second (FEV$_1$) A measurement that is reflective of flow in the large or central airways in adults in 1 second; however, in children, this measurement also reflects flow in the medium to small airways because their lungs are smaller and empty more quickly.

forced vital capacity (FVC) The volume of air that can be exhaled from the lungs after taking the deepest breath possible and then forcibly exhaling as much air as possible.

functional residual capacity (FRC) The volume of air present in the lungs at the end of passive expiration.

G

geometric standard deviation A measurement of how spread the size of aerosol particles are around the mass median aerodynamic diameter.

gestational age The amount of time that a fetus grows inside the mother's uterus, which is usually measured in weeks, that is the time period between the first day of the mother's last menstrual period and the day of delivery.

gestational diabetes mellitus (GDM) A form of diabetes that first occurs in women during a pregnancy.

Glasgow Coma Scale (GCS) A numeric scoring system used to evaluate patient alertness following a head injury. The scale ranges from 3 to 15. A lower score indicates a decreased level of consciousness and more severe head trauma; a score of 8 or less indicates a congenital condition in which there is downward displacement or retraction of the tongue and the patient will likely be in a coma and the outcome is poor.

glossoptosis An abnormal formation in which the base of the tongue is positioned upward and posterior toward the pharynx; it is often associated with Pierre Robin Syndrome and Trisomy 21 and can result in airway obstruction.

granulomas A small area of inflammation in tissue that is produced due to infection, inflammation, or the presence of a foreign substance.

grasp reflex An involuntary action of neonates; when placing a finger in a neonate's open palm results in the neonate closing their hand around the finger and tightening their grasp when the finger is moved within the palm. This is a normal reflex that is present until about 4 months of age.

gravida A term used to indicate the number of times the mother has been pregnant.

growth charts A series of percentile curves in which the selected body measurements of a particular child are plotted against the known percentile of other children.

grunting The sound an infant makes when expiring against a partially closed glottis. It is not a normal finding; rather, it is a compensatory mechanism to maximize gas exchange and is a hallmark sign of respiratory distress.

guided imagery Any of various techniques (as a series of verbal suggestions) used to guide another person or oneself in imagining sensations and especially in visualizing an image in the mind to bring about a desired physical response (as a reduction in stress, anxiety, or pain).

Guillain-Barré syndrome (GBS) A rare neurologic disorder in which the body's immune system attacks the nerves. Tingling and weakness in the legs are usually the first symptoms. Over the course of hours, days, or weeks, symptoms can spread to the upper body and lead to paralysis of the respiratory muscles.

H

head bobbing A condition that occurs when the sternocleidomastoid muscles, which are also used to stabilize the head, are being used to assist with respiration.

heart murmur A sound heard when there is turbulent or abnormal blood flow in or around the heart. A common finding in neonates usually resolves within the first 48 hours following birth. Murmurs are evaluated for their intensity or loudness, with descriptions that range from barely audible, soft, loud, to loud enough to hear with the stethoscope off of the chest.

heated high-flow nasal cannula (HHFNC) An oxygen-delivery device that provides a flow of heated, humidified gas through nasal prongs at flow rates that meet and/or exceed the patient's incubator.

heliox A mixture of helium and oxygen used to treat acute asthma as well as upper airway obstruction.

helium dilution One of three techniques to measure the functional residual capacity of the lung in which a patient breathes through a spirometer containing a known concentration of helium.

HELLP syndrome A syndrome characterized by *H*emolysis (H), *E*levated *L*iver enzymes (EL), and *L*ow *P*latelet count (LP) that occurs during pregnancy; it presents serious morbidity concerns and is managed similarly to preeclampsia.

hemoptysis Expectoration of blood from the larynx, trachea, or lungs.

hemothorax A condition in which there is the presence of blood in the pleural space. The source of blood may be the chest wall, lung parenchyma, heart, or great vessels, secondary mainly to a blunt trauma, iatrogenic causes, or a spontaneous occurrence.

high-frequency chest wall oscillation (HFCWO) A form of airway clearance therapy in which the child wears a garment or vest that delivers compression pulses to the chest wall. The alternating pulses quickly compress and release the chest wall, helping to loosen and thin mucus so that it is more easily removed from the lungs.

high-frequency jet ventilation (HFJV) A nonconventional mode of ventilation often used as a primary proactive strategy to limit exposure to excessive alveolar stretch and prevent lung injury when volutrauma exists; it is microprocessor controlled and capable of delivering and monitoring between 240 and 660 humidified breaths per minute. HFJV provides small pulses of fresh gas using high-velocity flow interruption during inspiration.

high-frequency oscillatory ventilation (HFOV) A nonconventional mode of ventilation often used as a primary proactive strategy to limit exposure to excessive alveolar stretch and prevent lung injury when volutrauma exists; a high-flow CPAP system with superimposed pressure oscillations. The pressure oscillations are created by an electronically driven diaphragm. HFOV incorporates a recruitment strategy by applying mean airway pressure to inflate the lung at or beyond the opening pressure and a lung protective strategy that uses rapid shallow delivery of active oscillation to provide minute ventilation, resulting in attenuated pressure delivery of gas to the lungs.

high-level disinfection (HLD) A process of cleaning the medical devices for complete elimination of all microorganisms.

high-risk delivery The delivery of a neonate as a result of a pregnancy that threatened the health or life of the mother or her fetus.

high-risk pregnancy A pregnancy that places the mother and/or her fetus at high risk for having complications that threaten the health of the mother or neonate.

history of present illness (HPI) A thorough description of relevant symptoms listed in chronological order and including any previous treatment.

home evaluation An assessment of a home to determine if the environment is safe and accessible for a child who has respiratory equipment needs at home.

home medical equipment company The company that provides medical equipment that can be used in the home.

home nursing agency A nursing agency that provides nursing support in the home.

home ventilator A mechanical ventilator that is capable of providing ventilation in the home setting.

hospice care End-of-life care in which a cure is no longer an option. To be eligible for hospice care, a physician must attest that the child's life expectancy is approximately 6 months or less.

hospitalized children The confinement of a child or infant in a hospital for diagnostic testing or therapeutic treatment.

huff coughing A type of deep breathing and coughing exercise in which a patient inhales deeply while leaning forward and exhale sharply while making a "huff" sound to mobilize secretions in the airway.

hypoplastic left heart syndrome A complex congenital heart disease in which the left side of the heart does not develop correctly in utero. This leaves the heart without the ability to effectively pump blood to the rest of the infant's body.

I

impedance pneumography A noninvasive method to monitor changes in the breathing activity of infants and children. Electrodes are placed on the infant's or child's chest wall and are typically held in place by a soft wrap. The electrodes are attached to a monitor by leads and a cable, similar in appearance to those used for electrocardiogram monitoring.

impeller A rotating device used in centrifugal pumps that are magnetically paired with an electric motor; the rotation of the motor causes a pressure differential that urges the forward flow of blood.

impulse oscillometry (IOS) A method to measure airway resistance in the preschooler. The child breathes through a pneumotach with a mouthpiece and nose clip in place. Downstream from the pneumotach is a miniature loudspeaker that produces forced oscillations generated by soundwaves with a range of frequencies into the airway.

incentive spirometry Also referred to as sustained maximal inspiration; a device that uses a visual aid to encourage children to take a deep breath, with the spirometer providing feedback on the child's inspiratory volume.

incubator A Plexiglas enclosure device that encompasses the infant's entire body and is capable of delivering a range of low concentrations of oxygen in a temperature- and humidity-controlled environment.

infant pulmonary function test (IPFT) A test that collects lung flow and volume and then adjusts the measurements for the lower lung volumes and flows of infants; comparable to spirometry and plethysmography in older children and adults.

influenza An extremely contagious respiratory illness caused by influenza A or B viruses; commonly known as "flu" and appearing most frequently in winter and early spring.

inhaled carbon dioxide A specialty gas used to allow for mild hypercapnea that will limit pulmonary blood flow in single ventricle congenital heart defects.

inhaled corticosteroids (ICSs) Medications used for asthma control that contains corticosteroids.

inhaled nitric oxide (iNO) A specialty gas that is inhaled to produce pulmonary vasodilation. Exogenous iNO enters the alveoli, diffuses across the alveolar–capillary membrane to the pulmonary smooth muscle cells, and results in vasodilation. iNO has a high affinity for hemoglobin, where it is bound and deactivated.

inspiratory capacity (IC) The total volume of air that can be drawn into the lungs after normal expiration.

inspiratory positive airway pressure (IPAP) The positive airway pressure delivered to the lungs during inspiration. It is applied above expiratory positive airway pressure and directly controls volume delivery to the patient.

inspiratory time The amount of time devoted to inspiration.

inspired carbon dioxide A specialty gas used to induce hypercarbia and increase pulmonary vascular resistance, which limits pulmonary blood flow in congenital heart defects such as hypoplastic left heart syndrome.

insufflation-exsufflation See cough assistance therapy.

intermittent mandatory ventilation (IMV) A mode of mechanical ventilation in which mandatory breaths are delivered at a set rate while spontaneous breaths can be taken between the mandatory breaths.

intraosseous (IO) An effective route through marrows of the bone for fluid resuscitation, drug delivery, and laboratory evaluation; an acceptable route for vascular access.

intraosseous (IO) needle A needle used to inject fluids or medication directly into the marrows of the bone.

intrapartum The period from the onset of labor to the end of the third stage of labor.

intrapulmonary percussive ventilation (IPV) An airway clearance therapy that delivers small, rapid, high-flow bursts of air directly into the airway. These bursts of air oscillate, causing a wedge of pressure to get behind secretions, loosening them so that they can then move to the large airways where they are expectorated or removed through suctioning. This provides airway clearance as well as hyperinflation.

invasive mechanical ventilation A method that requires the use of an artificial airway (e.g., endotracheal tube, tracheostomy tube) to provide continuous or intermittent mechanical ventilatory support.

isoflurane An anesthetic gas used in the treatment of status asthmaticus for its bronchial dilation properties.

ivacaftor The first available CFTR modulator therapy drug that targets the underlying cause of cystic fibrosis (CF). It is an oral medication approved for use in patients with cystic fibrosis who are 6 years of age and older with the CFTR gene mutation G551D. This medication is classified as a "potentiator" because it improves (potentiates) the function of the CFTR protein on the cell surface by allowing chloride absorption in the sweat gland, decreasing sweat chloride concentration.

J

jet nebulizers A type of nebulizer that uses a gas source to convert a solution/suspension into a mist. The gas is forced through a very small orifice, resulting in a decrease in pressure at the sides of the high-velocity jet stream (Bernoulli effect). Solutions/suspensions present in the nebulizer cup are drawn up the capillaries and aerosolized.

K

kyphoscoliosis A deformity of the spinal vertebrae that is a combination of kyphosis and scoliosis.

kyphosis A spinal vertebrae deformity due to excessive outward curvature of the spine, causing a hump-like appearance of the back.

L

lactate Any salt of lactic acid or the anion of lactic acid.

large for gestational age (LGA) Neonates having birth weights that are above the 90th percentile for their gestational age.

large-volume nebulizers Continuous output nebulizers used for continuous aerosol delivery of bronchodilators in the treatment of status asthmaticus. They have a favorable cost–benefit ratio over small-volume nebulizers. In general, the nebulizer reservoir can hold 200 to 240 mL of solution and produce an aerosol for 8 hours.

laryngeal mask airway A widely used supraglottic airway device; a small, elliptically shaped mask designed to fit in the hypopharynx and to provide a conduit that bypasses the upper airway and allows positive pressure ventilation.

laryngotracheal groove A furrow that develops in the foregut endoderm during the embryonic stage, which lasts from about 3 to 7 weeks' gestation, that develops into the lungs.

Laryngotracheobronchitis (LTB) An inflammatory process that affects the larynx, trachea, and occasionally the bronchi, resulting in edema and varying degrees of airway narrowing. It is the most common cause of upper airway obstruction due to infection in young children

lateral decubitus Position of the patient while doing radiography examination that is used to evaluate the presence of air or fluid in the pleural space.

lecithin-to-sphingomyelin (L:S) ratio A marker for fetal lung maturity; ratio between the lecithin and the amount of sphingomyelin in amniotic fluid.

left ventricular outflow tract obstruction A congenital heart defect that results from a series of stenotic areas between the left ventricular outflow tract and the descending aortic arch. This can lead to left ventricular hypertrophy and left ventricular failure.

leukotriene modifiers Medication used for the prophylaxis and chronic treatment of asthma in adults and children.

ligation A surgical procedure of tying a ligature tightly around a blood vessel or other duct or tube in the body for treating diseases such as patent ductus arteriosus.

long-acting beta2-agonists (LABAs) Also commonly called "long-acting beta-agonists"; medications used for asthma maintenance therapy in conjunction with inhaled corticosteroids to relieve bronchospasm and reduce airway inflammation. These inhaled medications have a slightly longer onset of action but provide bronchodilation for a longer duration of time (e.g., 12 hours).

looping A process in which the heart undergoes dramatic changes through differential cellular growth by the 4th gestational week.

lung biopsy A procedure performed by inserting biopsy forceps through the working channel of a bronchoscope to obtain a sample of transbronchial lung tissue.

lung bud A pouch that appears as the laryngotracheal groove, formed during the development of lungs in the embryonic stage, separates from the primitive esophagus.

lung clearance index (LCI) A measure of the cumulative expired volume needed to clear a tracer gas from the lungs divided by the functional residual capacity; it is measured by performing a gas washout using a low concentration of an inert gas.

M

machine-triggered A mechanical ventilation breath initiated after a preset time has elapsed.

macrocephaly A head circumference that is greater than two standard deviations above the mean for a given age, gender, and gestation.

macroglossia An enlarged tongue that can create chewing, speech, and airway management problems and can be associated with dentomusculoskeletal deformities as well as other disorders, including Beckwith Wiedemann and Down syndrome.

magnetic resonance imaging An imaging technique that uses a combination of magnetism, radio waves, and computer processing to create detailed anatomical images.

mandatory minute ventilation (MMV) An automatic weaning mode that involves setting a target minute ventilation that is the reference point for support. The ventilator predicts the minute ventilation over 8 to 10 breaths and provides support based on that prediction.

mandibular hypoplasia A craniofacial disorder in neonates, also known as micrognathia, strawberry chin, or hypognathia, characterized by an undersize facial jaw, specifically a small mandible and receding chin.

mannitol challenge Optional testing to assess bronchial hyperresponsiveness for individuals who cannot achieve and/or maintain the recommended target heart rate and ventilation to evaluate exercise-induced bronchospasm.

mass median aerodynamic diameter (MMAD) The particle diameter at which half of the mass of the particles in an aerosol are smaller and the other half of the particles are larger.

massive hemoptysis The expectoration of a large amount of blood originating from the tracheobronchial tree or lung parenchyma and is regarded as a life-threatening situation.

maximal expiratory pressure (MEP) A measurement made when the patient expires maximally against an occlusion for 1 to 3 seconds. The measured pressure is recorded in cm H_2O. MEP measures the accessory muscles and elastic recoil of the lungs.

maximal inspiratory pressure (MIP) A measurement made when the patient inspires maximally against an occlusion for 1 to 3 seconds. The measured pressure is recorded in cm H_2O. MIP primarily measures inspiratory muscle strength.

mean blood pressure Also referred to as "mean arterial pressure" or "MAP." An average blood pressure in arteries during one cardiac cycle. For a neonate it is calculated as follows: adequate mean blood pressure = gestational age in weeks + 5.

meconium aspiration syndrome (MAS) A condition in which the infant aspirates meconium (fetal bowel content) prior to or during birth.

meconium ileus An intestinal obstruction resulting from the impaction of thick, tenacious meconium in the distal small bowel of a newborn infant.

membrane oxygenator A silicone sheet arranged in a spool with separated blood and gas compartments. Gas exchange across the silicone sheet is dependent on the driving pressures of oxygen and carbon dioxide and is influenced by the composition of the supply gas, referred to as sweep gas; the degree of desaturation of the blood; and the rate at which it flowed through the membrane.

meninges The three connective tissue layers that protect the brain and spinal cord. It contains cerebrospinal fluid and supports the blood vessels that run throughout the central nervous system.

mesoderm The middle of the three germ layers of an embryo formed by the 3rd week of life; it contributes to the blood; endothelium; heart; kidneys; reproductive organs; bones; skeletal tissues; and smooth and connective tissue, such as tendons, ligaments, dermis, and cartilage.

methacholine challenge A test to assess bronchial or airway hyperresponsiveness in which a patient is given increasing inhaled doses of methacholine followed by spirometry to determine changes in the FEV_1.

methemoglobin (MetHb) An abnormal hemoglobin formed when inhaled nitric oxide binds with hemoglobin (Hb), which reduces the hemoglobin's affinity for oxygen and ability to transport O_2.

methylxanthines Medications indicated for asthma, neonatal apnea, and status asthmaticus. They inhibit phosphodiesterase and histone deacetylase-2 activation, causing an increase in cAMP and resulting in the deactivation of inflammatory genes, which leads to bronchodilation.

microcephaly A head circumference that is two or more standard deviations below the mean for a given age, gender, and gestation.

minor hemoptysis The expectoration of a small amount of blood, less than 200 ml, originating from the tracheobronchial tree or lung parenchyma.

minute ventilation A product of respiratory rate and tidal volume; it is the amount of air inhaled or exhaled in one minute and expressed as liters per minute.

mitochondrial disorders A group of neuromuscular diseases that occur when there is damage to the mitochondria in the cells. Enzymes within the mitochondria change nutrients into cellular energy; mitochondrial failure leads to death of the cells and ultimately organ failure. These disorders can be caused by genetic mutation or may be acquired following the adverse effects from drugs or infections.

mitomycin C An antibiotic that inhibits cell division, protein synthesis, and fibroblast proliferation, resulting in reduced granulation formation in patients undergoing nasal reconstruction; a topical agent aid used intraoperatively to prevent the formation of scar tissue and restenosis following choanal atresia repair.

modified Allen's test The test used to verify the presence or absence of collateral circulation.

Moro reflex A reflex action of a neonate when it is held and the head allowed to drop slightly but suddenly; a normal response is to be startled, with the arms extended and abducted outward and the palms open. This is quickly followed by the neonate bringing the arms inward in an embracing posture with the hands clenched into fists, and is often associated with a momentary cry.

morula A solid ball of blastomeres formed when the zygote undergoes cellular division.

mucociliary escalator A mechanism involving ciliary action by which the mucus layer in the airway is moved from bronchioles through the bronchi and trachea to the larynx.

mucolytics Medications that change the biophysical properties of secretions. They are capable of modifying mucus production, secretion, nature and composition, and interactions with mucociliary epithelium.

mucus hypersecretion The increased production of mucus in the airways; a key pathophysiologic feature in many patients with asthma, cystic fibrosis, and bronchiectasis.

multiple breath washout (MBW) A method that has gained considerable interest in identifying lung disease in children with cystic fibrosis and is thought to be more sensitive than spirometry in accomplishing this. MBW is used to measure functional residual capacity and to assess distribution of ventilation.

multiple gestation A pregnancy with twins, triplets, or more.

Murphy eye An additional orifice on the side of the endotracheal tube (ETT) at the distal tip. It will allow bilateral lung ventilation when the tip of the ETT sits close to the carina; gas is able to pass to one lung out of the distal orifice of the ETT and to the other lung through the Murphy eye.

muscular dystrophy (MD) A group of genetic disorders that are characterized by progressive muscular degeneration and weakness. This weakness is usually due to abnormalities in muscle proteins caused by genetic mutations. There are more than 30 forms of muscular dystrophy.

myasthenia gravis A chronic autoimmune neuromuscular disease that causes varying degrees of muscle weakness. The body's own antibodies block, alter, or destroy acetylcholine receptors, which in turn disrupts the transmission of nerve impulses to the muscles. The most commonly affected muscles are those that control the eyes, face, speech, and swallowing.

N

nasal cannula A commonly used variable performance oxygen delivery device that delivers low concentrations of oxygen to infants and children. It consists of small-bore oxygen tubing connected to two short prongs. The prongs are inserted in the nares and angled down to conform to the anatomic features of the nares.

nasal flaring A term used to describe the widening of the nares or nostrils with each breath during inspiration. It is a sign of respiratory distress and is the result of the neonate or child attempting to move more air through the nares and to decrease airway resistance.

nasopharyngeal airway A soft, flexible device placed inside the nares of the nose designed to maintain or improve upper airway patency by creating a conduit from the tip of the nose to the hypopharynx. This device often bypasses an upper airway obstruction.

near infrared spectroscopy (NIRS) A noninvasive, spectroscopic tool, which uses the near-infrared region of the electromagnetic spectrum, and provides real-time continuous monitoring of regional tissue oxyhemoglobin saturation (rSO_2).

nebulizers Devices used in aerosol therapy that convert a solution/suspension into an inhalable mist.

negative pressure ventilation A type of mechanical ventilation. To generate ventilation, these ventilators apply a negative pressure to the outside of the chest and abdomen during inspiration.

neurodisability disorders Conditions associated with impairment involving the brain and/or nervous system.

neuromuscular blocking agents (NMBAs) Medications used for the induction of neuromuscular blockade and that provide skeletal muscle relaxation during surgery or mechanical ventilation.

neutral thermal environment Maintenance of ambient temperatures in an incubator within 0.5°C of the newborn's body temperature to avoid heat or cold stress and to optimize energy use and oxygen consumption.

neutrally adjusted ventilatory assist ventilation (NAVA) A spontaneous mode of ventilation that is available on the Servo-I and Servo-U ventilators (Maquet, Rastatt, Germany). Similar to pressure support, the patient's own respiratory drive controls the rate of ventilation. This uses an orogastric catheter embedded with special sensors that detect electronic signals from the phrenic nerve to the diaphragm, sensing diaphragmatic contraction.

New Ballard Score A system that determines gestational age of a neonate through the assessment of six physical and six neuromuscular features. The system works on the presumption that fetal skin, subcutaneous tissues, and the neuromuscular system mature at predictable rates, and a numeric score is determined for each of the 12 features.

nitric oxide (NO) A colorless, odorless gas, consisting of one nitrogen and one oxygen atom, normally found in exhaled air, can be useful in monitoring airway inflammation. Also a free radical and highly reactive gas that is unstable in the presence of air and an endothelial-derived vasodilator and a pulmonary vasodilator that is inhaled to treat atrioventricular canal defect.

nitrogen dioxide (NO_2) A toxic environmental pollutant formed by the oxidation of nitric oxide (NO) that it is associated with airway damage and inflammation.

nitrogen washout One of three techniques to measure the functional residual capacity of the lungs in which the patient breathes in 100% oxygen after which the nitrogen concentration of the exhaled gas is measured.

nonaccidental trauma (NAT) Trauma due to abuse or self-harm that imposes a significant physical, psychological, emotional, and financial burden on children and their families.

noncardiogenic pulmonary edema An accumulation of fluid within the lungs caused by increased permeability of the alveolar–capillary membrane.

noncommunicable Diseases not able to be transmitted from one sufferer to another, such as leukemia.

noninvasive biphasic positive pressure ventilation See continuous positive airway pressure (CPAP).

noninvasive positive pressure ventilation (NPPV) A mode of ventilation for older children who are stable and require support only during sleep.

noninvasive ventilation (NIV) A technique that delivers intermittent or continuous assisted ventilation or provides continuous positive pressure during spontaneous breathing to enhance lung expansion by restoring or improving functional residual capacity (FRC) and/or improving minute ventilation without the use of an artificial airway.

non-rapid eye movement (NREM) A stage in the sleep state during which dreams do not occur.

nonrebreathing mask An oxygen reservoir device; it has a circular flap or valve at the juncture where the reservoir bag attaches to the disposable plastic mask. Oxygen is delivered in this device through small-bore, smooth lumen tubing below the flap or valve at the junction between the mask and the reservoir bag. The flap or valve between the reservoir bag and the mask prevents exhaled gas from entering the reservoir bag and diluting the concentration of oxygen available for delivery.

nonstress test (NST) A noninvasive test in which a monitor measures the fetal heart rate (FHR) in response to fetal movement, generally over a 20-minute period, and records a tracing of the FHR and uterine activity.

normoxemic hypoxia The presence of tissue hypoxia in spite of having a normal PaO2 or SpO2.

nuchal cord An umbilical cord that becomes coiled around the fetus's body, usually the neck.

O

oblique A radiographic position that is halfway between anteroposterior (AP) or posterioanterior (PA) and lateral positions that gains an additional perspective of the lungs. The oblique rotation will place the anatomic structures in a different position to provide further evaluation of areas previously superimposed on the anteroposterior/posteroanterior image. This position also elongates the ribs to allow for better determination of fracture.

obstructive sleep apnea A disorder of breathing during sleep characterized by prolonged partial upper airway obstruction and/or intermittent complete obstruction that disrupts alveolar gas exchange and normal sleep patterns.

occipitofrontal circumference A measurement around the largest area of the head; it is used as a measurement of head growth.

oligohydramnios A condition occurring most often during the last trimester in pregnancy characterized by a decreased amount of amniotic fluid.

oropharyngeal airway A rigid, c-shaped device that is inserted through the mouth to provide a clear passage of airflow past the obstruction of the tongue and upper airway tissue to the level of the supraglottic area.

oscillatory positive expiratory pressure therapy Also known as vibratory PEP, this airway clearance therapy uses the resistance during exhalation while creating vibrations or oscillations at the airway opening to sher mucus from the surface of the airways.

oxygen hoods Enclosure devices that encompass the infant's head and neck, typically to the shoulder area. An oxygen blender is used to provide the ordered or specified FiO_2, ranging from 0.21 to 1.0, which can be connected directly to the hood or to a circuit capable of providing heat and humidity. An oxygen analyzer is typically used to verify the oxygen concentration delivered to the infant.

oxygenation index (OI) A calculation that helps gauge disease severity. Mean airway pressure (mPaw) and FiO_2 information obtained from the mechanical ventilator are used to calculate the oxygenation index (OI), which is determined as follows: OI × mPaw / (FiO_2/PaO_2) × 100. An OI in excess of 40 while using conventional mechanical ventilation has been associated with mortality risk great than 80%.

P

palliative care Specialized care for patients who have a life-limiting or terminal illness. It includes comprehensive medical, psychosocial, and spiritual care aimed at relieving symptoms and suffering, slowing the progression of the disease, and achieving the best possible quality of life for the patient, while also providing emotional support to the family.

paradoxical cyanosis Cyanosis that is relieved when an infant cries; most often occurring when there is relief of an airway obstruction such as choanal atresia.

paradoxical respirations A breathing pattern in which the chest moves in on inspiration and out on expiration; also called seesaw breathing or thoracoabdominal asynchrony, a condition that may be noted during respiratory distress of any cause.

parallel play Playing alongside other children but not engaging.

parity A term used to indicate the number of pregnancies that went beyond 20 weeks' gestation or to viability. The number of fetuses does not affect the parity.

partial rebreathing mask A reservoir device used to deliver oxygen to children; it has a reservoir bag attached to the disposable plastic mask. Oxygen is delivered in this device through small-bore, smooth lumen tubing at the junction between the mask and the reservoir bag. It has exhalation ports on either side of the mask to allow exhaled gas to escape, and to provide a mechanism for the patient to entrain air should the oxygen source fail.

patent ductus arteriosus (PDA) An acyanotic heart defect in which the ductus arteriosus fails to close after birth. The ductus arteriosus is a channel that connects the aortic arch to the pulmonary arteries and is a normal and essential fetal structure. Closure typically occurs within the first few hours to first few days of life.

Patient Protection and Affordable Care Act (PPACA) Also known as the Affordable Care Act or ACA; the health care reform law enacted in March 2010 that has three primary goals: to make affordable health insurance available to more people, to expand the Medicaid program to cover all adults with income below 138% of the federal poverty level, and to support innovative medical care delivery methods designed to lower the costs of health care generally.

patient-triggered During mechanical ventilation, the inspiration begins or is initiated by the patient and not by the mechanical ventilator. patient has an inspiratory effort that starts or initiates a mandatory breath.

peak flow meter A hand-held device used to measure the peak expiratory flow rate.

pectus carinatum Also known as pigeon chest, a condition in which there is anterior or outward protrusion of the sternum.

pectus excavatum The most common chest malformation, and often referred to as funnel chest, in which the chest has a sunken appearance and remains sunken even during inhalation.

Pediatric Assessment Triangle (PAT) A rapid, strategic primary assessment of a child's severity of illness; it uses a visual and auditory assessment of the child, including evaluation of the child's appearance, work of breathing, and circulation. It allows the clinician to quickly form an accurate initial impression of the child as "sick" or "not sick" and, therefore, to prioritize as appropriate.

Pediatric Risk of Mortality Score (PRISM) A prognostic scoring system used to determine the risk for mortality. This tool, derived from 14 physiologic variables, assesses mortality risk for pediatric patients during their first 24 hours of care in the intensive care unit (ICU).

percent predicted Spirometry values are generally expressed as percent predicted. It is calculated as follows: percent predicted = (observed value ÷ Predicted Value) × 100.

percussion A rhythmic clapping made by percussing the chest using a cupped hand or a device made for percussion, focusing on the various segments of the lungs, to mobilize secretions.

periodic breathing A sequence of three or more consecutive respiratory pauses lasting 3 or more seconds, with 20 seconds or less of normal respiration between pauses. In premature neonates, an irregular breathing pattern of intermittent respiratory pauses that last longer than 5 seconds.

peripheral artery catheter A small catheter placed through the skin into an artery of the arm or leg. It is used when frequent sampling of arterial blood is required or when cannulation of the umbilical artery is not a viable option.

peripheral IV A catheter placed into a vein to give fluids or medications.

peripherally inserted central catheter (PICC) A catheter inserted into the superior vena cava through a peripheral vein. It is threaded percutaneously through a superficial vein and can be used to administer vasoactive medications and parenteral nutrition. It allows concentrated solutions to be delivered with less risk of complications.

permissive hypercapnia A lung-protective strategy used with mechanical ventilation in which the $PaCO_2$ is maintained at 45–55 mm Hg and the pH is maintained at greater than 7.2.

persistent pulmonary hypertension of the newborn (PPHN) A neonatal condition in which there is interference with the normal change from fetal to postnatal circulation and the usual reduction in pulmonary vascular resistance does not occur; it is usually due to hypoxia associated with parenchymal lung disease, such as respiratory distress syndrome and bronchopulmonary dysplasia.

personal protective equipment (PPE) Protective clothing that must be worn by all staff involved at the bedside during certain procedures, including the flexible airway endoscopy. This includes face masks and eye protection, nitrile gloves, and gowns.

phospholipids Lipids that are the dominant component of lung surfactants, comprising nearly 80% of the surfactant complex.

photoplethysmography A simple and low-cost optical technique that uses light to analyze variations in volume changes in tissue during pulsatile blood flow to distinguish between arterial and venous blood flow.

Pierre Robin syndrome A set of facial abnormalities, consisting of mandibular hypoplasia, cleft palate, and glossoptosis. This triad of deformities may potentially contribute to respiratory distress, airway obstruction, and hypoxia.

placenta The pancake-shaped organ that attaches, during pregnancy, to the mother's uterus. By way of the umbilical cord it supplies the fetus with oxygenated blood and nutrients and removes waste products, including carbon dioxide, from the fetus.

placenta previa A condition in which the placenta is implanted abnormally low in the uterus, partially or completely covering the cervix.

placental abruption A condition in which the placenta either partially or completely separates from the uterine wall, also known as abruptio placentae.

placental circulation Circulation between the mother and fetus, established to provide gas exchange necessary to sustain life. It consists of the left umbilical vein and umbilical artery.

pleural effusion Any abnormal collection of fluid in the pleural space. It is the most common manifestation of pleural disease.

pleurodesis A medical procedure that is performed to prevent recurrent accumulation of pleural effusions.

pneumomediastinum A condition that occurs when free air traverses from the ruptured alveolus along the pulmonary vasculature to the mediastinum.

pneumopericardium A condition in which air leaks into the pericardial space, which can lead to acute, life-threatening symptoms as air accumulates and comes under tension within the limited pericardial space.

pneumothorax A condition that occurs when air escapes from the airway and enters the space bounded by the parietal pleura of the chest wall and the visceral pleura of the lung.

polyhydramnios A condition in pregnancy characterized by an abnormally high level of amniotic fluid.

Polysomnography (PSG) The most commonly used test for the evaluation and diagnosis of sleep disorders. It includes monitoring of the patient's airflow through the nose and mouth, blood pressure, electrocardiographic activity, blood oxygen level, brain wave pattern, eye movement, and the movement of respiratory muscle and limbs.

positive airway pressure A mode of ventilation used in the treatment of sleep apnea.

positive end-expiratory pressure (PEEP) The positive pressure that exists in the lungs at the end of an expiration during mechanical ventilation.

post accident incident plan (PAIP) A plan developed to guide staff, management, dispatch, and local law enforcement in the event of an accident or incident.

postductal Placement of a pulse oximeter probe on a neonate's left hand or on either foot measures oxygen saturation distal to the aortic opening of the ductus arteriosus.

posteroanterior (PA) A position in which the patient either is in a prone position or is standing and the radiographic beam enters from back to front.

postterm pregnancy A pregnancy that extends past 42 weeks.

postural drainage An airway clearance technique that uses gravity in moving secretions from the lung. The patient is placed in various positions to target drainage of specific lung segments.

pre- and post-bronchodilator testing A spirometry test that provides information regarding reversibility of bronchoconstriction or airway hyperresponsiveness, as seen in asthma.

preductal Placement of a pulse oximeter probe on a neonate's right hand measures oxygen saturation proximal to the aortic opening of the ductus arteriosus.

preeclampsia A condition in which the mother develops elevated blood pressures and proteinuria after the 20th week of pregnancy.

premature rupture of membranes Rupture of membranes (breakage of the amniotic sac) prior to the onset of labor.

prenatal care The comprehensive medical care and monitoring that a woman receives during pregnancy; it involves the physical assessment of the mother and fetus, screening and treatment for medical conditions, and emotional support and counseling.

pressure control ventilation (PCV) A mode of ventilation used in preterm infants. PCV results in the delivery of a predetermined pressure during inspiration, at a predetermined time and rate.

pressure support ventilation (PSV) A spontaneous mode of ventilation in which breaths are supported by an operator-set pressure target. The breath can be initiated by pressure or flow triggering.

pressure-triggered breath To initiate a breath, the patient must make sufficient effort to generate an airway pressure drop below end-expiratory pressure larger than the operator-set sensitivity threshold.

pressurized metered dose inhalers (pMDIs) A device that delivers a specific amount of medication to the lungs when inhaled; medication is delivered in an aerosol form.

preterm Before completion of the full term (not more than 37 weeks of pregnancy).

preterm labor Regular contractions of the uterus that occur between 20 and 37 weeks' gestation and are of sufficient frequency and intensity to cause effacement and dilation of the cervix.

primary assessment A systematic approach to determine what life-threatening conditions may exist. The assessment is based on the mnemonic ABCDE, which is as follows: *Airway, Breathing, Circulation, Disability, Exposure.*

primary caregiver The person who takes primary responsibility for the daily care and rearing of a child.

prostaglandin A hormone-like substance that participates in a wide range of body functions, such as the contraction and relaxation of smooth muscle, the dilation and constriction of blood vessels, control of blood pressure, and modulation of inflammation.

provocation dose (PD$_{20}$) The dose of methacholine given to the patient in a methacholine challenge test at which a drop of 20% or greater from baseline value of FEV$_1$ is documented.

pseudomacroglossia A condition in which the tongue may be normal in size but is forced to sit in an abnormal position due to anatomical associations.

ptosis The drooping of one or both eyelids.

pulmonary agenesis A very rare congenital anomaly of the lung that is also commonly associated with other congenital malformations of the cardiovascular, skeletal, gastrointestinal, or urinary systems; characterized by the total absence of bronchus and lung with no vascular supply to the affected area.

pulmonary air leak syndromes Common syndromes that occur when there is a rupture of the trachea, bronchi, or smaller airways, leading to an escape of air into the surrounding tissue; caused by positive pressure applied during mechanical ventilation, especially with high alveolar pressures and/or volumes. It occurs more frequently in the newborn period than at any other time of life.

pulmonary aplasia A rare congenital malformation that is usually associated with other congenital abnormalities and characterized by the presence of a bronchus without any lung tissue.

pulmonary artery catheters Also known as Swan Ganz catheters; insertion of a catheter into a pulmonary artery for direct monitoring of pulmonary and intracardiac pressures and measurement of mixed venous oxygen tensions and cardiac output.

pulmonary artery hypertension (PAH) A condition in which blood pressure in the arteries is high.

pulmonary atresia A rare congenital heart defect in which the pulmonary valve fails to develop between the 6th and 9th weeks of gestation and results in a valve that is small and lacks an opening.

pulmonary composite A set of factors applicable to neurodisability patients with pulmonary complications.

pulmonary function testing A group of noninvasive tests that measure lung volume, capacity, flow rate, and gas exchange.

pulmonary hypertension (PH) The condition of elevated systolic pulmonary artery pressure.

pulmonary hypoplasia A condition in which there is inadequate development of the fetal lung characterized by a

decreased number of airways, cells, and alveoli; decreased size and weight of lungs; causes include impaired fetal breathing, decreased production of amniotic fluid, and fetal or maternal conditions that limit fetal lung growth.

pulmonary interstitial emphysema (PIE) A condition that occurs when air leaks into the pulmonary interstitial space.

pulmonary sequestration A congenital disorder in which the lung tissue has no connection to the bronchial tree or pulmonary arteries.

pulmonary stenosis (PS) A congenital heart condition characterized by obstruction to blood flow from the right ventricle into the pulmonary artery; stenosis at one or more locations from the right ventricular outflow tract causes the obstruction. The stenosis may be subvalvular (before the valve), supravalvular (after the valve), valvular, or in the pulmonary artery.

pulmonary surfactant A complex mixture of lipids and proteins that is secreted into the alveolar space, whose deficiency leads to lung immaturity and is the primary causes of respiratory distress syndrome in neonates and older infants; it functions to lower surface tension at the air–liquid interface in the lung and in turn to stabilize the alveoli.

pulmonary vascular resistance The resistance blood faces when flowing across the pulmonary vascular bed; ejection of blood through the pulmonic valve against the low pressure of the pulmonary circulation in the right ventricle.

pulse contour analysis A minimally invasive technique that uses pressure measurements obtained from a pulmonary artery or central venous catheter to continuously calculate cardiac output.

pulse oximetry Widely used it means to noninvasively monitor oxygenation status and to provide objective data to guide care. It provides continuous, instantaneous monitoring of heart rate and hemoglobin oxygen saturation, reported as SpO$_2$.

pulse pressure The difference between the systolic and diastolic blood pressures. A narrow pulse pressure occurs when cardiac output is low and there is an increase in systemic vascular resistance.

Q

Qp/Qs ratio The ratio of pulmonary blood flow to systemic blood flow.

quality of life A person's general well-being, including mental status, health status, stress level, freedom from disease, and ability to pursue daily activities.

R

radiolucent Allowing the passage of X-rays or other radiation; not radiopaque.

raised volume rapid thoracoabdominal compression technique (RV/RTC) A pulmonary function technique to obtain measurements similar to forced vital capacity in which the infant's inspiratory effort is augmented by 30 cm H$_2$O positive pressure applied to the breathing circuit.

ramp time The period in mechanical ventilation during which the inspiratory pressure is gradually increased. Adjustments in ramp time are made to assist with patient tolerance and comfort.

rapid eye movement (REM) A stage in sleep state in which there is random, rapid eye movement beneath the lids.

recirculation The tendency of reinfused oxygenated blood to mix with venous blood, reducing the overall amount of oxygen delivered.

reservoir device A device that provides a continuous flow of oxygen; it allows the patient to breathe in the flow of oxygen provided by the flowmeter in addition to the gas contained within the device.

residence time A measure of how long aerosol particles remain in the lung, in particular the last six generations of the airways.

residual volume (RV) The amount of air remaining in the lungs after a full exhalation.

respirable fraction The fraction of the aerosol that is highly likely to deposit in the lungs.

respiratory distress syndrome (RDS) A problem for premature infants born at fewer than 28 weeks' gestation, also known as hyaline membrane disease (HMD), due to a surfactant deficiency.

respiratory failure The inability of the lungs to perform their basic task of gas exchange, which is the transfer of oxygen from inhaled air into the blood and the transfer of carbon dioxide from the blood into exhaled air.

respiratory inductance plethysmography A method to determine respiratory movements or effort.

respiratory resistance (Rint) A noninvasive measurement used to determine airway resistance.

respiratory syncytial virus (RSV) A virus that is the leading cause of lower respiratory tract infections in infants and young children and the most common cause of bronchiolitis and pneumonia in children younger than 1 year of age. It occurs primarily during the fall, winter, and spring seasons.

retinopathy of prematurity (ROP) An eye disease that occurs in premature infants; caused by an aberrant development of the blood vessels supplying the retina within the eye and can lead to blindness; formerly known as retrolental fibroplasia.

retractions The inward movement or sucking in of the skin covering the chest during inspiration.

review of systems A list of questions, arranged by organ system, that provides a systematic overview of the child's health.

Reynold's equation The product of the velocity of gas flow, diameter of the tube the gas is flowing through, and the gas density, divided by the viscosity of the gas. Solving this mathematical equation will yield a Reynold's number (Re), whose value will determine whether flow is laminar or turbulent.

Reynold's number (Re) Solving Reynold's equation will yield a Reynold's number (Re), whose value will determine whether flow is laminar or turbulent. An Re >4000 describes turbulent flow through a tube while an Re <2000 represents laminar flow through a tube.

rigid bronchoscopy A procedure used to immediately remove a foreign body in children presenting with partial obstruction and clinical compromise.

rima glottides The elongated opening between the true vocal cords and the arytenoid cartilages.

rise time A parameter available on a mechanical ventilator that enables improved breath synchrony. It reflects how quickly inspiratory flow is delivered. It is the amount of time required to reach the maximum flow during pressure support ventilation (PSV) or pressure control ventilation (PCV) and should be set to maximize patient comfort.

roller pumps Occlusive mechanical pumps used for the displacement of blood through an extracorporeal membrane oxygenation (ECMO) circuit.

rooming-in A period of time in which caregivers stay in the room with their child assuming all medical care with supervision from the medical team to determine if they are ready and competent to provide safe care at home.

rooting reflex An action seen in normal neonates, when the cheek is stroked and the neonate turns toward the stroked side and begins making sucking motions.

rotor wing The helicopter used to transport critically ill children.

S

safety management system (SMS) A commonly used transport tool, vital to creating a culture of safety that supports risk assessment, accountability, professionalism, and organizational dynamics. It integrates safety risk management and safety assurance concepts into repeatable, proactive systems.

scoliosis A spinal vertebra deformity causing a sideways curvature of the spine.

secondary caregiver Other persons who also provide assistance to a child but without having the primary responsibility.

septum primum A wall or partition between the right and left chambers in the embryonic heart; originating in the roof of the common atria, it stretches to connect with the fused endocardial cushion of the atrioventricular canal.

short-acting beta2-agonists (SABAs) Also commonly called "short-acting beta-agonists"; the quick-relief drugs used for acute exacerbations of asthma and to prevent exercise-induced bronchospasm. The onset of action is rapid, or within 3 to 5 minutes following administration, and the effects last for 4 to 6 hours.

siblings Each of two or more children or offspring having one or both parents in common; a brother or sister.

Silverman Score A tool that assesses and grades or scores a neonate; it is used to quantify respiratory distress and lung disease.

simple mask An oxygen reservoir device; a lightweight plastic mask designed to fit over the nose and mouth. The mask has exhalation ports located on either side that also allow the patient to entrain air to meet their total flow needs. The mask is held in place by a small, adjustable elastic band attached to the device's peripheral ends. A flexible metal strip, located at the proximal end of the mask, allows the caregiver to conform the mask to the contours of the nasal bridge to prevent the flow of oxygen from escaping and to minimize irritation to the eyes.

skeletal muscle relaxants See neuromuscular blocking agents.

skills validation A tool used to document ongoing competency. Caregivers are informed that the skills validation will be performed at an upcoming clinic visit and are instructed to bring their home equipment with them. During the visit, they are asked to set up the equipment and to perform therapy as they do at home. If any deficiencies are identified during the skills validation session, remedial education can be provided at that time.

sleep architecture The basic structural organization of normal sleep characterized by several measures, which include sleep time, sleep efficiency, sleep onset latency, awake time after sleep onset, and percentage of sleep time spent in non-rapid eye movement stage and in rapid eye movement sleep.

sleep hygiene Also called routine sleep practice; different practices and habits that are necessary to have good nighttime sleep that include evening routine, time to go to bed, bedtime behavior, sleep environment, nocturnal and morning behavior, and daytime functioning.

sleep-disordered breathing A group of disorders characterized by abnormal respiratory patterns (e.g., the presence of apneas or hypopneas).

small for gestational age (SGA) Neonates having birth weights that are below the 10th percentile for their gestational age.

smart care An automatic mechanical ventilation weaning mode that adjusts pressure support levels based on tidal volume (Vt), respiratory rate, end-tidal carbon dioxide, and patient condition.

smart nebulizers Nebulizers that incorporate technology to allow control of drug delivery and to record adherence to therapy. This type of nebulizer is more precise because it interacts with the patient's breathing pattern and is ideal for the delivery of expensive drugs with low therapeutic index. The system also allows a distal and proximal airway delivery mode by releasing the aerosol at the beginning or middle of the inspiratory cycle. It is bulky and expensive.

sniffing position A head position in which the patient is supine and the neck slightly extended; aligning the posterior pharynx, larynx, and trachea.

soft mist inhalers Propellant-free devices that use the mechanical energy generated by a tensioned spring to generate the aerosol. This aerosol delivery to the patient is slower and the mist lasts longer than the one generated by a pressurized metered dose inhaler; therefore, it is recommended to be used without a spacer or valved holding chamber.

spacers Valveless tubes that provide distance between the pressurized metered dose inhaler and the patient's mouth. It allows deceleration of the aerosol and impaction of the large particles against their walls. This results in a decrease in oropharyngeal deposition effects.

Spaulding Classification Scheme A system that classifies medical devices as noncritical, semicritical, or critical. The classification is based on the amount of risk the patient has of being contaminated by the device.

specific airway conductance (sGaw) A measure of intrinsic airway resistance, to determine airway function or dysfunction.

specific airway resistance (sRaw) A spirometry method to measure airway resistance that requires the child to be seated in the body plethysmograph with the door closed. A mouthpiece with a nose clip in place is used to breathe through a pneumotach. During tidal volume breathing, flow is measured by the pneumotach and the change in pressure is measured by pressure transducers in the plethysmograph. The sRaw is calculated from the change in volume divided by the change in flow.

spectrophotometry A tool to determine the SpO_2 based on the Beer-Lambert law, which states that every substance has its own pattern of light absorption.

spina bifida A disorder involving incomplete development of the brain, spinal cord, and/or their protective coverings. This occurs during the first month of pregnancy, when the fetal spine fails to close properly. The result is permanent nerve damage with varying degrees of paralysis of the lower limbs.

spinal muscular atrophy (SMA) A group of hereditary diseases that progressively cause muscle weakness and wasting of muscle (atrophy). They are the second most common autosomal-recessive inherited disorders (cystic fibrosis being the most common). The disorders are caused by a mutation in a gene known as the survival motor neuron gene 1 (SMN1). The abnormal gene causes motor neurons in the spinal cord to degenerate and die.

spirometry The most common pulmonary function test performed in both children and adults. It can test for lung volumes and airway resistance.

spontaneous mode A patient-triggered mode of mechanical ventilation that provides an inspiratory pressure assist without a backup rate. When choosing this mode, the patient must have a good respiratory drive and be able to effectively trigger breaths.

spontaneous/timed mode A patient-triggered mode of mechanical ventilation that provides inspiratory pressure assist with a backup time-based rate. This mode may offer a combination of patient safety and patient comfort, provided that triggering is effective.

STABLE The mnemonic used to represent the six parameters essential to newborn assessment in the aftermath of resuscitation. The core assessment parameters include blood *Sugar* monitoring and treatment, *Temperature* stabilization and maintenance, maintaining a patent *Airway*, normalizing *Blood* pressure, obtaining *Lab* work to assess acid–base and electrolyte balance, and providing the family with *Emotional* support.

steatorrhea The presence of excessive amounts of fat in feces.

stertor A heavy, snoring sound heard during inspiration upon auscultation of breath sounds.

stridor An abnormal, high-pitched breathing sound caused by a blockage or narrowing in the upper airways; it occurs during inspiration, expiration, or both, and is indicative of upper airway edema and/or obstruction.

subambient gas mixtures Gas mixtures that deliver an FiO_2 in the range of 0.14 to 0.20; these mixtures are provided to increase pulmonary vascular resistance by inducing hypoxic vasoconstriction.

suctioning The manual removal of secretions from a patient's airway; it is commonly performed in patients with an artificial airway.

supraglottic airway (SGA) A device that provides an unobstructed airway from the mouth to the supraglottic area and a 15-mm connector to provide positive pressure ventilation.

surfactant A mixture of lipids and proteins that reduces surface tension at the alveolar interface in the lung and that is composed of phospholipids and four surfactant proteins: A, B, C, and D.

surface tension The cohesive forces between liquid molecules within the alveoli that cause the lungs to have a tendency to collapse.

surfactant protein Proteins present in surfactant. There are four types: surfactant proteins A and D are hydrophilic proteins that are members of a family of collagenous carbohydrate binding proteins, known as collectins, or calcium-dependent (C-type) lectins and are primarily related to the innate immune response in the alveolar barrier; surfactant proteins B and C are the hydrophobic proteins, essential for the biophysical activity of pulmonary surfactant.

surfactant protein deficiencies Congenital disorders caused by mutations in the gene proteins, which are critical for the production and function of pulmonary surfactant.

sweat chloride test Considered the gold standard for diagnosing cystic fibrosis (CF), it provides evidence of CFTR dysfunction; it can be performed in children older than 6 months. A minimum of 75 mg of sweat over a 30-minute interval must be collected to perform the analysis. A chloride concentration of more than 60 mmol/L on two or more occasions is suggestive of CF. Sweat chloride values may be elevated (i.e., between 60–80 mmol/L) in non-CF-related diseases, such as atopic dermitis and anorexia nervosa. Values between 40 and 60 mmol/L are considered borderline and are more suggestive of CF in infants.

swine flu (H1N1) A respiratory infection caused by the highly contagious swine influenza A virus.

synchronized intermittent mandatory ventilation (SIMV) A spontaneous mode of ventilation that provides a preset number of mandatory breaths and allows the patient to take a spontaneous breath between the mandatory breaths. Spontaneous breaths can be unsupported or augmented with the addition of pressure support.

systemic vascular resistance (SVR) The resistance that must be overcome for blood to flow through the circulatory system.

T

technology-dependent child A child who requires both a life-sustaining medical device and ongoing nursing care.

term A definite period, especially the period of gestation (not less than 37 weeks of pregnancy).

therapeutic lavage A process of systematically instilling large volumes of solutions throughout the lungs or into a particular area of interest followed by thorough suctioning to remove mucous plugs and airway clots and to help relieve atelectasis.

thoracentesis A procedure done to remove excessive fluid in the pleural space.

thoracic gas volume (TGV) The volume of gas contained within the chest during body plethysmography when the mouth shutter is closed.

tidal volume (Vt) The amount of air inhaled during a normal breath that is measured in milliliters. It is correlated to body weight and is reported in milliliters per kilogram (mL/kg).

timed mode A mode of mechanical ventilation in which a set pressure is delivered at a preset mandatory rate that allows additional patient-triggered breaths as needed. This mode can lead to asynchrony when patient breathing efforts conflict with the preset rate.

titration study A type of sleep study in which positive airway pressure (PAP) is adjusted or titrated to find the optimal pressure that will prevent upper airway obstruction. Education about PAP therapy should be provided prior to a titration study.

tocolytic agents Medications given to mothers to reduce uterine contractions, delay delivery for 48 hours, and allow glucocorticoids to improve lung maturity when the fetus has reached a point of viability, which is usually by 24 weeks' gestation.

total anomalous pulmonary venous return (TAPVR) A congenital heart defect in which the pulmonary veins fail to return to the left atrium; instead they enter either the right atrium or another site in the systemic venous system. This causes oxygenated blood to flow into the right atrium instead of the left atrium for systemic circulation and oxygenation.

total lung capacity (TLC) The amount of gas contained in the lung at the end of a maximal inhalation.

trach go bag Every tracheostomy-dependent child must have a bag, or any type of portable satchel or backpack, that contains all the necessary supplies to perform an emergency tracheostomy tube change; the bag should be transported with the child at all times.

tracheoesophageal fistula A congenital miscommunication between the trachea and esophagus.

tracheostomy tube A tube placed into the trachea via an opening in the neck known as a stoma.

transcutaneous carbon dioxide tension (PtcCO$_2$) A heated sensor attached to the skin increases perfusion of the capillaries and uses an electrode to electrochemically provide a continuous measurement of the carbon dioxide tension in the blood.

transcutaneous oxygen tension (PtcO2) A heated sensor attached to the skin increases perfusion of the capillaries and uses an electrode to electrochemically provide a continuous measurement of the oxygen tension in the blood.

transient tachypnea of the newborn (TTN) A parenchymal lung disease of a neonate caused by pulmonary edema, resulting from delayed reabsorption of fetal lung fluid; it has also been known as transient respiratory distress syndrome (RDS), type II RDS, wet lungs, and retained fetal lung liquid syndrome.

transilluminating light A device that uses a light to localize an artery or vein for cannulation.

transillumination A noninvasive procedure in which a high-intensity light probe is placed against an infant's chest wall near the axilla. A diffuse bright light illuminating the chest suggests the absence of underlying lung tissue, which is displaced by extrapleural air, suggesting a pneumothorax is present.

transition to adult care The purposeful, planned movement of adolescents and young adults with chronic physical and medical conditions from child-centered to adult-oriented healthcare systems.

transition to adulthood A period of growth and accomplishment (after adolescence) after which a person is considered an adult and the process in which adolescents who have been dependent on parents throughout childhood start taking definitive steps to become independent.

transposition of the great arteries (TGA) A congenital heart defect in which the pulmonary artery and the aorta are misplaced, or transposed, across the ventricular septum. Specifically, the pulmonary artery leaves the left ventricle and the aorta rises from the right ventricle, so there is no communication between the systemic and the pulmonary circulation.

transthoracic cannulation Venous-arterial extracorporeal membrane oxygenation support that can also be accomplished through the femoral vein and artery or direct cannulation of the aorta and right atrium.

transudate The fluid that accumulates within a pleural effusion that consists of a low protein count and few cells; usually associated with an imbalance between the hydrostatic and oncotic pressures due to fluid overload or congestive heart failure.

transverse myelitis A neurodisability disorder caused by inflammation of an area across the spinal cord, resulting in damage to the myelin that covers nerve cells.

traumatic brain injury Injury caused by an external force to the brain, resulting in loss of consciousness, memory loss, dizziness, and confusion and in some cases leading to long-term health effects.

Treacher Collins syndrome (TCS) A genetic disorder that affects the ears, eyes, cheekbones, and chins of infants. This congenital deformity alters the development of facial bones and tissues and is generally associated with a bilateral cleft palate and craniofacial disease. The primary clinical characteristics of TCS include prominent eye dysmorphia, middle and external ear deformity, distinctive midfacial malformations, and maxillamandibular abnormalities.

tricuspid atresia A congenital heart defect in which the tricuspid valve fails to develop; it results in a complete right-to-left shunt at the atrial level with no communication between the right atrium and the right ventricle.

trigger The initiation of an inspiratory breath.

trigger sensitivity A parameter available on the intensive care unit ventilator that enables improvement in breath synchrony; trigger sensitivity should be set so that the patient can easily trigger a spontaneous or assisted breath.

trophoblast The outermost layer of the blastocyst that contains approximately 80 cells and forms the chorionic sac and fetal components of the placenta.

truncus arteriosus A congenital heart defect in which a distinct aorta and pulmonary artery do not develop but instead there is only one large single vessel leaving the heart, giving rise to the coronary, systemic, and pulmonary arteries and containing only one valve.

U

ultrasonic nebulizers Nebulizers that use a piezoelectric crystal to create acoustic vibrations that cause the liquid or medication immediately above the transducer to disrupt the air–liquid interface and form droplets. The higher the vibration frequency, the smaller the particle size generated by the nebulizer. The nebulization process is generally noiseless and produces an aerosol particle size larger than those produced by jet nebulizers.

umbilical artery Artery that carries deoxygenated blood from the fetus to the placenta.

umbilical artery catheter (UAC) A catheter inserted into the umbilical artery of a neonate.

umbilical cord prolapse (UCP) An obstetric emergency in which the umbilical cord passes through the cervix in front of or alongside the fetal presenting part.

umbilical vein Vein that carries oxygenated blood from the placenta to the fetus.

umbilical venous catheter (UVC) A catheter inserted into the umbilical vein of a neonate.

upper airway resistance syndrome A condition characterized by intermittently high negative airway pressures during inspiration that lead to arousals and sleep fragmentation. It is also associated with increased upper airway collapsibility during sleep.

V

valved holding chamber (VHC) An add-on, tubelike device used with pressurized metered dose inhalers that minimizes coordination problems between actuation and inhalation of the inhaler and facilitates medication delivery.

valvuloplasty A surgical procedure performed during cardiac catheterization in which a balloon is used to open or widen a stenotic heart valve. Successful valvuloplasty produces a tear in the valve, which widens the track and reduces resistance to blood flow.

valvulotomy A surgical procedure performed to enlarge a narrowed heart valve, often the surgical management for aortic stenosis, pulmonary stenosis, and pulmonary atresia; it consists of making surgical slits.

variable performance An oxygen device that provides a portion of the total flow of gas a patient inhales per breath. These devices do not satisfy the patient's total flow needs; the patient entrains air as well as the flow of oxygen from the device.

venous-arterial (VA) The original approach to extracorporeal membrane oxygenation (ECMO) support; cannulation of the right internal jugular vein, from where deoxygenated blood is drained, and the right common carotid artery, where oxygenated blood is returned. Because the patient's blood exits in the body on the venous side and reinfuses on the arterial or systemic side, this type of ECMO provides both cardiac and respiratory support.

venous-venous A form of extracorporeal membrane oxygenation support that involves the drainage and reinfusion of blood by way of the venous system or right side of the heart. This mode provides pulmonary support only and requires the patient to have sufficient cardiac function.

ventricular septal defect (VSD) A congenital heart defect in which there is a hole in the septum between the lower chambers of the heart, the ventricles; the defect may be a single hole, a series of small holes, or an absent septum.

vibrating mesh nebulizers Nebulizers in which the liquid is forced through a membrane with laser-drilled holes. A piezoelectric crystal vibrates either a plate (active mesh), generating an upward/downward movement of the plate, or a horn (passive mesh), which generates an upward/downward movement of the liquid. The diameter and shape of the holes, as well the characteristics of the medication (viscosity and surface tension), determine the aerosol particle size. These devices are quiet, efficient, and have a low residual volume.

vibration An airway clearance technique of chest physiotherapy to mobilize secretions in which pressure and a shaking movement of the hand are applied to various segments of the lungs.

vitelline circulation Circulation between the embryo and the yolk sac that develops as the precursor to future liver circulation; consists of the vitelline artery and vein.

vocal cord dysfunction (VCD) A disorder with asthma-like symptoms caused by abnormal closure of the vocal cords.

volume control ventilation (VCV) A mode of ventilation that delivers a consistent tidal volume (Vt) and flow at a set mandatory breath rate. Pressure is not held constant and is dependent on lung compliance and airway resistance.

volume expander A type of intravenous therapy that uses crystalloids or red blood cells to add volume to the circulatory system when blood loss is suspected. Isotonic saline may also be used as a volume expander.

volume targeted ventilation Also known as adaptive ventilation; a ventilation technique that uses algorithmic technology that monitors volume delivery and provides automatic pressure adjustment to maintain the preset targeted tidal volume (VT). As a safety measure, the algorithm does not allow for pressure delivery changes that exceed 2 to 3 cm H_2O per breath.

volutrauma A lung injury caused by any uneven distribution of ventilation that can potentially lead to regional overdistention of the lungs.

Z

zygote The single-celled earliest stage of human development formed within 12 to 24 hours of fertilization and containing all the genetic material needed to form a human embryo.

Index

Note: Page numbers followed by *b*, *f*, or *t* indicate material in boxes, figures, or tables, respectively.

Chapter 1

Question 1

Behaviors and tasks that most children can do by a certain age are known as _____ .

Chapter 1

Question 2

The result of frequently laying supine for prolonged periods of time is known as _____ .

Chapter 1

Question 3

At what age does crawling, a motor function developmental milestone, normally occur?

Chapter 1

Question 4

Injury prevention strategies aimed at preventing unintentional injury should be targeted at which chronological age group?

Question 1 Answer:

Developmental milestones

Developmental milestones are behaviors and tasks that most children can do by a certain age. Like growth, developmental milestones are built with the experience and mastery of the behaviors before them.

Question 2 Answer:

Deformational plaigiocephaly

Deformational plaigiocephaly is a physical condition whereby the soft bones of the head become flat on the back of the head as a result of frequently laying supine for prolonged periods of time.

Question 3 Answer:

9 months

An infant's gross motor functions, developing throughout the 1st year of life, are categorized in 3-month increments. As the muscles develop and strengthen, head control occurs at 3 months of age, sitting independently at 6 months of age, crawling at 9 months of age, and walking by 12 months of age.

Question 4 Answer:

Adolescents

Risk taking during adolescence can result in injuries from high-risk behaviors and can mask self-harm tendencies.

Chapter 1
Question 5

Accidental drowning most commonly occurs with which chronological age group?

Chapter 1
Question 6

At which chronological age does the developmental milestone of sitting independently occur?

Chapter 1
Question 7

Playing alongside other children but not engaging is known as _____.

Chapter 2
Question 1

What is the term used to describe a respectful partnership between a child's family, specifically the parents or primary caregivers, and the clinical practitioners and professionals caring for that child?

Question 5 Answer:

Toddlers

Toddlers are very curious and learn many things from their environment by seeing and touching. Vigilant supervision of the toddler's activity is very important to the child's safety. Drowning is the leading cause of injury and death for toddlers, so activities around water, including bathtubs, pools, ponds, lakes, whirlpools, or the ocean, must be supervised at all times.

Question 6 Answer:

6 months

An infant's gross motor functions, developing throughout the 1st year of life, are categorized in 3-month increments. As the muscles develop and strengthen, head control occurs at 3 months of age and sitting independently at 6 months of age.

Question 7 Answer:

Parallel play

Toddlers move from watching children play to parallel play, which is playing alongside other children but not engaging. They also begin pretend play at this age.

Question 1 Answer:

Family-centered care

The concept of family-centered care is based on the assumption that the family is the constant in a child's life. A child's illness can affect the entire family. Family-centered care is a respectful partnership between a child's family, specifically the parents or primary caregivers, and the clinical practitioners and professionals caring for that child.

Chapter 2

Question 2

Due to family constraints, a 2-week-old infant hospitalized with respiratory syncytial virus is separated from her family. What can nurses and respiratory therapists do to develop a trusting relationship with this infant?

Chapter 2

Question 3

Toddlers have a difficult time distinguishing realities from fantasies. When a toddler is hospitalized, what challenge does this developmental consideration present to direct care providers?

Chapter 2

Question 4

A 7-year-old patient with leukemia is scheduled for a bone marrow transplant. List one method the interprofessional team can use to educate the child on the procedure.

Chapter 2

Question 5

A 16-year-old male is hospitalized with an exacerbation of cystic fibrosis. What can the medical team do to promote normalization within the hospital environment?

Question 2 Answer:

Have continuity of care among the nurses and therapists; attempt to maintain a schedule similar one the infant uses at home

In situations where the family is unable to be present all the time, having continuity of care among the nurses and therapists can aid in the infant developing trusting relationships with medical caregivers. Although it may be difficult to do, attempting to maintain a schedule similar to one the infant uses at home can be beneficial in maintaining the sleep, wake, and feeding cycles.

Question 3 Answer:

The developmental consideration may contribute to the toddler's misunderstanding of medical-related explanations

Toddlers have a difficult time distinguishing realities from fantasies, which may contribute to their misunderstanding of medical-related explanations. Many times, especially in an unfamiliar environment like a hospital, toddlers become fearful and develop stranger anxiety when their family is not present.

Question 4 Answer:

Use puppets or dolls when educating the child on what they will experience during the procedure

Because of their imaginative thinking, using puppets or dolls for education concerning a procedure or medical equipment is appropriate for this age.

Question 5 Answer:

Permit and encourage visits from friends and activities with peers

To promote normalization within the hospital environment, visits from friends are encouraged, as are activities with peers. Many hospitals have a teen room or lounge where adolescents can meet.

Chapter 2

Question 6

Describe one way a respiratory therapist can provide the psychosocial support and assurance a family needs while the therapist is providing care to their hospitalized child.

Chapter 3

Question 1

List the five stages of lung development.

Chapter 3

Question 2

Which stage of lung development continues after birth?

Chapter 3

Question 3

During development, a fetus does not have adequate breathing movements and the amount of fetal lung fluid in the airways is decreased. What condition should the respiratory therapist anticipate after birth?

Question 2 Answer:

Alveolar

The first four stages occur prenatally, and the alveolar stage continues after birth. Each stage gradually transitions to the next, with some overlap between stages. A disruption in any stage can profoundly affect lung development and result in a number of pulmonary defects.

Question 3 Answer:

Pulmonary hypoplasia

For lung development to proceed normally, the fetus must have adequate breathing movements and an appropriate amount of fetal lung fluid in the airways. Pulmonary hypoplasia can occur if fetal breathing movement is impaired or fluid production is decreased.

Question 6 Answer:

Be a good listener for the family; guide the family to the member of the multidisciplinary team who can provide them with the ongoing resources they need

Being a good listener for the family is critical, as is as guiding them to the member of the multidisciplinary team who can provide them with the ongoing resources they need.

Question 1 Answer:

Embryonic, pseudoglandular, canalicular, saccular, alveolar

Lung development proceeds in an organized manner and is typically divided into five distinct stages: (1) embryonic, (2) pseudoglandular, (3) canalicular, (4) saccular, (5) alveolar.

Chapter 3

Question 4

List two functions of fetal lung fluid.

Chapter 3

Question 5

List the condition that results in an abnormal opening or hernia in the diaphragm that occurs early in fetal lung development.

Chapter 3

Question 6

What is the term used to describe an abnormally high level of amniotic fluid?

Chapter 4

Question 1

During which gestational week is the heart fully developed?

Question 4 Answer:

Maintains lung expansion; directly affects growth, including the size and shape of the developing airways

Fetal lung fluid is secreted by the pulmonary epithelium at a rate of 4 to 5 ml/kg/hour. The presence of this fluid in the fetal lung maintains lung expansion and directly affects growth, including the size and shape of the developing airways.

Question 6 Answer:

Polyhydramnios

Polyhydramnios, an abnormally high level of fluid, occurs in approximately 1% of all pregnancies and is associated with preterm labor and delivery as well as with several fetal anomalies.

Question 5 Answer:

Congenital diaphragmatic hernia

Congenital diaphragmatic hernia (CDH) is the most common condition associated with restricted growth due to lung compression. In CDH, an abnormal opening, or hernia in the diaphragm, occurs early in fetal lung development. The hernia allows abdominal contents to move into the chest and compress the developing lung.

Question 1 Answer:

8th

At the beginning of the 8th gestational week, the formed structure of the heart will persist for the remainder of intrauterine life.

Chapter 4

Question 2

What are the three shunts that serve to enhance the efficacy and distribution of blood flow to the developing fetus?

Chapter 4

Question 3

What is the germ layer that produces the cecum, intestine, stomach, thymus, liver, pancreas, thyroid, prostate, and lungs?

Chapter 4

Question 4

What is the term used to describe a single-celled earliest stage of human development, is formed within 12 to 24 hours of fertilization, and contains all the genetic material needed to form a human embryo?

Chapter 4

Question 5

What is the term used to describe the germ layer that forms the nervous system, skin or epidermis, glandular tissue, and many of the sensory organs?

Question 2 Answer:

Ductus venosus, ductus arteriosus, and foramen ovale

From the blood entering the right atrium, approximately 80% of blood flow is directed through either of two adaptive anatomical shunts: the foramen ovale or the ductus arteriosus.

Question 3 Answer:

The endoderm

The endoderm produces the cecum, intestine, stomach, thymus, liver, pancreas, thyroid, prostate, and lungs.

Question 4 Answer:

Zygote

The zygote, or the single-celled earliest stage of human development, is formed within 12 to 24 hours of fertilization and contains all the genetic material needed to form a human embryo.

Question 5 Answer:

The ectoderm

The ectoderm forms the nervous system, skin or epidermis, glandular tissue, and many of the sensory organs.

Chapter 4

Question 6

At what postmenstrual gestational age do the heart chambers begin to form?

Chapter 5

Question 2

What is the term used to describe the number of times the mother has been pregnant?

Chapter 5

Question 1

A respiratory therapist is called to the delivery of an infant whose mother did not receive prenatal care during pregnancy. What can the respiratory therapist anticipate?

Chapter 5

Question 3

What is the term used to describe the number of pregnancies that went beyond 20 weeks or to viability?

Question 6 Answer:

Week 4

By the 4th gestational week, the heart undergoes dramatic changes through differential cellular growth in a process called looping, which is the beginning of heart chamber development.

Question 1 Answer:

The infant may be born with potentially serious problems that can harm the mother or the baby

The focus of prenatal care is early identification and treatment of potentially serious problems that can harm the mother or fetus. Women who do not receive prenatal care or whose care is delayed until late in the pregnancy have an increased risk of preterm birth, low birthweight, and neonatal death.

Question 2 Answer:

Gravida

Gravida is the term used to indicate the number of times the mother has been pregnant.

Question 3 Answer:

Parity

Parity refers to the number of pregnancies that went beyond 20 weeks or to viability. The number of fetuses does not affect the parity.

Chapter 5

Question 4

A mother is pregnant for the 6th time, has delivered 3 term children and 2 preterm children, and has had 1 miscarriage. What is her gravida?

Chapter 5

Question 6

After maternal use, how long will it take opioids to transfer to the placenta?

Chapter 5

Question 5

Which maternal viral infection may present as chronic with liver cirrhosis or liver failure?

Chapter 6

Question 1

Provide the name of the scoring system that determines the gestational age of a neonate through physical and neuromuscular assessment.

Question 6 Answer:

60 minutes

Heroin and methadone are the most commonly used opioids among pregnant women. Opioids rapidly transfer to the placenta within 60 minutes of use.

Question 4 Answer:

Gravida 6

Gravida is the term used to describe the number of times the mother has been pregnant. Because she has been pregnant 6 times, she is gravida 6.

Question 1 Answer:

Ballard Scoring System

The New Ballard Score is a system that determines the gestational age of a neonate through physical and neuromuscular assessment. It uses six physical and six neuromuscular features to estimate a certain gestational age.

Question 5 Answer:

Hepatitis B

Hepatitis is a viral infection with the potential for lifelong impact on the fetus. Although there are numerous types of hepatitis, hepatitis B (HBV) results in maternal and neonatal consequences, and infection can be severe. Mothers infected with HBV may or may not be symptomatic. Their disease may be acute with no sequelae or may be chronic with liver cirrhosis or liver failure.

Chapter 6
Question 2

What is the normal range for heart rate in a neonate?

Chapter 6
Question 4

A term infant weighed shortly after birth was determined to be above the 90th percentile for birth weight. What maternal condition should the respiratory therapist anticipate contributed to this finding?

Chapter 6
Question 3

A male infant has a gestational age of 30 weeks estimated by the New Ballard Score. What is the value for an adequate mean blood pressure the respiratory therapist should anticipate?

Chapter 6
Question 5

Upon examination, an infant is noted to have a sunken or hollowed appearance of the abdominal cavity. What condition is this finding highly suggestive of?

Question 2 Answer:

100 to 160 beats per minute

The normal range of heart rate for a neonate varies from 100 to 160 beats per minute.

Question 3 Answer:

35 mm Hg

An adequate mean blood pressure (MBP) value can be calculated if the neonate's gestational age is known. Calculation of MBP = gestational age + 5.

Question 4 Answer:

Maternal diabetes

Neonates who are above the 90th percentile for birth weight are considered large for gestational age. This is most often due to maternal diabetes.

Question 5 Answer:

Congenital diaphragmatic hernia

The neonate with a sunken or hollowed appearance of the abdominal cavity is described as having a scaphoid abdomen. This is highly suggestive of congenital diaphragmatic hernia, a defect in which the diaphragm allows the abdominal contents to enter the chest cavity.

Chapter 7
Question 1

During the care of an infant following a high-risk delivery, what device allows for decompression of the stomach during ventilatory support with a resuscitator and mask?

Chapter 7
Question 2

List a device that is capable of delivering positive pressure ventilation, continuous positive airway pressure, and/or supplemental oxygen in the delivery room.

Chapter 7
Question 3

When evaluating the function of a mechanical suction device, what is the range the suction pressure should be set between?

Chapter 7
Question 4

What position should a respiratory therapist place an infant in to prevent airway obstruction and to facilitate the initiation of assisted ventilation if needed?

Question 1 Answer:

8 Fr feeding tube

During bag-mask ventilation, air can enter the stomach. An 8 Fr feeding tube allows for decompression of the stomach during ventilatory support with a resuscitator and mask.

Question 2 Answer:

T-piece resuscitator and flow-inflating bag

Flow-inflating resuscitators lack a nonrebreathing valve and are capable of providing free-flow oxygen, assisted ventilation, or continuous positive airway pressure (CPAP). A t-piece resuscitator can be automatically set to deliver a set pressure and FiO_2 for CPAP and positive pressure ventilation and FiO_2 for supplemental oxygen delivery.

Question 3 Answer:

80 to 100 mm Hg

Evaluate the negative pressure of the suction apparatus by occluding the end suction tubing used to attach a suction catheter. While occluded, suction pressure should range between 80 to 100 mm Hg. Pressure should return to zero when the occluded end of the tubing is released.

Question 4 Answer:

Sniffing

The sniffing position, or positioning the infant supine with the neck slightly extended, aligns the posterior pharynx, larynx, and trachea. This position prevents airway obstruction and facilitates the initiation of assisted ventilation if needed. Neck flexion or hyperextension may partially or fully restrict air from entering the trachea from the upper airway.

Chapter 7

Question 5

An infant requires tracheal suctioning in the delivery room. What equipment should the respiratory therapist use to perform this procedure?

Chapter 8

Question 1

Describe the radiologic features common to infants with respiratory distress syndrome.

Chapter 8

Question 2

How long do symptoms associated with transient tachypnea of the newborn generally last?

Chapter 8

Question 3

What is the mainstay treatment for newborns with mild meconium aspiration syndrome?

Question 5 Answer:

An endotracheal tube with suction directly applied through a connector, such as a commercially available meconium aspiratory adaptor

For an infant requiring direct laryngotracheal suctioning, intubate the trachea with an endotracheal tube (ETT) and directly apply suction to the ETT. A commercially available meconium aspirator adaptor enables the suction source to easily attach to the ETT.

Question 1 Answer:

Ground-glass appearance of the lungs with air bronchograms

The chest radiographic features classically described as "ground-glass appearance of the lungs with air bronchograms" demonstrates low lung volume. This radiographic pattern results from alveolar atelectasis contrasting with aerated airways.

Question 2 Answer:

72 hours

Symptoms associated with transient tachypnea of the newborn (TTN) generally last for less than 72 hours. Infants with TTN do not frequently require an FiO_2 above 0.60 or mechanical ventilatory support. Characteristic findings on chest radiographs include increased lung volumes with flattened diaphragms, interstitial edema appearing as fluffy infiltrates, and prominent vascular markings with streaky perihilar markings. Pleural effusions and mild cardiomegaly can also be present. Radiologic findings are symmetrical and typically resolve in approximately 48 hours.

Question 3 Answer:

Supplemental oxygen therapy

The treatment of mild meconium aspiration syndrome may involve only supplemental oxygen therapy to minimize hypoxemia. The targeted SpO_2 is as high as 99% to help in the prevention of hypoxia and associated airway obstruction and vascular remodeling of the pulmonary bed.

Chapter 8

Question 4

What is the gradient between pre- and postductal arterial PO_2 that confirms the presence of a ductal shunt?

Chapter 8

Question 6

List one therapy used in the treatment strategy for persistent pulmonary hypertension of the newborn.

Chapter 8

Question 5

Provide the calculation for oxygen index.

Chapter 9

Question 1

Name the congenital disorder in which there is a narrowing of the back of the nasal cavity, resulting in a lack of continuity between the nasal cavity and the pharynx.

Question 6 Answer:

Maintain adequate systemic blood pressure, decrease pulmonary vascular resistance, maintain adequate oxygenation, minimize lung injury

The treatment strategy for persistent pulmonary hypertension of the newborn is aimed at maintaining adequate systemic blood pressure, decreasing pulmonary vascular resistance, ensuring adequate oxygenation, and minimizing complications caused by high levels of inspired oxygen and ventilator high-pressure settings.

Question 1 Answer:

Choanal atresia

Choanal atresia is a congenital disorder in which there is a narrowing of the back of the nasal cavity (choanae), resulting in a lack of continuity between the nasal cavity and the pharynx. Choanal atresia is the most common form of congenital nasal obstruction, and infants often present with difficulty breathing. This development problem of the neonatal airway can consist of a bony or membranous obstruction, but in the majority of cases, the obstruction is caused by a combination of both obstructions.

Question 4 Answer:

10 to 20 mm Hg

After birth or generally within 12 hours, arterial blood gas analysis will show a low PaO_2 frequently even with high FiO_2 administration. Preductal (right radial artery) and postductal (umbilical artery and arteries in lower extremities) blood gas analysis that shows a greater than 10 to 20 mm Hg difference will confirm the presence of a ductal shunt. SpO_2 monitoring comparing the right hand with either foot may also be used, and a difference of 5% to 10% is considered significant and consistent with ductal shunting.

Question 5 Answer:

$(MAP \times FiO_2 / PaO_2) \times 100$

The oxygen index (OI) is calculated by the following formula: OI = $(MAP \times FiO_2 / PaO_2) \times 100$. A high OI will indicate severe hypoxemic respiratory failure. A term or late term infant with an OI of ≥ 25 should be receiving care in a center that has the availability of high-frequency ventilation, inhaled nitric oxide, and extracorporeal membrane oxygenation.

Chapter 9

Question 2

List the four main anomalies associated with choanal atresia.

Chapter 9

Question 3

Describe mandibular hypoplasia.

Chapter 9

Question 4

List the postnatal management strategies used to treat congenital diaphragmatic hernia.

Chapter 9

Question 5

List two complications associated with congenital diaphragmatic hernia.

Question 2 Answer:

Narrowing of the nasal cavity, lateral obstruction by the atretic plate, medial obstruction by the vomer (nasal septum), and membranous obstruction

With choanal atresia, the nasal openings are not formed, which causes lack of communication between the nasopharynx and the remainder of the infant's airway. There are four main anomalies associated with choanal atresia: narrowing of the nasal cavity, lateral obstruction by the atretic plate, medial obstruction by the vomer (nasal septum), and membranous obstruction.

Question 3 Answer:

A condition characterized by an undersize facial jaw, specifically a small mandible and receding chin

Mandibular hypoplasia is a congenital syndrome, also known as micrognathia, strawberry chin, or hypognathia. It is characterized by an undersize facial jaw, specifically a small mandible and receding chin. This disorder has varying degrees of severity. Infants with markedly hypoplastic mandibles are at high risk for potential abnormalities, including glossopteris, or retraction of the tongue, and upper airway obstruction.

Question 4 Answer:

Invasive ventilation with lung protective strategies and permissive hypercapnia, inhaled nitric oxide, high-frequency ventilation, or extracorporeal membrane oxygenation

Postnatal management has evolved to include lung protective strategies during invasive ventilation, permissive hypercapnia, the use of inhaled nitric oxide, high-frequency ventilation, or extracorporeal membrane oxygenation to stabilize the infant prior to surgical repair.

Question 5 Answer:

Pulmonary hyperplasia and persistent pulmonary hypertension of the newborn

Despite the continuous improvement in knowledge and management of this disease, congenital diaphragmatic hernia (CDH) still carries a mortality rate of greater than 50%. Pulmonary hyperplasia and persistent pulmonary hypertension of the newborn are chief complications following the repair of CDH.

Chapter 10

Question 1

What method is used to diagnose retinopathy of prematurity?

Chapter 10

Question 3

List two factors that contribute to the development of bronchopulmonary dysplasia.

Chapter 10

Question 2

List a complication common to infants who develop more significant retinopathy of prematurity.

Chapter 10

Question 4

Pulmonary edema is seen on the chest radiograph of an infant with bronchopulmonary dysplasia. What medication would the respiratory therapist recommend to improve lung mechanics?

Question 1 Answer:

Visualization of the retinal vasculature using indirect ophthalmologic examination

The diagnosis of retinopathy of prematurity is made through visualization of the retinal vasculature using indirect ophthalmologic examination. Infants can be placed in a number of diagnostic categories, from no signs of this disease to severe impairment.

Question 2 Answer:

Severe myopia and glaucoma

Severe myopia and glaucoma are common complications for infants who develop more significant retinopathy of prematurity.

Question 3 Answer:

Prematurity, ventilator-induced lung injury, oxygen toxicity, patent ductus arteriosus, excessive fluid and sodium intake, inflammatory responses, and nutritional imbalance or malnutrition

There are several factors that contribute to the development of bronchopulmonary dysplasia. These include prematurity, ventilator-induced lung injury, oxygen toxicity, patent ductus arteriosus, excessive fluid and sodium intake, inflammatory responses, and nutritional imbalance or malnutrition.

Question 4 Answer:

A diuretic

When pulmonary edema occurs in infants with bronchopulmonary dysplasia, diuretics are commonly used to improve lung mechanics, especially in infants on chronic mechanical ventilation or those with established disease. Improved airway resistance, lung compliance, oxygenation, and quicker ventilator weaning occurs when loop diuretics, such as furosemide, are used.

Chapter 10
Question 5

List two factors that contribute to the risk for air leaks in a neonate requiring mechanical ventilatory support?

Chapter 11
Question 2

After birth, a patient is considered to have a patent ductus arteriosus if the ductus arteriosis does not close within how many hours?

Chapter 11
Question 1

List the four defects present in Tetralogy of Fallot.

Chapter 11
Question 3

In intubated and mechanically ventilated infants, what intervention can greatly improve cardiac output in single ventricle patients?

Question 5 Answer:

Use of long inspiratory times; use of high peak ventilating pressures

The use of long inspiratory times contributes to alveolar overdistention. The use of high peak ventilating pressures contributes to barotrauma.

Question 1 Answer:

Ventricular septal defect, overriding aorta, pulmonary stenosis, right ventricular hypertrophy

Tetrology of Fallot is a heart defect that features four problems: (1) a hole between the lower chambers of the heart, (2) an obstruction from the heart to the lungs, (3) the aorta (blood vessel) lies over the hole in the lower chambers, and (4) the muscle surrounding the lower right chamber becomes overly thickened.

Question 2 Answer:

72

Once the baby is born and begins to breathe on their own using the lungs, the partial pressure of oxygen in the arterial blood is increased and there is a decrease in pulmonary vascular resistance. This process causes the ductus arteriosus and foramen ovale to close. When the ductus doesn't close within 72 hours after birth it is called a patent ductus arteriosus.

Question 3 Answer:

Early extubation

Early extubation minimizes the propensity for ventilator associated morbidity, including ventilator induced lung injury and healthcare acquired lung infections.

Chapter 11

Question 4

Name the congenital heart defect characterized by a narrowing of the aortic valve obstructing blood flow to the rest of the body as well as causing left ventricular hypertrophy.

Chapter 11

Question 5

Name the congenital heart defect characterized by obstruction to blood flow from the right ventricle to the pulmonary artery.

Chapter 11

Question 6

List the congenital heart defect characterized by failure of the tricuspid valve to develop.

Chapter 11

Question 7

A pulmonary valve that does not form correctly, is sealed, and can't open is known as _____ .

Question 4 Answer:

Aortic stenosis

Aortic stenosis is a congenital heart defect characterized by a narrowing of the aortic valve. This obstructs blood flow to the rest of the body and contributes to the development of ventricular hypertrophy.

Question 5 Answer:

Pulmonary stenosis

Pulmonary stenosis is a condition characterized by obstruction to blood flow from the right ventricle into the pulmonary artery. The stenosis may be subvalvular (before the valve), supravalvular (after the valve), valvular, or in the pulmonary artery.

Question 6 Answer:

Tricuspid atresia

Tricuspid atresia occurs when the tricuspid valve fails to develop. Without a tricuspid valve, there is a complete right-to-left shunt at the atrial level and there is no communication between the right atrium and the right ventricle.

Question 7 Answer:

Pulmonary atresia

The pulmonary valve is an opening on the right side of the heart that helps prevent blood from leaking back into the heart between beats. In pulmonary atresia, the pulmonary valve does not form correctly: it's sealed and can't open.

Chapter 12
Question 1

What is the term used to describe the health problem or concern described in the child's or parent's own words that caused the individual to seek medical attention?

Chapter 12
Question 2

At what stage of development are the intercostal muscles fully developed?

Chapter 12
Question 3

A respiratory therapist assesses a 3-month-old infant in the emergency department. The infant is noted to have head bobbing and nasal flaring. What should the respiratory therapist conclude about the infant's work of breathing?

Chapter 12
Question 4

A 2-year-old child presents to the emergency department with the inability to swallow following a choking episode. The child is drooling and has suprasternal retractions. List a diagnosis that the medical team should consider based on the child's clinical presentation.

Question 1 Answer:

Chief complaint

The history begins with a discussion of the child's current illness, including the chief complaint and the history of present illness. The chief complaint is the health problem or concern described in the child's or parent's own words that caused the individual to seek medical attention.

Question 2 Answer:

School age

The ribs in infants and young children are more horizontally oriented, which lessens the ability of the intercostal muscles to lift the rib cage, especially when lying flat on the back. The intercostal muscles don't reach full development until school age.

Question 3 Answer:

Work of breathing is increased

Both head bobbing and nasal flaring are signs of increased respiratory effort and accessory muscle use as well as an increased work of breathing. Head bobbing occurs when the sternocleidomastoid muscles are used to assist with breathing.

Question 4 Answer:

Swallowing disorder; upper airway obstruction (foreign body aspiration, airway edema)

Drooling or the inability to swallow secretions or liquids can indicate swallowing disorders. It can also be indicative of an impairment or obstruction of the upper airway, either by the presence of a foreign body or by swelling within the airway.

Chapter 12

Question 5

List two causes of paradoxical breathing in children.

Chapter 12

Question 7

During auscultation of the chest of a 3-month-old infant, what should the respiratory therapist do to minimize the chance of auscultating distorted breath sounds?

Chapter 12

Question 6

What is the term used to describe a breathing pattern in which the respiratory frequency and tidal volume are completely irregular and feature irregular pauses that are accompanied by increasing episodes of apnea ensue?

Chapter 13

Question 1

What is the most common cause of cardiopulmonary arrest in children?

Question 5 Answer:

Poor muscle tone, respiratory muscle fatigue, chest trauma, multiple rib fractures

Paradoxical breathing is an inward motion of the abdomen as the chest wall moves inward during inhalation; asynchrony between the rib cage and the abdomen creating a seesaw-type motion. This occurs when an infant or child has poor muscle tone or when respiratory muscle fatigue, chest trauma, or multiple rib fractures are present.

Question 6 Answer:

Ataxic respirations

Ataxic respiration is a term used to describe a breathing pattern in which there is a completely irregular breathing frequency and tidal volume that is accompanied by irregular pauses and increasing episodes of apnea. This breathing pattern is common among children with the following conditions: head trauma, stroke, cerebral palsy, and brain tumor.

Question 7 Answer:

Clear the nasal passages (suction the nares)

During auscultation, the respiratory therapist should clear the nasal passages, if needed, to prevent nasal sounds from distorting breath sounds.

Question 1 Answer:

Respiratory failure

Unlike adults, where the most common cause of cardiopulmonary arrest is underlying coronary artery disease that often develops into sudden ventricular fibrillation cardiac arrest, respiratory failure is the primary cause of pediatric cardiorespiratory arrest. Following which, the pediatric patient will experience significant hypoxia or circulatory shock that will then lead to cardiac arrest.

Chapter 13

Question 2

During the assessment of a child with respiratory distress, what sign would alert the respiratory therapist to suspect the child has increased airways resistance?

Chapter 13

Question 4

What audible finding will children whose disease process causes edema and/or upper airway obstruction often exhibit?

Chapter 13

Question 3

What audible finding will children whose disease process reduces their functional residual capacity often exhibit?

Chapter 13

Question 5

List two components essential to the rapid assessment of the circulatory system.

Question 2 Answer:

The presence of suprasternal, intercostal, or even substernal retractions; nasal flaring

The chest wall of infants and small children is very compliant. Increases in airways resistance often manifest in the presence of suprasternal, intercostal, or even substernal retractions. Retractions signify increased work of breathing. In younger pediatric patients, nasal flaring may be noted as the child attempts to inspire maximal air with each breath. Nasal flaring may be a subtle sign but is indicative of a child in distress.

Question 3 Answer:

Grunting

The sounds an infant or child produces as they breathe can provide the clinician with valuable information. Just as adults perform purse lip breathing to stint open narrowed airways and/or increase functional residual capacity by creating autoPEEP, infants often make a grunting noise. Grunting describes the sound an infant makes when expiring against a partially closed glottis. Grunting is not a normal finding. Rather, it is a compensatory mechanism to maximize gas exchange and is a hallmark sign of respiratory distress.

Question 4 Answer:

Stridor

Stridor is the sound an infant or child produces on inspiration and is indicative of upper airway edema and/or obstruction. Stridor may be present following extubation or associated with an infectious process or aspiration of a foreign body. Wheezing may be audible as well. It may be present on inspiration or expiration and is typically due to bronchospasm, secretions, or inflammation of the lower airways. Auscultation of breath sounds follows visual assessment of the patient's breathing. The lateral neck and lungs are assessed for the presence and symmetry of air entry as well as for the occurrence of adventitious breath sounds.

Question 5 Answer:

Mental status, capillary refill, pulses, blood pressure

Rapid assessment of the systemic perfusion is an essential part of pediatric resuscitation. It is accomplished by evaluating mental status, capillary refill, pulses, and blood pressure. The presence and character or volume of peripheral pulses provides an indication of systemic vascular resistance and the degree of shunting that is necessary to maintain blood pressure and end-organ perfusion.

Chapter 13
Question 6

What is normal capillary refill time?

Chapter 14
Question 1

List two pathogens commonly associated with bronchiolitis.

Chapter 13
Question 7

Following intubation, what should the respiratory therapist use to confirm tracheal intubation?

Chapter 14
Question 2

What is the mode of transmission for bronchiolitis?

Question 6 Answer:

Less than 2 seconds

Capillary refill is normal if color returns in less than 2 seconds. Volume depletion or hypotension can cause a delay in capillary refill of more than 3 seconds.

Question 7 Answer:

Capnography or colorimetric CO_2 devices

Capnography confirms tracheal intubation rapidly and reliably. The capnograph provides a numeric value for end-tidal CO_2, as well as a waveform, which is of diagnostic value. Colorimetric devices may also be used to confirm tracheal placement. These devices display a color change, typically from purple to yellow when CO_2 is detected. However, there are conditions that can lead to false positive or false negative readings.

Question 1 Answer:

Respiratory syncytial virus, influenza, parainfluenza viruses, human metapneumovirus, adenovirus

The majority of cases with bronchiolitis result from a viral pathogen, such as respiratory syncytial virus (RSV), influenza and parainfluenza viruses, human metapneumovirus, or adenovirus. RSV is the most common pathogen responsible for bronchiolitis. Approximately 90% of children are infected with RSV in the first 2 years of life, 40% of whom will experience lower respiratory tract infection during the initial infection.

Question 2 Answer:

Direct contact

Bronchiolitis is highly contagious. The responsible virus can easily spread from person to person through direct contact with nasal secretions, airborne droplets, and fomites.

Chapter 14

Question 3

A steeple sign is a classic radiologic finding associated with which pediatric condition?

Chapter 14

Question 4

What causative factors are associated with spasmodic croup?

Chapter 14

Question 5

A thumb sign is a classic radiologic finding associated with which pediatric condition?

Chapter 14

Question 6

What is the recommended treatment for parapneumonic effusions?

Question 3 Answer:

Laryngotracheobronchitis

The steeple sign is a classic radiologic sign associated with laryngotracheobronchitis. This sign represents edema at the subglottic area, or the narrowest region of the larynx in infants and children. Edema, even a slight degree, causes a significant reduction in the cross-sectional area of the subglottic region.

Question 4 Answer:

Allergies and gastroesophageal reflex

Spasmodic croup (recurrent croup) typically presents at night with the sudden onset of a croupy or barky cough and stridor. Spasmodic croup is mostly allergic in nature but has been reported in children with gastroesophageal reflux. Children will recover fully from recurrent croup within 3 to 6 hours.

Question 5 Answer:

Epiglottitis

Chest radiographs may be used to make a diagnosis of epiglottitis. Findings on a lateral neck radiograph include the classic thumb sign of an enlarged epiglottis, loss of the vallecular air space, thickened aryepiglottic folds, a distended hypopharynx, and straightening of the cervical spine.

Question 6 Answer:

Antibiotics

Parapneumonic effusions will improve clinically within 1 week with the appropriate antibiotic treatment. Parapneumonic effusions that cannot be drained adequately by needle or small-bore catheters may require surgical intervention.

Chapter 15

Question 1

What is the triad of events associated with variable recurring symptoms of an acute exacerbation of asthma?

Chapter 15

Question 2

Which diagnostic test is instrumental to the diagnosis and management of asthma in children ≥5 years of age?

Chapter 15

Question 3

The respiratory therapist is reviewing the spirometry results for a 10-year-old child with asthma who is symptom-free. What range should the respiratory therapist anticipate the FEV_1/FVC to be in?

Chapter 15

Question 4

What % decrease in FEV_1 is required for a bronchial provocation test to be positive?

Question 1 Answer:

Airflow obstruction, bronchial hyperresponsiveness, and ongoing underlying inflammation

The interaction between the inflammation in the airway causes variable and recurring symptoms: airflow obstruction, bronchial hyperresponsiveness, and ongoing underlying inflammation. The airways react to certain stimuli—smooth muscles that wrap around the airways tighten, the airway wall becomes inflamed, and thick mucus is produced.

Question 2 Answer:

Spirometry

Spirometry is essential for the diagnosis and management of asthma in children ≥ 5 years of age. The forced vital capacity (FVC), forced expiratory volume in 1 second (FEV_1), and the ratio of forced expiratory volume in 1 second to forced vital capacity (FEV_1/FVC%) are most commonly used.

Question 3 Answer:

Normal range

Typically, when the child is not having an exacerbation of asthma and is free of asthma exacerbation symptoms, the FEV_1/FVC should be within the normal range. The FEV_1/FVC% should also be within the normal range of the child's age, which is at least 85% of predicted.

Question 4 Answer:

20% reduction of FEV_1

A bronchial provocation test is performed in a clinic setting using either methacholine or mannitol. Following baseline spirometric testing, the child repeatedly inhales a dose of methacholine by aerosol mist or dry powder in increasing concentration until hyperreactivity of the small airways is noted. Spirometry is performed after each dose to evaluate response, or a reduction in FEV_1. A 20% reduction of FEV_1 is considered a positive test.

Chapter 15
Question 5

A 9-year-old child presents with a severe exacerbation of asthma and requires 3 beta2-agonist treatments spaced 15 minutes apart. In addition to the short-acting bronchodilator, what other medication should the child receive to alleviate symptoms?

Chapter 15
Question 6

Immunoreactive trypsinogen is used in newborns to screen for which disorder?

Chapter 16
Question 1

List two findings that suggest a muscular dystrophy is adversely affecting the muscles of the respiratory system.

Chapter 16
Question 2

What is the most severe form of spinal muscle atrophy known as?

Question 5 Answer:

Administration of systemic corticosteroids, inhaled ipratropium bromide

Children presenting to the emergency department with a severe exacerbation require care escalation, which includes additional beta2-agonist treatments, typically 3 treatments spaced 15 minutes apart, the addition of inhaled ipratropium bromide, and administration of systemic corticosteroids.

Question 6 Answer:

Cystic fibrosis

In the United States, all newborns are screened for cystic fibrosis (CF). As with all newborn screenings, within the first few days of life, blood is taken for analysis from the baby's heel. Although not used in all states, the immunoreactive trypsinogen (IRT) screens for CF in the newborn. In those states in which the IRT is not used, genetic screening is performed.

Question 1 Answer:

Difficulty with swallowing, ineffective cough, respiratory failure

Several muscular dystrophies can affect the muscles of the respiratory system, causing difficulty with swallowing, ineffective cough, and respiratory failure.

Question 2 Answer:

Spinal muscle atrophy Type I or Werdnig-Hoffman disease

There are four types of spinal muscle atrophy: Type I, II, III, and IV. Prognosis depends upon the type, with Type I (also known as Werdnig-Hoffman disease) being the most severe form. The onset of symptoms is between birth and 6 months of age. Muscle weakness is severe, and this form is often fatal.

Chapter 16

Question 3

What is the most common cause of excessive airways secretions in a child with a neurodisability?

Chapter 16

Question 5

List the indications for mechanical ventilatory support for a child with a neurodisability.

Chapter 16

Question 4

What is the primary cause of recurrent acute infection, mucus plugging, and atelectasis, leading ultimately to bronchiectasis and chronic pulmonary insufficiency in a child with a neurodisability?

Chapter 16

Question 6

List two nonpulmonary problems that are essential to address in the management of a child with a neurodisability.

Question 3 Answer:

Ineffective cough

A major beginning point in the progression of excessive airway secretions to chronic lung disease is the presence of an ineffective cough. This is one of the most commonly seen factors in the pulmonary composite regardless of the primary diagnosis. An ineffective cough, which is most closely linked to hypotonia and the ambulatory status of the patient, sets the stage for secretion retention.

Question 4 Answer:

The presence of chronic bacterial colonization

The presence of chronic bacterial colonization may result in recurrent acute infection, mucus plugging, and atelectasis, leading ultimately to bronchiectasis and chronic pulmonary insufficiency, and is a significant factor in the progression of chronic lung disease and respiratory failure.

Question 5 Answer:

Daytime hypercapnia (pCO$_2$ greater than 45 torr) and nocturnal hypoventilation (SaO$_2$ less than 88% for 5 consecutive minutes)

Daytime hypercapnia (pCO$_2$ greater than 45 torr) and nocturnal hypoventilation (SaO$_2$ less than 88% for 5 consecutive minutes) are established indications for the initiation of ventilator support. Patient symptoms, including fatigue, respiratory accessory muscle use, tachypnea, dyspnea, and recurrent pulmonary exacerbations requiring frequent hospital admissions, are all common indicators for the need for mechanical ventilation.

Question 6 Answer:

Seizures, spasticity, drooling

Although daily respiratory therapies can often take up the greater part of the day, especially in the patient with significant chronic pulmonary disease, the caregiver also has responsibility in most cases for all activities of daily living. This includes providing for enteral nutrition and managing multiple medications for nonpulmonary problems, including seizures, spasticity, and drooling.

Chapter 17
Question 1

List a simple screening algorithm developed to assess sleep-related disorders in the primary care setting.

Chapter 17
Question 2

What is the term used to describe a disorder of breathing during sleep characterized by prolonged partial upper airway obstruction and/or intermittent complete obstruction during sleep that disrupts alveolar gas exchange and normal sleep patterns?

Chapter 17
Question 3

What is the term used to describe a pattern of persistent partial upper airway obstruction associated with gas exchange abnormalities, including CO_2 retention?

Chapter 17
Question 4

Describe the typical presentation of hypertrophic adenoids, or adenoid facies.

Question 1 Answer:

BEARS

BEARS is a simple screening algorithm developed to assess sleep-related disorders in the primary care setting. This tool asks questions regarding sleep problems in five different domains, each represented by a letter:

- Bedtime problems
- Excessive daytime sleepiness
- Awakenings during the night
- Regularity and duration of sleep
- Snoring

Question 2 Answer:

Obstructive sleep apnea

The American Thoracic Society defines obstructive sleep apnea as a disorder of breathing during sleep characterized by prolonged partial upper airway obstruction and/or intermittent complete obstruction during sleep that disrupts alveolar gas exchange and normal sleep patterns.

Question 3 Answer:

Obstructive hypoventilation

Obstructive hypoventilation is a pattern of persistent partial upper-airway obstruction associated with gas exchange abnormalities, including CO_2 retention.

Question 4 Answer:

A long, open-mouthed face with hyponasal speech

Typical presentation of hypertrophic adenoids, or adenoid facies, is a long, open-mouthed face with hyponasal speech.

Chapter 17

Question 5

According to the American Academy of Pediatrics, which diagnostic test is the gold standard for the diagnosis of ostructive sleep apnea in children?

Chapter 18

Question 1

What is the primary cause of acute respiratory distress syndrome among children?

Chapter 17

Question 6

What is often needed to improve adherence with positive airway pressure therapy in children with obstructive sleep apnea?

Chapter 18

Question 2

List the PaO_2-to-FIO_2 criteria used to define acute respiratory distress syndrome.

Question 5 Answer:

Polysomnography

According to the American Academy of Pediatrics, polysomnography (PSG) is indicated for the diagnosis of obstructive sleep apnea (OSA) in children. Overnight PSG performed in a laboratory is considered the gold standard for diagnosis of OSA because it provides an objective, quantitative evaluation of disturbances in respiratory and sleep patterns.

Question 6 Answer:

Extensive behavioral conditioning

Although positive airway pressure therapy is safe and effective in children, extensive behavioral conditioning is needed to achieve satisfactory adherence.

Question 1 Answer:

Infection

Although exposure to noxious gases such as chlorine, aspiration of gastric contents, pneumonia, and pulmonary contusions caused by chest trauma, are all among the possible causes of acute respiratory distress syndrome (ARDS), infection, specifically pneumonia, is the primary cause of ARDS in pediatrics.

Question 2 Answer:

PaO_2-to-FiO_2 ratio of <200

The PaO_2/FiO_2 is used to quantify the degree of oxygenation impairment. The diagnosis of acute respiratory distress syndrome is made by a combination of chest radiograph and arterial blood gas information.

Chapter 18

Question 3

Describe the radiologic features common to acute respiratory distress syndrome.

Chapter 18

Question 5

List two signs of cold shock.

Chapter 18

Question 4

According to the Pediatric Acute Lung Injury Consensus Conference Group, what is the goal SpO_2 range for children with acute respiratory distress syndrome requiring supplemental oxygen to address hypoxemia?

Chapter 18

Question 6

The administration of what sedative is recommended prior to intubating a child with severe sepsis?

Question 3 Answer:

Noncardiogenic pulmonary edema with bilateral pulmonary infiltrates on chest X-ray

The diagnosis of acute respiratory distress syndrome (ARDS) is made by a combination of chest radiograph (CXR) and arterial blood gas information. ARDS is defined as acute, noncardiogenic pulmonary edema with bilateral pulmonary infiltrates on chest X-ray (CXR).

Question 4 Answer:

88% to 92%

The literature supports maintaining an SpO_2 of 88% to 92%, which is the recommendation from the Pediatric Acute Lung Injury Consensus Conference Group.

Question 5 Answer:

Low cardiac output and elevated systemic vascular resistance

Pediatric patients with sepsis often display signs of profound volume depletion. Typically, these patients present with a low cardiac output (CO) and elevated systemic vascular resistance (SVR), or cold shock. However, CO and SVR will fluctuate throughout the course of illness, necessitating changes to vasopressor therapy. Because of the decreased CO, oxygen delivery to tissues is decreased.

Question 6 Answer:

Ketamine

Prior to intubation or central venous catheter placement, sedation with ketamine is recommended.

Chapter 19
Question 1

When initiating pulse oximetry on a newborn infant to obtain a pre-ductal SPO$_2$ value, where should the respiratory therapist place a pulse oximeter probe?

Chapter 19
Question 2

When using transcutaneous CO$_2$ monitoring for an infant receiving ventilatory support by high-frequency oscillation, how often should the respiratory therapist change the site of a transcutaneous CO$_2$ probe?

Chapter 19
Question 3

What is the term used to describe the noninvasive monitoring tool that provides real-time continuous monitoring of regional tissue oxyhemoglobin saturation?

Chapter 19
Question 4

List two locations for placement of a near infrared spectroscopy sensor.

Question 1 Answer:

Right hand

Studies have shown that the fastest and most reliable SpO$_2$ readings have been measured using the right hand because this extremity has a higher blood pressure, is well perfused, and represents the pre-ductal oxygenation status during the first several minutes of life.

Question 2 Answer:

Every 3 to 4 hours

Depending on the skin thickness of the patient and the temperature used to heat the skin, the probe is removed every 3 to 4 hours and the site changed. Localized erythema may be present at the site when the sensor is initially removed. The redness should dissipate shortly after the sensor is moved. It is important to follow the manufacturer's recommendations for use, which include setting the temperature according to patient type (neonate, infant, child, adolescent, etc.), sensor location, and the maximum time a sensor can be left in one location.

Question 3 Answer:

Near infrared spectroscopy

Near infrared spectroscopy (NIRS) is a noninvasive tool that provides real-time continuous monitoring of regional tissue oxyhemoglobin saturation. NIRS uses the Beer-Lambert law to determine the absorption of NIR light by oxyhemoglobin, which it translates to tissue oxygenation. NIRS are most commonly used in infants and children who have undergone cardiac surgery or who are critically ill and at risk for low cardiac output syndrome.

Question 4 Answer:

Forehead, abdomen, low back at T-10 to L-2

Common locations for placement of the sensors are the forehead and the abdomen or low back at T-10 to L-2. Because the skull is easily penetrated by near infrared light, sensors placed on the forehead provide a real-time assessment of regional cortical oxygenation.

Chapter 19

Question 5

What is the position of the tip umbilical arterial catheter in the high- and low-lying position?

Chapter 19

Question 6

List two complications associated with the use of peripherally inserted arterial catheters.

Chapter 20

Question 1

In relation to the spine, at which vertebra would tracheal bifurcation into the right and left mainstem bronchi be seen on a chest radiologic in infants and children?

Chapter 20

Question 2

Which radiologic position would the respiratory therapist recommend to evaluate the position of the endotracheal tube within the trachea?

Question 5 Answer:

The 6th through the 8th thoracic vertebrae in the high-lying position and the 3rd to 4th lumbar vertebrae in the low-lying position

The tip of the umbilical artery catheter overlies the 6th through the 8th thoracic vertebrae in the high-lying position and the 3rd to 4th lumbar vertebrae in the low-lying position.

Question 6 Answer:

Infection, bleeding, thrombosis

The insertion of a peripherally inserted arterial catheter carries a risk for catheter-associated infections. To minimize the risk for infection, adherence to aseptic technique and catheter-related bloodstream infection bundles is essential. Bleeding and thrombosis are also complications associated with indwelling arterial catheters. The risk of thrombosis increases proportionally with the size and duration of catheter placement. Younger children, less than 5 years of age, carry a higher risk for complications and should be closely monitored for signs of thrombosis.

Question 1 Answer:

At T4 in infants and T6 in children

The trachea bifurcates at the carina into the right and left main stem bronchi at the 6th thoracic vertebra (T6) in children and 4th thoracic vertebra (T4) in neonates.

Question 2 Answer:

The AP/PA frontal view

The AP/PA frontal view is the primary choice to evaluate the distance of the endotracheal tube to the carina.

Chapter 20

Question 3

List two interventions that are used to obtain useful clear CT images of an infant or child.

Chapter 20

Question 5

The radiologic finding of air trapping during expiration in a confined or isolated area is suggestive of what clinical condition?

Chapter 20

Question 4

List three general pediatric conditions in which MRI is the imaging modality of choice.

Chapter 20

Question 6

Which radiologic position would the respiratory therapist recommend to evaluate the presence of an aspirated foreign body?

Question 3 Answer:

Conscious sedation and general anesthesia

CT, while delivering useful information, can be difficult to obtain. CT imaging requires the patient to lie extremely still, which often requires sedation or general anesthesia to obtain adequate images.

Question 4 Answer:

Neurologic, musculoskeletal, and cardiovascular diseases

Unlike imaging techniques generated with ionizing radiation, with MRI there is no exposure to radiation. MRI is the imaging modality of choice in a vast array of pediatric conditions, particularly in neurologic, musculoskeletal, and some cardiovascular diseases. Advantages of MRI include excellent image quality, superior soft tissue contrast, and lack of ionizing radiation.

Question 5 Answer:

A complete bronchial obstruction

Air trapping during expiration in a confined or isolated area is suggestive of a complete bronchial obstruction. Normally the lung loses volume during expiration. However, when a foreign body lodges in the airway and completely obstructs it, air is unable to escape from that area, and the affected portion of the lung will remain inflated.

Question 6 Answer:

The lateral decubitus position

The lateral decubitus position is most frequently requested to determine the presence of a foreign body aspiration. Proper positioning is critical for a good image. Arms and chin must be raised and remain out of range of the image. Elevating an infant on a radiolucent sponge prevents the chest from sinking into the cart pad. When the body sinks into the cart pad, artifact lines superimpose over the lateral lung field, obscuring the image.

Chapter 21

Question 1

At what age are most children able to perform spirometry with good technique and repeatability?

Chapter 21

Question 2

What type of equipment is used to test for lung volumes and airway resistance?

Chapter 21

Question 3

List the four variables that normal lung volumes and spirometric values are based upon.

Chapter 21

Question 4

What measurement is used as a surrogate for obtaining height in children who are unable to stand and be measured by a calibrated stadiometer?

Question 1 Answer:

5 years of age

By 5 years of age, most children can perform spirometry with good technique and repeatability, although this may require practice and more than one visit or training session.

Question 2 Answer:

Body plethysmograph

Testing for lung volumes and airway resistance can be done using a body plethysmograph. This equipment should meet or exceed the equipment performance standards set by the American Thoracic Society.

Question 3 Answer:

Height, age, sex, and race

Lung function is directly correlated to height, age, sex, and race.

Question 4 Answer:

Arm span

A calibrated stadiometer is used to obtain the height at each testing session. The measurement is done with the shoes removed and the child standing straight and looking forward. Measuring the arm span may be used in children who are unable to stand for a height measurement.

Chapter 21

Question 5

Describe what forced expiratory volume in 1 second, or FEV_1, is reflective of in children.

Chapter 21

Question 6

List the maneuver that can provide information regarding an extra thoracic obstruction.

Chapter 22

Question 1

List the airway adjunct that is indicated for an unconscious child when spontaneous ventilation is partially or fully obstructed or mask ventilation is inadequate despite optimal facemask position, mask fit, and mask seal.

Chapter 22

Question 2

When properly placed, describe the position where the distal aperture of a nasopharyngeal airway should rest.

Question 5 Answer:

Medium to small airways

The forced expiratory volume in 1 second, or FEV_1, also measured in liters, is reflective of flow in the large or central airways in adults. However, in children this measurement also reflects flow in the medium to small airways because their lungs are smaller and empty more quickly.

Question 6 Answer:

Maximal inspiratory measurements

Maximal inspiratory measurements can provide information regarding extra thoracic obstruction.

Question 1 Answer:

Oropharyngeal airway

An oropharyngeal airway is indicated when spontaneous ventilation is partially or fully obstructed or mask ventilation is inadequate despite optimal facemask position, mask fit, and mask seal. When correctly positioned, the oropharyngeal airway displaces the tongue forward, away from the palate and the posterior wall of the pharynx. The distal portion rests just above the larynx.

Question 2 Answer:

Just superior to the epiglottis

When properly placed, the distal aperture should rest just superior to the epiglottis.

Chapter 22

Question 3

Prior to inserting a laryngeal mask airway, how should the respiratory therapist position the patient?

Chapter 22

Question 5

For cuffed tracheal tubes, at what pressure will mucosal ischemia occur?

Chapter 22

Question 4

List one absolute contraindication for tracheal intubation.

Chapter 22

Question 6

List three methods with which the cuff on a tracheostomy tube can be inflated.

Question 3 Answer:

Supine in the sniffing position

Prior to insertion of the laryngeal mask airway (LMA), the patient is placed in the sniffing position. The cuff of the LMA is fully deflated, ensuring that the posterior surface of the mask is smooth and wrinkle-free. Some recommend having a slight amount of air in the cuff. The tip of the LMA should be deflected backward, away from the aperture, encouraging the LMA to slide posterior to the epiglottis without pushing it over the glottic opening.

Question 4 Answer:

Airway collapse from a mediastinal mass

Caution should be used when tracheal intubation with positive pressure ventilation is used to bypass an airway obstruction because of the risk of the intrathoracic airways collapse. Therefore, tracheal intubation is contraindicated for patients with airway collapse from a mediastinal mass.

Question 5 Answer:

> 25 mm Hg

Cuff pressures that exceed 25 mm Hg will produce mucosal ischemia that may heal with scar tissue, producing subglottic stenosis.

Question 6 Answer:

Air, water, and foam

Cuffed tracheostomy tubes reduce the risk of aspiration and are also used when high-ventilation pressures are required. There are currently three methods of cuff inflation: Air is injected into the pilot tubing to inflate the cuff, sterile water is used to inflate the cuff, or the foam is contained within the cuff and when the pilot tube opens, ambient air pressure inflates the cuff.

What is the term used to describe when tissue hypoxia is present despite normal arterial pO_2 or SpO_2?

For a standard nasal cannula, what is the prong-to-nare ratio that should not be exceeded?

A child is receiving 35% oxygen by air-entrainment mask following surgery. Upon assessment, the respiratory therapist discovers that the air-entrainment ports are inadvertently covered by the bed linens. What affect will this have on the oxygen concentration delivered to the child?

List three positive effects associated with the use of a heated high-flow nasal cannula.

Question 1 Answer:

Normoxemic hypoxia

Normoxemic hypoxia is when tissue hypoxia is present despite normal arterial pO_2 or SpO_2. Cyanide poisoning is an example of normoxemic hypoxia.

Question 2 Answer:

50%

The prong-to-nare ratio describes the amount of space the prong occupies in the nare. For a standard nasal cannula, the literature reports that the prong-to-nare ratio should not exceed 50%.

Question 3 Answer:

Higher oxygen concentration delivered to the child

Inadvertent occlusion of the air-entrainment ports can alter the oxygen concentration delivered to the child. Bed linens, such as blankets and sheets, can block the flow of ambient air through the air-entrainment ports. Depending on the patient's inspiratory flow demands, a higher FiO_2 will be delivered if the total flow delivered to the patient still meets or exceeds the patient's inspiratory demands.

Question 4 Answer:

Reduced work of breathing, improved lung compliance, enhanced mucociliary clearance, increased functional residual capacity by providing a continuous positive airway pressure effect

The use of a heated high-flow nasal cannula is reported to reduce work of breathing, improve lung compliance, enhance mucociliary clearance, and increase functional residual capacity by providing a continuous positive airway pressure effect.

Chapter 23

Question 5

An infant in an incubator is receiving 24% oxygen. What device should the respiratory therapist recommend to continue oxygen therapy during kangaroo care?

Chapter 23

Question 6

In order to prevent cold stress, at what temperature should an incubator be maintained?

Chapter 24

Question 1

What is the term used to describe the dispersion measurement, or a measure of how spread out the particles are in relation to their size?

Chapter 24

Question 2

A respiratory therapist is delivering 70:30 heliox to a 2-year-old child. An oxygen calculated flowmeter set at 8 L/minute is used to deliver the gas mixture. What is the total flow delivered to the child?

Question 5 Answer:

Nasal cannula

Kangaroo care can't be accomplished in an incubator and requires the use of an alternate delivery device, such as a nasal cannula, to provide this type of care.

Question 6 Answer:

The infant's neutral thermal environment

The temperature in an incubator should be monitored and maintained within the infant's neutral thermal environment to minimize the propensity for exposing the infant to overheating and/or cold stress.

Question 1 Answer:

Geometric standard deviation

The dispersion measurement is the geometric standard deviation, or a measure of how spread out the particles are in relation to their size. Generally, particles with a mass median aerodynamic diameter between 3 μm and 5 μm are deposited in the airways.

Question 2 Answer:

12.8 L/minute

Total flow for a 70:30 mixture of helium and oxygen through an oxygen calibrated flowmeter = 1.6 × the set flow:

1.6 × 8 L/min = 12.8 L/min

Chapter 24

Question 3

A respiratory therapist is switching from a standard jet nebulizer to a breath-enhanced nebulizer to deliver albuterol to a 12-year-old child with an acute exacerbation of asthma. What is one adjustment the respiratory therapist may consider recommending to the physician before administering the therapy?

Chapter 24

Question 4

Why should a respiratory therapist avoid using an ultrasonic nebulizer to deliver budesonide?

Chapter 24

Question 5

A physician orders aerosolized administration of Cayston™ to an adolescent with an exacerbation of cystic fibrosis. What class of drug will the respiratory therapist be delivering?

Chapter 24

Question 6

The respiratory therapist is administering a medicated aerosol by jet nebulizer and mask to a 1-year-old child. The child's mother is holding her son during the therapy. The respiratory therapist notices that the blanket the child is wrapped in is occluding the holes on either side of the mask. What should the respiratory therapist conclude?

Question 3 Answer:

Adjust the dose or the nebulization time

Breath-actuated nebulizers use a one-way valve to deliver aerosol only during inspiration. Therefore, there is no drug wasted to the atmosphere. The trade-offs associated with the use of breath-enhanced nebulizers are an increase in the nebulization time and the need to either adjust the dose or the nebulization time to avoid overdosing the patient.

Question 4 Answer:

The ultrasonic nebulizer causes the medication suspension/aerosol solution to heat up over time, which could lead to denaturalization of proteins

The suspension/aerosol solution heats up over time, which could lead to denaturalization of proteins. These factors limit the type of medication that can be delivered by an ultrasonic nebulizer. For example, this technology is inefficient and should not be used to deliver budesonide.

Question 5 Answer:

An antibiotic

Cayston™ is an aerosolized antibiotic commonly used in the treatment of patients with cystic fibrosis. This medication is delivered by a proprietary vibrating mesh device.

Question 6 Answer:

The child is at risk for rebreathing CO_2

Face masks have holes that allow air entrainment when the inspiratory flow exceeds the nebulizer flow. Occluding these holes does not improve drug delivery and has the potential of creating CO_2 rebreathing.

Chapter 25
Question 1

List two goals of airway clearance therapy.

Chapter 25
Question 3

What is the term used to describe a form of airway clearance therapy that uses a cycle of controlled breathing exercises at varying depths to loosen secretions in different areas of the lungs?

Chapter 25
Question 2

To reduce the risk of vomiting and aspiration, what length of time should food be withheld or tube feedings stopped prior to chest physiotherapy?

Chapter 25
Question 4

List two absolute contraindications to the use of high-frequency chest wall oscillation.

Question 1 Answer:

Clear greater volumes of excess secretions from the lungs, improve cough, improve mucociliary escalator function, reduce air trapping, and improve ventilation

Airway clearance therapy (ACT) is a general term that refers to several modalities having one goal: to clear retained pulmonary secretions from the airways. There are four goals of ACT: (1) clear greater volumes fo excess secretions from the lungs, (2) improve cough, (3) improve mucociliary escalator function, and (4) reduce air trapping and improve ventilation.

Question 2 Answer:

30 to 60 minutes

To reduce the risk of vomiting and aspiration, food should be withheld and tube feedings stopped for 30 to 60 minutes prior to chest physiotherapy, or treatment should be delayed for 1 to 2 hours after eating.

Question 3 Answer:

Active autogenic drainage

Autogenic drainage is a form of airway clearance therapy that uses a cycle of controlled breathing exercises at varying depths to loosen secretions in different areas of the lungs. The exercises consist of three phases, with the depth of inspiration increasing with each phase.

Question 4 Answer:

Active hemoptysis or pulmonary hemorrhage and unstable head or neck injury

There are two absolute contraindications to the use of high-frequency chest wall oscillation: active hemoptysis or pulmonary hemorrhage and unstable head or neck injury.

Chapter 25

Question 5

A child with muscular dystrophy has a weak cough and is having difficulty clearing secretions. What airway clearance therapy should the respiratory therapist recommend?

Chapter 25

Question 6

At what age can children effectively perform autogenic drainage?

Chapter 26

Question 1

What is the term used to describe the delivery of intermittent/continuous assisted ventilation or providing continuous positive pressure during spontaneous breathing to enhance lung expansion by restoring or improving functional residual capacity and/or improving minute ventilation without the use of an artificial airway?

Chapter 26

Question 2

List two goals for the use of noninvasive ventilation for preterm infants with surfactant deficiency.

Question 5 Answer:

Cough assist

Children who will benefit most from cough assistance therapy are those with an ineffective cough or absent cough or ineffective secretion removal. This is often seen in neurodisabilities, such as muscular dystrophy, myasthenia gravis, and disorders with paralysis of the respiratory muscles, as well as those with an artificial airway in place.

Question 6 Answer:

10 to 12 years of age

In comparison to other forms of airway clearance therapy, autogenic drainage is a slightly complex, time-consuming technique to learn and requires more training to effectively perform. Younger children may have difficulty understanding and performing it correctly. By the time they are 8 to 12 years of age, most children can effectively perform the therapy.

Question 1 Answer:

Noninvasive ventilation

Noninvasive ventilation refers to the delivery of intermittent or continuous assisted ventilation or providing continuous positive pressure during spontaneous breathing to enhance lung expansion by restoring or improving functional residual capacity and/or improving minute ventilation without the use of an artificial airway.

Question 2 Answer:

Increase the functional residual capacity, decrease the work of breathing, improve pulmonary compliance, and improve the ventilation-to-perfusion ratio to enhance gas exchange

The goals of noninvasive ventilation for preterm infants with surfactant deficiency are to increase the fuctional residual capacity, decrease the work of breathing, improve pulmonary compliance, and improve the ventilation-to-perfusion ratio to enhance gas exchange.

Chapter 26
Question 3

A 32-weeks' gestation infant is receiving continuous positive airway pressure at 4 cm H_2O at an FiO_2 of 0.40. The following arterial blood gases are available:

pH 7.23

PCO_2 68

pO_2 49

HCO_3 24

BE −7

What should the respiratory therapist conclude?

Chapter 26
Question 5

Provide the name of the ventilator setting that adjusts how aggressive inspiratory flow is delivered.

Chapter 26
Question 4

A respiratory therapist is preparing to deliver noninvasive ventialtion to an infant who is 30 weeks' gestation. What is the inspiratory time setting range the respiratory therapist should use?

Chapter 26
Question 6

Describe the method a respiratory therapist should use to adjust the amplitude setting for an infant during the initiation of high-frequency oscillatory ventilation.

Question 3 Answer:

The infant has failed continuous positive airway pressure

Continuous positive airway pressure is defined as $PaCO_2$ >65 mm Hg; pH <7.25: frequent and severe apneas.

Question 4 Answer:

0.3 to 0.6 seconds

Inspiratory time determines the length of time inspiration occurs, or the time that inspiratory pressure is delivered to the lungs. Inspiratory time should be sufficient for breath delivery (typically 0.3–0.6 seconds). Excessively long inspiratory times will be uncomfortable for patients and may increase the work of breathing if patients are forced to exhale against inspiratory flow.

Question 5 Answer:

Rise time

The rise time reflects how aggressive inspiratory flow is delivered. Rise time should be set to meet the patient's inspiratory demands and to maximize comfort.

Question 6 Answer:

Amplitude is increased until the pressure is sufficient to produce a chest wall wiggle

Amplitude is adjusted while observing chest wall movement. Amplitude is increased until the pressure is sufficient to produce a chest wall wiggle.

Chapter 27

Question 1

A child requires long-term invasive ventilation at home. Before transitioning from an intensive care unit ventilator to a portable ventilator, the respiratory therapist verifies the child's weight. What is the minimum weight limit approved by most portable ventilator manufacturers?

Chapter 27

Question 2

At what continuous positive airway pressure and FiO_2 settings are children generally transitioned to oxygen therapy with no positive pressure support?

Chapter 27

Question 3

What ventilator parameter should the respiratory therapist adjust to minimize the risk for prolonged inspiratory times when large or significant endotracheal tube leaks are present?

Chapter 27

Question 4

What pH range should be maintained when permissive hypercapnia is ordered?

Question 1 Answer:

≥5 kg

If noninvasive ventilation is required for use outside the pediatric intensive care unit, in long-term care facilities, or in the home, portable ventilators approved for patients ≥5 kg are usually employed. The weight limit is provided because of inspiratory time and tidal volume constraints during volume control ventilation.

Question 2 Answer:

Continuous positive airway pressure level of 5 to 6 cm H_2O with an FiO_2 of less than or equal to 40%

Continuous positive airway pressure (CPAP) may be discontinued when the patient has been stable on a level of 5 to 6 cm H_2O with an FiO_2 of less than or equal to 40%. Patients are commonly transitioned to high-flow nasal cannula first, as an intermediate step following CPAP, before transitioning to a standard nasal cannula.

Question 3 Answer:

Cycle sensitivity

To minimize the risk for prolonged inspiratory times when large or significant endotracheal tube leaks are present, the clinician can increase the cycle sensitivity, which in turn will synchronize the transition from inspiration to expiration with the patient's breathing pattern.

Question 4 Answer:

A pH of 7.20 to 7.25 or greater

Permissive hypercapnia is a strategy that allows $PaCO_2$ levels to rise above normal values while maintaining a pH of 7.20 to 7.25 or greater.

Chapter 27

Question 5

List the values for plateau pressure and oxygen index that indicate conventional ventilation has failed.

Chapter 28

Question 1

At what gestational age does synthesis of the surfactant lipid and the lipophilic proteins SP-B and SP-C begin?

Chapter 27

Question 6

List two factors a respiratory therapist should consider when recommending postextubation care.

Chapter 28

Question 2

Prior to attending a high-risk delivery, the respiratory therapist notes the results of a lecithin-to-sphingomyelin ratio in the maternal medical record as 1.6. What should the respiratory therapist conclude?

Question 5 Answer:

Plateau pressures of greater than 28 cm H_2O or oxygenation index of greater than 12 to 15

Indicators that conventional ventilation has failed include plateau pressures of greater than 28 cm H_2O or oxygenation index (OI) of greater than 12 to 15 (OI = $mP_{AW} \times FiO_2/PaO_2$).

Question 6 Answer:

The child's ability to maintain functional residual capacity, the child's minute ventilation, the child's oxygenation status

The postextubation intervention will depend on the patient's ability to maintain functional residual capacity, minute ventilation, or oxygenation status.

Question 1 Answer:

22 weeks' gestation

Earlier in fetal development, around 22 weeks' gestational age, surfactant lipid and the lipophilic proteins SP-B and SP-C begin to be synthesized and aggregated into lamellar bodies in the maturing type II cells.

Question 2 Answer:

Immature fetal lungs

In utero, the ratio of lecithin to sphingomyelin (L:S ratio) is used to determine lung maturity. An L:S ratio of greater than 2.0 to 2.5 is indicative of fetal lung maturity in most assays.

Chapter 28

Question 3

List the two main strategies for preventing neonatal respiratory distress syndrome when a preterm delivery is eminent.

Chapter 28

Question 5

A respiratory therapist is preparing to administer surfactant to an intubated and mechanically ventilated infant. How should the infant be positioned during surfactant administration?

Chapter 28

Question 4

At what time intervals are repeat doses of surfactant administered?

Chapter 28

Question 6

Define the INSURE technique.

Question 3 Answer:

Administration of antenatal steroids prior to delivery and prophylactic administration of exogenous surfactant shortly after birth

Two main strategies are available for the prevention of neonatal respiratory distress syndrome in cases of preterm delivery: antenatal administration of corticosteroids (i.e., dexamethasone and betamethasone) that accelerate fetal lung maturation and prophylactic treatment with surfactant soon after birth.

Question 4 Answer:

6- to 24-hour intervals

Repeat doses of surfactant are contingent upon the continued diagnosis of neonatal respiratory distress syndrome. The frequency with which surfactant replacement is performed should depend upon the clinical status of the patient and the indication for performing the procedure. Additional doses of surfactant, given at 6- to 24-hour intervals, may be indicated in infants who experience increasing ventilator requirements or whose conditions fail to improve after the initial dose.

Question 5 Answer:

Supine

Improved homogeneity is achieved when the patient is positioned supine during surfactant administration.

Question 6 Answer:

An acronym for Intubation, Surfactant Administration, and Extubation

The INSURE technique (INtubation, SURfactant, and Extubation) is a very effective and useful method that reduces the need for mechanical ventilation, decreases side effects, shortens the hospitalization time, and eliminates extra hospital expenses. When the INSURE technique is used, the infant is intubated to administer the surfactant, then extubated to either continuous positive airway pressure or noninvasive ventilation.

Chapter 29

Question 1

List two methods for administering heliox therapy to a spontaneously breathing child.

Chapter 29

Question 2

A respiratory therapist is delivering a 70:30 heliox mixture to a child with asthma who is intubated and receiving pressure control ventilation. What parameters would the respiratory therapist use to noninvasively monitor how well the patient is being ventilated and to evaluate intrinsic PEEP (positive end-expiratory pressure)?

Chapter 29

Question 3

What is the approved Food and Drug Administration indication for inhaled nitric oxide?

Chapter 29

Question 4

Define a pulmonary hypertensive crisis.

Question 1 Answer:

Nonrebreathing mask and heated high-flow nasal cannula

For spontaneous breathing patients, a nonrebreathing mask is a reliable delivery device that can reduce room air entrainment and prevent an increase in gas density. Nonrebreathing masks are capable of delivering sufficient gas flow to meet a child's inspiratory flow demands. High-flow nasal cannula (HFNC) is another method of heliox delivery. The primary advantage of using HFNC to deliver heliox is based on this device's ability to meet or exceed the patient's inspiratory flow demand.

Question 2 Answer:

Respiratory mechanics and end-tidal or volumetric carbon dixoide

End-tidal or volumetric carbon dioxide monitoring, as well as respiratory mechanics, are helpful in determining intrinsic PEEP and how well an intubated child receiving heliox is being ventilated.

Question 3 Answer:

Term and near-term neonates (>34 weeks' gestation) with hypoxic respiratory failure associated with persistent pulmonary hypertension of the newborn and/or echocardiographic diagnosis of pulmonary hypertension

Inhaled nitric oxide has been approved by the Food and Drug Administration only for therapy in term and near-term neonates (> 34 weeks' gestation) with hypoxic respiratory failure associated with persistent pulmonary hypertension of the newborn and/or echocardiographic diagnosis of pulmonary hypertension.

Question 4 Answer:

The mean pulmonary artery pressure acutely exceeds the mean systolic arterial pressure

Pulmonary hypertension is described as the ratio of systolic pulmonary artery pressure relative to systolic systemic artery blood pressure (e.g., more than half of the systemic blood pressure). A pulmonary hypertensive crisis occurs when the mean pulmonary artery pressure acutely exceeds the mean systolic arterial pressure.

Chapter 29
Question 5

An intubated and mechanically ventilated infant is receiving inhaled nitric oxide. List one factor that would increase this infant's risk for developing methemoglobinemia.

Chapter 30
Question 1

List the two main modes of extracorporeal membrane oxygenation (ECMO) support.

Chapter 29
Question 6

An infant with congenital heart disease is receiving invasive ventilatory support and inhaled nitric oxide (iNO) at 20 ppm. The infant failed three attempted iNO weaning trials. What pharmacologic agent should the respiratory therapist recommend to ameliorate rebound pulmonary hypertension prior to the next weaning attempt?

Chapter 30
Question 2

List the two types of pumps that can be used to displace blood through an extracorporeal membrane oxygenation (ECMO) circuit.

Question 5 Answer:

Concurrently using high concentrations of both inhaled nitric oxide and FiO$_2$ and inhaled nitric oxide doses >20 ppm

Methemoglobin is formed when inhaled nitric oxide (iNO) binds with hemoglobin (Hb), which reduces the availability of Hb available to transport oxygen. Factors associated with an increased risk for the development of methemoglobinemia include concurrently using high concentrations of both iNO and FiO$_2$ and iNO doses >20 ppm.

Question 6 Answer:

Sildenafil

Sildenafil has been shown to ameliorate rebound pulmonary hypertension during weaning and discontinuation of inhaled nitric oxide (iNO) therapy for neonates with congestive heart disease who previously failed iNO weaning trials.

Question 1 Answer:

Venous–arterial and venous–venous

Extracorporeal membrane oxygenation (ECMO) is typically described by the route of drainage that is always the venous system and the route of reinfusion that can be either the venous system or the arterial system; accordingly, the two main modes of ECMO support are venous–arterial and venous–venous.

Question 2 Answer:

Mechanical or roller pumps and centrifugal pumps

The displacement of blood through an extracorporeal membrane oxygenation (ECMO) circuit is achieved by two types of mechanical pumps—roller pumps, which are occlusive, and centrifugal pumps, which are nonocclusive.

Chapter 30

Question 3

Describe the purpose of the membrane oxygenator.

Chapter 30

Question 5

A respiratory therapist is adjusting the dose of unfractionated heparin for a child receiving venous–arterial extracorporeal membrane oxygenation (ECMO) support. What target range should the respiratory therapist maintain the activated clotting time within?

Chapter 30

Question 4

A child with acute respiratory distress syndrome is receiving venous–arterial extracorporeal membrane oxygenation (ECMO) support. List two tests that can be used to monitor anticoagulation with this patient.

Chapter 30

Question 6

List two patient complications associated with extracorporeal membrane oxygenation (ECMO) support.

Question 3 Answer:

It exchanges oxygen and carbon dioxide to blood exiting the patient

Blood traverses the extracorporeal membrane oxygenation (ECMO) circuit in a continuous and closed loop, with venous blood entering the circuit by gravity if a roller pump is being used, or actively by the negative draw of a centrifugal pump. Blood then passes through the membrane oxygenator where oxygen and carbon dioxide are exchanged, which occurs by the driving pressures and gradients between gas and blood compartments.

Question 4 Answer:

Clotting time, prothrombin time, activated partial thromboplastin time, and anti-factor Xa assay

Managing anticoagulation is an important aspect of monitoring the extracorporeal membrane oxygenation (ECMO) circuit as areas of stagnation may be prone to clotting. Anticoagulation has been monitored through a variety of tests, including activated clotting time, prothrombin time, activated partial thromboplastin time, and the anti-factor Xa assay.

Question 5 Answer:

160 to 180 seconds

The activated clotting time (ACT) is one of the most common tests used to adjust unfractionated heparin dosages, typically to maintain an ACT range of 160 to 180 seconds.

Question 6 Answer:

Bleeding, neurologic sequale, and infection

Bleeding continues to be the most prevalent complication. Neurologic complications may occur during extracorporeal membrane oxygenation (ECMO), particularly in the neonatal population as the risk of intracranial hemorrhage is higher. Infection is another complication to be considered during extracorporeal support, highest in patients who require ECMO for >14 days.

Chapter 31

Question 1

A child has a foreign body partially obstructing the intra-arytenoid portion of the glottis. Prior to assisting the physician with foreign body removal, what type of bronchoscope would the respiratory therapist prepare?

Chapter 31

Question 3

A 10-year-old child with cystic fibrosis has mucus plugging resulting in a right upper lobe collapse. The respiratory therapist is preparing to assist the physician with a bronchoscopy. What type of bronchoscope would the respiratory therapist prepare?

Chapter 31

Question 2

What is the largest size (outer diameter) flexible airway endoscope feasible for use in children?

Chapter 31

Question 4

A 15-year-old child with cystic fibrosis is hospitalized with an acute exacerbation. On hospital day 2, the child expectorates approximately 300 mL of bright-red blood following airway clearance therapy. The respiratory therapist is preparing to assist the physician in a bronchoscopic procedure. What blood test would the respiratory therapist anticipate to be performed prior to the procedure?

Question 1 Answer:

A rigid bronchoscope

Rigid bronchoscopy allows evaluation of suspected lesions in the intra-arytenoid portion of the glottis and better visualization of the subglottic region. Rigid bronchoscopy is indicated mainly for retrieval of a foreign body and for control of massive hemoptysis.

Question 2 Answer:

4.4 mm outer diameter

Flexible endoscopes range from 2.8 mm outer diameter (OD) to 6.3 mm OD, with internal working channels ranging from 1.2 mm to 3.2 mm. An endoscope with a 4.4 mm OD may be the largest size practical in pediatrics.

Question 3 Answer:

A flexible airway endoscope

According to the American Academy of Pediatrics, the most common indications for flexible airway endoscopy are stridor or noisy breathing, chronic wheezing, persistent atelectasis, and recurrent radiographic densities.

Question 4 Answer:

Prothrombin time

Arterial blood gases and clotting factor (prothrombin time) are often obtained during the evaluation of a child prior to performing a bronchoscopy. Because this child has massive hemoptysis, evaluation of clotting time is crucial to the medical management of this child prior to, during, and after the procedure.

Chapter 31

Question 5

List two patient interfaces with which a flexible airway endoscope can be inserted during a bronchoscopy.

Chapter 31

Question 6

A respiratory therapist is assisting a physician during a bronchoscopy. What medication would the respiratory therapist recommend to reduce the incidence of cough and/or bronchospasm during the procedure?

Chapter 32

Question 1

A respiratory therapist is assessing a 7-year-old child with asthma during a high-risk asthma visit. The child's asthma action plan specifies the use of four actuations of an albuterol inhaler when the patient is symptomatic and budesonide 0.25 twice daily management. The patient reports he uses his albuterol inhaler 2 to 3 times daily. The dosimeter confirms the child is adherent with budesonide use. What should the respiratory therapist recommend?

Chapter 32

Question 2

A 3 kg infant presents with stridor following extubation. What medication and dose range should the respiratory therapist recommend?

Question 5 Answer:

Endoscopy mask, laryngeal mask airway, tracheostomy tube, endotracheal tube

Insertion of the endoscope into the child's airways may be accomplished through the nose or mouth (with a bite block in place), an endoscopy mask, laryngeal mask airway, tracheostomy tube, or endotracheal tube.

Question 6 Answer:

Lidocaine

Injectable 1% or 2% lidocaine may be applied to the vocal cords and/or carina to reduce the incidence of cough and/or bronchospasm.

Question 1 Answer:

The addition of a long-acting bronchodilator

Long-acting bronchodilators should be used as adjunctive therapy in patients who are uncontrolled with an inhaled corticosteroid.

Question 2 Answer:

Racemic epinephrine 2.25% solution, 0.05 mL/kg up to a maximum of 0.5 mL per dose

Racemic epinephrine stimulates alpha-adrenergic receptors, leading to the constriction of precapillary arterioles, reducing airway edema. Typically, a 2.25% solution is used. Side effects include difficulty speaking, hoarse voice, oral candidiasis, and cough.

Chapter 32

Question 3

A 14-year-old child is admitted for an exacerbation of cystic fibrosis. The order for dornase alpha is incomplete and does not include the dose or frequency for administration. What dose and frequency of administration should the respiratory therapist recommend?

Chapter 32

Question 5

What is the recommend dose of montelukast for a 6-year-old child?

Chapter 32

Question 4

List an indication for zafirlukast.

Chapter 32

Question 6

List two side effects associated with the administration of skeletal muscle relaxants.

Question 3 Answer:

2.5 mg by nebulizer once daily

Dornase alfa is available for nebulization as a preservative-free solution that should be kept refrigerated prior to use. Dosage is 2.5 mg administered by nebulizer once per day.

Question 4 Answer:

Prophylaxis and chronic treatment of asthma

Zafirlukast is a leukotriene modifier and is indicated for the prevention and chronic treatment of asthma in pediatric patients 5 years of age and older.

Question 5 Answer:

5 mg once daily

The dosage of montelukast, a leukotriene receptor antagonist, is 5 mg once daily for children 6 to 14 years of age. Typically, the child/family is instructed to administer the medication in the evening.

Question 6 Answer:

Flushing, bradycardia, hypotension, tachyarrhythmia, and rash

Flushing, bradycardia, hypotension, tachyarrhythmia, and rash are side effects seen with administration of skeletal muscle relaxants.

Chapter 33

Question 1

List an important skill taught during crew resource management training for the staff of an air and ground neonatal/pediatric specialty transport team.

Chapter 33

Question 2

List three essential components incorporated into transport team safety training.

Chapter 33

Question 3

A physician in the emergency room contacts a tertiary care center to transport a child requiring intubation and mechanical ventilation. Outline the role of the medical control physician during the initial triage of a critically ill child.

Chapter 33

Question 4

List the four functional components of a transport safety management system.

Question 1 Answer:

Communication

Communication skills are taught through a crew resource management (CRM) course in addition to practicing with closed-loop communication in simulation and certification courses. CRM has a focus on leadership, interpersonal communication, and decision making.

Question 2 Answer:

Vehicle breakdown, scene safety, and survival training

Despite mature safety management systems, safety events may still occur. Safety training should include vehicle breakdown, scene safety, and survival training.

Question 3 Answer:

Oversight of the clinical management of the care for the transferred patient

After the initial triage communication between the referring facility and the medical control physician or accepting physician, the role of the medical control physician transitions to the oversight of the clinical management of the care for the transferred patient.

Question 4 Answer:

Safety policy, safety risk management, safety assurance, and safety promotion

The four functional components of a transport safety management system include (1) safety policy, which establishes senior management's commitment to continually improve safety and also defines the methods, processes, and organizational structure needed to meet safety goals; (2) safety risk management, which determines the need for and adequacy of new or revised risk controls based on the assessment of acceptable risk; (3) safety assurance, which evaluates the continued effectiveness of implemented risk control strategies and supports the identification of new hazards; and (4) safety promotion, which includes training, communication, and other actions to create a positive safety culture within all levels of the workforce because promotion of safety is everyone's responsibility.

Chapter 33
Question 5

List three pieces of equipment important for the respiratory therapist to include in the airway management transport bag.

Chapter 34
Question 1

List three goals defined by the American Association for Respiratory Care of home mechanical ventilation.

Chapter 33
Question 6

What is the importance of using an isolette during the transport of an infant born at 32 weeks' gestation from a community hospital to a Level 3 neonatal intensive care unit?

Chapter 34
Question 2

List two key components of family education and training prior to discharging a child with a tracheostomy who requires mechanical ventilatory support.

Question 1 Answer:

Sustain and prolong life, enhance quality of life, reduce morbidity, improve or maintain physical and psychological function, and provide cost-effective care

The American Association for Respiratory Care defines the goals of home mechanical ventilation as (1) to sustain and prolong life, (2) enhance quality of life, (3) reduce morbidity, (4) improve or maintain physical and psychological function, and (5) provide cost-effective care. Specifically for pediatrics, there is an additional goal to enhance growth and development.

Question 2 Answer:

Caregiver instruction in operating and troubleshooting equipment specific to the ventilator; tracheostomy care

Operating and troubleshooting equipment specific to the ventilator. Although the ventilator is considered life support equipment, tracheostomy education and training is perhaps the most vital element that must be mastered to safely care for these children in the home setting.

Question 5 Answer:

Resuscitation bag and masks, laryngoscope blades and handles, endotracheal tubes, airway adjuncts, and medications for rapid sequence intubation

A pouch or bag specific to airway management should include a resuscitation bag and masks, laryngoscope blades and handles, endotracheal tubes, airway adjuncts, and medications for rapid sequence intubation.

Question 6 Answer:

Temperature control

An isolette is used during air and ground transport to provide thermal environment control. Keeping the infant within their neutral thermal environment during transport can reduce the propensity for harm from cold stress.

Chapter 34

Question 3

List three benefits to providing care to a medically complex child requiring invasive ventilatory support in the home rather than continuing care in an acute care facility.

Chapter 34

Question 4

List two risks associated with caregivers providing medical care to their child with invasive mechanical ventilatory needs in the home.

Chapter 34

Question 5

What is the role of the respiratory therapist in transitioning a child with a tracheostomy home on continuous ventilatory support?

Chapter 34

Question 6

A respiratory therapist is planning the discharge of a child with a tracheostomy tube requiring continuous mechanical ventilatory support. According to the American Association for Respiratory Care Clinical Practice Guideline regarding long-term invasive mechanical ventilation in the home, is a second ventilator required for this child?

Question 3 Answer:

Risk of infection, decreased cost, and improved quality of life

The child's home is preferred over the hospital for several reasons, including a reduced risk of infection, decreased cost, and improved quality of life. The home also provides a better atmosphere for addressing psychosocial and developmental needs.

Question 4 Answer:

Stress and fatigue, financial loss, and lack of community and financial resources

Risks associated with caregivers providing medical care to their child with invasive mechanical ventilatory needs in the home include stress and fatigue, financial loss, and lack of community and financial resources. Attending to the ventilator-dependent child is demanding and can consume the caregiver as it is a 24-hours-a-day, 7-days-a-week, continuous occupation. The care burden can impact families by creating marital discord, draining financial resources, and enhancing sibling rivalry.

Question 5 Answer:

Provision of bedside care to the child in the hospital prior to discharge and providing patient and family or caregiver education

The role of the respiratory therapist is multifaceted in caring for the ventilator-dependent child. Not only do they generally provide direct care at the bedside but also may be involved in training and education for the family.

Question 6 Answer:

Yes

The American Association for Respiratory Care Clinical Practice Guideline regarding long-term invasive mechanical ventilation in the home recommends a second ventilator for those patients who are unable to maintain spontaneous ventilation for 4 or more consecutive hours, those residing in an area where a replacement device cannot be provided within 2 hours, and those requiring ventilation during mobility.

Chapter 35
Question 1

What is the essential difference between adult and pediatric palliative care?

Chapter 35
Question 3

List three adjunctive therapies that can be used with or in lieu of medication for pain or symptom management during palliative care.

Chapter 35
Question 2

What factor influences how a child understands their illness and death?

Chapter 35
Question 4

List the eligibility criteria for pediatric hospice care.

Question 1 Answer:

How consent is obtained

The essential difference between adult and pediatric palliative care is the age of the patient. In adult medicine, typically the patient (adult) provides consent. In pediatric medicine, consent is provided by the child's primary caregiver(s)—typically one or both parents.

Question 2 Answer:

The child's level of development

How a child understands their illness and death depends upon their level of development. A child's developmental age and chronological age may be altered due to an illness. If an illness begins at infancy, the child may not reach developmental milestones as would be expected with normal development.

Question 3 Answer:

Therapeutic play, aromatherapy, guided imagery, massage, and music therapy

The palliative care team provides a thorough assessment of pain and can assist with recommendations for the route most appropriate for medication administration and compounded medicine preparations as well as adjunctive therapies that can be used with or in lieu of medication for pain or symptom management. Adjunctive therapies include therapeutic play with a child life specialist, aromatherapy, guided imagery, massage, and music therapy.

Question 4 Answer:

The child's life expectancy is approximately 6 months or less

Palliative care is open-ended, and although support is ongoing during palliative care, it may be sought alongside goals of a cure. In a typical hospice setting, however, a cure is no longer an option. To be eligible for hospice care, a physician must attest that the child's life expectancy is approximately 6 months or less.

Chapter 35

Question 5

What is the term used to describe curative care that is provided to the child to treat a disease or to normalize an underlying health condition while the child also receives hospice care for pain and symptom management and psychosocial end-of-life needs?

Chapter 35

Question 6

A child with severe traumatic brain injury has a positive apnea test. The family's decision was to terminally extubate the child. What element of care is essential to the child and family during and after the extubation?

Question 5 Answer:

Concurrent curative care

Concurrent curative care occurs when a child receives curative care to treat a disease or to normalize an underlying health condition while also receiving hospice care for pain and symptom management and psychosocial end-of-life needs.

Question 6 Answer:

Psychosocial and emotional care/support

When the family questions current medical management and requests to redirect the plan of care, a family-centered approach that includes discussion with the multidisciplinary team is imperative. Withdrawal of medical devices and technology, including mechanical ventilatory support and an endotracheal tube, may take place simultaneously with an increase in delivery of psychosocial and emotional care.